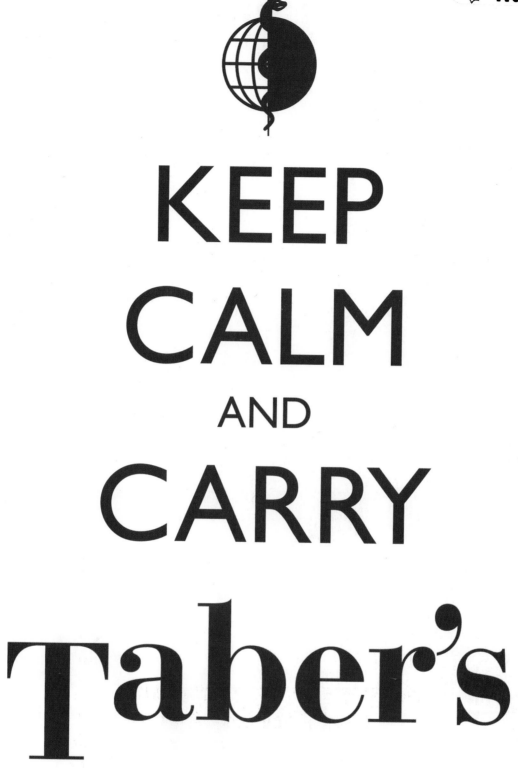

KEEP
CALM
AND
CARRY
Taber's

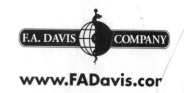

Classroom to Clinical
to Professional *Success!*

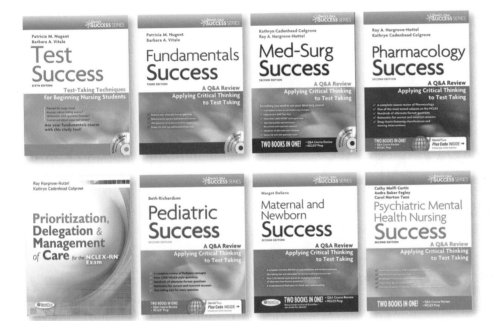
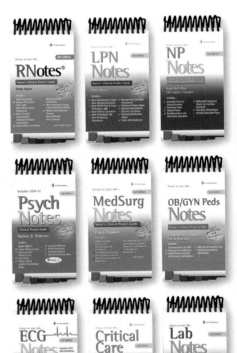
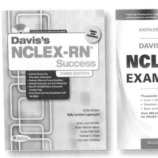
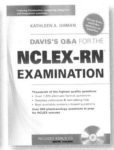
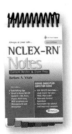
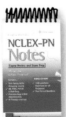
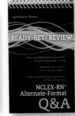
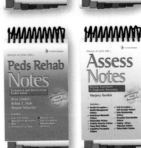
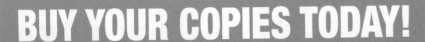
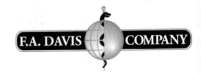

Nutrition *and* Diet Therapy

SIXTH EDITION

Carroll A. Lutz, MA, RN
Associate Professor Emerita
Jackson College
Jackson, Michigan

Erin E. Mazur, MSN, RN, FNP-BC
Assistant Professor of Nursing
Jackson College
Jackson, Michigan

Nancy A. Litch, MS, RD
Supervisory Dietitian
VA Medical Center
Ann Arbor, Michigan

F.A. Davis Company • Philadelphia

F. A. Davis Company
1915 Arch Street
Philadelphia, PA 19103
www.fadavis.com

Printed in the United States of America

Last digit indicates print number: 10 9 8 7 6 5 4 3 2 1

Publisher, Nursing: Joanne Patzek DaCunha, RN, MSN
Director of Content Development: Darlene D. Pedersen
Content Project Manager: Elizabeth Hart, Christina Snyder
Electronic Project Manager: Katherine Crowley
Illustration and Design Manager: Carolyn O'Brien

As new scientific information becomes available through basic and clinical research, recommended treatments and drug therapies undergo changes. The author(s) and publisher have done everything possible to make this book accurate, up to date, and in accord with accepted standards at the time of publication. The author(s), editors, and publisher are not responsible for errors or omissions or for consequences from application of the book, and make no warranty, expressed or implied, in regard to the contents of the book. Any practice described in this book should be applied by the reader in accordance with professional standards of care used in regard to the unique circumstances that may apply in each situation. The reader is advised always to check product information (package inserts) for changes and new information regarding dose and contraindications before administering any drug. Caution is especially urged when using new or infrequently ordered drugs.

Library of Congress Cataloging-in-Publication Data

Lutz, Carroll A., author.
  Nutrition and diet therapy / Carroll A. Lutz, Erin Mazur, Nancy A. Litch. — Sixth edition.
     p. ; cm.
  Includes bibliographical references and index.
  ISBN 978-0-8036-3718-4
  I. Mazur, Erin, author. II. Litch, Nancy A., author III. Title.
  [DNLM: 1. Diet Therapy. 2. Diet. 3. Nutritional Physiological Phenomena. WB 400]
  RM217
  613.2—dc23
                              2014003146

*D*edications

To my coauthor of 22 years, Karen R. Przytulski, RD, an exceptional and steadfast colleague throughout the first five editions of this text, to Gail Ladwig, RCV, who recommended me to F. A. Davis company in 1989 and led me to Nancy in 2011, and to my nephew, Bob Weber, my trusted source of information and encouragement for all six editions.

—Carroll A. Lutz

To Carroll, thank you for your guidance and wisdom throughout this process. To Jeff, Spencer, and Carter, thank you for your encouragement and patience; you are loved!

—Erin E. Mazur

To Carroll, for your wealth of knowledge and experience, thank you for this opportunity. To Paul and Evan, thank you for your support and understanding.

—Nancy A. Litch

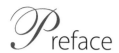

Preface

The sixth edition of *Nutrition and Diet Therapy* is designed to provide the beginning student with knowledge of the fundamentals of nutrition related to the promotion and maintenance of optimal health. Practical applications and treatment of pathologies with nutritional components are stressed. In addition, basic scientific information is introduced to enable students to begin to understand nutritional issues reported in the mass media. The sequential introduction of material continues to be a unique feature of this text. The authors resist the temptation to introduce concepts and examples of applications before the underlying basic science and vocabulary have been covered. The sixth edition has been extensively updated with new information (the FODMAP diet) incorporating new illustrations and tables (a more detailed vitamin K-controlled diet). Increased attention is paid to feeding the hungry and global issues involving nutrition. Within the boundaries of a beginning course, enough specific information is included to enhance understanding of the "why" of nutritional care, not only the "what."

This book was written to meet the educational needs of nursing students, dietetic assistants, diet technicians, and others. Support materials for the student include case studies with examples of care plans, including referrals to other members of the health-care team, followed by Critical Thinking Questions designed to provoke imaginative thought and to foster discussion. Each chapter has review questions and clinical analysis study questions. Additional student study aids listed in this Preface are available online through DavisPlus.

As researchers discover new and more effective treatments for nutrition-related disorders and health maintenance, the ability to think critically becomes increasingly important for professional growth and development. Students need not only to grasp the facts but also to apply the information in a clinical environment. This text has been developed to facilitate acquiring these skills.

The text can be used to teach a complete course in nutrition or as a desk reference for practitioners. The student using this book needs no previous grounding in anatomy, physiology, or medical terminology. Subjects are fully supported by diagrams, illustrations, figures, and tables. Depending upon the curriculum, chapters may be omitted or presented in a different sequence. We recognize that this text contains an immense amount of data

and information. We hope this rich store of information permits instructors to adapt the text to the objectives of their courses while serving as a reference and directory for students, satisfying their curiosities or completing solo or group projects whether in preclinical or in clinical courses.

The content of *Nutrition and Diet Therapy,* sixth edition, is organized into three units.

Unit 1, **The Role of Nutrients in the Human Body,** covers basic information on nutrition as a science and how this information is applied to nutritional care. All the essential nutrients are covered, including definitions and descriptions of functions, effects of excesses and deficiencies, and food sources. Nutritional standards, including the Dietary Reference Intakes, are explained and incorporated into discussions of nutrients. Information on the use of food in the body and how the body maintains energy balance completes the unit.

Unit 2, **Family and Community Nutrition,** provides an overview of topics such as nutrition throughout the life cycle covering pregnancy, lactation, infancy, childhood, adolescence, and adulthood. Lastly, issues in food management are addressed.

Unit 3, **Clinical Nutrition,** focuses on the care of clients with pathologies caused by or causing nutritional impairments. General topics include nutrient delivery via oral, enteral, and parenteral routes, and interactions among foods, nutrients, medications, and supplements. Pathological conditions include diabetes mellitus and hypoglycemia, cardiovascular disease, renal disease, digestive diseases, and cancer. Other pertinent topics include weight control, nutrition in critical care and during stress, diet affecting inflammation and infections, and care of the client with a terminal illness.

Special features are used throughout the text to facilitate the teaching and learning process. All of the chapters include the following:

Boxes and Tables contain summaries, assessment tools, commonly prescribed diets used in medical nutrition therapy, and research findings.

Clinical Applications stimulate the interest of the beginning student by showing how the information is pertinent to providing health care.

Clinical Calculations isolate and explain many of the mathematical calculations that are used in nutritional science.

Dollars & Sense items focus on costs associated with commonly used foods and supplements. Occasionally, budget-sparing recipes are given to exemplify principles in the chapters.

Genomic Gems highlight links between a person's genetic makeup and utilization of nutrients and dietary substances.

Illustrations reinforce important points in the text or graph statistical data for clarity.

Flowcharts of physiological and pathological processes lead the student to an understanding of the relationship between nutrition and health.

A **Case Study** with a proposed **Care Plan** allows the student to see how the nutrition principles described in the chapter are applied in a specific clinical situation. The case studies were written to incorporate elements that are likely to occur in practice.

Teamwork following the care plan illustrates continuing care of a client by various members of the health-care team.

Study Aids, Chapter Review Questions, and Clinical Analysis Questions help the student to focus on essential concepts. Answers to the Study Aids questions are printed in Appendix C.

Critical Thinking Questions invite the student to think holistically with compassion and creativity. They can be used as a basis for class discussion.

Appendices of Dietary Reference Intakes (Appendix A) and the Academy of Nutrition and Dietetics Exchange Lists for Diabetes (Appendix B) serve as readily available sources of information for students in class discussions or group assignments.

A **Glossary** (Appendix D) of more than 1000 entries assists the reader to recall definitions of terms boldfaced in the text.

The **Bibliography** (Appendix E) supports the text with data sources and introduces the student to the scientific literature.

In addition to the text resources, students can access online resources via DavisPlus:

Student Study Questions are different from the in-book questions and provide the student with additional content review. All 360 questions are broken down by chapter, include a rationale, and have print and e-mail capabilities.

Flash Cards developed from the book glossary provide students an online resource for key term review.

Additional Web Resources are compiled in one place to provide the student easy access to nutrition content, including links to MyPlate resources, U.S. Department of Agriculture resources, and nutrition management tools.

Electronic Updates will be added as new information becomes available. Updates will be posted under the link for "Content Updates."

Accompanying the text for instructors who adopt it for their classes are:

An **Instructors' Guide** with suggestions for course organization, classroom activities, and student assignments.

PowerPoint Presentations for all the chapters of the book. These presentations provide a ready source of material to select for classroom use.

An **Electronic Test Bank** containing an additional 200 questions, arranged by chapter.

We believe that *Nutrition and Diet Therapy,* sixth edition, provides the clinical information necessary for a fuller understanding of the relationship between the knowledge about nutrition and diet and its clinical application. This text balances direct explanations of the underlying science with an introduction to the clinical responsibilities of the health-care professional.

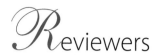

Reviewers

Chanda D. Beaty, MSN, RN/NP
Nursing Instructor
Upper Cape Regional Technical School
Bourne, Massachusetts

Stephanie Bruce, MS, RN
Assistant Professor
Alverno College
Milwaukee, Wisconsin

Patricia Davis-Scott, MS, RN
Assistant Professor
Cumberland University
Lebanon, Tennessee

Diane Dembicki, PhD, LMT, CYT
Clinical Associate Professor and Director of MS
    Nutrition Program
College of Nursing and Public Health
Adelphi University
Garden City, New York

Holly Doogs, RN, MSN
Nursing Faculty
State Fair Community College
Sedalia, Missouri

Cathleen Dowe, MSN, RN
Adjunct Instructor
Jefferson Community College
Watertown, New York

MaryAnn Edelman, RN, MS, CNS
Associate Professor
Kingsborough Community College
Brooklyn, New York

Tonia Grant, MSN, RN
Assistant Professor
Medgar Evers College—CUNY
Brooklyn, New York

Coleen Kumar, RN, MS
Associate Professor/Deputy Chairperson
Kingsborough Community College
Brooklyn, New York

Cathleen E. Kunkler, MSN, RN, ONC, CNE
Associate Professor, Nurse Education
Corning Community College
Corning, New York

Karen A. Lindale Potts, RN, BC, MSN, CDE
Nursing Director
Delaware Skills Center Practical Nursing Course
Wilmington, Delaware

Gayla Love, MSN Ed, BSN, RN, COI, CCM
Program Administrator
Southern Crescent Technical College
Griffin, Georgia

Jane Lucht, RN, MSM
Associate Professor
Edgewood College
Madison, Wisconsin

Anjeleigh L. Partridge, RN, MSN
Nurse Educator and LPN Instructor
Southern Crescent Technical College
Griffin, Georgia

Sharon Todd, MSN NIS, BSN, ASN, RN
Practical Nursing Instructor
Southern Crescent Technical College
Griffin, Georgia

Susan Wessel, RN, MSN
Professor of Nursing
Southwestern Illinois College
Belleville, Illinois

Shawn White, MSN, BSN, RN
Nurse Educator
Southern Crescent Technical College
Griffin, Georgia

Acknowledgments

Writing a book, even a sixth edition, is a huge task, requiring the assistance of many people. Of particular note are the two new coauthors who accepted ownership of the project right from the beginning. All of our colleagues and family members contributed to this project, sometimes with information and critiques, sometimes by being supportive, sometimes just by leaving us alone to work.

We thank all the organizations and publishers that gave permission for the use of their materials for this and previous editions. Our editorial and production staff at F.A. Davis Company, including Joanne DaCunha, Elizabeth Hart, Christina Snyder, Katherine Margeson, and Bob Butler, shared their knowledge and expertise throughout joint project. Our developmental editor, Jennifer Schmidt, and production editors, Kelly Boutross and Chris Waller, kept us focused on our common goal of excellence. To all of them and the countless others who did not have to deal with us directly go our heartfelt thanks.

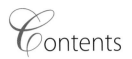

Contents

Unit 3

Clinical Nutrition   305

Appendices

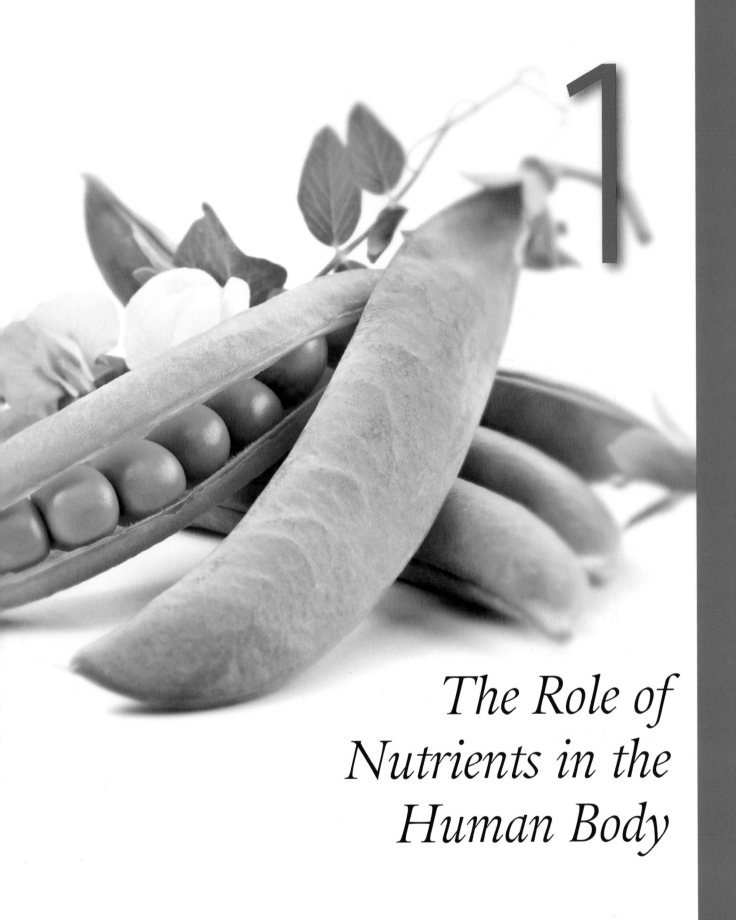

The Role of Nutrients in the Human Body

1

Nutrition in Human Health

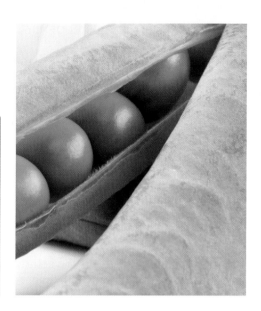

LEARNING OBJECTIVES

After completing this chapter, the student should be able to:

- Describe the relationship between nutrition and health.
- Identify the six classes of nutrients, their functions, and their essentiality.
- Recognize the possible relationship of genetics to the adequacy of nutrition.
- Compare dietary intakes in the United States with the U.S. Department of Agriculture Dietary Guidelines.
- Discuss issues related to food insecurity on local and global levels.
- List and describe the steps in providing nutritional care.
- Explain the intended use of the Dietary Reference Intakes.
- Relate the underlying concept of the Exchange Lists to overall healthful eating.
- Give an example of a provider's use of, and respect for, cultural beliefs having a favorable impact on a health outcome for a client.
- State the preferences and dietary restrictions of several cultural and religious groups.

Food is essential to life. Choosing food wisely can contribute to a healthy, satisfying life. This chapter introduces concepts and practices that underlie the nourishment of human beings as well as some barriers to achieving optimal nutrition. Information on the influence of culture on nutrition concludes the chapter.

The Language of Nutrition

Nutrition is the science of food and its relationship to health. Nutrition involves the processes of taking in and utilizing nourishment. It includes natural and artificial feeding.

According to the World Health Organization, **health** is the state of complete physical, mental, and social well-being and not merely the absence of disease or infirmity. How nutrition influences human health is the subject of this textbook.

That food or its lack affects physical health is readily seen. For example, both motor and mental development are suboptimal in young children with iron deficiency **anemia** (Stoltzfus, 2011). On occasion, social well-being may be developed to the detriment of physical well-being as when social occasions are accompanied by foods that may not contribute to the best possible health.

Certainly, human beings should take nourishment daily. What an individual chooses to eat may affect his or her health that day but also well into the future.

Disease Prevention

The general prevention of disease is categorized on three levels: primary, secondary, and tertiary. Application of the principles of nutrition can contribute to prevention of disease on each of these levels.

Primary prevention is the implementation of practices that are likely to avert the occurrence of disease. Many nutritional changes have been promoted to thwart particular diseases, but most, with the exception of actual vitamin deficiency diseases, lack solid evidence of effectiveness. Excessive body weight is clearly related to heart disease, stroke, type 2 diabetes mellitus, some cancers, joint diseases, and some fertility disorders. The difficulty lies in motivating people to change behavior today for possible benefits in the perhaps distant future. Maintaining a healthy body weight is a primary prevention strategy.

Secondary prevention is the institution of monitoring techniques to discover incipient diseases early enough to enhance the opportunity to control their effects. If a person's risk for diabetes is found in the prediabetes stage by testing blood sugar levels, noninvasive treatments such as weight loss and diet modification can successfully derail or delay the development of the disease.

Tertiary prevention is the use of treatment techniques after a disease has occurred to prevent complications or to promote maximum adaptation. For example, clients with various diseases that cause swallowing disorders can be helped to maintain nourishment and to avoid choking incidents with nutritional interventions (see Chapter 14).

Nutrients

Historically, the science of nutrition has been based on the nutrients in food. **Nutrients** are the chemical substances supplied by food that the body needs for growth, maintenance, and repair.

Classes and Essentiality

Nutrients are divided into six classes, each of which is discussed in subsequent chapters:

1. Carbohydrates (often abbreviated as CHO for carbon, hydrogen and oxygen; these elements are also those in lipids but an abbreviation is not used for lipids.)
2. Fats (lipids)
3. Proteins
4. Minerals
5. Vitamins
6. Water

Nutrients are considered essential, nonessential, or conditionally essential, depending on whether the body can or cannot manufacture them.

■ An **essential nutrient** is one that the human body requires but cannot manufacture in sufficient amounts to meet bodily needs. Thus, essential nutrients must be supplied by foods in the diet. Vitamin C, vitamin A, and calcium are three of the more than 40 essential nutrients.

■ **Nonessential nutrients** are not needed in the diet because the body can make them from other substances. For example, the amino acid alanine is a nonessential nutrient because the body can manufacture it from other raw materials.

■ **Conditionally essential nutrients** are those that, under most circumstances, a healthy body can manufacture in sufficient quantities. In certain situations of physiological status or disease, the body cannot produce optimal amounts. The amino acid tyrosine is an example of a conditionally essential nutrient (see Chapter 4).

Functions

All nutrients perform one or more of the following functions:

1. Serve as a source of energy or heat
2. Support the growth and maintenance of tissue
3. Aid in the regulation of basic body processes

These three life-sustaining functions collectively are part of **metabolism,** the sum of all physical and chemical changes that take place in the body. Nutrients have specific metabolic functions and interact with one another to maintain the body.

SOURCE OF ENERGY

Energy is defined in the physical sciences as the capacity to do work. Energy exists in a variety of forms: electric, thermal (heat), chemical, mechanical, and others.

All food enters the body as chemical energy. The body processes the chemical energy of food and converts it into other energy forms. For example, chemical energy is transformed into electric signals in nerves and into mechanical energy in muscles.

Carbohydrates, fats, and proteins, the nutrients that supply energy, are referred to as the **energy nutrients.** The energy both in foods and in the body is measured in **kilocalories,** abbreviated kcal (see Glossary). Because energy cannot be seen, heard, or felt, it is one of the most difficult biological concepts to understand. For this reason, it warrants its own chapter (see Chapter 5).

GROWTH AND MAINTENANCE OF TISSUES

Some nutrients provide the raw materials for building body structures, and they participate in the continued growth and maintenance of necessary tissues. Water, proteins, fats, and minerals are the nutrient classes that contribute in a major way to building body structures.

REGULATION OF BODY PROCESSES

Some nutrients control or regulate chemical processes in the body. For example, certain minerals and proteins help regulate how water is distributed in the body. Vitamins are necessary in the series of reactions involved in generating energy. Vitamins themselves are not energy sources, but if the body lacks a particular vitamin, it will not produce energy efficiently.

Functional Foods

In addition to the nutrients listed above, foods contain other physiologically active substances from plant (**phytochemical**), animal, and microbial sources, some of which reputedly promote health. Phytochemicals identified thus far number in the tens of thousands, including 8000 polyphenolic compounds (Gropper and Smith, 2013). It is small wonder that pinning down the health effect of one component in a food is daunting. Therefore, the amount and quality of evidence for the usefulness of functional foods varies.

Definitions of functional foods are equally varied by source and are not officially recognized as a food category by the U.S. Food and Drug Administration (FDA). One of the simplest definitions is as follows:

> **Functional foods** are foods or food ingredients that have additional health or physiological benefits over and above the normal nutritional value they provide (Nicoletti, 2012).

The Academy of Nutrition and Dietetics (formerly the American Dietetic Association) categorizes functional foods as indicated in Table 1-1. Several examples of functional foods being studied appear in Table 1-2. Bear in mind that a given food may contain thousands of phytochemicals that differ under divergent cultivation and storage methods. The extent to which foods

TABLE 1-1 ■ Functional Foods

CATEGORY	SELECTED EXAMPLES
Conventional foods (whole foods)	Blueberries Cranberry juice (see Chapter 21) Cruciferous vegetables: broccoli, cabbage, cauliflower, Brussels sprouts (see Chapter 21) Green tea Mushrooms Some nuts Oatmeal as part of heart healthy diet Tomatoes (see Chapter 21)
Modified foods, fortified	Omega-3 fatty acids in eggs and margarines (For definition, see Chapter 6.)
Synthesized food ingredients	Oligosaccharides functioning as prebiotics (see Chapter 20)

Adapted from Crowe and Francis, 2013; Milner, Toner, and Davis, 2014.

TABLE 1-2 ■ Selected Functional Foods, Bioactive Components, and Reported Health Benefits

FUNCTIONAL FOODS	BIOACTIVE COMPONENTS UNDER STUDY	REPORTED HEALTH BENEFIT
Apples, tea, onions	Flavonoids	Prevention of cardiovascular disease
Berries	Polyphenols	Protection against cancer through abilities to counteract, reduce, and repair damage from oxidative stress and inflammation
Cruciferous vegetables (broccoli, cauliflower, cabbage)	Isothiocyanates	Reduction of prostate cancer risk
Green Tea	Polyphenols	Inhibition of cancer initiation and blockage of cancer progression
Oats	Beta-glucan (soluble fiber)	Reduction of blood cholesterol levels
Purple grape juice or red wine	Resveratrol	Reduction of heart disease risk by decreasing blood platelet aggregation
Soy products	Isoflavones	Reduction in incidence of hormone-related cancers

Sources: American Dietetic Association, 2009; Kanwar, Taskeen, Mohammad, Huo, et al, 2012; Li, Kong, Bao, Ahmad, et al, 2011; Liu, Mao, Cao, and Xie, 2012; Majewska-Wierzbicka and Czeczot, 2012; Othman, Moghadasian, and Jones, 2011; Seeram, 2008; Zhang, 2012.

may be labeled with a health claim is discussed in Chapter 15. Specific examples of functional foods with the best **efficacy** are provided as the subject matter dictates in other chapters.

Nutritional Genomics

In April 2003, the Human Genome Project announced that the actual sequence of the human genetic code had been transcribed. In simple terms, the genetic code is the human body's software instructions for manufacturing proteins (see Genomic Gem 1-1). It is now possible to cheaply and quickly sequence the parts of genes that encode **amino acids** of all 22,000 human genes (Brunner, 2012).

A subfield of nutritional genomics, **nutrigenetics,** detects **gene** variants within an individual to identify environmental factors that trigger dysfunction or disease. Examples of gene variants conveying susceptibility for dysfunction include those for food allergies and celiac disease (Gropper and Smith, 2013). The trigger in food allergy is the offending food (see Chapter 11). In celiac disease, it is the gluten in wheat, rye, or barley (see Chapter 20).

Another subfield of nutritional genomics is **nutrigenomics,** the study of the interaction between one's diet and his or her genes, which can markedly influence digestion, absorption, and elimination as well as influence their sites of actions (Riscuta and Dumitrescu, 2010). A

Genomic Gem 1-1

Genetic Code as Software

To visualize the relationships among the human body, genetic code, and diet, think of the body as a machine similar to a personal computer. Software provides directions to the computer; a person's genetic code provides instructions to the body. Just as a personal computer cannot operate without software, the human body cannot operate without instructions from the genetic code. Think of data input by the operator as much like food that is taken in or eaten.

For years, scientists have studied the effects of nutrients and phytochemicals on our body's hardware, or structure. Only recently have researchers begun the study of nutrients and phytochemicals on the body's software, or genetic code. Almost everyone has software on their computers that is never used. The human body also has instructions that are similarly never used.

What causes a software program or gene in the human body to be turned on or expressed? Some scientists are beginning to understand that the activation is partly due to the food we eat or do not eat. The premise underlying nutrigenomics is that diet's influence on health depends on an individual's genetic makeup, thereby suggesting that not all individuals respond identically to a given diet. Thus, one person would be more susceptible to the negative effects of a suboptimal diet than another person would be. More research is needed to identify those who will benefit most from dietary change and those who might be placed at risk because of an adjustment (Riscuta and Dumitrescu, 2010).

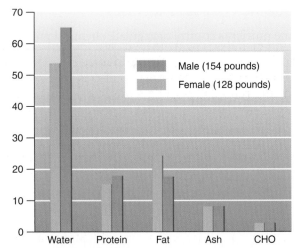

FIGURE 1-1 Approximate body composition as a percent of body weight of a 25-year-old man weighing 154 pounds and woman weighing 128 pounds. Note that the typical woman has more fat and less protein than the man because of differences in muscle. The percentage of ash content is equal in both sexes. The human body has minimal carbohydrate content.

possible application of nutrigenomics in a person susceptible to chronic inflammation is to ensure adequate omega-3 fatty acids intake (see Chapter 3) to reduce the expression of genes that encode for inflammatory **cytokines** (Gropper and Smith, 2013).

Body Composition

Nutrient intake can affect body composition, which in turn can affect health. The human body is composed of five types of substances:

1. Water
2. Protein
3. Fat
4. Ash (mineral content as in the skeleton)
5. Carbohydrate

Figure 1-1 shows these substances as a percentage of body weight in young adults. Because of its increased muscle, the male body contains more protein than the female body. With age, body composition typically becomes higher in fat and lower in protein.

Health-care providers are often concerned that their clients retain their muscle, particularly when losing weight (see Chapter 16). When the body loses protein, it is losing muscle tissue, organ mass, the protein stored in body substances, or combinations thereof. Preservation of body protein is necessary for optimal health.

A person's body fat and protein content can be modified by food intake, exercise, or both. Exercise increases body protein content by increasing muscle. Eating too much food increases the fat content of the body because fat is stored for future use as energy. Excessive body fat, both in amount and location, has health consequences.

Food Choices

Often unconscious and automatic, more than 220 food decisions may be made daily with emotional cues, habit, and peer pressure playing major roles in food choices. A French study found that price was most often cited as the primary factor influencing food choice decisions followed by eating habits, and taste (Jacquier, Bonthoux, Baciu, and Ruffieux, 2012). Note the lack of attention to nutritional composition. Undoubtedly, the French are not unique in ranking nutritional composition tenth of the most frequently cited factors used in food choice decisions.

Despite the complexity of food decisions, many governments worldwide have published well-researched, rational, and practical dietary and food guidelines. This text discusses only the U.S. recommendations, which are revised periodically to incorporate new research findings into advice promoting healthy dietary behaviors.

What We Should Eat

Poor diet and physical inactivity are the most important factors producing the **epidemic** of overweight and **obesity** in this country that affects men, women, and children in all segments of society. Even in persons of normal weight, poor nutrition and physical inactivity are associated with heart disease, diabetes, thinning bones, and some forms of cancer. In addition, certain racial and ethnic groups have disproportionate rates of excessive body weight and associated **chronic illnesses.** Current dietary advice from the U.S. government attempts to remedy that unhealthy state of affairs. The *Healthy People 2020* Web site has a section on Nutrition and Weight Status at www.healthypeople.gov/2020/topicsobjectives2020/overview.aspx?topicid=29.

Dietary Guidelines

Every 5 years since 1980, the U.S. Department of Agriculture (USDA) and the U.S. Department of Health and Human Services (HHS) have published *Dietary Guidelines for Americans* based on the latest scientific and medical information. Traditionally, the focus has been on *healthy individuals* aged 2 years and older. In 2010, the *Guidelines* were also aimed at *those at risk for chronic disease* to encourage proper dietary habits to promote health and reduce risk for major chronic diseases. These recommendations accommodate the food preferences, cultural traditions, and economic resources of many diverse groups who live in the United States.

The *Guidelines* are intended to evaluate several days' intake of food, not to rate individual food items or a single meal or 1 day's intake. Government policymakers, nutrition educators, and health providers are expected to use the advice to improve the health of the nation. For example, the *Guidelines* would be used to create menus for school lunch programs, nursing home residents, and prisoners.

The *Dietary Guidelines for Americans, 2010* also recognizes that in recent years, nearly 15% of American households have been unable to acquire adequate food to meet their needs. This dietary guidance can help them maximize the nutritional content of their meals. Many other Americans consume less than optimal intake of certain nutrients even though they have adequate resources for a healthy diet. Published materials encompass printed and electronic versions of *Dietary Guidelines for Americans,* and interactive Internet materials are available at www.choosemyplate.gov/print-materials-ordering.html.

Of note, the guidelines do not apply to individuals who have diseases or conditions that alter normal nutritional requirements. Clinical Application 1-1 summarizes the key recommendations for the general population and certain subsets of the population. Many of the terms may be unfamiliar but will become so in later chapters.

1-1

Clinical Application

Key Recommendations of 2010 Dietary Guidelines

BALANCING CALORIES TO MANAGE WEIGHT
- Prevent and/or reduce overweight and obesity through improved eating and physical activity behaviors.
- Control total calorie intake to manage body weight. For people who are overweight or obese, this will mean consuming fewer calories from foods and beverages.
- Increase physical activity and reduce time spent in sedentary behaviors.
- Maintain appropriate calorie balance during each stage of life—childhood, adolescence, adulthood, pregnancy, breastfeeding, and older age.

FOOD AND FOOD COMPONENTS TO REDUCE
- Reduce daily sodium intake to less than 2300 milligrams (mg) and further reduce intake to 1500 mg among persons aged 51 and older and those of any age who are African American or have hypertension, diabetes, or chronic kidney disease. The 1500 mg recommendations applies to about half of the U.S. population, including children, and the majority of adults.
- Consume less than 10% of calories from saturated fatty acids by replacing them with monounsaturated and polyunsaturated fatty acids.
- Consume less than 300 mg per day of dietary cholesterol.
- Keep *trans* fatty acid consumption as low as possible by limiting foods that contain synthetic sources of *trans* fats, such as partially hydrogenated oils, and by limiting other solid fats.
- Reduce the intake of calories from solid fats and added sugars.
- Limit the consumption of foods that contain refined grains, especially refined grain foods that contain solid fats, added sugars, and sodium.
- If alcohol is consumed, it should be consumed in moderation—up to one drink per day for women and two drinks per day for men—and only by adults of legal drinking age.

(Continued)

1-1

$\mathscr{C}$linical $\mathscr{A}$pplication—cont'd

FOODS AND NUTRIENTS TO INCREASE

Individuals should meet the following recommendations as part of a healthy eating pattern while staying within their caloric needs.

- Increase fruit and vegetable intake.
- Eat a variety of vegetables, especially dark-green and red and orange vegetables and beans and peas
- Consume at least half of all grains as whole grains. Increase whole grain intake by replacing refined grains with whole grains.
- Increase intake of fat-free or low-fat milk, and milk products, such as milk, yogurt, cheese, or fortified soy beverages.
- Choose a variety of protein foods, which include seafood, lean meat and poultry, eggs, beans and peas, soy products, and unsalted nuts and seeds.
- Increase the amount and variety of seafood consumed by choosing seafood in place of some meat and poultry.
- Replace protein foods that are higher in solid fats with choices that are lower in solid fats and calories and/or sources of oils.
- Use oils to replace solid fats where possible.
- Choose foods that provide more potassium, dietary fiber, calcium, and vitamin D, which are nutrients of concern in American diets. These foods include vegetables, fruits, whole grains, and milk and milk products.

RECOMMENDATIONS FOR SPECIFIC POPULATION GROUPS

Women capable of becoming pregnant:

- Choose foods that supply heme iron, which is more readily absorbed by the body, additional iron sources, and enhancers of iron absorption such as vitamin C-rich foods.

- Consume 400 micrograms (mcg) per day of synthetic folic acid (from fortified foods and/or supplements) in addition to food forms of folate from a varied diet.

Women who are pregnant or breastfeeding:

- Consume 8 to 12 ounces of seafood per week from a variety of seafood sources.
- Because of their high methyl mercury content, limit white (albacore) tuna to 6 ounces per week, and do not eat the following four types of fish: tilefish, shark, swordfish, and king mackerel.
- If pregnant, take an iron supplement, as recommended by an obstetrician or other health-care provider.

Individuals aged 50 years and older:

- Consume foods fortified with vitamin B_{12}, such as fortified cereals, or dietary supplements.

BUILDING HEALTHY EATING PATTERNS

- Select an eating pattern that meets nutrient needs over time at an appropriate calorie level.
- Account for all foods and beverages consumed and assess how they fit within a total healthy eating pattern.
- Follow food safety recommendations when preparing and eating foods to reduce the risk of foodborne illnesses.

SOURCE: *Dietary Guidelines for Americans, 2010.* www.cnpp.usda.gov/DietaryGuidelines.htm

MyPlate

The latest educational food guidance system promoted by the USDA is called MyPlate, available online at www.choosemyplate.gov/print-materials-ordering/getting-started.html (Fig. 1-2). The intent of the MyPlate icon is to reduce risks for obesity, diabetes, cardiovascular disease, cancer, and other chronic diseases by helping consumers to eat correct proportions of healthy foods meal by meal.

The interactive Web site offers sections for consumers and professionals, sample menus and recipes, tips for vegetarians, and many links to other resources. A page to personalize goals and record progress is located at www.choosemyplate.gov/SuperTracker.

What We Actually Eat

The government periodically surveys food intake of the population to monitor progress toward meeting dietary goals. Information from two such investigations is discussed next.

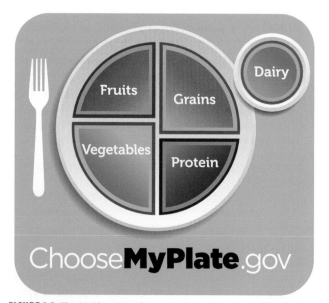

FIGURE 1-2 The MyPlate icon shows relative proportions of five food groups to permit consumers to more easily visualize an ideal meal. The ChooseMyPlate.gov interactive Web site offers dietary assessment tools, nutrition education resources, and clear actionable information about how to make better food choices. (From U.S. Department of Agriculture, 2011, with permission.)

The What We Eat in America Survey

Each year, more than 5000 U.S. residents are interviewed about what they ate and drank for 24-hour periods on 2 nonconsecutive days. The data is part of the HHS National Health and Examination Survey (**NHANES**) that also includes physical examinations.

Among the recent findings concerning foods consumed by Americans are the following:

1. Most people reported eating less than 2 ounces of whole grains per day compared with the 1.5 to 5 ounces recommended according to age and gender.
2. Grain-based desserts (cakes, cookies, pies, cobblers, sweet rolls, pastries, and doughnuts) accounted for a greater proportion of daily kilocalories than did any other food group.
3. Average intake of fluid milk in persons 9 years of age and older was about three-quarters of a cup compared with the recommended amount of 3 cups. Adolescents reporting milk consumption on a given day was 49% compared with 76% 30 years ago.
4. Snacks provided 32% of all daily kilocalories from solid fats and added sugars for women and 31% for men (Bliss, 2012).

Thus, eating healthier foods to maintain a healthy weight is still an unachieved goal for most Americans. Much more information on this topic appears in Chapter 16.

State-Specific Trends in Fruit and Vegetable Consumption

Reflecting the importance of fruit and vegetable intake to a healthy diet (encompassing one-half of the MyPlate graphic), the Centers for Disease Control (CDC) monitors dietary intake through a telephone survey. Results show that much behavior change will be needed to increase to 75% of the population those who consume two or more servings of fruit daily and to 50% those who consume three or more servings of vegetables daily. In the 2009 survey:

1. An estimated 32.5% of U.S. adults consumed fruit two or more times per day with the highest percentage in Washington, DC (40.2%) and the lowest in Oklahoma (18.1%).
2. Above average consumption of fruit was reported by women, adults over the age of 55 years, Black and Hispanic people, and college graduates.
3. An estimated 26.3% of adults consumed vegetables three or more times per day with the highest percentage in Tennessee (33.0%) and the lowest in South Dakota (19.6%).
4. Above average consumption of vegetables was reported by women; adults over the age of 45 years; White, non-Hispanic people; and individuals who had attended or graduated from college (Centers for Disease Control, September 10, 2010).

Effectiveness of Policy

Nutritional public policies have had a limited impact on consumer behavior probably because the mechanisms of food choice decisions are poorly understood. Decision-making not only involves rationality but also feelings, emotions, and memories (Jacquier et al, 2012).

Analysis of the effectiveness of policy interventions in the European Union found that although diet quality had improved across countries, it still fell short of the World Health Organization dietary guidelines. This review divided interventions into measures providing information and those targeting the market environment.

Information measures included

1. Reduced or banned unhealthy food advertisements—generally produced a weak positive effect on improving diets.
2. Public information campaigns—raised awareness of unhealthy eating but failed to translate the message into action.
3. Nutritional labeling—allowed for informed but not necessarily healthier choices.

Interventions targeting the market environment included

1. Fiscal measures and
2. Nutrient, food, and diet standards.

The last two are rarer and generally more effective than information measures, although admittedly more intrusive (Brambila-Macias, Shankar, Capacci Mazzocchi et al, 2011).

Unbalanced Nutrition

Ingesting too much or too little of a nutrient can interfere with health and well-being. Each nutrient has a beneficial range of intake; an intake below or above that range is incompatible with optimal health.

Malnutrition

Malnutrition (faulty nutrition) can be caused by inadequate or unbalanced intake of food or nutrients or to ineffective processing by the body due to malfunction or disease. The result in the body's cells is an excess or deficiency of one or more nutrients that can lead to physical abnormalities and possibly mental dysfunction.

Ideally, a person should consume a diet marked by balance, moderation, and variety.

1. Balance is displayed in the MyPlate icon that shows the proportions of foods in a meal.
2. Moderation is exemplified by judicious portion sizes such as are used on the Nutrition Facts labels found on many food items (see Chapter 13).
3. Variety is characterized by selection of many different foods rather than always eating one's favorites or those easiest to prepare.

If those three qualities of a good diet are consistently absent, health may suffer and recovery from illness may be prolonged. For instance, ambulatory adults who were at nutritional risk when admitted to the hospital had inpatient stays almost twice as long (13 versus 7 days) as those not at nutritional risk when admitted (Caccialanza, Klersy, Cereda, Cameletti et al, 2010).

Malnutrition involving protein is addressed in Chapter 4. Vitamin and mineral deficiency diseases are found in Chapters 6 and 7. Effects of other nutritional imbalances are considered in other chapters as appropriate.

Food Insecurity

Food insecurity is the limited or uncertain availability of nutritionally adequate and safe foods or doubtful ability to acquire food, whether some of the time or always. Food insecurity, often associated with poverty and low income, has important implications for the health and nutrition of individuals and nations.

In the United States

The *2010 Dietary Guidelines for Americans* acknowledged the extent of food insecurity in the country. One objective of the *Guidelines* was to assist residents with limited resources to maximize the nutritional content of their meals.

EXTENT OF THE PROBLEM

An estimated 14.5% (17.2 million) of American households were food insecure at some time during 2010. These households had difficulty at some time during the year providing enough food for all their members due to a lack of resources.

Rates of food insecurity were higher than the national average for households with incomes near or below 185% of the federal poverty level, households with children headed by single women or single men, and Black and Hispanic households. Food insecurity was more prevalent in households with children than those with no children. Elderly people living alone or with others had the least food insecurity of the households described.

Food insecurity was also more common in large cities and rural areas than in the suburbs. Regionally, the prevalence of food insecurity was higher in the South and West than in the Midwest and Northeast. See Figure 1-3 to compare the percentage of the household groups categorized as food insecure. It is apparent that a household fits into several of the subgroups simultaneously. For instance, a single Hispanic mother living in the West below the federal poverty line is at risk on all those levels. The degree of compounded risk is not discernible from these statistics.

FOOD COSTS AND RESOURCES

In 2010, all U.S. households spent a **median** of $43.75 per week per person on food. Households with low food security and very low food security spent $34.00 per week per person (Coleman-Jensen, Nord, Andrews, and Carlson, 2011).

Fifty-nine percent of the food-insecure households received assistance from one or more of the federal food and nutrition assistance programs during the

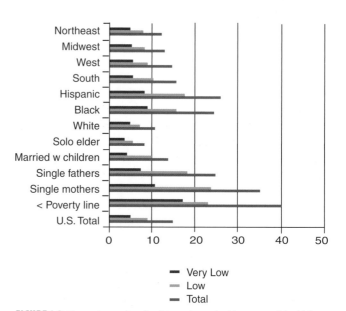

FIGURE 1-3 Percentage of each of these household groups of the U.S. population experiencing very low food security, low food security, and the total of the two. Forty percent of the poor households and 35% of households headed by single mothers faced the most food insecurity according to the survey (data from Coleman-Jensen, Nord, Andrews, and Carlson, 2011).

month before the survey (Coleman-Jensen et al, 2011).

1. The Supplemental Nutrition Assistance Program (SNAP, formerly the Food Stamp Program) provided benefits to 40.9% of food-insecure households while serving 46 million individuals overall in 2011 (Gunderson, 2014).
2. Children in 32.4% of the food-insecure households received free or reduced-price school lunches. In 2009, more than 31 million students participated in the National School Lunch Program with 16.3 million receiving free lunches (Gunderson, 2014).
3. Women and children in 13.6% of the food-insecure households received food vouchers from the **Women, Infants, and Children's** program (WIC). Currently WIC serves 45% of all infants who are born in the United States (Gunderson, 2014).

Despite that assistance, poor people's food intake overall is concentrated in inexpensive, high-kilocalorie food of low nutritional quality. Low-cost, high-kilocalorie foods containing added sugar and fat comprise almost 40% of the daily kilocalorie intake of people with low resources because their communities offer little else. The lack of full service supermarkets with fresh produce and low-fat dairy products led to the descriptor of *food deserts* for such neighborhoods.

Redefining obesity more broadly as a food security problem rather than an individual choice problem may generate better solutions. Some communities have provided incentives for convenience stores to stock fresh produce. Farmers' markets have opened in some localities. Large food retailers have opened stores in poor neighborhoods as the result of public-private partnerships (Center for School, Health, and Education, 2011). A model of a mobile market distribution system to serve in-need neighborhoods shows that, with relatively few resources, these residents' access to healthy food could be increased (Widener, Metcalf, and Bar-Yam, 2012).

On the other hand, availability of fast food and convenience outlets versus purveyors of healthier food does not independently explain weight gain over time in elementary school–age children (Lee, 2010). Greater supermarket availability was generally unrelated to diet quality and fruit and vegetable intake. Relationships between grocery store availability and diet outcomes were mixed, suggesting that access to food stores alone is insufficient to produce behavior change, which may require complementary or alternative strategies (Boone-Heinonen, Gordon-Larsen, Kiefe, Shikany, et al, 2011).

Worldwide

If access to food was not dependent on income but on need, the food available globally would be sufficient to meet the needs of humankind. Economic disparities are evident in consumption patterns. The amount of animal protein foods consumed by the wealthiest 20% of the world's population is fourfold that of the poorest 20% (Uauy, Hawkesworth, and Dangour, 2014).

In 2011, an estimated 925 million people suffered chronic **hunger.** Almost all the world's undernourished live in developing countries, with 578 million in Asia and the Pacific and 239 million in sub-Saharan Africa. (See the map at www.wfp.org/hunger/map.) Five of the top 10 cost-effective solutions for development focus on nutrition (World Food Program, 2011). Multiple organizations, both governmental and private, are working to feed the hungry (See Box 1-1).

AGRICULTURAL INNOVATIONS TO COMBAT HUNGER

At least half the world's food-insecure people are poor, small farmers working marginal lands without modern productivity enhancements (Fanzo and Pronyk, 2011). Scientists are working to improve plants, animals, and food products. The goals are to discover sustainable changes to agricultural practices in developing countries and to increase the nourishment in the food raised. Plant genetics remains a key component of global food security. Millions of lives depend on the extent to which crop genetic improvement can keep pace with the growing global population, changing climate, and shrinking environmental resources (Ronald, 2011). Following are some examples of work being accomplished.

Diversifying Crops. In Kenya, just 10 of 210 species of leafy vegetables were marketed at baseline. A project in Nairobi to educate farmers, to stimulate demand for the

---

Box 1-1 ■ *Feeding the Famished*

Global food aid deliveries in 2010 totaled 5.4 million tons, two-thirds of it delivered by the United Nations' World Food Program. One ton of mixed commodities will feed about 1800 persons for one day (World Food Program, 2011).

A new fully cooked food-aid product has been developed to be used as a supplemental food ration for delivery overseas for humanitarian feeding programs. Uncooked blends were subject to spoilage and tended to have uneven distribution of vitamins and minerals. The processing of this instant corn-soy blend uses high heat and high pressure to cook the mixture completely in less than two minutes; it is then milled to a powder to be added to **potable water** and eaten as porridge (Bliss, 2011).

"other" vegetables, and to distribute the produce effectively was successful. Within 3 years, produce delivery to market swelled from 31 to 400 tons per month, and increased the incomes of the monitored farmers 2- to 20-fold (Fanzo and Pronyk, 2011).

Controlling Plant and Animal Diseases. Mapping the human genome is not the only genetic breakthrough affecting nutrition. Both plants and animals are under investigation for their potential to minimize losses from diseases.

Rice is the main dietary staple for more than half the world's population. It is grown in 114 countries on six continents (Ronald, 2011). A Japanese variety was the first rice genome to be sequenced, thus permitting researchers to determine which genes control certain traits such as disease resistance. Just as microorganisms develop immunity to antibiotics given to humans, plant **pathogens** also evolve so that the plant needs multiple genes to confer resistance (Durham and Avant, 2011). Rice blast, caused by a fungus, affects the plants in all stages of development. Geneticists at the USDA Agricultural Research Service developed molecular markers to screen for resistance genes (Yao and Flores, 2010). See Chapter 7 for information about arsenic in rice.

Corn has been genetically engineered to produce proteins from the soil bacterium *Bacillus thuringiensis* which kills some key caterpillar and beetle pests. Consequently, lower amounts of chemical insecticides are used, thus reducing costs while protecting the environment (Ronald, 2011).

Scientists are looking for areas in the cattle genome that support tolerance to tickborne diseases. A particular breed of South African cattle has such tolerance but has other traits that keep it from becoming the most marketable steer. If the desirable genes can be discovered, breeders will have sound knowledge to use when selecting animals for reproduction.

A second objective of the Agricultural Research Service in South Africa is to help select breeds of cattle best suited for dairy ranching. In this operation, cows and calves graze together during the day but the calves are separated from their mothers at night so that the cow can be milked in the morning for daily income for the farmer. The calves still receive enough milk to grow and stay healthy (O'Brien, 2011).

Enhanced Nutritional Content. Only a small percentage of corn varieties have naturally high levels of **carotenoids,** precursors of vitamin A. Researchers have discovered two genes in corn linked to higher **beta-carotene** levels as well as a faster, less expensive method to screen corn plants for more genes to produce even higher levels of the nutrient. Ultimately, the levels of carotenoids in Africa's corn could be at least tripled (O'Brien, 2010).

More than 250 million Africans rely on the starchy root crop cassava as their staple source of calories. A typical cassava-based diet, however, provides less than 30% of the minimum daily requirement for protein and only 10 to 20% of that for iron, zinc, and vitamin A. Efforts to develop genetically engineered cassava with increased amounts of those nutrients are underway. Additional goals are to increase shelf life, boost resistance viral disease, and reduce toxic cyanogenic glycosides (see Chapter 4) to safe levels (Sayre, Beeching, Cahoon, Egesi, et al, 2011).

Progress toward the United Nations' Millennium Development Goal of reducing the proportion of people who suffer from hunger by half between 1990 and 2015 has been mixed. Of the 117 countries analyzed by UNICEF, 63 are on track to meet the target. Of the 20 countries that made no progress toward the goal, most are in Africa (Fanzo and Pronyk, 2011).

The scientific advance of incorporating genes from other plants and bacteria into the rice gene, creating Golden Rice by adding beta-carotene, had not reached the poor farmers who desperately need it 14 years after its invention. Despite the donation of the technology by its inventors to the poor of the world, political and regulatory burdens plagued its dissemination. Fears of harm have been discredited by the United Nations' Food and Agriculture Organization. Academies of science throughout the world have declared genetic modification of plants to be no more hazardous to people or the environment than are conventional plant breeding techniques (Dubock, 2012). See Chapter 6 for information on vitamin A deficiency that Golden Rice promises to cure.

Nutritional Care

Nutritional status refers to the body's condition related to the intake and use of nutrients. All members of the health-care team have roles in the effective evaluation of a client's nutritional status. See Team Work 1-1.

Dietary status describes what a client has been eating. Although a client's dietary status may be adequate, his or her nutritional status may be poor. An evaluation of a client's dietary status can help to determine the reason for this poor nutritional status, or it may rule out poor diet as the source of the client's problem.

Providing nutrition care usually involves several health-care providers to conduct the four steps of the process: assessment, analysis/diagnosis, planning/intervention, and monitoring/evaluation. Fictional case studies throughout this book integrate the steps to provide nutritional care for the described clients with commonly encountered problems.

1-1

Health-Care Providers in Nutrition Delivery

A client's health-care team may include more than 15 members. The following are the respective titles and responsibilities of the major members of the health-care team.

Registered nurses (RNs) are often the first team members to interview a client, and they communicate important nutritional information such as a client's response to food, including intake and tolerance, to other team members. In addition, they identify and refer clients at high nutritional risk to other team members, and they provide some nutritional information to clients.

Licensed practical nurses/licensed vocational nurses (LPNs/LVNs), supervised by RNs, feed clients, monitor food consumption, measure intake and output, and record data.

Registered dietitians (RDs) and physicians are responsible for meeting clients' nutritional needs. Dietitians interpret the physician's diet order in terms of clients' food habits and food choices, calculate clients' nutritional requirements, evaluate clients' response to therapeutic diets, recommend the best route for nutrient administration, **enteral** or **parenteral**, and provide in-depth nutrition education and counseling to clients. Among team members, the registered dietitian usually has the most education and training in the nutritional sciences.

Dietetic technicians (DTs) assist dietitians by taking nutrition histories and body measurements, reviewing records, and monitoring clients' food intake. They are often responsible for screening clients for nutritional risk and referring clients at risk to the registered dietitian.

Physicians are responsible for the diagnosis and treatment of medical conditions. They manage medical care, order laboratory tests, and prescribe medications and diets. Physicians are responsible for communicating the diagnosis and explaining treatment options to clients. Treatment options should always be presented to clients at the same time they are given bad news. Only the physician or the designee can order diagnostic tests, medications, and other treatments.

Medical assistants are responsible for taking vital signs and measuring a client's height and weight. When this information is not available, a complete nutritional assessment is not possible.

Clinical pharmacists (RPhs) prepare, preserve, and compound medicines and **parenteral nutrition** preparations and dispense them according to the prescriptions of physicians. They function as valuable resources for all team members and may also counsel clients about food–drug and drug–drug interactions.

Speech pathologists diagnose and treat swallowing disorders along with other nonnutrition-related disorders. Diagnosis involves determining the type of **dysphagia** the client manifests (see Chapter 9). Treatment for swallowing disorders may include exercises, positions, and strategies such as changing food and liquid textures for easier and safer swallowing.

Occupational therapists recommend strategies to assist clients with disabilities attain maximum functioning in activities of daily living; regarding nutrition, they may provide assistive feeding devices or help modify food preparation areas.

Social workers assess the family support system and link clients with services to help with care; they also provide assistance with financial concerns related to health care and with obtaining appropriate levels of care.

Other health-care personnel who may be involved in client care include medical technologists, nurse practitioners, and psychologists. Many health-care personnel have advanced training and certification in one specific area. For example, both RNs and RDs may elect to obtain Certified Diabetes Educator (CDE) certification.

Identifying a problem but having insufficient resources to address it is more likely than having too much assistance from other team members. Many functions of health-care personnel overlap to avoid missing a client's problem (see Dollars & Sense 1-1).

Assessment

Initiation of nutrition assessment in a timely manner is a requirement of accrediting and licensing agencies. Two levels of methodology are commonly used to identify clients at nutritional risk. Institutions are likely to select a screening technique expected to identify nutritional problems common in their clientele. Although no nutritional screening tool is considered the gold standard for identifying nutritional risk, a comparison of four such tools found that each identified such clients at risk. Moreover, those at nutritional risk indeed developed

TABLE 1-3 ■ Sample Subjective and Objective Nutritional Data	
SUBJECTIVE	OBJECTIVE
Usual diet and fluid intake	Measured height and weight
Number of meals per day	**Edema**, severity, location
Last meal: time, foods, beverages, and amounts	Skin **turgor** and/or dryness
Food and nutrient supplements	Condition of teeth and gums
Appetite	Hair quantity and quality
Problems with digestion and/or elimination	Body fat measurements
Allergies or food intolerances	Complete blood count
Usual alcohol consumption	Serum **albumin**
Chewing and swallowing problems	Serum **electrolytes**
Use of dentures	
Usual weight and recent changes	
Food Likes and Dislikes	

from 48% to 280% more complications during hospitalization and had a 1.6-day to 2.2-day longer hospital stay than those not identified to be at nutritional risk (Velasco, Garcia, Rodriguez, Frias, et al, 2011).

A nutritional screening should be brief enough that the information can be gathered quickly. The time to administer the tool may be extremely brief because if a key factor is found to be present, the screening is stopped, and the client is declared at nutritional risk and referred to a dietitian.

More comprehensive than screening, a **nutritional assessment** is the second level of methodology. It is an evaluation of a client's nutritional status (nutrient stores) based on a physical examination, **anthropometric measurements**, laboratory data, and food intake information. Many members of the health-care team are involved in a comprehensive nutritional assessment, including the physician, dietitian, nurse, social worker, and laboratory staff.

Because it requires considerable resources, this second level of nutritional assessment is usually completed only in the cases of clients at high nutritional risk. For example, a surgeon may order a comprehensive nutritional assessment before surgery to determine whether the client could tolerate a procedure better after nutritional rehabilitation.

Assessment involves an organized and systematic search for pertinent subjective (what the client reports) and objective (what the health-care provider measures) data. (See samples in Table 1-3.) Note the difference between a client's reported height and weight as subjective data and the health-care provider's measured height and weight as objective data. Sometimes they may be identical, but not always. A conscientious search for accurate data creates a sound foundation on which to build nutritional care.

Subjective Data

Subjective data as they relate to nutrition include the client's history from an interview, or questionnaire, or food diary. Information on of the five techniques listed in Table 1-4 may be used. Some of the advantages and disadvantages of each are listed in the table. Of special concern are the food frequency questionnaires, food records, and dietary recalls are based on self-reported data. Any of them can contain errors because of inadequate recall and serious underreporting of kilocalorie intake by **obese** people (Rasmussen, Winning, Savorani, Toft, et al, 2012).

Neither reported dietary intake nor any other item of assessment data is suitable to use as the sole criterion of nutritional status.

Objective Data

A physical examination can include general appearance, anthropomorphic measurements, and laboratory or other diagnostic tests.

GENERAL APPEARANCE

Well-nourished people generally look healthy and usually have an optimistic perspective. Table 1-5 compares the appearance of a well-nourished individual with that of an individual who is less well nourished. A person need not display all of the abnormal signs listed to be regarded as malnourished.

ANTHROPOMETRIC DATA

For clinical purposes, body size, weight, and proportions are determined by **anthropometry,** the science of measuring the body. Such measurements are used to determine growth, body composition, and nutritional status. The body's energy and protein stores also can be derived from these measurements. Underwater weighing and dual-energy x-ray absorptiometry (DEXA) are considered the gold standards for body composition assessment (Wang, Lim, and Caballero, 2014).

TABLE 1-4 ■ Commonly Used Techniques to Obtain Food Intake Information

TECHNIQUE	ADVANTAGES	DISADVANTAGES
Comparison With the MyPlate Model Health-care provider asks client what he or she eats and compares this reported food intake with MyPlate Model.	Can be used to screen many clients quickly. Requires a minimally trained interviewer.	Is not comprehensive. May overlook some clients who would benefit from nutritional care.
Food Frequency Questionnaire Health-care provider requests client fill out a questionnaire asking about **usual food intake** during specified times, such as, "What do you usually eat for breakfast?"	Questionnaire can be tailored to particular nutrients of interest (e.g., lactose, gluten). May assess food usage for any length of time: day, week, month, weekends versus weekdays, summer versus winter, etc. Initial client contact does not require a highly trained interviewer.	May require special resources (e.g., computerized database) to evaluate the information collected. Provides limited information on a client's food behaviors such as shopping and preparation, meal spacing, length of usual mealtime, etc.
Food Records Health-care provider asks client to record his or her food intake for a specified length of time (1, 3, or 7 days).	A motivated client will provide reasonably accurate information. Research shows some clients will change their food habits while keeping a food record; therefore, this technique works well when a behavior change is desired.	A less highly motivated client will "forget to keep" part or all of the food record or record questionable amounts. Thus, this technique could yield inaccurate data to determine a client's actual dietary and/or nutritional status. May require special resources (e.g., a computerized database) to evaluate the information obtained. Requires a follow-up visit to review the evaluated food records. Analysis of data is time-consuming.
24-Hour Dietary Recall Health-care provider asks client what he or she has eaten during the previous 24 hours.	Technique is fairly simple. Interviewer should be trained not to ask leading questions.	Yields limited information. The previous 24 hours may not have been usual for the client. Typically, clients may not remember what they ate and the amounts they ate. Estimates of amounts are frequently inaccurate.
Diet History Health-care provider conducts an in-depth interview to obtain information about usual food intake, drug and medication usage, alcohol and tobacco use, financial and physical ability to obtain food, special dietary needs, food allergies and intolerances, weight history, cultural and religious preferences that may influence food selection, ability to chew and swallow foods, previous dietary instructions received, client knowledge about nutrition, and elimination patterns.	Technique is comprehensive. Requires a highly trained interviewer, usually a dietitian. An analysis of the results obtained can usually be provided on the same day the information is collected. Is a good technique for high-risk clients when information is needed to evaluate the need for nutritional support and the likelihood of dietary prescriptions being implemented.	Is highly dependent on the willingness of the client to reveal information to the interviewer. Client must be a good historian. Technique is time-consuming.

The collection of anthropometric data on height and weight—triceps skinfold, midarm circumference, abdominal circumference, waist measurements, and body density measures—is described briefly in the following sections. Other measurements may also be selected.

Height and Weight. These are the most widely used anthropometric measurements, and their derivative, the **body mass index** is the most commonly used indirect indicator of obesity and body adiposity (Wang et al, 2014). Height may be measured in inches or centimeters. Adults and older children are measured standing with head erect; infants and young children are measured lying on a firm, flat surface.

Weight may be recorded in pounds or kilograms. The agency policy regarding calibration of the scale should be followed. Each time the client is weighed, it should be on the same scale at the same time of the day, and the client should be wearing the same kind of clothing.

Triceps Skinfold. Because skin is typically only 0.5 to 2 millimeters thick, skinfolds can be used as a measure of underlying fat. For this site, the tissue over the triceps muscle in the back of the upper arm is measured with calibrated calipers (Gropper and Smith, 2013). The **triceps skinfold** measurement helps to differentiate between a person who is heavy because of muscle mass and one who is heavy because of excess fat.

Dietitians usually take skinfold measurements, a skill requiring much practice. All measurements should be repeated two or three times with the average recorded as the skinfold value. A skilled provider may achieve accuracy within 5% (Gropper and Smith, 2013). Body areas other than the triceps can also be used to measure skinfolds. When measuring extremities, if U.S. survey data are the standard of comparison, the right side of the body is used. In the United Kingdom and some other locales, the left side is used (Gropper and Smith, 2013).

TABLE 1-5 ■ General Appearance as an Indicator of Nutritional Status		
	NORMAL	**ABNORMAL**
Demeanor	Alert, responsive Positive outlook	Lethargic Negative attitude
Weight	Reasonable for build	Underweight Overweight, obese
Hair	Glossy, full, firmly rooted Uniform color	Dull, sparse; easily, painlessly plucked
Eyes	Bright, clear, shiny	Pale conjunctiva Redness, dryness
Lips	Smooth	Chapped, red, swollen
Tongue	Deep red Slightly rough One longitudinal furrow	Bright red, purple Swollen or shrunken Several longitudinal furrows
Teeth	Bright, painless	Painful, mottled, or missing, **dental caries**
Gums	Pink, firm	Spongy, bleeding, receding
Skin	Clear, smooth, firm, slightly moist	Rashes, swelling Light or dark spots Dry, cracked
Nails	Pink, firm	Spoon shaped or ridged Spongy bases
Mobility	Erect posture Good muscle tone Walks without pain or difficulty	Muscle wasting Skeletal deformities Loss of balance

Midarm Circumference. Because 50% of the body's protein stores are located in muscle tissue, the circumference (the outside edge of a circle) of the midarm provides information about body protein stores. The upper arm is measured between the shoulder and the elbow. The **midarm circumference** measurement is easily obtained and can be used to monitor a client's nutritional progress.

Waist Measurements. A standard procedure should be used for waist measurements that are recorded in inches or centimeters according to agency procedure. In general, with the person standing, the waist is measured at the narrowest site. The tissue should not be compressed.

Abdominal circumference or girth is also used to monitor growth of a fetus or of abnormal tissue within the abdomen. The measure is also valuable when an individual is accumulating fluid in the abdominal cavity, a condition called **ascites.**

Body Density Measures. Muscle and fat tissue have different rates of metabolism. Therefore, the proportions of each in the body influence whether a person is overweight. These proportions can be determined by several techniques, including underwater weighing, dual-energy x-ray absorptiometry (DEXA), and bioelectrical impedance.

Underwater weighing compares the person's scale weight with his or her weight underwater. After correcting for lung volume, the examiner calculates the proportion of body fat. Underwater weighing provides the most accurate assessment of the amount of fat in the body. It is not easily determined, however. Even in research studies, several measurements must be taken and averaged to obtain a value that minimizes error. Because the technique is cumbersome, time-consuming, and requires special equipment, its main use is in research.

In **DEXA,** two x-ray beams are passed through the body. The amount of energy detected after the beams pass through the body varies with bone, fat, and muscle tissue, and the percentage of those tissues in the body can be calculated. The x-ray exposure is relatively low: 1 to 10% of that used for a chest x-ray (Gropper and Smith, 2013), and unlike bioelectrical impedance, discussed next, DEXA is not affected by the client's hydration status (Moran, Lavado-Garcia, and Pedrera-Zamorano, 2011).

In clinical practice, DEXA is used to measure bone mineral density as an indicator of conditions marked by bone loss, such as **osteopenia** and **osteoporosis** (see Chapter 7). A screening test to determine a person's level of risk for those conditions can be conducted with an **ultrasound bone densitometer** that involves no radiation exposure.

In the **bioelectrical impedance test,** electrodes on the extremities are stimulated with a small amount of electrical current, which is then measured at the exit electrodes. Muscle tissue, organs, and blood, rich in water and **electrolytes,** allow an electrical current to pass with greater ease than does denser fat tissue. The greater electrolyte content and conductivity of the body's **fat-free mass** is compared with that of fat. Currents are not painful and usually are not felt because of the small amount of current used.

Body composition is predicted from equations developed on specific populations and may not be valid for tests performed on other groups. The client's fat-free mass is predicted, and his or her percentage of body fat is determined by comparing body weight with the predicted fat-free mass. The three measurements obtained are percentages of the following:

1. Body water
2. **Lean body mass**
3. Body fat

Because bioelectrical impedance is based on total body water, any factors disturbing water balance may alter the results. Examples are diuretic use, excessive sweating, hemodialysis, premenstrual edema, and alcohol consumption within the 24 hours before the test.

This technology is the basis for the bathroom scales that measure body fat. Because the feet are the only contact places for the current to enter and exit, the scales are limited to estimating the fat in the lower body (Buzzell and Pintauro, 2012).

LABORATORY TESTS

Laboratory tests analyze body fluids and excretions. These data include results from blood, urine, and stool tests. From these tests, much information can be obtained concerning what a person has eaten, what his or her body has stored, and how the body is using nutrients.

Blood can be analyzed for glucose, protein, or fat content. Vitamin and mineral status can be determined directly by examining the blood or indirectly by examining enzymes related to the vitamin or mineral. Many experts doubt, however, that vitamin or mineral body stores can be accurately determined by blood samples. The uncertainty lies in whether the nutrient in the blood reflects body stores, a transport form of the nutrient, or the amount in one specific body compartment.

Also circulating in the blood are **metabolites** that are formed in and by the body as it processes food and nutrients. An international project documented 84% of the human **serum** metabolites and electronically published a catalog of 4229 of them for the use of scientists. In the future, a person's metabolic fingerprint might reliably evaluate his or her health and risk for certain diseases (Wood, 2012), fine-tuning present-day measures of cholesterol, for instance, which is an imperfect predictor of health or illness.

Good clinical judgment must be used in selecting tests and interpreting results. Reliance on a single test or single reading is not recommended.

Analysis/Diagnosis

The health-care provider uses subjective data, objective data, or both to identify the level of the client's wellness regarding nutrition. The client's physical findings are compared with standard nutritional parameters. His or her dietary intake is compared with that recommended for his or her age and activity level.

Physical Standards

The data gathered for a client is compared with expected results for similar clients. Commonly used standards include body mass index and waist measurements.

BODY MASS INDEX

The BMI, also known as the **Quetelet Index,** is derived from weight and height and was designed to provide a measure of weight independent of height. Although the BMI has been used as an indicator of obesity, it fails to distinguish **adipose tissue** from muscle or water weight. For very athletic individuals, BMI charts may falsely indicate obesity when the major body mass is not fat but muscle. Because the BMI is noninvasive, easily

assessed at low cost, and has a strong association with body fat and health risks, it is regarded as the best choice of available measures of body fatness (Wang et al, 2014).

Clinical Calculation 1-1 shows the calculations using metric and American measurements. Although not identical, the results are close when calculated without rounding until the final result at three decimal places. For an approximate value using whole numbers, see Table 16-2. Internet calculators can be found at www.nhlbi.nih.gov/guidelines/obesity/BMI/bmicalc.htm. and www.cdc.gov/healthyweight/assessing/bmi

Having derived a value for BMI, what meaning does it have for one's health? In general, the following classifications are used:

- BMI of 18 or less: Underweight
- BMI of 19 to 24: Normal
- BMI of 25 to 29: Overweight
- BMI of 30 to 39: Obese
- BMI of 40 or greater: Morbidly obese

Those standards were developed using Caucasian subjects. Alternative cutoff points recommended for Southeast Asians and Asian Americans to optimize diabetes care are as follows:

- BMI less than 18.5: Underweight
- BMI of 18.5 to 22.9: Normal
- BMI of 23 to 24.9: Overweight
- BMI of 25 to 29.9: Obese
- BMI of 30 or greater: Extremely obese (Mechanick, Marchetti, Apovian, Benchimol, et al, 2012).

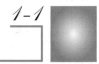

1-1

𝒞linical 𝒞alculation

Body Mass Index

Consider a person 5 feet, 10 inches tall who weighs 170 pounds.

To calculate this body mass index using metric measures:

$$BMI = \text{weight in kilograms}/(\text{height in meters})^2$$

1. Convert 70 inches to meters:
   Divide 70 by 39.37 (inches/meter) = 1.778 meters
2. Convert pounds to kilograms:
   Divide 170 by 2.2 (pounds/kilogram) = 77.273 kg
3. Insert values into BMI formula:

$$BMI = \text{weight in kilograms}/(\text{height in meters})^2$$
$$77.273/1.778 \times 1.778$$
$$77.273/3.161 = 24.446$$

Using the same values in an alternative American measures formula:

Weight in pounds × 705; Divide by height (in inches); divide result by height in inches
$$170 \times 705 = 119,850/70 = 1712.143/70 = 24.459$$

The minimum survivable body weight in humans is a BMI of approximately 13. The maximum survivable body weight is a BMI of about 150 (Going, Hingle, and Farr, 2014).

WAIST CIRCUMFERENCE

Waist circumferences of more than 40 inches in non–Asian American men and 35 inches in non–Asian American women are related to increased risks of diabetes and cardiovascular diseases. In Asian men the risks increase with a waist measurement of 36 inches; in Asian women, 32 inches.

Although relatively insensitive as a measure of the fatness of the **viscera,** waist circumference is widely used as a surrogate for visceral adipose tissue. In combination with BMI, waist circumference predicts disease risk better than either measure alone (Going et al, 2014).

Dietary Intake

A client's reported or recorded food intake can be grouped according to the classifications in MyPlate or individual foods can be analyzed using a computerized diet analysis program.

ANALYSIS BY FOOD GROUPS

A simple method of comparing a client's reported intake with that recommended for him or her is to focus on the food groups found in MyPlate. Online calculation is available at www.choosemyplate.gov/supertracker-tools/supertracker.html. Omitting entire food groups raises serious concerns about the adequacy of dietary intake and merits further investigation.

Remember the phrase "Garbage In, Garbage Out" pertaining to computer user fallibility; the same can be applied to dietary intake—errors are likely if amounts consumed are estimated rather than measured.

ANALYSIS OF NUTRIENTS

More detailed information can be obtained by examining foods for their component nutrients and comparing the client's data to Dietary Reference Intakes (described later). This process can be performed manually or electronically.

The USDA publishes National Nutrient Database for Standard Reference and updates it annually. It contains data on nearly 8000 food items and up to 146 food components. It serves as the foundation for most food composition databases in use such as those in ChooseMyPlate.gov, commercial weight-loss firms, and apps for mobile hand-held devices. The food industry, commercial businesses, government groups, research and academic institutions, and local schools and hospitals all use the information copyright-free, provided as a public service (Bliss, 2012). Search for nutrient content of individual foods at http://ndb.nal.usda.gov.

One user-friendly Web site with many nutrition management and calculation tools is found at http://nutritiondata.self.com/. Owned by Condé Nast Publications and based on the USDA National Nutrient Database for Standard Reference, its goals are to provide accurate, comprehensive, accessible, and understandable nutrition analysis. Its tool to rank foods by highest or lowest concentrations of nutrients can be found at http://nutritiondata.self.com/tools/nutrient-search.

Whether analyzed manually or electronically, care must be taken when selecting food items. For example, selection of "orange juice concentrate" instead of "orange juice" will skew the analysis badly.

Regardless of the process used, the data accumulated need correct interpretation. The only scientifically correct statement justified when intake falls short of recommended levels is that the intake for a given period does not meet whatever standard is being used as a measuring stick. It is inappropriate to base a judgment of nutritional or dietary status solely on one piece of information.

Planning/Intervention

The next step in providing nutritional care is to plan a strategy that addresses identified problems to treat or strengths to reinforce. Depending on the availability of resources, the strategy often involves referral to a dietitian.

Prioritizing Problems

To be successful in stimulating behavior change, the health-care provider and the client must prioritize the problems and select acceptable interventions. Making one or two changes may be easier for the client to sustain than overhauling the client's entire diet. For that reason, selecting the interventions most likely to make a major difference in the client's health status is important.

Except for teaching basic nutritional information, a nurse is likely to refer the client to a dietitian when one is available, particularly if the nutritional problem is severe or complex. Nurses with advanced training in nutrition, such as Certified Diabetes Educators, may assume the responsibility for a client's nutrition as part of comprehensive care. Referral to a dietitian has two functions:

1. Ensuring comprehensive care.
2. Increasing the client's awareness of the need for and benefits of nutritional services.

Using Dietary Reference Intakes

To focus care more finely than the broad approach using food groups, a client's dietary intake can be compared with **Dietary Reference Intakes (DRIs).** One of the categories retains an old title, Recommended Dietary Allowances (RDAs). For a brief history of the origin of the RDAs, see Box 1-2.

When first introduced, the RDAs focused on preventing deficiency diseases. Recent research supports a role for certain nutrients in reducing the risk of chronic diseases. This information has been factored into the standards for North America since 1997. In addition to RDAs for vitamins and minerals, DRIs have been established for the macronutrients (carbohydrate, fat, and protein) and for water and electrolytes.

The DRIs are composed of five nutrient-based reference values that can be used for assessing and planning diets for groups according to life stage and gender. The DRIs are intended to apply to the healthy general population and refer to average daily intakes for 1 or more weeks. The components of the DRIs are as follows:

- **Estimated Average Requirements (EARs):** Intake that meets the estimated nutrient needs of 50% of the individuals in the defined group. EAR is used to set the RDA and to assess or plan the intake of groups.
- **Recommended Dietary Allowances (RDAs):** Intake that meets the needs of 97 to 98% of individuals in the defined group. RDA is intended for use as a goal for daily intake by individuals, not for assessing the adequacy of an individual's nutrient intake.
- **Adequate Intakes (AIs):** Average observed or experimentally determined intake that appears sufficient to meet individuals in the stated group. AI is used if an EAR or RDA cannot be set because of lack of information.

- **Acceptable Macronutrient Distribution Range (AMDR):** Percentage of kilocalories (see Chapter 5 for information on kilocalories) from carbohydrate, fat, and protein associated with reduced risk of chronic disease while still providing sufficient intake of essential nutrients. Only the AMDR for protein has been set with the certainty of the RDA (see Appendix A). Figure 1-4 illustrates a single meal that complies with the AMDR.
- **Tolerable Upper Intake Levels (ULs):** Highest average daily intake by an individual that is unlikely to pose risks of adverse health effects in 97 to 98% of individuals in the defined group. Ordinarily the UL refers to intake from food, fortified food, water, and supplements; exceptions are footnoted in the table in Appendix A. The UL is designed for the general population and may be exceeded under medical supervision in clients with special needs.

Because the RDAs and AIs represent the quantities of nutrients found in typical diets in the United States and Canada, caregivers must adjust their planning for clients who take supplements or follow unusual diets. Table 1-6 compares and gives examples of these components of the DRIs. The DRIs, except the EARs, are listed in Appendix A.

Implementation

After assessment, diagnosis, and planning, the next step is implementation. It may take time and patience to select appropriate interventions for an individual client

---

Box 1-2 ■ *The Birth of the RDAs*

In 1940, as the United States geared up for its inevitable entrance into World War II, concern was raised about the nutritional status of military recruits and of the population in general. On the basis of studies conducted in the 1930s, an estimated one-third of the populace was not well nourished. Although the quantity of food was sufficient, the number of nutrient deficiencies documented indicated that the quality was inadequate (Yates, 2006).

The U.S. National Academy of Sciences convened the Food and Nutrition Board, which first met in November 1940. It proposed the first set of RDAs in April 1941 covering the nine nutrients known to be essential for human health at the time: protein; calcium; iron; vitamins A, C, and D; thiamin; riboflavin; and niacin. Kilocalories were listed in 1941 but had been delisted by 1989.

To help to remedy nutritional deficiencies, during World War II, bread was subject to a war food order mandating enrichment with thiamin, niacin, and iron and eventually riboflavin (U.S. Food and Drug Administration, 2009; Yates, 2006).

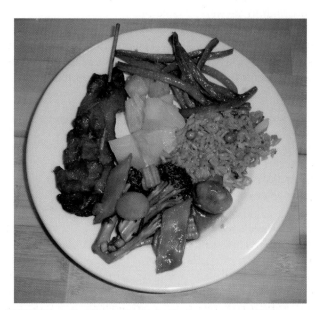

FIGURE 1-4 A plate from a Chinese buffet shows an acceptable distribution of macronutrients; however, the Acceptable Macronutrient Distribution Range and all the Dietary Reference Intakes are recommendations for a week or longer.

TABLE 1-6 ■ **Dietary Reference Intake (DRI) Components**

DRI	PERCENTAGE OF HEALTHY POPULATION INCLUDED	USE	EXAMPLES
EAR	50	Set RDAs Assess/plan for groups	Not applicable to individuals
RDA	97–98	Goal for individual daily intake	290 mcg of iodine for lactating women
AI	Unknown	Goal for individuals Tentative goals for groups	Vitamin K amounts for all ages Most nutrients for infants
UL	97–98	Monitor potential excesses	45 mg of iron for all older than 14 years of age
AMDR	Not specified	Suggested allocation of kilocalories to optimize health	Protein should contribute 10%–35% of daily kilocalories for adults

AI, Adequate Intake; AMDR, Acceptable Macronutrient Distribution Range; EAR, Estimated Average Requirement; RDA, Recommended Dietary Allowance; UL, Tolerable Upper Intake Level.

or family. Eating wisely or unwisely involves choices every day, several times a day, that affect the budget as well as health (see Dollars & Sense 1-2).

A given diet prescription may be implemented in various ways, but finding the approach a client will use faithfully is not only a challenge but also the key to success. Two food-based, as opposed to nutrient-based, interventions include (1) ChooseMyPlate and (2) Food Exchange Lists.

ChooseMyPlate

Much assistance, including budget advice, tips for choosing healthy foods, menus, recipes, games and activities for children, as well as guidance for parents appear on this Web site. For clients who wish to use it, the USDA interactive Web site offers a personalized nutrition and physical activity plan that also permits tracking of a person's progress at www.choosemyplate.gov/SuperTracker.

$ Dollars & Sense 1-2

Choosing Snacks Wisely

Veggies as snacks are not only healthier than salty munchies but also less costly and less kilocalorie dense.

Item	Price	Serving Size	Kilocalories	Cost/Serving
Potato chips, national brand	$3.99/9.5 oz	1 oz, about 11 chips	160	$0.42
Baby cut carrots, store brand	$1.69/lb	3 oz, about 13 carrots	35	$0.32

Food Exchange Lists

For the person who desires more information about food choices besides "fill half your plate with fruits and vegetables," the use of Food Exchange Lists offers the opportunity to combine nutrition education with day-to-day practice.

Few foods contain just one nutrient; rather, most are combinations of nutrients. Originally the basis for **medical nutrition therapy** for people with diabetes, **Food Exchange Lists** sort foods into equivalent groups to allow swapping of foods within the group.

The Food Exchange Lists are used to calculate a client's food intake, to educate a client about nutrition and meal planning, and to counsel a client about food choices. The lists are often adapted for weight loss programs and are sometimes used on labels for prepared meals.

UNDERSTANDING THE EXCHANGE LIST SYSTEM

The system is composed of six exchange lists of foods grouped by nutrient composition. For example, corn is on the starch list because it is closer in composition to a slice of bread than to green beans. The six basic lists are:

1. Starch
2. Fruit
3. Milk in three groups: fat-free/low-fat, reduced-fat, and whole
4. Nonstarchy Vegetable
5. Meat and Meat Substitutes in four groups: lean, medium-fat, high-fat, and plant-based proteins
6. Fat in three groups: monounsaturated, polyunsaturated, and saturated

Depending on the variety, cheese can be a lean, medium-fat, or high-fat meat exchange. Similarly, different cuts of pork can be a lean, medium-fat, or high-fat meat exchange. For the complete lists, as well as combination foods that are counted in several lists, see Appendix B or the online resource at www.eatright.org/search.aspx?search=Exchange%20lists.

Table 1-7 identifies typical foods in each exchange list. In addition, some foods are considered "free" and are permitted in large amounts because they contain little energy (few kilocalories). Free foods are on a separate list. Some free foods have limitations on the amount to be consumed in a day or at one time. In addition, combination foods (soups, casseroles) and selected fast foods appear on separate lists. Table 1-8 displays the amount of carbohydrate, protein, fat, and kilocalories (energy) for one exchange on each list. As the table shows, one exchange on the fruit list is

TABLE 1-7 ■ Typical Foods in Each Exchange List	
EXCHANGE LIST	**FOOD ITEMS**
Starch	Cereals, grains, pasta, dried beans, peas, lentils, starchy vegetables, bread, crackers
Meat and Meat Substitutes	Beef, pork, veal, poultry, fish, wild game, cheese, eggs, tofu, peanut butter
Fruit	Fresh, frozen, or unsweetened canned fruit; dried fruit; fruit juice
Vegetable	Raw or cooked nonstarchy vegetables, vegetable juices
Milk	Milk, yogurt, evaporated milk, powdered milk
Fat	Avocado, margarine, butter, mayonnaise, nuts, seeds, oil, salad dressing, bacon, coconut, cream, sour cream, whipped cream, cream cheese, olives

See the complete Exchange Lists in Appendix B (reprinted with permission of the American Dietetic Association, 2008) or access additional information at www.eatright.org/search.aspx?search=Exchange%20lists.

not equal to one exchange on the vegetable list. To use this method of meal planning correctly, clients must choose the correct number of items from each appropriate list.

In this context, *exchange* means a defined quantity of food within a list that can be interchanged with other foods in the same list. Portion sizes in the lists for various items have been adjusted to make each exchange approximately equal. Table 1-9 shows items equal to one starch exchange. Clearly, 1 ½ cup of puffed cereal would take longer to eat and be more filling than ⅓ cup of cooked rice.

USING THE EXCHANGE LISTS

Exchange lists can be adapted for any prescribed kilocalorie, protein, fat, or carbohydrate level. A specific meal plan for a client should be given with the exchange lists.

A meal plan is a food guide that shows the number of choices or exchanges the client should eat at each meal or snack. Table 1-10 illustrates meal plans for two kilocalorie levels. The table also illustrates how the exchanges might be distributed among meals.

In summary, exchange lists and meal plans:

■ Provide food choices that necessitate minimal calculation,
■ Control the distribution of nutrients throughout the day, and
■ Incorporate balance, variety, and moderation into special diets.

Evaluation and Documentation

After implementing a nutritional plan, the health-care provider and the client decide to what extent the objective has been met. If progress has been unsatisfactory, they explore the reasons, such as

1. unrealistic expectations,
2. insufficient time allotted,
3. interventions not appropriate
4. interventions incorrectly implemented or not implemented.

Documentation of services provided is a basic requirement for all health-care providers. Nurses may use the Nursing Process; dietitians the Nutrition Care Process. The employing agency dictates the format for documentation.

One system was designed for use by several disciplines. Employing such a universal format facilitates

TABLE 1-8 ■ Energy Composition of the Six Exchange Lists				
FOOD LIST	**CARBOHYDRATE (GRAMS)**	**PROTEIN (GRAMS)**	**FAT (GRAMS)**	**KILOCALORIES**
Starch	15	0-3	0-1	80
Fruits	15	—	—	60
Milk				
Fat-free (skim)/low- fat (1%)	12	8	0-3	100
Reduced fat (2%)	12	8	5	120
Whole	12	8	8	160
Nonstarchy Vegetables	5	2	—	25
Meat and meat substitutes				
Lean meat	—	7	0-3	45
Medium fat meat	—	7	4-7	75
High fat meat	—	7	8+	100
Plant-based protein	Varies	7	Varies	Varies
Fats	—	—	5	45

Source: Choose Your Foods: Exchange Lists for Diabetes, American Dietetic Association, 2008. Used with permission.

TABLE 1-9 ■ Examples of One Starch Exchange

Puffed cereal	1 ½ cups
Plain shredded wheat	½ cup
Bread, white, whole grain, rye	1 slice
Corn, whole kernel Green peas Sweet potato	½ cup
Rice, cooked	⅓ cup

See the complete Exchange Lists in Appendix B (reprinted with permission of the American Dietetic Association, 2008) or access additional information at www.eatright.org/search.aspx?search=Exchange%20lists.

TABLE 1-10 ■ 1500- and 1800-kcal Meal Plan Using Exchanges for 1 Day

	1500 KCAL	1800 KCAL
Starch	7	7
Meat, lean	1	3
Meat, medium	3	3
Vegetable	4	5
Fruit	3	5
Milk, skim	2	2
Fat	6	7

DISTRIBUTION OF EXCHANGES THROUGHOUT THE DAY

1500-KCAL MEAL PLAN

	BREAKFAST	LUNCH	DINNER	SNACK
Starch	2	2	2	1
Meat, lean	0	1	0	0
Meat, medium	0	0	3	0
Vegetable	0	2	2	0
Fruit	1	1	1	0
Milk, skim	1	0	0	1
Fat	2	2	2	0

communication among providers. An example is the system using SOAP notes. The letters stand for:

S: Subjective data (explained earlier)
O: Objective data (explained earlier)
A: Analysis or diagnosis based on S and O data
P: Plan of action or treatment

Within an agency, the client's problems may be numbered sequentially, and each SOAP note is numbered to correspond to a specific problem. In other systems, each encounter with the client is treated separately.

The Teamwork Notes following the Case Studies in this text are written in the SOAP format even though that may not be the required documentation format in the clinical facilities used by students studying nutrition. SOAP notes have the advantage of simplicity and

focus on problems that should assist the student to begin to think critically as well as to see the potential for comprehensive nutritional care.

Impact of Culture on Nutrition

Culture refers to all the socially transmitted behavior patterns (attitudes, beliefs, and customs) shared by most members of a particular group that guide their thoughts and actions. Although nation of origin, ethnic identity, and religious affiliation are prime examples of culture, other alliances such as colleges, corporations, professions, political parties, and service clubs also imbue people with values and behavioral norms.

Health practices draw together people of similar habits, such as athletes or vegetarians. Thus, some aspects of culture are passed on from birth, but other aspects are voluntarily selected. All aspects of culture, including the family's food ways, ethnicity, and religion, may influence an individual's food choices. Figure 1-5 shows a multigenerational birthday party shaped in part by culture.

Even among individuals of similar cultural heritage, differences exist. Dietary preferences, for example, differ among people of Hispanic descent from such diverse places as Cuba, Puerto Rico, and Mexico. Just because a person belongs to a certain ethnic or religious group does not mean that he or she has adopted its traditional lifestyle and practices.

Caution is advised before replacing traditional food preparation techniques that have succeeded for generations; changes can sometimes foster disease. For example, botulism outbreaks were traced to substituting

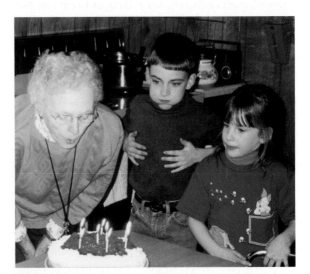

FIGURE 1-5 Different cultures have their own ways to observe life's milestones: births, birthdays, weddings, deaths. These children are sharing a birthday tradition with their 88-year-old great-grandmother.

plastic bags for clay pots in preparing a Native American dish in Alaska and to swapping similar bags for waxed paper and wooden crates to ship smoked fish in Michigan. The plastic bags excluded air and permitted the botulism organism to produce its toxin. Another example is mad cow disease spreading widely after changes in feed production in England.

Relation to Longevity

Life expectancy is the prospect of a certain mean length of life at a specified age based on current **mortality** rates in the population being considered. In 2007, the disparities in life expectancy in the United States by gender and race were the smallest ever recorded (Centers for Disease Control, September 17, 2010). As shown in Figure 1-6, life expectancy at birth has risen for Whites and Blacks in the United States since 1970, but not equally for all.

Certain groups display exceptional longevity that relates to nutrition. Although a single dietary pattern promoting longevity has not been recognized, kilocalorie restriction seems to play a role in persons surviving to the age of 100 years. Populations with an unusually high prevalence of centenarians all tended to be (or were) physically active, nonobese, and small in stature (Hausman, Fischer, and Johnson, 2011). Furthermore, in the United States, persons with slender or medium body builds at age 30 years had 2.6 times the chance of surviving to age 100 than did persons with "stout" body builds (Gavrilova and Gavrilov, 2010).

Long-lived Okinawans ascribe to the dietary mantra of "eat until you are only 80% full." They consume large amounts of fruits and vegetables with soy as the major

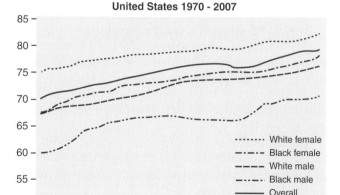

QuickStats: Life Expectancy at Birth, by Race* and Sex United States 1970 - 2007

*Includes Hispanics and non-Hispanics.

FIGURE 1-6 Life expectancy at birth for U.S. Blacks and Whites, 1970 to 2007. Although all segments of the population gained some expected years of life, the ascent is steadier for Whites than for Blacks (Centers for Disease Control, September 17, 2010).

protein component. Compared with other diets, their kilocaloric intake is less, resulting in low BMIs. No single factor explains exceptionally long life. Centenarians escaped infant mortality, infectious diseases before antibiotics were available, and age-associated diseases through combinations of genes, environment, and chance that vary with culture and geography (Pignolo, 2010).

Basic Terminology

To provide sensitive health-care services to people different from oneself requires some introspection as to one's own values and attitudes. Knowledge of a few terms from the study of culture will help to arrive at a level of self-understanding and perhaps increased respect for others.

Ethnocentrism

The belief that one's own group's view of the world is superior to that of others is **ethnocentrism.** Historically, the dominant cultural group in the United States has been White descendants of northern Europeans who are middle class and Protestant. As a result, our health-care system reflects the important values of this culture:

- Education
- Work
- Punctuality
- Independence
- A future orientation

Health-care providers have tried, often unsuccessfully, to deliver this version of health care to clients without regard to the clients' cultures. Hence, clients who failed to achieve goals imposed on them were labeled "noncompliant." Clients unable to communicate in the dominant culture's language were defined as having "altered communication."

Acculturation

The process of adopting the values, attitudes, and behavior of another culture, **acculturation,** often encourages less desirable health behaviors than were previously practiced. For example, using preference for the Spanish language to signify less acculturation, the prevalence of breastfeeding by Hispanic women was significantly higher among less acculturated than among highly acculturated mothers. Those who were more acculturated, responding to the survey in English, were 12% less likely to initiate breastfeeding, 23% less likely to breastfeed for 10 weeks or more, and 30% less likely to report exclusive breastfeeding for 10 weeks or more than the less acculturated group (Ahluwalia, D'Angelo, Morrow, and McDonald, 2012).

Another adverse effect of acculturation is the increase in various diseases in native populations. A major disease affecting widely scattered indigenous populations undergoing acculturation is type 2 diabetes mellitus. Before the 20th century, diabetes was virtually unknown among native people, but by 1987, most indigenous peoples had diabetes prevalence and mortality rates several times higher than comparable Caucasian populations (Ely, Zavaskis, and Wilson, 2011). The Pima Indians in Arizona currently have the highest recorded prevalence of diabetes in the world. On average, American Indian and Alaska Native adults are 2.6 times more likely to have diabetes than non-Hispanic Whites of similar age (Centers for Disease Control, 2011). Adopting the modern lifestyle, including dietary changes leading to obesity, is credited with contributing to the worsening the health status of native peoples.

Acculturation can have positive as well as negative effects on dietary patterns. More than half the Chinese immigrants to Canada surveyed reported more awareness and knowledge of healthy foods, increased consumption of fruits and vegetables, and decreased deep fat frying of foods compared with their previous practices in China. Compared with more recently arrived immigrants, those who lived in Canada the longest however, reported consuming increased portion sizes, dining out more frequently, and using more convenience foods (Rosenmoller, Gasevic, Seidell, and Lear, 2011)

Culturally Competent Care

Knowledge and acceptance of and respect for other cultures underpin culturally competent care, which is a willingness and ability to deliver culturally congruent and acceptable care to clients. Employing institutions can assist health-care providers by attending to demographic, cultural, and epidemiological characteristics of their service areas to plan for and implement services appropriate for the cultural and language needs of their clients (U.S. Department of Health and Human Services, 2007).

Even though health-care providers cannot be experts on every cultural group they encounter, they can develop openness to learning the client's perspective. The goal is a treatment plan that successfully blends the client's cultural beliefs with the practices of modern medicine. Clients learn their attitudes about health, the causes of illness, and their abilities to control outcomes as part of their maturation within their cultures. Those with high **self-efficacy** will believe they can perform a given task or behavior and will be more amenable to nutritional prescriptions and change than someone with less faith in her or his abilities or a more fatalistic view of life. Clinical Application 1-2 illustrates the adaptation of diabetic teaching to Native American mythology and beliefs.

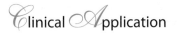

Clinical Application

1-2

Using Ojibway Mythology in Diabetic Teaching

A Toronto program capitalized on Ojibway mythology to provide diabetes self-care instruction. The program was organized at the request of Native Canadians and included day-long educational workshops conducted by an elder. All participants sat in a circle, which confers equal status on every individual and represents harmony with nature.

The beginning focus was on Nanabush, a legendary teacher of the Ojibway who symbolizes moderation and balance. Traditional narratives show him conversing with Diabetes. The moral of the story is to learn about "Diabetes," to live with him, and to control one's life through spiritual strength. Workshop activities included exercise breaks and a buffet lunch that allowed participants to choose their meals.

Practitioners learned that avoiding a rigid diet prescription would enhance the individual's freedom, which was highly valued among the Ojibway (Hagey, 1984).

Food Preferences of Ethnic Groups

Food items considered appropriate for human consumption vary widely by culture and reflect economic and geographic constraints. Rituals of preparation may be culturally determined, and allocation of food resources within a household may reflect the culture's values. Ethnic identity is important in determining staple foods, meal structure, and traditional holiday feasts.

Familiarity of cuisine may aid adaptation to unfamiliar circumstances. Among international postgraduate students in England, eating together was a popular leisure activity, with food of students' home countries being the most popular menu items. Eating home-country food offered emotional as well as physical sustenance (Brown, Edwards, and Hartwell, 2010).

In addition, certain foods may be culturally endorsed treatments for disease. For example, many cultures espouse variations of the "hot–cold" systems described in the sections that follow on Hispanic Americans and Chinese Americans. Also, foods traditionally given to children when they are sick may bring comfort to ill adults as well.

The following brief summaries describe traditional foods of four cultural groups and suggest possible applications for adapting nutritional needs to accommodate these preferences.

African Americans

Traditional African American cuisine began with the necessity of making do with ingredients available to slaves. One-pot dinners serve to tenderize meat and flavor vegetables. These stews often contain pork and greens such as dandelion, turnip, and collards. Other foods often served are dried beans, sweet potatoes, rice, grits, cornbread, and specialty gravies (red-eye, sausage, or cream).

Soul food signifies a shared heritage and loving preparation, not just favorite and familiar foods. African Americans who choose this type of food should be encouraged to use beans, rice, and sweet potatoes but to cook without a lot of fat, such as by

steaming. Traditional foods can be prepared by baking, braising, broiling, or grilling instead of frying. Fat-free broths can be substituted for rich gravies.

Hispanic Americans

The dietary pattern covered in this section is that of Mexican Americans. Table 1-11 lists characteristic foods consumed by Puerto Rican and Cuban people as

TABLE 1-11 ■ Characteristic Eating Patterns of Selected Cultural Groups

GROUP	GRAINS AND STARCHES	FRUITS	VEGETABLES	MEATS AND MEAT SUBSTITUTES	MILK AND MILK SUBSTITUTES	TO DECREASE FAT
LATINO Mexican	Tortillas, corn products, potatoes, corn		Chili peppers, tomatoes, onions, beets, cabbage, pumpkins, string beans	Meat, poultry, eggs; pinto, calico, garbanzo beans	Cheese; milk seldom consumed	Encourage: ■ Salsa as dip or topping ■ Baked corn tortillas, especially stuffed with chicken to make tamales, tostados, or enchiladas
Puerto Rican	Plantains (starchy vegetable that looks like a large banana), Puerto Rican bread (resembles Italian bread), rice, viands (starchy vegetable, the roots and tubers of which are peeled, boiled, and eaten as a side dish)	Guava, canned peaches, pears, fruit cocktail	Beets, eggplant, carrots, green beans, onions	Legumes (especially red kidney beans), eggs, pork, chicken, cod, fish, pigeon, peas, garbanzo beans	Flan (custard); milk seldom consumed	■ Rice with chicken or beans ■ Reduced-fat cheeses Discourage: ■ Fried tortillas ■ Sour cream and regular cheese as toppings ■ Refried beans that are cooked in lard ■ Deep-fried foods such as chimichangas
Cuban	Rice		Green peppers, onions, tomatoes	Black beans, pork, chicken, chorizo (a highly seasoned sausage)	Milk seldom used	
ITALIAN	Pasta, yeast breads, starchy root vegetables		Green peppers, onions, tomatoes	Spiced sausages, fish, tomato-based meat sauces	Cheese; milk seldom consumed (high incidence of lactose intolerance)	Encourage: ■ Salad with no-fat dressing ■ Minestrone soup ■ Pasta with tomato or clam sauce ■ Grilled meat or seafood Discourage: ■ White sauces made with cream, butter, or cheese ■ Breaded and fried meats and vegetables ■ Sausages and other fatty meats such as prosciutto (salt cured, dry aged ham)
SOUTHERN BLACK AMERICAN	Cornbread, biscuits, white bread, butter beans, corn, sweet potatoes, grits, rice, white potatoes, yams	Melons, bananas, peaches	Kale, collards, mustard greens, okra, tomatoes, cabbage, summer squash	Catfish, pork, chicken, black-eyed peas, other dried beans and peas	Buttermilk, evaporated milk, ice cream (high incidence of lactose intolerance)	Encourage: ■ Baked fish and chicken ■ Steamed vegetables ■ Fresh melon ■ Grilled foods
ASIAN Southern Chinese	Rice	All	Mushrooms, bean sprouts, Chinese greens, bok choy	Beef, pork, poultry, seafood	Limited except for ice cream	Encourage: ■ Hot and sour soup; wonton soup ■ Steamed (not fried) dumplings

(continued)

TABLE 1-11 ■ **Characteristic Eating Patterns of Selected Cultural Groups** (Continued)

GROUP	GRAINS AND STARCHES	FRUITS	VEGETABLES	MEATS AND MEAT SUBSTITUTES	MILK AND MILK SUBSTITUTES	TO DECREASE FAT
Northern Chinese	Wheat, millet seed used in noodles, bread, dumplings		Chinese greens, bamboo, alfalfa sprouts, bok choy	Beef, poultry, seafood, eggs, tofu, soybeans	None (high incidence of lactose intolerance among all Chinese)	■ Lightly stir-fried chicken or seafood ■ Steamed whole fish ■ Steamed vegetables and steamed rice
Japanese	Rice, most other complex carbohydrates		All	Fish, beef, pork, eggs, poultry, shellfish, soybean products	None (high incidence of lactose intolerance)	Discourage: ■ Egg rolls ■ Crispy fried noodles ■ Fried rice ■ Deep-fried entrees ■ Spareribs ■ Tempura
Asian Indian	Rice, wheat, millet, barley, maize, ragi (Old World cereal grain)	Mangoes, bananas	Cabbage, cauliflower, onions, chilies, tomatoes, potatoes, green leafy vegetables, okra, green beans, root vegetables	Legumes, nuts (Many vegetarians depending upon region)	Yogurt, buttermilk, milk added to coffee and tea	Encourage: ■ Broiled, poached, or steamed lean meats and poultry if nonvegetarian and religious practice permits ■ Steamed, stir fried, baked, or roasted vegetables ■ Olive oil, canola oil ■ Low-fat dairy products Discourage: ■ Deep fried breads and snacks ■ Coconut oil
EUROPEAN Middle Eastern	Pita bread, rice, couscous, bulgur wheat	Figs, peaches, dates	Grape leaves, tomatoes, peppers, olives, eggplant, onions, squash, fennel, okra, peas	Lamb, chicken, goat, legumes, fish, squid	Yogurt, feta cheese	Encourage: ■ Baked or grilled lean meats and vegetables, legumes ■ Fresh fruit ■ Yogurt dressings Discourage: ■ Fried meats and fish, excess cheese, butter between layers of phyllo (pastry) ■ Sour cream
Northern European	Dark breads, wheat breads, potatoes	All	All, especially onions, carrots, beans	Beef, pork, poultry, fish, shellfish, eggs, sausages	All cheese and milk products	Encourage: ■ Broiled, poached, or steamed lean meats ■ Wine- and tomato-based sauces ■ Consommé Discourage: ■ Creamed soups and sauces ■ Sausages ■ Whole milk and whole-milk products ■ Fried potatoes ■ Sour cream
NATIVE AMERICAN	Corn, wild oats and rice, Indian biscuits (Bannock bread)	Wild berries, choke cherries, black cherries, crab apples	Wild rhubarb, Indian celery, wild mushrooms and roots	Game, seafood, acorns, hazelnuts, pine nuts	Few used (high incidence of lactose intolerance)	Encourage: ■ Game with visible fat removed ■ Broiled, poached, or steamed meats Discourage: ■ Excessive fish oil ■ Fried food ■ Lard in cooking

well as other ethnic groups. The table also suggests means of decreasing fat intake.

Corn is the staple crop of Mexico. Vegetables and meat are characteristically incorporated into a main dish and served with salsa. Foods are typically stewed or fried in oil or lard. Fruits are popular. Sweet foods, such as yeast pastries, are common in the traditional Mexican diet, and sugar is commonly added to foods.

A health belief that may influence a Mexican American's food choices is the hot–cold system. Illness and physiological conditions are categorized as "hot" or "cold." Foods of the opposite category are eaten in an attempt to return balance to the body. Because these categories vary widely from region to region, it is best simply to ask clients what foods they would like to eat.

The traditional Mexican diet can be adapted to the recommendations of the Dietary Guidelines with some changes in preparation. Beans can be boiled, for example, instead of refried; beef can be grilled instead of fried; diet drinks can be substituted for lemonade or soda. The starches and fruits that are part of the Mexican American diet can still be used. Despite being low in milk and milk products, the usual diet provides calcium from the long-established practice of treating corn with calcium carbonate before incorporating it into tortillas. In many areas of the United States, however, tortillas are made with flour, bypassing this traditional compensatory mechanism that increased calcium intake (Purnell, 2013).

Native Hawaiians

Before the arrival of Westerners, native Hawaiians consumed a diet based on taro (a starch root similar to potato), sweet potatoes, breadfruit, fruit, greens, and seaweed. Fat content was approximately 10% of kilocalories. Foods were eaten raw or steamed.

Adopting a Western diet has been detrimental to native Hawaiians' health. Among all of the population groups in the United States, the prevalence of obesity among native Hawaiians is second only to that of the Pima Indians. Longevity is greater in Hawaii than in any other state, except among native Hawaiians, who have the shortest life span of the state's ethnic groups. Native Hawaiians also have the highest mortality rates dues to cardiovascular disease compared with all ethnic groups in the United States (Fong, Braun, and Tsark, 2003; Shintani, Beckham, Tang, et al, 1999; Shintani, Hughes, Beckham, and O'Connor, 1991).

An experimental diet was introduced to native Hawaiians to determine whether short-term dietary changes could alter their risk factors for cardiovascular disease. At the start, these individuals had an average BMI of 39.6. All of the food was provided in two on-site meals and take-home snacks. The evening meal included a cultural or health education session.

During the 3-week experiment, the participants were encouraged to eat as much of the traditional Hawaiian foods as they wanted but limited amounts of fish and chicken. Participants' average energy intake decreased 41%, and their serum cholesterol decreased 14% (Shintani, Hughes, et al, 1991). An average weight loss of 15.1 pounds was maintained for an average of 2.8 years of follow-up (Shintani, Beckham, et al, 1999).

As detailed in later chapters, total fat and cholesterol intakes are linked to an increased risk of chronic disease. For these native Hawaiians, adopting an ancestral diet dramatically altered risk factors for diabetes mellitus and heart disease. Some of the program's success was attributed to inspiring pride in their heritage, but another theory is presented in Genomic Gem 1-2.

Chinese Americans

As is common of cultures throughout the world, Chinese cooking is based on the availability of foodstuffs. Wheat is produced in northern China, where noodles and dumplings are a major part of the cuisine, whereas rice grown in the south is the staple grain of that area.

A common cooking technique involves cutting meats into bite-sized pieces in the kitchen. Experience with diseases resulting from poor sanitation led to avoidance of cold water and raw fruits and vegetables. Fruits and vegetables are cooked quickly to retain a crisp texture.

Chinese medicine views sickness as an imbalance between *yin* and *yang* forces, a system that some compare to the parasympathetic and sympathetic nervous systems that control involuntary bodily functions. Certain illnesses, foods, and medicines are categorized as *yin* or *yang*. *Yin,* or cold, foods include pork, most vegetables, boiled foods, foods served cold, and white foods. *Yang,* or hot foods, include beef, chicken, eggs,

---

Genomic Gem 1-2
Ancestral Foods

Much about the occurrence of diseases is still unknown, particularly why some populations seem to be more at risk than others and why certain dietary practices are more protective of some people than others. Perhaps the correct combination of genetic, cultural, and socioeconomic factors is needed to achieve the desired health benefit.

If the metabolism of a group of people evolved to work optimally on an ancestral diet rather than with a modern diet, possibly the **alleles** that are associated with increased disease risk may be silenced in the presence of the more ancestral and traditional diet and lifestyle (Ordovas, Kaput, and Corella, 2007).

fried foods, foods served hot, and red foods. Noodles and soft rice are neutral, neither *yin* nor *yang*.

To maintain fluid intake, Chinese Americans prefer hot tea to ice water. Dairy products are rarely used. A caregiver interested in increasing a Chinese American's calcium intake would probably achieve better results advocating green leafy vegetables or tofu rather than milk.

Family members may cook food at home to provide the hospitalized client with hot or cold foods. Because *yin* and *yang* cover various categories of foods, cooking methods, and colors, the perceptive nurse or dietitian can suggest items or procedures that also fit the diet prescribed by Western medicine. Clinical Application 1-3 relates such a case.

Food Restrictions by Religious Customs

Certain religious practices may promote healthy lifestyles. Among Thai persons with type 2 diabetes, higher scores for Buddhist values were significantly correlated with better medication self-care and better dietary self-care than among those with lower scores (Sowattanangoon, Kochabhakdi, and Petrie, 2008).

Table 1-12 lists selected religious customs that affect food intake, but practices change with locale and over time. Individuals also vary in the extent to which they implement dietary restrictions.

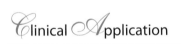

Bridging *Yin* and *Yang* Beliefs and the Germ Theory of Disease

A Chinese infant experienced repeated bouts of diarrhea. Several tests were performed, and changes were made in the child's formula to no avail. Finally, a nurse made a home visit. She discovered several bottles of home-prepared formula on the windowsill, whereas others were in the refrigerator. The family lived in a New York City apartment without air-conditioning, and it was midsummer.

When the nurse asked about the procedure used to store the formula, the mother stated that childbirth is regarded as a cold condition, so she should avoid cold. Her husband, therefore, removed the day's bottles from the refrigerator before he left for work every morning so the bottles would be warm for the mother's condition.

The nurse explained that storing the formula at room temperature permitted bacteria to grow in it and that these organisms were causing the baby's diarrhea. Together, the mother and nurse searched for another procedure to bridge the cultural belief and the germ theory of disease. The mother decided to don a coat, hat, and gloves before opening the refrigerator to retrieve each bottle at feeding time. The nurse wisely guided the mother to a solution that left the mother's belief system intact, and the infant's diarrhea was cured (Jackson, 1993).

TABLE 1-12 ■ Selected Religious Customs That Affect Food Intake	
RELIGION	**RESTRICTED FOODS AND BEVERAGES**
Buddhism	1. All meat
Catholicism	1. Meat prohibited by some denominations on holy days such as Good Friday and Ash Wednesday 2. Alcoholic beverages by some denominations
Hinduism	1. Vegetarianism common 2. Regional avoidance of some meat, poultry, fish, eggs, and cheese
Islam	1. All pork and pork products 2. All meat must be slaughtered according to ritual letting of blood 3. Carnivorous animals, birds of prey, and land animals without external ears 4. Blood and blood byproducts 5. Alcohol and intoxicants 6. Shellfish (some shellfish by some members)
Orthodox Judaism	1. All pork and pork products 2. All fish without scales and fins 3. Dairy products should not be eaten at the same meal that contains meat and meat products 4. All meat must be slaughtered and prepared according to biblical ordinances; because blood is forbidden as food, meat must be drained thoroughly. 5. Bakery products and prepared food mixtures must be prepared under acceptable kosher standards 6. Leavened bread and cake are forbidden during Passover
Seventh-Day Adventist	1. All pork and pork products 2. Shellfish 3. All flesh foods (some members) 4. All dairy products and eggs (some members) 5. Blood 6. Highly spiced foods 7. Meat broths 8. All alcoholic beverages 9. Coffee and tea

Jewish Americans

Orthodox Jews interpret dietary laws stringently. These are the three key characteristics of strict **kosher** food preparation:

1. Only designated animals may be eaten.
2. Some of those animals must be ritually slaughtered and dressed.
3. Dairy products and meats must not be eaten at the same meal.

Separate cooking and serving utensils are used for dairy meals and meat meals. Fruits, vegetables, and starches need no special preparation and can be served with either meat or dairy meals.

When a preplanned kosher meal is unavailable, a cottage cheese fruit plate is a good choice for an Orthodox Jew. The cottage cheese should be transferred to a paper plate with new disposable plastic utensils to avoid the possibility of the utensils having ever touched meat. If bread or crackers are served, labels must indicate that they contain no meat products.

Muslim Americans

One of the key health-care accommodations reported as necessary by American Muslims is the provision of **halal** food, which is seen as health promoting and integral to healing (Padela, Gunter, Killawi, and Heisler, 2012). Islam has a strict set of dietary prescriptions, including ritual slaughter of poultry, beef, and lamb to make the meat halal. Strict Muslims avoid pork and alcohol; some avoid shellfish (Purnell, 2013).

Figure 1-7 illustrates the multiple factors impinging on food choice and physical activity decisions. Modifying one's own eating behavior, much less assisting someone else to do so, entails much more than simply knowing which foods are recommended and which should be restricted.

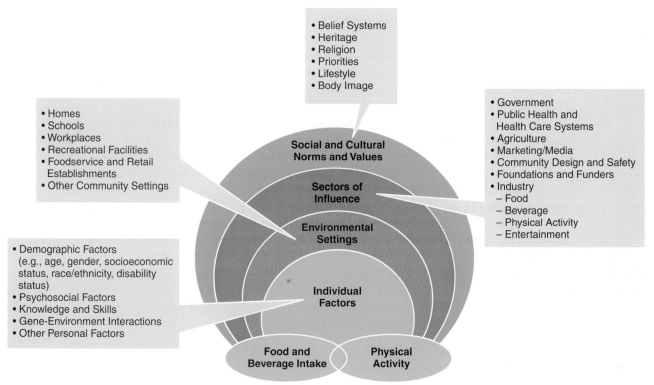

FIGURE 1-7 A Social-Ecological Framework for Nutrition and Physical Activity Decisions. Social and cultural norms and values, sectors of influence, environmental settings, and individual factors all contribute to decisions to eat, drink, and exercise. (Adapted from (1) Centers for Disease Control and Prevention. Division of Nutrition, Physical Activity, and Obesity. State Nutrition, Physical Activity and Obesity (NPAO) Program: Technical Assistance Manual. January 2008, page 36. Accessed April 21, 2010. www.cdc.gov/obesity/downloads/TA_Manual_1_31_08.pdf. (2) Institute of Medicine. Preventing Childhood Obesity: Health in the Balance, Washington (DC): The National Academies Press; 2005, page 85. (3) Story M, Kaphingst KM, Robinson-O'Brien R, Glanz K. Creating healthy food and eating environments: Policy and environmental approaches. Annu Rev Public Health 2008;29:253-272. Reprinted from *Dietary Guidelines for Americans, 2010*. 7th Edition, Figure 6-1, Washington, DC: U.S. Government Printing Office, December 2010 with permission. www.health.gov/dietaryguidelines/dga2010/DietaryGuidelines2010.pdf)

Keystones

■ Health is a state of complete physical, mental, and social well-being, not just the absence of disease or infirmity. Optimal health is not possible with an inferior diet.

■ The six classes of nutrients are carbohydrates, fats (lipids), proteins, vitamins, minerals, and water. Nutrients provide fuel, support tissue growth and maintenance, and regulate body processes. Essential nutrients are those that must be supplied by the diet or artificially because the body cannot manufacture sufficient amounts for health.

Keystones—cont'd

- New genetic knowledge offers the potential to personalize nutrition prescriptions to avoid interactions between one's diet and his or her genes, which can adversely affect the body's use of nutrients.
- According to the USDA Dietary Guidelines, most people do not consume enough whole grains, milk, or fruit and ingest too many solid fats and added sugars in grain-based desserts and snacks.
- Food insecurity in the United States, affecting certain demographic groups, is addressed with information measures and market strategies with a mixed record of success. Globally, food assistance and improved agricultural techniques have helped many countries, but hunger is still widespread in Africa.
- Nutritional care begins with assessment followed by analysis, planning, implementation, and evaluation. Assessment compiles subjective and objective data that are then analyzed to identify strengths and weaknesses. Planning with the client is essential to maximize the possibility of effective implementation and a favorable evaluation.
- The Dietary Reference Intakes (DRIs) encompass five nutrient-based reference values that can be used for assessing and planning diets for groups according to life stage and gender. The DRIs are intended to apply to the healthy general population and refer to average daily intakes for 1 or more weeks, not to judge adequacy of an individual's intake that necessitates a broader prospective.
- Exchange lists categorize foods by specific amounts according to similar nutrient composition, which permit substituting within the category and may be used to teach a client about healthful eating by illustrating that all foods are not equally desirable or satisfying choices.
- It is possible to achieve modern medicine's goal of minimizing bacterial proliferation in baby formula while maintaining a client's hot–cold cultural belief, as was done in accommodating a Chinese mother's need for protection from cold following childbirth with winter clothing when opening the refrigerator.
- Milk is likely not favored in cultural groups with a high prevalence of lactose intolerance, including African Americans, Asians, Italians, Latinos, and Native Americans. Religious convictions may restrict all meat for persons practicing Buddhism; pork for those practicing Islamic tenets, strict Judaism, and Seventh Day Adventist beliefs; as well as beef, pork, and fowl for Hindu adherents.

CASE STUDY 1–1

A student in a beginning nutrition course is showing a friend the textbook. "You could help me improve my diet," the friend says. "I know I am not eating right." At the time, the friend was eating a chocolate bar. She described herself as 18 years old and sedentary. The student asks the friend to list what she had eaten during the past 24 hours. From the friend's list, the student gathers the following data:

Breakfast: 8 ounces of reconstituted frozen orange juice, 2 cups of black coffee
Lunch: 6 ounces of low-fat fruit yogurt and 6 square graham crackers
Midafternoon snack: Mr. Goodbar, 1.2 ounces
Dinner: 1 medium baked pork chop, lean only eaten, 2 cups of green salad, 2 tablespoons reduced-calorie French dressing, 12 ounces of diet Coke

Opening a profile on ChooseMyPlate.gov, and inserting the friend's height and weight (5 ft 4 in., 163 lbs), the student finds her friend's BMI is 28.0 (overweight) and her 1-day intake compares with the recommended 1800 kilocalorie intake as follows:

	Friend's Intake	ChooseMyPlate
Oils	3 tsp	5 tsp
Milk	¾ cup	3 cups
Meat and beans	4 oz	5 oz
Vegetables	1 cup	2½ cups
Fruits	1 cup	1½ cups
Grains	1 ½ oz	6 oz
Discretionary kilocalorie allowance	327	161

In this situation, the student probably would not formalize a nutritional care plan for the friend, but the following plan illustrates the thought process involved in developing a care plan for this case.

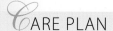# ARE PLAN

Subjective Data

Expressed need for instruction in healthy diet. Twenty-four hour recall shows less than the recommended ChooseMyPlate intake for all food groups but excessive discretionary kilocalories.

Overweight from reported height and weight

Objective Data

Observed eating a chocolate bar at 3 P.M.

Analysis

Self-reported need to improve nutrition

Plan

DESIRED OUTCOMES EVALUATION CRITERIA	ACTIONS/INTERVENTIONS	RATIONALE
Friend will keep a food record for 3 days.	Instruct friend to list everything she eats or drinks for 3 days.	Food record will gather facts about the friend's food intake to use as an instructional tool.
Friend will read the section on ChooseMyPlate in student's textbook by this evening.	Lend friend textbook to read.	Providing literature uses expert opinion to reinforce student's teaching. Reading and seeing illustrations elicits active participation and employs senses other than hearing.
Friend will meet with student in 4 days to compare food record to ChooseMyPlate profile and design a plan of action.	Meet with friend in 4 days to sort and analyze food record data. Provide apples at meeting to model healthy snack food.	Setting follow-up visit just after food record is completed will maintain the friend's interest. Modeling desirable behavior is a technique to encourage change.

After 4 days, the two friends met in the college library to access ChooseMyPlate on the Internet. The friend says she has not been keeping the requested food diary. "I'm hopeless. I'll never be able to change," she moans. They sat outdoors and ate the apples that the nutrition student provided, but her friend washed hers down with another Mr. Goodbar. At that point, thinking her friend required more professional help than her friendship could provide, the student recommended the free clinic run by the college's nursing department. They walked to the clinic together so the friend could make an appointment.

1-2

Clinic's Notes

The following Clinic's Notes are representative of the documentation found in a client's medical record.

Subjective: Requesting assistance with diet planning. Shared dietary recall from last week. Not inclined to keep food diary. Denies chronic illness. Has attempted weight control on her own with little success due to splurging on sweets. Recognizes need for lifestyle changes as well as dietary improvement. Unsure of social support for lifestyle changes.

Objective: Ht 5 ft; 4 in. Wt 163 lbs. BMI 28.0. VS WNL (vital signs within normal limits)

Analysis: Overweight due to unbalanced diet and sedentary lifestyle.

Plan: Instruct in basic nutrition. Suggest private use of ChooseMyPlate.gov site to track diet and activity. Recommend participation in daily walking group that meets in the Physical Education Department to achieve 150 minutes of physical activity weekly along with the possibility of social support from fellow walkers. Follow-up visit in 1 week.

Critical Thinking Questions

1. The 24-hour dietary recall in Case Study 1-1 tallies just 987 of the 1800 kilocalories recommended for the individual, yet she has been unsuccessful with weight control. What possible factors might explain the discrepancy?

2. When the nutrition student met with the friend after 4 days, what other options might have been chosen instead of referral to the nursing clinic?

3. You have a friend or relative who displays food intake similar to that described in Case Study 1-1. You care deeply for this person. How might you approach the subject of healthy eating if the person does not ask for assistance?

Chapter Review

1. Which of the following is an energy nutrient?
   a. Phytochemicals
   b. Vitamins
   c. Minerals
   d. Carbohydrates

2. Which of the following techniques is used to estimate the body's protein stores?
   a. Weighing the person under water
   b. Measuring midarm circumference
   c. Calculating the body mass index
   d. Determining triceps skinfolds

3. Which of the following is true of the traditional Chinese *yin* and *yang* health belief system?
   a. A cold, or *yin*, condition is balanced by consuming hot, or *yang*, foods.
   b. A hot condition is flushed with large quantities of cold water.
   c. Rice is considered magical and is consumed at every meal.
   d. *Yang*, or hot, foods include only foods served hot.

4. Which of the following adheres to strict kosher regulations?
   a. Avoiding cheese and cheese products
   b. Eating only certain cuts of pork
   c. Keeping separate utensils and dishes for meat and dairy meals
   d. Serving lobster, clams, and shrimp only on festive occasions

5. Intake that meets the needs of 97 to 98% of individuals in a defined group is called
   a. Acceptable macronutrient distribution range
   b. Adequate intakes
   c. Estimated average requirements
   d. Recommended dietary allowances

Clinical Analysis

1. Ms. G has just been diagnosed with type 2 diabetes. She is a Native American who has left her reservation for employment in town. Which of the following actions by the nurse shows respect for Ms. G's culture?
   a. Instructing her to increase her intake of vegetables
   b. Telling her to lose weight and avoid alcohol and fast-food restaurants
   c. Giving Ms. G an instruction sheet based on the Food Exchange Lists
   d. Asking Ms. G how she "sees" or perceives diabetes in her life

2. Mr. P is a 65-year-old man, recently widowed, whose physician is recommending weight loss. Mr. P has had little experience with grocery shopping or cooking. Which of the following systems for instructing Mr. P would the nurse select to offer the best chance of success?
   a. A computerized diet analysis program
   b. ChooseMyPlate
   c. Exchange lists
   d. The RDA/AI tables

3. Ms. E attended a community health fair where she entered her recalled intake for the previous 24 hours into a computer for analysis. On the basis of the printout she was given, she now thinks she should begin taking vitamin and mineral supplements. A friend who is a nurse correctly bases her advice on the following:
   a. A 1-day diet recall offers inadequate data on which to base supplementation.
   b. A hand recalculation should be done to verify the accuracy of the computer printout.
   c. The RDAs on which computer programs are based are intended for only the 50% of the population who are obsessed with health.
   d. Undoubtedly, the operators of the computer at the fair had a product to sell: "Let the buyer beware."

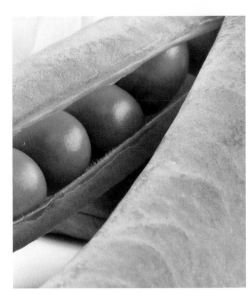

2

Carbohydrates

LEARNING OBJECTIVES

After completing this chapter, the student should be able to:

- Describe the types of carbohydrates, identify food sources of each, and indicate their functions in the body.
- List the major functions of carbohydrates and methods through which the body stores them.
- Discuss dietary fiber and list its functions; identify dietary food sources.
- Describe the relationship between carbohydrates and dental health.
- List the carbohydrate content (in grams) of each appropriate exchange list.
- Discuss dietary recommendations related to fiber, added sugar, and total carbohydrate intake.

Carbohydrates, fats, and proteins all meet the body's basic energy needs. Carbohydrates are the major source of energy because they break down rapidly and are readily available for use. This chapter defines basic terminology related to carbohydrates and discusses the body's use of carbohydrates and the way carbohydrates relate to the other energy nutrients.

Green plants manufacture carbohydrates during a complex process called **photosynthesis.** In this process, carbon dioxide from the air and water from the soil are transformed into sugars and **starches.** Sunlight and the green pigment **chlorophyll** are necessary for this conversion. All the food we eat is a product of photosynthesis. If this process did not occur, the whole food chain would collapse, and life would cease. Figure 2-1 illustrates this process.

On the basis of their chemical structure, carbohydrates are divided into two major groups: sugars and starches. Sugars have a simple structure; starches are more complex. Therefore, sugars are often called simple carbohydrates, and starches are called **complex carbohydrates.**

Composition of Carbohydrates

Understanding the composition of carbohydrates involves understanding three structures: molecule, element, and atom:

1. A **molecule** is the smallest quantity into which a substance may be divided without loss of its characteristics. For example, the formula for water is H_2O. If the hydrogen atoms are pulled from the oxygen atom, the resulting products are hydrogen and oxygen, which bear no resemblance to water. Molecules are made of elements. In the case of water, H_2O, the elements are hydrogen and oxygen.
2. An **element** is a substance that cannot be separated into simpler parts by ordinary means.
3. An **atom** is the smallest particle of an element that retains its physical characteristics.

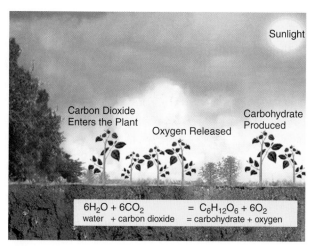

FIGURE 2-1 Photosynthesis is a vital process that transforms carbon dioxide and water into carbohydrates.

Basic Terminology

Carbohydrates are composed of the elements carbon, hydrogen, and oxygen. The ratio of hydrogen to oxygen is the same as that for water: two parts of hydrogen to one part of oxygen. The simplest carbohydrates have the formula $C_6H_{12}O_6$. Carbohydrates are frequently abbreviated CHO.

Simple carbohydrates (sugars) include monosaccharides and disaccharides (*mono-* means one, *di-* means two, and *-saccharide* means sweet). Starches are called **polysaccharides.**

Simple Carbohydrates

Simple carbohydrates are of two types: monosaccharides and disaccharides.

1. A **monosaccharide** contains one molecule of $C_6H_{12}O_6$.
2. A **disaccharide** is composed of two molecules of $C_6H_{12}O_6$ joined together (minus one unit of H_2O).

When the body joins two monosaccharide molecules, a molecule of water is released in the process.

Monosaccharides

Monosaccharides are the building blocks of all other carbohydrates. The three monosaccharides of importance in human nutrition are glucose, fructose, and galactose. Note the -ose ending in the name of each of these sugars. All monosaccharides and disaccharides end with the letters -ose.

Glucose

The monosaccharide glucose in the body is commonly called blood sugar. It is the major form of sugar in the blood. Normal **fasting blood sugar (FBS)** is 70 to 100 milligrams per 100 milliliters of serum or plasma. **Impaired fasting glucose (IFG)** is 100 to 125 milligrams per 100 milliliters of serum or plasma (www.care.diabetesjournal.org). Regardless of the form of sugar consumed, the body readily converts it to glucose.

Another name for glucose is **dextrose** (abbreviated D). Clients in health-care facilities often receive intravenous feedings. **Intravenous** simply means within or into a vein. The most common intravenous feeding is D_5W (5% dextrose in water), used primarily to deliver fluids to the client.

Fructose

Fructose is found in fruits and honey. It is the sweetest of all the monosaccharides. Fructose is used extensively in soft drinks, canned foods, and various other processed foods. High-fructose corn syrup (HFCS) is very sweet because the cornstarch has been treated with an enzyme that converts some of the naturally present glucose to the sweeter fructose. The human body readily converts fructose to glucose. HFCS has become increasingly controversial in its use by the food industry. A possible link has been identified with HFCS consumption and diabetes. Countries using HFCS in their foods have a 20% higher prevalence of diabetes than those that do not use it. It is estimated that in the United States, 55 lb per person of HFCS are ingested annually. Many countries, including Australia, China, Denmark, France, Italy, Sweden, and the United Kingdom, have a per capita consumption of approximately 1 lb annually (Goran, 2012).

Galactose

The monosaccharide galactose comes mainly from the breakdown of the milk sugar lactose. Yogurt and un-aged cheese may contain free galactose. It is the least sweet of all the monosaccharides. The body converts galactose into glucose after ingestion.

Disaccharides

When two monosaccharides are linked, a disaccharide is formed. The three important disaccharides are:

1. Sucrose
2. Lactose
3. Maltose

Sucrose

The most prevalent disaccharide, sucrose, is ordinary white table sugar made commercially from sugar beets and sugar cane. Brown, granulated, and powdered sugars are all forms of sucrose. Sucrose is also found in molasses, maple syrup, fruits, and vegetables. The two monosaccharides joined to form sucrose are glucose and fructose. See Box 2-1 for more information on sugar in the U.S. diet. Clinical Calculation 2-1 provides information on converting grams of sugar into teaspoons of sugar.

Lactose

Because lactose occurs naturally only in milk, it is commonly referred to as milk sugar. Lactose is the least sweet of the disaccharides. The two monosaccharides that make up lactose are glucose and galactose.

Maltose

Maltose is a double sugar that occurs primarily during starch digestion. The disaccharide maltose is produced when the body breaks starches into simpler units. Smaller amounts of this disaccharide are present in malt, malt products, beer, some infant formulas, and sprouting seeds. Maltose consists of two units of glucose.

Sugar in Foods

The amount of sugar that is in a food product can be found on its label. The total amount of sugar in grams can be found on the Nutrition Facts portion of the label.

Clinical Calculation   *2-1*

Converting Grams of Sugar Into Teaspoons of Sugar

An added sugar intake of 60 grams does not mean much to average American consumers because most Americans are not familiar with the metric system. Food labels use the metric system to list the nutritional content of a product. To enhance understanding of label reading, let us convert grams of sugar into teaspoons. One teaspoon of sugar contains 4 grams of CHO. Therefore, 60 grams of sugar is equal to 15 teaspoons.

Distinguished from the natural sugars such as lactose in milk and fructose in fruits, added sugars are those incorporated into foods and beverages during production. Major sources of added sugar include the following:

- Candy
- Soft drinks
- Fruit drinks
- "Energy" and sports drinks
- Grain-based desserts such as cookies, cakes, and pastries

In the 2010 Dietary Guidelines, the U.S. Department of Agriculture estimates that most Americans consume a diet of 16% added sugars. This contributes to a diet high in calories and low in nutrients.

Sugar is both present naturally in foods and added to foods. For example, fruits contain fructose, and fructose can be added to soft drinks to enhance sweetness.

The federal government regulates the use of terms such as *sugar free, reduced sugar, less sugar* for food products that have added sugar. Terms such as these can be located anywhere on the package's label. Table 2-1 lists the standards, or definitions, for legally defined label descriptors.

Sugar Alcohols

Some food products contain **sugar alcohols.** Sugar alcohols have various names, such as sugar replacers, polyols, nutritive sweeteners, and bulk sweeteners.

Box 2-1 ■ *Added Sugar in the U.S. Diet*

Added sugars contribute to dental caries, reduce the intake of essential micronutrients when sugar in the diet displaces more nutritious items such as milk, and may lead to an increased incidence of cognitive impairment in the elderly.

The increased consumption of added sugars is linked to a decreased intake of essential micronutrients and an increase in body weight. Data from the National Health and Nutrition Examination Survey, 2005–2010, indicate that children and adolescents obtain approximately 16% of their total kilocalories from added sugars, and adults 13% (Ervin, 2013).

What is an appropriate amount of added sugar in a healthful diet? According to the American Heart Association, no more than 100 kilocalories for women and 150 kilocalories for men should consist of added sugars per day (Academy of Nutrition and Dietetics, 2012).

Currently, the largest contributor of added sugar in the diet is sweetened carbonated beverages and other sweetened beverages, which provide 37% of added sugars (Bachman, 2008). The second largest contributor is table sugar and candy at 16.1% (U.S. Department of Agriculture, 2005).

TABLE 2-1 ■ Approved Definitions for Food Label Terms	
TERM	**STANDARD**
Sugar-free	Contains less than one-half gram of sugars per serving
Reduced sugar or less sugar	At least 25% less sugar or sugars per serving than a standard serving size of a traditional food
No added sugar or without added sugar	No sugars added during processing or packing, including ingredients that contain sugar, such as juice or dry fruit
Low sugar	May not be used as a claim on a food label

From Food and Drug Administration (2009).

Lactitol, maltitol, isomalt, sorbitol, xylitol, and mannitol are all sugar alcohols and currently are approved for use in the United States.

Sugar alcohols are commonly used on a one-for-one replacement basis for sugars in recipes. For example, 1 cup of sugar would be replaced with 1 cup of isomalt in a recipe. Sugar alcohols add not only sweetness but also bulk to recipes. Sugar alcohols have the following characteristics:

- Generally do not promote tooth decay
- Commonly have a cooling effect on the tongue
- Are slowly and incompletely absorbed from the intestine into the blood
- May have a laxative effect for some people if consumed in excess

Nonnutrative Sweeteners

Nonnutrative sweeteners (NNS) are sugar substitutes, providing intense sweetness. Unlike sugar replacers, NNS do not add bulk or volume to a food product; they add only sweetness. They are 150 to 500 times as sweet as sugar and are mostly artificial, or synthetic. There are seven NNS approved for use in the United States, the most common of which are shown in Table 2-2 (Academy of Nutrition and Dietetics, 2012).

Complex Carbohydrates

Chemically complex carbohydrates are called polysaccharides. *Poly-* means many, and polysaccharides consist of many molecules of $C_6H_{12}O_6$ joined and many molecules of water released in the process. Polysaccharides can be composed of various numbers of monosaccharides and disaccharides. The three types of complex carbohydrates of nutritional importance are starch, glycogen, and fiber. Table 2-3 summarizes the composition of carbohydrates.

Starch

Starch, the major source of carbohydrate in the diet, is found primarily in grains, starchy vegetables, and legumes and in foods made from grains—cereals, breads, and pasta. Box 2-2 lists the many kinds of

TABLE 2-3 ■ Composition of Carbohydrates	
Elements	C (carbon)
	H (hydrogen)
	O (oxygen)
Molecule	$C_6H_{12}O_6$
Monosaccharide (simple)	One unit of $C_6H_{12}O_6$
Disaccharide (simple)	Two units of $C_6H_{12}O_6$ minus one unit of H_2O
Polysaccharide (complex)	Many units of $C_6H_{12}O_6$ minus many units of H_2O

Box 2-2 ■ *Legumes*

Legumes include these dried peas and beans:

- Black beans
- Pinto beans
- Kidney beans
- Navy beans
- Soybeans
- Black-eyed peas
- Split peas
- Yellow peas
- Chick peas (garbanzo)
- Lentils

TABLE 2-2 ■ Nonnutritive Sweeteners		
ARTIFICIAL SWEETENER	**TRADE NAME**	**COMMENTS**
Aspartame	Nutrasweet	Used in sweetened products such as puddings, gelatins, frozen desserts, yogurt, hot cocoa mixes, powdered soft drinks, carbonated beverages, teas, breath mints, chewing gums, some vitamins, and cold preparations. Also used as a tabletop sweetener. Reviewed by such regulatory agencies as the Centers for Disease Control and Food and Drug Administration and found to be safe. Should not be used by individuals with a rare genetic disease called phenylketonuria (www.aspartame.org).
Saccharin	Equal	Artificial sweetener.
	Sweet'N Low	Carbonated beverages, toothpaste, cold remedies, dietetic puddings, cakes, cookies.
	Sugar Twin	Saccharin was banned in Canada in 1977. The U.S. Food and Drug Administration also proposed a ban on saccharin, but Congress passed a moratorium on the ban. Although high doses of saccharin were shown to cause bladder cancer in male rats, numerous human studies have shown no association between saccharin and cancer at human levels of consumption.
Sucralose	Splenda	The only noncaloric sweetener made from sugar. Approved for use by the Food and Drug Administration.
Rebaudioside A & stevioside purified from Stevia leaves	Stevia	Only the forms listed have been granted approval by the FDA, not whole stevia leaves (which are sold as dietary supplements).

Adapted from Academy of Nutrition and Dietetics, 2012.

legumes available. Strictly speaking, all starches yield simple sugars on digestion; starchy foods are mostly low in fat and high in carbohydrates, and some starchy foods have the advantage of containing much fiber.

Glycogen

Glycogen represents the body's carbohydrate stores. Glucose is stored in liver and muscle tissue as the polysaccharide **glycogen.** Glycogen is crucial to the function of the human body. During intense physical activity, the body utilizes blood glucose for energy. When blood glucose is depleted, muscle glycogen is broken down to provide immediate fuel in the form of glucose. Glycogen is built up and stored in muscle and the liver when blood glucose levels are high after infusion from the diet. Liver glycogen helps sustain blood glucose levels during sleep.

The typical human body has an available store of glucose in the form of glycogen for about 1 day's energy needs. Because the body's ability to store carbohydrates in the form of glycogen is limited, an adequate intake of dietary carbohydrates is essential. When glycogen is stored, water is also stored. Each glycogen molecule attracts many molecules of water because of the way the elements are arranged. When glycogen stores are completely filled, the average person weighs about 4 lb more than when glycogen stores are empty.

Dietary Fiber

Dietary fiber refers to foods, mostly from plants, that the human body cannot break down to digest and that is eliminated in intestinal waste. Sometimes called roughage or bulk, fiber adds almost no fuel or energy value to the diet, but it does add volume. Bulk fills the stomach, and most experts believe a full stomach contributes to a feeling of **satiety,** so further eating ceases.

The recommended daily **adequate intake (AI)** for fiber is based on 14 grams of fiber per 1000 kcalories consumed or:

- Men: 38 grams
- Women: 25 grams

In the United States, the average person consumes less than the recommended amount of dietary fiber, and few people consume the recommended levels. Research has indicated the average fiber intake for U.S. adults is only 15 grams per day (American Diabetes Association Position Paper, 2008). Whole grains are an excellent source of dietary fiber. Dollars & Sense 2-1 provides a recipe for an economical, easy-to-prepare vegetable soup.

$ Dollars & Sense 2-1

Vegetable Soup

Plan your meals around whole grains. Start with whole-wheat pasta, precooked brown rice, and beans (kidney, chick peas, white, etc.) and add other ingredients (leftover meats, seafood, quinoa, tofu, etc.) as your budget allows.

Pack several containers, freezing some as desired, of this economical, easy-to-fix lunch or dinner for those super busy times.

16-ounce can beans (any kind—kidney, chick peas, white, etc.), drained

2 15-ounce cans tomatoes, stewed, low sodium

28 ounces vegetable broth, low sodium

16 ounces vegetables, mixed, frozen (any kind—plain, no sauce)

1 cup whole-wheat pasta, quinoa, pre-cooked brown rice (frozen or packaged)

½ cup onion, chopped

1 teaspoon olive oil

2 cloves garlic, to taste (optional)

dash pepper, to taste (optional)

dash cayenne pepper or red pepper flakes, to taste (optional)

1. Sauté onion in olive oil for approximately 5 minutes or until slightly soft.
2. Combine all ingredients, except the whole-wheat pasta or pre-cooked brown rice.
3. Bring to a boil.
4. Add whole-wheat pasta or pre-cooked brown rice (along with optional ingredients, if desired) to the pot and simmer, covered, for approximately 10 minutes or until the pasta (if using) and/or vegetables are tender.

Makes approximately 6 servings.

Eating too much fiber can cause problems. Much evidence suggests that eating more than 50 grams of fiber a day can interfere with mineral absorption, which can lead to conditions such as anemia and osteoporosis. Healthy people should achieve a desirable fiber intake by consuming fiber-rich fruits, vegetables, legumes, and whole-grain cereals, which also provide minerals, vitamins, and **phytochemicals,** instead of adding fiber concentrates (such as psyllium) to their diet.

Fiber is classified as either soluble or insoluble. **Solubility** is the ability of one substance to dissolve in another. For example, oil does not dissolve in water, so oil is insoluble in water. Insoluble fiber does not dissolve in water, whereas soluble fiber does. Soluble fiber and insoluble fiber react differently in the body and are needed for different reasons.

Soluble Fiber

Sources of soluble fibers include beans, oatmeal, barley, broccoli, and citrus fruits; oat bran is a particularly good source of soluble fiber. Soluble fibers dissolve in water and thicken to form gels. The reported health benefits of soluble fibers include reduced cholesterol levels, regulated blood sugar levels, and weight loss (by helping dieters control their appetites).

Insoluble Fiber

Examples of sources of insoluble fibers include the woody or structural parts of plants, such as fruit and vegetable skins, and the outer coating (bran) of wheat kernels. Insoluble fibers have been reported to promote regularity of bowel movements and reduce the risk of diverticular disease and some forms of cancer. The mechanism of these effects for insoluble fiber is due to decreased intestinal transit time and decreased intestinal pressure. Table 2-4 lists the food sources of each type of fiber and their reported health benefits.

Functions of Carbohydrates

Carbohydrates play the following roles in the body:

- Provide fuel
- Spare body protein
- Help prevent ketosis
- Enhance learning and memory processes

Provide Fuel

Carbohydrates, fats, and proteins provide the body's energy needs. **Energy** is the capacity to do work. To understand the concept of energy, think of the human body as a machine. Just as gasoline is a car's fuel, so carbohydrates, proteins, and fats are the human machine's fuel. Without fuel, a car powered by gas ceases to operate. Without fuel sources over an extended time, the human machine dies from starvation. Just as a person cannot efficiently substitute something other than gasoline to fuel a car with a gasoline engine, a person cannot efficiently substitute something other than carbohydrate, protein, and fat for fuel in the human body.

Carbohydrate is a primary source of fuel for all cells in the body. The brain is a carbohydrate-dependent organ and must have an uninterrupted, ongoing source. The Recommended Dietary Allowance for carbohydrate is 130 g/d for adults and children based on the minimum amount of glucose used by the brain. The diet should be composed of 45% to 65% carbohydrates (Academy of Nutrition and Dietetics, 2012).

Spare Body Protein

When too few carbohydrates are eaten, the body suffers. A continuous supply of glucose is required for all cells to function, particularly those of the central nervous system. Body glycogen stores are limited, and after they are depleted, the body can convert protein to glucose. The body will break down internal protein stores (muscle tissue) before fat stores if carbohydrate intake is inadequate. An adequate supply of dietary carbohydrates spares body protein stores from being partially converted into glucose and allows protein to be used for growth and repair of body tissue. This principle has important ramifications, which are discussed throughout the text.

Help Prevent Ketosis

A balanced intake of energy nutrients is vital. If carbohydrate intake is too low, the body will break down both stored fat and internal protein to meet its fuel needs. The body cannot handle the excessive breakdown of stored fat because the body lacks the necessary equipment. As a result, partially broken-down fats accumulate in the blood in the form of ketones, and the person is said to be in a state of **ketosis.** Survival is possible on a very low carbohydrate diet, but good health is not.

Fatigue, nausea, and lack of appetite are some of the undesirable consequences of ketosis. Coma and death have occurred in severe cases. The presence of ketosis is easily determined by testing for the presence of acetone or diacetic acid in the urine. **Acetone** and **diacetic acid** are ketone bodies. One hundred thirty grams of carbohydrate each day is usually enough to prevent ketosis (National Institutes of Health, 2009).

TABLE 2-4 ■ Foods and Reported Benefits of Fiber		
	INSOLUBLE FIBER	**SOLUBLE FIBER**
Solubility	Does not dissolve in water	Dissolves in water
Food sources	Wheat bran	Oatmeal
	Corn bran	Oat bran, barley
	Vegetables	Some fruits such as apples, oranges
	Nuts	
	Fruit skins	Broccoli
	Some dry beans*	Some dry beans*
Benefit	Promotes regularity	May help reduce cholesterol levels
	May help reduce risk of some forms of cancer	May assist in regulating blood sugar levels
	May reduce risk of diverticular disease	May promote weight loss by increasing satiety†

*Current laboratory methods to assay soluble fiber content of individual foods are imprecise. This is the subject of much research.
†Satiety is defined as the sensation of fullness after eating.

Enhance Learning and Memory

Considerable evidence exists that blood glucose concentrations regulate neural and behavioral processes. Glucose enhances learning and memory in humans throughout the life cycle. Findings across many laboratories demonstrate that glucose consumed early in the morning facilitates specific forms of cognitive function, particularly verbal declaration memory (intentional memory for words and narratives). Children score higher on tests when they eat breakfast. Improvements include both enhanced memory and retrieval of information from long-term memory. Glucose enhanced cognitive function in elderly test subjects who had some mild age-related memory deficits (Korol, 2002). However, elevated blood glucose, as seen in individuals with impaired glucose tolerance, has an increased incidence for a decline in mental function (Valeo, 2009; Yaffe, 2004). There have been studies that indicate that diets high in carbohydrate increase the incidence of mild cognitive impairment or dementia in the elderly (Roberts, 2012).

Health and Carbohydrates

The kinds of carbohydrates eaten are important to health. Epidemiological data support the association between a high intake of vegetables and fruits and low risk of chronic disease. Legumes are low in fat and are excellent sources of protein, dietary fat, micronutrients, and phytochemicals. Numerous studies have linked regular consumption of whole grains with a lower risk of certain cancers and heart disease. Many nutrition experts attribute these health benefits to the fiber contained in whole grains.

Sugary foods also often displace other more nutritious foods in the diet. For example, carbonated beverages may be consumed instead of milk and fruit juices. The 2010 Dietary Guidelines for Americans recommends reducing the calories consumed from added sugars. The American Heart Association recommends that women should eat or drink no more than 100 calories/d from added sugars (25 grams or 6 teaspoons) and men 150 calories/d (38 grams or 10 teaspoons; Academy of Nutrition and Dietetics, 2012).

Consumption Patterns

Most of the world's population subsists primarily on carbohydrates. Foods rich in carbohydrates are easily grown in most climates, low in cost, and easily stored. Many carbohydrates do not require refrigeration or electricity, and their shelf life (the time a product can remain in storage without deterioration) may stretch to years. In Asia, where rice is a dietary staple, carbohydrates provide as much as 80% of the fuel in the diet. In the U.S. population as a whole, the largest source of added sugar is regular soft drinks, which accounts for one-third of intake (Academy of Nutrition and Dietetics, 2012).

The USDA's (2005) Continuing Survey of Food Intake by Individuals finds that:

- U.S. adults averaged only one serving per day of whole grains.
- Two percent of adults consumed no whole grain.
- Consumption of milk has decreased by 16% since the late 1970s, whereas consumption of carbonated soft drinks has increased by 16%.
- Only 54% of individuals ate fruit on a given day.

The 2010 Dietary Guidelines for Americans recommendations include:

- Reduction in the foods and drinks with added sugars or energy containing sweeteners.
- Drink few or no regular soda pop, sports drinks, and fruit drinks.
- Eat fewer grain-based or dairy-based desserts, other desserts, and candy or eat smaller portions less frequently.
- Drink water, fat-free milk, or 100% fruit juice instead of fruit-flavored drinks.
- Eat fruit for dessert.
- Use the Nutrition Facts label to choose breakfast cereals and other packaged foods with less sugar, and use the ingredients list to choose foods with little or no added sugars.

Dental Caries

Several studies have shown a relationship between carbohydrate consumption and dental caries. Dental caries is the gradual decay of the teeth. A dental cavity is a hole in a tooth caused by dental caries. Dental caries results from the interaction of four factors: a genetically susceptible tooth, bacteria, carbohydrate, and time. All four must occur simultaneously for a cavity to form, as Figure 2-2 illustrates. Some people are more genetically susceptible to caries than other people, as Genomic Gem 2-1 discusses.

Food Sources

Carbohydrates fall into two general groups: sugars and starches. All starches contain fiber; however, all starches do not provide equal amounts of fiber.

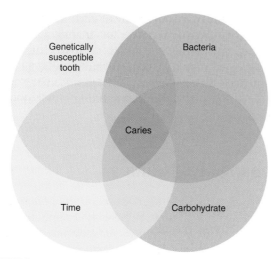

FIGURE 2-2 Interactions necessary for dental cavity formation.

Genomic Gem 2-1

Caries

Genetic susceptibility is an individual's likelihood of developing a given trait as determined by heredity. We cannot control our genetic susceptibility for cavities, and bacteria are always present in our mouths and difficult to eliminate. However, we can control the length of time carbohydrate-containing foods are in our mouths and the kinds of carbohydrates we eat.

Risk Factors for Cavity Formation
Bacteria, carbohydrate-containing foods, and the length of time that teeth are exposed to sugars influence cavity formation. Bacteria normally present in the mouth interact with dietary carbohydrates and produce acids. The acids, not the sugar, cause decay. All types of sugars can promote cavity formation, including fructose, glucose, maltose, lactose, and sucrose.

A strong relationship exists between the length of time sugars are present in the mouth and the development of caries. For example, sticky foods such as caramels and raisins, which adhere to the tooth surface for long periods, are more likely than other foods to lead to tooth decay in susceptible people. Sipping sweetened beverages continually throughout the day can lead to tooth decay.

Eating Right to Prevent Cavities
Certain foods may help counteract the effects of the acids produced by oral bacteria. Aged cheese (cheddar, Swiss, blue, Monterey jack, brie, gouda), as well as processed American cheese, may inhibit tooth decay. Cheese stimulates the production of saliva. Chewing fibrous foods such as apples or celery stimulates the production of generous amounts of saliva. Saliva helps clear the mouth of food and counteracts acid production. Because saliva production is increased during a meal, sugars eaten with a meal are less likely to cause decay than those eaten between meals.

Clinical Application 2-1

Nursing-Bottle Syndrome

Nursing-bottle syndrome is a dental condition caused by the frequent and prolonged exposure of an infant's or young child's teeth to liquids containing sugars. Milk, formula, fruit juice, and other sweetened drinks can all cause rampant dental cavities.

Typically, nursing-bottle syndrome occurs when a caretaker habitually puts a baby to bed with a bottle of milk, juice, or other sweetened liquid. During sleep, the flow of saliva decreases, which allows liquids from the nursing bottle to pool around the teeth, undiluted for extended periods. Parents need to be cautioned against this practice.

The main ways to maintain oral health include these steps:

- Reduce consumption and especially frequency of food and drink containing sugar.
- Consume sugar only as part of a meal.
- Snacks and drinks should be sugar-free.
- Avoid frequent consumption of acidic drinks.

Sugars

Table sugar contains approximately 4 grams of carbohydrates per teaspoon. When determining a person's sugar consumption, we consider not only the simple sugars such as honey, jam, and jelly but also the sugars present in carbonated beverages, ice cream, sherbet, cakes, pies, cookies, and donuts. Sugar alcohols contain on average about 2 grams of carbohydrate per teaspoon.

Starches

Starches are complex carbohydrates and are important sources of fiber and other nutrients. Figure 2-3 illustrates a typical cereal grain. Its main parts are the germ, bran, and endosperm. Most of the nutrients in cereal are in the bran and germ.

Whole grains are more nutritious than refined grains, in which nutrients are removed during the **milling** process. During the milling of grain, the germ and bran are removed from the grain kernel. White flour results from the milling of wheat and white rice from the milling of rice. Oat products are not normally milled. The nutritive value of cereal depends on the amount of bran and germ retained during the milling process. For this reason, the use of whole grains should be encouraged whenever possible. Examples of whole grains include the following:

- Cornbread made from whole ground cornmeal
- Ground cornmeal
- Cracked wheat bread
- Oatmeal and oatmeal bread

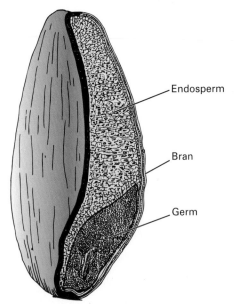

FIGURE 2-3 The most nutritious parts of wheat germ are the bran and endosperm, which are removed during the milling of grain.

- Pumpernickel bread (when made from whole grain flours)
- Rye bread (when made from whole grain flours)
- Whole-wheat bread
- Breads made from bran
- Barley
- Graham crackers

MyPlate

The USDA rolled out MyPlate in 2010 as a way to help consumers learn the messages of the 2010 Dietary Guidelines. The emphasis is on portion control, eating more fruits and vegetables (half the plate), drinking fewer sugary drinks, choosing low-fat dairy products, and ensuring that half of grain consumption (a quarter of the plate) is from whole grains (ChooseMyPlate.gov). See Figure 1-2 to review.

Carbohydrate Counting

In health care, carbohydrate counting helps teach clients about the carbohydrate content of foods and healthful portion sizes, which helps manage blood glucose levels. A serving is not the amount commonly eaten but a defined amount of a particular food according to nutrition experts. One serving or exchange of milk, fruit, grain, cereal, bread, or starchy vegetable is considered to be 15 grams of carbohydrate (American Diabetes Association and American Dietetic Association, 2009). Eating

45 to 60 grams of carbohydrate at each meal is recommended as a starting point for managing diabetes (Diabetes.org). Eating too much of any of the energy nutrients can result in unhealthful weight gain and uncontrolled blood glucose. Perhaps no other concept is more important to understanding nutrition than healthful portion sizes.

Exchange List Values

Exchange lists were introduced in Chapter 1. This section focuses on exchange lists that contain carbohydrates. Exchanges that include carbohydrates are the starch/bread, vegetable, fruit, and milk lists (Appendix B).

Starch/Bread Exchange List

One American Diabetes Association (ADA) exchange of starch contains approximately 15 grams of carbohydrates. For example, each of the food items in Figure 2-4 is equal to one starch exchange. Some foods are higher in fiber than other foods. See Table 2-5.

Vegetable Exchange List

Raw and cooked vegetables are also good sources of carbohydrates. Vegetables contain between 2 and 3 grams of fiber per serving. One vegetable exchange contains approximately 5 grams of carbohydrate. One-half cup of cooked vegetables or one cup of raw vegetables equals one vegetable exchange. Vegetables also contribute vitamins and minerals to the diet.

Fruit Exchange List

Fruits are another source of carbohydrates. One ADA exchange of fruit contains approximately 15 grams of carbohydrates (Table 2-6). Many fruits are excellent sources of fiber and contain vitamins and minerals. Figure 2-5 illustrates one serving or exchange of fruit.

Milk Exchange List

Milk, with its lactose content, is an important source of carbohydrates. One cup of milk contains 12 grams of carbohydrates. Skim, whole, and 2% milk all contain approximately the same amount of carbohydrates. Box 2-3 lists milk equivalents.

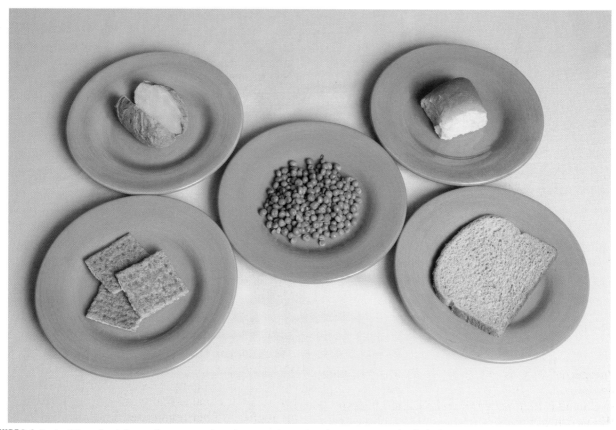

FIGURE 2-4 Each of these foods is equal to one starch exchange and contains about 15 grams of carbohydrates (see Appendix B).

TABLE 2-5 ■ Selected Starch Exchanges	
Bran cereal*	½ cup
Cooked cereal	½ cup
Ready-to-eat, unsweetened cereal	¾ cup
Sugar-frosted cereal	½ cup
Beans (cooked)*	½ cup
Corn, whole kernel	½ cup
Potato, baked	1 small (3 ounces)
Whole-wheat bread	1 slice (1 ounce)

General rule: ½ cup of cereal, grain, or pasta or 1 ounce of a bread product is equal to one starch exchange.
*Higher in fiber.

TABLE 2-6 ■ Selected Fruit Exchanges	
Apple (raw, 2 in. across)	1 (4 ounce) apple
Banana (small)	1 (4 ounce) banana
Blueberries*	¾ cup
Grapefruit (medium)	Half grapefruit
Orange (2½ in. across)	1 (6½ ounce) orange
Orange juice	½ cup
Prunes (dried)*	3 medium
Raspberries*	1 cup
Strawberries (raw whole)*	1¼ cup

*Contains 3 grams or more of fiber.

Dietary Recommendations

The Food and Nutrition Board of the National Academy of Sciences, Institute of Medicine, issued dietary recommendations for carbohydrates in 2005. To meet the body's daily energy and nutritional needs while minimizing risk for chronic disease, adults should get 45% to 65% of their calories from carbohydrates.

The committee reasoned that because carbohydrates, fat, and protein all serve as energy sources and can substitute for one another to some extent to meet caloric needs, the recommended ranges for consuming energy nutrients should be useful and flexible for dietary planning, hence the wide 45% to 65% range. The ranges for children are similar to those for adults in respect to carbohydrates.

The Recommended Dietary Allowance for children older than 1 year of age and most adults younger than 70 years of age is 130 grams of CHO/day. The RDA is 175 grams of CHO per day for pregnant women and 210 grams per day for lactating women. According to the 2010 Dietary Guidelines for Americans, no more than 6% of total calories eaten should comprise added sugars (Academy of Nutrition and Dietetics, 2012). This suggested maximum stems from evidence that people with diets high in added sugars have lower intakes of essential nutrients.

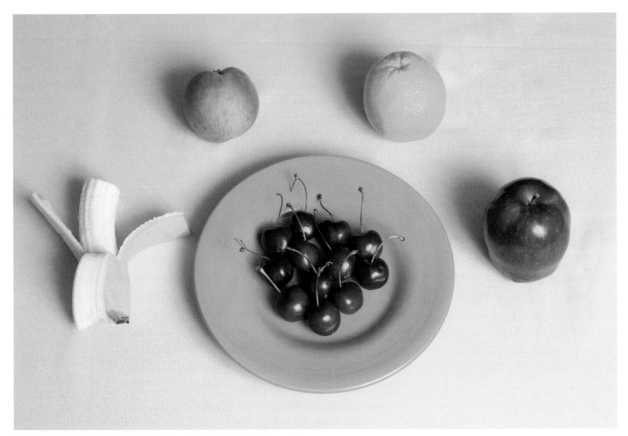

FIGURE 2-5 Each of these foods is equal to one fruit exchange (see Appendix B).

Box 2-3 ■ *Milk Equivalents*

Each of the following is equal to one exchange.

- Eight ounces of plain low-fat yogurt (with added nonfat milk solids)

- ⅓ cup dry nonfat milk
- ½ cup evaporated milk
- 1 cup of buttermilk

Keystones

- Carbohydrates are composed of sugars and starches.
- The average American's intake of sugars is considered excessive, whereas the intake of starches is considered low.
- Many Americans would benefit from increasing their fiber intake through the consumption of more whole-grain starches, fruits, and vegetables.
- Dietary carbohydrates promote tooth decay in susceptible individuals.
- The American Diabetes Association exchange lists that contain carbohydrates are the starch, vegetable, fruit, and milk lists.
- Strong evidence exists that a minimum of 130 grams of carbohydrates per day is necessary for adequate brain and body function.
- When there is no or little carbohydrate in the diet and the body uses protein or fat as a fuel source, the body in effect cannibalizes itself for glucose. Muscle and organ mass is lost in the process.
- The RDA for CHO is 130 grams of carbohydrates a day. Pregnant and lactating women have a higher Recommended Dietary Allowance for CHO.

CASE STUDY *2-1*

K. L. is a 19-year-old college student. He is interested in bodybuilding and spends much of his time on strength conditioning. He lifts weights or uses an elliptical machine daily. He is 6 feet tall and weighs 175 lb. For the past 3 weeks, he has been drinking a powdered protein supplement (that contains no carbohydrate) instead of eating the dorm food, which he states "isn't any good anyway." He also takes a high-stress vitamin and mineral tablet. He arrived at the clinic today with complaints of fatigue, nausea, a lack of appetite, lightheadedness, and memory loss. His urine tested positive for ketones. The client is willing to talk to a registered dietitian.

CARE PLAN

Subjective Data

The client has chosen not to eat any foods that contain carbohydrates for approximately 3 weeks.

Objective Data

Urine positive for ketones.

Analysis

Inadequate intake of CHO, related to erroneous ideas about healthy eating as evidenced by verbal statements that he has not been eating CHO-containing foods and by urine positive for ketones.

Plan

DESIRED OUTCOMES EVALUATION CRITERIA	ACTIONS/INTERVENTIONS	RATIONALE
Client will state one reason why he needs CHO by the end of the appointment.	Encourage client to consume foods from MyPlate, including milk, starches, fruits, and vegetables. Refer to the dietitian for instruction on normal nutrition and protein needs for athletes.	Explaining why carbohydrates are necessary in the diet may motivate the client to eat carbohydrates. Milk, vegetables, fruits, and starches are all good sources of CHO. The nurse may need to educate the client about dietary sources of carbohydrates.
Schedule the client for a return visit in 1 week. Client will keep a food record for the dietitian.	On next visit, ask client to demonstrate knowledge gained. (For example, "How many servings of starch, fruits, and vegetables do you need daily?") Test the urine for ketones at the next visit.	

 2-1

Dietitian's Note

The following Dietitian's Notes are representative of the documentation found in a client's medical record.

Dietitian's Notes

Subjective: Client states he wants to be able to lift more weight. Food records for 4 days show an average daily intake of 18 meats, 12 fats, 1 starch, 1 fruit, and 1 vegetable, and 1 low-fat milk. Client states he has just recently added starch, fruit, and milk to his diet per nurse's recommendation. Patient continues to complain of fatigue and constipation. He finds it difficult to concentrate and study.

Objective: Ketones in urine, weight 175 lb (81 kg) height: 6 ft

Analysis: Ideal body weight 178 ± 10%; estimated protein needs 81–97 grams. Estimated kcal need based on 81 kg and 25–35 kcal/kg = 2025–2835. Food records show an approximate intake of 2111 kcal and 25% protein, 66% fat, and 8% carbohydrate.

Inadequate carbohydrate intake related to food and nutrition-related knowledge deficit as evidenced by ketone smell on breath, complaints of fatigue and difficulty concentrating, and food records.

Continued

2-1

Dietitian's Note—cont'd

Client appears open to learning and prefers written and oral instructions.

Plan

1. Client to substitute CHO kcal for fat kcal by eliminating bacon, olives, soy nuts, and fatty meats from diet.

2. Client agreed to try adding 3 cups low-fat milk, 4 vegetables, 3 fruits, and 6 whole grains to diet.
3. Appointment scheduled for follow-up in 1 week.
4. Copy of MyPlate given to client.

Critical Thinking Questions

1. At the client's next visit, what would you do if the food records showed a recorded carbohydrate intake of only 30 grams for most days? What if the client said, "I don't want to eat any more because I feel better"?

2. At the next client visit, what would you do if the food records showed that the client ate only sugar to increase his carbohydrate intake because "Sugar is a quick energy food"?

3. At the next client visit, what would you do if he made no changes to his diet?

Chapter Review

1. Which of the following is a disaccharide?
   a. Glucose
   b. Lactose
   c. Fructose
   d. Galactose

2. A healthy adult needs _____ grams of fiber each day.
   a. 5 to 11
   b. 12 to 20
   c. 21 to 38
   d. More than 50

3. Twelve grams of simple carbohydrate is equal to _____ teaspoon(s) of sugar.
   a. 1
   b. 2
   c. 3
   d. 8

4. One slice of bread contains approximately _____ grams of carbohydrates.
   a. 5
   b. 8
   c. 10
   d. 15

5. Which of the following may cause diarrhea?
   a. A medication that contains sorbitol
   b. A lack of dietary fiber
   c. A lack of exercise
   d. An insufficient fluid intake

Clinical Analysis

1. Ms. C is concerned about the dangers associated with the consumption of artificial sweeteners and wants to know if they are safe. As a health-care worker, it is appropriate for you to:
   a. Ignore Ms. C's comments because you think she is overly concerned.
   b. Assure her that the government wouldn't allow a food or herbal product to be sold if it was hazardous to her health.
   c. Explain to her that no food is guaranteed to be 100% safe, and it is best to avoid artificial sweeteners if she is not comfortable with these products.
   d. Refer her to the local health food store.

2. Mr. J claims he is trying to lose weight, and his urinalysis shows that his urine contains ketones (ketonuria). You should ask him:
   a. When he ate last
   b. How much milk, fruit, and starch he usually eats
   c. What else he usually eats
   d. All of the above

3. Mr. P complains of constipation. As his nurse, you would like to teach him to eat more insoluble fiber to help alleviate his discomfort. You should encourage the intake of:
   a. Wheat and corn bran, nuts, fruit skins, and dried beans
   b. Eggs, cheese, and chicken
   c. Milk, yogurt, and ice cream
   d. Oatmeal, barley, and broccoli

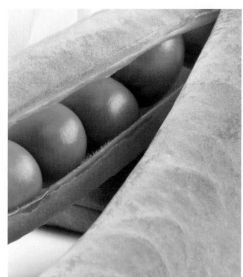

3

Fats

LEARNING OBJECTIVES

After completing this chapter, the student should be able to:

- Identify how fats are classified and discuss their physical properties.
- List the major functions of fats both in the diet and in the body.
- Discuss the relationships to health of cholesterol, saturated fat, polyunsaturated fat, *trans*-fatty acids, and monounsaturated fat.
- List three current recommendations of the Food and Nutrition Board of the National Research Council that pertain to fat.

This chapter presents an introduction to lipids for students without a chemistry background. Chapter 18 expands on this chapter and discusses clinical nutrition in more detail. The descriptive name for fats of all kinds, lipids, is used in clients' medical records. **Lipids** include true fats and oils as well as related fatlike compounds such as **lipoids** and **sterols.** Fats are a major source of fuel for the body. Dietary fat is found in both animal and plant products. Animal fats, which consist of a larger content of saturated fats, tend to have a higher melting point and are solid at room temperature. Plant-derived fats are normally in the form of oils, having a lower melting point and comprising more unsaturated fats than animal products.

Lipids are **insoluble** in water and are greasy to the touch. When two insoluble substances are mixed together, such as vinegar and oil, they separate readily. You can shake the vinegar and oil combination repeatedly, but it will still separate after the agitation stops.

Basic Terminology

Lipids are composed of the elements carbon, hydrogen, and oxygen. These are the same three elements that make up carbohydrates, but the proportion of oxygen to carbon and hydrogen is lower in fats. The basic structural unit of a true fat is one molecule of **glycerol** joined to one, two, or three fatty acid molecules. Glycerol is thus the backbone of a fat molecule.

A **fatty acid** is composed of a chain of carbon atoms with hydrogen and a few oxygen atoms attached. The fatty acid chains joined to the glycerol molecule vary in length (depending on the number of carbon atoms present) and composition. The different taste, smell, and physical appearance of each fat results from the variety of fatty acids and their physical arrangement in the fat molecules. Beef fat tastes, smells, and looks different from that of chicken mostly because of the difference in fatty acid composition. All fats contain fatty acids.

A fat can have from one to three fatty acids, and the number of fatty acids a fat contains has important implications for both diet and health.

Monoglycerides and Diglycerides

When a single fatty acid is joined to a glycerol molecule, the resulting fat is called a **monoglyceride.** When two fatty acids are joined to a glycerol molecule, the fat is called a **diglyceride.** The terms *monoglyceride* and *diglyceride* are commonly seen on food labels.

Triglycerides

When three fatty acids are joined to a glycerol molecule, a **triglyceride** is formed. Most of the fat found in our diets and in the body is in the form of triglycerides. Excess triglycerides are stored in the specialized **adipose cells** that make up adipose tissue. The human body has a virtually unlimited capacity to store fat. Figure 3-1 illustrates the structure of monoglycerides, diglycerides, and triglycerides.

Length of Fatty Acid Chain

Fatty acids vary in the length of their fatty acid chains: Each chain is determined by the number of carbon atoms present, which can vary from 2 to 24. The length of the chain determines how the body transports the fat in the body; fatty acid chains of short length (<6 carbon atoms) and medium length (8–12 carbon atoms) are processed differently than longer chains are. The chain length has dietary implications in many diseases. For example, in certain diseases of malabsorption, the client cannot tolerate foods with long-chain fatty acids. This problem is discussed in more detail in later chapters.

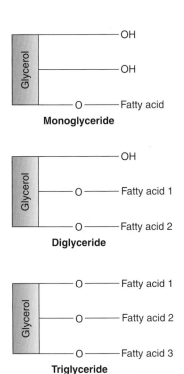

FIGURE 3-1 Monoglycerides, diglycerides, and triglycerides. A monoglyceride has one fatty acid attached to the glycerol molecule, a diglyceride has two fatty acids attached to the glycerol molecule, and a triglyceride has three fatty acids attached to the glycerol molecule.

Degree of Saturation

The terms *saturated, trans-fats, unsaturated, monounsaturated,* and *polyunsaturated* have become household words. Consumers and clients ask sophisticated questions about fats and expect health-care professionals to define and explain the terminology. Technically, all of these terms refer to the chemical structure of fatty acids, based on the degree or nature of the hydrogen atom saturation.

The degree of saturation of a fatty acid depends on the extent to which hydrogen is joined to the carbon atoms present. A **saturated fatty acid** is filled with as many hydrogen atoms as the carbon atoms can bond with and has no double bonds between carbons. In this case, a **double bond** describes the type of chemical connection between two neighboring carbon atoms, each lacking one hydrogen atom. In an **unsaturated fatty acid,** the carbon atoms are joined together by one or more of such double bonds.

Wherever a double bond occurs, another hydrogen atom could potentially join the chain. In other words, the fatty acid chain is lacking hydrogen atoms and is thus less saturated than a chain that is completely filled. A fatty acid with only one carbon-to-carbon double bond is **monounsaturated.** A fatty acid with more than one carbon-to-carbon bond is **polyunsaturated.** See Figure 3-2 for a structural comparison of saturated, monounsaturated, and polyunsaturated fatty acids.

In addition to the fats in the body, the fats found in foods are combinations of saturated and unsaturated fatty acids. They are designated as follows:

- Saturated fat: Composed mostly of saturated fatty acids
- Unsaturated fat: Composed mostly of unsaturated fatty acids
- Monounsaturated fat (MUFA): Composed mostly of monounsaturated fatty acids
- Polyunsaturated fat (PUFA): Composed mostly of polyunsaturated fatty acids
- *Trans*-fatty acids: Composed of partially hydrogenated fatty acids

Figure 3-3 shows the mixtures of fatty acids in dietary fats.

Physical Properties and Food Sources

Terms such as *saturated fats, unsaturated fats,* and *hydrogenation* are commonly used. This section of the text introduces these terms and discusses food sources.

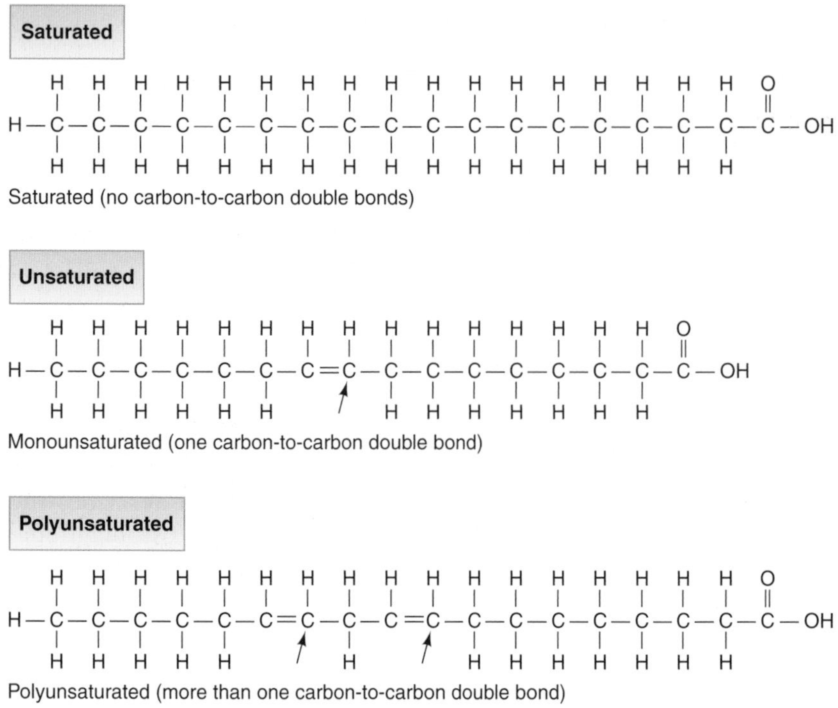

Saturated

H—C—C—C—C—C—C—C—C—C—C—C—C—C—C—C—C—C—C—OH

Saturated (no carbon-to-carbon double bonds)

Unsaturated

H—C—C—C—C—C—C=C—C—C—C—C—C—C—C—C—C—OH

Monounsaturated (one carbon-to-carbon double bond)

Polyunsaturated

H—C—C—C—C—C=C—C—C=C—C—C—C—C—C—C—C—OH

Polyunsaturated (more than one carbon-to-carbon double bond)

FIGURE 3-2 Saturated, monounsaturated, and polyunsaturated fatty acids. A saturated fatty acid has no carbon-to-carbon double bonds. A monounsaturated fatty acid has one carbon-to-carbon double bond. A polyunsaturated fatty acid has more than one carbon-to-carbon double bond.

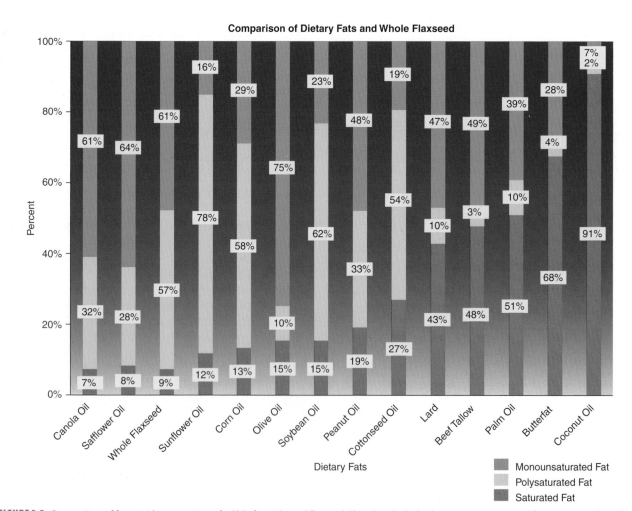

Comparison of Dietary Fats and Whole Flaxseed

FIGURE 3-3 Comparison of fatty acid composition of edible fats, oils, and flaxseed. The oil with the highest monounsaturated fat content is olive oil. The oil with the lowest saturated fat content is canola.

Saturated Fats

Saturated fats, which are likely to be solid at room temperature, are usually found in animal products such as meat, poultry, and whole milk. The exceptions are tropical coconut and palm-kernel oils and cocoa butter, which are vegetable sources of saturated fat. See Tables 3-1 and 3-2 for a more complete list of foods containing saturated fat.

Saturated fats are more chemically stable than unsaturated fats. For this reason, saturated fats become rancid slowly because the chemical bond between carbon and hydrogen is stable. A rancid fat has an offensive odor and taste caused by the partial chemical breakdown of the fat's molecular structure. Consumers usually discard **rancid** foods because of the highly offensive odor.

Products made with saturated fats have a fairly long shelf life because the fat in the product is fairly stable. However, saturated fats have been targeted for reduction in the average American's diet by health authorities because these fats have unhealthful effects when ingested in excess of the body's needs.

Unsaturated Fats

Unsaturated fats are likely to be liquid at room temperature and of plant origin; they tend to become rancid more quickly than saturated fats. The double carbon bonds in unsaturated fatty acids are unstable and therefore easily broken. For this reason, many convenience products have traditionally been made with saturated fats to lengthen their shelf life. The food industry is changing this practice; increasingly, more convenience products are made with unsaturated fats. Examples of unsaturated fats are corn, cottonseed, safflower, soybean, and sunflower oils. See Table 3-3 for a more complete list of unsaturated fats.

Hydrogenation

Commercial food processing frequently involves hydrogenation—adding hydrogen to a fat of vegetable origin (unsaturated) either to extend the fat's shelf life or make the fat harder. This process of adding hydrogen to a fat is called **hydrogenation.** If only some of the fat's double bonds are broken by the hydrogenation, the product becomes partially hydrogenated. If all of the double bonds are broken, the product becomes completely hydrogenated.

Completely hydrogenated fats are highly saturated fats; that is, they have no carbon-to-carbon double bonds. For example, a completely hydrogenated corn oil is closer to lard in saturation than a partially hydrogenated corn oil. All vegetable spreads, such as corn oil margarine, have been hydrogenated to some extent. If these spreads had not been hydrogenated, they would be liquids (except for the saturated tropical oils). Clients are usually advised to avoid products that contain completely hydrogenated fats when the therapeutic goal is to decrease saturated fat intake.

A health consequence of hydrogenation is the formation of *trans*-**fatty acids.** *Trans*-fatty acids are produced by the partial hydrogenation of unsaturated

TABLE 3-1 ■ Food Sources of Saturated Fats

Meat products	Visible fat and marbling in beef, pork, and lamb, especially in prime-grade and ground meats, lard, suet, salt pork
Processed meats	Frankfurters Luncheon meats such as bologna, corned beef, liverwurst, pastrami, and salami Bacon and sausage
Poultry and fowl	Chicken and turkey (mostly beneath the skin), Cornish hens, duck, and goose
Whole milk and whole-milk products	Cheeses made with whole milk or cream, condensed milk, ice cream, whole-milk yogurt, all creams (sour, half-and-half, whipped)
Plant products	Coconut oil, palm-kernel oil, cocoa butter
Miscellaneous	Fully hydrogenated shortening and margarine, many cakes, pies, cookies, and mixes

TABLE 3-2 ■ Selected Foods High in Cholesterol and/or Saturated Fat

FOOD	AMOUNT	CHOLESTEROL (MG)	SATURATED FAT (MG)
Liver	3 oz	410	2.4
Cream puff	1	228	10.0
Baked custard	1 cup	213	7.0
Egg, hard cooked	1	215	5.0
Waffles, homemade	2	204	8.0
Coconut custard pie	1 piece	183	8.0
Cheesecake	3.25 oz	170	10.0
Shrimp, boiled	6 large	167	0.2
Eggnog, commercial	1 cup	149	11.0
Bread pudding/raisins	1 cup	142	4.5
Whole milk	1 cup	124	5.0
Ground beef, 21% fat	3 oz cooked	76	7.0

TABLE 3-3 ■ Food Sources of Unsaturated Fats

FOODS HIGH IN MONOUNSATURATED FATTY ACIDS	FOODS HIGH IN POLYUNSATURATED FATTY ACIDS
Canola, olive, peanut oils	Corn, cottonseed, mustard seed, safflower, sesame, soybean, and sunflower seed oils
Almonds, avocados, cashews, filberts, olives, and peanuts	Halibut, herring, mackerel, salmon, sardines, fresh tuna, trout, whitefish

vegetable oils. As illustrated in Figure 3-4, a *cis* config-uration double bond between carbon atoms in a fatty acid has a kink or bend. A *trans* configuration double bond between carbon atoms in a fatty acid is straighter.

During hydrogenation, many of the fatty acids are converted from the *cis* to the *trans* configuration. Evi-dence indicates that the *trans* configuration is detrimental to health. If the dietary goal is to decrease consumption of *trans*-fatty acids, the client must decrease consumption of hydrogenated foods. Foods that may be high in *trans*-fatty acids include the following:

- Commercially baked goods
- Fried foods in restaurants
- Hard margarines and shortenings
- Crackers
- Biscuit and some cake mixes
- Some candy
- Animal crackers and cookies
- Frozen waffles and pancakes
- Microwave popcorn

The food industry has reformulated many of these products to decrease their *trans*-fatty acid content.

Functions of Fats

Lipids are important in the diet and serve many func-tions in the human body.

Fats in Food

Fats serve several functions in food including serving as a fuel source and acting as a vehicle for fat-soluble vitamins.

Fuel Source

Fats are the major dietary source of fuel. Because fats have proportionately more carbon and hydrogen and less

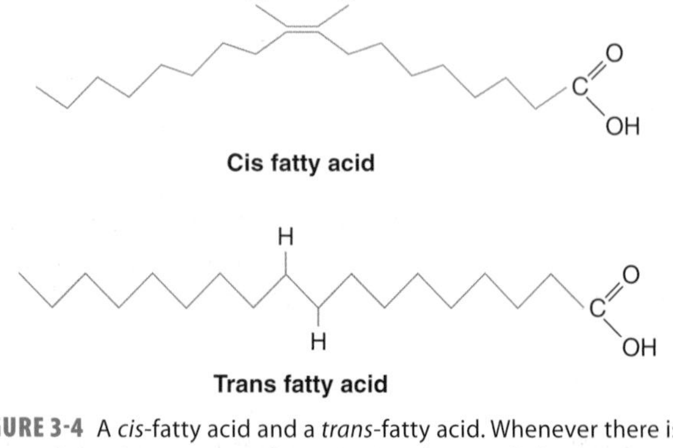

FIGURE 3-4 A *cis*-fatty acid and a *trans*-fatty acid. Whenever there is a change from *cis* to *trans* configuration in a fatty acid, the three-dimensional shape of the molecule is altered.

oxygen than carbohydrates, fats have a greater potential for the release of energy. In practical terms, this means that fats are a concentrated source of fuel or kilocalories.

Fats furnish more than twice as many kilocalories, gram for gram, as carbohydrates. Each gram of fat yields 9 kilocalories, so 1 teaspoon of fat, which is equivalent to 5 grams of fat, yields 45 kilocalories. Compare these numbers with those for carbohydrates, each gram of which yields only 4 kilocalories. A teaspoon of sugar contains 4 grams of carbohydrates and therefore yields only 16 kilocalories.

Vehicle for Fat-Soluble Vitamins

In foods, fats act as a vehicle for vitamins A, D, E, and K. In the body, fats assist in the absorption of these fat-soluble vitamins.

Satiety Value

Fats also contribute flavor, satiety value, and palatability to the diet. They supply texture to food, trap and in-tensify its flavor, and enhance its odor. Satiety is a per-son's feeling of fullness and satisfaction after eating. Fat contributes to the sensation of satisfaction because it leaves the stomach more slowly than carbohydrates.

Consider for a moment the sensations felt when eating 2 cups of ice cream versus 2 cups of chopped apples. Ice cream has a high fat content, and apples have no fat. An individual may feel full after eating 2 cups of apples but complain of a bloated feeling and a lack of gratification. Satiety is feeling full, completely satisfied, and that enough or too much food has been eaten.

Sources of Essential Fatty Acids

An essential nutrient is one that must be supplied by the diet because the body cannot manufacture it in sufficient amounts to prevent disease. Fat contains the essential fatty acids linoleic, arachidonic, and linolenic. Linolenic acid is subdivided into two groups, alpha and gamma. Figure 3-5 shows the pathways of these fatty acids.

Although the body can manufacture gamma-linoleic (linolenic) acid and arachidonic acid from linoleic acid, all three of these fatty acids are considered essential. Linoleic is called an omega-6 fatty acid. Omega is the last letter in the Greek alphabet and is used by chemists for naming fatty acid classes by their chemical structure. The six designation means that the first double bond is located six carbons down the chain (counting from the omega end).

Linoleic acid strengthens cell membranes and has a major role in the transport and metabolism of choles-terol. The omega-6 fatty acids together prolong blood-clotting time, hasten fibrolytic activity, and are involved

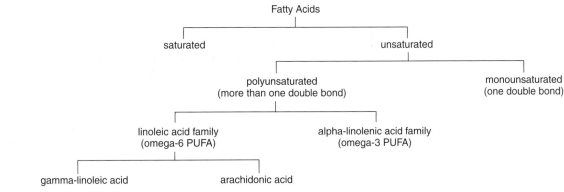

FIGURE 3-5 Classification of fatty acids.

in the development of the brain. **Prostaglandins,** compounds with extensive **hormone-**like actions, require arachidonic acid for synthesis.

Another name for alpha-linolenic fatty acid is omega-3 polyunsaturated fatty acid (PUFA). The omega-3 PUFA has a variety of biological effects that may influence the risk of cardiovascular disease. Mono- and polyunsaturated fatty acids may reduce the risk of cognitive decline in dementia, but more research is needed (Frisardi, Panza, Seripa, Imbimbo, et al, 2010; Roberts, Cerhan, Geda, Knopman, et al, 2010; Solfrizzi, Panza, Frisari, Seripa et al, 2011).

Linoleic acid deficiency was first observed in the medical community during the middle of the 20th century with the introduction and widespread use of infant baby formulas. Initially, the formulas were deficient in linoleic acid, and infants fed formula subsequently developed dry and flaky skin. When linoleic acid was added to formula recipes, the infants' symptoms ceased (Wiese, Hansen, and Adam, 1958). There are global standards for the composition of infant formula, which more closely mimic human breast milk (HBM) to include linoleic acid (Koletzko, Baker, Cleghorn, Neto, et al, 2005).

Linoleic acid deficiency was observed in the early 1970s in hospitalized clients fed exclusively with intravenous fluids containing no fat. Symptoms included scaly skin, hair loss, impaired wound healing, increased susciptibility to infection, and immune dysfunction. When lipids were introduced into intravenous feedings, such symptoms ceased.

Fats in the Body

The major functions of fat in the human body include the following:

1. Supply fuel to most tissues
2. Function as an energy reserve
3. Insulate the body
4. Support and protect vital organs
5. Lubricate body tissues
6. Form an integral part of cell membranes
7. Carrier for the absorption of fat soluble vitamins

Fuel Supply

Fat serves as a fuel that supplies body tissues with needed energy.

Fuel Reserve

Fat also functions as the body's main fuel or energy reserve. Excess kilocalories consumed are stored in specialized cells called adipose cells. When an individual does not eat enough food to meet the energy demands of the body, the adipose cells release fat for fuel.

Lubrication

Fats also lubricate body tissue. The human body manufactures oil in structures called sebaceous glands. Secretions from the sebaceous glands lubricate the skin to retard loss of body water to the outside environment.

Organ Protection

Fatty tissue cushions and protects vital organs by providing a supportive fat pad that absorbs mechanical shocks. Examples of organs supported by fat are the eyes and kidneys.

Insulation

The subcutaneous layer of fat beneath the skin helps to insulate the body by protecting it from excessive heat or cold. A sheath of fatty tissue surrounding nerve fibers provides insulation to help transmit nerve impulses.

Cell Membrane Structure

Fat serves as an integral part of cell membranes and in this capacity plays a vital role in drug, nutrient, and metabolite transport and provides a barrier against water-soluble substances.

Carrier for Fat Soluble Vitamins

Fat is a carrier of the fat soluble vitamins A, D, E, and K and carotenoids so that they may be adsorbed by the body.

Cholesterol

Cholesterol is not a true fat but belongs to a group called sterols. Cholesterol is a component of many of the foods in our diet. In addition, the human body manufactures about 1000 milligrams of cholesterol a day, mainly in the liver. See Genomic Gem 3-1. The liver also filters out excess cholesterol and helps eliminate it from the body.

Functions

Cholesterol has several important functions. It is:

1. A component of bile salts that aid digestion
2. An essential component of all cell membranes
3. Found in brain and nerve tissue and in the blood
4. A precursor for the production of steroid hormones

Cholesterol is also necessary for the production of several hormones, including:

■ Cortisone
■ Adrenaline
■ Estrogen
■ Testosterone

A **hormone** is a substance produced by the endocrine glands and secreted directly into the bloodstream. Hormones stimulate functional activity of organs and cells or stimulate secretion of other hormones to do so.

Food Sources

Cholesterol is present only in animal foods. When animal products are ingested, one also ingests the cholesterol the animal made. The 2010 Dietary Guidelines for Americans states that because dietary cholesterol has been shown to raise blood cholesterol, an intake of less than 300 milligrams per day can help maintain normal blood cholesterol levels. For individuals who are at a high risk of developing cardiovascular disease, an intake of less than 200 milligrams per day is recommended.

Table 3-2 lists selected foods high in cholesterol. Note that one large egg supplies about 186 milligrams of cholesterol. According to the 2010 Dietary Guidelines for Americans, evidence suggests that one egg per day does not result in increased blood cholesterol levels or increase the risk of cardiovascular disease in healthy individuals.

The current thinking among most nutrition experts is that total diet should be evaluated for risk prevention. An overall healthy eating pattern that includes fruits, vegetables, and whole grains are important for risk reduction. No one food, even if it contains cholesterol, is unhealthy if eaten in appropriate amounts.

Fat Intake as a Worldwide Concern

The combination of underweight in children and overweight in adults, frequently coexisting in the same family, is a phenomenon in developing countries undergoing nutrition transition (Caballero, 2005). Changes in diet, food availability, and lifestyle are all components of transition as countries modernize. However, obesity in adults has been linked to the availability of cheap, energy-dense foods (including those from street vendors and fast-food restaurants) that facilitate the consumption of more fat. In addition, the introduction of low-cost vegetable oils from industrialized countries greatly increases the amount of fat in the average diet.

Genomic Gem 3-1

Client Response to Dietary Modification

A great deal of evidence indicates a relationship between cholesterol intake (especially one component of cholesterol called low-density lipoprotein cholesterol) and increased risk of coronary heart disease. In addition, increasing evidence shows genetic factors influence a person's response to both increases and decreases in cholesterol intake. For example, one study found defects in two different genes can lead to markedly increased absorption of both cholesterol and plant sterols (Food and Nutrition Board, 2005).

Another gene has been found to attenuate the plasma cholesterol response to dietary cholesterol in diets high in polyunsaturated fat but not in diets high in saturated fat (Food and Nutrition Board, 2005). These studies have been done in animals, but to date human data are lacking. The goal of this research is to be able to predict exactly which factors will lead to a disease in a particular individual. Genetics is the branch of biology that studies heredity and variation in both plants and animals. Genetics may also explain why one client may respond to diet modification but another client may not respond.

Healthier foods, including fruits and vegetables, have long been thought to be more expensive to the poorest people. A 2012 report examined purchasing foods based on the 2010 Dietary Guidelines for Americans using food groups and portions found in the MyPlate recommendations. The conclusion was that if foods were purchased to fulfill the MyPlate recommendations, even individuals receiving government assistance through the Supplemental Nutritional Assistance Program (SNAP) could afford to eat healthy foods (Carlson and Frazao, 2012).

Dietary Recommendations Concerning Fat

The National Academy of Science report on Dietary Reference Intakes for Macronutrients issued guidelines pertaining to fats in 2005 (Food and Nutrition Board, Institute of Medicine, 2005). Box 3-1 discusses the acceptable macronutrient distribution range (AMDR) for fats.

Before this recommendation, most government health authorities and professional groups recommended that the fat content of the U.S. diet not exceed 30% of caloric intake. The rationale for the change is that carbohydrates, fat, and protein all serve as fuel sources and can substitute for one another to some extent to meet fuel needs. Therefore, the recommended ranges for consuming these nutrients should be useful and flexible for dietary planning (Food and Nutrition Board, Institute of Medicine, 2005). Table 3-4 lists the recommended ranges in grams of fat for various calorie levels. See Clinical Calculation 3-1 as well.

The Food and Nutrition Board of the Institute of Medicine stated that saturated fat and cholesterol provide no known beneficial role in preventing chronic diseases and are not required at any level in the diet. However, the complete elimination of saturated fat and cholesterol from the diet would make it difficult to meet other nutritional guidelines. Some monounsaturated and polyunsaturated fatty acids are required to provide the essential fatty acids. See Box 3-2 and Dollars and Sense 3-1.

Box 3-1 ■ *Acceptable Macronutrient Distribution Range for Fats*

A range of intake for a particular energy source that is associated with a reduced risk of chronic disease and that provides adequate intakes of essential nutrients is called the acceptable macronutrient distribution range (AMDR; Hise and Brown, 2007). The AMDR for adults is 20% to 35% of kilocalories from fat. The AMDR for infants and young children is 25% to 40% of kilocalories from fat.

TABLE 3-4 ■ Recommended Range of Fat Intake at Selected Kilocalorie Levels

KILOCALORIE LEVEL	TOTAL FAT (GRAMS)
1200	26–46
1500	33–58
1600	35–62
1800	40–70
2000	44–78
2200	49–85
2400	53–93
2500	55–97

Clinical Calculation 3-1

Percent of Kilocalories from Fat

The following formula can be used to determine the percentage of kilocalories from fat in many packaged foods:

Kilocalories from fat per serving/kilocalories* × 100 = percent kilocalories from fat per serving

Example: kilocalories from fat = 30
Kilocalories per serving = 90
% kilocalories from fat = 30%

*Food labeling regulations require manufacturers to list both the number of kilocalories in a serving and the number of kilocalories from fat.

The 2010 Dietary Guidelines for Americans recommends that people eat less than 10% of calories from saturated fats by replacing them with monosaturated and polyunsaturated fatty acids, consume less than 300 milligrams per day of dietary cholesterol, reduce the intake of calories from solid fats, and limit *trans-fats* as much as possible in the diet because they are not essential in the diet and may be linked to increasing the risk of cardiovascular disease. The American Heart Association's Nutrition Committee recommends that trans-fats should comprise less than 1% of the diet (www.heart.org).

Dietary Fat Intake and Health

Fat plays a key role in diet and health. A diet too low in fat not only lacks satiety and palatability but may also lack adequate levels of the essential fatty acids; a diet with excessive fat may result in increased risk of disease.

Box 3-2 ■ *Essential Fatty Acids*

AI FOR ESSENTIAL FATTY ACIDS FOR ADULTS 19–51 YEARS OLD*	KIND	FOOD SOURCES
Men: 17 grams Women: 12 grams	Omega-6 fatty acids Linoleic acid	■ Vegetable oils such as safflower, corn, soybean, cottonseed ■ Poultry fat ■ Nuts and seeds
Men: 1.6 grams Women: 1.1 grams	Omega-3 fatty acids Linolenic acid	■ Human milk ■ Fatty fish ■ Vegetable oils such as soybean, flax, canola ■ Wheat germ ■ Soybeans

AI, adequate intake.
*Refer to dietary reference intakes tables for other age groups.

$ Dollars & Sense 3-1

Dietary Guidelines for Fat

The Dietary Guidelines for Americans 2010, American Heart Association, and The National Heart, Lung, and Blood Institute (NHLBI) recommend that most dietary fats come from sources of polyunsaturated and monounsaturated fatty acids. One way to obtain these fats is to incorporate nuts in the diet.

Nuts also provide other essential nutrients such as linolenic acid, vitamins A and E, magnesium, dietary fiber, copper, and zinc. Many nuts are also high in phytonutrients.

The best method of incorporating nuts into the diet on a daily basis is to practice good portion control. For example, an exchange or serving of nuts contains about 5 grams of fat and 45 kilocalories. One pound of shelled pistachios may seem expensive, but if eaten in exchange serving sizes of 16 nuts, that pound should yield 60 servings. Add a daily serving of nuts to oatmeal, a whole grain waffle, or a low-fat yogurt parfait at breakfast or brown rice dishes later in the day to enhance the food, bringing it crunch and essential nutrients.

Dietary Fat

A diet that has an appropriate balance of fat and carbohydrate is important for optimal health. Chronic consumption of either a low-fat/high-carbohydrate or a high-fat/low-carbohydrate diet may result in the inadequate intake of nutrients (Food and Nutrition Board, 2005). A diet too low in fat not only lacks satiety and palatability but may also lack adequate levels of the essential fatty acids, zinc, and certain B vitamins (Food and Nutrition Board, 2005). Excessive dietary fat has been associated with an increased risk of cardiovascular disease, the development of obesity and diabetes, and an increased risk of certain cancers.

The in 2011 the U.S. Department of Agriculture (USDA) reviewed the literature published from 2004 through 2009 regarding studies of saturated fatty acids and cardiovascular disease risk. It was concluded that by replacing 5% of total calories of saturated fatty acids with polyunsaturated or monounsaturated fatty acids, there is a decreased risk of nonfatal myocardial infarction and coronary death.

The USDA reported that in 2011, 11% of calories in the American diet were comprised of saturated fatty acids, which it recommended be reduced to no more than 10%. Lowering this percentage to 7% can further reduce the risk of cardiovascular disease. The top foods consumed by Americans that contribute to the high saturated fatty acid intake are pizza, grain-based desserts, dairy desserts, chicken and chicken mixed dishes, and beef and beef mixed dishes (USDA, 2011).

Monounsaturated Fats

Monounsaturated fats are a form of unsaturated fat. Most health educators recommend increasing intake of monounsaturated fats while decreasing intake of saturated fats. Evidence suggests that individuals with a higher intake of monounsaturated and polyunsaturated fats, a low intake of saturated fats, and a low total fat intake may have a decreased risk of coronary heart disease.

Monounsaturated fats are found in nuts, avocado, canola, olive, and peanut oil. Many nutrition experts advocate the consumption of fats derived from plant sources, such as those shown in Figure 3-6, because those foods also contribute fiber, antioxidants, and phytochemicals to the diet.

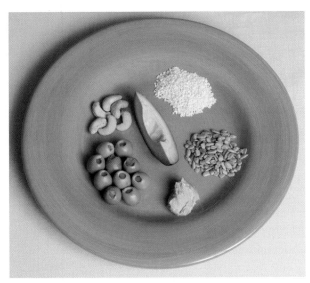

FIGURE 3-6 Plant sources of fats include avocado, nuts, olives, peanut butter, and some seeds such as sesame and flax.

Polyunsaturated Fats

Polyunsaturated fats come in the form of omega-6 and omega-3 PUFAs. Food sources of omega-6 PUFA include nuts and vegetable oils such as soybean, safflower, and corn. Good food sources of omega-3 PUFA include walnuts, flaxseeds, fatty fish, and some oils including soybean, canola, flax, and fish.

Body Fat

Both the amount of body fat a person carries and its distribution on the body are related to health risk. Many experts feel that the ratio of body fat to total weight is more important than total weight. Healthy ranges for body fat are 15% to 19% for men and 18% to 22% for women. A high percentage of body fat has been associated with increased risk of disease, even when total body weight is normal.

The location of excess body fat is also important. Excessive fat on the lower body, specifically on the hips and thighs, seems to be less dangerous than excessive fat on the abdomen and upper body, which is associated with a much higher risk of diseases such as cancer, heart disease, and diabetes. The exchange lists in the next section can be used to assist in planning meals low in fat and teach clients about food composition.

Exchange Lists

Exchange lists can be used to learn food composition and portion control and assist in planning lower-fat meals. For example, many people do not know that sugar and fruit contain no fat and oil contains no carbohydrate. Exchange categories that include fat are the

milk, meat, and fat lists. The amount of fat in one exchange of meat or milk varies within the list. Some foods not listed on the exchange lists are also high in fat. Many of these foods may be found in the nutritive values of foods tables.

Milk Exchange List

The fat content of milk varies according to the type of milk—whole, 2%, 1%, or nonfat. Table 3-5 shows the grams of fat and percentage of kilocalories from fat in one milk exchange for each kind of milk. Although whole milk and 2% milk contain saturated fat and cholesterol, the protein, carbohydrate, vitamin, and mineral contents of whole, 2%, 1%, and nonfat milk are comparable. Nonfat milk contains only a trace of fat and is thus a nutritional bargain.

Meat and Meat Substitute Exchange List

The meat exchange list is divided into four subgroups:

■ *One lean* meat exchange contains 0 to 3 grams of fat.
■ *One medium*-fat meat exchange contains 4 to 7 grams of fat.
■ *One high*-fat meat exchange contains 8 or more grams of fat.

Table 3-6 lists selected food examples from each of the meat exchanges.

Many clients have misconceptions about meat. Some clients avoid all red meat because they think it contains excessive fat. In fact, some beef and pork products are not excessively high in fat. Many consumers are not aware of the lean cuts of beef or pork. Conversely, not all fish and poultry items are lean meat exchanges. Nurses and other health educators can help clients by providing correct information about meats.

Different methods of food preparation can greatly influence the fat content of meats. Those that are baked, broiled, grilled, or roasted contain fewer kilocalories than fried versions. Some clients have the misconception that if they eat only lean meats, they can eat large quantities prepared in any manner, but preparation really does count. For example, a 3-ounce breaded fried chicken breast contains more fat than a grilled hamburger patty.

TABLE 3-5 ■ Grams of Fat in One Milk Exchange		
TYPE	FAT (GRAMS)	PERCENTAGE OF KILOCALORIES FROM FAT
Whole milk	8	48
2% (low fat)	5	38
Nonfat milk	Trace	<1

TABLE 3-6 ■ Examples of Lean, Medium-Fat, and High-Fat Meat Exchanges

Each of the following is one lean meat exchange and contains less than 1 gram of fat:		
Poultry	Chicken or turkey (white meat, no skin)	1 oz
Fish	Fresh or frozen cod, flounder, haddock	1 oz
Game	Venison	1 oz
Cheese	Nonfat cottage cheese	¼ cup
	Fat-free cheese	1 oz
Other	Egg whites	2
	Hot dogs with less than 1 g of fat	1 oz
	Egg substitute	¼ cup
Each of the following is one lean meat exchange and contains 3 grams of fat:		
Beef	Round, sirloin, or flank steak	1 oz
Fish	Salmon (fresh or frozen)	1 oz
Pork	Tenderloin	1 oz
Veal	Lean chop or roast	1 oz
Poultry	Chicken, dark meat, no skin	1 oz
Game	Goose, no skin	1 oz
Cheese	4.5% fat cottage cheese	¼ cup
	Cheeses with less than 3 g of fat per oz	1 oz
Other	Hot dogs with less than 3 g of fat per oz	1 oz
	Processed lunch meat with less than 3 g of fat per oz	1 oz
Each of the following is one medium-fat meat exchange and contains 5 grams of fat:		
Beef	Ground beef, corned beef	1 oz
Pork	Chops	1 oz
Poultry	Chicken, dark meat, with skin	1 oz
Fish	Any fried fish product	1 oz
Cheese	Mozzarella	1 oz
Other	Egg (high in cholesterol)	1
	Tofu	½ cup
Each of the following is one high-fat meat exchange and contains 8 grams of fat:		
Pork	Spareribs, pork sausage	1 oz
Cheese	All regular cheeses such as cheddar, Swiss, and American	1 oz
Other	Bologna	1 oz
	Knockwurst, bratwurst	1 oz
	Bacon	3 slices

Meat exchanges are usually 1 ounce, but a usual portion is 3 ounces, about half a chicken breast. Table 3-7 shows the total fat content of three meat exchanges. Typically, Americans eat large amounts of meats such as prime rib (from 6-ounce to 16-ounce servings). Therefore, teaching clients about meat portion sizes is usually indicated when the goal is to decrease fat intake and decrease total kilocalorie intake.

Whether the meat is classified as a lean, medium-fat, or high-fat meat exchange, the grams of fat in each exchange are calculated based on the following assumptions:

■ Visible fat on meat is not consumed.
■ Meat is weighed after cooking.
■ Meat is cooked by a low-fat method—baked, boiled, broiled, grilled, or roasted (unless otherwise indicated).

TABLE 3-7 ■ Total Fat in Three Meat Exchanges

MEAT	SUBGROUP	GRAMS OF FAT/EXCHANGE	GRAMS OF FAT PER SERVING
Cod	Lean	1	3
Sirloin steak	Lean	3	9
Hamburger patty, broiled*	Medium fat	5	15
Spareribs†	High fat	8	24

*About 4 oz raw.
†Boneless.

Since 1994, food-labeling regulations have allowed two definitions for the fat content labeling of meat, poultry, seafood, and game meats: *lean* and *extra lean.*

■ *Lean* can be used on meat, poultry, seafood, or game meat products only if the product contains less than 10 grams of fat, less than 4.5 grams of saturated fat, and less than 95 milligrams of cholesterol per 100-gram serving (3.5 ounces). The legal term *lean* thus equals the ADA exchange list definition for a lean meat exchange.

■ *Extra lean* can be used only if the product contains less than 5 grams of fat, less than 2 grams of saturated fat and *trans* fat combined, and less than 95 milligrams of cholesterol per serving and per 100 grams (3.5 ounces).

Some clients may choose not to eat animal products. Health-care workers should always accommodate their client's religious, ecological, and ethical beliefs and values. See Appendix B for brief exchange list information, which includes some meat substitutes. Many low-fat meat substitutes including dried beans, peas, and lentils are not derived from animals. Medium-fat vegetarian meat exchanges include soymilk, tempeh, and tofu. Peanut butter, which contains 8 grams of fat per exchange (2 tablespoons), is a high-fat meat exchange.

Fat Exchange List

Each fat exchange provides 5 grams of fat. Figure 3-7 illustrates three fat exchanges. The fat list is subdivided into two groups: unsaturated fats (monounsaturated and polyunsaturated) and saturated fats. Table 3-8 lists selected exchanges from each group.

Additional Food Sources of Fat

It is important to advise clients that snack foods, including crackers, cakes, pies, donuts, and cookies, may be high in both total fat and *trans*-fatty acids. Often, potato chips, gravies, cream sauces, soups, pizza, tacos, and spaghetti are high in fat. Microwave

TABLE 3-8 ■ Examples of Monounsaturated, Polyunsaturated, and Saturated Fat Exchanges

Each of the following is one fat exchange high in monounsaturated fatty acids and contains 5 g of total fat:

Olives	5 large
Canola oil	1 tsp
Peanut butter	2 tsp
Pecans	4 halves

Each of the following is one fat exchange high in polyunsaturated fatty acids and contains 5 grams of total fat:

Margarine, stick or tub	1 tsp
Mayo, regular	1 tsp
Corn oil	1 tsp
English walnuts	4 halves

Each of the following is one fat exchange high in saturated fatty acids and contains 5 grams of total fat:

Bacon	1 slice (20 slices/lb)
Butter, stick	1 tsp
Cream cheese, regular	1 tbsp (½ oz)
Cream cheese, reduced-fat	2 tbsp (1 oz)
Sour cream, regular	2 tbsp
Sour cream, reduced-fat	3 tbsp

popcorn is higher in fat than air-popped popcorn (without added fat).

Consumers who desire low-fat foods need not avoid eating out, but they do need to make wise food choices, especially if they eat most meals in restaurants. Many of the specialty fast-food hamburgers are high in fat; therefore, a small hamburger is the best burger choice. A small side salad with low-fat dressing is a better low-fat choice than French fries. Nonfat milk is lower in fat than either a milkshake or whole milk. A grilled chicken breast salad with a fat-free dressing is also a good choice. See Box 3-3.

Box 3-3 ■ *Food Label Terms*

Food labeling regulations spell out what terms may be used to describe the level of fat in a food and how the labels can be used. These are the terms:

■ *Fat-free* on a food label means that the food contains no more than 0.5 grams of fat per serving. Synonyms for *free* include *without, no,* and *zero. Nonfat* is another synonym for *fat-free.* These terms legally can be used on a food label only if the product contains no amount of—or only trivial or "physiologically inconsequential" amounts of—fat, saturated fat, and cholesterol.

■ *Low-fat* is legally defined as a food that contains no more than 3 grams of fat in a serving.

■ *Low saturated fat* is legally defined as a food that contains no more than 1 gram of saturated fat per serving.

■ *Low cholesterol* is defined as a food that contains less than 20 milligrams of cholesterol per serving. Synonyms for *low* include *little, few,* and *low source of.*

In addition, serving sizes listed on food labels are standardized to make nutritional comparisons of similar products easier.

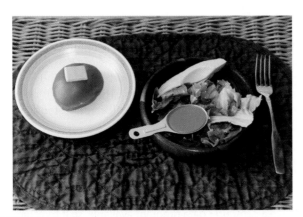

FIGURE 3-7 One teaspoon of margarine, one tablespoon of regular French dressing, and ⅛ of an avocado are each equal to one fat exchange and contain about 5 grams of fat.

Plant Stanols and Sterols

Foods that contain plant stanols and sterols have been shown to reduce blood cholesterol levels (USDA, 2000). Plant sterols and stanols work by blocking dietary cholesterol's entrance into the body. Foods that contain plant stanols and sterols include certain margarine spreads and salad dressings. Benecol®, Take Control®, and Smart Balance® are brand names currently available in grocery stores. Minute Maid Premium Heart Wise® orange juice was the first orange juice to contain plant sterols.

Keystones

- The group name for all fats is *lipids*.
- Hydrogen, oxygen, and carbon are the primary elements in fats.
- Gram for gram, fats contain more than twice the kilocalories of carbohydrates.
- Fats are labeled according to the amount and type of fatty acids they contain as saturated, unsaturated, monounsaturated, polyunsaturated, and *trans*-fatty acids.
- Fats serve many important functions in our diets and our bodies.
- A balanced intake of carbohydrate and fat is essential for optimal health. Excess fats in our diets are associated with cardiovascular disease, obesity, diabetes, and some types of cancer.
- Cholesterol is a fatlike substance that is present in animal food sources and produced by the human body.
- Many Americans would benefit from decreasing their intake of cholesterol, *trans*-fatty acids, and saturated fat.
- The National Academies of Science on Dietary Reference Intakes for Macronutrients recommends that adults consume between 20% and 35% of their kilocalories from fat (Food and Nutrition Board, 2005).
- *Dietary Guidelines for Americans* recommends a saturated fat intake of less than 10% of kilocalories and dietary cholesterol intake of less than 300 milligrams per day.
- The ADA exchanges that contain fat are the milk, meat, and fat lists.

CASE STUDY *3-1*

Mr. D had a physical examination by his family physician, who also treated the client's brother and his father. His father had died of a stroke, and his 35-year-old brother recently had a myocardial infarction (heart attack). The physician noted several xanthomas (fat build up under the skin) around his eyes. His height was 5 feet 6 inches, and his weight was 180 lb. The client reported consuming frequent or large portions of high-fat foods. The client agreed to speak with the student nurse directly after the appointment. The student is doing a practicum in the doctor's office. The registered nurse supervising the student nurse (Mike) requested that he do the following:

1. Schedule the client for follow-up with the physician.
2. Develop a nursing care plan that addresses the client's nursing problem to complement the medical diagnosis.

Because the student was assigned only one client, he had the time to complete his assigned tasks in greater detail than a nurse normally would. The student did not have a computer data program available, so it took him several hours to complete this assignment.

CASE STUDY *(Continued)*

Mike, the student nurse, scheduled the follow-up appointment with the physician for 2 days later (just before the client was leaving for a cruise). Mr. D was instructed by the student to write down all food he consumed for 1 day before the appointment. The client was advised to choose a typical day to record his food intake to provide a more accurate analysis of his usual diet.

Two Days Later

Mr. D arrived on the appropriate day and handed his food record to the student for review. Mike calculated the grams of fat in Mr. D's food record based on a combination of ADA exchanges and a table of food composition. Mr. D's food record and Mike's calculations follow.

The physician has just seen the client at his follow-up appointment and reviewed Mr. D's food record and Mike's calculations. Mr. D's total cholesterol was 350 mg/dL (normal for laboratory test is <200 mg/dL). His low-density lipoprotein (LDL) cholesterol was elevated to 150 mg/dL (normal for laboratory test is <100 mg/dL).

Mr. D told the doctor "I cannot understand why my cholesterol is elevated. My weight is stable. I always select the salad bar for lunch, avoid sweets, and drink low-fat milk." The client agreed to meet with the dietitian after his cruise.

11:00 AM	
Food	Grams of Fat
Salad Bar	
Assorted vegetables and lettuce	0
4 tbsp blue cheese dressing (cup)	20 (4 fats)
4 oz shredded cheese	32 (4 high-fat meat)
1 oz diced ham	3 (1 lean meat)
1 cup potato salad	14*
Dinner roll	0
4 tsp butter	20 (4 fat)
1 cup clam chowder	7*

7:00 PM Restaurant	
Food	Grams of Fat
4 oz hamburger, checked weight	20 (4 medium-fat meats)
2 oz cheese	16 (2 high-fat meat)
2 tbsp mayo	30 (6 fats)
Bun	0
6 onion rings	15*
Tossed salad	0
4 tbsp blue cheese dressing	20 (4 fats)

11:00 PM Home	
Food	Grams of Fat
1 cup 2% milk	5
1 orange	0
Total fat for the day	202 g of fat

*Values obtained from a table of food composition.

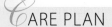ARE PLAN

Subjective Data

Admitted knowledge deficit. Food record for 1 day contained 202 grams of fat.

Objective Data

Cholesterol level: 350 mg/dL and LDL level was 150; height: 5 ft, 6 in.; weight: 160 lb

Analysis

Client's dietary intake of cholesterol is related to elevated blood cholesterol levels.

(Continued on the following page)

Plan

DESIRED OUTCOMES EVALUATION CRITERIA	ACTIONS/INTERVENTIONS	RATIONALE
Client will keep a food record for 1 day.	Instruct the client on the recording of his food intake.	Keeping food records will remind the client of the importance of decreasing his or her fat intake. Reviewing them with the client permits positive reinforcement and correction of misperceptions.
Client will decrease his fat intake by 50%.	Encourage client to first cut the major sources of fat in his diet: salad dressings and cheese.	50% of client's fat intake is from cheese, mayo, and salad dressings.
Encourage the client to meet with the dietitian after his cruise.	Offer the client a referral to the dietitian so that his estimated nutritional needs can be calculated and receive tips on long-term compliance.	A student nurse cannot be expected to follow client long term.
	Tell the client to call the nurse if he is having trouble interpreting dietary instructions at home.	Offers the client support between visits.

3-1

Dietitian's Note

The following dietitian's notes are representative of the type of documentation found in the narrative portion of a client's medical record.

Six Weeks Later

Subjective: Met with the client and his significant other. Although the client has made a recent change to substitute fat-free mayo and salad dressings for regular dressings, he was not able to give up cheese. Admits to sedentary lifestyle. The 24-hour dietary recall cross-checked with a food frequency showed a three-meal-per-day pattern with a salad for lunch and the evening meal in a restaurant.

Objective: Most recent cholesterol was 330 mg/dL, and LDL was 142 mg/dL. Height: 5 ft 6 in.; weight 158 lb.

Analysis: Ideal body weight at 106 lb for the first 5 ft and 6 lb for each additional inch = 128–156. Estimated caloric need at 10 to 11 kilocalories/lb at 156 lb (maximum body weight) = 1560 to 1760 kilocalories. Maximum recommended kilocalories from fat at 35% of total kilocalories = 546 to 616 kilocalories and 60 to 68 grams. Clients estimated fat intake from 24-hour recall and food frequency showed an intake of 110 to 115 grams of fat.

Excessive fat intake as evidenced by food- and nutrition-related knowledge and elevated cholesterol (330) and LDL (142) and reported food intake.

Plan

1. Encourage client to attend group class "Healthy Heart."
2. Monitor weight and blood lipid levels.
3. Recommend the client substitute nonfat cheese for regular cheese and consider packing his lunch.
4. Encourage the client to record his food intake 3 days per week.
5. Congratulate the client on his recent weight loss and the slight drop in his blood lipid levels.

Critical Thinking Questions

1. Do you think this client will respond to diet therapy? What would you do if after 3 months a client's food diary shows greatly reduced dietary fat but his or her cholesterol has not dropped? The physician would probably decide to prescribe medication to lower the cholesterol. How would you explain this therapy to the client?

2. What would you do if, at the following visit, the food diary shows that the client has returned to his former eating habits, thinking fat consumption no longer matters because he is taking medication?

Chapter Review

1. Monoglycerides and diglycerides are names of lipids commonly seen:
   a. In clients' medical records
   b. On laboratory reports
   c. On food labels
   d. On clients' skin

2. Cholesterol is found:
   a. Only in saturated fats
   b. Only in foods of animal origin
   c. Mostly in eggs
   d. Only in triglycerides

3. Saturated fats are:
   a. Liquid at room temperature
   b. More likely to become rancid than other types of fats
   c. Primarily of animal origin
   d. Composed of many double carbon bonds

4. According to most health authorities, the average American would benefit by increasing his or her intake of which of the following fats while decreasing intake of other fats?
   a. Corn oil
   b. Olive oil
   c. Safflower oil
   d. Lard

5. One ounce of very lean meat contains 1 gram of fat and 35 kilocalories. What percentage of kilocalories comes from fat?
   a. 9
   b. 20
   c. 26
   d. 49

Clinical Analysis

1. Mrs. S, 50 years old, has a cholesterol level of 233 mg/dL. She weighs 125 lb and is 5 ft, 5 in. tall. The dietitian has estimated her body fat content to be 35%. When taking a nursing history, the nurse asks Mrs. S if she eats any foods that may be related to her elevated cholesterol level. Which of the following groups of foods are most related to an elevated cholesterol level?
   a. Vegetable oils such as corn, cottonseed, and soybean
   b. Fruits and vegetables
   c. Starches such as bread, potatoes, rice, and pasta
   d. Animal fats such as butter, meats, lard, and bacon

2. Mr. B buys as many low-fat foods as possible. He eats fat-free muffins for breakfast, eats low-fat brownies or cookies for lunch each day, uses only fat-free ice cream, and buys fat-free salad dressings. He eats little meat and chooses fat-free dairy products. He wonders why he hasn't lost more weight. The best advice is to encourage him to:
   a. Consider the amount of soda and sugar he consumes
   b. Eat even less meat
   c. Consume fewer dairy products
   d. Quit trying to lose weight

Clinical Analysis—cont'd

3. When Mrs. L describes her regular intake of foods, you observe that her diet is especially low in monounsaturated fats. Which of the following oils would you recommend be used in place of corn oil to increase her intake of monounsaturated fats?
   a. Sunflower seed
   b. Soybean
   c. Olive
   d. Cottonseed

4

Protein

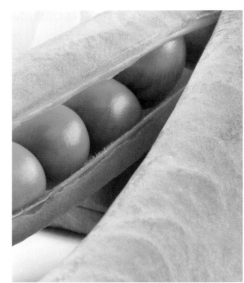

LEARNING OBJECTIVES

After completing this chapter, the student should be able to:

■ Distinguish protein from the other energy nutrients.

■ Contrast essential and nonessential amino acids.

■ Define and give two examples of conditionally essential amino acids.

■ Relate nitrogen balance to conditions in which anabolism or catabolism predominate.

■ Describe causes and symptoms of two types of protein energy malnutrition.

■ Explain the difference between complete and incomplete proteins and give examples of food sources of each.

■ List the grams of protein in each exchange list generally containing protein.

■ Identify two serious genetic conditions caused by metabolic malfunctions affecting nutrition.

■ Describe two ways in which protein is essential to circulation.

■ Explain the principle of complementation and its application to meal planning.

Along with carbohydrate and fat, protein is an energy nutrient, but in many ways, it is paramount. Even the term *protein,* which is derived from the Greek *proteos,* means primary or taking first place. Protein makes unique contributions to the body's health that cannot be duplicated by carbohydrate or fat. This chapter covers the functions, composition, and dietary sources of protein, plus clinical implications of dysfunctional protein metabolism.

Protein can also be used as an auxiliary source of energy if kilocaloric intake is inadequate. As is true of carbohydrates and fats, protein eaten in excess can contribute to body fat stores.

Proteins are the building blocks of the body's tissues and organs. Skeletal muscle contains 40% of the body's protein, its organs 25%, and more than half the solid content of the body's cells is protein (Gropper and Smith, 2013). It is second only to water in amounts present in the body. Descriptions of

some of the tissues composed of protein appear in Box 4-1.

Composition of Proteins

To understand the functions of protein in the body, it is necessary first to comprehend their basic structure: their chemical **elements** and the arrangement of those elements.

Proteins are composed of four elements:

1. Carbon
2. Hydrogen
3. Oxygen
4. Nitrogen

These elements are arranged in building blocks called amino acids. Nitrogen is the element that distinguishes

---

Box 4-1 ■ *Examples of Proteins in the Human Body*

People need a steady intake of protein for normal body maintenance because most cells require periodic replacement. Even
bone tissue undergoes change and renewal in healthy adults.
However, the body cannot effectively repair tooth enamel
destroyed by decay, hence the need for dental restoration, or fill-
ings. When a person is growing or has diseased or injured
tissue to repair, the need for protein is even greater than usual.

Scar Tissue

Wound healing requires proteins. Many blood-clotting factors,
such as the protein prothrombin, form a blood clot. The fibrin
threads that form the mesh to hold the scar tissue in place are
composed of protein. Wound-healing requires much energy
that is usually released from body energy stores and protein reserves, a major challenge for undernourished and malnourished
clients (Wild, Rahbarnia, Kellner, et al., 2010). In hip-fracture
clients, delayed wound healing was predicted preoperatively
by total white blood counts and the Geriatric Mini Nutrition

Assessment tool shown in Chapter 12 (Guo, Yang, Qian, et al.,
2010).

Hair

Hair cells are dead. Hence, haircuts are not painful. The new growth
of hair does require protein building blocks, however. One sign of
malnutrition is hair that can be easily and painlessly plucked.

Blood Albumin

Albumin is a transport protein that carries nutrients or elements. In
addition to carrying substances to body cells, albumin has functions
relating to water balance (see Chapter 8) and plays a significant role
in medication absorption and metabolism (see Chapter 15).

Hemoglobin

Another transport protein, **hemoglobin,** is the oxygen-carrying
part of the red blood cell. The **globin** part of this molecule is a
simple protein.

---

the structure of proteins from that of carbohydrates
and fats as described in previous chapters. Sometimes
sulfur and other elements also form part of the protein
molecule.

Box 4-2 discusses dire consequences of inadequate
protein intake in remote, poverty-stricken areas of the
word. Neurologic crippling results from inadequate
dietary protein along with incorrect food processing
techniques.

Box 4-2 ■ *Cyanide in Food*

In parts of Africa, a staple of the diet is flour made from bitter
cassava root, a hardy, drought-resistant plant that thrives in poor
soil and produces cyanide as a defense mechanism for itself. If
the roots are not adequately processed and a person's diet is low
in sulfur-containing amino acids (methionine and cysteine) that
the body uses to detoxify the cyanide, a permanent, but not progressive, paralytic disease of the legs called **konzo** can result.

Growing cassava requires little labor but correct processing
is labor-intensive. Common methods to reduce the cyanogenic
glycosides in the roots include soaking, sun drying, heap fermentation, and grating plus roasting (Nzwalo and Cliff, 2011).
A newer method (wetting and drying the flour made from the
roots) reduces its cyanide content by three-to sixfold and is
promulgated by free posters in multiple languages (Bradbury,
Cliff, and Denton, 2011).

Children older than 3 years and women of childbearing age
are most often affected by this terrible consequence of inadequate nutrition, possibly because they process the roots and
may eat the fresh roots. In drought and wartime, cassava may
be the only source of food for poverty-stricken people (Nzwalo
and Cliff, 2011). A broader solution than simply teaching correct
processing methods would foster agricultural development to
increase food security in the chronically affected areas (Cliff,
Muquingue, Nhassico, et al., 2011). Genetically improving cassava to increase its sulfur-containing amino acids is suggested
as a long-term preventive technique (Ngudi, Kuo, Van Montagu,
and Lambein, 2012).

Amino Acids

Amino acids are linked by **peptide bonds** in an exact
order to make a particular protein. A chain of two or
more amino acids joined together by peptide bonds is
called a **polypeptide**. A single protein may consist of a
polypeptide comprising from 50 to thousands of amino
acids. Scientists have estimated that the human body
contains up to 50,000 proteins, of which only about
1000 have been identified. Thus, an enormous variety
of combinations is possible.

Think of the elements as the letters of the alphabet
and amino acids as words. The letters (the elements)
can make countless words (amino acids). Words put
into a certain order make up sentences that have a
specific and unique meaning. In this comparison,
a sentence is a protein. Each protein has a specific and
unique sequence of amino acids. To complete the anal-
ogy of language to anatomy, see Table 4-1.

Animal and vegetable proteins that we eat are dis-
assembled in the digestive process into component
amino acids. Absorption occurs throughout the small

TABLE 4-1 ■ Comparison of Language and Anatomy

COMPONENT OF LANGUAGE	COMPONENT OF ANATOMY
Letters	Elements
Word	Amino acid
Sentence	Protein
Paragraph	Cell
Chapter	Tissue
Book	Organ
Books on a subject	System
Library	Human body

intestine, predominantly the **duodenum** and proximal **jejunum** with essential amino acids being absorbed more rapidly than nonessential ones. Uptake of amino acids by skeletal muscles occurs readily after the ingestion of a protein-containing meal. Between meals or in a fasting situation, muscle tissue releases amino acids for use by other tissues (Gropper and Smith, 2013). Whether from ingested protein or **endogenous** sources, the amino acids are reassembled into human proteins. Precision is necessary to manufacture proteins. A slight genetic error in the construction of a protein, such as occurs in sickle cell disease, can have severe consequences (see Clinical Application 4-1).

Twenty-three amino acids have been identified as important to the body's metabolism. These amino acids are classified as essential, conditionally (or acquired) essential, or nonessential.

Essential Amino Acids

An amino acid is classified as essential if the body is unable to make it in sufficient amounts to meet metabolic needs. All **essential amino acids** must be available in the body simultaneously and in sufficient quantity for the synthesis of body proteins (Figure 4-1). These amino acids may come from recently ingested food or from the body's own cells as they age and are broken down and replaced. Structural proteins and plasma proteins have relatively long lifetimes; enzymes and hormones have shorter lifetimes and higher rates of synthesis. Approximately 340 grams of amino acids enter the free pool each day, but only about 90 grams are derived from the diet (Matthews, 2014).

Inability to metabolize three essential amino acids causes maple syrup urine disease. The disease is so named because of the characteristic odor of urine and sweat, particularly strong in earwax (Fong, 2010). See Genomic Gem 4-1.

A person's physiological state influences the need for essential amino acids. Thus, for infants and young children, 30% of the protein requirement should be constituted of essential amino acids. That figure drops to 20% in later childhood and to 11% in adulthood (Matthews, 2014).

Conditionally (Acquired) Essential Amino Acids

Other amino acids are conditionally essential or can become essential, depending on the biochemical needs of the body and the health of its organs. For example, cysteine and proline are indispensable for premature infants. In **phenylketonuria (PKU**; see Clinical Application 4-2) tyrosine becomes essential

4-1

ℭlinical 𝒜pplication

Sickle Cell Disease

Hemoglobin (Hgb) consists of 146 amino acids combined in a specific order. In the hemoglobin of a person with sickle cell disease, one amino acid, glutamic acid, has been replaced by valine at one specific location on the protein chain. In sickle cell disease, the body has 99.3% of the amino acids in the correct sequence in the red blood cell, but early death can result from the 0.7% error.

Sickle cell disease, with an **autosomal recessive** inheritance pattern (Figure 4-1), is most common among black people but also occurs in Mediterranean people, affecting approximately 1 in 400 African American newborn infants each year in the United States compared with about 1 in 2400 of all newborns (Debaun and Telfair, 2012). To have the disease, an individual has to be **homozygous** for the defective gene affecting an estimated 70,000 to 100,000 people in the United States. Someone who is **heterozygous** is a carrier of the trait, affecting approximately 2 million persons in the United States (Centers for Disease Control, 2010). Since May 1, 2006, all states have required and provided universal newborn screening for sickle cell disease (Benson and Therrell, 2010).

In sickle cell disease the red blood cells (RBCs) have a life span of 10 to 12 days compared with the normal 120 days, leading to chronic **anemia.** In addition, the RBCs become rigid and crescent shaped. These abnormal cells tend to clump together and block small blood vessels in many organs, leading to strokes, acute chest syndrome (a life-threatening, pneumonia-like illness), and pain crises (Figure 4-2).

The only cure for sickle cell disease is a bone marrow or stem cell transplant from a compatible donor. Some autosomal recessive disorders such as sickle cell disease are good candidates for gene therapy because a normal **phenotype** can be restored in diseased cells with only a single normal copy of the mutant gene. Much research is still needed, however, because no randomized or quasi-randomized clinical trials of gene therapy for sickle cell disease were available for evaluation (Olowoyeye and Okwundu, 2010).

Being heterozygous for the sickle cell trait is not completely benign. Of 20 sudden deaths due to medical causes in National Collegiate Athletic Association (NCAA) athletes in 2004 through 2008, 25% were associated with sickle cell trait and all occurred in black Division I football players (Harmon, Drezner, Klossner, and Asif, 2012). Although such association does not prove causality, in 2010, the NCAA began mandatory sickle cell screening for Division I athletes (National Collegiate Athletic Association, 2010).

An association with a tropical disease suggests the sickle cell trait might provide adaptation to the environment. The people at risk for sickle cell trait originated in areas of the world where malaria is (or was) **endemic.** It is thought that carriers of the trait are less likely to have the severe forms of malaria (Centers for Disease Control, 2011).

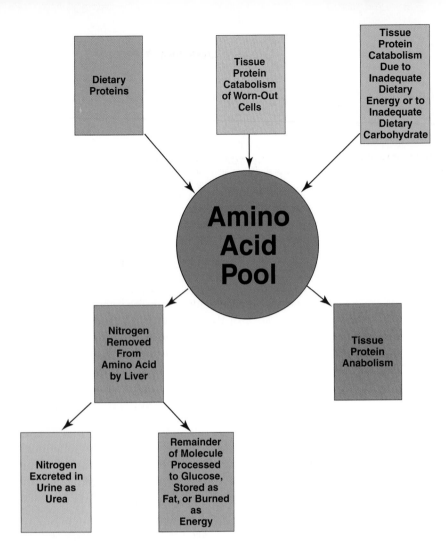

FIGURE 4-1 Anabolism/catabolism of protein. The body obtains amino acids from dietary protein and the catabolism of body tissue, enzymes, and secretions. The body uses amino acids to build new tissue or for immediate or future energy use. Every meal or snack does not have to contain every essential amino acid to permit anabolism. To maximize an adult's health, all essential amino acids should be supplied in adequate amounts by diet daily or at least every 2 to 3 days.

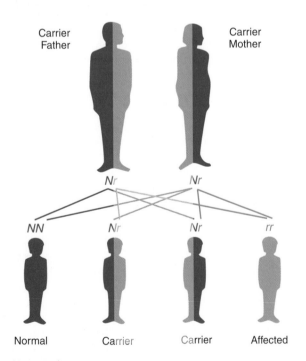

N : normal
r : recessive

FIGURE 4-2 Autosomal recessive inheritance pattern. Be aware that the chance of normal, carrier, or affected child is the same with every pregnancy. Having had one affected child does not mean the offspring of next three pregnancies will be normal or carriers.

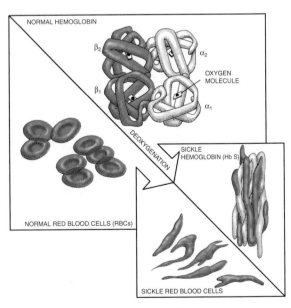

SICKLE CELL ANEMIA

FIGURE 4-3 Normal red blood cells (RBCs) and hemoglobin (Hgb) compared with those in sickle cell anemia. (Reprinted with permission from Venes, D., editor: *Taber's cyclopedic medical dictionary,* 21st ed. FA Davis, Philadelphia, 2009, p. 119.)

Genomic Gem 4–1

Maple Syrup Urine Disease

This disease with an autosomal recessive inheritance pattern (Figure 4-2), caused by defective metabolism of branched chain amino acids, affects 1 in 225,000 persons worldwide but 1 in 150 in the Mennonite population of the United States (Gropper and Smith, 2013).

The most severely affected infants present with overwhelming illness in the first days of life, beginning with vomiting and lethargy, and progressing to seizures, coma, and death within 10 days if untreated. Irreversible brain damage may occur within the first week of life (Elsas and Acosta, 2014). Those with milder forms of the disease because of partial enzyme activity may manifest symptoms only with protein loading or

during stress such as infection or surgery (Elsas and Acosta, 2014; Fong, 2010). Normal development is expected if dietary isoleucine, leucine, and valine are restricted to 20% to 40% of the Recommended Dietary Allowance during infancy (Elsas and Acosta, 2014).

Besides the restriction but not elimination of the branched chain amino acids through medical foods designed for this disease, treatments may include exchange transfusions and peritoneal dialysis. Liver transplantation is an effective long-term treatment for classical maple syrup urine disease and may arrest brain damage, but will not reverse it (Mazariegos, Morton, Sindhi, et al., 2012).

Clinical Application 4–2

Phenylketonuria Essentials

Persons with **phenylketonuria (PKU)** are unable to convert the essential amino acid **phenylalanine** to tyrosine because the enzyme *phenylalanine hydroxylase (PAH)* is lacking or defective. Phenylalanine occurs in all protein foods, including milk. Once feedings start, affected infants are at risk of accumulating high blood levels of phenylalanine and consequent mental retardation. Irreversible brain damage occurs if treatment is not initiated before the second week of life (Elsas and Acosta, 2014).

In the United States, screening tests performed 24 to 48 hours after birth, using a few drops of blood from an infant's heel, are mandated by all states. If a test is done before the infant is 24 hours old, retesting is recommended at 1 to 2 weeks of age to ensure adequate intake of milk to cause a reaction.

DIETARY TREATMENT

Immediate and lifelong avoidance of excess phenylalanine is the principal treatment. Because phenylalanine is an essential amino acid, small amounts of breast milk or infant formula are given to provide just the amounts of phenylalanine the infant needs and can use for growth and metabolism without excessive accumulation. Special phenylalanine-free formulas (the unpalatable taste of which hinders compliance with the regimen) provide the remaining amino acids. In addition, about 8% to 10% of protein prescribed should be as tyrosine because tyrosine supplements alone will not prevent mental retardation in classic PKU. Nonprotein sources of kilocalories such as corn syrup, sugar, and pure fats can satisfy the child's hunger without affecting blood phenylalanine levels (Elsas and Acosta, 2014). Later solid foods may include carefully selected amounts of fruits, vegetables, and low-protein breads and pastas but no high-protein foods (Widaman, 2009).

The artificial sweetener **aspartame** (Equal®, NutraSweet®), which is composed of aspartic acid and phenylalanine, bears a warning label regarding PKU. This disease requires frequent monitoring of growth and blood levels of phenylalanine and tyrosine that should be provided by specialists in the field.

MATERNAL PHENYLKETONURIA

Until the 1980s, dietary restrictions were relaxed as the client grew, so that now pregnant women with PKU may be eating protein foods during the 8 weeks after the woman's last menstrual period—a critical

developmental period for the central nervous system and heart. Consequently, their infants may be born with microcephaly, mental deficiency, and congenital heart disease. Because most of these infants have not inherited PKU but instead were injured in utero by their mothers' high blood levels of phenylalanine, even the rigorous standard treatment for PKU cannot help them. Here, a gene defect in one organism (the mother) can, through interaction with the environment (an unrestricted diet), result in a toxic environment that can have **teratogenic** effects on another organism (the fetus) and effects that mimic those in infants with PKU who receive an unrestricted diet (Widaman, 2009).

Tragically, a case review found 64% of women with PKU are not treated during their pregnancies, resulting in neonatal damage significantly related to mean phenylalanine concentration in each trimester (Prick, Hop, and Duvekot, 2012). A world literature review showed that since 1990, 60 women with previously undiagnosed PKU, most with relatively normal intellectual function, produced 119 offspring, virtually all profoundly damaged (Hanley, 2008). In a recent case, a 33-year-old woman was not diagnosed with PKU until after she delivered an affected infant (Bouchlariotou, Tsikouras, and Maroulis, 2009).

Careful history-taking may reveal a family history of mental retardation or the fact that a woman was on a special diet as a small child and thus may need to have phenylalanine levels tested and PKU treatment resumed at least 3 months before attempting pregnancy (Elsas and Acosta, 2014). Unfortunately, identifying persons with PKU through newborn screening does not guarantee optimal lifetime treatment because of inconsistent third-party payer coverage (Camp, Lloyd-Puryear, and Huntington, 2012).

ADJUNCT THERAPY

A tablet formulation of sapropterin dihydrochloride is approved for therapeutic use in Europe and the Unites States (Trefz and Belanger-Quintana, 2010). It is a synthetic cofactor of phenylalanine hydroxylase that reduces phenylalanine levels in a significant proportion of clients with PKU. Thus, in one clinic, 26.7% of clients with higher baseline phenylalanine levels but 100% of those with lower baseline levels responded to the drug, presumably because of varying amounts of residual enzyme function. Even severely affected middle-aged and older adults showed

(Continued)

4-2

Clinical Application—cont'd

Phenylketonuria Essentials

behavioral and symptom improvement with individualized diet and/or medication therapy. An extremely important outcome for clients with lower baseline phenylalanine levels was a carefully monitored liberalization of their diets (Vernon, Koerner, Johnson, et al., 2010). One woman treated with the drug and diet during pregnancy delivered a normal infant (Koch, Moseley, and Guttler, 2005) whose IQ at age 4 was 132 (Koch, 2008).

Possible future treatments include enzyme substitution with phenylalanine ammonia lyase, which degrades phenylalanine, and gene therapy to restore phenylalanine hydroxylase activity (Blau, van Spronsen, and Levy, 2010). Medical therapies are probably many years away because multiple gene mutations suggest that a "one size fits all" treatment is unlikely (Widaman, 2009). For other information on genetic implications of PKU, see Genomic Gem 4-2.

Genomic Gem 4-2
Phenylketonuria Genetics

An autosomal recessive disorder, PKU occurs most commonly in Whites for whom the incidence is about 1 in 14,000 live births compared with 1 in 132,000 Black infants. As an indication of the complexity of PKU, more than 500 mutations on the phenylalanine hydroxylase gene on chromosome 12 have been identified (Elsas and Acosta, 2014). Molecular genetic testing of the phenylalanine hydroxylase gene is available for prenatal testing and for genetic counseling to determine carrier status of at-risk relatives (Mitchell, Trakadis, and Scriver, 2011).

TABLE 4-2 ■ Essential, Conditionally and/or Acquired Essential, and Nonessential Amino Acids

ESSENTIAL	CONDITIONALLY AND/OR ACQUIRED ESSENTIAL*	NONESSENTIAL
Histidine	Arginine	Alanine
Isoleucine‡	Cysteine*†	Asparagine
Leucine‡§	Glutamine	Aspartic acid
Lysine	Proline	Glutamic acid
Methionine†	Tyrosine	Glycine
Phenylalanine		Serine
Threonine		
Tryptophan		
Valine‡		

*Gropper and Smith, 2013. Classification varies in references.
†Sulfur-containing amino acids.
‡Branched chain amino acids.
§Unique role in muscle protein synthesis (Seyler and Layman, 2012).

because normally it is produced from phenylalanine by the same **enzyme** that is lacking in PKU clients. In addition to tyrosine, cysteine becomes essential in clients with **cirrhosis** of the liver (Gropper and Smith, 2013).

Nonessential Amino Acids

Nonessential amino acids are those that the body ordinarily can build in sufficient quantities to meet its needs. Typically, they are derived from other amino acids. Nonessential amino acids are necessary for good health, but under normal conditions, adults do not have to obtain them from food. Table 4-2 lists the amino acids that have been classified as essential, conditionally and/or acquired essential, and nonessential.

Functions of Proteins in the Body

Protein serves six major functions in the body, as shown in Table 4-3.

TABLE 4-3 ■ Functions of Protein

FUNCTION	EXAMPLE
Provide structure	Muscle mass
Maintain and build cells	Hair growth
Regulate body processes	**Glucagon** (actions opposite those of insulin)
Produce immunity	Antibodies
Substitute as fuel	If adequate carbohydrate and fat are lacking
Maintain blood volume and pressure	**Albumin** draws fluid back into capillaries from interstitial (between the cells) spaces

Provision of Structure

Proteins provide much of the body's mass. Contractile proteins, actin and myosin, are found in skeletal, smooth, and cardiac muscles. Fibrous proteins, such as **collagen,** elastin, and keratin, are found in blood vessels, bone, cartilage, hair, nails, tendons, skin, and teeth.

Maintenance and Growth

Because protein is a part of every cell (half the dry weight), adults as well as growing children require adequate protein intake. As cells of the body wear out, they must be replaced.

Anabolism and Catabolism

Anabolism is the building up of tissues as occurs in growth or healing. **Catabolism** is the breaking down of tissues into simpler substances that the body can reuse or eliminate.

Both processes occur simultaneously in the body. For example, tissue proteins are constantly being broken down into amino acids, which are then reused for building new tissue and repairing old tissue. Anabolism and catabolism, however, are not always in balance; at times, one process may dominate the other.

Nitrogen Balance

Foods or artificial feedings containing protein are the body's only external sources of nitrogen. Nitrogen is excreted in the urine, feces, and sweat; nitrogen is also sometimes lost through bleeding or vomiting. A person is in nitrogen equilibrium or nitrogen balance when the amount of nitrogen taken in equals the amount excreted (Clinical Calculation 4-1). A healthy adult at a stable body weight is usually in nitrogen equilibrium. Under certain circumstances, however, nitrogen balance may be either positive or negative.

POSITIVE NITROGEN BALANCE

A person consuming more nitrogen than he or she excretes is in positive **nitrogen balance.** The body is building more tissue than it is breaking down, a normal state during periods of growth such as infancy, childhood, adolescence, and pregnancy.

NEGATIVE NITROGEN BALANCE

A person consuming less nitrogen than he or she excretes is in negative nitrogen balance. Such a person is receiving insufficient protein and/or the body is breaking down more tissue than it is building. Situations marked by negative nitrogen balance include undernutrition, illness, and trauma. More than half the cases of diarrhea, acute respiratory infection, malaria, and measles in children younger than 5 years of age have undernutrition as the underlying cause (Ramirez-Zea and Caballero, 2014).

Bed Rest

One of the most consistent effects of prolonged bed rest is an increase in nitrogen excretion derived from skeletal muscle. Prolonged bed rest for multiple conditions results in decreased muscle mass, strength, and function predominantly caused by decreased muscle protein synthesis. Providing nutrition support with high-quality protein and encouraging appropriate muscle-loading exercise can reduce these deleterious effects (Evans, 2010). During 4 weeks of bed rest and programmed energy deficit in healthy middle-aged men, administration of 15 grams of essential amino acids pre- or post-resistance training attenuated losses in muscle mass and strength by approximately two-thirds compared with only essential amino acid without resistance training (Benton, Whyte, and Dyal, 2011; Brooks, Cloutier, Cadena, et al., 2008).

Muscle Nutrition

Counteracting muscle loss involves more than providing protein because muscle protein synthesis proceeds intermittently regardless of amino acid supply. Despite ongoing elevated plasma levels of essential amino acids, human muscle protein synthesis returned to basal rates about 2.25 hours after protein intake whether provided intravenously or orally. This suggests that muscle possesses a mechanism to gauge its capacity to synthesize new proteins, a "muscle full" hypothesis in which an upper limit exists beyond which muscle protein synthesis does not occur (Atherton, Etheridge, Watt, et al., 2010).

Research also indicates that the amino acid leucine acts as a key anabolic signal in muscle protein synthesis (Breen and Phillips, 2012) in many cell culture and animal studies. Whether supplemental leucine exerts a unique stimulatory effect, compared with other essential amino acids, on muscle anabolism in humans has not been clearly demonstrated (Pasiakos and McClung, 2011).

In particular situations, attention to individual amino acid intake and timing of protein intake may

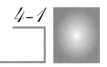

Clinical Calculation 4-1

Nitrogen Balance Studies

To calculate a client's nitrogen balance, the dietitian compares the amount of nitrogen in the foods the client consumes with the amount of nitrogen excreted in the urine. Other potential losses are estimated.

Protein is approximately 16% nitrogen, so the amount of protein consumed (in grams) is multiplied by 0.16. Thus, a person who ingests 50 grams of protein has a nitrogen intake of 8 grams. If he is in nitrogen equilibrium, he would be expected to excrete or lose 8 grams of nitrogen.

Good clinical judgment is required to interpret the results. A client may be in nitrogen balance but in amino acid imbalance (Gropper and Smith, 2013).

be helpful. To optimize muscle health, Seyler and Layman (2012) suggested the following practice: consumption of three daily meals each containing 30 grams of high-quality protein with 2.5 grams of leucine. This is twice the Recommended Dietary Allowance (RDA) for protein and three times the leucine RDA for a 59-kg client (Gropper and Smith, 2013). If each meal includes animal products, it probably contains enough leucine. For instance, 8 ounces of milk *plus* 3 ounces of tuna, pork chop, chicken, *or* beef contain 2.6 grams of leucine. Vegetarians and athletes will need to eat more total protein to obtain adequate leucine (Seyler and Layman, 2012). Such a meal pattern is unusual in the United States but may have value for individuals attempting to build muscle or retard its loss. For additional information, see Chapter 15.

Long-term nutritional intervention studies do not confirm the clinical efficacy of leucine as a pharmaconutrient (van Loon, 2012), but study of supplemental leucine during conditions such as endurance exercise, caloric deprivation, and aging may be warranted (Pasiakos and McClung, 2011). Foods highest in leucine can be found at http://nutritiondata.self.com/foods-000082000000000000000.html

Malnutrition

Clients who receive inadequate food, sometimes for days, because of treatments or diagnostic tests are at risk for malnutrition. An alert health-care provider intervenes in such cases to rearrange meal schedules or obtain food supplements.

Institutionalized clients are susceptible to **protein–energy malnutrition (PEM),** also termed **protein–calorie malnutrition (PCM),** when they are unable to feed themselves. In the developed world, PEM most often accompanies a disease process. **Lean body mass,** chiefly skeletal and visceral (internal organs) muscle, is the critical element that is lost in PEM.

Among the laboratory tests that are used to measure protein status and monitor malnutrition are:

- Albumin—half-life of 14 to 20 days; a low result suggests chronic malnutrition
- Prealbumin—half-life of 12 to 48 hours; reflects recent intake and visceral protein status; useful to monitor effectiveness of therapy (Gropper and Smith, 2013)

Two subtypes of PEM are marasmus and kwashiorkor. **Marasmus** occurs when the victim consumes too few kilocalories and insufficient protein. The person appears to be wasting away. Marasmus is commonly seen in children in developing countries, but it also occurs in debilitating diseases such as cancer or AIDS.

Kwashiorkor classically occurs in a child shortly after weaning from breast milk. The child receives more kilocalories than one with marasmus but not enough protein to support growth. Clinically, he or she may look chubby, especially in the abdominal area, but the cause of this swelling is fluid retention, not fat (Figure 4-4). Kwashiorkor is **endemic** in areas where the staple diet has a low protein to energy ratio. A nutrient-dense supplement is available to some children suffering from malnutrition (Box 4-3), but refeeding must be carefully managed to prevent precipitating a crisis (see refeeding syndrome in Chapter 22).

Clinical Application 4-3 presents a firsthand account of the desperate situation of people in a developing country. Although rare, kwashiorkor also occurs in industrialized nations, not because of lack of food but because of parental ignorance about nutrition. In recent reports, five children developed kwashiorkor after subsisting mainly on a rice beverage with inadequate protein content (Carvalho, Kenney, Carrington, and Hall, 2001; Fourreau, Peretti, Hengy, et al., 2012; Katz, Mahlberg, Honig, and Yan, 2005; Tierney, Sage, and Shwayder, 2010). Kwashiorkor has even been documented in a child abuse fatality case for which the parents were imprisoned (Piercecchi-Marti, Louis-Borrione, Bartoli, et al., 2006).

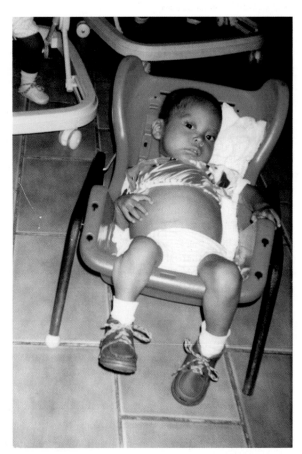

FIGURE 4-4 A child with kwashiorkor at the Nutrition Rehabilitation Center in San Carlos, Bolivia.

Box 4-3 ■ *The Plumpy'nut Saga*

Acute malnutrition affects an estimated 20 million children worldwide. Enter Plumpy'nut, a therapeutic food made with dried, high-energy milk, peanuts, sugar, and oil, successfully used to treat acutely malnourished children at home. Distributed in 500 kilocalorie foil packets, tasting like the filling of Reese's Peanut Butter cups, it does not require **potable water** or refrigeration. Children receiving the product can recover from near death to relative health in a month. Compared with inpatient tube feeding, the standard practice in which 20% to 60% of children die, treatment of 60,000 children with Plumpy'nut in Niger cut the mortality rate to 3%.

The manufacturing and distribution of Plumpy'nut have been embroiled in multinational legal, ethical, and financial arguments:

■ A French company, Nutriset, registered Plumpy'nut as a trademark and holds the patent on the product until 2017. In 2009, its French factory supplied 90% of UNICEF's purchases of the product.

■ One nonprofit company, Edesia, manufactures Plumpy'nut under license in Rhode Island to comply with domestic sourcing regulations for U.S. government aid.

■ India restricted importation of the product, calling it an unproven colonialist import.

■ Haitian manufacturers have ignored the patent to produce similar products.

Plumpy'nut is not free to humanitarian aid groups. It costs about $50 per child for a 6-week supply. In 2011, Nutriset and partner's sales exceeded $100 million. UNICEF planned to purchase 32,000 metric tons of Plumpy'nut in 2013.

Nutriset has aggressively defended its patent in developed countries while licensing producers in developing countries with the philosophy of helping local people. In countries without local sources of peanuts, other legumes are substituted. For example, in Pakistan, the paste is made from chickpeas. A 2012 Google search for the Plumpy'nut recipe returned 14 entries, some of which had no peanut butter or paste and contained oatmeal and dried fruits.

Adapted from Rice, 2010; Wells, 2012.

4-3

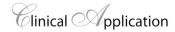

Clinical Application

A Letter From Valle de Sacta, Bolivia

By Constance O'Connor BSN, RN

Your letter arrived January 17th, the first mail since a week before Christmas. Mail here is an event... no TV, no newspapers. Shortwave BBC is about it for input. Much of what I do is aimed at keeping us healthy, such as ironing all line-dried clothes to get rid of any tiny insects or larvae. All fruits and vegetables are washed in chlorine bleach solution before use. Water we consume is either bottled or boiled for 20 minutes.

The people here are very poor, most living out in the bush, clearing land to grow bananas, pineapples, oranges, lemons, and coca. They usually construct a two-story hut on stilts so they can get out of the water with the rains. There are half-walls, if any, no screens, no toilets, rarely a well. It is a hard life. Few people survive past 55 and many children die at birth or in the first year.

Statistics are hard to obtain, as reporting even of births and deaths is minimal. A study done in our area in 1998 found 38.9% of children younger than 5 years of age suffered from chronic malnutrition, and 0.6% from acute malnutrition.

One acute case we saw, an 18-month-old boy, was so jaundiced and had such swelling in his lower extremities, we thought he had a kidney or liver problem. We did get care for him and learned the doctors here call that edema "the edema of hunger." These parents were motivated to get treatment as their first child died at 18 months with the same symptoms. When we visited a center for disnutrition about 50 miles from us, we learned that of the 54 children there, all younger than 3 years old, 21 had kwashiorkor.

Today I am taking a 3-year-old child to a malnutrition center about a 3-hour drive from us, hoping that it is not too late to save her life. The parents refused care for her up to this point though our pueblo elders, neighbors, and other family members pleaded with them. She has protein-energy malnutrition with kwashiorkor syndrome.

We personally pay for the children we send to these centers. Obviously, if the parents had money their children would not be starving. Most poor parents just accept that the children will die. They will dress them in their nicest clothes, hold them almost constantly during this dying process, and bury them soon after death. No funeral, no coffin.

Malnutrition is a factor in many of the measles, pneumonia, shigellosis, staphylococcal disease, and of course, tuberculosis cases Jim and I care for here. On our first Christmas here we were in the middle of a yellow fever outbreak. I have had to cope with children dying from malnutrition, dehydration, infections that did not get treated in time. I think I will always see their faces.

I hope to see you in March when I'm home begging for medicines and supplies. Many thanks for your letters.

Regulation of Body Processes

Protein contributes to the regulation of body processes. Hormones and enzymes are prime examples. Table 4-4 lists some of these regulators and gives examples of each. Nucleoproteins, also containing protein, are essential to normal body functioning.

Hormones

Hormones are chemicals secreted by various organs to regulate body processes. Hormones are secreted directly into the bloodstream rather than into a duct or an organ. **Insulin** and **glucagon** are two important hormones that help control glucose metabolism. Growth

TABLE 4-4 ■ Examples of Regulators of Body Processes			
REGULATOR	EXAMPLES	SOURCE	ACTION
Hormones	Growth hormone	Anterior pituitary	Increases transport of amino acids into cells
Increases rate of protein synthesis
	Glucagon	Pancreas	Raises blood glucose by stimulating its release from liver glycogen
	Insulin	Pancreas	Lowers blood glucose by increasing its uptake by cells
Enzymes	Lipase	Pancreas	Breaks down emulsified fats into fatty acids and glycerol
	Peptidase	Small intestine	Splits polypeptides into amino acids
	Sucrase	Small intestine	Splits sucrose into glucose and fructose

hormone regulates cell division and protein synthesis. The hormone **melatonin** that influences sleep–wake cycles is produced in the brain from the amino acid tryptophan.

Enzymes

Enzymes are crucial to many body processes, such as digestion. The breakdown of foods in the stomach and small intestine involves enzymes, which act as **catalysts** (chemicals that influence the speed at which a chemical reaction takes place but do not actually enter into the reaction). Chapter 9 details the enzymes listed in Table 4-4. Without the aid of enzymes, many of the processes in the body would proceed too slowly to be effective.

An enzyme provides a place (its surface) for two substances to meet and react with each other. The new substance is then released, and the enzyme catalyzes a new reaction. If it were not for enzymes, the two substances would be less likely to encounter one another, and basic body functioning would be impossible. The lack of an effective enzyme can have devastating effects on health as was shown in Clinical Application 4-2 about phenylketonuria.

Nucleoproteins

Nucleoproteins are regulatory complexes that include proteins. These complexes are located in the cell nucleus, where they direct the maintenance and reproduction of the cell. **Deoxyribonucleic acid (DNA)** and **ribonucleic acid (RNA)** are nucleoproteins that control the protein synthesis in the cell.

A **gene** is a part of the DNA that carries the code to direct the synthesis of a single protein. The kinds of proteins the cell makes vary with the nature of the cell—for example, whether an intestinal or skin cell or an ovum or sperm cell.

Immunity

A protein called an **antibody** is produced in the body in response to the presence of a foreign substance or a substance that the body senses to be foreign. Antibodies provide **immunity** to certain diseases and other toxic conditions. A specific antibody is created for each foreign substance.

If a person is exposed to a certain kind of disease-producing organism, the body designs an antibody that neutralizes the harmful effects of only that particular species or strain of organism. For some diseases, once the body has produced many copies of a given antibody, it can respond quickly to another attack, making the individual immune to that disease.

Circulation

The main protein in blood is albumin. It helps to maintain blood volume by drawing fluid back into the veins from body tissues. Thus, it plays a major role in maintaining blood pressure. In addition, some proteins aid in maintaining the body's acid–base balance. This buffering action is described in Chapter 8.

Some proteins in cell membranes carry nutrients into and out of cells. Proteins also attach to fats to become **lipoproteins** for moving lipids in the bloodstream. Drugs bind with albumin in the bloodstream. The term *protein-bound* refers to the portion of a drug dose that is inactive because it is attached to albumin. Chapter 15 elaborates on this process and its implications.

Energy Source

Glucose is the most efficiently used source of energy, but fat and protein can be adapted as backup sources. Most other body systems use fat for energy more readily than the nervous system does. The brain comprises just 2% of the body's weight but consumes 20% of its energy without any storage capability (Matthews, 2014). When the body has insufficient glucose available for nervous system energy needs (as in a carbohydrate dietary deficit of longer than 12 hours for instance, in an overnight fast), the body will utilize body protein tissue to meet the energy needs of the brain and spinal cord.

Thus, adequate carbohydrate intake is necessary to:

1. Spare protein for its unique contribution to tissue building
2. Avoid the undesirable consequences—**ketosis** and muscle loss—of obtaining energy from the less efficient sources: fat and protein

Once liver glycogen stores are depleted, less than 24 hours into a fast, the glucose needs of the brain are derived by **gluconeogenesis** by sacrificing amino acids from protein. Without a change in the process, the use of the body's protein for glucose production would cause death within days. Fortunately with a week of the onset of starvation, the muscles use free fatty acids and the brain uses ketone bodies for energy (Matthews, 2014).

The amount of energy obtained from a gram of protein is the same as the amount obtained from a gram of carbohydrate: 4 kilocalories. Loss of more than about 30% of body protein is likely to be fatal due to reduced muscle strength for breathing, impaired immune function, and decreased organ function (Matthews, 2014). Total starvation is fatal in 8 to 12 weeks. Thus, certain symptoms of protein energy malnutrition do not have time to develop (Morley, 2012).

Classification of Food Protein

Few foods are composed solely of protein. The white of an egg comes close, with 92% of its kilocalories derived from protein. Most foods contain various combinations of protein, fat, and carbohydrates. Some foods, however, are better sources of protein than others.

Protein foods are classified by the number and kinds of amino acids they contain:

- **Complete proteins** are foods that supply all nine essential amino acids in sufficient quantity to maintain tissue and support growth.
- **Incomplete proteins** lack one or more of the essential amino acids.

Complete Protein

With few exceptions, single foods containing complete protein come from animal sources such as meat, poultry, fish, eggs, milk, and cheese. Based on the absorption of amino acids, animal protein foods are 90% to 99% digestible. Of the dairy group, butter contains no protein; sour cream and cream cheese only 1 gram per serving. Although gelatin is an animal product, it is an incomplete protein because it lacks the essential amino acid tryptophan. Soybeans are one plant source of complete protein that is

processed into several products. Compared with milk protein at 100, soybean's protein digestibility corrected amino acid score is 94 (Gropper and Smith, 2013).

Meat and most milk products are both good sources of complete protein. An adult requiring 2000 kilocalories per day following MyPlate guidelines would consume the equivalent of 5 to 6½ ounces from the meat group and three cups of milk daily. Dollars & Sense 4-1 illustrates a means to stretch meat resources and to bolster protein content in sauces with readily available products.

Each meat and meat substitutes exchange contains 7 grams of protein, but the lists are subdivided into lean, medium-fat, high-fat, and plant-based sections. All beef is not high in fat, just as all fish and poultry is not low in fat. Figure 4-5 shows a 3-ounce portion of beef tenderloin equal to three lean meat exchanges providing 21 grams of protein.

Each milk exchange furnishes 8 grams of protein with the lists subdivided into fat free, reduced-fat, and whole milk sections. All of these milk exchanges offer equal protein nutrition but are not nutritionally equivalent because of their varied fat content.

$ Dollars & Sense 4-1
Stretching the Meat Budget

Here is a suggestion to stretch leftover (or planned-over or deli) cooked chicken with a new look. Adding dry powdered milk boosts the protein content of the sauce and can be used in other similar sauces or puddings.

Curried Chicken

If using raw rice, prepare first. Note suggested method in Chapter 7 under arsenic.
Brown rice, 1.5 servings/person
    Prepare as above or substitute quick rice after making sauce
3 tablespoons canola, olive, or peanut oil
1 teaspoon curry powder
    Sauté.
3 tablespoons flour
¼ teaspoon pepper
    Add. Bubble 1 minute. Remove from heat.
2 cups milk
⅓ cup powdered dry milk
    Add. Cook over low heat, stirring until thick.
2 cups (more or less, about 10 oz) cooked diced chicken
    Add. Heat. Serve over rice.
4 tablespoons chopped, slivered, or sliced almonds
    Top each serving.
    4 servings, 34 grams protein each
Total cost, assuming oil, flour, and pepper are available in pantry and a bottle of curry powder had to be purchased and charged to this meal = $9.06 which amounts to $2.27 per serving.

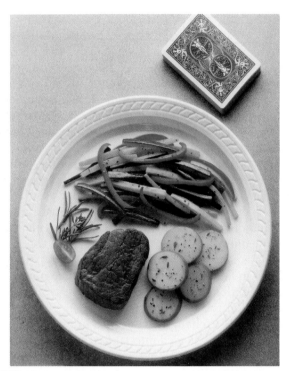

FIGURE 4-5 The 3-oz beef tenderloin pictured equals three lean meat exchanges. A standard deck of playing cards is shown for size comparison. (From the National Live Stock and Meat Board, 444 North Michigan Avenue, Chicago, IL 60611, used with permission.)

Incomplete Protein

Most plant foods that contain protein lack the amounts of one or more essential amino acids necessary to maintain tissue and support growth. Thus, the protein of plants is called incomplete, but the term *incomplete* does not mean these foods are undesirable. Different types of plant foods can be combined to provide all the essential amino acids. Grains, vegetables, legumes, nuts, and seeds contain incomplete protein and are 70% to 90% digestible (Gropper and Smith, 2013).

The vegetable, starch, and fat exchanges are sources of incomplete protein.

■ One vegetable exchange usually contains 2 grams of protein.
■ One starch exchange contains 0 to 3 grams of protein.
■ One fat exchange contains 0.3 grams of protein in coconut (almost all saturated fat) and 4.6 grams of protein in roasted pumpkin seeds (American Dietetic Association, 2007).

It is important to note the size of the item; specialty bagels and muffins may be much larger than the referenced item on the exchange list. See Box 4-4 for examples of foods in multiple exchange lists. Table 4-5 lists the protein content of the exchange lists and gives examples of foods in each list.

Box 4-4 ■ *Special Exchanges of Protein-Containing Plant Foods*

Dried beans, peas ($^1/_2$ cup cooked) are counted as 1 lean meat *plus* 1 starch exchange and include

■ Black, garbanzo, pinto, kidney, lima, navy, and white beans
■ Split and black-eyed peas

Nuts appear on the fat exchange lists.

■ One monounsaturated exchange equals 6 almonds or cashews or 10 peanuts, providing 1.4 to 2.4 grams of protein
■ One polyunsaturated exchange equals 4 walnut halves or 1 tablespoon of pumpkin or sunflower seeds providing 1.2 to 4.6 grams of protein.

Peanut butter appears on two exchange lists:

■ Plant-based protein equal to 1 high-fat meat (1 tablespoon) providing 4 grams of protein
■ Monounsaturated fat (1.5 teaspoons) providing 2 grams of protein.

Sources: American Dietetic Association, 2007 and 2008. See the complete Exchange Lists in Appendix B (reprinted with permission of the American Dietetic Association, 2008) or access additional information at www.eatright.org/search.aspx?search=Exchange%20lists.

TABLE 4-5 ■ Grams of Protein per Exchange

EXCHANGE	GRAMS OF PROTEIN	EXAMPLES
Milk	8	
Fat-free		1 cup 1% milk
Reduced fat		1 cup 2% milk
Whole milk		$^1/_2$ cup evaporated whole milk
Meat and Meat Substitutes	7	
Lean		1 oz Canadian bacon
Medium-fat		1 egg
High-fat		1 oz cheddar cheese
Plant-based proteins		$^1/_2$ cup cooked kidney beans
Starch	2.7	1 slice of whole wheat bread
	4.2	2 slices reduced calorie wheat bread
	3.0	$^1/_2$ cup cooked oatmeal
	1.2	$^1/_3$ cup cooked barley
	2.0	$^1/_2$ cup potato mashed with milk
	4.1	$^1/_2$ cup green peas
Nonstarchy Vegetable	2.1	$^1/_2$ cup cooked broccoli
	2.8	$^1/_2$ cup cooked Brussels sprouts
	1.1	1 cup raw carrots

Sources: American Dietetic Association, 2007 and 2008. See the complete Exchange Lists in Appendix B (reprinted with permission of the American Dietetic Association, 2008) or access additional information at www.eatright.org/search.aspx?search=Exchange%20lists.

Limiting Amino Acids and Complementation

Plants are classified as incomplete protein sources because they lack one or more essential amino acids. This undersupplied amino acid is called the **limiting amino** acid. In cereal grains, the limiting amino acid is **lysine;** in legumes, **methionine** and **cysteine** (Gropper and Smith, 2013).

On the basis of animal studies, the principle of **complementation** was promoted, recommending every meal contain a combination of plant foods that provide all the essential amino acids. Later human studies showed that adults are adequately nourished by consuming assorted plant proteins throughout the day. As shown in Figure 4-1 supplying the amino acid pool is a dynamic process, not completely dependent on diet. **Endogenous** protein sources from the digestive tract include shed mucosal cells yielding about 50 grams and enzymes and glycoproteins delivering about 17 grams of protein daily (Gropper and Smith, 2013). Neither is combining of complementary proteins in each meal thought to be necessary for children who eat frequently throughout the day (Amit, 2010).

Vegetable Sources of Protein

For vegetarians or other individuals who limit their intake of animal foods, **legumes** are an important protein source. Legumes are plants having roots containing **nitrogen-fixing bacteria** that lock nitrogen into the plant's structure, thus increasing its nitrogen content.

Commonly consumed legumes are peas, beans, lentils, and peanuts. Not all peas and beans are legumes. Figure 4-6 compares the protein content of peas, beans, and nuts. Many legumes are not only low in fat but also high in fiber. Box 4-4 locates some legumes and nuts in the exchange lists.

Instructions at ChooseMyPlate.gov for people who seldom eat meat, poultry, or fish permit counting some peas and beans as part of the protein group, ¼ cup cooked equaling 1-ounce equivalent of protein. Types of these plant foods containing significant amounts of protein are:

- Beans—black, garbanzo (chickpeas), kidney, lima, pinto, white
- Peas—black-eyed, split
- Lentils (U.S. Department of Agriculture, June 22, 2011)

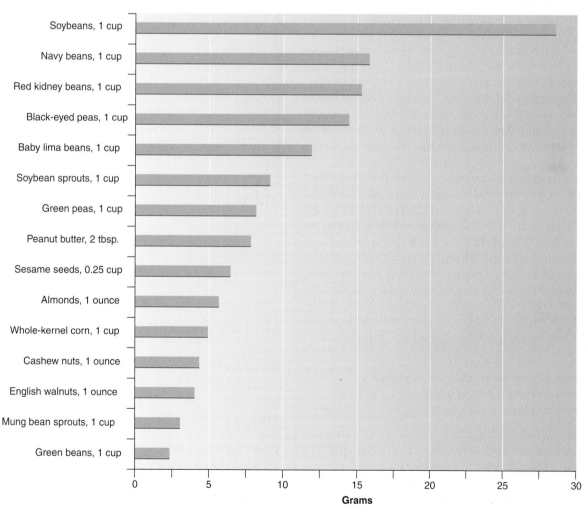

FIGURE 4-6 Protein content of selected plant foods. Notice that all foods named peas or beans are not legumes. Green beans offer just 2 grams of protein, whereas navy beans contain 16 grams.

Also, ½ ounce of nuts or seeds equals 1 ounce equivalent of protein. Examples include:

■ Nuts—12 almonds, 24 pistachios, or 7 walnut halves
■ Seeds—½ ounce of pumpkin, squash, or sunflower, hulled and roasted (U.S. Department of Agriculture, June 4, 2011)

Soy protein is recognized as a high-quality plant protein (Hughes, Ryan, Mukherjea, and Schasteen, 2011) that can be processed into textured soy protein for use as a meat analog or extender. In the United States, such meat alternatives rank third in sales in the soy food marketplace (Katayama and Wilson, 2008).

Vegetarianism

There are many degrees of vegetarianism, depending on the beliefs of the individual or family. Some reasons frequently offered include long-term health benefits, religious convictions, environmental concerns, and economic necessity. Some vegetarians eat fish or poultry occasionally. Clinical Application 4-4 distinguishes various vegetarian diets. The more restrictive the diet, the more care is required to ensure adequate nutrition.

Pregnant women, infants, children, and elderly people who are vegetarians may need special assessment and instruction in the use of fortified foods and supplements. A well-balanced lacto-ovo–vegetarian diet, including eggs and dairy products, can satisfy all nutritional needs of the growing child. In contrast, a vegan diet, excluding all animal food sources, at least has to be supplemented with vitamin B_{12}, with special attention to adequate sources of vitamin D, calcium, zinc, and energy-dense foods containing enough high-quality protein for young children. The more restricted the diet and the younger the child, the greater the risk for deficiencies (Van Winckel, Vande Velde, De Bruyne, and Van Biervliet, 2011).

Embracing a healthful vegetarian lifestyle encompasses more than just eliminating foods derived from animals. It is necessary to find appropriate substitutes for the nutrient-dense animal products. Many traditional regional or ethnic dishes combine a grain with a legume, with each supplying the other's limiting amino acid, for example:

■ A peanut butter and whole wheat bread
■ Baked beans with brown bread
■ A bean burrito

Similarly, eliminating meat does not necessarily decrease fat intake. Vegetable oils and cheeses used in sauces to enhance flavor are high in fat.

Usually hospital or care facility dietitians can provide balanced vegetarian diets. Rather than expect the client to select acceptable items from a general menu, it is better to inform the dietitian of the client's wishes. Dollars

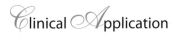

Clinical Application   4-4

Vegetarian Diets

Vegetarians practice different degrees of strictness. From most liberal to most restrictive, the vegetarian diets are ovolactovegetarian, lactovegetarian, ovovegetarian, and strict vegetarian or vegan. The prefixes *ovo-* and *lacto-* mean eggs and milk, respectively. Persons following macrobiotic diets consume unrefined/unprocessed grains; small amounts of fruits, vegetables, and legumes; and sometimes milk products. A fruitarian consumes only raw fruits, nuts, seeds, and berries.

Foods Chosen in the Various Vegetarian Diets

	MEAT, FISH, POULTRY	DAIRY PRODUCTS	EGGS
Ovolactovegetarian	No	Yes	Yes
Lactovegetarian	No	Yes	No
Ovovegetarian	No	No	Yes
Strict vegetarian (vegan)	No	No	No

Nutrients Vegetarians May Need to Obtain From Supplements or Designated Food Sources

NUTRIENT	SITUATION TO CONSIDER SUPPLEMENTATION
Vitamin B_{12}	Individuals consuming few or no animal products; infants of vegan mothers
Vitamin D	Individuals consuming few or no animal products, living in northern latitudes, and those with dark skin or limited sun exposure; vitamin D_2 may be preferred source (see Chapter 6)
Calcium	Individuals not consuming dairy products
Iron	Individuals consuming few or no animal products
Omega-3 fatty acids	Adequate sources of linolenic acid (flaxseed and canola oils, walnuts, and soy) provide the precursor to **DHA** and **EPA** (see Chapter 18)
	Vegetarian sources of DHA from microalgae available

Source: Amit, 2010.

& Sense 4-2 offers an easily made, economical vegetarian main dish using readily available grocery items.

Dietary Reference Intakes

Dietary reference intakes are provided in Appendix A. On the basis of body weight (grams per kilogram of body weight per day), infants synthesize more than twice the whole body protein that adults do. Infants less than 6 months of age are given an Adequate Intake (AI) based on mean intake of healthy full-term breastfed infants because protein deficiencies have not been reported in such infants. Individuals older than 6 months have assigned Recommended Dietary Intakes (RDAs).

The RDAs for protein assume adequate intake of the other energy nutrients to avoid the use of protein for

Dollars & Sense 4-2

Pantry Vegetarian Chili

This suggestion could help to wean an apartment-living college student away from processed prepared foods. Although it specifies dried seasonings to be consistent with the pantry theme, fresh ones could be substituted if available. About 4 times the amount of fresh ingredients should substitute well for dried ones. The chili could be cooked and stirred in a large pot, but the slow cooker is much more convenient.

Pantry Vegetarian Chili

Place all ingredients in 3-quart electric slow cooker. Cook on low about 8 hours.
1 qt unsalted vegetable broth
1 can (15.5 oz) drained reduced sodium black beans
1 can (15.5 oz) drained reduced sodium kidney beans
1 can (15.5 oz) drained reduced sodium pinto beans
1 can (15 oz) drained no added salt whole kernel corn
1 can (14.5 oz) no-added-salt diced tomatoes
2 tablespoons dried onion
3 tablespoons chili powder
1 teaspoon oregano
1 teaspoon coriander or caraway seeds
2 tablespoons sugar or sugar substitute
1 teaspoon garlic powder
¼ teaspoon black pepper
2 tablespoons dark chocolate chips
1 tablespoon dried orange peel
¼ cup corn meal
Makes 12 cups, 7.3 g protein/cup
Six 2-cup servings, 14.6 g protein/serving
Total cost if all the ingredients except sugar and pepper must be purchased = $27.05. Cost per 2 cup serving = $4.51, which is not cheap. The next time the chili is made using the seasonings however, the cost for the broth and vegetables would = $8.15 or $1.36 per 2-cup serving.

energy. The Acceptable Macronutrient Distribution Range (AMDR) of 10% to 35% of kilocalories offers a broad goal for protein intake but severely restricting kilocalorie intake as well as choosing the 10% value as a benchmark for protein energy intake would not be sufficient to maintain nitrogen balance in an adult (Gropper and Smith, 2013). See Appendix A and Clinical Calculation 4-2. Higher intakes may be prescribed for elderly clients and athletes (see Chapters 12 and 15).

Wise Protein Choices

Some protein foods are much less expensive than others. Dollars & Sense 4-3 lists equivalent sources of 10 grams of protein by price. Typical regular prices of nationally advertised brands were used, except for

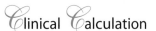 *4-2*

Clinical Calculation

Individualized Protein Requirement

The standard on which the adult RDA is based is 0.8 grams of protein per kilogram of body weight.

$$\frac{\text{Weight in pounds}}{2.2 \text{ lb/kg}} = \text{Weight in kilograms} \times 0.8 = \text{protein RDA in grams}$$

$$\frac{154 \text{ lb}}{2.2} = 70 \text{ kg} \times 0.8 = 56 \text{ grams of protein}$$

 Dollars & Sense 4-3

Comparative Sources of 10 Grams of Protein

Although the prices listed are only a snapshot depending on the day selected for price checking, it is worth noting that tuna has been in the top three of these 10 foods in low cost per gram of protein for 20 years.

Food	Portion	Kcalories	Price/Amount	Cost/10 gram of Protein
1% milk	1¼ cups	128	$2.89/gal	$0.226
Tuna, canned in water	1.4 oz	46	$0.85/5 oz	$0.2380
Large eggs, poached	1.7	133	$1.68/doz	$0.2380
Cottage cheese, 1% low fat	6 tbsp	65	$2.64/24 oz	$0.248
Boneless top round steak, lean only	1.0 oz	59	$4.69/lb	$0.29312
Peanut butter	2.5 tbsp	238	$3.29/16.3 oz	$0.29375
American cheese	1.7 oz	177	$5.98/2 lb	$0.318
Whole wheat bread	2 slices	220	$3.99/24 oz	$0.499
Bean soup, condensed, prepared with water	1¼ cups	213	$1.59/11.5 oz	$0.69
Bologna	2.9 oz	261	$4.79/lb	$0.868

bread, cottage cheese, eggs, milk, and steak. Substituting store brands, buying on sale, and using home-prepared foods lessen the cost.

Whether high-protein diets are detrimental to health is controversial but no Tolerable Upper Intake Level (UL) has been established for protein. Concerns focus on the following:

■ Risk of dehydration because the kidneys must excrete large amounts of nitrogenous waste products

■ Risk to bones from acidity produced by protein metabolism and consequent leeching of minerals from bone to **buffer** the acid if adequate sources of **bicarbonate,** mostly from fruits and vegetables, are unavailable

Dehydration is avoidable with adequate fluid intake. Little evidence supports the hazard of high protein intake in healthy individuals, but kidney damage may be an issue for individuals with existing kidney dysfunction (Tipton, 2011).

Both the **catabolic** effects on bone and **anabolic** effects have been reported, and thus additional research is needed on the long-term effects of a high protein diet on bone health (Gropper and Smith, 2013). Note that the scenario with inadequate sources of bicarbonate described earlier requires an *unbalanced* diet. See Chapter 7 regarding calcium's interfering factors and Chapter 8 on acid–base balance for additional information.

Amino acid supplements are not recommended for the following reasons:

■ Potential imbalanced absorption caused by competition for common carrier systems
■ Nitrogen assimilation from protein-containing foods is superior to that from free amino acids
■ Expense
■ Unpalatability
■ Possible gastrointestinal distress (Gropper and Smith, 2013)

Environmentally and socially conscious consumers may choose to decrease the amounts of animal proteins they ingest to conserve resources. Because meat production requires many pounds of plant protein per pound of meat obtained these consumers believe such plant protein could be better used to feed people directly.

Keystones

■ All three energy nutrients contain carbon, hydrogen, and oxygen, but protein also contains nitrogen and sometimes sulfur and uniquely serves to build and maintain tissue.
■ Essential amino acids must be obtained externally because the body cannot produce a sufficient supply to meet metabolic needs. Nonessential amino acids can usually be manufactured by the body from other amino acids.
■ Conditionally essential amino acids are nonessential amino acids that must be obtained externally because of the condition of the client. Examples are cysteine in the premature infant and tyrosine in a client with phenylketonuria.
■ Someone who is building tissue for growth and obtaining more than sufficient protein for those needs is in positive nitrogen balance. Someone in negative nitrogen balance is not receiving enough protein to replace tissue that is being broken down because of malnutrition or illness.
■ Protein energy malnutrition may involve
   ■ insufficient kilocalories and insufficient protein (marasmus) in which the person displays generalized wasting or
   ■ adequate kilocalories and insufficient protein (kwashiorkor) in which the client may appear chubby because of edema related to deficient albumin levels.
■ Complete protein foods are those that supply all nine essential amino acids in sufficient quantities to maintain tissue and support growth. Animal products except gelatin are complete protein foods. Most plant foods lack one or more essential amino acids but can still be part of a healthy diet. Many soy products are sources of complete protein.
■ Meat exchanges contain 7 grams of protein each, milk 8 grams, starch 0 to 3 grams, and vegetables 2 grams. Legumes are counted as a lean protein and a starch exchange.
■ Two autosomal recessive diseases that have a serious impact on nutrition and life itself because of defective or lacking enzymes are phenylketonuria (PKU), affecting phenylalanine and tyrosine and maple syrup urine disease, affecting the branched chain amino acids isoleucine, leucine, and valine.

Keystones—cont'd

■ The protein globulin is part of the hemoglobin molecule, which transports oxygen in the bloodstream. The major protein in the blood, albumin, aids the return of fluid from the cells and tissues to the bloodstream to maintain blood volume and pressure.

■ The complementation principle relates to balancing the intake of plant foods lacking a particular amino acid with foods providing it but lacking another amino acid. Although not regarded as crucial for people consuming animal foods, complementation may play a role in planning vegetarian diets.

CASE STUDY 4–1

Mrs. F is a 72-year-old widow who eats independently in her family home. Her usual meals are tea and toast for breakfast, canned fruit and a muffin for lunch, and frozen potpie or canned hash for dinner. She complains that she has been having trouble chewing with her old dentures and has not been eating as much food as she usually does. She does not like milk.

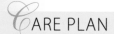 ## CARE PLAN

Subjective Data

Food deficit as evidenced by usual food intake information ■ Has trouble chewing. ■ Does not like milk.

Objective Data

Height: 5 ft 4 in. ■ Weight: 103 lb ■ Loose-fitting dentures

Analysis

Inadequate intake of protein and kilocalories, related to difficulty chewing, as evidenced by stated usual intake of 28 to 32 grams of protein per day and body mass index of 17.73, classified as underweight.

Plan

DESIRED OUTCOMES EVALUATION CRITERIA	ACTIONS/INTERVENTIONS	RATIONALE
Client will gain 1 lb per week during the next 2 weeks.	Encourage easily chewed sources of complete protein: cottage cheese, eggs, ground meat, and fish.	Complete protein foods contain all essential amino acids necessary for tissue building.
Client will increase her total protein intake by 14–18 grams per day by 2-week follow-up.	Create a model meal plan with Mrs. F using the exchange group system to count grams of protein.	Mrs. F's RDA is 46 grams of protein. The meal plan she described in her history contains only 28–32 grams depending on dinner selection.
Client will call for dental appointment within next 2 weeks.	Explore sources of financial assistance for dental care if necessary or refer to social worker.	Better-fitting dentures would permit Mrs. F a wider variety of foods.

When following up after 2 weeks, the nurse finds that Mrs. F has gained one-half pound instead of 2 as set in the desired outcome. She has increased her intake of eggs and cheese on occasion but says she feels full before finishing her meal.

She has not made a dental appointment. Her dentist retired, and she is embarrassed to have to negotiate payment with a new one. The nurse refers the client to the agency social worker.

4-1

Social Worker's Notes

The following Social Worker's Notes are representative of the documentation found in a client's medical record.

Subjective: Client's resources are mainly Social Security payments. She does not have dental insurance.

Objective: Demonstrable ill-fitting dentures.

Analysis: Financial issues preclude private dental care.

Plan: Refer to Family Health Center dental clinic.

Critical Thinking Questions

1. What other food groups or nutrients are lacking in Mrs. F's usual diet? Would you have given any of them a higher priority than protein? Why or why not?

2. Speculate on the reasons Mrs. F has developed her present meal pattern. What additions could you make to the care plan to take those reasons into consideration?

3. If Mrs. F added one egg and one ounce of Swiss cheese per day without changing the other components of her meal plans, to what extent would she have met her protein needs? What additional interventions would you suggest?

Chapter Review

1. For which of the following functions of protein can other nutrients be substituted?
   a. Energy source
   b. Immunity
   c. Maintenance and growth
   d. Regulation of body processes

2. Which of the following foods is a complete protein?
   a. Baked beans
   b. Broccoli
   c. Beef kabobs
   d. Bread sticks

3. If a person has difficulty purchasing meat to serve every day, which of the following foods should the nurse suggest as offering the best source of protein?
   a. Bran muffins with raisins
   b. Red beans and rice
   c. Green bean, onion, and mushroom casserole
   d. Sweet potatoes and cornbread

4. How much protein would a person receive from a glass of milk?
   a. 7 grams
   b. 8 grams
   c. 14 grams
   d. 21 grams

5. Which of the following people would the nurse regard as being in a catabolic state?
   a. Adolescent boy who is into bodybuilding
   b. Lactating mother
   c. Pregnant woman in the second trimester
   d. Surgical client, first day after a stomach resection

Clinical Analysis

Mr. P, a 65-year-old man, widowed for 6 months, has been referred to your home health agency for assistance in managing his nutritional intake. He has lost 10 pounds over the past 6 months. A physical examination within the past month revealed no disease processes requiring treatment.

1. In assessing Mr. P, which of the following data would the nurse gather first?
   a. List of current medications the client takes
   b. Blood protein levels analyzed during the recent physical examination
   c. A description of the procedure Mr. P uses to weigh himself
   d. Dietary recall of Mr. P's food and fluid intake

2. Which of the following plans would be most appropriate to increase Mr. P's protein consumption immediately?
   a. Refer client to nutrition education program.
   b. Have Mr. P apply for home-delivered meals.
   c. Recommend that Mr. P supplement his meals with one of the milk-based liquid breakfast products.
   d. Suggest to Mr. P that he sign up for cooking lessons at the local high school or community college.

3. Which of the following outcomes would indicate achievement of the nutritional objective for Mr. P?
   a. A gain in weight of 2 pounds in 2 weeks
   b. An invitation to the nurse to join him for a dinner he has learned to cook
   c. A report by Mr. P that he is eating better
   d. A visual inspection of Mr. P's refrigerator revealing fresh meat and milk products in abundance.

5

Energy Balance

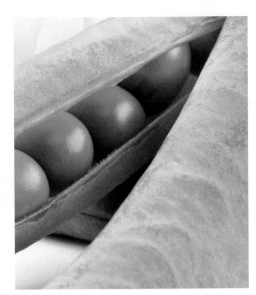

LEARNING OBJECTIVES

After completing this chapter, the student should be able to:

■ Describe energy homeostasis. List two reasons the body needs energy.

■ Describe how energy is measured both in foods and in the human body.

■ Discuss the effect of body composition on energy output.

■ Name the energy nutrient that has the highest kilocalorie density and identify two substances usually found in foods with a low kilocalorie density.

complete understanding of the human body's energy balance system eludes experts. In approximately 40% of the U.S. population, the human body regulates energy intake and expenditure automatically to maintain an **energy balance.** This balance occurs even when the amount of energy needed varies and food intake is erratic. The body can also compensate during food restriction or starvation by conserving energy. Maintenance of a reduced or elevated body weight is associated with compensatory changes in energy expenditure, which oppose the maintenance of a body weight that is different from the usual body weight.

Most experts agree that the human body's energy balance system is the most complex of all the biological systems. This text provides an introduction to this fascinating research.

A basic understanding of what is known about energy balance is necessary for understanding energy imbalance. This chapter therefore focuses on energy balance (Chapter 16 on weight management focuses on energy imbalance), and in particular on the effects of energy intake and expenditure on energy balance. Topics include the following:

■ Energy measurements
■ Factors influencing the body's energy need
■ Energy consumption patterns
■ The kilocaloric content and nutrient density of foods

■ Energy allowances
■ Current recommendations concerning energy consumption

Homeostasis and Survival

The human body seeks homeostasis—that is, equilibrium, or balance. Homeostasis, in terms of energy balance, occurs when the number of kilocalories eaten equals the number used to produce energy. An individual who maintains a stable body weight is usually in energy balance.

However, the human body has developed biological mechanisms allowing it to survive at the cost of maintaining energy balance. Throughout human history, periods of feast or famine were common. The human body developed numerous redundant systems to safeguard against death by starvation. In the event that one metabolic pathway malfunctioned, another evolved to compensate. However, in modern times—when food is often plentiful—these evolutionary survival mechanisms have proved to be a detriment for many people. This disadvantage is evident by the increasing number of people who are overweight or obese. Obesity has nearly double worldwide since 1980 (World Health Organization, 2013).

Energy Intake

The typical adult eats 500,000 to 850,000 kilocalories per year. Eating an excess of only 1% or 15 extra kilocalories per day would result in a weight gain of 1.5 pounds per year—the kilocalories in ⅓ teaspoonful of butter or a quarter of a small apple. Individuals at a stable, healthy weight give little thought to the amount of food that they eat each day, yet their body weight remains constant.

Eating appears to be a voluntary act influenced by the external environment, but it is regulated internally as well. The internal regulation of energy balance involves the gastrointestinal tract, the endocrine system, the brain, and body fat stores. Physiologic regulation is evidenced by the constancy of body weight in adults and the fact that, after weight gain or loss, this constant body weight is reestablished. Over the long term, food energy intake is regulated to balance energy expenditure. See Box 5-1 for a discussion on appetite and hunger.

Energy Expenditure

Energy expenditure, which varies daily, is measured by the number of kilocalories used to meet the body's demand for fuel. A person uses many more kilocalories to run a marathon than to sleep. Physical activity accounts for 25% to 50% of human energy expenditure (Walpole et al., 2012).

Adaptive Thermogenesis

Energy expenditure frequently adapts to large increases or decreases in food intake of several days' duration by means of a process called **adaptive thermogenesis.** Adaptive thermogenesis is one example of how the human body evolved to cope with feast-or-famine conditions. Energy expenditure decreases during food restriction or starvation. Kilocalories are burned more efficiently. Adaptive thermogenesis causes an individual trying to lose weight either to lose at a slower rate or to stop losing weight. As a result, losing weight is difficult for many people but not impossible.

However, overeating for several days will cause an increase in energy expenditure. Energy expenditure has been found to be higher than predicted during the refeeding of previously starved patients, such as in those with eating disorders (Sum, Mayer, and Warren, 2011).

Measuring Energy

Both the energy (fuel) foods contain and the amount of energy the body uses can be measured. The methods used to measure energy are fairly universal.

Units of Measure

The energy content of food is measured in calories and, increasingly, in joules.

A **calorie** is the amount of energy required to raise or lower 1 kilogram of water 1°C. In chemistry, a calorie is the amount of heat required to raise 1 gram of water 1°C. One kilocalorie, as used in the nutritional sciences, contains 1000 times as much energy as 1 calorie used in chemistry. In summary, one calorie is equal to 1000 calories or 1 kilocalorie. Understanding the difference is important. *Kilocalorie (abbreviated kcalorie or kcal)* or *Calorie* are the terms used throughout this text because these terms are used in the medical literature, including patients' medical records. Using kcalories for nutritional measurement eliminates the large numbers that using the chemical term would necessitate.

The **joule** is another unit used to measure energy. One **kilojoule** is the amount of energy required to move a mass of 1 kilogram with an acceleration of 1 meter per second. The kilojoule is equal to 0.239 kilocalorie; a kilocalorie equals 4.184 kilojoules.

Energy Nutrient Values

The energy nutrients are carbohydrates, fat, and protein. Alcohol (ethanol) also yields energy. A food's kcalorie value is determined by its content of protein, fat, carbohydrates, and alcohol.

- 1 gram of carbohydrate equals 4 kilocalories (or 17 kilojoules)
- 1 gram of protein equals 4 kilocalories (or 17 kilojoules)
- 1 gram of fat equals 9 kilocalories (or 37.6 kilojoules)

Box 5-1 ■ *Appetite versus Hunger*

Appetite is different from hunger.

Appetite is a strong desire for food or a pleasant sensation, based on previous experience, that causes one to seek food for taste and enjoyment.

Hunger is a sensation that results from a lack of food, characterized by a dull or acute pain around the lower part of the chest. A truly hungry person will most likely eat anything and take drastic action to acquire food.

Unfortunately, eating is not always the result of hunger. People eat or do not eat in response to stress, time of day, boredom, physical activity, and other reasons. In short, people can override the internal biological signals for eating.

■ 1 gram of alcohol equals 7 kilocalories (or 29.3 kilojoules).

Water, fiber, vitamins, and minerals do not provide kilocalories. Clinical Calculation 5-1 demonstrates how to determine the energy content of a food item.

Determining Energy Values

Energy, whether in foods or the body, is measured as a form of heat.

Foods

The energy content of individual foods is measured by a device called a bomb calorimeter, illustrated in Figure 5-1. A bomb calorimeter is an insulated container that has a chamber in which food is burned. The amount of heat (kcalories) produced by the burning of the food is determined by the change in the temperature of a measured amount of water that surrounds the chamber. All energy in food is in the form of chemical energy. In a bomb calorimeter, the chemical energy stored in the food sample is transformed into heat energy. The following equation may facilitate understanding of this concept:

Protein + oxygen = heat energy + water + carbon dioxide

(Carbohydrate or fat may be substituted for protein in the equation.)

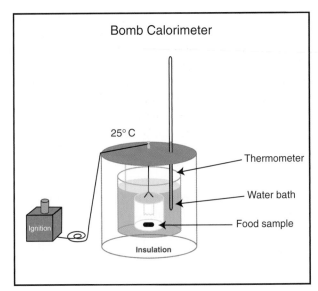

FIGURE 5-1 Illustration of a bomb calorimeter. The food sample is ignited and burned. The heat produced is absorbed by the known volume of water in the surrounding section. Change in temperature provides a measure of the heat produced.

The Human Body

A process similar to the combustion of food in the bomb calorimeter occurs in the body. The amount of energy the human body uses can be measured directly or indirectly.

Direct measurement of energy used by the human body requires expensive equipment that is used only in scientific research. Energy is measured directly by placing a person in an insulated heat-sensitive chamber and measuring the heat emitted by the body.

Indirect measurement of energy (also called indirect calorimetry) is discussed in Clinical Application 5-1.

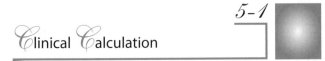

Clinical Calculation   *5–1*

Calculating the Energy Content of a Food Item

If you know the carbohydrate, fat, and protein content of a food item, you can readily calculate the food's kcalorie content. Two examples are shown here. One starch exchange contains 3 grams of protein and 15 grams of carbohydrate. Adding the protein and carbohydrate content in the starch exchange equals 18.

	Carbohydrate (grams)		Protein (grams)		Fat (grams)		Total (grams)
One starch exchange	15	+	3	+	0	=	18

Each gram of carbohydrate and protein has 4 kcal, so to obtain the kcalorie content of the starch exchange, multiply 4 by 18. Thus, one starch exchange has 72 kcal.

One fat exchange contains 5 grams of fat.

	Carbohydrate (grams)		Protein (grams)		Fat (grams)		Total (grams)
One starch exchange	0	+	0	+	5	=	5

A gram of fat has 9 kcal. To obtain the kilocaloric content of one fat exchange, multiply 5 by 9. Thus, one fat exchange contains 45 kcal.

Clinical Application   *5–1*

Measurement of Resting Energy Expenditure by Indirect Calorimetry

The process of measuring resting energy expenditure (REE) with indirect calorimetry is the clinical gold standard of REE measurement (O'Riordan, Metcalf, Perkins, & Wilkin, 2010). Indirect involves measuring oxygen and carbon dioxide concentrations in expired air during a prescribed period of time. The amount of oxygen that is utilized and the amount of carbon dioxide produced is entered into a scientific formula that will calculate energy expenditure. This method can be used with spontaneous breathing or with a mechanically ventilated individual, such as a patient in an intensive care unit.

In clinical practice an estimation of the resting energy expenditure (REE) can be made using formulas such as the Harris-Benedict equation (see Table 5-1). REE is estimated on the basis of the height, weight, age, and sex of the individual. There are separate formulas for men and women. Although developed more than 90 years ago, the Harris-Benedict formula continues to prove as accurate as more recently developed formulas (Kreymann, Adolph, and Mueller, 2009). When only weight is available, the following estimate for REE can be used:

- 20 to 30 year olds: 25 kcalories/kg body weight/day
- 30 to 70 year olds: 22.5 kcalories/kg body weight/day
- >70 years old: 20 kcalories/kg body weight/day (Kreymann et al., 2009).

Components of Energy Expenditure

The human body requires energy to meet its resting energy expenditure needs, satisfy its physical activity requirements, and process nutrients. REE, which includes all involuntary activities, is the kcalories a person burns under controlled conditions and lying comfortably. Voluntary physical activity includes the energy needed for voluntary activities—which are consciously controlled, such as running, walking, and swimming. The third component of energy expenditure is the energy expended to digest, absorb, transport, and utilize nutrients.

Resting Energy Expenditure

REE represents the energy expended or used by a person at rest. In most people, REE requires more total kcalories than physical activity. Clinical Application 5-1 discusses the measurement of REE in clients. The term REE is generally associated with the use of a respirometer or a device that measures oxygen consumption. The kcalories necessary to support the following contribute to resting energy expenditure:

- Contraction of the heart
- Maintenance of body temperature
- Repair of the internal organs

- Maintenance of cellular processes
- Muscle and nerve coordination
- Respiration (breathing)

REE accounts for 60% to 70% of total energy expenditure but varies between individuals (O'Riordan et al., 2010). Body composition influences resting energy expenditure. Individuals of similar age, sex, height, and weight with a higher percentage of muscle (lean body mass) have a higher REE than those with less muscle. It takes more energy, or kcalories, to support lean body mass (protein) than to support body fat. Muscle tissue requires more kcalories than does fat tissue, even when muscle tissue is resting. Therefore, the higher a person's body protein content, the more kcalories he or she can eat and still maintain a stable body weight.

Age

REE varies with lean body mass, which varies with age. The highest rates of energy expenditure per pound of body weight occur during infancy and childhood. In adults, REE declines about 1% to 2% per decade after age 20 because of a decline in lean body mass. The result is a reduced need for kcalories. Individuals can slow the decline in lean body mass somewhat by increasing their exercise. An individual who fails either to decrease kilocaloric intake to compensate for this reduced need or to increase physical activity may experience a slow weight gain.

Sex

Differences in body composition between men and women occur as early as the first few months of life. The differences are relatively small until the child reaches age 10. During adolescence, body composition changes radically. Men develop proportionately greater lean muscle mass than women, who deposit fat as they mature. Consequently, REE differs by as much as 10% between men and women.

Growth

Human growth is most pronounced during the growth spurts that take place before birth and during infancy and puberty. Kcalories required per kilogram of body weight are highest during these growth spurts because the kilocaloric cost of anabolism is greater than the kilocaloric cost of catabolism.

Body Size

People with large bodies require proportionately more energy than smaller ones. A tall individual uses more energy because he or she has a greater skin surface through which heat is lost than does a shorter person.

TABLE 5-1 ■ Harris-Benedict Equation to Calculate REE
To convert weight in pounds to kilograms (kg): 1 kg = 2.2 pounds; divide body weight in pounds by 2.2.
To convert height in inches to centimeters (cm): 1 inch = 2.54 cm; multiple height in inches by 2.54.
■ REE for men: $66.5 + (13.8 \times \text{weight in kg}) + (5 \times \text{height in cm}) - (6.8 \times \text{age in years})$
■ REE for women: $655 + (9.6 \times \text{weight in kg}) + (1.8 \times \text{height in cm}) - (4.7 \times \text{age in years})$

A shorter person also has less muscle tissue or lean body mass than a taller person.

Most health-care professionals are surprised at the large volume of food needed to maintain a tall male's body weight (greater than 6 feet tall) and how small a volume of food is needed to maintain weight in a short female (less than 5 feet tall). In proportion to total body weight, the infant has a large surface area, loses more heat through the skin, and therefore has a proportionately high REE.

Climate

Climate affects REE because kcalories are needed to maintain body temperature. This fact pertains to extreme differences in external temperatures, whether cold or hot. In the United States and Canada, most people do not need to eat more kcalories during colder months because most living environments range from 68°F to 77°F. Outside, people usually protect themselves from extreme cold and shivering, which causes an increase in REE, by wearing warm clothes.

Genetics

REE is strongly influenced by individual genetic patterns; see Genomic Gem 5-1.

Thermic Effect of Food

After a meal, the heat produced by the body is called the **thermic effect of food** (TEF). An older term for this energy cost is specific dynamic action (SDA). Energy is needed to chew, swallow, digest, absorb, and transport nutrients. Metabolism increases after eating. As metabolism increases, more kcalories are used.

The consumption of protein and carbohydrates results in a larger thermic effect than the consumption of fat. Fat is metabolized efficiently as compared with

glucose. Studies are demonstrating that there is greater variability in energy use when smaller molecules, like glucose, are broken down compared to larger molecules of fat (Scott, 2012). If an individual eats as many kcalories from carbohydrate or protein as from fat, he or she will store fewer of the nonfat kcalories as body fat.

Kcalories do count, however, regardless of the source. Consumers need to read food labels carefully. Sometimes a regular version of a food may actually contain fewer kcalories than the fat-free or reduced-fat version. For example, a regular fig cookie contains 50 kcalories, and one fat-free version contains 70 kcalories. One-half cup of regular ice cream contains 180 calories, and the same amount of one kind of reduced-fat ice cream contains 190 kcalories. Sometimes consumers are under the illusion that because the food they are eating is low-fat, they can eat unrestricted amounts and maintain body weight (Dollars and Sense 5-1).

Physical Activity

For most of the world's population, physical activity uses fewer kcalories than those required for resting energy expenditure. Physical activity accounts for 25%-50% of human energy expenditure (Walpole et al, 2012). Very few people are active enough to burn more kcalories as a result of physical activity than as a result of their resting energy expenditures; however, some very active individuals do expend more kcalories as a result of physical activity (Fig. 5-2). For example, professional athletes may burn a large number of kcalories as a result of training and engaging in competition.

As Table 5-2 shows, the intensity and duration of any physical activity enormously influences kcalorie expenditure. For example, a 154-pound man who trains by running vigorously at a speed of 5 miles per hour will expend almost 600 kcalories in a 1-hour training

---

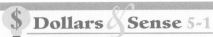

Genomic Gem 5-1
Resting Energy Expenditure

REE is strongly influenced by individual genetic patterns. Each person appears to be programmed with a need to burn a certain number of kcalories to maintain energy balance. This fact becomes apparent to health-care workers when counseling two very similar clients. Both clients may be of the same sex, of equal weight, perform similar types of physical activity, and have about the same body fat content. Yet each client may need to eat a different number of kcalories to maintain a stable body weight. Many individuals have little control over the number of kcalories required to meet the needs of REE.

$ Dollars & Sense 5-1
Kcalorie Control

Kcalorie control = Portion control = Fewer dollars spent at the grocery store.

Here's why: Some nutrients are needed daily because the body is unable to store them. Vitamin C is one example. Orange juice is high in vitamin C and is best consumed in ½ cup serving sizes to meet the daily need for vitamin C. If a food purchaser drinks an entire quart of orange juice daily, he or she will need to buy this item frequently.

Because fruits and fruit juices are becoming increasingly more expensive, think of expensive food items primarily as sources of nutrients to be eaten in recommended serving sizes.

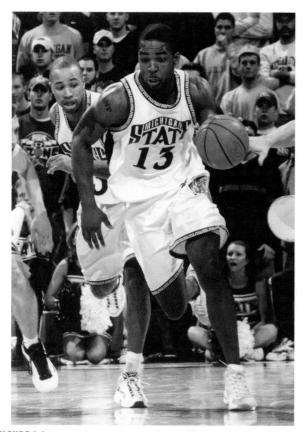

FIGURE 5-2 A trained athlete may burn more kcalories as a result of physical activity than as a result of resting energy expenditure. (Courtesy of Kevin Fowler, Sports Information, Michigan State University.)

session. The energy cost of physical activity is frequently referred to as the thermic effect of exercise (TEE).

Daily fluctuations in physical activity can greatly influence an individual's energy requirements (Table 5-3). For example, a 38 year old man of normal weight may require only 2200 kcalories on a sedentary day and as many as 2800 kcalories on a very active day. A 38 year old woman of normal body weight may require only 1800 kcalories on a sedentary day and as many as 2200 kcalories on a very active day.

The Institute of Medicine of the National Academies (2005) put together a report on Dietary Reference Intakes that describes a method to estimate energy needs that includes both those needed for REE and activity (www.nal.usda.gov/fnic/DRI/DRI_Energy/energy_full_report.pdf). This method to estimate kcaloric need is often used in wellness programs to give clients some idea of their approximate energy need. The most accurate method for determining a client's kcalorie requirement is to monitor both food intake and body weight over time. Sometimes in clinical settings, obtaining weight and food intake information is impossible during a client's assessment. In the critical care chapter, we provide a formula that takes into account age, sex, weight, and height for estimating kcal need.

Thermic Effect of Exercise

Energy expended during exercise is only a portion of the total energy cost of physical activity. Exercise may

TABLE 5-2 ■ Kcalories Expended in 30 Minutes and 1 Hour		
ACTIVITY	**KCALORIES EXPENDED BY A 154-POUND MAN IN 60 MINUTES**	**KCALORIES EXPENDED BY A 154-POUND MAN IN 30 MINUTES**
Moderate Activity		
Walking (3½ miles per hour)	140	280
Light gardening/ yard work	165	330
Golf (walking and carrying clubs	165	330
Dancing	165	330
Vigorous Activity		
Running/jogging (5 miles per hour)	295	590
Cycling (more than 10 miles per hour)	295	590
Walking (4½ miles per hour)	230	510
Swimming (slow freestyle laps)	255	510

SOURCE: United States Department of Agriculture, www.choosemyplate.gov/food-groups/physicalactivity_calories_used_table.html

TABLE 5-3 ■ Energy Needs Based on Age and Activity			
ENERGY NEEDS IN KCALORIES BASED ON ACTIVITY LEVEL			
	Sedentary*	**Moderately Active****	**Active*****
18-year-old males	2000	2400	2800
18-year-old females	1800	2000	2400
19- to 30-year-old males	2400	2600	3000
19- to 30-year-old females	1800	2000	2400
31- to 50-year-old males	2200	2400	2800
31- to 50-year-old females	1800	2000	2200
51+ males	2000	2200	2400
51+ females	1600	1800	2000

Male reference is 5 feet 10 inches tall and weighs 154 pounds and female reference is 5 foot 4 inches tall and weighs 126 pounds.
* Sedentary is defined as lifestyle that includes light activity associated with day-to-day life.
** Moderately active defined as activity that includes walking 1.5 to 3 miles per day at 3 to 4 miles per hour with typical day-to-day light activity.
*** Active defines as lifestyle that includes physical activity that includes walking more than 3 miles per day at 3 to 4 miles per hour, in addition to day-to-day light activity.
SOURCE: Adapted from U.S. Department of Agriculture and U.S. Department of Health and Human Services (2010), www.Dietaryguidelines.gov.

also affect both resting energy expenditure (REE) and the thermic effect of exercise (TEF). Some clients' REE increases for up to 48 hours after exercise. Although the exact reason for this increase is unknown, the most plausible explanation is that glycogen stores need to be refilled. Because exercise depletes glycogen stores, energy is used to provide glycogen stores pre-exercise and to refill these stores during the postexercise periods.

Adaptive Response to Exercise

An individual with well-developed muscles performs more efficiently—uses fewer kcalories to perform a given amount of physical work—than an individual with less well-developed muscles. As exercise is repeated, the body learns how to get the job done with the least effort (the body's adaptive response to exercise). If an individual has a weight loss due to increased exercise, he or she will eventually use fewer kcalories to do a specific activity. This is the reason body builders need to continually increase the amount of weight lifted to achieve maximum results. Lighter people require fewer kcalories for a given amount of exercise than heavier people do; it takes fewer kcalories to move a smaller mass than a larger one.

Although heavier people, who move more weight, burn more kcalories than lighter people when they exercise, a heavy body is a disincentive for movement and physical activity. Heavier people tend to do fewer energy-demanding activities. Studies have indicated that exercise may be difficult for obese patients due to poor exercise tolerance and lack of enjoyment (Dalle-Grave et al., 2011).

Exercise and Appetite

Many exercise researchers think that exercise decreases appetite—that is, a person may be satisfied with less food after exercise. Exercise at a sufficient intensity and duration release a chemical in the brain called beta-endorphin and leads to increased circulating concentrations (Jamurtas et al., 2011). Beta-endorphin has an effect similar to that of natural morphine; it produces a state of relaxation. In effect, exercise can be a safe substitute for overeating in some individuals who eat to decrease stress and tension. However, an individual with a severe eating disorder may exercise compulsively to relax.

Aerobic Exercise

Aerobic exercise is any activity during which the energy metabolism needed is supported by the amount of increase in oxygen inspired. Aerobic exercises increase physical fitness and involve large muscle groups. Vigorous workouts that last at least 30 minutes require an increase in the amount of oxygen inspired. Box 5-2

Box 5-2 ■ *Examples of Aerobic Exercise*

These are some popular forms of aerobic exercise:

Fast walking
Cycling
Swimming
Skating
Jumping rope
Dancing
Hiking
Jogging
Rowing

---

provides examples of aerobic exercise. Aerobic exercise provides many health benefits, including the following:

■ Decreased risk of cardiovascular disease
■ Improved blood sugar control for people with diabetes
■ Decreased risk of obesity
■ Reversal or prevention of varicose veins
■ Decreased risk of osteoporosis
■ Improved quality of sleep
■ Improved hypertension control

Anaerobic Exercise

Exercise during which energy is provided without an increase in the use of inspired oxygen is **anaerobic exercise.** Short bursts of vigorous activity, such as resistance or muscle strength training (e.g., weight lifting), are forms of anaerobic exercise. Anaerobic exercise allows for:

■ Muscle toning
■ The building of muscular strength and endurance
■ Building of bone mass

This kind of training provides added strength and toughness, which help to reduce injury during aerobic exercise, prevents lower back problems, and allows for a more muscular appearance.

Balance and Stretching

Balance and stretching exercises such as yoga, t'ai chi, and martial arts promote:

■ Increased physical stability
■ Increased flexibility
■ Decreased risk of injury

Bone Strengthening

Exercises that place force on the bone, such as jumping rope and running, will promote growth and strength of bone. This form of exercise is recommended to be included in the weekly exercise program of children.

Diet and Activity

A healthy lifestyle depends on much more than diet. Physical activity makes a vital contribution to health, function, and performance. The greatest benefit derived from physical activity is gained when a person moves from sedentary to moderate levels of activity. The combination of a balanced diet and regular physical activity has a stronger effect on energy balance than either strategy alone.

The Centers for Disease Control and Prevention (CDC) and the World Health Organization (2011) currently recommend the following minimum activity guidelines for adults aged 18 to 65 years:

- 150 minutes of moderate-intensity aerobic activity every week and muscle-strengthening activities on 2 or more days a week or;
- 75 minutes of vigorous-intensity aerobic activity every week and muscle-strengthening activities on 2 or more days per week or;
- A combination of moderate- and vigorous-intensity aerobic activities and muscle-strengthening activities on 2 or more days a week. One minute of vigorous-intensity activity is equivalent to about 2 minutes of moderate-intensity activity (CDC, 2011).

For additional health benefits, adults should increase their moderate-intensity aerobic activities to 300 minutes per week or engage in 150 minutes of vigorous-intensity aerobic physical activities per week, or an equivalent combination of moderate- and vigorous-intensity activities. Muscle-strengthening activities should include all major muscle groups—legs, hips, back, abdomen, chest, shoulders, and arms. The activity need not be continuous but may be broken up into short sessions. For example, six brisk 10-minute walks would meet the minimum requirement. A 154-pound man performing this activity for 60 minutes expends 280 total kcalories. In general, the more time a person spends exercising each week will increase the total number of kcalories expended and increase overall health benefits. For complete activity guidelines visit: www.cdc.gov/physicalactivity/everyone/guidelines/index.html.

Energy Intake

Between 2009 and 2010, the mean reported energy intakes for men aged 20 to 59 was 2482 to 2736 kcalories per day averaging 2512 kcalories for men over age 20 years (U.S. Department of Agriculture [USDA], 2012). The mean reported energy intakes for women aged 20 to 59 was between 1759 to 1949 kcalories per day averaging 1778 kcalories for women over age 20 years (USDA, 2012). The average reported intakes for women are of special concern because of the difficulty of incorporating all nutrients at recommended levels in a diet so low in kcalories. The average woman's need to increase energy output or physical activity is well documented.

Many experts attribute increased obesity to decreased energy expenditure. America is becoming an increasingly sedentary society. The current recommendation is that the average person increase physical activity rather than decrease kcalorie intake below their estimated energy requirements (EER) to achieve energy balance. If the average reported intakes for both sexes are compared with the EER, the need for more physical activity in most people becomes clear. For specifics, refer to the dietary reference intakes in Appendix A.

Kilocaloric Density of Foods

Some foods are more kilocalorically dense than other foods. Density is the quantity per unit volume of a substance. **Kilocaloric density** refers to the kcalories contained in a given volume of a food generally, the number of calories in a gram. Foods with a high water and fiber content tend to have a lower kcaloric density. Fruits and vegetables such as lettuce, watermelon, and celery are high in water content and low in kcalories. A given volume of grapes has fewer kcalories than an equal volume of raisins because grapes contain more water than raisins.

Fats or foods high in fat have the highest kcaloric density (see Fig. 5-3). Whole-milk products, high-fat meat exchanges, fat exchanges, and foods made with these ingredients all contain appreciable amounts of fat. Box 5-3 lists several tips for decreasing the kcaloric density of a diet.

Studies have demonstrated that diets with high energy density lead to increased kcalorie consumption

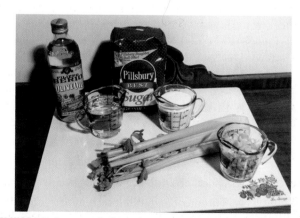

FIGURE 5-3 One cup of celery contains 17 kcalories, 1 cup of sugar contains 770 kcalories, and 1 cup of oil contains 1925 kcalories. Celery is the least kcalorically dense of the foods pictured, and oil is the most dense. Sugar is between celery and oil in kcaloric density.

Box 5-3 ■ *Tips for Decreasing the Kilocaloric Density of a Diet*

- Use low-fat or nonfat dairy products including skim milk, cheese, and yogurt.
- Brown meats by broiling or cooking in nonstick pans with little or no fat. Avoid fried foods.
- Chill soups, stews, sauces, and broths. Lift off and discard hardened fat.
- Add extra vegetables to casseroles, chili, lasagna, or other hot dishes.
- Trim all visible fat from meat before cooking.
- Use water-packed, canned foods such as fruits and tuna.
- Use fresh fruits and vegetables often. Try to eat at least 2½ cups of these foods each day.
- Use low-kcalorie salad dressings.
- When you eat out, do not look at the menu. Instead, have an idea of what you would like to eat before you arrive at the restaurant. Explain to the waitress or waiter what you would like to eat.
- Eat smaller portion sizes of all foods, but particularly sandwiches.
- Limit consumption of sweetened carbonated beverages and other empty kcalorie foods.

and increased risk of obesity and low energy density diets have the opposite effect (Shrapnel, 2010).

Nutrient Density of Foods

Kilocaloric content alone should not be the criterion to decide whether to include a food in one's diet. The nutrient density of a food—the concentration of nutrients in a food compared with the food's kilocaloric content—is also an important consideration. If a food is high in kcalories and low in nutrients, the nutrient density of the food is low. **Empty kcalories** means that the food contains kcalories and almost no nutrients; table sugar is an example of such a food. If a food is low in kcalories and high in nutrients, the nutrient density of the food is high.

Cantaloupe is an example of a food with a high nutrient density—it is low in kcalories and high in vitamin C and contains a moderate amount of vitamin A. Skim milk and whole milk are similar in nutrient content; both types of milk contain about the same amounts of protein, calcium, vitamin D, and riboflavin. Eight ounces of skim milk provides about 90 kcalories compared with 150 kcalories in 8 ounces of whole milk. Skim milk thus has a higher nutrient density than whole milk.

In 2005, the federal government issued the Dietary Reference Intake (DRI) for EER Values for Energy for Active Individuals (see the full report at www.nal.usda.gov/fnic/DRI/DRI_Energy/energy_full_report.pdf). Note that the values for pregnant and lactating women are higher than for nonpregnant and nonlactating women.

Dietary Recommendations

All the major national health organizations recommend that individuals maintain a healthy body weight. The American Heart Association recommends maintaining a healthy body weight to decrease the risk of heart and circulatory diseases. The American Cancer Society cites numerous studies suggesting that lower kilocaloric intake may lower an individual's risk of cancer. Most individuals would benefit by monitoring their weight and increasing their energy expenditure or decreasing their energy intake as necessary to maintain a healthy body weight.

Current guidelines for the distribution of macronutrients and daily caloric intake for adults, aged 19 years old and older, are:

- Carbohydrate 45% to 65%
- Protein 10% to 35%
- Fat 20% to 35%

Keystones

- Energy balance exists when energy intake equals energy output. A person whose body weight remains stable is usually in energy balance.
- A person's appetite can overrule the body's ability to maintain homeostasis.
- A hungry person will most often be willing to eat almost anything.
- When an individual is not in energy balance, he or she is gaining or losing weight.
- The most accurate method for determining kcalorie need is to monitor both food intake and body weight over time.
- Foods high in water and fiber (fruits and vegetables) are low in kilocaloric density.

Keystones—cont'd

- Foods high in fat (fatty meats, oils, spreads, salad dressings, and food made with those ingredients) are high in kilocaloric density.
- Foods that are low in kcalories and contain substantial amounts of one or more nutrients are high in nutrient density.
- The recommended range of energy nutrient intake is:
  - 45% to 65% for carbohydrate
  - 20% to 35% for fat
  - 10% to 35% for protein
- The current recommendation is that individuals who gain weight while consuming their energy EER should increase their activity to maintain energy balance.
- Most Americans are eating too much of one, two, or three of the energy nutrients to maintain energy balance.

CASE STUDY *5-1*

The Fairview Nursing Home holds a weekly client care conference. Nursing care plans for all of the facility's residents are reviewed on a rotating basis, with each client's nursing care plan reviewed once every 3 months. All members of the health-care team are often present at the conference. Team members include the administrator, the physician, the director of nursing, the staff nurse, the nursing assistant, the activities director, the social worker, the dietitian, and the client or a family member representing the client.

Mr. G has been experiencing a slow weight gain. His weight history follows:

2/08	169 lb (77 kg)
6/08	172 lb (78 kg)
9/08	175 lb (80 kg)
12/08	180 lb (82 kg)
03/09	183 lb (83 kg)

Mr. G is 5 ft, 8 in. tall and 79 years old. He is alert, feeds himself, and has normal bowel and bladder function. Mr. G walks to the dining room three times a day. His favorite activity is watching television. He has good dentition and is on a regular diet. According to the appetite records kept by the nurse's aide, Mr. G's intake is good to excellent. He accepts all of the major food groups. He admits to overeating at social activities, especially those sponsored by the facility in the evenings. Mr. G is concerned with his slow weight gain but claims he does not know what to do. To address the slow weight gain problem, the health-care team and Mr. G developed the following nursing care plan.

*C*ARE PLAN

Subjective Data

Client expressed concern about his slow weight gain.

Objective Data

Height is 5 ft, 8 in. Weight:

2/08 169 lb ■ 03/09 183 lb

Analysis

Weight gain related to sedentary activity level and eating in response to external cues.

(Continued on the following page)

CASE STUDY *(Continued)*

Plan

DESIRED OUTCOMES EVALUATION CRITERIA	ACTIONS/INTERVENTIONS	RATIONALE
Client will select fresh fruits at social activities.	Request that Foods and Nutrition Department serve fresh fruit at social functions	Replacing kilocalorically dense cakes, pies, and cookies with fresh fruit will promote weight maintenance
Refer client to registered dietitian (RD)	Reinforce dietitian's teaching	The dietitian will generally be able to spend more time with client than the floor nurse
Refer client to activities director	Reinforce activities director's teaching	The activities director will be able to discuss opportunities to exercise with client as well as order appropriate foods for activities

5-1

Dietitian's Notes

The following Dietitian's Notes are representative of the documentation found in a client's medical record.

Subjective: Client states he would like to lose weight but can't resist treats served at social functions. Loves cakes, pie, donuts, and cookies and admits to lack of self-control. Client would appreciate having more healthful snacks available at social functions. Admits to being unaware of what he actually eats every day. Admits he avoids body movement.

Objective: Height 5 ft 8 in. 02/08 weight 169 lb, 03/09 weight 183 lb. Appetite records show a food intake of 100% of all food served plus second portions.

Analysis: Ideal body weight 148 to 180 lb

Estimated kcal needs at 12 kcal/pound = 2280 (between sedentary and moderately active).

Excessive energy intake related to failure to adjust for lifestyle changes and decreased metabolism as evidenced by body weight and client history. Client expressed verbal desire to manage his weight.

Plan:

1. Client will keep a food record for 3 of every 7 days to enable him to be more conscious of food choices (self-monitor behavior). Will evaluate food records for 2 weeks.
2. Client's goal is to maintain weight and perhaps lose a few pounds.
3. Will encourage activities director to order fresh fruit at facility functions and evaluate client for physical activity opportunities.

5-2

Activity Director's Note

The following Activities Director's Notes are representative of the documentation found in a client's medical record.

Met with client and discussed activities calendar including those with an exercise component. Will order a fresh fruit option at social activities that serve food.

Critical Thinking Questions

1. What would you do at the next client care conference if Mr. G changed his mind about weight control and said, "All I have left in life is food. I don't want to lose weight"?

2. What would you do at the next client care conference if Mr. G had done everything asked but only managed to maintain his weight.

3. What types of exercise would be appropriate to suggest to Mr. G?

Chapter Review

1. The components of energy expenditure are:
   a. Mental activity and physical activity
   b. Thermic effects of exercise and foods
   c. Resting energy expenditure, physical activity, and to a lesser extent the thermic effect of foods
   d. Thermic effect of foods, physical activity, and thermic effect of exercise

2. Energy homeostasis exists when:
   a. Kcalories from food intake equal kcalories used for energy expenditure.
   b. Kcalories used for physical activity equal kcalories used for energy expenditure.
   c. An individual is gaining weight.
   d. Kcalories from food intake equal kcalories used for resting energy expenditure.

3. A kilocalorie is used to measure both:
   a. Weight and percentage body fat
   b. Height and weight
   c. The units of energy used in the body and contained in foods
   d. Leanness and body-fat content

4. Kilocalories required per kilogram of body weight are highest during:
   a. Starvation
   b. Growth
   c. Weight loss
   d. Old age

5. Which of the following foods is the most kilocalorically dense?
   a. 1 cup of sugar
   b. 1 cup of celery
   c. 1 cup of skim milk
   d. 1 cup of margarine

Clinical Analysis

1. Monitoring a resident's weight is a government requirement in long-term care facilities. The goal is to prevent a slow weight loss, which, over time, can have health consequences. Mr. I, resident of Sunnybrook Nursing Home, has been experiencing an undesirable slow weight loss. His weight history is as follows:

   Feb   180 lb (82 kg)
   June   175 lb (80 kg)
   Oct   ~170 lb (77 kg)

   As Mr. I's nurse, you should first:
   a. Encourage Mr. I to eat only twice a day
   b. Call the doctor
   c. Wait for the next client care conference to act on this problem
   d. Monitor Mr. I's food intake and physical activity

2. A teacher noticed that many students in her fifth-grade class were overweight. As a school project, the class kept food records for 3 days. A computer software program analyzed the records. Many students were eating less than their recommended dietary allowance for kcalories but gaining weight nonetheless (a common problem among our nation's young). The teacher asked the class by a show of hands what they did after school and on weekends. Many of the same children who were overweight raised their hands when asked if they played mostly video games and watched television when not in school. The teacher shared this information with the school nurse and asked her to speak to the class. The school nurse correctly decided that:
   a. The teacher is overly concerned because the percentage of overweight students approximates the percentage of overweight adults in the community.
   b. The computer program must be in error.
   c. All the students need to increase their total intake, including foods from the major food groups.
   d. Many students would benefit from an increase in physical activity.

3. A client appears to be totally concerned with the kilocaloric density of foods and not at all concerned with the nutrient density of foods. You need to encourage the consumption of both types of foods. Which of the following behaviors do you need to discourage?
   a. The substitution of skim milk for 2% milk
   b. The avoidance of all meat, fish, and poultry
   c. The inclusion of dark green and yellow fruits and vegetables in the diet
   d. The inclusion of whole grains in the diet

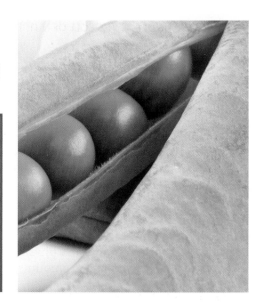

6

Vitamins

LEARNING OBJECTIVES

After completing this chapter, the student should be able to:

- Define vitamins.
- Differentiate between fat- and water-soluble vitamins.
- Describe the diseases caused by deficiencies of vitamins A and D.
- List four diseases caused by specific water-soluble vitamin deficiencies.
- Identify two vitamins with good food sources limited to the fruit and vegetable group.
- Differentiate enrichment from fortification.
- Distinguish two vitamins with associated toxicities from natural or fortified foods, emphasizing persons with increased risk.
- Name three good food sources of provitamin A and vitamin C.
- Describe the prudent use of vitamin supplements.
- Relate two large population groups for whom supplements or fortified foods are recommended to the specified vitamin for each group.

The importance of vitamins was first recognized by the effects of their absence. Some deficiency diseases have been known for centuries, but it was not until the early 20th century that vitamins were isolated in the laboratory. This chapter considers the importance of vitamins in the body and diet, the general functions of vitamins, the classification of vitamins, and the use of vitamin supplements. It also includes information on metabolism, functions, sources, deficiencies, toxicities, and factors affecting stability.

The Nature of Vitamins

Vitamins are organic substances needed by the body in small amounts for normal metabolism, growth, and maintenance. Organic substances are derived from living matter and contain carbon. Vitamins are not sources of energy nor do they become part of the structure of the body. Vitamins act as regulators or adjusters of metabolic processes and as **coenzymes** (substances that activate enzymes) in enzymatic systems.

Specific Functions

Vitamin functions are specific. With few exceptions, bodily processes do not permit substitutes. Thus, vitamins are similar to keys in a lock. All the notches in a key have to fit the lock, or the key will not turn. Overall, one vitamin cannot perform the functions of another. If a person does not consume enough vitamin C, for instance, taking vitamin D will not correct the deficiency. Vitamin D is the wrong key for that lock.

Classification

A major distinguishing characteristic of vitamins is their solubility in either fat or water. This physical property is used to classify vitamins and is also significant for storage and processing of foods that contain vitamins and for the utilization of the vitamins in the body. Vitamins A, E, D, and K are fat-soluble. The eight B-complex vitamins and vitamin C are water-soluble.

Dietary Reference Intakes

The amounts of vitamins recommended in the United States to meet the needs of almost all healthy individuals are listed by age and physiological status in Appendix A. Recommended amounts vary in other countries.

Vitamins A, D, and E historically have been measured in **International Units (IUs),** a dosage amount that still appears on some labels. The Recommended Dietary Allowances (RDAs) and Adequate Intakes (AIs), however, are listed using the metric system: **micrograms** and milligrams. There are no generic units that can be converted directly to the metric system. The amount designated by a unit is specific for each vitamin. The principles used to convert IUs to the metric system are given in Clinical Calculation 6-1.

Fat-Soluble Vitamins

More or less of a vitamin may be retained in a food, depending on the methods of processing and storing. New information on the effects of thermal extrusion showed fat-soluble vitamins to be more vulnerable to losses than previously noted (Riaz, Asif, and Ali, 2009). A summary of factors affecting stability of vitamins appears as Table 6-2. See Box 6-1 for an explanation of oxidation.

Sources of the fat-soluble vitamins with examples of foods containing the RDA/AI of each are listed

6-1

Clinical Calculation

The Elusive International Unit

Formerly, fat-soluble vitamins were measured in international units (IUs), as defined by the International Conference for Unification of Formulae. *A unit of vitamin A is not an equal measure of vitamin D or of vitamin E.* Because that system still appears in laws, on labels, and in research reports, the principles used to convert IUs to metric measures are given here. These equivalents incorporate recent changes in the calculation of provitamin A using **retinol activity equivalents (RAEs)** to compensate for varying amounts of vitamin A obtainable from animal versus plant sources and beta-carotene versus other plant based carotenoids.

VITAMIN A*

Animal Foods: 1 IU = 0.3 microgram of retinol
Plant Foods: 1 IU =
3.6 micrograms of beta-carotene
7.2 micrograms of RAEs from other provitamin A carotenoids[†]

VITAMIN D

40 IU =1 microgram of cholecalciferol

VITAMIN E[†]

Natural form: 1 IU =
0.67 milligram of alpha-tocopherol
Synthetic form: 1 IU =
0.45 milligram of alpha-tocopherol

*A vitamin A calculator is available at www.nutrisurvey.de/vac/vac.htm.
[†]Gropper and Smith, 2013.

in Table 6-3. Fat-soluble vitamins are absorbed from the intestine in the same way as fats, and like fats, they can be stored in the body for varying lengths of time, giving the potential for health problems due to excessive intake. Toxicity from vitamins A and D can be fatal.

Vitamin A

For DRIs, see Appendix A. For food and other sources, see Table 6-3. To investigate the vitamin content of a particular item, go to http://ndb.nal.usda.gov or to http://nutritiondata.self.com. For stability information, see Table 6-2.

Ancient Greeks and Egyptians used liver to cure **night blindness,** but vitamin A was not synthesized until the 1930s. Finally, in the 1950s, **retinal** was identified as the essential light-absorbing component of **rhodopsin** (Ross, 2014).

Vitamin A comes in two forms: preformed vitamin A (**retinol**) and **provitamin A** (found in **beta-carotene** and other **carotenoids,** 50 of which have some provitamin A activity). A **preformed vitamin** is already

TABLE 6-1 ■ Classification of Vitamins	
FAT SOLUBLE	**WATER SOLUBLE**
Vitamin A	Vitamin C
Vitamin D	Thiamin
Vitamin E	Riboflavin
Vitamin K	Niacin
	Vitamin B_6
	Folic acid
	Vitamin B_{12}
	Biotin
	Pantothenic acid

TABLE 6-2 ■ Factors Affecting Stability of Vitamins

VITAMIN	STABLE TO				
	OXYGEN	HEAT	LIGHT	ACIDS	ALKALIES
Fat Soluble					
A	No	No	No	No	*
D	No	Yes	Yes	*	*
E	No	No	No	Yes	No
K	No	No	No	No	No
Water Soluble					
C	No	No	No	Yes	No
Thiamin	No	No	No	Yes/No†	No
Riboflavin	Yes	Yes	No	Yes	No
Niacin	Yes	Yes	Yes	Yes	Yes
B₆	No	Yes	No	Yes	No
Folate	No	No	No	No	Yes
B₁₂	Yes	Yes	Yes	No	No
Pantothenic acid	*	No	*	No	No

*Data unavailable.
†Destroyed by tannic and caffeic acid; protected by ascorbic and citric acid.
Sources: Gropper and Smith, 2013; Riaz, Asif, and Ali R, 2009; Trumbo, 2014.

Box 6-1 ■ *Oxidation*

The process through which a substance combines with oxygen is called **oxidation.** Several substances can be destroyed by oxidation, including all the fat-soluble vitamins. Of the water-soluble vitamins, only riboflavin and niacin are stable to oxidation.

Tissues with cell membranes especially susceptible to oxidation include the lungs, brain, and red blood cells. Some **molecules** become very unstable when they are oxidized. Their accelerated movements can damage nearby molecules.

in a complete state in ingested foods, whereas a **provitamin** requires conversion in the body to be in a complete state. Provitamin A is converted to retinol mainly in the intestine. The term *precursor* is often used interchangeably with the term *provitamin*. A **precursor** is a substance from which another substance is derived.

Absorption, Metabolism, and Excretion

Retinol absorption is relatively unregulated, even when intake is very high (Ross, 2014). Of preformed vitamin A, 70% to 90% is absorbed if consumed with at least 10 grams of fat. Beta-carotene absorption ranges from 20% to 50%, but less than 5% of carotenoids are absorbed from raw vegetables (Gropper and Smith, 2013). Retinol transport in the blood requires a retinol-binding protein and prealbumin, both of which are synthesized in the liver. Consequently, poor nutritional protein status interferes with the transportation and usage of vitamin A. About 40% of vitamin A metabolites are excreted via the bile in feces, and about 60% is excreted in urine unless intake is high, when fecal excretion generally exceeds that in urine (Gropper and Smith, 2013).

Up to a year's supply of retinol is stored in the liver. Excessive carotene, which is apparently harmless for most people, is stored in adipose tissue, giving fat a yellowish tint. (See Vitamin A Toxicity in this chapter and Chapter 21 for information on exceptional situations.)

Functions

Several crucial body functions depend on vitamin A, or retinol: vision, bone growth, and maintenance of epithelial tissue. In addition, provitamin A serves as an antioxidant (see Vitamin E in this chapter).

TABLE 6-3 ■ Fat-Soluble Vitamins

VITAMIN	ADULT RDA/AI AND FOOD PORTION CONTAINING IT*	FUNCTIONS	DEFICIENCY DISEASE	SIGNS AND SYMPTOMS OF DEFICIENCY	SOURCES
A	700–900 mcg 0.5–0.8 cups cooked sliced carrots	Dim light vision Differentiation of epithelial cells	Night blindness Xerophthalmia	Night blindness Dry and thick outer covering of eye Blindness Growth retardation Increased susceptibility to infections Increased intracranial pressure Infertility	*Preformed:* Liver Egg yolk Fortified milk Fish *Provitamin:* Carrots Sweet potatoes Squash Apricots Cantaloupe Spinach Collards Broccoli Cabbage

(continued)

TABLE 6-3 ■ Fat-Soluble Vitamins (Continued)

VITAMIN	ADULT RDA/AI AND FOOD PORTION CONTAINING IT*	FUNCTIONS	DEFICIENCY DISEASE	SIGNS AND SYMPTOMS OF DEFICIENCY	SOURCES
D	15–20 mcg (600–800 IU) 5.2–6.9 cups 1% fortified milk	Increases intestinal absorption of calcium Stimulates bone production Decreases urinary excretion of calcium	Rickets Osteomalacia	Bowlegs, knock-knees, misshapen skull Tetany in infants Soft fragile bones, especially of spine, pelvis, lower extremities	Sunlight on skin Fortified milk Cod liver oil Salmon Herring Tuna Eggs Liver Fortified cereals
E	15 mg 3.3 tbsp safflower oil	Antioxidant Protects polyunsaturated fatty acids in red blood cell membranes from oxidation in lungs	No specific term	Muscle pain and weakness Hemolytic anemia Degenerative neurological problems (peripheral neuropathy, **ataxia**) Anemia in premature infants	Sunflower, safflower, and canola oils Almonds, hazelnuts, and peanuts Broccoli, cooked spinach Fortified ready-to-eat cereals
K	90–120 mcg 0.6–0.8 cup raw chopped spinach	Used in synthesis of several clotting factors, including prothrombin Assists vitamin D to synthesize a regulatory bone protein	No specific term	Prolonged clotting time	Collards Spinach Brussels sprouts Cabbage Broccoli Soybean and canola oils Synthesis in intestine

AI, Adequate Intake; RDA, Recommended Dietary Allowances.
*Example; not suggested as sole source of the vitamin

VISION

In many ways, a camera mimics the eye: both have a dark layer to keep out excess light, a lens to focus light, and a light-sensor. In the eye, the sensor is a light-sensitive layer at the back of the eye, called the **retina.** In the retina, light rays are changed into electrical impulses that travel along the **optic nerve** to the back of the brain. The vitamin A metabolite **retinal** is part of a chemical in the retina responsible for this electrical conversion. The body can synthesize this retinal chemical, **rhodopsin** (or visual purple), only if it has an appropriate supply of vitamin A.

When the eye is functioning in dim light, rhodopsin is broken down into a protein **(opsin)** and vitamin A. In darkness or during sleep, opsin and vitamin A reunite to become rhodopsin. Figure 6-1 shows this reaction. The body can keep reusing the vitamin A, but some of the vitamin is depleted during each visual cycle so that a dietary deficiency produces night blindness, or impaired dim-light vision. Clinical Application 6-1 relates a common method for conserving rhodopsin for night vision.

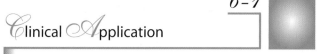

FIGURE 6-1 Vitamin A and the protein opsin combine during sleep to form rhodopsin. When we need to see in dim light, the rhodopsin breaks down into vitamin A and opsin.

MAINTAINING EPITHELIAL TISSUE

Epithelial tissue covers the body and lines the organs and passageways that open to the outside of the body. Skin is epithelial tissue, as are the surface of the eye and the lining of the gastrointestinal tract. Epithelial tissue has a protective function, often producing mucus to wash out foreign materials. Vitamin A helps to keep epithelial tissue healthy by aiding the differentiation of specialty cells. This function, control of gene expression, has led some scientists to believe that vitamin A may play a role in cancer prevention. See Clinical Application 6-2 for more information on vitamin A and cancer.

OTHER FUNCTIONS

Vitamin A participates in bone metabolism in an undefined manner in that deficiency causes excessive

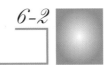

Clinical Application

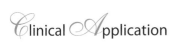

Vitamin A and Cancer

Cancers begin with abnormal differentiation and rampant proliferation of cells. Vitamin A plays a hormone-like role in normal cell differentiation throughout the body. In studies of populations, lower intakes of vitamin A have been associated with higher risk of certain cancers, particularly those of epithelial origin. In experimental animals, vitamin A deficiency increased tumor incidence and susceptibility to chemical **carcinogens** (Ross, 2014).

The provitamin also functions as an antioxidant to neutralize **free radicals.** These highly reactive **atoms** or **molecules** can damage **DNA,** with resultant abnormal cell growth. Intervention studies using beta-carotene were not protective, however, but actually resulted in increased cancers in susceptible individuals (see Chapter 21).

Evidence does not support a benefit for consuming more than the RDA for vitamin A (Ross, 2014). Health claims have been approved by the U.S. Food and Drug Administration for carotenoid-rich foods that also are low in fat and are good sources of fiber (Gropper and Smith, 2013). See dietary supplements in Chapter 15.

deposition of bone by **osteoblasts** and reduced bone degradation by **osteoclasts.** Excessive vitamin A, in contrast, stimulates osteoclasts and inhibits osteoblasts, resulting in decreased bone mineral density and increased fracture risk (Gropper and Smith, 2013). Vitamin A is recognized as an important regulator in several types of immune cells (Ross, 2014). Vitamin A also contributes to blood formation and to normal reproduction, but less is understood about the physiology involved in those areas.

Deficiency

Even though vitamin A is effectively stored in a healthy body when intake is adequate, deficiencies can occur. Vitamin A deficiency is a public health problem in more than 100 countries, especially in Africa and Southeast Asia, affecting mostly pregnant women and young children. Worldwide, more than 124 million children are estimated to be vitamin A–deficient, and nearly 8 million preschool-age children die each year as the result of this deficiency (Ronald, 2011).

Globally, the prevalence of vitamin A deficiency has been declining, which may be due to widespread vitamin A supplementation in conjunction with measles immunization in at-risk populations (Sherwin, Reacher, Dean, and Ngondi, 2012). Vitamin A supplementation in children has been proven to be effective in reducing mortality among children between 6 months and 5 years of age, making further placebo trials in this age group unnecessary; however, studies comparing different doses and delivery mechanisms (for example,

fortification) are needed. Furthermore, until alternate sources are available, vitamin A supplements should be given to all children at risk of deficiency, particularly in low- and middle-income countries (Mayo-Wilson, Imdad, Herzer, et al, 2011).

Vitamin A deficiency in the United States is most often due to disease. For example, clients with long-lasting infectious disease, fat absorption problems, or liver disease are at risk of vitamin A deficiency. Vitamin A deficiency is common after **bariatric surgery** and is associated with a low serum concentration of prealbumin. Vitamin A status should be assessed in patients who have undergone gastric bypass surgery, and deficiency should be suspected in those with evidence of protein-calorie malnutrition (Zalesin, Miller, Franklin, et al, 2011). Prevention of deficiencies requires lifelong vitamin supplementation after bariatric surgeries (Stroh, Weiher, Hohmann, et al, 2010).

SIGNS AND SYMPTOMS

Lack of vitamin A as retinal causes night blindness. In this condition, the resynthesis of rhodopsin is too slow to allow quick adaptation to dim light. Approximately 10 million pregnant women around the world develop night blindness annually (Pandev, Lin, Collier-Tenison, and Bodden, 2012), but treating fertile women is complicated because of the hazard preformed vitamin A presents to the fetus (see Toxicity).

All epithelial tissue suffers because of vitamin A deficiency. The most serious effect is the thickening of the epithelial tissue covering the eye. **Xerophthalmia,** an abnormal thickening and drying of the outer surface of the eye, is a leading cause of preventable blindness in some developing countries (Sherwin, Reacher, Dean, and Ngondi, 2012) and the leading cause of childhood blindness (Dubock, 2012). Figure 6-2 shows a characteristic lesion caused by accumulation of shed cells that

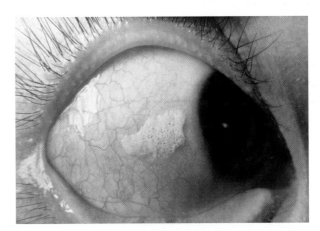

FIGURE 6-2 Bitot spot, a triangular shiny gray spot on the conjunctiva seen in vitamin A deficiency. (From McLaren and Frigg [2001]. Reproduced with permission of Sight and Life.)

may be caused by present or previous vitamin A deficiency or trauma (Heimburger, 2014).

Other signs and symptoms of vitamin A deficiency include anorexia, growth retardation, increased susceptibility to infections, and disorders of the skin and hair follicles (Gropper and Smith, 2013). Likewise, taste impairment, balance disturbances, bone changes that impinge on the cranial nerves, increased intracranial pressure, and infertility may result from vitamin A deficiency (Ross, 2014).

TREATMENT AND PREVENTION

Providing vitamin A by any of the strategies below is the treatment for night blindness. Although they did not know the responsible component, ancient Greek and Roman physicians recognized that liver cured the condition.

Active corneal xerophthalmia is a medical emergency demanding high-dose vitamin A orally. If vomiting or diarrhea precludes oral dosing, a water-miscible injection is given, a form that can also be used to provide adequate vitamin A to individuals with fat absorption disorders.

Prevention of vitamin A deficiency involves multiple strategies:

- Breastfeeding
- Vitamin A supplementation
- Fortification of foods
- Genetic modification of crops (see Golden Rice in Chapter 1)
- Diet diversification

Often these strategies are combined to fit local needs. Work in Kenya demonstrated that fresh or dried mangoes, popular food items and a significant source of provitamin A, should be included in food-based approaches to reduce vitamin A deficiency. In amounts acceptable to children and women, fresh and dried mangoes can supply 50% or more of the daily required retinol equivalent for children and women (Muoki, Makokha, Onyango, and Ojijo, 2009).

An international humanitarian effort to eliminate vitamin A deficiency by DSM Nutritionals provides free vitamin A capsules as well as free educational materials (wall posters, books, videos, PowerPoint slides) in English, French, German, Spanish, and other languages. For free downloadable materials, see www.sightandlife.org/media.html. Sight and Life can be contacted at P.O. Box 2116, CH 4002 Basel, Switzerland, or accessed at www.sightandlife.org.

Sources and Interfering Factors

Preformed vitamin A is found in animal foods with the highest levels occurring naturally in liver, fish liver oils, and other organ meats. Good sources include egg yolk, fish, and fortified milk products.

The body converts the provitamin A carotenoids present in fruits and vegetables to retinol. The best-utilized sources are yellow, orange, and red brightly colored fruits and cooked yellow tubers, followed by dark green leafy vegetables.

Carotene, a yellow pigment found mostly in fruits and vegetables, is readily visible in yellow and orange foods such as carrots, sweet potatoes, squash, apricots, and cantaloupe. Although not as noticeable because chlorophyll masks the yellow color, carotene is also present in dark leafy green vegetables, including spinach, collards, broccoli, and cabbage.

Carotene content of a species of vegetable can vary with the vegetable's maturity, handling, and preparation. Carrots packaged in plastic bags are better protected from light and air than the bouquets secured by a rubber band. **Beta-carotene** is more available to the body in carrots cooked with a small amount of fat than in raw carrots, an exception to the general rule that cooking depletes vitamins.

Individuals with higher than normal requirements for vitamin A include those with:

- Fat absorption disorders
- Chronic kidney disease
- Acute protein deficiency
- Intestinal parasites
- Acute infections (Gropper and Smith, 2013)

Conditions that interfere with fat digestion may reduce the efficiency of vitamin A absorption (Ross, 2014). Even with adequate vitamin A stores, zinc deficiency is associated with decreased plasma retinol-binding protein and with decreased mobilization of retinol from the liver (Gropper and Smith, 2013).

Any combination of preformed and provitamin A is sufficient to meet a person's needs. In the United States, about 66% of vitamin A intake is preformed, partly derived from nutritional supplements. In the developing world, vitamin A is consumed mainly as carotenoids (Ross, 2014).

Toxicity

Fetal malformations can be caused by either deficiency or excess of vitamin A. Although most other vitamin toxicities are a result of supplementation, hypervitaminosis A can be caused by foods. For instance, liver contains 27,720 micrograms of retinol (91,476 IU) in a 3-ounce serving. Even when intake is high, about 70% of dietary vitamin A is absorbed. Some experts caution against frequent consumption of foods very high in vitamin A by pregnant or potentially pregnant women (Ross, 2014).

In addition, vitamin A derivatives are often prescribed to control severe acne, which presents a threat to unborn children. The risk of fetal malformations was significantly higher among women who consumed more than 3000 micrograms (10,000 IU) of retinol in early pregnancy. This information was considered in establishing the Tolerable Upper Intake Level (UL) at 3000 micrograms (Ross, 2014). See also Chapter 10.

CAROTENEMIA

Beta-carotene is recognized by the Food and Drug Administration as Generally Recognized as Safe (**GRAS**) as a dietary supplement and a colorant. Nevertheless carotene can be consumed to excess, causing **carotenemia.** The person's skin becomes yellow, similar to that shown in jaundice, but with carotenemia, the palms of the hands and the soles of the feet are also affected. Also in contrast to jaundice, the whites of the eyes do not become yellow in carotenemia. A common cause of carotenemia in infants is consumption of too much squash and carrots. The skin returns to normal within 2 to 6 weeks after stopping the excessive intake.

Occasionally carotenemia can be problematic. A 3-month-old infant with classic skin discoloration, dry skin, and pruritus had high levels of serum carotenoids but normal serum vitamin A. Because the usual causes of carotenemia were absent, the condition was attributed to a defect in an enzyme involved in vitamin A production. The child was placed on a low-carotenoids diet for 6 months, resulting in decreased serum carotenoid levels and regression of cutaneous signs and symptoms, especially pruritus (Maruani, Labarthe, Dupré, et al, 2010). The assumption that carotene is harmless was challenged by studies in which beta-carotene supplementation was associated with icreased occurrence of lung cancer in particularly susceptible clients. See Chapter 21.

HYPERVITAMINOSIS A

Vitamin A toxicity is called **hypervitaminosis A.** An acute case can result from even a single dose of 50,000 IU of vitamin A. Symptoms of vitamin A toxicity are similar to those of a brain tumor, such as headaches and blurred vision or **diplopia** and other signs of increased pressure within the skull, as well as skin and muscle abnormalities (Gropper and Smith, 2013). One 18-year-old female developed headache, vomiting, back pain, and diplopia after ingestion of a high dose (about 10 million IU) of vitamin A in response to family problems (Khasru, Yasmin, Salek, et al, 2010). Other symptoms of hypervitaminosis A include pain in the bones and joints, dry skin, and poor appetite.

Individuals with chronic hypervitaminosis A may present with the foregoing symptoms as well as hair coarseness or loss; **ataxia;** bone, muscle, abdominal, and eye pain; and liver damage. Self-prescribed vitamin A supplements have produced liver disease. For one such client, the hepatic signs and symptoms did not appear

until 10,300 IU daily for 17 years and 270,000 IU daily for 1 year had been ingested (Miksad, de Ledinghen, McDougall, et al, 2002). Another client died after consuming 25,000 IU (2.5 times the UL) daily for 6 years (Kowalski, Falestiny, Furth, and Malet, 1994).

One hazard of excessive vitamin A intake is unique to the Arctic. Polar bear liver has made both men and dogs sick. Acute toxicity can result from ingesting more than 300,000 IU, which is only about 10 to 15 g of polar bear liver. At that rate, a 3-ounce serving contains 181 times the UL for adults. Other Arctic game poses similar hazards.

Vitamin D

For DRIs, see Appendix A. For food and other sources, see Table 6-3. To investigate the vitamin content of a particular item, go to http://ndb.nal.usda.gov. Because of improved analytical techniques, vitamin D values for 3000 foods were recently added to the U.S. Department of Agriculture National Nutrient Database (Bliss, 2012). For stability information, see Table 6-2.

Vitamin D deficiency diseases were recognized by Dutch and English physicians in the 17th century. By the turn of the 20th century, rickets reached almost epidemic proportions in the industrialized cities of northern Europe because of air pollution and long indoor working hours. In 1922, vitamin D was named as the factor in cod liver oil that prevented rickets (Jones, 2014).

Vitamin D is not a true vitamin because there are sources other than diet. Instead, this key nutrient is a pro-hormone, which can be synthesized from a steroid precursor if not obtained from diet (Shin, Choi, Longtine, and Nelson, 2010). **Vitamin D,** long known to be essential for bone growth, targets more than 200 human genes in a wide variety of tissues. One of the most important genes vitamin D upregulates is for *cathelicidin*, a naturally occurring broad-spectrum antibiotic (Cannell, Zasloff, Garland, et al, 2008). Vitamin D receptors have been found in more than 30 organs not usually associated with bone metabolism such as breast, brain, colon, heart, lung, muscle, pancreas, and prostate (Gropper and Smith, 2013).

Absorption, Metabolism, and Excretion

Two forms of vitamin D are metabolically active. Vitamin D_2, **ergocalciferol,** is formed when ergosterol (provitamin) in plants is irradiated by sunlight. Vitamin D_3, **cholecalciferol,** is formed when 7-dehydrocholesterol (another provitamin) in the skin of animals or humans is irradiated by ultraviolet light or sunlight. Firm conclusions about different effects of these two forms of vitamin D cannot be drawn: at nutritional doses, vitamins D_2 and D_3 appear to be equivalent, but at high doses vitamin D_2 is less potent (National Institutes of Health, June 24, 2011b).

Both forms are absorbed into the blood. About 50% of dietary vitamin D_3 is absorbed, most rapidly in the duodenum but the greatest amount in the distal small intestine (Gropper and Smith, 2013). Intestinal absorption of vitamin D decreases with age, as does the capacity of the skin to synthesize cholecalciferol. Like other fat-soluble vitamins, it is transported in the blood bound to protein. The liver alters the vitamin to **calcidiol,** an inactive form of vitamin D. By enzyme action, the kidney converts the calcidiol to calcitriol, the active form of vitamin D. Some calcitriol production from calcidiol also occurs in immune cells, the skin, the placenta, and other tissues (Shin, Choi, Longtine, and Nelson, 2010), but the synthesis of *circulating* calcitriol in the normal nonpregnant mammal appears to be the exclusive domain of the kidney (Jones, 2014). Figure 6-3 diagrams the path of these processes.

Functions

Vitamin D has long been recognized as essential to proper bone metabolism. Recent findings suggest a role in preventing a wide range of chronic diseases.

BONE METABOLISM

Vitamin D promotes normal bone mineralization by stimulating:

- DNA to produce transport proteins to increase intestinal absorption of calcium and phosphorus
- Bone cells to build and maintain bone tissue with calcium and phosphorus
- The kidneys to return calcium to the bloodstream rather than excreting it in the urine

An opposite effect is caused by **parathyroid hormone** that is secreted in response to a low serum calcium level. Parathyroid hormone causes the **catabolism** of bone to raise the serum calcium level. The body's priority goal is maintenance of correct serum calcium for blood clotting, nerve function, and muscle contraction. Without this mechanism to sustain vital functions, a person would not live long enough to develop rickets, the bone disease of vitamin D deficiency.

POSSIBLE PREVENTION OF CHRONIC DISEASES

Although clear mechanisms have not been delineated, vitamin D intake may partly explain the north–south disparity in the occurrence and prognosis of many diseases. For instance:

- North American and northern European countries exhibit the highest incidence of breast cancer, whereas women in southern regions are relatively protected (Suba, 2012).

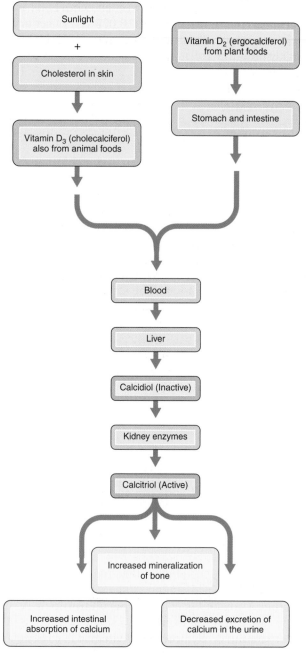

FIGURE 6-3 Vitamin D, whether from food or synthesis in the skin, is metabolized by the liver and the kidneys to its active form.

- The more northern the location of an adoptive country, the higher the breast cancer risk for dark skinned immigrants (Suba, 2012).
- People residing in the highest-latitude countries had the highest rates of leukemia in both men and women; countries with low ultraviolet B irradiance had higher age-adjusted incidence rates of leukemia (Mohr, Garland, Gorman, et al, 2011).
- Multiple sclerosis rates correlate positively with distance from the equator and inversely with altitude, which permits more intense solar radiation (Schwalfenberg, 2012).

Those correlations infer the protective value of vitamin D synthesized in the skin. The U.S. Preventive Services Task Force concluded that evidence is not sufficiently robust to draw conclusions regarding the benefits or harms of vitamin D *supplementation* for the prevention of cancer (Chung, Lee, Terasawa, et al, 2011). Obviously, much remains to be determined about vitamin D's actions in cell differentiation and immune system functioning. See Genomic Gem 6-1.

Deficiency

One difficulty with setting an RDA for vitamin D is the multiple sources of the vitamin. Some people, particularly outdoor workers, may achieve optimal serum levels without supplements. Overall, skin synthesis of vitamin D contributes somewhat to the body's supply because serum vitamin D levels are generally higher than would be predicted on the basis of vitamin D intakes alone. In contrast, homebound or institutionalized individuals, women who wear long robes and head coverings for religious reasons, and people with occupations that limit sun exposure are unlikely to obtain adequate vitamin D from sunlight (National Institutes of Health, June 24, 2011b).

Genomic Gem 6-1
Vitamin D and Tuberculosis

Tuberculosis (TB), caused by infection with *Mycobacterium tuberculosis*, is one of the major bacterial infections worldwide resulting in approximately 2 million fatalities annually (Saiga, Shimada, and Takeda, 2011). Among racial and ethnic groups born in the United States, the greatest racial disparity in TB rates occurred among non-Hispanic Blacks, whose rate was six times the rate for non-Hispanic Whites (Centers for Disease Control, March 23, 2012). Because of their dark skins, African Americans also have decreased serum levels of vitamin D.

Toll-like receptors (TLRs) have been found to be critical for the body's recognition of pathogenic microorganisms including mycobacteria. Several molecules, including active vitamin D₃ induced by TLR stimulation, direct the body's immune responses to mycobacteria (Saiga et al, 2011).

Furthermore, stimulation of **macrophages** induces an enzyme that catalyzes the conversion of calcidiol to calcitriol, which upregulates production of antimicrobial peptides, including *cathelicidin*, which is needed to help fight the tubercle bacillus (Gropper and Smith, 2013).

Although not the only mechanisms at work in resisting microbes, **polymorphisms** in vitamin D receptors may contribute to susceptibility to tuberculosis. Investigators have hypothesized that increased risk of tuberculosis is associated with a lack of appropriate vitamin D receptor–dependent antimycobacterial activity (Tang, Smit, and Semba, 2014).

These findings shed light on the success of Southwestern U.S. sanitariums, before the advent of antibiotics, of using sun exposure to treat tuberculosis.

A body mass index of 30 or greater is associated with lower serum vitamin D levels compared with nonobese individuals. Obesity does not affect the skin's capacity to synthesize vitamin D, but greater amounts of subcutaneous fat sequester more of the vitamin and alter its release into the circulation. Obese individuals who have undergone gastric bypass surgery may become vitamin D deficient over time without a sufficient intake of this nutrient from food or supplements because part of the upper small intestine where vitamin D is absorbed is bypassed. Any vitamin D mobilized into the serum from fat stores may not compensate over time (National Institutes of Health, June 24, 2011b). The Endocrine Society Clinical Practice Guideline suggests that obese children and adults be given at least two to three times more vitamin D than the RDA for their age group to satisfy their need for the vitamin (Holick, Binkley, Bischoff-Ferrari, et al, 2011).

A varying percentage of the population is vitamin D deficient, at any time, during any season, at any latitude, although the percentage is higher in the

- Winter
- Aged
- Obese
- Sun-deprived
- Dark-skinned
- Populations farther from the equator

Seasonal variation of vitamin D levels even occur around the equator, and widespread vitamin D deficiency can occur at equatorial latitudes, probably due to sun avoidance, rainy seasons, and air pollution (Cannell, Zasloff, Garland, et al, 2008).

Besides lack of sunshine, low vitamin D intake, fat malabsorption disorders, chronic liver or kidney disease, and rare genetic disorders cause vitamin D deficiency. Vitamin D–deficient diets are associated with milk allergy, lactose intolerance, ovo-vegetarianism, and veganism (National Institutes of Health, June 24, 2011b). Children whose bones are still growing are most vulnerable to this deficiency.

RICKETS

Vitamin D deficiency in children is called **rickets.** Although nutritional rickets is preventable, it still occurs in developed countries. Vitamin D deficiency rickets was confirmed in 104 Canadian children from July 1, 2002, to June 30, 2004. Incidence rates were highest among children residing in the north (Ward, Gaboury, Ladhani, and Zlotkin, 2007).

In 2000 and 2001, cases of rickets among children living in North Carolina, Texas, Georgia, and the mid-Atlantic region, prompted a wider search for additional cases. Between 1986 and 2003, 166 cases of rickets were reported among U.S. children. Approximately 83% of children with rickets were described as African

American or Black, and 96% were breastfed. Among children who were breastfed, only 5% of records confirmed vitamin D supplementation (Weisberg, Scanlon, Li, and Cogswell, 2004). Although breast milk is the best single source of food for infants, it contains less than 25 to 78 IU/L of vitamin D and thus, by itself, is insufficient to provide adequate levels of vitamin D for infants (Perrine, Sharma, Jefferds, et al, 2010). A 16-month-old child with advanced rickets had received a vegan diet and an unfortified soy beverage after weaning from the breast at 10 months of age (Carvalho, Lenney, Carrington, and Hall, 2001). To prevent such deficiency diseases or to diagnose them early, health-care providers should assess the client's total situation and not just focus on the immediate reason for the visit.

Rickets can occur without vitamin D deficiency. Children in equatorial Africa exposed to plenty of sunshine have developed rickets due to lack of dietary calcium and were cured by calcium supplementation alone (Wolpowitz and Gilchrest, 2006). Rickets can also be caused by defects in the vitamin D receptors. See Genomic Gem 6-2.

OSTEOMALACIA

Vitamin D deficiency in adults is called **osteomalacia.** This deficiency disease occurs most often in women who have insufficient calcium intake and little sunlight exposure. It occurs frequently among those who are pregnant or lactating.

Environmental causes for osteomalacia are similar to those for rickets. And people with low exposure to sunlight are at increased risk—for example, cloistered nuns, office workers, residents of smoggy areas, and institutionalized elderly people.

Because of the complex processes involved in vitamin D metabolism, liver or kidney disease can lead to bone deterioration. Chronic kidney failure has caused osteomalacia because of the inability of the kidneys to convert vitamin D to its active form. Clients with kidney disease are commonly prescribed pharmaceutical vitamin D supplements.

SIGNS AND SYMPTOMS

Children with rickets have soft, fragile bones. Classic deformities include bowlegs, knock knees, and misshapen skulls. Vitamin D deficiency may cause **tetany** in infants due to low levels of blood calcium. A 1-week-old, full-term male infant presented to the emergency department with generalized seizures. He was exclusively breastfed since birth. Both parents were vegetarians, of Asian origin, and the mother dressed with most of her body covered. She did not take vitamin supplements during pregnancy. The baby's seizures ceased within 3 days of starting treatment with vitamin D and calcium. At 6 months of age, he had normal serum levels of the two nutrients and was developing according to his chronological age (Camadoo, Tibbott, and Isaza, 2007).

Adults with osteomalacia also have increasing softness of the bones, causing deformities due to loss of calcium. The bones most commonly affected are those of the spine, pelvis, and lower extremities.

DRIs and Sources

In 2010, because of increased information on which to base recommendations, the Institute of Medicine revised the DRIs for vitamin D. The AIs for infants were doubled. The AIs for all other age groups were upgraded to RDAs: the amounts tripled for those up to the age of 50 and increased by smaller amounts for those older than 50 years. ULs were also increased except for infants younger than 6 months of age. DRIs for vitamin D are based on skeletal outcomes only and assume minimal exposure to sunlight. For sources of vitamin D, see Table 6-4. Two sources are readily available to most people: synthesis by the skin and fortified milk, which is widely available in the United States.

SKIN SYNTHESIS

A major source of vitamin D is the body itself. Vitamin D is manufactured in the skin. Children with low

---

Genomic Gem 6-2
Vitamin D–Resistant Rickets

Hereditary vitamin D–resistant rickets is a rare **autosomal recessive** disease caused by mutations in the vitamin D receptor (VDR). One young girl displayed clinical and radiographic features of rickets, hypocalcemia, and elevated serum concentrations of calcitriol. A single heterozygous mutation was found in the VDR gene that substituted alanine for glutamic acid in a specific amino acid (Malloy, Zhou, Wang, et al, 2011).

TABLE 6-4 ■ Selected Food Sources of Vitamin D		
FOOD AND PORTION	**IUs**	**MICROGRAMS**
Swordfish, cooked, dry heat, 3 ounces	566	14.2
Salmon, pink, canned, total contents, 3 ounces	465	11.6
Salmon (sockeye), cooked, 3 ounces	447	11.2
Tuna fish, canned in water, drained, 3 ounces	154	3.9
Milk, nonfat, reduced fat, and whole, vitamin D–fortified, 1 cup	100	2.5
Liver, beef, cooked, 3 ounces	42	1.1
Egg, one large (vitamin D is found in yolk)	41	1.0
Shitake mushrooms, ½ cup, cooked	20	0.5

Sources: Gropper and Smith, 2013; National Institutes of Health, June 24, 2011b; U.S. Department of Agriculture Nutrient Database, Release 25.

dietary intakes may escape rickets if their exposure to sunlight is adequate. Some researchers suggest that approximately 5 to 30 minutes of sun exposure between 10 a.m. and 3 p.m. at least twice a week to the face, arms, legs, or back without sunscreen usually leads to sufficient vitamin D synthesis. Complete cloud cover reduces ultraviolet (UV) energy by 50%; shade (including that produced by severe pollution) by 60%, and window glass by 100%. Sunscreens with a sun protection factor (SPF) of 8 or more appear to block vitamin D–producing UV rays, although in practice people generally do not apply sufficient amounts, cover all sun-exposed skin, or reapply sunscreen regularly. Therefore, skin likely synthesizes some vitamin D even when protected by sunscreen as typically applied (National Institutes of Health, June 24, 2011b).

Aging diminishes the effectiveness of skin synthesis illustrated by serum levels of vitamin D that were three times lower in people aged 62 to 80 than in people aged 22 to 30 given the same sunlight exposure (University of Washington, 2009). Exposure of the face is not recommended at any age because precancerous *actinic keratoses* are related to sun exposure. The body regulates skin synthesis of vitamin D to avoid overdosing from this source.

FOOD

For people not exposed to sunshine, food sources of vitamin D become increasingly important. Dietary sources are critical at latitudes above 43 degrees north (the level of the Nebraska-South Dakota border) between October and April when UVB light does not penetrate the atmosphere resulting in insignificant skin synthesis of vitamin D (Jones, 2014).

Few commonly consumed foods naturally provide vitamin D. The flesh of fatty fish such as swordfish, salmon, and tuna are among the best sources. Smaller amounts of vitamin D are found in beef liver and egg yolks. Vitamin D in these foods is primarily in the form of vitamin D_3. Some mushrooms provide vitamin D_2 in variable amounts, and mushrooms with enhanced levels of vitamin D_2 from being exposed to UV light under controlled conditions are also available. Food labels, however, are not required to list vitamin D content unless a food has been fortified with this nutrient (National Institutes of Health, June 24, 2011b).

Fortified foods provide most of the vitamin D in the American diet. In the United States, the major food source of vitamin D is fortified milk. Milk is the ideal food to link with vitamin D because it also contains calcium and phosphorus, which are necessary for bone **anabolism.** Almost all of the U.S. milk supply is voluntarily fortified with 100 IU (2.5 micrograms) per cup. Other dairy products made from milk, such as cheese and ice cream, are generally not fortified. Ready-to-eat breakfast cereals often contain added vitamin D, as do some brands of orange juice, yogurt, margarine, and other food products. In a review of research needs, note was made of the lack of reliable data on the practice and impact of discretionary fortification (Cashman and Kiely, 2011).

In Canada, milk is fortified by law with 35 to 40 IU/100 mL, as is margarine at 530 IU/100 grams or higher. Both the United States and Canada mandate the fortification of infant formula with vitamin D: 40 to 100 IU/100 kcal in the United States and 40 to 80 IU/100 kcal in Canada (National Institutes of Health, June 24, 2011b).

See Box 6-2 and Clinical Application 6-3 on the **fortification** of foods. For other food sources, see Table 6-4 and Table 6-3.

SUPPLEMENTS

Historically, the means to obtain vitamin D was cod liver oil, which contains 453 IU (11.3 micrograms) of vitamin D_3 per teaspoonful. Although a natural product, cod liver oil is a supplement, not a food. In various forms, vitamin D supplements are used by 37% of the U.S. population (National Institutes of Health, June 24,

---

Box 6-2 ■ *Enrichment and Fortification*

Enrichment is the replacing of nutrients lost in processing or during storage. Enriched flour is an example. Not all the nutrients are replaced; therefore, whole grain products are recommended.

Fortification is the addition of nutrients not normally present in a given food to increase its nutritional value, for example, vitamins A and D in milk.

6-3
Clinical Application

Fortification of Foods: Use and Misuse

Fortification is the addition of nutrients to foods in amounts greater than normally present. Many cereals are fortified with vitamins and minerals not normally found in grains. Occasionally, intentions are better than practices. Between 1985 and 1991, 56 cases of hypervitaminosis D were identified in Massachusetts. Two individuals died as a result, and nine were discharged from the hospital with residual effects. Although state law required an upper limit of 500 IU (12.5 micrograms) of vitamin D per quart, the implicated dairy's milk exceeded this by 70 to 600 times (Blank, Scanlon, Sinks, et al, 1995).

Even without considering errors in processing, experts are concerned that voluntary fortification of multiple foods by the producers could lead to excessive intakes. Currently, foods permitted to be fortified with vitamin D include milk products, cereals, fruit juices, and drinks. Maximum levels of added vitamin D are specified by law.

2011b). The form that many vegans prefer is vitamin D_2 because of its plant origin. Intake from multiple fortified and supplemental sources should be monitored to avoid toxicity. Supplemental vitamin D can be taken without regard to food intake because it does not require dietary fat for absorption (Holick, Binkley, Bischoff-Ferrari, et al, 2011).

Interfering Factors

Little special handling of foods is necessary but a high-fiber diet interferes with the vitamin's absorption. Abnormalities of absorption such as diarrhea, fat malabsorption, and biliary obstruction also may lead to vitamin D deficiency. See Chapter 15 for drug–nutrient interactions.

Toxicity

Although excessive sun exposure is a risk factor for skin cancer, it does not result in acute vitamin D toxicity. Whether individuals with high levels of calcidiol from sun exposure (e.g., lifeguards, outdoor workers) suffer from more renal stones or higher cancer or mortality rates than persons with lower levels has yet to be determined (Jones, 2014).

Intakes of vitamin D from food that are high enough to cause toxicity are unlikely. Toxicity is much more likely to occur from high intakes of dietary supplements containing vitamin D (National Institutes of Health, June 24, 2011b).

DOSAGE

More than any other vitamin, a high consumption of vitamin D is likely to cause toxicity from excess. Doses of 10,000 IU daily for several months have caused **hypercalcemia** and calcification of soft tissues (Gropper and Smith, 2013). The use of supplements of both calcium (1000 mg/day) and vitamin D (400 IU) by postmenopausal women was associated with a 17% increase in the risk of kidney stones over 7 years in the Women's Health Initiative (National Institutes of Health, June 24, 2011b).

Infants and children face increased risk from multiple fortified foods and supplements. For example, a 16-month-old previously healthy boy presented to the emergency department with refractory hypercalcemia due to an overdose of an over-the-counter vitamin supplement. He was successfully treated, but the case highlights the potential danger of giving children high-dose vitamin supplements (Chatterjee and Speiser, 2007).

SIGNS AND SYMPTOMS

Clinical manifestations of hypervitaminosis D include loss of appetite, nausea, vomiting, polyuria, muscular weakness, and constipation. More serious consequences of vitamin D overdose result from calcium deposits in the heart, kidneys, and brain.

Vitamin E

For DRIs, see Appendix A. For food and other sources, see Table 6-3. To investigate the vitamin content of a particular item, go to http://ndb.nal.usda.gov or to http://nutritiondata.self.com. For stability, see Table 6-2.

In 1922, fetal resorption in rats was identified as resulting from a deficient diet. In 1936, vitamin E was isolated from wheat germ and named alpha-tocopherol from the Greek *tokos* (offspring) and *pherin* (to bear) (Traber, 2014).

An RDA of 15 milligrams was set for both men and women because the latter, despite generally weighing less, have more body fat needing the antioxidant protection that vitamin E provides (Traber, 2014). Persons who smoke may have higher requirements for vitamin E, but specific recommendations for smokers have not been published. More information on interpretation of research findings is provided in Chapter 21.

Absorption, Metabolism, and Excretion

The primary site of absorption of vitamin E is the **jejunum,** where fat and bile are required for optimal uptake. Absorption rates vary widely, from 20% to 80% with higher intakes reducing absorption rates (Smith and Gropper, 2013). Excretion is via bile in the feces. More than 90% of the body's pool of vitamin E is stored in adipose tissue (Traber, 2014).

Functions

The major function of vitamin E is to protect the integrity of cell membranes. To do this, vitamin E serves as an **antioxidant** by accepting oxygen instead of allowing other molecules to become unstable. In this role, vitamin E protects provitamin A and unsaturated fatty acids from oxidation. It also preserves the stability of the polyunsaturated fatty acids in the red blood cell membranes, protecting them from oxidation in the lungs. The vitamin E in lung cell membranes provides an important barrier against air pollution.

Available data do not support supplementation with vitamin E to prevent cancer, cataracts, Parkinson disease, or Alzheimer disease. Regarding cardiovascular disease, not only is there a lack of benefit to supplementing with vitamin E, but also the incidence of stroke was increased significantly in individuals who received vitamin E (Gropper and Smith, 2013). Similarly, vitamin E supplements taken for 5.5 years significantly increased the risk of prostate cancer by 17% (Klein, Thompson, Tangen, et al, 2011). An exception to those findings is the decreased occurrence of venous thromboembolism in persons receiving vitamin E supplements (Traber, 2014).

Evidence is accumulating that refutes the usefulness of vitamin E or beta-carotene supplements in preventing or delaying the onset of age-related macular degeneration (Evans and Lawrenson, June 2012), but antioxidant vitamin and mineral supplementation may delay in its progression in people already diagnosed with the disease (Evans and Lawrenson, November 2012).

Deficiency

No particular disease is caused by vitamin E deficiency. Vitamin E deficiency is rare, virtually never resulting from dietary deficiency, but rather is usually related to lipid metabolism disorders. Premature infants are at risk because of impaired fat utilization. Diseases characterized by fat malabsorption such as cystic fibrosis and hepatobiliary diseases can lead to deficiencies. Also, persons with genetic defects in lipoproteins or the *a*-tocopherol transfer protein are at risk (Gropper and Smith, 2013).

Signs and symptoms include muscle pain and weakness, hemolytic anemia, and degenerative neurological problems such as peripheral **neuropathy, ataxia,** and loss of coordination of the limbs (Gropper and Smith, 2013). Serum vitamin E levels may fall within 1 to 2 years of diagnosis with lipid malabsorption disorders. The appearance of the progressive, peripheral, sensory neuropathy that is the first sign of vitamin E deficiency in humans may be delayed 10 or 20 years because of adequate stores of vitamin E and its slow depletion from nervous tissue (Traber, 2014).

Premature infants with inadequate reserves of vitamin E develop anemia. Without sufficient vitamin E, the membranes of the red blood cells break down easily when exposed to oxygen or an oxidizing agent. Vitamin E supplements have become routine care for premature infants (Chitambar and Antony, 2014).

Persons with peripheral neuropathies or retinitis pigmentosa of unknown causes as well as those with ataxia should be evaluated for vitamin E deficiency (Traber, 2014).

Sources, Stability, and Interfering Factors

The best sources of vitamin E are vegetable oils and nuts. Selected food sources of vitamin E are listed in Table 6-5. All vegetable oils are not equal in vitamin E content. Those highest in alpha-tocopherol are sunflower and safflower oils. In contrast, corn and soybean

TABLE 6-5 ■ Selected Sources of Vitamin E

	MG
Wheat germ oil, 1 tablespoon	20.3
Sunflower seeds, dry roasted, unsalted, 1 ounce	7.4
Almonds, dry roasted, 1 ounce (22 kernels)	6.8
Sunflower oil, 1 tablespoon	5.6
Safflower oil, 1 tablespoon	4.6
Hazelnuts, 1 ounce	4.3
Peanut butter, smooth, 2 tablespoons	2.9
Canola oil, 1 tablespoon	2.4
Peanuts, 1 ounce	2.2

Sources: Gropper and Smith, 2013; U.S. Department of Agriculture Nutrient Database, Release 25.

oils have a greater proportion of gamma-tocopherol, which no longer is counted as contributing to vitamin E intake (see Table 6-3 for other good resources).

Vitamin E and selenium (see Chapter 7) have a complementary relationship. Higher concentrations of one can compensate for lower concentrations of the other. Another antioxidant, vitamin C, can regenerate vitamin E following its oxidation (Gropper and Smith, 2013).

Vitamin E is stable to acid, but heat and light lead to destruction. Thus, roasting of nuts reduces their vitamin E content. High beta-carotene intake may decrease plasma vitamin E concentrations, but vitamin E inhibits the absorption and metabolism of both beta-carotene and vitamin K (Gropper and Smith, 3013). Persons who limit fat in their diets are likely limiting their vitamin E intake also.

Toxicity

Toxicity from natural vitamin E from food is unknown. Excessive supplemental vitamin E can cause gastrointestinal symptoms, muscle weakness, double vision, and increased bleeding tendencies. Thus clients taking anticoagulant drugs should not exceed the UL for vitamin E. Clinical Application 6-4 describes a client with vitamin E toxicity.

Vitamin K

For DRIs, see Appendix A. For food and other sources, see Table 6-3. To investigate the vitamin content of a particular item, go to http://ndb.nal.usda.gov or to http://nutritiondata.self.com. For stability, see Table 6-2.

In 1929, hemorrhagic diseases in chickens were associated with a low-fat, cholesterol-free diet. The 1941 Nobel Prize in medicine was awarded to two researchers for identifying vitamin K (from Dutch—*koagulation*) to be responsible for delayed clotting (Gropper and Smith, 2013).

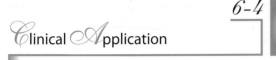

Vitamin E Toxicity

A client was admitted to the hospital for **narcolepsy,** a disorder characterized by recurrent, uncontrollable, brief periods of sleep from which the individual is easily awakened. This client would fall asleep while driving his car.

Narcolepsy can be a sign of uremia, hypoglycemia, diabetes, hypothyroidism, increased intracranial pressure, tumors of the brain stem or hypothalamus, or absence **epilepsy.** If all of these causes are ruled out, the medical diagnosis is either classical or independent narcolepsy.

During her assessment, the dietitian discovered one unusual nutritional practice: After a clerk in a health foods store had recommended vitamin E, the client had begun and continued to take this supplement. The dietitian investigated vitamin E's adverse effects and suggested to the physician that the narcolepsy could be caused by excessive vitamin E. After the client discontinued taking vitamin E, the narcolepsy disappeared.

In this case, a thorough nutritional assessment and an inquiring attitude eliminated the need for extensive diagnostic tests.

Vitamin K is frequently prescribed as a medication. Its intake has an impact on the effectiveness of the commonly prescribed anticoagulant **warfarin,** which interferes with the synthesis of vitamin K. Vitamin K can also serve as an antidote for warfarin overdose. Instructions regarding food intake for clients taking warfarin are given in Chapter 15.

Absorption, Metabolism, and Excretion

Two naturally occurring forms of vitamin K can meet the body's needs. Vitamin K_1, or **phylloquinone,** is found in plant foods. Vitamin K_2, or **menaquinone,** is synthesized by intestinal bacteria. A synthetic, water-soluble pharmaceutical form of vitamin K_1, **phytonadione,** can be administered orally or by injection. An aqueous oral preparation is available for people with fat malabsorption disorders. The intravenous route is rarely used and requires extreme caution because of life-threatening reactions (Vallerand, Sanoski, and Deglin, 2013).

Phylloquinone is absorbed primarily in the jejunum, and menaquinone is absorbed in the distal small intestine and the colon. Absorption and utilization of menaquinone vary considerably from person to person. Within the body, vitamin K is stored primarily in cell membranes of the lungs, kidneys, bone marrow, and adrenals. The total amount in the body is estimated to be only 50 to 100 milligrams. Turnover of vitamin K in the body occurs about every 1.5 days. Most of vitamin K_1's metabolites are excreted in feces via bile with some also excreted in the urine (Gropper and Smith, 2013).

Functions

The actions of vitamin K in blood clotting have been known since 1941 when its discoverers received the Nobel Prize in medicine. A vitamin K–dependent protein in bone that helps regulate serum calcium levels requires both vitamin K and vitamin D for synthesis. In addition, vitamin K–dependent proteins have been found in heart, kidney, and smooth muscle, although the mode of action there remains to be discovered (Gropper and Smith, 2013).

BLOOD CLOTTING

Vitamin K is necessary for the liver to make factors II (**prothrombin**), VII, IX, and X. Four additional coagulation proteins are vitamin K dependent. These factors and proteins plus calcium are key links in the chain of events producing a blood clot.

BONE METABOLISM

Two vitamin K–dependent proteins have been identified in bone, cartilage, and dentine, but evidence that dietary vitamin K is protective of bone health is equivocal (Gropper and Smith, 2013). A vitamin K–dependent protein, **osteocalcin,** is the second most abundant protein in bone, but its function is not yet clearly defined (Suttie, 2014; see also Vitamin A).

Deficiency

Individuals at risk of vitamin K deficiency include newborn infants as well as adults who avoid green leafy vegetables or are undergoing long-term antibiotic therapy. Clients with fat malabsorption syndromes are also at risk. Careful assessment of dietary factors in these clients is warranted.

Infants are at risk because inadequate amounts of vitamin K cross the placenta and because the intestinal tract of a newborn infant is sterile. For this reason, the baby is unable to produce vitamin K until the intestine is colonized with bacteria from the environment, usually within 24 hours, when he can begin to synthesize vitamin K. To prevent vitamin K deficiency bleeding of the newborn, the American Academy of Pediatrics (2009) recommends an intramuscular dose of vitamin K be administered to the baby immediately after birth. In a sad outcome, a pregnant woman with complications of bariatric surgery delivered an infant who suffered extensive cerebral hemorrhage due to maternal vitamin K deficiency (Van Mieghem, Van Schoubroeck, Depiere, et al, 2008).

Deficiencies, uncommon in healthy adults, have been associated with disease and with drug therapy. For example, fat absorption problems from gastrointestinal diseases may hinder vitamin K absorption, resulting in prolonged blood clotting time. In addition, antibiotics, which kill normal bacteria—some of which produce vitamin K—along with the infectious organisms can cause low levels of vitamin K.

Sources

The human body is capable of manufacturing some vitamin K, and many common foods contain adequate amounts.

INTESTINAL SYNTHESIS

The amount of bacterially produced vitamin K that is absorbed and utilized varies from one individual to another. Nevertheless, bacterial synthesis alone will not maintain adequate vitamin K status in healthy children or adults (Gropper and Smith, 2013).

FOOD

Green leafy vegetables and vegetables of the cabbage family are the best sources of vitamin K (see Table 6-3). Limited studies suggest that phylloquinone from vegetable sources has a **bioavailability** that is about 15% to 20% of that from a supplement (Suttie, 2014). With two vegetables, lesser bioavailability would be no problem, but preparation mode has an impact:

- Cooked spinach has 889 micrograms per cup, but raw 145 mcg.
- Cooked collards have 836 micrograms per cup, but raw 184 mcg.

In some situations, that rich a source would be problematic. Controlling intake of vitamin K is part of the treatment plan for clients receiving a common anticoagulant drug, warfarin (see Chapter 15).

Stability and Interfering Factors

Vitamin K is susceptible to significant destruction by light and heat (Gropper and Smith, 2013) and is unstable in the presence of oxygen, alkalis, and strong acids. In addition, overconsumption of vitamins A and E can interfere with the absorption of vitamin K, and excess vitamin E may also interfere with vitamin K's metabolism (Gropper and Smith, 2013). The anticoagulant warfarin interferes with the liver's use of vitamin K, but that is the desired effect of the medication.

Toxicity

The naturally occurring forms of vitamins K_1 and K_2 have not been associated with adverse effects, but caution is warranted, particularly if high doses are taken. Phytonadione, the pharmaceutical preparation of vitamin K_1, causes fewer adverse effects than earlier, stronger formulations but because of life-threatening reactions, intravenous administration is not recommended except in emergencies. As always, special care must be taken when administering any medication, including vitamin K, to infants.

Table 6-3 summarizes the fat-soluble vitamins. See Clinical Application 6-5 for a description of two conditions that mimic deficiencies of fat-soluble vitamins.

Water-Soluble Vitamins

Vitamins that dissolve in water are vitamin C, or **ascorbic acid,** and the B vitamins (**thiamin, riboflavin, niacin,** vitamin B_6, **folate,** vitamin B_{12}), as well as **pantothenic acid, biotin,** and choline, the last strictly speaking not a vitamin.

Vitamin C

For DRIs, see Appendix A. For food and other sources, see Table 6-6. To investigate the vitamin content of a particular item, go to http://ndb.nal.usda.gov or to http://nutritiondata.self.com. For stability, see Table 6-2. Rose hip, a seed capsule found in roses, contains vitamin C and is used to manufacture vitamin C supplements but does not appear to be superior to other sources (Gropper and Smith, 2013).

Scurvy, the deficiency disease caused by lack of vitamin C, was described by the Egyptians in 3000 B.C. In 1753, James Lind proved that citrus fruits cured scurvy, but not until 1795 did the Royal Navy mandate issuing citrus juice to sailors after 2 weeks at sea,

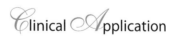
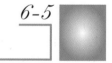

6-5

𝒞linical 𝒜pplication

Conditions Mimicking Fat-Soluble Vitamin Deficiencies

PROTEIN DEFICIENCY

Water and fat do not mix. To circulate fats in the water-based blood, the liver attaches fat-soluble vitamins to protein carriers. Sometimes a protein deficiency hinders the use of the fat-soluble vitamins.

ZINC DEFICIENCY

A zinc-containing protein carries vitamin A from storage in the liver to tissues. Zinc deficiency is associated with both decreased mobilization of retinol from the liver, even with adequate vitamin A stores in the liver, as well as decreased plasma retinol-binding protein concentrations (Gropper and Smith, 2013). For this reason, a zinc deficiency can mimic a vitamin A deficiency.

TABLE 6-6 ■ Water-Soluble Vitamins

VITAMIN	ADULT RDA AND FOOD PORTION CONTAINING IT*	FUNCTIONS	DEFICIENCY DISEASE	SIGNS AND SYMPTOMS OF DEFICIENCY	SOURCES
C Ascorbic Acid	75–90 mg 0.8–0.9 cup of orange juice, prepared from frozen concentrate	Formation of collagen Antioxidant Facilitation of iron absorption	Scurvy	Bleeding mucous membranes Poor wound healing or reopening of scars Softened ends of long bones Teeth loosen, may fall out Death probably due to internal bleeding	Citrus fruit and juice Broccoli, Brussels sprouts Green and red peppers Cantaloupe, Strawberries Kiwi fruit Papayas
B_1 Thiamin	1.1–1.2 mg 4.1–4.5 oz pork loin, roasted, lean only	Coenzyme in CHO and amino acid metabolism	Beriberi	Anorexia, Weight loss Muscle weakness and wasting Peripheral neuropathy Right heart failure Wernicke's encephalopathy	Pork Beef liver Salmon Black beans Wheat germ Fortified cereals
B_2 Riboflavin	1.1–1.3 mg 2.2–2.6 cups 1% milk	Coenzyme in protein metabolism; need increases as protein needs increase	Ariboflavinosis	Lesions on lips and in mouth Seborrheic dermatitis Normochromic, normocytic anemia	Milk and dairy products Eggs Meats, especially liver Fortified cereals
B_3 Niacin	14–16 mg niacin equivalents 3.8–4.3 oz water-packed light tuna	Coenzyme in energy production Participant in synthesis of fatty acids and steroid hormones	Pellagra	Bilaterally symmetrical dermatitis on face, neck, hands, and feet Diarrhea Dementia	Liver Tuna Meats, fish, poultry Whole, enriched, or fortified grains Coffee Tea
B_6 Pyridoxine	1.3–1.7 mg 2.2–2.8 cups sliced banana	Coenzyme in metabolism of amino acids	No specific term	Mouth lesions Peripheral neuropathy Confusion Hypochromic, microcytic anemia Convulsions in infants	Sirloin steak Salmon Chicken breast Whole grains, fortified cereals Bananas
Folate Folic Acid	400 mcg 2.8 cups canned pinto beans	Essential to the formation of DNA Participant in formation of heme	No specific term	Bright red tongue Fatigue, weakness Shortness of breath Heart palpitations Megaloblastic anemia	Liver Dried peas, beans, lentils Wheat germ Peanuts Asparagus Endive Lettuce Brussels sprouts Broccoli Spinach Fortified grain products Liver
Cobalamin	2.4 mcg 1.9 oz canned salmon	Synthesis of DNA, RNA, metabolism of amino and fatty acids Synthesis and maintenance of myelin	Pernicious anemia (lack of intrinsic factor, not dietary) Vitamin B_{12} deficiency (avoidance of animal products)	Fatigue Pallor Shortness of breath Heart palpitations Megaloblastic anemia Numbness and tingling of extremities Abnormal gait Possible memory loss Dementia	Meat Fish Poultry Milk Cheese Eggs Vitamin B_{12}-fortified soymilk or tofu
Pantothenic Acid	5 mg 1 cup cooked shiitake mushrooms	Coenzyme in fatty acid metabolism Many other metabolic and regulatory processes	No specific term	*Burning feet syndrome*	Liver Chicken Egg yolk Yogurt Legumes Mushrooms Potatoes Broccoli Whole grain cereal

TABLE 6-6 ■ Water-Soluble Vitamins (Continued)

VITAMIN	ADULT RDA AND FOOD PORTION CONTAINING IT*	FUNCTIONS	DEFICIENCY DISEASE	SIGNS AND SYMPTOMS OF DEFICIENCY	SOURCES
Biotin	30 mcg 3 large eggs	Coenzyme is the synthesis of fat, glycogen, and amino acids	No specific term	**Alopecia** Scaly, red rash around the eyes, nose, and mouth **Paresthesias** of the extremities Depression, and hallucinations	Liver Eggs Salmon Peanuts Milk Sweet potato Soybeans
Choline	450–550 mg 3.6–4.4 large eggs	Liver and brain function Lipid metabolism Cell membrane structure	No specific term	Liver and muscle damage	Liver Eggs Beef Pork Milk, yogurt Baked beans Broccoli Wheat germ

*Example; not suggested as sole source of the vitamin.

leading to the term "limey" for a British sailor. Diffusion of the citrus mandate to merchant vessels in 1854 happened 101 years after Lind's work. The Nobel Prize in 1937 was awarded to the scientists who isolated the antiscorbic principle, determined its structure, and named it ascorbic acid (Gropper and Smith, 2013; Levine and Padayatty, 2014).

Most animals manufacture vitamin C in their livers. Humans, along with other primates, guinea pigs, some birds, and fruit-eating bats, cannot synthesize vitamin C. Humans and primates have an inactive form of an encoding gene for the last enzyme in the chain reaction for vitamin C synthesis and therefore must obtain vitamin C from the diet (Levine and Padayatty, 2014).

Absorption, Metabolism, and Excretion

Vitamin C is absorbed from the small intestine. As the amount of vitamin C consumed increases, the proportion of the vitamin absorbed decreases. At usual intakes from food of 30 to 180 milligrams, 70% to 90% of vitamin C is absorbed. At intakes greater than 1 gram, typically less than 50% of vitamin C is absorbed (Gropper and Smith, 2013).

Absorbed vitamin reaches the liver through the hepatic vein and then is accumulated in almost all human tissues. The pituitary and adrenal glands have the highest concentrations of vitamin C, but the greatest total amount is found in the liver. The maximal vitamin C pool is estimated to be about 2 grams (Gropper and Smith, 2013). Excretion is via the urine. After doses of less than 100 milligrams in men and 60 milligrams in women, no vitamin C was detected in the urine. However, after intravenous doses of 500 or 1250 milligrams, virtually all the vitamin C was excreted (Levine and Padayatty, 2014).

Functions

Vitamin C has diverse functions in the body. It contributes to wound, burn, and fracture healing; serves as an antioxidant; enhances the absorption of iron; and assists in the synthesis of hormones and neurotransmitters.

COLLAGEN SYNTHESIS

Vitamin C is necessary in the formation of **collagen,** the strong fibrous protein in connective tissue. Bone, skin, blood vessels, soft dental structures, and scar tissue all contain collagen. Without vitamin C, collagen molecules are inadequately cross-linked, resulting in weak tissue.

ANTIOXIDANT

Vitamin C is a powerful antioxidant. By preventing the uptake of oxygen by other molecules, it deters the destruction of tissue by unstable molecules. It also has been shown to regenerate other antioxidants in the body, including vitamin E (National Institutes of Health, 2011a).

IRON ABSORPTION FACILITATOR

Vitamin C facilitates iron absorption by acting with hydrochloric acid to keep iron in the more absorbable **ferrous** form. Four ounces of orange juice, for instance, nearly quadruples the iron absorbed from the plant foods eaten with it.

OTHER FUNCTIONS

High concentrations of vitamin C are found in the **adrenal glands.** These are the organs that secrete adrenalin, the "fight-or-flight" hormone, in times of stress. Vitamin C also aids in the synthesis of norepinephrine and **serotonin.**

Vitamin C has not been shown to prevent common colds in the general population, but prophylactic use has reduced the duration of colds by 8% in adults and 14% in children. In marathon runners, skiers, and soldiers on subarctic exercises, prophylactic vitamin C in doses of 250 to 1000 milligrams per day reduced the risk of common cold by 50%. When taken after the onset of symptoms, however, vitamin C did not affect cold duration or symptom severity (National Institutes of Health, June 24, 2011a). Nevertheless, given the consistent effect of vitamin C on the duration and severity of colds in the regular supplementation studies, and the low cost and safety, it may be worthwhile for individuals to test the benefits of therapeutic vitamin C for themselves (Hemilä and Chalker, 2013).

Deficiency

Signs of scurvy can appear within 1 month of vitamin C intake of less than 10 milligrams per day (National Institutes of Health, 2011a), but a genetic component has also been suggested (see Genomic Gem 6-3).

SIGNS AND SYMPTOMS

Early signs of scurvy are tender, sore gums that bleed easily and small skin hemorrhages due to weakened blood vessels. The late manifestations of scurvy relate to the breakdown of collagen. Wound healing is delayed; even healed scars may separate. The ends of long bones soften and become malformed and painful, and fractures appear. Teeth loosen in their sockets and fall out. Hemorrhages occur about the joints, stomach, and heart. Untreated scurvy often progresses to sudden death, probably from internal bleeding.

Diagnosis is generally made on the basis of clinical features, corroborated by a history of dietary inadequacy, and the subsequent rapid resolution of symptoms with the restoration of an adequate vitamin C intake (Ben-Zvi and Tidman, 2012). If untreated, scurvy is fatal, and treatment should not be delayed awaiting laboratory confirmation (Levine and Padayatty, 2014).

TREATMENT

An initial intravenous dose may be given. Moderate doses of vitamin C, 100 milligrams orally three times a day, will cure scurvy. With this regimen, symptoms will disappear in about 3 months (Gropper and Smith, 2013). With prompt diagnosis and treatment, permanent damage can be prevented (Levine and Padayatty, 2014).

RISK FACTORS AND CONTEMPORARY CASES

A diagnosis of scurvy may not be considered initially because scurvy today exists primarily within certain populations: the elderly, those with neurodevelopmental disabilities or psychiatric illnesses, or persons with unusual dietary habits (Cole, Warthan, Hirano, et al, 2011).

Case reports still appear in medical journals describing scurvy in developed countries. Recent reports have come from Canada, France, Italy, and Japan, but for cases occurring in the United States. Often the client or the parents sought treatment for symptoms suggestive of diverse conditions, and a dietary deficiency was

---

Genomic Gem 6-3

Possible Genetic Susceptibility to Scurvy

Modern laboratory techniques reveal that vitamin C intake explains only 17% of the variance in vitamin C serum levels (Delanghe, Langlois, De Buyzere, and Torck, 2007). A possible explanation may be related to polymorphisms in the gene for haptoglobin (Hp), a plasma hemoglobin–binding protein, that result in Hp 1 and Hp 2 alleles. Three **phenotypes** could be inherited:

- Hp 1-1 and Hp 2-2 which are **homozygous**
- Hp 1-2 that is **heterozygous** for the affected allele

The proteins formed by each of the three phenotypes are structurally and functionally different with Hp 1-1 the most effective at binding free hemoglobin and suppressing inflammatory responses associated with it (Cahill and El-Sohemy, 2010). Individuals with the Hp 2-2 phenotype show not only significantly lower ascorbic acid concentrations but also decreased stability of vitamin C in their serum (Delanghe et al, 2007). Furthermore, lower serum ascorbic acid levels have been observed in European and Chinese persons with the Hp 2-2 phenotype. During explorations and wars, Asians had a higher mortality rate from scurvy than Europeans whose death rate roughly parallels the frequency of the Hp 2-2 phenotype in European populations (Delanghe et al, 2007).

Serum ascorbic acid is inversely associated with risk of cardiovascular disease, diabetes, and all-cause mortality. In particular, oxidative stress is a feature of cardiovascular disease where the Hp 2-2 phenotype is overrepresented in whites diagnosed with it (Delanghe et al, Langlois, De Buyzere, and Torck, 2007).

The reason prevention studies show inconsistent results may be because of individual genetic variation in serum ascorbic acid response to dietary vitamin C. In addition to Hp, other genes contain common polymorphisms shown to be potential determinants of serum ascorbic acid (Cahill and El-Sohemy, 2010).

not included in the differential diagnosis until late in the process.

- Investigation of rheumatologic symptoms in three clients seen in a large urban medical center in Minnesota over a 6-month period (Mertens and Gertner, 2011)
- Rapid-onset enlargement of upper and lower gums in a 48-year-old Pennsylvania woman whose diet was nearly void of fruits and vegetables (Li, Byers, and Walvekar, 2008)
- Clinical skin changes initially thought to represent inflammation of small blood vessels in an Alabama inpatient (Swanson and Hughey, 2010)
- Painful swollen leg with purplish discoloration and difficulty breathing in a 57-year-old man in Alabama whose diet consisted primarily of TV dinners and canned vegetables (Velandia, Centor, McConnell, and Shah, 2008)
- Regression to crawling in a 20-month-old Florida boy whose fruit and vegetable intake was limited due to refusal, allergies, and maternal rejection of nutritional advice (Popovich, McAlhany, Adewumi, and Barnes, 2009)
- Bruising and leg swelling after an injury to his left leg with a surfboard in a 10-year-old boy with autism and slight developmental delay (Cole et al, 2011)

The case of the 10-year-old autistic boy is not unique in its convoluted path to the diagnosis of scurvy. The child was evaluated in an urgent care center 4 weeks after the injury, fracture ruled out, and ibuprofen recommended for pain. A few days later, the boy forcefully removed 3 loose teeth causing significant bleeding, was seen by a dentist who prescribed mouthwash. When the child's right leg developed bruises, he was twice seen by an orthopedist who ruled out fractures but on the second visit referred the boy to primary care for blood work and follow-up because by then the boy refused to walk. The pediatrician admitted the child to the hospital for laboratory tests, MRIs of the knees, and a chest x-ray that showed mild diffuse osteoporosis. At this time, a dermatologist was consulted, who diagnosed scurvy from skin and mouth changes when it was revealed that the boy consumed only hamburgers, Wheat Chex, Pop-Tarts, oyster crackers, pancakes, and water (Cole et al, 2011). Clinical improvement was seen within 24 hours of ascorbic acid administration.

Scurvy is rare but, as these cases indicate, not unheard of in the United States. Some authors suggest that in children with musculoskeletal symptoms, the possibility of vitamin C deficiency be considered before undertaking an extensive and expensive search for more frequently occurring pathologies (Popovich, McAlhany, Adewumi, and Barnes, 2009).

Three foods that are high in both vitamins A and C are shown in Figure 6-4.

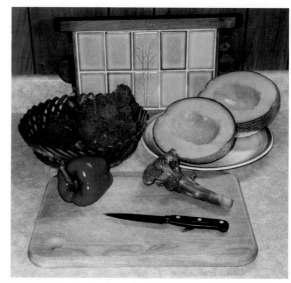

FIGURE 6-4 Broccoli, cantaloupe, and red pepper are excellent sources of both vitamins A and C.

Stability and Preservation

Boiling, cooking, and canning fruits and vegetables lower the vitamin C content by 33% (Velandia, Centor, McConnell, and Shah, 2008). During juice processing, temperature and oxygen are the main factors responsible for vitamin C losses. In regard to packaging, the vitamin C in fruit juice is quite stable when stored in metal or glass containers, whereas the vitamin C content in juice stored in plastic bottles has a much shorter shelf life (Martí, Mena, Cánovas, et al, 2009).

Orange juice from frozen concentrate contains more vitamin C than ready-to-drink juices. Frozen orange juice concentrates have

- 86 milligrams per cup when prepared and
- 39 to 46 milligrams per cup after 4 weeks of storage.

In contrast, ready-to-drink juices have

- 27 to 65 milligrams per cup on opening and
- 0 to 25 milligrams at expiration 4 weeks later (Johnston and Bowling, 2002).

In contrast, the same effects in the body were not observed. Changes in plasma vitamin C levels in the 2-hour period following consumption of commercial orange juices on day 1 versus day 8 of storage were analyzed. The ascorbic acid content decreased significantly after storage of juice reconstituted from frozen concentrate but did not change with chilled juice (Johnson and Hale, 2005).

Easily implemented food preparation procedures can minimize loss of vitamin C:

- Store orange juice in a metal or glass opaque container that holds no more than an amount that can be consumed in a short time.

- Buy ready-to-drink orange juice 3 to 4 weeks before expiration and use within 1 week (Johnston and Bowling, 2002).
- Eat vegetables raw when possible or cook them as quickly as possible; crisp-cooked is better than limp-cooked for retaining the vitamin C content.
- Boil the cooking water for 1 minute before adding the food to eliminate the dissolved oxygen that would otherwise oxidize the vitamin C.

In years past, many food establishments routinely added baking soda to vegetables to enhance their color, but the alkali also destroyed the vitamin C. Fortunately, this practice is now illegal.

Increased Needs

Individuals who smoke require an additional 35 milligrams of vitamin C, and those exposed to secondhand smoke should obtain the RDA daily. Secondhand smoke was strongly associated with lower blood vitamin C levels in children in Puerto Rico (Preston, Rodríguez, and Rivera, 2006). Increased utilization may account for low vitamin C concentrations in smokers and critically ill persons (Levine and Padayatty, 2014).

Blood vitamin C concentration falls after uncomplicated surgery and decreases further after surgery in surgical intensive care unit clients (Fukushima and Yamazaki, 2010). Based on measured blood concentrations and urine excretions of vitamin C after gastrointestinal surgery, an intravenous vitamin C dose of 500 milligrams (but not 100 milligrams) per day is adequate (Yamazaki, Horikawa, and Fukushima, 2011).

Food Processing Use

Vitamin C is used to mitigate undesirable reactions in food. For example, sodium or potassium nitrite is widely used in cured meat products because it inhibits outgrowth and neurotoxin formation by *Clostridium botulinum,* delays the development of oxidative rancidity, develops the characteristic flavor of cured meats, and reacts with myoglobin to stabilize the red meat color. Nitrite that has not reacted with myoglobin is the residual nitrite level (Viuda-Martos, Fernández-López, Sayas-Barbera, et al, 2009). In the small intestine, nitrates combine with amino acids to form nitrosamines, which have been linked to some cancers (See Chapter 21). These health concerns relating to the use of nitrates and nitrites in cured meats have led to decreased use to alleviate the potential risk to the consumers from formation of **carcinogenic** compounds (Viuda-Martos et al, 2009). Because vitamin C blocks the formation of nitrosamines from nitrates, some meat packers add vitamin C to their products to protect against nitrosamine formation.

Toxicity

A dose 10 times the RDA is called a **megadose.** The most common side effects of large amounts (2 grams) of vitamin C are abdominal pain and osmotic diarrhea from bacterial metabolism of the vitamin in the colon Theoretically, large doses disbursed throughout the day could make toxicity more likely than if the same amount were ingested as a single dose because more would be absorbed in divided doses (Gropper and Smith, 2013).

Because vitamin C increases the amount of non-heme iron absorbed (see Chapter 7), persons with diseases characterized by iron overload such as sickle cell anemia (see Chapter 4) and **hemochromatosis** (see Chapter 7) should avoid large doses of vitamin C but not fruits and vegetables (Levine and Padayatty, 2014).

Individuals prone to kidney stones are sometimes advised not to take megadoses of vitamin C because it is metabolized to oxalate, and kidney stones are often composed of calcium oxalate. By a different mechanism of competing with uric acid for reabsorption by the kidney, megadoses of vitamin C theoretically could increase the risk of urate stones but the actual clinical importance of uricosuria with regard to stone formation is unknown (Gropper and Smith, 2013). In healthy persons without prior kidney stones, vitamin C from food and supplements did not increase stone formation (Levine and Padayatty, 2014).

Excessive vitamin C causes false readings in two common laboratory tests. Some urine glucose tests will read falsely positive. Stool tests for occult blood will read falsely negative.

A purported consequence of chronic high intake of vitamin C that is abruptly discontinued is **rebound scurvy.** The body cannot adjust quickly enough and continues to absorb a meager proportion of the now smaller dose. Rebound scurvy has been observed in animals but its existence in human populations has not been determined (Touger-Decker, Radler, and DePaola, 2013) although anecdotal evidence has been reported (Gropper and Smith, 2013). Even without megadose supplements, however, plasma vitamin C levels fall to deficiency levels in healthy humans (who began the experiment saturated with vitamin C) within 30 days of removal of vitamin C from the diet (Levine and Padayatty, 2014).

B-Complex Vitamins

The B-complex group encompasses six traditionally recognized vitamins: thiamin, riboflavin, niacin, vitamin B_6, folate, and vitamin B_{12}. Recently added to the list are the vitamins pantothenic acid and biotin as well as the essential nutrient choline. Some diseases, including beriberi and pellagra, are associated with deficiencies of a single B vitamin.

Thiamin

For DRIs, see Appendix A. Differences in DRIs for men and women are based on body size and energy needs (Gropper and Smith, 2013). For food and other sources, see Table 6-6. To investigate the vitamin content of a particular item, go to http://ndb.nal.usda.gov or to http://nutritiondata.self.com. For stability, see Table 6-2.

Chinese medical texts refer to the condition later labeled beriberi as early as 2700 B.C. In 1884, a Japanese naval surgeon pinpointed the cause as dietary deficiency. Another military doctor in the Dutch East Indies observed that fowl fed polished rice became paralyzed. The vitamin, originally named vitamin B_1, was isolated from rice bran in 1912 and synthesized in 1936 (Bemeur and Butterworth, 2014).

ABSORPTION, METABOLISM, AND EXCRETION

The human body contains about 30 milligrams of thiamin, about one-half of it located in the skeletal muscles, but the liver, heart, kidneys, and brain also have relatively high concentrations. Thiamin is absorbed in the small intestine, primarily in the jejunum and ileum. With high intakes, absorption is by passive diffusion; with lower intakes, through two thiamin transporters (Gropper and Smith, 2013). As a person's energy expenditure increases, the need for thiamin increases. Excess thiamin is mainly excreted in the urine.

FUNCTIONS

Thiamin is an essential coenzyme in the metabolism of glucose and branched-chain amino acids (see Genomic Gem 4-1). It also plays a role in nerve conduction (Gropper and Smith, 2013).

DEFICIENCY

Beriberi is the deficiency disease due to a lack of **thiamin.** The enrichment of food products has almost eliminated this disease, but it is still seen even in developed countries. The need for thiamin increases as kilocaloric consumption increases. Individuals whose thiamin status is marginal may become deficient when an increased need for energy is caused by strenuous activity, pregnancy, a growth spurt, or fever. Parenteral nutrition without thiamin or with excessive glucose can cause thiamin deficiency within a few weeks (Gropper and Smith, 2013).

Despite what is known about the functions of thiamin on a cellular level, that knowledge does not explain all the manifestations of the deficiency disease. *Dry beriberi* is seen mostly in adults with chronic low thiamin intake especially if coupled with high carbohydrate intake. It is characterized by muscle weakness and wasting, particularly in the lower extremities and symmetrical sensory and motor conduction problems affecting the distal limbs. Progression to *wet beriberi* involves the cardiovascular system, culminating in right-sided **heart failure** (Gropper and Smith, 2013). Cardiac beriberi has occured in healthy young adults in the tropics following strenuous exercise (Roman, 2014). In *infantile beriberi*, often presenting between the ages of 2 and 6 months, the child may have a loud, piercing cry and convulsions. Death may result if thiamin is not administered promptly (Bemeur and Butterworth, 2014), as happened to 2 of the 20 infants in Israel diagnosed with thiamin deficiency. Their nondairy, soy-based infant formula, designed and manufactured for the Israeli market, was ultimately found to contain undetectable levels of thiamin (Fattal-Valevski, Kesler, Sela, et al, 2005).

Recent cases of beriberi have been reported in the developed world associated with heavy alcohol intake:

■ In Japan, a 49-year-old man admitted in heart failure and a 70-year-old man who ate mainly polished rice (Imai, Kubota, Saitou, et al, 2012)
■ In Germany, a 67-year-old male patient with reversible cardiomyopathy (Reinhardt, Giambarba, and Raimondi, 2011)
■ In the United Kingdom, a 44-year-old man with a 15-year history of alcoholic binges but with regular food intake until the week before his illness when he ate next to nothing (Murphy, Bangash, and Varma, 2009)

Surgery altering the gastrointestinal tract has been followed by beriberi in:

■ A 49-year-old man in the Netherlands 4 months after bariatric surgery (Goselink, Harlaar, Vermeij, et al, 2012)
■ A 25-year-old woman in Pennsylvania after bariatric surgery (Becker, Ingala, Martinez-Lage, et al, 2012)
■ A 70-year-old man in Ohio with a history of a **Whipple procedure** for pancreatic cancer (Essa, Velez, Smith, et al, 2011)
■ In Italy, two fatal cases:
  ■ A 47-year-old man with a history of gastric resection 10 months earlier
  ■ A 43-year-old man operated on for severe ulcerative rectocolitis followed by 3 weeks of intravenous nutrition without multivitamins (Bello, Neri, Riezzo, et al, 2011)

In developed countries, thiamin deficiency is often associated with alcoholism because of

1. Inadequate food intake
2. Increased requirements because liver damage impairs use of the vitamin

3. Decreased absorption because alcohol inhibits intestinal expression of the two thiamin transporters (Gropper and Smith, 2013)

The following two neurological disorders are often associated with thiamin deficiency in alcoholism. Clients with **Wernicke encephalopathy,** a neurological disorder caused by thiamin deficiency, display many motor and sensory deficits often involving eye muscles, balance, and memory. Although thiamin deficiency is common in clients with alcoholism, only about 10% to 12% of persons with alcoholism develop Wernicke encephalopathy (Bemeur and Butterworth, 2014). Some clients develop **Korsakoff psychosis** characterized by amnesia and impaired conceptual functions. These disorders have also been reported in clients with severe gastrointestinal disease, HIV/AIDS, and pregnant women with **hyperemesis** (Bemeur and Butterworth, 2014). (See Chapters 10 and 20.) In these conditions, thiamin must be administered by injection to raise plasma levels sufficiently to traverse the blood–brain barrier (Gropper and Smith, 2013). Response to thiamin is complete in only 25% of cases of Wernicke-Korsakoff syndrome (cerebral beriberi) and partial in 50% (Heimburger, 2014). Thiamin treatment for cardiac beriberi and Wernicke encephalopathy must be initiated based on suspicion alone (Roman, 2014).

STABILITY AND INTERFERING FACTORS

Air and heat destroy thiamin levels, especially in the presence of alkalis. For this reason, adding baking soda to green vegetables to retain their color or to dried beans to soften them inactivates the thiamin in the vegetables. Also, an enzyme in raw fish, raw shellfish, and ferns, **thiaminase,** destroys thiamin, but cooking inactivates the enzyme. Regular consumption of foods containing thiaminase is a risk factor for thiamin deficiency (Bemeur and Butterworth, 2014). Tannic and caffeic acids found in coffee, tea, blueberries, black currants, Brussels sprouts, and red cabbage are also thiamin **antagonists,** but their actions may be prevented by vitamin C and citric acid (Gropper and Smith, 2013).

TOXICITY

No adverse effects associated with thiamin from food or supplements have been reported. Neither have side effects have been reported from oral intakes of 500 milligrams daily. Thiamin in amounts of 100 times recommendations by injection, however, has been associated with adverse effects, including convulsions, cardiac arrhythmias, and anaphylactic shock (Gropper and Smith, 2013).

Riboflavin

For DRIs, see Appendix A. For food and other sources, see Table 6-6. To investigate the vitamin content of a particular *item, go to http://ndb.nal.usda.gov or to http://nutritiondata. self.com. For stability, see Table 6-2.*

Riboflavin, vitamin B_2, was encountered late in the 19th century when laboratory workers observed a yellow-green fluorescent pigment that formed crystals. Not until the 1930s was riboflavin isolated and eventually named for a sugar it contains (ribose) and the color yellow (Latin: *flavus*).

ABSORPTION, METABOLISM, AND EXCRETION

Most absorption of riboflavin occurs in the proximal small intestine facilitated by bile. About 95% of the riboflavin from foods is absorbed, up to a maximum of about 27 milligrams per single meal or dose. Normal bacteria in the large intestine synthesize riboflavin, producing larger amounts when a person consumes a vegetable-based diet rather than a meat-based diet. The exact contribution of **endogenous** riboflavin to overall nutrition requires further study (Said and Ross, 2014).

Small amounts of the vitamin are found in many tissues, with the greatest concentrations in the liver, kidneys, and heart. Body stores are estimated to suffice for 2 to 6 weeks. The kidneys contribute to riboflavin **homeostasis** by excreting the excess. Even an intake of 1.7 milligrams of riboflavin (the amount in a multivitamin tablet) imparts a bright orange-yellow color to urine (Gropper and Smith, 2013). Excretion is enhanced with **diabetes mellitus,** trauma, stress, and oral contraceptive use (Said and Ross, 2014).

FUNCTIONS AND PHARMACEUTICAL POTENTIAL

Riboflavin is a coenzyme in the metabolism of protein and of other vitamins. Thyroid and adrenal hormones accelerate the conversion of riboflavin to its active coenzymes, which are involved in many oxidative enzyme systems. Riboflavin needs increase as protein needs increase. Clients undergoing major healing processes, such as those with extensive burns, require more riboflavin than the average person.

A proposed use for riboflavin is the inactivation of pathogens in blood products. Such a system is in development and utilizes riboflavin and ultraviolet light to provide pathogen reduction and white blood cell inactivation. The effectiveness of the system against a variety of pathogens has been established (Reddy, Doane, Keil, et al, 2013). Research is continuing because riboflavin is likely to be safe for this use.

DEFICIENCY

Riboflavin deficiency commonly occurs with thiamin and niacin deficiencies. A person who avoids all dairy products, however, may be deficient in riboflavin alone, a condition called **ariboflavinosis.** Signs of this deficiency that may appear after 4 months of inadequate intake include painful lesions on the outside of the lips and in the corners of the mouth, redness and swelling in the mouth, inflammation of the skin, anemia, and peripheral nerve dysfunction (Gropper and Smith, 2013). Other individuals at risk besides those who avoid dairy products are those with congenital heart disease, some cancers, and excessive alcohol intake (because of limited dietary intake and diminished absorption). Also, riboflavin metabolism is impaired in hypothyroidism and adrenal insufficiency (Said and Ross, 2014).

STABILITY AND INTERFERING FACTORS

Riboflavin is fairly resistant to heat, oxygen, and acid but is sensitive to UV light. Thus, cardboard milk cartons or opaque plastic bottles are more protective of the vitamin than clear glass bottles. Even light therapy used to treat hyperbilirubinemia in newborns causes riboflavin destruction (Gropper and Smith, 2013).

TOXICITY

Large oral doses have not yielded reports of toxicity. High doses (400 milligrams) have been used in clinical trials as migraine prophylaxis without adverse effects (Gropper and Smith, 2013). Among other complementary therapies, riboflavin is listed at probably effective for migraine prevention by the American Academy of Neurology and the American Headache Society (Holland, Silberstein, Freitag, et al, 2012).

Niacin

For DRIs, see Appendix A. Niacin allowances are related to energy intake. For food and other sources, see Table 6-6. To investigate the vitamin content of a particular item, go to http://ndb.nal.usda.gov or to http://nutritiondata.self.com. For stability, see Table 6-2.

Use of corn as a staple food in the southeastern United States in the early 1900s caused **niacin** deficiency to reach epidemic proportions: 170,000 cases per year from 1910 to 1935 (Roman, 2014). Corn contains a relatively unavailable form of niacin that Native Americans counteracted by treating their maize with alkalis. That procedure was not conveyed to Europeans with the corn that Columbus introduced there, resulting in outbreaks of **pellagra** in Spain, Italy, and Egypt in the 1700s and 1800s (Kirkland, 2014). The disease was described in Spain in 1735 and named pellagra, from the Italian for "rough skin" in 1771 (Oldham and Ivkovic, 2012). In 1915, Dr. Joseph Goldberger conducted a clinical trial, inducing pellagra in prison populations and curing it with balanced diets or yeast supplements.

Niacin, vitamin B_3, is a generic term for nicotinic acid and nicotinamide, both of which provide the vitamin's actions (Gropper and Smith, 2013). Nicotinic acid was isolated in 1867, but its role as an active vitamin was not identified until 1937 (Kirkland, 2014).

ABSORPTION, METABOLISM, AND EXCRETION

Preformed niacin can be absorbed in the stomach but is more easily absorbed in the small intestine by carrier-mediated diffusion. Pharmaceutical doses (3 to 4 grams) are absorbed almost completely by passive diffusion (Gropper and Smith, 2013). Metabolism by the liver and excretion of excess in the urine is the usual pathway. The body does not have any appreciable stores of niacin (Oldham and Ivkovic, 2012).

Not all of the body's niacin has to come from preformed niacin in food. The liver can convert the essential amino acid tryptophan to niacin. The process also requires riboflavin, vitamin B_6, and iron so that deficiencies of those nutrients could impact niacin synthesis (Gropper and Smith, 2013). When tryptophan levels are low, protein synthesis is given a higher priority than niacin formation (Kirkland, 2014).

FUNCTIONS

Requisite for more than 200 enzymes, niacin is a coenzyme required for energy metabolism. Niacin also participates in the synthesis of steroid hormones and fatty acids.

Persons with schizophrenia display a diminished flushing response to topical niacin, which may indicate abnormalities in phospholipid metabolism. Those abnormalities may play a role in the etiology of schizophrenia, and possibly other psychiatric and neurological diseases (Nadalin, Buretić-Tomljanović, and Rubesa, 2010). Also, among patients with schizophrenia, reduced niacin sensitivity is associated with greater functional impairment (Messamore, 2012). New studies, controlling adequately for age, sex, drug abuse, diet, as well as genetic factors that may influence the intensity and reaction time, are necessary to clarify the usefulness of niacin testing in psychiatry (Nadalin et al, 2010).

DEFICIENCY

Pellagra is the deficiency disease caused by the lack of niacin. Symptomatic niacin deficiency can present as soon as 60 days after insufficient dietary intake. Currently, pellagra occurs most frequently in people with risk factors for malnutrition such as chronic alcohol intake, homelessness, AIDS, or absorption problems. Recently, three clients displayed delirium due to pellagrous **encephalopathy** presenting as alcohol withdrawal delirium, also known as delirium tremens or DTs (Oldham and Ivkovic, 2012). Pellagra has also occurred in clients with **anorexia nervosa** (Jagielska, Tomaszewicz-Libudzic, and Brzozowska, 2007; MacDonald and Forsyth, 2005). One case of pellagra-like dermatitis occurred in a 32-year-old woman 3 months after bariatric surgery (Ashourian and Mousdicas, 2006). See Box 6-3 for the clinical signs and symptoms of pellagra.

To have a deficiency, a person must consume a diet lacking in both niacin and tryptophan. Pellagra has serious effects and is fatal if untreated. With treatment, the dermatologic and gastrointestinal symptoms generally resolve within 48 hours, which can confirm the diagnosis. Neurocognitive symptoms may resolve within days or may persist (Oldham and Ivkovic, 2012).

SOURCES AND STABILITY

Food composition tables report only preformed niacin (Gropper and Smith, 2013). Certain assumptions were made in devising the DRIs to allow for niacin from preformed sources and from protein sources providing tryptophan to be converted to niacin. The measurement derived is a **niacin equivalent** (see Clinical Calculation 6-2). The conversion is not easily predictable because of low overall efficiency of the process in the liver as well as lesser efficiency with lower tryptophan intake (Kirkland, 2014). Likewise, liver function, supplies of riboflavin, vitamin B_6, and iron, and the body's need for protein synthesis would impact the conversion of tryptophan to niacin. Nevertheless, tryptophan provides about 50% of the niacin intake in the United States (Gropper and Smith, 2013). See Genomic Gem 6-4 for another impediment to tryptophan conversion to niacin.

Coffee and tea contain niacin and can prevent pellagra in cultures with low protein diets but high intakes of these beverages. A compound in coffee is converted to niacin by heat (with roasting) and acid (Gropper and Smith, 2013).

Box 6-3 ■ *Pellagra*

The "three Ds" are pellagra's major symptoms: dermatitis, diarrhea, and dementia. The fourth D is death. Diarrhea is certainly not unique to niacin deficiency but contributes to worsening nutritional status. The more characteristic symptoms of dermatitis and dementia can vary markedly from person to person, complicating the diagnostic process.

The sun-sensitive dermatitis is a red rash on exposed skin: the face, neck, arms, hands, and feet. The rash is bilaterally symmetrical with a definite border marking its beginning: on the hands and arms, the rash sometimes resembles gloves, on the feet, boots.

Clients may have hallucinations and display paranoid, suicidal, and aggressive behaviors. In epidemics of pellagra, it is likely that inmates in asylums were merely niacin deficient, without the dermatitis, and kept malnourished by the poor food provided. Eleven such residents of the Georgia State Sanitarium were cured of their dementia with a nutrient-rich diet, reported in a 1915 journal. Beginning in 1937, numerous reports of dramatic recoveries from dementia nearly overnight upon receiving nicotinic acid therapy, indicating niacin deficiency disrupts a short-term process such as neural transmission rather than causing degeneration of brain tissue (Kirkland, 2014).

Clinical Calculation 6-2

Niacin Equivalents (NEs)

1 NE = 1 milligram preformed niacin = 60 milligrams tryptophan

1 gram of complete protein is assumed to provide 10 milligrams of tryptophan.

For example, 1% milk fortified with vitamins A and D contains:

0.227 mg preformed niacin
8.22 g protein.

Then:

8.22 g protein × 10 mg tryptophan/g protein = 82.2 mg tryptophan

$$\frac{82.2 \text{ mg tryptophan}}{60 \text{ mg per NE}} = 1.37 \text{ NEs from tryptophan}$$

0.227 mg preformed + 1.37 NE *possible* from tryptophan = 1.6 NE per cup of milk

---

Genomic Gem 6-4

Hartnup Disease

This rare autosomal recessive disease was first described in 1956. Four of the eight family members of the Hartnup family of London had aminoaciduria, a skin rash resembling pellagra, and cerebellar ataxia (Patel and Prabhu, 2008).

The disease is caused by a mutation in a transporter gene that results in small bowel malabsorption of tryptophan, phenylalanine, methionine, and other amino acids. Amino acids retained within the intestinal lumen are converted by bacteria to compounds toxic to the nervous system (Patel and Prabhu, 2008).

Although the disorder is present from birth, it may not be manifested until childhood or early adulthood and may be precipitated by sunlight, fever, drugs, or other stressors. Poor nutritional intake nearly always precedes appearance of symptoms that result from niacin deficiency and resemble those of pellagra particularly the rash on parts of the body exposed to the sun. Neurologic manifestations include cerebellar ataxia and mental abnormalities. Intellectual disability, short stature, headache, and collapsing or fainting are common. The treatment is niacin supplements, and the prognosis is good (Brazy, 2010).

One case detailed a 10-year-old girl from a **consanguineous marriage,** who displayed all "three Ds." Initially she had *diarrhea* but then became confused and agitated (*dementia*) with a characteristic glove and boot *dermatitis*. Her skin, psychiatric symptoms, and diarrhea responded dramatically to niacin, and she was discharged after 7 days (Patel and Prabhu, 2008).

Despite its water solubility, only small amounts of niacin are lost in cooking water. Cooking accounts for no more than a 25% reduction in niacin owing to niacin's heat stability (Oldham and Ivkovic, 2012). It is the most environmentally stable vitamin.

TOXICITY

Pharmacological doses of niacin, given to lower blood cholesterol, cause flushing and over the long term can cause liver damage. Although serious hepatic toxicity from niacin administration has been reported, it is largely confined to the use of slow-release formulations given as unregulated nutritional supplements. Overall, the perception of pharmaceutical niacin side effects is often greater than the reality (Guyton and Bays, 2007).

Even reformulation of breakfast cereal to 100% of the RDA of vitamins, including niacin, has caused flushing and a rash in a person who consumed six cupsful for breakfast that contained almost 3.5 times the UL (Morse, Morse, and Patterson, 1999). A case of niacin toxicity from food is reported in Clinical Application 6-6. It explains how food poisoning outbreaks are investigated and how to preserve evidence.

Vitamin B₆

For DRIs, see Appendix A. For food and other sources, see Table 6-6. To investigate the vitamin content of a particular item, go to http://ndb.nal.usda.gov or to http://nutritiondata.self.com. For stability, see Table 6-2.

Vitamin B₆ was first reported in 1934, isolated in 1938, and synthesized 1939 (da Silva, Mackey, Davis, and Gregory, 2014). Vitamin B₆ serves in many roles, but no deficiency disease is associated with it. The name for the pharmaceutical preparation of vitamin B₆ is **pyridoxine.**

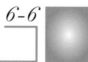

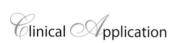

Clinical Application   6-6

Niacin Toxicity

In late 1980, almost half the residents of a small nursing home became flushed or developed a rash 15 to 30 minutes after breakfast. To diagnose the problem, the foods consumed were compared. Which food was eaten by all those who became ill but by none of those who did not become ill? The answer was cornmeal mush.

Careful observation and documentation of the sequence of signs and symptoms, which commonly disappear before the physician arrives, may steer the investigators in the right direction. In this nursing home, the signs and symptoms lasted only an average of 50 minutes.

If food poisoning is suspected, none of the food should be discarded before health authorities take samples to examine in the laboratory. The Food and Drug Administration tested the cornmeal from the nursing home's kitchen. It contained more than 1000 milligrams of niacin per pound compared with the recommended amount of 16 to 24 milligrams per pound. In this case, the offending food was identified but the method of contamination was never positively determined (Bartlett, Morris, and Spengler, 1982).

ABSORPTION, METABOLISM, AND EXCRETION

The body contains from 45 to 185 milligrams of vitamin B₆, 75% to 80% of it in the muscles. The vitamin is absorbed in the small intestine, mainly in the jejunum, with an overall absorption rate from the average U.S. diet of 75% (Gropper and Smith, 2013). The liver is the primary site for vitamin B₆ metabolism, which also requires riboflavin, niacin, and zinc (da Silva et al, 2014). Most excess vitamin is excreted in the urine, with little eliminated via the feces.

FUNCTIONS

Vitamin B₆ is a coenzyme in the metabolism of amino acids. It is involved in the metabolism of more than 100 enzymes, including those that synthesize niacin from tryptophan and heme for hemoglobin (Gropper and Smith, 2013). The importance of adequate vitamin B₆ status for proper immune function has been known for many years (da Silva et al, 2014).

DEFICIENCY

A deficiency of B₆ is unlikely in healthy people because large amounts are present in the general diet. Based on **NHANES** (National Health and Nutrition Examination Survey) plasma vitamin B₆ findings, however, certain subgroups of the population are at risk of suboptimal vitamin B₆ intake and status:

- Women of childbearing age
- Current and former oral contraceptive users
- Smokers
- Non-Hispanic Blacks
- Elderly individuals (Morris, Picciano, Jacques, and Selhub, 2008).

Furthermore, factors such as disease, drug interactions, or errors in food processing may cause an actual deficiency. In the 1950s, severe heat treatment of commercial infant formula produced vitamin B₆ deficiency–induced convulsive seizures that were cured by pyridoxine. As a result, fortification of infant formulas with pyridoxine became routine (da Silva et al, 2014).

Vitamin B₆ deficiency may become apparent in 2 to 3 weeks but may take up to 2½ months to appear. Clinically, a person with a vitamin B₆ deficiency may present with these signs and symptoms:

- Rash on face, neck, shoulders, and buttocks
- Mouth lesions
- Fatigue and weakness
- Confusion
- Peripheral neuropathy

Interference with heme production may lead to a hypochromic, microcytic anemia (see Chapter 7). Infants are prone to seizures and convulsions (Gropper and Smith, 2013), as are adults with liver disease. Three such men did not respond to conventional antiepileptic medications, but their seizures resolved within 2 days of pyridoxine supplementation (Gerlach, Thomas, Stawicki, et al, 2011). Vitamin B_6 deficiency may also cause niacin deficiency because of impaired tryptophan metabolism (Roman, 2014).

SOURCES AND STABILITY

Vitamin B_6 is widely distributed in foods. Those of animal origin are the best sources but whole grains, vegetables, some fruits, nuts, and fortified cereals are major contributors of vitamin B_6 to the diet. Much of the vitamin can be lost through prolonged heating (sterilizing and canning) and through milling and refining of grain (Gropper and Smith, 2013).

TOXICITY

No adverse effects of vitamin B_6 from foods have been reported. Long-term intake of pharmacologic doses of pyridoxine, greater than 500 milligrams per day, is associated with a risk of sensory neuropathies (da Silva et al, 2014). High intakes also appear to cause degeneration of neurons in the spinal cord (Gropper and Smith, 2013).

Folate

For DRIs, see Appendix A. For food and other sources, see Table 6-6. To investigate the vitamin content of a particular item, go to http://ndb.nal.usda.gov or to http://nutritiondata.self.com. For stability, see Table 6-2.

Folate (also known as vitamin B_9) and vitamin B_{12} were discovered during the search for the reason that eating liver cured **megaloblastic anemia.** Folic acid was discovered as a factor in yeast in 1931 and was later isolated from spinach leaves and named from the Italian for "foliage." By 1945, folic acid had been synthesized (Stover, 2014).

The term for this nutrient as it occurs in foods and body tissues is **folate.** The oxidized and more stable form used to fortify foods and in supplements is **folic acid.** Total body folate levels are estimated to range from 11 to 28 milligrams, about half of which is stored in the liver. Because red blood cells (RBCs) acquire folate only when being formed, RBC folate concentrations reflect longer-term (2 to 3 months) folate status than plasma levels do (Gropper and Smith, 2013).

ABSORPTION, METABOLISM, AND EXCRETION

The **bioavailability** of folate from a mixed diet is approximately 50% but rises to about 85% when fortified foods are included. Folic acid supplements are 100% bioavailable if consumed on an empty stomach (Gropper and Smith, 2013). Enzymes in the jejunal and pancreatic secretions and bile convert the folate in foods to the absorbable form used in fortified foods

and supplements, which is then absorbed in the acid environment of the upper small intestine and transported to the liver. In the liver, some of the folate is processed for storage in the tissues or the liver and some is secreted into bile.

When the gallbladder releases bile into the duodenum, folate may again be split off and absorbed. This recycling process, which may account for 100 micrograms of reabsorbed folate daily, is important in allowing folate stores to be adequate for 2 to 4 months, compared with 1 to 4 weeks for thiamin stores. Excretion of folate occurs via the urine and a minimal amount through the bile into feces. Most of the folate found in feces is of bacterial origin (Gropper and Smith, 2013).

FUNCTIONS

Folate is involved in protein synthesis, including that of amino acids, **DNA, RNA,** and heme. Thus, folate participates in the reproduction of every cell and is particularly necessary for rapidly growing cells, including those in the gastrointestinal tract, blood, and fetal tissue where the absence of adequate amounts becomes clinically and often catastrophically apparent. See the Toxicity section for a relationship to cancer.

DEFICIENCY

Poor dietary intake is the most common cause of folate deficiency especially when coupled with abuse of alcohol that causes intestinal malabsorption, decreased hepatic uptake, and increased excretion, mainly via the urine. Decreased serum folic acid may occur in 80% of persons with alcoholism (Cylwik and Chrostek, 2011).

Other clients at risk are those with gastrointestinal diseases marked by malabsorption and with increased losses due to hemodialysis. In addition, five inborn errors affecting folate transport and metabolism have been identified (Watkins and Rosenblatt, 2012).

Folate deficiency results in impaired cell division and protein synthesis, including the faulty synthesis of red blood cells. Concentrations in the RBCs are diminished after about 3 to 4 months of low folate intake, and in about 4 to 5 months, megaloblastic anemia occurs (Gropper and Smith, 2013). In addition to laboratory blood changes, a client may have these signs and symptoms of folate deficiency:

- Bright red tongue
- Fatigue and weakness
- Headaches, irritability
- Shortness of breath
- Heart palpitations

DIETARY REFERENCE INTAKES

Folate RDAs and AIs are given in dietary folate equivalents (DFEs).

One DFE equals

- 1 microgram of food folate
- 0.6 microgram of folic acid from fortified food or as a supplement consumed with food
- 0.5 microgram of a supplement taken on an empty stomach (Gropper and Smith, 2013)

Foods that provide at least 40 micrograms of folate per serving are permitted by the FDA to make the health claim: "Healthful diets with adequate folate may reduce a woman's risk of having a child with a neural tube (brain or spinal cord) defect."

SOURCES AND STABILITY

Green, leafy vegetables, for which the nutrient is named, are good sources as are fruits, legumes, and liver that started the search for the vitamin because of its curative powers (see Table 6-6).

In 1998, the United States and Canada began mandatory fortification of flours, grains, and cereals with folic acid (140 micrograms per 100 grams of product) to prevent neural tube defects (see Chapter 10). Those products are now major sources of the vitamin (Gropper and Smith, 2013). By 2009, 51 countries had mandatory wheat flour fortification programs that included folic acid. In the United States and Canada, estimates show that the additional intake of about 100 to 150 micrograms per day of folic acid through food fortification has been effective in reducing the prevalence of neural tube defects and increasing blood folate concentrations (Berry, Bailey, Mulinare, et al, 2010). Still, the mechanism through which folate affects neural tube development is unclear (Gropper and Smith, 2013).

From 50% to 80% of folate in foods is lost through processing and preparation (Gropper and Smith, 2013). Folate is destroyed by heat, oxidation, ultraviolet light, and acids. To minimize losses, folate-rich foods should be eaten raw or cooked quickly in small amounts of water.

INTERFERING FACTORS

Folic acid does not require digestion, but folate does. Zinc deficiency impairs an enzyme that digests folate. Alcohol ingestion and inhibitors in legumes, lentils, cabbage, and oranges also diminish digestive enzyme activity, hence the absorption of folate (Gropper and Smith, 2013). Folate can also be impaired by deficiencies of nutrients required for its metabolism: riboflavin and vitamins B_6 and B_{12} (Stover, 2014).

Methotrexate, an anticancer drug, is a folate antagonist. Its purpose is to interfere with DNA in cancer cells, but it simultaneously affects normal cells. Other anticancer (5-fluorouracil) and antimicrobial agents that target folate-requiring enzymes have been developed (Stover, 2014). See Chapter 15 for details on the interaction of folic acid and medications.

TOXICITY

No adverse effects of folate from food or folic acid from supplements have been reported. The UL of 1000 micrograms of synthetic folic acid from supplements and fortified foods, not natural foods, has been set to avoid masking signs of pernicious anemia (Gropper and Smith, 2013). See vitamin B_{12} discussion.

Folate intakes of 15 times the UL (15,000 micrograms) have been associated with insomnia, irritability, and gastrointestinal distress. Supplemental folic acid at doses from 800 to 5000 micrograms have been shown to increase cancer risk and cancer mortality (Gropper and Smith, 2013).

Vitamin B_{12} (Cobalamin)

For DRIs, see Appendix A. Persons older than 50 years are counseled to obtain vitamin B_{12} from fortified foods or supplements because 10% to 30% of older people have changes in the gastrointestinal tract that limit the absorption of the vitamin from foods. For food and other sources, see Table 6-6. To investigate the vitamin content of a particular item, go to http://ndb.nal.usda.gov or to http://nutritiondata.self.com. For stability, see Table 6-2.

In 1926, eating large amounts of liver was shown to effectively treat **pernicious anemia,** but **vitamin B_{12}** was not isolated until 1948 (Gropper and Smith, 2013). Both of those achievements obtained Nobel Prizes for the scientists (Carmel, 2014). Vitamin B_{12}, also called cobalamin, is an essential coenzyme in the synthesis of DNA, RNA, and **myelin** and is necessary for normal red blood cell formation. Vitamin B_{12} is stored to a greater extent than the other B vitamins, but diverse causes can precipitate vitamin B_{12} deficiency.

ABSORPTION, METABOLISM, AND EXCRETION

Cobalamins in foods must be liberated from the proteins to which they are attached in foods, a digestive process using gastric acid and pepsin in the stomach. Efficient absorption of vitamin B_{12} also requires an explicit protein-binding factor called **intrinsic factor (IF),** secreted by the gastric mucosal cells in the stomach. Intrinsic factor combines with vitamin B_{12}, also called **extrinsic factor,** in the proximal small intestine to protect vitamin B_{12} from digestive enzymes and intestinal bacteria until the complex reaches the ileum, where the vitamin is absorbed about 4 hours after ingestion. If the intrinsic factor system is working, more than 50% of the cobalamin in a typical meal will be absorbed, but the intrinsic factor system is limited to about 2 micrograms of cobalamin at a time. Larger doses such as those found in supplements are absorbed by passive diffusion at a rate of about 1% to 2% (Carmel, 2014).

Vitamin B_{12} is not freely absorbed. The amount absorbed depends on the body's storage levels and the amount ingested. At low levels of intake, a large amount of the vitamin is absorbed and vice versa. In addition, in healthy persons, the vitamin can be recycled from bile and intestinal secretions before the remainder is excreted in feces. The intestinal-liver recycling provides about 3 to 8 micrograms of vitamin B_{12} per day (Gropper and Smith, 2013). Thus, a person's stores of vitamin B_{12} last from 3 to 5 years. The principal storage site is the liver, which contains 50% of the body's estimated 2500 microgram supply (Carmel, 2014).

FUNCTIONS

Vitamin B_{12} is a coenzyme in the synthesis of DNA and RNA and the metabolism of amino acids and fatty acids. Vitamin B_{12} is also essential for the synthesis and maintenance of myelin, the fatty insulation that permits speedy transmission of impulses along the nerves.

SOURCES

Vitamin B_{12} is synonymous with animal products that have derived their cobalamins from microorganisms. Healthy young adults who regularly consume meat, fish, poultry, milk, cheese, or eggs are not at risk of vitamin B_{12} deficiency. Bioavailability from meals varies from 40% to 89% (Gropper and Smith, 2013). Milk and cobalamin-fortified cereals are efficient sources in the United States diet and fish in the Norwegian diet, all three exceeding meats in bioavailability of the vitamin (Carmel, 2014).

Plants are negligible sources of cobalamin, but dried green and purple algae may contain bioavailable vitamin (Carmel, 2014). Some plant foods may contain vitamin B_{12} from bacterial contamination or, in the case of legumes, from the nitrogen-fixing bacteria on their roots. For strict vegetarians, nutritional yeast and vitamin B_{12}-fortified products (soymilk or tofu) are more appropriate food sources than reliance on bacterial contamination.

The vitamin is fairly stable, resistant to light, heat, and oxidation (Gropper and Smith, 2013). Products that list vitamin B_{12} rather than cobalamin as an ingredient may include nonbioavailable sources (Centers for Disease Control, 2003).

DEFICIENCY

Sixteen percent of healthy individuals aged over 65 years have been shown to have a deficiency of vitamin B_{12} (Wagner, Schatz, Coston, et al, 2011). Deficiency of Vitamin B_{12} is a common cause of neuropsychiatric symptoms in elderly persons, with most cases caused by malabsorption (Lachner, Steinle, and Regenold, 2012). Persons may be at increased risk of vitamin B_{12} deficiency because of gastrointestinal or dietary causes.

Gastrointestinal Causes

AFFECTING ALL COBALAMIN. When a person lacks intrinsic factor, the result is a condition called **pernicious anemia,** a complex, autoimmune, multifactorial disease (Banka, Ryan, Thomson, and Newman, 2011). The prevalence of this **autoimmune disease** increases with age and is attributed to autoimmune antibodies against both gastric parietal cells and intrinsic factor. Its prevalence is 0.1% in the general population and 1.9% in persons over the age of 60 years. Of vitamin B_{12} deficiencies in adults, 20% to 50% are caused by pernicious anemia (Andres and Serraj, 2012).

Susceptibility appears to be genetically determined, although the mode of inheritance remains unknown. Evidence for the role of genetic factors includes familial occurrence of pernicious anemia and its association with other autoimmune diseases (Andres and Serraj, 2012). Pernicious anemia usually is manifested after middle age, especially in persons with prematurely gray hair and blue eyes (Heimburger, 2014).

Pernicious anemia can also occur after the surgical removal of the stomach or a large portion of the stomach. In those cases, the cause is not autoimmune interference but missing tissue to produce intrinsic factor. Only 15% to 30% of these clients display clinical deficiency of vitamin B_{12}, however, and most postgastrectomy deficiencies are limited to food-bound cobalamin (Carmel, 2014) as detailed subsequently.

Intestinal diseases can cause severe intrinsic-factor-related malabsorption of vitamin B_{12} in the ileum. Some of those acquired causes are intestinal parasites, surgical alteration of the ileum, radiation therapy, **celiac disease,** and **Crohn disease** (see Chapter 20).

AFFECTING FOOD-BOUND COBALAMIN. The chief etiology of vitamin B_{12} deficiency in elderly persons is food-cobalamin malabsorption (Andres and Serraj, 2012). In this condition, cobalamin's release from food is impaired. Because gastric acid facilitates separation of vitamin B_{12} from the foods containing it, vitamin B_{12} deficiency can be caused by conditions that decrease gastric acid such as gastric or bariatric surgery. Similarly, prolonged use of medications that neutralize gastric acid or block its production can impair vitamin B_{12} status.

Dietary Causes

Vitamin B_{12} deficiency can be caused by a diet devoid of animal products. People particularly at risk are the elderly who choose tea and toast for meals, persons with alcoholism who eat poorly, and vegetarians. The latter develop B_{12} depletion or deficiency regardless of demographic characteristics, place of residency, age, or type of vegetarian diet and should regularly take supplements containing cobalamin (Pawlak, Parrott, Raj, et al, 2013).

Of particular concern are vegan mothers with subclinical vitamin B_{12} deficiencies whose breastfed babies have developed severe neurological problems. Two breastfed children in Georgia, aged 15 and 30 months, were initially evaluated for failure to thrive, which was eventually diagnosed as neurological impairment due to maternal cobalamin deficiency (Centers for Disease Control, 2003). In Italy, an exclusively breastfed 5-month-old male infant presented with anemia, poor growth, and developmental delay. He was born after a normal full-term pregnancy to a vegan mother who took a multivitamin oral preparation during the second and third trimesters but not during lactation. The infant was treated with packed red blood cells, intramuscular vitamin B_{12} injections, and iron supplementation. Within a few days, his hematological parameters rapidly improved, but his development was still retarded 7 months after beginning treatment (Guez, Chiarelli, Menni, et al, 2012).

In an adult case, a 33-year-old man who had been a strict vegetarian for many years without taking vitamin supplements became irreversibly blind as a result of severe bilateral optic neuropathy. The condition was attributed to deficiencies of vitamin B_{12} and thiamin (Milea, Cassoux, and LeHoang, 2000).

SIGNS AND SYMPTOMS

Symptoms of vitamin B_{12} deficiency can be seen in the circulatory and nervous systems; however, some clients display only one or the other. Circulatory symptoms include megaloblastic anemia and result in these signs and symptoms:

- Fatigue
- Pallor
- Shortness of breath
- Heart palpitations

Neurological manifestations include these signs and symptoms that may be irreparable:

- Numbness and tingling in the extremities
- Abnormal gait and poor coordination of movements
- Memory loss, disorientation
- Psychosis and dementia (Gropper and Smith, 2013)

The neurological problems occur in 75% to 90% of clients with vitamin B_{12} deficiency, but the mechanism for many of the neurologic changes is not clear (Gropper and Smith, 2013). A case of acute dementia in a 52-year-old client caused by vitamin B_{12} deficiency without other symptoms led the researchers to recommend screening psychiatric clients for vitamin B_{12} and folate deficiencies regardless of age or previous health status (Lerner and Kanevsky, 2002).

Diagnosing vitamin B_{12} deficiency by examining red blood cells is difficult in persons consuming ample folate because folate enables the continued manufacturing of red blood cells in the correct size and number. Folic acid cannot maintain myelin, however. As a result

of the inability to diagnose the deficiency quickly, the neurological deterioration of pernicious anemia continues unabated.

Data are insufficient to determine whether fortification of grains with folic acid has compromised early diagnosis of cobalamin deficiency or worsened its neurological pathology (Carmel, 2014). An additional concern that has been raised is the increased risk of cognitive impairment in U.S. subjects older than 59 years who have high serum folate concentrations combined with low vitamin B_{12} status (Brouwer and Verhoef, 2007).

Folic acid supplementation in a person with sickle cell anemia, however, did result in a delayed diagnosis of pernicious anemia that had progressed to neuropsychiatric symptoms before being identified (Dhar, Bellevue, and Carmel, 2003). In all, four cases of pernicious anemia complicating sickle cell disease have been reported leading to a suggestion to reconsider routine folate supplementation in sickle cell disease in the era of folic acid fortification. At the least, periodic screening of cobalamin levels in patients taking folic acid is prudent (Carmel, Bellevue, and Kelman, 2010).

TREATMENT

In most countries, treatment of vitamin B_{12} deficiency related to pernicious anemia is intramuscular injections of cobalamin particularly for clients with severe neurological forms of the disease (Andres and Serraj, 2012). The pharmaceutical names for vitamin B_{12} are **cyanocobalamin** and **hydroxocobalamin.** Allergic reactions have occurred rarely but can be severe (Carmel, 2014).

Oral cobalamin should be reserved for clients with only hematological manifestations of vitamin B_{12} deficiency and can be useful in patients undergoing anticoagulant or antiplatelet agent therapy in whom intramuscular injections are contraindicated (Andres and Serraj, 2012). An intranasal product is also available (Vallerand, Sanoski, and Deglin, 2013).

INTERFERING FACTORS

Excessive intake of alcohol or vitamin C interfere with vitamin B_{12} absorption and utilization. The body's use of vitamin B_{12} is also impaired by a deficiency of vitamin B_6 and by antacids.

TOXICITY

No toxicity from vitamin B_{12} has been recorded from food or supplements or from parenteral doses to clients with pernicious anemia. Neither has any benefit been noted from excessive intake in persons with adequate vitamin status (Gropper and Smith, 2013).

Table 6-2 lists factors affecting the stability of the 13 vitamins described thus far. Table 6-6 summarizes the information on the nine water-soluble vitamins.

Other Essential Nutrients

Three additional nutrients are so widely distributed in foods that only special circumstances have produced deficiencies. Long-term **parenteral nutrition (PN)** is one such situation. That therapy is detailed in Chapter 14. Two are vitamins and the third technically is not a vitamin, but all three appear in the DRI tables for vitamins.

For DRIs, see Appendix A. To investigate the pantothenic acid or choline content of a particular item, go to http:// nutritiondata.self.com/tools.nutrient-search or to www.nal .usda.gov/fnic/foodcomp/Data/Choline/Choline.html. Partial data on biotin content of foods is available at www.ncbi. nlm.nih.gov/pmc/articles/PMC1450323.

PANTOTHENIC ACID

This vitamin's name is derived from Greek for "everywhere" because it is widely found in nature. **Pantothenic acid** was isolated in 1931, its structure determined in 1939, and it was synthesized in 1940. Not until 1954 was it categorized as essential to human nutrition (Carmel, 2014).

Pantothenic acid serves as a coenzyme in fatty acid metabolism and many other metabolic and regulatory processes. Because it is present to some extent in all foods, pantothenic acid deficiency is rare except in severe malnutrition. No cases of deficiency have been documented in people who eat a variety of foods, but deficiencies have occurred in prisoner-of-war camps and have been produced experimentally (Trumbo, 2014). *Burning feet syndrome* with numbness and burning sensation in the feet is thought to result from pantothenic acid deficiency because it is corrected by supplementation (Gropper and Smith, 2013).

Most adults in the United States consume 4 to 7 milligrams per day, of which about 50% is absorbed, principally in the jejunum. The vitamin is excreted intact, primarily in the urine. People with diabetes mellitus (Chapter 17), alcoholism, and inflammatory bowel diseases (Chapter 20) may have an increased need for pantothenic acid. Animals' intestinal microorganisms synthesize pantothenic acid, but this source in humans is unknown (Trumbo, 2014), Good food sources include meats, egg yolk, yogurt, and mushrooms. No toxicities have been reported, but intakes of 15 to 20 grams have been associated with mild intestinal distress (Gropper and Smith, 2013).

BIOTIN

In 1931, a substance in liver was recognized as curing a syndrome called *egg white injury*. In the early 1940s, the structure of biotin was determined (Gropper and Smith, 2013). As a coenzyme is the synthesis of fat, glycogen, and amino acids, **biotin** is an essential nutrient because bacterial synthesis in the large intestine is insufficient to meet a person's needs. Dietary biotin is absorbed primarily in the jejunum, and small amounts are stored in the muscle, liver, and brain. Smoking seems to accelerate catabolism in women, and excretion mainly occurs via the urine (Gropper and Smith, 2013).

Biotin deficiency appears to be common during normal human pregnancy with fetal concentrations six times higher than the mother's. In animals, biotin deficiency causes birth defects, particularly cleft palates. Yet biotin is one of few essential nutrients omitted from prenatal vitamins (Perry and Caudill, 2012).

Meat, fish, poultry, eggs, and dairy products are rich dietary sources of biotin, but accuracy in estimating dietary biotin is limited both by data gaps in food composition tables and by inaccuracies in published data (Staggs, Sealey, McCabe, et al, 2004). Table 6-7 lists good food sources of biotin.

Deficiencies have been caused by parenteral nutrition that omitted biotin but also in children with an autosomal recessive inborn error of biotin metabolism. Biotin deficiency may develop in persons with alcoholism or gastrointestinal diseases and those on long-term anticonvulsant therapy or kidney dialysis. Symptoms include **alopecia,** a scaly, red rash around the eyes, nose, and mouth, **paresthesias** of the extremities, depression, and hallucinations (Gropper and Smith, 2013). Before biotin was permitted to be added to infant formulas in Japan beginning in 2003, infants affected with biotin deficiency developed intractable chronic diarrhea. Exact mechanisms producing the signs and symptoms in deficiency states are not clear. Bioavailability of pharmaceutical biotin is approximately 100% (Mock, 2014).

Toxicity has not been reported. Use of biotin as a hair and skin conditioner has been judged to be safe (Gropper and Smith, 2013).

Avidin, a protein in raw egg white that is thought to serve as a **bacteriostat,** interferes with biotin absorption by irreversibly binding with it. Excessive consumption of raw egg whites has caused biotin deficiency. Cooking the egg white inactivates avidin and thus eliminates the risk (Mock, 2014).

TABLE 6-7 ■ Selected Food Sources of Biotin	
	MICROGRAMS
Chicken liver, cooked, 3 oz	159
Beef liver, cooked, 3 oz	35.5
Egg, whole, cooked, 1 large	10
Salmon, pink, canned in water, 3 oz	5.03
Peanuts, roasted, salted, 1 oz	5.01
Pork chop, cooked, 3 oz	3.82
Sweet potato, cooked, 1 cup	3.33

Source: Data from Perry and Caudill, 2012.

CHOLINE

Choline was discovered in 1862, synthesized in 1866, but not recognized as essential for humans until 1998 because investigators thought the body manufactured sufficient amounts of the substance. Although the liver synthesizes choline, the gene for the enzyme catalyzing the synthesis is induced by estrogen. Thus **endogenous** production is inadequate for most men and post-menopausal women (Zeisel, 2014).

Choline is essential for liver and brain function, lipid metabolism, and cellular membrane composition and repair. It plays a critical role throughout the life cycle, beginning with fetal brain and spinal cord development (Caudill, de Costa, Zeisel, and Hornick, 2011). Choline is a part of the neurotransmitter **acetylcholine** and of **phospholipids** that are structural components of all human cell membranes. Although not a vitamin by strict definition, choline has been given an AI and is listed in the DRIs with the vitamins. Choline is widely distributed in foods, with the best sources being liver, eggs, beef, and pork. A varied diet should provide enough choline for most people, but vegetarians who consume no milk or eggs may be at risk of inadequate choline intake (Linus Pauling Institute, 2009). Although choline is available as a supplement, many multivitamins and prenatal vitamins do not contain choline (Caudill, de Costa, Zeisel, and Hornick, 2011).

Deficiency of choline produces liver and muscle damage that is resolved when choline is restored to the diet (Zeisel, 2014).

Effects of excessive intake (10 to 16 grams per day) include sweating, salivation, vomiting, and a fishy body odor. The last is due to excessive production and excretion of trimethylamine, a metabolite of choline (Linus Pauling Institute, 2009).

Analysis of the vitamins in foods at http://nutrition-data.self.com may list betaine, a choline metabolite, which cannot be converted to choline but may reduce choline requirements. Plant-derived foods can be rich sources of betaine (named after beets), but only membrane-rich plant components such as wheat germ contain significant amounts of choline (Zeisel, 2014).

Table 6-8 lists the sources of vitamins by food groups to clarify the potential for inadequate intake if a person excludes an entire food group.

Vitamin Supplements

Vitamin supplements are not intended as substitutes for a healthy diet mainly because foods contain many nutrients and phytochemicals in addition to vitamins.

TABLE 6-8 ■ Good Sources of Vitamins by Food Groups

VITAMIN	SYNTHESIS/MISCELLANEOUS	MEATS	MILK	FRUITS/VEGETABLES	GRAINS
A		Liver Egg yolk	Fortified	Deep yellow, dark green leafy	
D	In skin	Saltwater fish	Fortified		Fortified cereals
E				Sunflower, safflower, canola oils Nuts Leafy vegetables	Wheat germ Whole grains Fortified cereals
K	In intestine			Green leafy Canola, soybean oils	
C				Fresh fruit, especially citrus Vegetables	
Thiamin		Pork Beef liver Salmon		Black beans	Wheat germ Fortified cereals
Riboflavin		Meats, esp. liver Eggs	Milk		Fortified cereals
Niacin	Coffee Tea	Meat Fish Poultry			Whole or enriched grains Fortified cereals
B6		Sirloin steak Salmon Chicken breast		Bananas Nuts Broccoli Carrots	Whole grains Fortified cereals
Folate Folic Acid		Liver		Dried peas, beans, lentils Dark green leafy Peanuts	Fortified grain products Whole grains Wheat germ

(continued)

TABLE 6-8 ■ Good Sources of Vitamins by Food Groups (Continued)

VITAMIN	SYNTHESIS/MISCELLANEOUS	MEATS	MILK	FRUITS/VEGETABLES	GRAINS
B$_{12}$		Meat Fish Poultry Eggs	Milk Cheese	Fortified soymilk, tofu	
Pantothenic Acid	Possibly in intestine	Liver Chicken Egg yolk	Yogurt	Mushrooms Broccoli Potatoes	Whole grain cereals
Biotin	In intestine	Liver Egg yolk Salmon		Soybeans Peanuts Sweet potato	
Choline	In liver	Liver Eggs Beef Pork	Milk Yogurt	Baked beans Broccoli	Wheat germ

Knowledge of vitamins and the foods containing them is constantly evolving. The single piece of advice given most frequently in the conclusions of researchers, however, is the admonition to eat five servings of fruits and vegetables every day. Fruit eaten out-of-hand is the original fast food (Fig. 6-5).

No U.S. government health agency, private health group, or health professional organization promotes regular use of a multivitamin/mineral supplement or individual nutrients without first considering the quality of a person's diet (National Institutes of Health, January 7, 2013). For certain groups of people, fortified foods or supplements are recommended. As indicated in this chapter, synthetic vitamins in fortified food or supplements are recommended for women capable of becoming pregnant (folic acid) and individuals older than 50 years (vitamin B$_{12}$). In addition, vegans should ensure that their intakes of vitamin B$_{12}$ from fortified foods or supplements are adequate (National Institutes of Health, January 7, 2013). The American Academy of Pediatrics recommends infants receive vitamin D supplements until consuming 1 liter per day of vitamin D–fortified milk or formula (Wagner and Greer, 2008). For community-dwelling adults aged 65 years or older who are at increased risk for falls, the U.S. Preventive Services Task Force recommends exercise or physical therapy and vitamin D supplementation to prevent falls (Moyer and U.S. Preventive Services Task Force, 2012).

Individuals wishing to take supplements should consider taking a multivitamin instead of a medley of single vitamins and should not exceed 100% of the RDA/AIs. The risks of using RDA-level multivitamins appear minimal and the cost is low, especially when compared with the price of fresh fruits and vegetables (Willett and Stampfer, 2014). An RDA/AI amount of multivitamins will prevent deficiency in healthy individuals, and toxicity is unlikely. When choosing a vitamin product, people should select one tailored to their age, gender, and situation (e.g., pregnancy). For instance, prenatal supplements generally provide no vitamin A as retinol (National Institutes of Health, January 7, 2013). In any event, vitamin taking should be reported to health-care providers along with medication history.

Although not a major expense for individuals, sales of multivitamin/mineral supplements in 2011 in the United States totaled $5.2 billion. Supplement users also tend to have higher micronutrient intakes from their diets than do nonusers. Consequently, the populations at highest risk of nutritional inadequacy who might benefit the most from multivitamin/ mineral supplements are the least likely to take them (National Institutes of Health, January 7, 2013). Multivitamins are sold in many formulations. Dollars & Sense 6-1 suggests considerations when shopping for multivitamins.

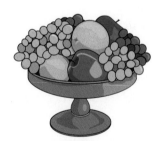

The Original Fast Food

FIGURE 6-5 Fruits eaten out-of-hand are the original fast foods and healthy choices.

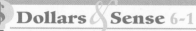

$ Dollars & Sense 6-1

Brand-Name versus Generic Multivitamins

Reading the label, although a necessary first step, does not automatically indicate the best choice of a supplement. Tests of 60 multivitamins sold in the United States and Canada found the following:

- Eight contained less of an ingredient than the label claimed
- Two contained more than claimed
- One failed to properly disintegrate
- Three listed ingredients in ways that did not comply with U.S. Food and Drug Administration requirements.

In addition, many products contained levels of vitamins or minerals that exceed Tolerable Upper Intake Levels, potentially increasing the risk of side effects. Surprisingly, there was almost no connection between price and quality (Consumer Lab, 2012). For reasons that will be clarified in Chapter 15, vitamin supplements produced by a pharmaceutical manufacturer are the best choices.

Centrum, recommended for adults under 50 years of age, sold for $8.99 for 100 tablets (9 cents each) on the same day that Walgreens A Thru Z Multivitamin/Multimineral sold for $7.29 for 130 tablets (5.6 cents each). At these prices, a year's supply of the Walgreen brand would save $12.41 for each person over the Centrum product. Greater savings might be had if larger quantities were purchased, but that is not always the case. Sometimes larger amounts of an item cost more per unit than smaller amounts. It pays to shop carefully.

Keystones

- Vitamins are organic substances required by the body in minute quantities and that do not become part of the structure of the body.
- Vitamins A, D, E, and K are fat soluble and require sufficient dietary fat intake and adequate fat digestion for proper utilization. The water-soluble vitamins, C and the B-complex vitamins, are not stored in the body in appreciable amounts, requiring more frequent intake than fat-soluble ones.
- Deficiency of vitamin A results in xerophthalmia and night blindness, and deficiency of vitamin D causes rickets and osteomalacia.
- Vitamins C, B_{12}, thiamin, and niacin have specific diseases associated with deficiency: scurvy, pernicious anemia, beriberi, and pellagra.
- Vitamin K is present in green leafy vegetables and canola and soybean oils; vitamin C in fresh vegetables and fruit, especially citrus.
- Enrichment is the restoration to a product of nutrients that were lost during processing. Fortification is the addition of nutrients not normally present in a food to increase its nutritional value.
- Pregnant women should avoid excessive intake of preformed vitamin A from foods or supplements because of risk to the fetus. Excessive vitamin D from supplements or multiple fortified foods may be hazardous to children.
- Good sources of vitamins A and C are broccoli, cantaloupe, and red pepper.
- People who take vitamins should limit their intake to 100% of the RDA in a multivitamin product, except individuals with special needs.
- Two large groups of people for whom synthetic vitamins in fortified food or supplements are recommended are women capable of becoming pregnant (folic acid) and individuals older than 50 years (vitamin B_{12}).

CASE STUDY *6-1*

Mr. J, a 79-year-old widowed man, prides himself on caring for himself during the past year since his wife died. His typical meal pattern is as follows:

- Breakfast—egg, toast, jam, coffee
- Lunch—cheese or lunchmeat sandwich, tea
- Dinner—canned stew or hash

Although Mr. J has a refrigerator, he avoids buying fresh fruits or vegetables. He says he has difficulty consuming produce before it spoils. He seldom goes out to eat.

For the past few months, Mr. J has noticed that his gums are tender. He stopped wearing his dentures when his gums began to bleed.

The visiting nurse confirmed inflammation of the gums. When the nurse took Mr. J's blood pressure, she noted a red, flat rash on Mr. J's forearm.

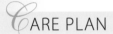ARE PLAN

Subjective Data

Sore gums   ■   Diet lacks fresh fruits and vegetables

Objective Data

Inflamed gums   ■   Erythematous **petechiae** related to blood pressure measurement

Analysis

Possible vitamin C deficiency related to lack of fresh fruit and vegetables as evidenced by sore bleeding gums and petechiae after sphygmomanometer use.

Plan

DESIRED OUTCOMES EVALUATION CRITERIA	ACTIONS/INTERVENTIONS	RATIONALE
Will consume foods containing 90 mg of vitamin C every day within 3 days	Teach the importance of daily vitamin C	Little vitamin C is stored in the body; should be consumed nearly every day
	Explore the acceptability of good sources of vitamin C; list amounts necessary to obtain 90 mg; recommend purchasing small quantities	Foods would be better sources than vitamin supplements because food also supplies other nutrients
	If the client selects frozen vegetables, teach to boil water 1 minute before adding vegetables and to cook quickly until crisp-tender	Heat and oxygen destroy vitamin C
	Follow up in 3 days; report to primary care provider if unimproved	

Three days later, the nurse determined that Mr. J had not been grocery shopping, and his bleeding gums and petechiae persisted. After telephone consultation with his physician, she instructed Mr. J to have the vitamin C blood test the physician ordered and to visit the doctor the following week.

6-1

Physician's Notes

The following Physician's Notes are representative of the documentation found in a client's medical record.

When the doctor saw Mr. J, he wrote the following:

Chief complaint: Referred by home health regarding possible vitamin C deficiency

Subjective: Unsure of reason for visit. "Sent by nurse."

Objective: Gingival hypertrophy and inflammation, recent bruising on extremities

Serum ascorbic acid level 0.15 milligrams per 100 milliliters

Analysis: Scurvy

Plan: Replete vitamin C levels with ascorbic acid: 1 gram per day for 5 days, then 500 milligrams per day until normal levels achieved.

Follow up in 2 weeks

Critical Thinking Questions

1. Is this the end of Mr. J's nutritional problems? What additional assessment data would be helpful as you continue to work with Mr. J?

2. Why do you think Mr. J did not follow the nurse's initial advice?

3. Even after the physician prescribes vitamin C, why is it important to improve Mr. J's food intake?

Chapter Review

1. Which of the following vitamins are water soluble?
   a. A and C
   b. A, D, E, and K
   c. B and C
   d. B, D, E, and K

2. The vitamin that is essential to the synthesis of several blood clotting factors is:
   a. Vitamin A
   b. Vitamin B$_6$
   c. Vitamin C
   d. Vitamin K

3. Which of the following groups of foods would be the best sources of carotene?
   a. Apricots, cantaloupe, and squash
   b. Asparagus, beets, and sweet potatoes
   c. Broccoli, lettuce, and lima beans
   d. Lemons, oranges, and strawberries

4. Deficiency of vitamin D causes:
   a. Rickets
   b. Pellagra
   c. Night blindness
   d. Beriberi

5. In general, individuals who elect to take a vitamin supplement should:
   a. Buy the most economical product
   b. Limit the amounts to 100% of RDA levels
   c. Obtain a physician's prescription
   d. Select the most advertised product

Clinical Analysis

1. Ms. C is bringing her 3-month-old baby girl to the well-baby clinic. Ms. C states that the baby is taking 6 ounces of a commercial baby formula every 4 hours. Ms. C has not added solid foods to the baby's diet. She was told to wait until the baby is 4 to 6 months old before adding cereal. Ms. C is giving the baby the multivitamin preparation prescribed. She also has added cod liver oil to the infant's diet. "It's only a teaspoonful," she said. Ms. C's grandmother gave Ms. C cod liver oil as a child. Ms. C credits her grandmother's care during her own childhood for her strong bones and teeth. She admires her grandmother, who at age 75 still stands straight and tall. Which of the following pieces of information should the nurse gather first to focus on the situation presented?
   a. The amount of vitamin C in the multivitamin supplement
   b. The conditions under which the vitamins are stored
   c. Ms. C's technique for measuring the vitamins
   d. The total amount of vitamin D the infant receives each day

2. Mr. S has expressed interest in improving his diet. The nurse assessed Mr. S's usual intake, noting the absence of citrus fruit. He stated that the acids upset his stomach. Which of the following suggestions to maximize vitamin C content in vegetables is appropriate?
   a. Adding baking soda to the cooking water
   b. Cooking thoroughly to kill any bacteria
   c. Eating good sources raw when possible
   d. Keeping food in a mesh bag to allow air to circulate

3. Ms. M is a Seventh-Day Adventist who has elected a vegan lifestyle and who lives an indoor life. For which of the following vitamin deficiencies would she be at greatest risk without professional dietary advice?
   a. Vitamins A, C, and E
   b. Vitamins B_{12}, D, and niacin
   c. Vitamin B_6, folate, and thiamin
   d. Vitamin K, riboflavin, and biotin

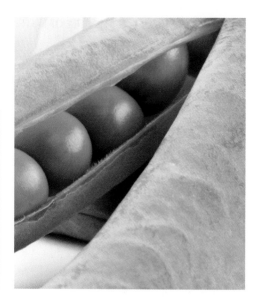

7

Minerals

LEARNING OBJECTIVES

After completing this chapter, the student should be able to:

■ Define minerals and state their functions in the human body.

■ Differentiate major and trace minerals and list three examples of each.

■ Discuss the importance of calcium to human health. List at least two natural food sources of calcium and one fortified food source.

■ Discuss the importance of iron to human health. List at least two natural food sources and one fortified food source of iron.

■ List three minerals that contribute to nerve and muscle function.

■ Identify the major effects of deficiencies of the following minerals: iodine, fluoride, and selenium.

■ Describe the relationship of minerals to anemia, cretinism, goiter, Keshan disease, Menkes disease, and Wilson disease.

■ Identify individuals at increased risk for mineral imbalances.

■ Relate reasons nutrient delivery, medical treatment, or storage methods can result in nutrient toxicities.

■ Suggest practices to prevent toxicities from one mineral with common and two with uncommon occurrences of toxicity.

$\mathcal{I}$n a broad sense, minerals are obtained from the Earth's crust. Through the effects of the weather, rocks that contain minerals are ground into smaller particles, which then become part of the soil. Growing plants absorb the minerals from the soil with the water they need. Animals eat the plants, and humans eat both the plants and the animals.

Water is the medium of absorption of nutrients for plants and the basis of the body's nutrient delivery system. In addition, certain forms of minerals are intricately bound to the distribution and movement of water in the body.

Minerals make vital contributions to growth and maintenance of the body's health. This chapter covers minerals important in human nutrition and the role each plays in the body. It describes some general functions of minerals and explains how minerals are classified in nutrition. It details the nutritional implications of the 7 major and 10 trace minerals.

Functions of Minerals

Minerals represent 4% of total body weight. Like vitamins, minerals help to regulate bodily functions without providing energy and are essential to good health. Unlike vitamins, minerals:

1. Are inorganic substances.
2. Become part of the body's composition.

133

For instance, calcium and phosphorus combine to give bones and teeth their hardness. Iron attaches to the protein globin to form hemoglobin. Iodine becomes part of the thyroid hormones.

Most minerals serve a variety of functions in the body's regulatory and metabolic processes. Sodium is essential for maintaining fluid balance. Sodium, potassium, and calcium have critical functions in nerve and muscle activity. Potassium and phosphorus play significant roles in acid–base balance. A disruption of the body's balance of any one of these minerals, albeit not necessarily caused by diet, can be life threatening.

Classification of Minerals

Three groups of minerals are considered in nutrition: major, trace, and ultratrace.

Major minerals (macrominerals) and **trace minerals** (microminerals) are differentiated by:

- Amounts present in the body:
  - Major: more than 5 grams (approximately 1 teaspoonful)
  - Trace: less than 5 grams
- Intake requirements:
  - Major: 100 milligrams (approximately $\frac{1}{50}$ teaspoonful) or more per day
  - Trace: less than 100 milligrams per day
  - Ultratrace: less than 1 milligram per day

Despite their small amounts, trace minerals make vital and often unique contributions to the body's functioning.

Ultratrace minerals appear in the Dietary Reference Intakes (DRI) tables (see Appendix A). The only values that have been set are Tolerable Upper Intake Level (ULs) for three of the five minerals in this category.

Major Minerals

The seven major minerals include calcium, sodium, and potassium, which are familiar to many people in a dietary context. The other four are phosphorus, magnesium, sulfur, and chloride.

Calcium

About 1.5% to 2% of total body weight is calcium, representing 40% of the body's mineral mass. The body of a 150-pound adult contains approximately 3 pounds of calcium, 99% in the bones and teeth. The remaining 1% of the calcium circulates in the body fluids.

Functions

Calcium, with phosphorus, forms the hard substance of bones and teeth. Ample calcium and phosphorus alone will not guarantee strong bones and teeth, however. Vitamin D is necessary for calcium absorption and protein serves as the matrix that determines the structure of the bone. Exercise, particularly weight-bearing exercise, is also essential for strong bones. Except for slightly demineralized areas, teeth cannot repair themselves so that dental restoration is needed.

Calcium also performs several vital metabolic functions in the nervous, muscular, and cardiovascular systems, for instance:

1. Calcium assists in manufacturing **acetylcholine,** a neurotransmitter (a chemical that enhances transmission of nerve impulses).
2. Calcium acts as a catalyst in initiating and controlling muscle contraction and relaxation. At the beginning of a muscle contraction, calcium is released from its storage area inside the muscle cell. At the end of a contraction, the calcium is gathered into its storage area.
3. Calcium is a catalyst in the clotting process: it aids in the conversion of platelets to thromboplastin and in the conversion of **fibrinogen** to **fibrin.**

Control Mechanisms

Remodeling of bone begins before birth and continues throughout life, such that the bone calcium pool turns over every 8 to 12 years on average in adults, but this turnover does not occur in the teeth (Weaver and Heaney, 2014). One reason for the changes in bone composition is to maintain the adult serum calcium concentration within the normal limits of 8.2 to 10.2 milligrams per 100 milliliters of serum.

Another reason for the movement of calcium in and out of the bones is to renew the bone tissue. Bone remodeling is the process through which bone is renewed to maintain bone strength and mineral homeostasis. The remodeling process resorbs old bone and forms new bone to prevent accumulation of bone microdamage (Clarke, 2008). In this process, bone cells called **osteoclasts** produce enzymes to destroy the protein matrix that holds the calcium phosphate in place. Other bone cells, called **osteoblasts,** produce new matrix protein, which chemically attracts calcium and other nutrients to rebuild the bone.

Several hormones work together to accomplish these activities. Vitamin D (see Chapter 6) is one of these hormones. **Parathyroid hormone** and calcitonin are the other two. Tiny glands behind the thyroid gland in the neck secrete **parathyroid hormone** when the serum calcium level is too low. The thyroid gland secretes **calcitonin** when the serum calcium level is too high.

Figure 7-1 illustrates the complementary actions of parathyroid hormone and calcitonin.

Other hormones also affect the body's use of calcium. One prominent one is estrogen that affects bone formation and resorption in ways that are incompletely understood but may involve prolonging the life span of osteoblasts (Bradford, Gerace, Roland, and Chrzan, 2010). Estrogen deficiency promotes bone resorption in all age groups and in adolescence prevents attainment of peak bone mass (Gropper and Smith, 2013).

Dietary Reference Intakes

For DRIs see Appendix A. In 2010, the values for calcium were upgraded from Adequate Intake (AIs) to Recommended Dietary Allowance (RDAs) for all ages except infants. For food and other sources, see Table 7-1. To investigate the mineral content of a particular item, go to http://ndb.nal.usda.gov or to http://nutritiondata.self.com.

Sources

Calcium can be obtained from animal or vegetable sources, but calcium from animal sources is more readily absorbed.

ANIMAL SOURCES

Milk and milk products are the best animal sources of calcium. In milk, calcium is accompanied by lactose, which increases absorption in infants but not in adults. Another advantageous component of milk is the protein the osteoblasts need to rebuild the bone matrix. In sum, milk is such an important source of calcium that it is virtually impossible to obtain adequate dietary calcium without dairy products. Figure 7-2 shows a child drinking milk with a "fast-food" meal.

See Table 7-2 to evaluate alternate sources of calcium compared to fluid milk. Note the cost in kilocalories.

Milk products supply other nutrients in addition to calcium, such as vitamins A and D, and are also a major source of riboflavin and protein (see Fig. 7-3). Supplements should not substitute for food but sometimes are necessary adjuncts. Clinical Application 7-1 describes some of the contaminants in "natural" calcium supplements and suggestions for choosing a supplement when necessary.

Calcium supplements should be taken:

- In doses of 500 milligrams or less for optimal absorption
- With meals if calcium carbonate (stomach acid enhances absorption)
- Without regard to meals if calcium citrate

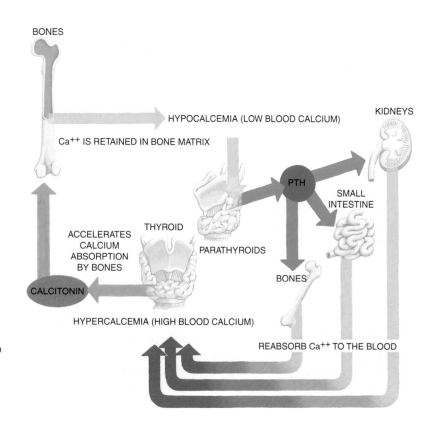

FIGURE 7-1 Parathyroid hormone raises serum calcium levels when they are too low. Calcitonin from the thyroid gland lowers serum calcium levels when they are too high. (Reprinted from Venes, D [Ed.]: *Taber's Cylcopedic Medical Dictionary*, 21st ed. FA Davis, Philadelphia, 2010, p. 338, with permission.)

TABLE 7-1 ■ Major Minerals

MINERAL	ADULT RDA/AI AND FOOD PORTION*	FUNCTIONS	SIGNS AND SYMPTOMS OF DEFICIENCY	SIGNS AND SYMPTOMS OF EXCESS	GOOD SOURCES IN COMMON FOODS
Calcium	1000–1200 mg 3.3–4 cups 1% milk	Structure of bones and teeth Nerve conduction Muscle contraction Blood clotting	Tetany Osteoporosis Rickets (premature infants)	Calcification of soft tissue	Milk products Salmon, sardines with bones Clams Oysters
Phosphorus	700 mg 8.9-oz sockeye salmon	Structure of bones and teeth Component of DNA and RNA Component of buffers and almost all enzymes Component of ADP and ATP	Increased calcium excretion Bone loss Muscle weakness	Tetany Convulsions Renal insufficiency	Lean meat Fish Poultry Milk Nuts Legumes
Sodium	1200–1500 mg 0.5–0.65 tsp salt	Fluid balance Transmission of electrochemical impulses along nerve and muscle membranes	Hyponatremia	Hypernatremia	Table salt Processed foods Milk and milk products
Potassium	4.7 g 4 cups canned white beans	Conduction of nerve impulses Muscle contraction	Hypokalemia (not usually dietary)	Hyperkalemia (not usually dietary)	Banana Cantaloupe Winter squash Green leafy vegetables Legumes Salt substitutes
Magnesium	310–420 mg 2.1–2.8 cups spinach	Associated with ADP and ATP Involved in DNA and protein synthesis Influences cardiac and smooth muscle contractility	Impaired CNS function Tetany	Weakness Depressed respirations Cardiac arrest	Green leafy vegetables Seafood Peanut butter Legumes Coffee Cocoa
Sulfur	Not established	Component of amino acids methionine and cysteine Gives shape to hair, skin, and nails	None known due solely to sulfur	None known due solely to sulfur	Complete protein foods
Chloride	1800–2300 mg 0.5–0.67 tsp salt	Component of hydrochloric acid Helps maintain fluid and acid base balance	In infants: neurological impairments	None known	Table salt Salty snacks Processed foods Eggs Meat Seafood

ADP, adenosine diphosphate; ATP, adenosine triphosphate; CNS, central nervous system.
*Examples only; not suggested for a sole source of a day's intake.

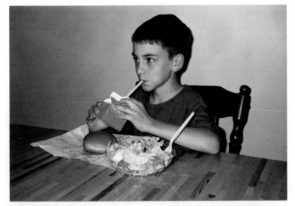

FIGURE 7-2 This child has a balanced meal from a fast-food restaurant: a small hamburger, a salad, and milk. Growing bones and teeth need calcium from milk products.

TABLE 7-2 ■ Food Containing Approximately 300 Milligrams of Calcium, Equal to 1 Cup of Milk

FOOD	AMOUNT	KILOCALORIES
Skim milk	1.0 cup	86
Plain low-fat yogurt	0.7 cup	101
Swiss cheese	1.1 oz	118
Whole milk	1.0 cup	150
Cheddar cheese	1.5 oz	171
Low-fat yogurt with fruit	0.9 cup	199
Cottage cheese, 2% low-fat	2.0 cups	410
Soft ice cream	1.3 cups	479
Cottage cheese, creamed, large curd	2.25 cups	529
Sherbet	2.9 cups	786

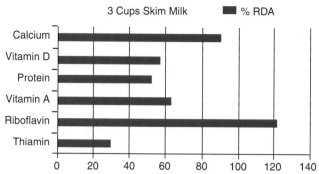

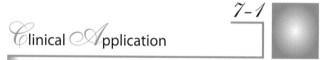

FIGURE 7-3 Milk supplies many nutrients in addition to calcium. Three cups of skim milk provide a woman between 19 and 50 years of age with these percentages of her RDAs: calcium, 90%; vitamin D, 58%; protein, 54%; vitamin A, 64%; riboflavin, 122%; and thiamin, 30%. The kilocaloric cost for all of these nutrients is a minuscule 249 kilocalories.

7-1
Clinical Application

Contents of Natural Calcium Supplements

Shells, dolomite, and bones are natural sources of calcium that are used as dietary supplements. Much of the calcium found in shells and bones is in the form of calcium phosphate, one of the most difficult calcium compounds to absorb. More important, shells and dolomite, a limestone product, may be contaminated with aluminum and lead, and the latter often contaminates bone meal preparations (Gropper and Smith, 2013).

Supplements labeled "USP" or "CL" (see Chapter 15) meet voluntary industry standards for quality, purity, and tablet disintegration or dissolution. To test the dissolvability of a calcium product, place a tablet in one-half cup of vinegar. Stir occasionally over one-half hour after which no particles should be visible. Dissolvability is only the first step in calcium absorption, however, because of the multiple factors affecting it.

PLANT SOURCES

Good plant sources of calcium include turnip and mustard greens, broccoli, cauliflower, kale, legumes, and dried fruits (Gropper and Smith, 2013). Some experts question how much calcium the body is actually able to absorb from plant sources because of multiple interfering factors.

Another good plant source that is readily available is calcium-fortified orange juice. A source of calcium for Navajo Americans is the ash derived from the branches and needles of the juniper tree. The ash is used to flavor various foods, such as cornmeal mush and pancakes and Navajo tea. One teaspoon of the ash supplies roughly the calcium in one glass of milk (Christensen et al, 1998), illustrating the wisdom of traditional ways.

Absorption and Excretion

Calcium is absorbed throughout the small intestine through two distinct processes. In the **duodenum** and proximal **jejunum,** the process is active, through

the intestinal cells, and involves vitamin D–dependent calcium-binding transport proteins. In the distal jejunum and ileum, the process is passive, between the intestinal cells. Lastly, bacteria in the large intestine appear to release calcium from some food fiber, permitting absorption of calcium through that site (Gropper and Smith, 2013).

Infants and young children absorb up to 60% of dietary calcium, compared with 20% to 30% absorbed by adults, however, that rate is increased during pregnancy (NIH Office of Dietary Supplements, August 1, 2012). With decreased estrogen in aging females, calcium absorption may shrink to 15% because of diminished calcitriol production (Gropper and Smith, 2013). Compounding the absorption issue is the fact that the average postmenopausal woman's diet contains just 700 milligrams of the 1200-milligram RDA. Even with calcium supplementation, just 38% of American women achieve recommended intake levels (Roush, 2011).

Excretion takes place in urine (average daily loss of about 170 milligrams) and feces, but also through the skin with an average daily loss of 60 milligrams (Gropper and Smith, 2013).

Interfering Factors

In general, the percentage of available calcium absorbed from vegetables is considerably less than that absorbed from milk. The exceptions from which calcium is as easily absorbed as that in milk include:

- Broccoli
- Cabbage
- Bok choy (Chinese cabbage)
- Collards
- Kale
- Mustard and turnip greens (Amit, 2010; Weaver and Heaney, 2014).

The difficulty becomes the volume of food necessary to provide the quantity of calcium equal to that in a glass of milk: 4.2 cups of cooked cabbage or 4.8 cups of chopped cooked broccoli.

Several factors can interfere with the absorption and retention of calcium, as described in Table 7-3.

TABLE 7-3 ■ Factors Affecting Calcium Absorption and Excretion		
INCREASE ABSORPTION	DECREASE ABSORPTION	INCREASE EXCRETION
Lactose (infants)	Oxalic acid	Excessive protein
Vitamin D	Phytic acid	Excessive sodium
	Zinc supplements coupled with low calcium intake	Caffeine coupled with low calcium intake

OXALATES

Some plants contain salts of oxalic acid called **oxalates** that bind with the calcium present in some vegetables to produce calcium oxalate, an insoluble substance excreted in the feces. These potent inhibitors are found in high concentrations in rhubarb and spinach and to a lesser extent in dried beans and sweet potatoes (Weaver and Heaney, 2014). Unusually high intake of some of these and other foods may cause oxalic acid poisoning (see Clinical Application 7-2). Low oxalate diets are sometimes recommended to lessen risk of calcium oxalate kidney stones (National Kidney Foundation, 2011).

PHYTATES

Cereals contain **phytic acid,** which forms an insoluble complex with calcium. Phytates are the storage form of phosphorus in seeds; however, only foods with heavy concentrations of phytate, such as extruded wheat bran cereal and dried beans, substantially reduce calcium absorption (Weaver and Heaney, 2014).

The overall effect of oxalic and phytic acids on calcium availability in most balanced diets usually is not significant. People who avoid dairy products, however, need careful attention to meal planning. Ovovegetarian and vegan clients should seek calcium-fortified products, such as orange juice and calcium-set tofu, to bolster their intake of the mineral.

PROTEIN

The impact of dietary protein on calcium absorption has been a subject of debate. High-protein diets increase urinary calcium excretion and make the urine more acidic. These two effects were suspected to produce a dietary environment favorable for demineralization of the skeleton. However, increased calcium excretion due to a high-protein diet does not seem to be linked to impaired calcium balance. In contrast, some data indicate that high-protein intakes increase intestinal calcium absorption. Moreover, no clinical data support the hypothesis of a detrimental effect of a high-protein diet on bone health, except in a context of inadequate calcium supply (Calvez, Poupin, Chesneau, et al, 2012). In a 2-year study of protein-replete healthy ambulant women, aged 70 to 80 years, 30 grams of supplemental protein had neither beneficial nor deleterious effects on bone mass or strength (Zhu, Meng, Kerr, et al, 2011). Using a high intake of fruits and vegetables to counter the theorized demineralization of bone by a high protein diet has not been substantiated. The benefits of fruit and vegetables on bone health remain unclear (Hamidi, Boucher, Cheung, et al, 2011). Furthermore, a meta-analysis uncovered no evidence to support the premise that an alkaline diet (heavy in fruits and vegetables) is protective of bone health (Fenton, Tough, Lyon, et al, 2011). See Chapter 8 for more information on acid–base balance.

OTHER MINERALS

Because calcium, magnesium, and zinc use the same absorption mechanism, magnesium and zinc can impair the absorption of calcium. Especially in situations when calcium intake is low and the zinc is taken as a supplement, the absorption of calcium is impeded (Gropper and Smith, 2013).

Sodium intake can also have a detrimental effect on calcium balance. For every 500-milligram increase in sodium intake, an additional 10 milligrams of calcium is spilled in the urine (Gropper and Smith, 2013)—a small amount compared with the RDA but the amount could be important in women consuming high-salt, low-dairy diets over a lifetime. Dietary sodium has a tremendous potential to influence bone loss at suboptimal calcium intakes in women. Each extra gram of sodium per day is projected to produce an additional rate of bone loss of 1% per year if the calcium loss in the urine comes from the skeleton (Weaver and Heaney, 2014).

CAFFEINE

Caffeine promotes the return of calcium from the blood to the gut (thereby increasing intestinal losses) and stimulates urinary excretion of calcium (Gropper and

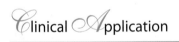

Clinical Application   7-2

Oxalic Acid Poisoning

Although rarely reported, poisoning is possible by ingesting too much of the foods containing oxalic acid. Lists are long and varied but may include these high oxalate foods:

- Peanuts, tree nuts
- Soybeans, soy milk
- Wheat germ and wheat bran
- Rhubarb, beets
- Spinach, sweet potatoes, most dried beans
- Black tea, instant tea, chocolate (National Kidney Foundation, 2011)

For example, one normal serving of rhubarb contains one-fifth the toxic dose. Rhubarb leaves contain three or four times as much as the stalks so a fairly small amount of leaf can poison a child.

One way to minimize the chance of oxalic acid poisoning is to consume foods that contain calcium with foods high in oxalic acid. The calcium combines with the oxalate, which then passes through the intestine harmlessly but also of necessity decreases calcium absorption.

Smith, 2013), which may become important when caffeinated beverages replace milk in the diet. Caffeine equal to 2 to 3 cups of coffee accelerated bone loss from the spine and total body in postmenopausal women who consumed less than 744 milligrams of calcium per day (Weaver and Heaney, 2014). Therefore, if a person's calcium intake is low or marginal, drinking many caffeinated beverages could adversely affect bone health.

OTHER FACTORS

In certain situations, calcium bioavailability may be reduced by diseases or medications to treat them. In individuals with digestive system diseases producing **steatorrhea,** the excess fat in the bowel combines with calcium, forming insoluble soap, which is then excreted in the feces. Because gastric acid is needed to solubilize calcium in the stomach, medications that decrease the amount of gastric acid may diminish calcium absorption (Gropper and Smith, 2013).

Deficiencies

Calcium deficiency in children can contribute to poor bone and tooth development. Rickets is typically more directly related to vitamin D deficiency than to calcium deficiency except in premature infants, whose skeletons still need much added mineral. Two other conditions related to calcium balance are osteoporosis and tetany.

OSTEOPOROSIS

According to the World Health Organization, **osteopenia** is bone mineral density 1 to 2.5 standard deviations below the mean of healthy young adults, whereas **osteoporosis** is bone mineral density more than 2.5 standard deviations below the mean. Osteoporosis permits minimal trauma to cause fractures commonly affecting the hip, wrist, or vertebrae and can be diagnosed following such a fracture such as one that occurs from a standing height (Grossman, 2011).

Two major factors in the development of osteoporosis are:

1. The bone mass developed from birth to age 30
2. The rate at which bone mass is lost in later life

In girls and women, 99% of total bone body mineral content is achieved by age 22. Total body bone mass remains fairly constant through the reproductive years but decreases in the aging adult, most markedly in postmenopausal women who lose bone most rapidly in the first 3 years after menopause (Weaver and Heaney, 2014). After the onset of menopause, bone loss occurs at 2 to 6 times premenopausal rates, gradually slowing to about 1% annually by 10 years postmenopause, the same rate of loss suffered by older men (Tucker and Rosen, 2014).

Intuitively, then, estrogen treatment might help prevent osteoporosis but is not first-line therapy because of increased risks of heart disease, pulmonary emboli, and deep vein phlebitis. *Raloxifene,* a selective estrogen receptor modulator, is approved for prevention and treatment of postmenopausal osteoporosis with the additional advantage of reducing risk of breast cancer but is contraindicated in clients with histories of thromboembolic events (Vallerand, Sanoski, and Deglin, 2013).

Osteoporosis is most common in postmenopausal, fair-complexioned white women; however, all are not equally affected (see Genomic Gem 7-1). Men and black women lose bone mass also, but because their skeletons are generally heavier, they are at lower risk of osteoporosis.

Figure 7-4 shows normal and osteoporotic cancellous bone. Generally, osteoporosis causes reduced bone mass, both matrix and mineral (Heaney, 2014). Figure 7-5 displays x-ray films of normal and osteoporotic bones. Clinical Application 7-3 details prevalence, major risk factors, diagnostic aids, and treatment approaches for osteoporosis.

Two lifestyle factors impacting bone include:

1. Smoking
2. Alcohol consumption

Alcohol abuse and smoking habits have adverse effects on bone health and are a risk factor for osteoporosis, fractures, and impaired fracture repair (Fini, Giavaresi, Salamanna, et al, 2011). The decrease in bone mass and strength following alcohol consumption is mainly due to a bone remodeling imbalance, primarily decreased bone formation (Maurel, Boisseau, Benhamou, and Jaffre, 2012), but there is also evidence for increased bone resorption in alcoholics (Ronis, Mercer, and Chen, 2011).

Genomic Gem 7-1

Osteoporosis Is Familial

About 80% of the variance in peak bone mass is an inherited trait. A family history of hip fracture may be predictive of a twofold increased risk of hip fracture.

An early marker of genetic influence on bone physiology entails the vitamin D receptor, which has been associated with low bone mineral density in several populations. Women with the low bone mineral density vitamin D receptor genotype not only displayed more rapid bone loss but also failed to increase calcium absorption if calcium intake was low.

Most of the known genes identified with osteoporosis encode components of pathways involved in bone synthesis or resorption. To date, only a small proportion of the total genetic variation implicated in osteoporosis has been ascertained. Progress in this area is expected to accelerate in the future (Tucker and Rosen, 2014).

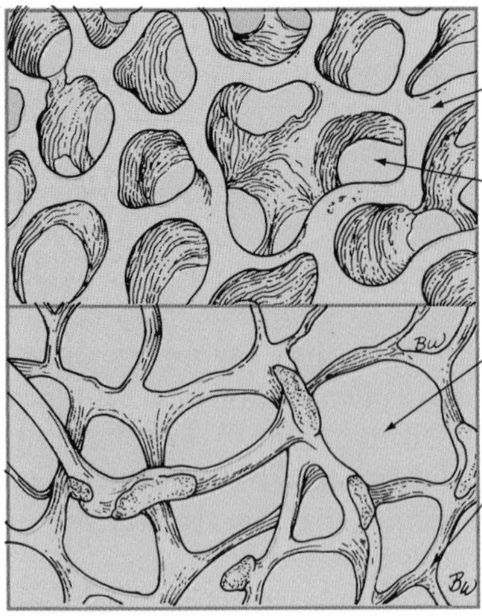

OSTEOPOROSIS

NORMAL CANCELLOUS BONE

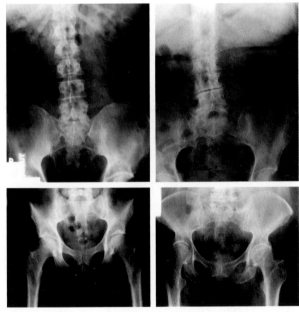

TRABECULAE
ARE THICK

SPACE BETWEEN
TRABECULAE IS SMALL

ENLARGED SPACE
BETWEEN TRABECULAE

THIN TRABECULAE
COMPARED TO NORMAL

AS OSTEOPOROSIS CONTINUES
THE TRABECULAE ARE
COMPLETELY RESORBED

OSTEOPOROTIC CANCELLOUS BONE

FIGURE 7-4 Sketch of normal and osteoporotic cancellous bone showing enlarged spaces and thinner bony structure in the latter. (Reprinted from Venes, D [Ed.]: *Taber's Cyclopedic Medical Dictionary*, 21st ed. FA Davis, Philadelphia, 2010, p. 1659, with permission.)

FIGURE 7-5 X-ray films of a normal bone on the left and an osteoporotic bone on the right. (Courtesy of Dr. Russell Tobe.)

Relatively minor risk factors for decreased calcium metabolism (alcohol, caffeine, high-protein intake, phytic acid– and oxalic acid–containing foods, sodium, and smoking), when combined, and especially when coupled with low-calcium and vitamin D intake or sunlight aversion, might make a decided difference in an individual's bone health. Dietary recommendations for calcium and vitamin D are an important cornerstone in the treatment of osteoporosis, which may

7-3

Clinical Application

Osteoporosis Prevalence, Risk Factors, Diagnosis, and Treatment

PREVALENCE
- An estimated 10 million people in the United States, 80% of them women, have osteoporosis, the major factor in fractures in the elderly.
- Estimated cost of osteoporosis-related fractures in 2005 was $19 billion (National Osteoporosis Foundation, undated).

MAJOR RISK FACTORS IN WHITE POSTMENOPAUSAL WOMEN
- Personal history of fracture as an adult. In a 2004 report, the U.S. Surgeon General called attention to the low (20%) treatment rate for osteoporosis following fragility fractures in elderly individuals. Subsequently the American Orthopedic Association designed a quality improvement program that was widely implemented in 2009. It features:
  - Communication with the client and primary care physician regarding diagnosis and treatment of osteoporosis
  - Counseling on nutrition, physical activity, and lifestyle changes (Bunta, 2011)
- History of fragility fracture in a first-degree relative.
- Low body weight (less than 127 pounds)
- Current smoking
- Use of corticosteroid therapy (even in low doses) for 3 or more consecutive months (International Osteoporosis Foundation, undated) through inhibition of osteoblast function (De Nijs, 2008)
- A risk assessment tool is available at www.iofbonehealth.org/one-minute-osteoporosis-risk-awareness-test

DIAGNOSIS
- History and physical examination including assessment for height loss and posture changes
- Measurement of bone mineral density (BMD) if postmenopausal. Until 30% to 40% of bone mass is lost, it is not detectable on x-ray film (see Figure 7-5), but dual-energy x-ray absorptiometry (DEXA) permits earlier diagnosis.

TREATMENT
- Optimize nutrition, including protein, vitamin D, and calcium. Supplements when indicated. High intakes of calcium reduce bone resorption by reducing parathyroid hormone secretion.
- Exercise to the extent fragility permits.
- Consider medications to affect bone metabolism in conjunction with, not instead of, nutrition and exercise. Optimal vitamin D status seems to be necessary to maximize the response to antiresorbers in terms of both BMD changes and antifracture efficacy (Adami, Giannini, Bianchi, et al, 2009). Correction of vitamin D insufficiency in clients with declining bone mineral density while receiving bisphosphonate drugs led to a significant rebound in BMD (Geller, Hu, Reed, et al, 2008).

also include pharmacologic agents (Tucker and Rosen, 2014).

TETANY

Despite the hormonal control of serum calcium and the large reservoir in the bones, serum calcium levels sometimes fall below normal. An actual lack of calcium or a lack of ionized (see Chapter 8) calcium may cause tetany. A serum calcium level that is too low is called **hypocalcemia.** If the signs and symptoms described here appear, the condition is called **tetany.** Causes include parathyroid deficiency, **alkalosis,** and (in infants) vitamin D deficiency (see Chapter 6).

Hypocalcemia is a major postoperative complication of total thyroidectomy caused by damage to, or impairment of blood supply to, one or more parathyroid glands during surgery. A marked decrease in blood calcium, immediately after surgery, was a sensitive predictor of hypocalcemia that permitted early preventive measures allowing most clients to escape symptomatic hypocalcemia (Tredici, Grosso, Gibelli, et al, 2011).

In **alkalosis,** because of the excessive alkalinity of body fluids, a greater number of calcium ions than usual are bound to serum proteins, effectively inactivating calcium and impairing nerve and muscle function (see Acid–Base Balance in Chapter 8). Alkalosis may be caused by:

- Losing acid (due to vomiting or gastric suction)
- Ingesting alkalis (e.g., sodium bicarbonate)
- Breathing too rapidly, either in response to fear or through mechanical ventilation

The result of rapid breathing is excessive loss of carbon dioxide. In the blood, carbon dioxide is transported as carbonic acid. Thus, when too much carbon dioxide is exhaled, the alkalinity of the blood increases and produces tetany.

Early symptoms of tetany are:

- Nervousness
- Irritability
- Numbness
- Tingling of the extremities and around the mouth
- Muscle cramps

Diagnostic signs of tetany are Trousseau sign and Chvostek sign.

In **Trousseau sign,** inflation of the blood pressure cuff above systolic pressure for 3 minutes causes ischemia of the peripheral nerves, increasing their excitability.

In **Chvostek sign,** a tap over the facial nerve in front of the ear causes a twitch of the facial muscles on that side. Figure 7-6 depicts these diagnostic signs.

Because of the many functions of calcium, tetany is a medical emergency. Untreated, tetany can progress to:

- blood clotting irregularities,
- heart dilatation,
- respiratory paralysis,
- seizures, and
- coma.

Toxicity

For basic information on mineral toxicity, see Table 7-4. A serum calcium level that is too high, above 11 milligrams per 100 milliliters of serum in adults, is called **hypercalcemia,** most often caused by cancer or hyperparathyroidism. Calcium-containing kidney stones are not usually caused by dietary calcium but by malfunctioning kidneys that permit too much calcium to be spilled into the urine (Weaver and Heaney, 2014).

Another condition, one that involves ingestion of large amounts of calcium along with absorbable alkali, is **milk-alkali syndrome,** currently the third most common cause of hypercalcemia, causing about 12% of cases (Grubb, Gaurav, and Panda, 2009). Historically, this syndrome was associated with the milk

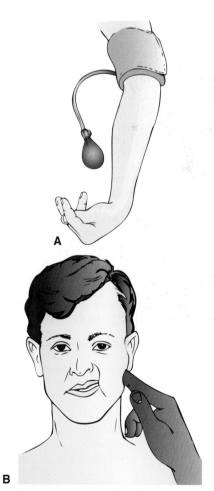

FIGURE 7-6 Indications of hypocalcemia. *A,* Positive Trousseau sign. *B,* Positive Chvostek sign. (Reprinted from Phillips, L: *Manual of I.V. Therapeutics,* 5th ed. FA Davis, Philadelphia, 2010, pp. 150–151, with permission.)

TABLE 7-4 ■ Mineral Toxicities

	SIGNS AND SYMPTOMS	NUTRITIONAL CAUSES	ASSOCIATED CONDITIONS
Calcium	Calcium deposits in the soft tissues of the body	Almost never	Hyperparathyroidism Vitamin D poisoning (most frequent in infants) Absorbable antacids Milk-alkali syndrome
Phosphorus	Calcifications in soft tissue	Dietary overload unusual Excessive phospholipids in parenteral nutrition Occurred in infants during the first few weeks of life from diet consisting solely of cow's milk	Kidney disease Overmedication with vitamin D Oral sodium phosphate bowel-cleansing drugs
Sodium	Hypernatremia (Table 7-6)	Healthy people excrete excess sodium without immediate adverse effects except in salt-sensitive individuals	Possible long-range adverse effects due to calcium loss
Potassium	Hyperkalemia (Table 7-6)	Rarely caused by excessive dietary intake Intravenous potassium should be given only to clients excreting urine	Diabetic acidosis Kidney failure Adrenal insufficiency Severe dehydration Transfusion with old blood (see Clinical Application 7-5)
Magnesium	Hypotension Nausea Vomiting Lethargy Confusion Slow pulse Depressed respirations Loss of patellar reflex	Not ordinarily seen	Kidney disease
Sulfur			Environmental causes such as air pollution with sulfur dioxide
Chloride			Environmental release of gas: industry, rail accidents

Iron	Accumulated mineral damages tissues
	Acute:
	  Gastroenteritis
	  Shock
	  Seizures
	  Liver failure
		Most people at little risk of iron toxicity from diet except with homemade beer in Africa
		Accidental overdosing with supplements
			Iron metabolism disorders
			Chronic alcoholism
			Iron poisoning can be fatal.

Iodine	Burning of mouth, throat, and stomach Brassy taste in mouth Increased salivation Nausea, vomiting, diarrhea Acne-like lesions Hypothyroidism Hyperthyroidism Thyroiditis	Asian infants: congenital hypothyroidism due to large amounts of iodine-rich seaweed consumed by their mothers during pregnancy and lactation (Emder and Jack, 2011).	Frequent exposure to x-ray contrast media Prescribed *amiodarone*

Fluoride	Mottled, discolored but sound teeth
	Bone and kidney dysfunction
	Acute toxicity:
	  Nausea, vomiting, diarrhea
	  Acidosis
	  Cardiac arrhythmias
		Drinking water with a fluoride concentration of <2 parts per million rarely problematic
		Overuse, swallowing of fluoridated dental products
		Drinking water with a fluoride concentration of four parts per million (EPA limit)
			Fluorosis possible in children up to 8 years of age
			Increased dental caries
			Rarely, skeletal fluorosis
			Acute toxicity can be fatal

Zinc	Nausea, vomiting
	Reduced immune response
	Acute toxicity:
	  Metallic taste
	  Bloody diarrhea
	Chronic toxicity:
	  Copper deficiency
	  Gait abnormalities (Gropper and Smith, 2013)
		Supplemental doses three times the Recommended Dietary Allowance can interfere with copper absorption leading to copper deficiency (Gropper and Smith, 2013)	Loss of sense of smell with zinc nasal products

TABLE 7-4 ■ **Mineral Toxicities** (Continued)

	SIGNS AND SYMPTOMS	NUTRITIONAL CAUSES	ASSOCIATED CONDITIONS
Copper	Accumulation of copper in the liver, kidneys, brain, and cornea of the eye	Consuming acidic foods stored in copper vessels Infants fed water high in copper Long-term overdosing with supplements	Wilson disease Clients treated with an artificial kidney that used copper tubing
Selenium	Fatigue Nausea, vomiting, diarrhea Nail and hair brittleness and loss (Gropper and Smith, 2013)	Overdosing with supplements Manufacturing error with supplements (see Chapter 15)	Miners
Chromium	Disagreeable metallic taste	Contaminated foods or parenteral nutrition solutions Overdosing with supplements	Inhalation of chromium in an industrial setting Possible wear debris from hip prostheses
Manganese	Signs/symptoms similar to Parkinson's disease Neurological abnormalities	Parenteral nutrition, especially in neonates Well water high in manganese	Decreased liver function Cholestasis Pica Miners exposed to manganese dust Welders exposed to manganese fumes
Cobalt	Heart, lung signs and symptoms		Occupational exposure in industry Possible wear debris from metal-on-metal hip prostheses
Molybdenum	Goutlike symptoms (Gropper and Smith, 2013)	Eating food from regions with high levels in the soil	Occupational exposure

and cream antacid treatment of peptic ulcers. In the 1970s, the syndrome accounted for just 1% of hypercalcemia cases. The 12-fold increase occurred because the introduction of nonabsorbable antacids and other new medications reduced gastric acidity (Waked, Geara, and El-Imad, 2009).

The recent resurgence in cases is attributed to the use of calcium carbonate to prevent or treat osteoporosis and hyperphosphatemia in clients with chronic kidney disease (Grubb et al, 2009). Examples of reported cases involved:

- A 26-year-old pregnant woman taking eight or nine calcium carbonate tablets daily for heartburn along with several glasses of milk and a calcium-containing prenatal supplement (Kolnick, Harris, Choma, and Choma, 2011)
- A 50-year-old man who was twice admitted for renal failure and metabolic acidosis (see Chapter 8) before his self-medication with a calcium carbonate product for heartburn was identified as causing milk-alkali syndrome (Swaminathan, 2011)
- A 81-year-old man, taking 25 calcium carbonate tablets daily to prevent osteoporosis, who presented in acute kidney failure, refused more than two kidney dialysis treatments, but whose kidney failure resolved spontaneously within 4 weeks after discharge and discontinuation of calcium carbonate tablets (Waked et al, 2009)

Some clients with milk-alkali syndrome present with confusion, which complicates the diagnostic process.

These cases emphasize the importance of carefully taking a client's dietary and medication history as well as teaching a client about over-the-counter and prescription medications. Just because a product is available over-the-counter does not make it safe regardless of amount or conditions. Early diagnosis of milk-alkali syndrome could limit permanent kidney dysfunction.

Phosphorus

Phosphorus occurs in bones and teeth as calcium phosphate. Second to calcium in amount present in the body, 0.8% to 1.2% of body weight, phosphorus is distributed:

- 85% in bone,
- 14% in soft tissue, and
- 1% in body fluids (Gropper and Smith, 2013).

Phosphorus is closely associated with calcium in both foods and interrelated metabolic body functions. Their control mechanisms are also entwined.

Phosphorus is a component of DNA, RNA, and the coenzyme forms of vitamins B_1 and B_6 (Gropper and Smith, 2013). The storage forms of energy, **adenosine diphosphate (ADP)** and **adenosine triphosphate (ATP),** contain phosphorus. It is also an essential mineral in **phospholipids,** which are structural components of cells. Lecithin, a part of cell membranes, and myelin, the insulating covering of many nerves, are phospholipids. Phosphorus is contained in almost all enzymes, and phosphorus compounds function as buffers to maintain the blood's pH as slightly alkaline.

Control Mechanisms

Between 50% and 70% of dietary phosphorus is absorbed primarily from the duodenum and jejunum with greater absorption occurring from animal products and less from phytic acid-containing foods. Vitamin D (calcitriol) is the chief enhancer of absorption. Excessive intakes of aluminum, calcium, and magnesium, often found in antacid medications, inhibit it (Gropper and Smith, 2013). Unabsorbed phosphorus is eliminated in the feces.

Low levels of serum phosphorus stimulate the kidney to produce more active vitamin D (calcitriol). Vitamin D increases the absorption of phosphorus from the intestinal tract and enhances phosphate resorption from the bones. In response to parathyroid hormone, the kidneys, the chief guardians of phosphate balance, excrete excess phosphorus, which can have far-reaching effects, as shown in Clinical Application 7-4.

Dietary Reference Intakes and Sources

For DRIs, see Appendix A. For food and other sources, see Table 7-1. To investigate the mineral content of a particular item, go to http://ndb.nal.usda.gov or to http://nutritiondata.self.com.

Deficiency

Although calcium and magnesium impair phosphorus absorption, deficiency is unlikely in healthy persons consuming a normal diet. Deficiency, however, has occurred in clients receiving parenteral nutrition (see Chapter 14) with insufficient phosphorus.

In addition, certain medications or diseases can produce **hypophosphatemia.** For example, persons ingesting a diet low in phosphorus while also taking a phosphate-binding drug, such as the antacid aluminum hydroxide, have experienced hypophosphatemia. Also, the following conditions have precipitated hypophosphatemia:

■ Malabsorption disorders
■ Severe burns
■ Uncontrolled diabetes mellitus

7-4

𝒞linical 𝒜pplication

Phosphorus Intake and Calcium Balance

In the past, the ratio of calcium to phosphorus was considered crucial to proper calcium balance. Now authorities think that the calcium-to-phosphorus ratio is less important than an adequate calcium intake for adults; however, both premature and term infants require carefully balanced intakes because of immature kidneys (see Chapter 11). In contrast, athletes and others with high energy expenditure often consume amounts of phosphorus greater than the UL with no apparent ill effects (Institute of Medicine, 2011).

Two related issues attract the attention of researchers:

■ Widespread inadequate calcium intake
■ Increasing amounts of phosphorus intake

In many countries, phosphorus intake is two to three times the RDA, while calcium intake is below the RDA. Complicating the issue is incomplete data on phosphate additives in processed foods (Kemi, Rita, Kärkkäinen, et al, 2009).

A high dietary phosphorus intake may have negative effects on bone through increased parathyroid hormone secretion because a high serum parathyroid hormone concentration increases bone resorption. In healthy females aged 21 to 40 years, given measured amounts of phosphorus and calcium, when phosphorus intake was 2.5 times the RDA, increasing the amount of calcium intake to 1.7 times the RDA did decrease serum parathyroid concentration compared with calcium intake at the RDA level (Kemi et al, 2008).

In addition, phosphate additives, because they are almost completely absorbed, may have more harmful effects on bone than other phosphorus sources. This is indicated by higher mean concentrations of serum parathyroid hormone among participants who consumed the most phosphate-containing food additives. Because of the high dietary phosphorus intake and current upward trend in consumption of processed foods in Western countries, these findings may have important public health implications (Kemi et al, 2009).

As an example, colas contain phosphoric acid along with caffeine, both of which may adversely affect bone. In the Framingham Osteoporosis Study, intake of cola but not of other carbonated soft drinks was associated with significantly lower bone mineral density at each hip site, but not the spine, in women but not in men. Similar results were seen for diet cola and, although weaker, for decaffeinated cola. Total phosphorus intake was not significantly higher in daily cola consumers than in nonconsumers; however, the calcium-to-phosphorus ratios were lower (Tucker, Morita, Qiao, et al, 2006). Depending on a person's habits, cola beverages (that contain 25–40 milligrams of phosphorus in 12 ounces) can contribute significantly to intake (Gropper and Smith, 2013). It is likely that regular exposure to phosphoric acid may cause small BMD losses, which accumulate to measurable losses over time (Tucker and Rosen, 2014).

While data are being gathered and researchers forge it into evidence, a simple solution to the issue of calcium-phosphorus balance is available. Dairy products, which provide large amounts of both nutrients, should be a mainstay of the diet, complemented by moderation in intake of processed foods and cola beverages. Once again, balance, moderation, and variety are keys to a healthy diet.

Additionally, **refeeding syndrome,** a condition related to imbalances in phosphorus, occurs when wasted or starved clients are given nutrients in excess of what their bodies can process (see Chapter 22).

Hyperparathyroidism is a disease causing excess excretion of phosphorus. In this disease, parathyroid hormone causes withdrawal of calcium from the bones. Because the two minerals, calcium and phosphorus, are combined in the bones, phosphorus is lost along with calcium. Chronic kidney disease often produces the same result.

An inherited, most commonly in an **X-linked dominant** pattern, hypophosphatemia causes vitamin D resistant rickets. In these individuals, a reabsorption defect in the kidneys causes excessive losses of phosphate in the urine (Gropper and Smith, 2013).

Reflecting the wide distribution and functions of phosphorus in the body, deficiency affects many organs and systems. Signs and symptoms of hypophosphatemia include the following:

- Impaired growth
- Osteomalacia
- Proximal muscle atrophy and weakness
- Cardiac arrhythmias
- Respiratory insufficiency
- Nervous system disorders

Toxicity

For basic information on mineral toxicity, see Table 7-4. Decreased renal excretion of phosphorus is the most common cause of **hyperphosphatemia.**

In 2006, the Food and Drug Administration (FDA) posted a warning regarding oral sodium phosphate bowel cleansing products that caused acute renal failure in 22 clients who used them. Since then an additional 20 cases were reported occurring within several hours to as long as 21 days after use. Equal concern was expressed regarding prescription or over-the-counter oral sodium phosphate products for bowel cleansing. The FDA recommends caution with prescription products for bowel cleansing in the following clients:

- Those older than 55 years
- Those with dehydration, kidney disease, acute colitis, or delayed bowel emptying
- Those taking medications that affect kidney function (U.S. FDA, 2008)

Previous cases of hyperphosphatemia causing serious neurological damage were attributed to sodium phosphate bowel cleansing products administered rectally to individuals with bowel diseases. Clients with conditions that increase the permeability of the intestine are at special risk when using these products.

Sodium

The body of a 154-pound adult contains about 105 grams (3.5 ounces) of sodium. Approximately 70% of the sodium in the body is in the blood and other extracellular fluids and in nerve and muscle tissue. The other 30% is on the surface of the bone crystals where it is available for release to counteract a low serum sodium level (Gropper and Smith, 2013).

Sodium has a major role in maintaining fluid balance in the body and contributes to maintaining acid–base balance as well (see Chapter 8). Sodium is also necessary for the transmission of electrochemical impulses along nerve and muscle membranes.

The intestine readily absorbs sodium. At most, 5% of dietary sodium travels within the intestine to remain in the feces. The remaining 95% of ingested sodium is absorbed into the bloodstream. To maintain a normal level of sodium in the blood, the kidney either reabsorbs sodium and returns it to the bloodstream or allows it to be spilled in the urine. The major hormone controlling sodium excretion, **aldosterone** from the adrenal cortex, stimulates the kidney to return sodium to the bloodstream (see Chapter 8).

Dietary Reference Intakes and Sources

For DRIs, see Appendix A. For food and other sources, see Table 7-1. To investigate the mineral content of a particular item, go to http://ndb.nal.usda.gov or to http://nutritiondata.self.com.

Table salt, the major dietary source of sodium, is 40% sodium and 60% chloride. One teaspoonful (5 grams) of salt contains 2.3 grams of sodium, the UL for adults younger than 50 years of age. Many foods, such as milk, milk products, and several vegetables, are naturally high in sodium.

The average sodium intake among persons in the United States aged 2 years and older is 3266 milligrams per day *excluding table salt.* The estimated distribution of intake is:

- 75% from packaged and restaurant foods
- 12% from natural sources
- 11% from salt added while cooking or eating a meal (Centers for Disease Control, 2012b)

See Figure 7-7, which compares mean sodium intake to recommended levels for everyone over age 2 years.

Despite the fact that salt is not so crucial to maintaining year-round food stocks as it was years ago, when, for instance, meat was salted to preserve it, food processors still find it a useful and inexpensive additive. Manufacturers add sodium for flavor, to alter the texture of the food, or to extend its shelf life. Consequently, food industry participation will be needed to achieve significant reductions in sodium intake. Table 7-5 compares the sodium content of relatively unprocessed foods with processed versions. Sodium-restricted diets and the legal definitions regarding the sodium content of foods are covered in Chapter 18.

Deficiency

Sodium deficiency is typically caused not by dietary deficiency (because of the abundance of sodium in foods) but by increased sodium loss from:

- Diarrhea
- Vomiting
- Kidney disease
- Heavy sweating that produces a loss of 3% of body weight (Smith and Gropper, 2013)

Hyponatremia is the technical name for low serum sodium, less than 135 **milliequivalent**s (see Chapter 8) per liter in adults. Low serum sodium because of excess retained water is called **dilutional hyponatremia.** It can result from disordered hormonal control (syndrome of inappropriate antidiuresis, **SIAD**) and from overhydration with plain water

by perspiring athletes or military trainees (see Chapter 8).

Because of the rigid confines of the skull, the brain is subject to dysfunction when it fails to control its water content effectively. Overall morbidity and mortality in hyponatremic encephalopathy is 42%, clearly categorizing the condition as a medical emergency (Ayus, Achinger, and Arieff, 2008). The impairment of brain function is evident in the signs and symptoms of abnormal sodium and potassium levels listed in Table 7-6.

At the opposite extreme, too rapid correction of hyponatremia presents a risk of **osmotic demyelinating disease** causing motor nerve dysfunction including quadriplegia (Bailey, Sands, and Franch, 2014). Thus, therapy must navigate between the possibility of fatal cerebral edema and the complications of excessive therapy, osmotic demyelinating disease (Sterns, Hix, and Silver, 2010).

Toxicity

For basic information on mineral toxicity, see Table 7-4. The reported 4 to 6 grams of sodium in the average American diet is probably an underestimate. Frequently such surveys do not account for all sources of sodium. An excess of sodium in the blood, greater than 145 milliequivalents per liter in adults, is called **hypernatremia.** Its signs and symptoms appear in Table 7-6.

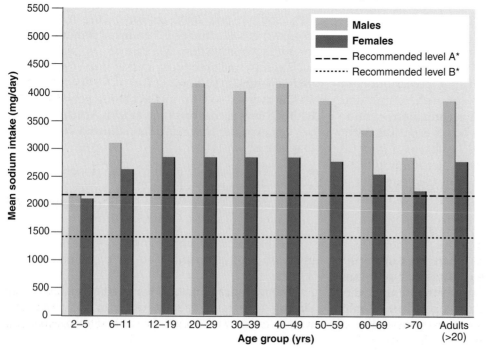

Mean sodium intake (excluding table salt), by age and sex, and recommended levels* - National Health and Nutrition Examination Survey, United States, 2007–2008

FIGURE 7-7 The bars in the graph show the mean sodium intake (excluding table salt), by age and sex, in the United States, during 2007–2008 according to National Health and Nutrition Examination Survey (**NHANES**). Current dietary guidelines recommend reducing consumption of sodium to less than 2300 mg/day (recommended level A), and that African Americans, persons aged ≥51 years, and persons of any age with hypertension, diabetes, or chronic kidney disease further reduce intake to 1500 mg/day (recommended level B). Regardless of age or sex, sodium intake by most U.S. residents considerably exceeds recommended levels. (*Source:* Centers for Disease Control, May 25, 2012b. Retrieved from www.cdc.gov/mmwr/preview/mmwrhtml/mm6105a2.htm?s_cid=mm6105a2_w#fig.)

TABLE 7-5 ■ Comparison of Sodium Content in Fresh and Processed Foods

FRESH FOOD	SODIUM (MG)	PROCESSED FOOD	SODIUM (MG)
Natural Swiss cheese, 1 oz	74	Pasteurized, processed Swiss cheese, 1 oz	388
Lean roast pork, 3 oz	65	Lean ham, 3 oz	930
Whole raw carrot, 1	25	Canned carrots, ½ cup	176
Tomato juice, canned without salt, 1 cup	24	Tomato juice, canned with salt, 1 cup	881

TABLE 7-6 ■ Signs and Symptoms of Abnormal Serum Sodium and Potassium Levels

	LOW	NORMAL	HIGH
Sodium			
Lab value	<135 mEq/L	135–148 mEq/L	>148 mEq/L
Condition	Hyponatremia		Hypernatremia
Symptoms	Weakness Headache Irritability Anxiety		Thirst Fatigue
Signs	Muscle twitching Fingerprinting over the sternum Altered consciousness Seizures Coma Permanent neurological damage Respiratory arrest		Flushed skin Sticky mucous membranes Agitation Coma
Potassium			
Lab value	<3.5 mEq/L	3.5–5.0 mEq/L	>5.0 mEq/L
Condition	Hypokalemia		Hyperkalemia
Symptoms	Nausea Paresthesias, especially lower extremities Disorientation		Irritability Abdominal cramps
Signs	Vomiting Decreased bowel sounds Diminished reflexes Muscle weakness Weak, irregular pulse Coma		Weakness, especially lower extremities Irregular pulse Characteristic electrocardiograph changes Cardiac arrest

Potassium

The body of a 154-pound adult contains about 245 grams of potassium, approximately 8.6 ounces. More than 85% of ingested potassium is absorbed from the small intestine and possibly the colon (Gropper and Smith, 2013). From 95% to 98% of the body's potassium is inside the cells, where it helps to control fluid balance.

In addition to fluid balance, potassium is essential for the conduction of nerve impulses and the contraction of muscles, including the heart. Potassium also helps maintain the body's **electrolyte** and acid–base balance (see Chapter 8) and can contribute to cardiovascular health. The U.S. FDA has approved this health claim: "Diets containing foods that are good sources of potassium and low in sodium my reduce the risk of high blood pressure and stroke." Qualifying foods must contain at least 350 milligrams of potassium, but no more than:

- 140 milligrams of sodium
- 3 grams of total fat
- 1 gram of saturated fat
- 20 milligrams of cholesterol
- 15% kilocalories from saturated fat (Gropper and Smith, 2013)

Dietary Reference Intakes

For DRIs, see Appendix A. For food and other sources, see Table 7-1. To investigate the mineral content of a particular item, go to http://ndb.nal.usda.gov or to http://nutritiondata.self.com.

Sources of Potassium

Potassium is present in all plant and animal cells, but the best sources are unprocessed foods. Only fats, oils, and white sugar have negligible amounts of potassium (see Table 7-1). Dietary instructions may focus on fruit sources because the client might also need to limit sodium, which frequently occurs in greater amounts in vegetables and dairy products than in fruits. Potassium might also be obtained from salt substitutes that often replace the sodium with potassium. Table 7-7 shows several good sources of potassium that, if prepared without salt, are also very low in sodium.

Deficiency

A potassium deficiency is related to diet only in cases of severe protein-energy malnutrition. **Hypokalemia,** a serum potassium of less than 3.5 milliequivalents per liter, can be fatal if prolonged or severe. Hypokalemia may be caused by:

■ Vomiting
■ Increased losses in urine, stool, or sweat (for cystic fibrosis, see Chapter 20)
■ Alkalosis
■ Potassium-wasting diuretics

It may also occur as part of refeeding syndrome (Gropper and Smith, 2013; see also Chapter 22). For signs and symptoms, see Table 7-6.

Toxicity

For basic information on mineral toxicity, see Table 7-4. A potassium level greater than 5.0 milliequivalents per liter is hyperkalemia. Signs and symptoms of hyperkalemia appear in Table 7-6.

Hyperkalemia is rarely caused by food but rather by impaired kidney function. It may also be caused by excessive destruction of cells in burns, crushing injuries, or severe infections. No symptoms may be apparent until blood levels of potassium are very high and skeletal muscle weakness is seen, followed by cardiac dysfunction that could prove fatal. One adverse effect of blood transfusion with old blood is elevated serum potassium. Clinical Application 7-5 covers that possibility. Other signs, such as results of electrocardiograms, assist in diagnosis of potassium imbalances, but cases of serum potassium greater than 7 mEq/L have displayed normal EKG tracings (Bailey, Sands, and Franch, 2014).

Dire consequences can result from hyper- or hyponatremia and hyper- or hypokalemia. If the nurse recognizes and reports early signs and symptoms, the need for drastic treatment measures and perhaps permanent damage may be averted.

Magnesium

The human body contains about 25 grams (0.9 ounce) of magnesium. About 50% to 60% of the magnesium is in bone, 39% to 49% in soft tissue, and 1% in body fluids (Gropper and Smith, 2013).

Absorption, Elimination, and Functions

Magnesium is absorbed throughout the small intestine, mostly in the distal jejunum and ileum and may be absorbed from the colon if disease has impaired small intestine absorption. Of usual intakes, from 30% to 60% is absorbed, with the smaller percentage absorbed at high intakes and the larger percentage at low intakes.

Excess magnesium is eliminated by the kidneys, where it competes with calcium for reabsorption sites. Excretion can be increased by protein, alcohol, and caffeine consumption but the exact homeostatic mechanism for magnesium is unclear (Gropper and Smith, 2013).

Magnesium is involved in more than 300 different enzymatic reactions. It is associated with ADP and ATP in energy metabolism. Magnesium is involved in DNA synthesis and degradation, in protein synthesis, and insulin action. It influences cardiac and smooth muscle

TABLE 7-7 ■ Good Sources of Potassium with Very Low Sodium and Moderate Kilocalories					
FOOD	PREPARATION	SERVING	Mg K+	Mg Na+	KILOCALORIES
Acorn squash	Baked Unsalted	1 cup cubes	896	8.2	115
White potato	Baked Unsalted	1 small (5 oz) with skin	738	13.8	128
Banana	Sliced	1 cup	537	1.5	133
Orange juice	Frozen, diluted 1:3	1 cup	473	2.5	112
Cantaloupe	Unsalted	1 cup cubes	427	25.6	54
Prunes	Uncooked, pitted	1/3 cup	425	1.2	139
Apricots	Canned in juice	1 cup	403	9.8	117

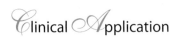

Clinical Application 7-5

Hyperkalemia After Blood Transfusion

Red blood cells (RBCs) do not survive as long in the blood bank as they do in the human body. Potassium is the major **cation** (see Chapter 8) in red blood cells. When the red blood cells die and their cell walls rupture, potassium is spilled into the surrounding liquid.

Blood that has been stored for a prolonged period may contain up to 30 mEq per liter of potassium due to the destruction of the red blood cells. This may not sound like a large amount, but potassium is usually administered intravenously at a concentration of 40 mEq per liter to a person who is potassium depleted. The person receiving a blood transfusion (or many units of blood) may have a serum potassium level that is nearly normal, and the old blood containing a higher concentration of potassium could precipitate hyperkalemia.

In a worse-case scenario, rapid transfusion of RBCs to critically ill clients has resulted in intraoperative transfusion-associated hyperkalemic cardiac arrest with a 12.5% in-hospital survival rate (Smith, Farrow, Ackerman, et al, 2008). The serum potassium level of one client in severe hemorrhagic shock (who received 18 units of red cell concentrate during surgery) increased from 4.05 to 8.24 mEq/L over a 7-minute period. The hemorrhage could not be controlled in surgery and the client expired after her second cardiac arrest (Tsukamoto, Maruyama, Nakagawa, et al, 2009).

The nurse should be aware of the age of blood products and identify clients at risk of hyperkalemia. Some promising strategies to prevent transfusion-related hyperkalemia include RBC washing and the use of in-line potassium filters (Vraets, Lin, and Callum, 2011), but such measures may not be feasible in emergency situations.

contractility directly and through calcium utilization (Gropper and Smith, 2013).

Dietary Reference Intakes and Sources

For DRIs see Appendix A. For food and other sources, see Table 7-1. To investigate the mineral content of a particular item, go to http://ndb.nal.usda.gov or to http://nutritiondata.self.com.

Magnesium is widely distributed in foods, especially green, leafy vegetables in which it is a component of chlorophyll. Removing the germ and outer layers of the wheat kernel can remove more than 75% of its magnesium content. Beverages such as coffee and cocoa also contain magnesium (Gropper and Smith, 2013).

Interfering Factors and Deficiency

Phosphorus can inhibit magnesium absorption especially when magnesium intake is low and that of phosphorus is high. The two are thought to combine in the intestinal tract, rendering both unavailable for absorption. Pure magnesium deficiency from inadequate dietary intake has not been reported (Gropper and Smith, 2013).

Diabetes mellitus is commonly associated with magnesium deficiency, presumably due to renal losses, and several studies have identified deficiencies in acutely or chronically ill clients (Rude, 2014). Deficiency may also result from the following:

- Malabsorption disorders causing vomiting or diarrhea
- Excessive alcohol use coupled with poor nutritional intake
- Chronic diuretic use (Gropper and Smith, 2013)

Magnesium deficiency is often associated with muscle cramps, and supplementation improved cramps in some clinical studies (Beier, Landes, Mohammad, and McClain, 2014). In a review of seven trials, however, only those of pregnant women presented sufficient conflicting evidence to suggest a need for further research. No randomized controlled trials evaluating magnesium for exercise-associated muscle cramps or disease state-associated muscle cramps (for example, amyotrophic lateral sclerosis/motor neuron disease) were found (Garrison, Allan, Sekhon, et al, 2012).

Serum magnesium in migraine clients was found to be significantly lower than in those without such a history and was related to the frequency of migraine attacks (Talebi, Savadi-Oskouei, Farhoudi, et al, 2011). The Canadian Headache Society recommended 11 drugs to prevent migraine headaches, including the nutrients magnesium and riboflavin (Pringsheim, Davenport, Mackie, et al, 2012), both of which are considered safe for pregnant women because they lack severe adverse effects (Airola, Allais, Castagnoli, Gabellari, et al, 2010).

Because of its safety, magnesium sulfate has been used for decades as an anticonvulsant for **preeclampsia** and **eclampsia** (see Chapter 10) and contributes to the low mortality rate from these conditions in developed countries. Magnesium's chief mode of action in these cases may be to stabilize nervous and vascular tissues rather than to correct electrolyte imbalances (Rude, 2014).

Because magnesium metabolism is intricately linked to calcium metabolism, magnesium-deficient clients display the signs of tetany. Other signs include the following:

- Personality changes
- Anorexia
- Nausea
- Vomiting (Heimburger, 2014)

Magnesium heptogluconate is useful as a supplement to correct hypomagnesemia without causing diarrhea (Jeejeebhoy, 2014).

Toxicity

For basic information on mineral toxicity, see Table 7-4. Ordinarily, magnesium levels do not build up in the blood except as a result of kidney disease. In fact, oral magnesium can cause diarrhea—Epsom salt is magnesium sulfate. Because of magnesium's close link to calcium, the effects of magnesium toxicity can be blocked by administering calcium.

Sulfur

The adult body contains approximately 175 grams of sulfur, a component of the cytoplasm of every cell. Sulfur is especially notable in hair, skin, and nails where it contributes to their shape. Sulfur is a component of thiamin, biotin, insulin, and heparin and of the amino acids methionine and cysteine. A protective function of sulfur is that of combining with toxins to neutralize them.

The major source of sulfate for humans is provided through the amino acid pool (see Fig. 4–2) by catabolism of the sulfur-containing amino acids methionine and cysteine. Dietary intake of foods containing these amino acids helps to replenish the supply (see Table 7-1). Cases of deficiency of sulfur alone are unknown. Only people with a severe protein deficiency lack this mineral. *For basic information on mineral toxicity, see Table 7-4.*

Chloride

Chloride plays a major role in maintaining fluid balance and acid–base balance. The body of a 154-pound adult contains approximately 105 grams of chloride. Of the body's chloride, 88% is found in extracellular fluids such as the hydrochloric acid in the stomach, and 12% is found in intracellular fluids. Chloride also is released by white blood cells as they fight substances foreign to the body. Chloride is almost completely absorbed through the small intestine and is excreted primarily by the kidney as a result of sodium regulation (Gropper and Smith, 2013).

For DRIs see Appendix A. For food and other sources, see Table 7-1.

The DRI levels were established proportionate to the AI for sodium because nearly all dietary chloride is derived from salt. Table salt, which is 60% chloride, contains about 3 grams of chloride per teaspoon (5 grams).

Normally, most chloride is excreted by the kidney; however, loss of gastrointestinal fluids through severe vomiting, nasogastric suctioning, or diarrhea is a common cause of chloride deficiency, typically causing convulsions (Gropper and Smith, 2013). Chloride deficiency has occurred in infants because chloride was omitted from their formulas. Long-term **sequelae** in some of these children included cognitive impairments, visuomotor difficulties, and attention-deficit

disorder (Kaleita, Kinsbourne, and Menkes, 1991). A genetic defect in chloride transport regulation causes **cystic fibrosis** (see Chapter 20).

Sodium and chlorine are so chemically active that in nature they are always found bound to each other or to other elements. Table salt is a compound of sodium (an unstable, silvery white, waxy, soft metal) and chlorine (a greenish yellow poisonous gas), which when accidentally released in industrial settings or train derailments, can cause fatalities (Centers for Disease Control, July 22, 2011; Van Sickle, Wenck, Belflower, et al, 2009).

Trace Minerals

Many trace minerals occur in such small amounts that they are difficult to measure and analyze; thus, their physiological functions and possible roles in nutrition are not completely understood.

Ten trace minerals have well-known bodily functions, and nine of them have been assigned RDAs or AIs. Four of them are commonly recognized for their relationship to health:

1. Iron
2. Iodine
3. Fluoride
4. Zinc

The other six are:

1. Selenium
2. Chromium
3. Copper
4. Manganese
5. Cobalt
6. Molybdenum

Five additional trace minerals, arsenic, boron, nickel, silicon, and vanadium, termed ultratrace minerals, appear in the UL tables, but RDAs or AIs are not determinable.

Iron

For a nutrient with functions as vital as those of iron, the amount in the body is slight—approximately 38 milligrams per kilogram of body weight for women and 50 milligrams per kilogram for men (Gropper and Smith, 2013). Thus a 154-pound (70 kilogram) man would have 3.5 grams of iron, less than the weight of a penny, in his body. The body conserves its supply of iron by recycling the mineral released from the catabolism of worn-out red blood cells.

Functions

Iron is essential to the formation of hemoglobin, the component of the red blood cell that transports approximately 98.5% of the oxygen in the blood. **Hemoglobin** is composed of **heme,** the nonprotein portion that contains iron, and globin, a simple protein.

Iron is also a component of **myoglobin,** a protein located in muscle tissue. Myoglobin stores oxygen within the muscle cells. When the body needs an immediate supply of oxygen, such as during strenuous exercise, myoglobin releases its stored oxygen.

Iron is also present in enzymes that support energy metabolism and the synthesis and catabolism of neurotransmitters. The iron content of parts of the brain is comparable to that in the liver and continues to increase until the third decade of life (Chitambar and Asok, 2014).

About 80% of the iron in a healthy body is available for carrying oxygen: hemoglobin contains 65%, myoglobin 10%, and iron-containing enzymes 3%. The balance is in the blood or stored in the liver, spleen, and bone marrow for future use. The primary storage form of iron in the body's cells is **ferritin,** a dynamic protein–iron compound that through constant degrading and resynthesis provides a supply for metabolic needs (Smith and Gropper, 2013).

Absorption

The body tightly conserves its supply of iron. Dietary iron is absorbed throughout the small intestine, most efficiently in the duodenum. When red blood cells are destroyed after their usual life span of 120 days, their iron is stored for reuse. Once iron is absorbed, there is no physiological mechanism for excreting the excess. Fortunately, under normal conditions, the body is selective about absorbing iron.

Perhaps the most exciting breakthrough in iron biology is the discovery of **hepcidin,** an iron regulatory hormone (Wessling-Resnick, 2014). The liver manufactures hepcidin, a hormone that regulates iron metabolism in the duodenum, liver, spleen, and bone marrow. When the body's iron levels are high, hepcidin is synthesized to inhibit iron transport in the duodenum and to prevent release of stored iron (Harrison-Findik, 2009, 2010).

FACTORS AFFECTING AMOUNTS

As the body's need for iron increases, so does the proportion absorbed. In a healthy person, about 10% of the iron in foods is absorbed whereas a person who is iron deficient may absorb as much as 35% (Gropper and Smith, 2013).

The amount of dietary iron that is absorbed is determined by the amount of ferritin present in the intestinal mucosa. The iron obtained from ingested food is bound to a protein called **apoferritin** in the intestinal mucosa to form ferritin. When the total supply of apoferritin has been bound to iron, any additional iron in the gut is rejected and eliminated in the feces. Similarly, iron within the apoferritin that is not needed remains in the intestinal cell to be sloughed off and excreted in the feces (Gropper and Smith, 2013).

Absorbed iron combines with a protein in the blood, **transferrin,** which transports iron to the bone marrow for hemoglobin synthesis, to the liver or spleen for storage, or to the body cells for use. Hemoglobin synthesis requires many other substances, including adequate protein and traces of copper, in addition to iron but the shortages most likely to impair synthesis of red blood cells are:

- Iron
- Cobalamin
- Folate (Chitambar and Asok, 2014)

FACTORS AFFECTING ABSORPTION RATES

Two types of iron are found naturally in food that are absorbed through different mechanisms:

1. Heme iron
2. Nonheme iron (Wessling-Resnick, 2014)

Heme iron is bound to the hemoglobin and myoglobin in meat, fish, and poultry. From 50% to 60% of the total iron in these animal sources is heme iron. Because heme iron is composed of **ferrous iron** (Fe^{2+}), it is rapidly transported and absorbed intact.

Nonheme iron is the other 40% to 50% of the total iron in meat, fish, poultry, and all the iron in plant sources (Gropper and Smith, 2013).

The absorption of nonheme iron is slow because it is closely bound to organic molecules in foods as **ferric iron** (Fe^{3+}). In the acidic medium of the stomach, oxygen is removed from ferric iron during a chemical reaction called reduction. The end product is ferrous iron, which is more soluble and bioavailable. See Figure 7-8 for an overview of the steps involved in the process of iron absorption.

FACTORS ENHANCING ABSORPTION

Several factors increase the absorption of nonheme iron through different mechanisms.

- Alcohol suppresses hepcidin synthesis by the liver, which then permits increased duodenal absorption of iron (Harrison-Findik, 2009).
- Acids, such as ascorbic and citric, increase absorption by combining with the iron in a soluble compound, thus preventing formation of insoluble iron complexes.

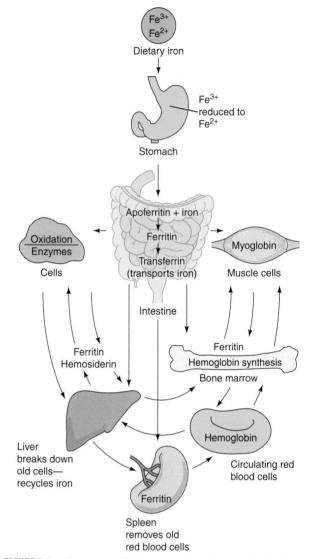

FIGURE 7-8 In the process of dietary iron absorption, iron is absorbed primarily in the small intestine but also is recovered from worn-out cells before being transported or stored to meet the body's needs.

■ MFP Factor (meat, fish, poultry) increases the absorption of nonheme iron when meat, fish, or poultry is consumed at the same time.

FACTORS INTERFERING WITH ABSORPTION

Other minerals compete with iron for absorption.

■ Calcium blocks uptake of both heme and nonheme iron (Wessling-Resnick, 2014).
■ Zinc or manganese may also decrease iron absorption by an undefined mechanism (Gropper and Smith, 2013).
■ Phytic acid from cereals (whole grains, legumes, and maize) forms insoluble complexes with iron.
■ Oxalic acid from certain berries and vegetables (see the calcium section) combines with iron, reducing its availability.

■ Decreased gastric acid, whether because of antacid medications or gastric resection, lessens the iron that is absorbed.
■ Polyphenols found in tea and coffee, when consumed with nonheme iron, can reduce iron absorption by more than 50%.
■ Coffee, taken with or just after a meal, may reduce iron absorption by 40% (Gropper and Smith, 2013).

Table 7-8 summarizes the factors that affect iron absorption. People who consume vegetarian diets should be especially careful to construct optimal menus not only because of the elimination of meat but also because of the increased amounts of phytates likely included in the diet. Practical suggestions to enhance iron and zinc nutrition in vegetarian diets are given in Table 7-9.

Excretion

No known mechanism exists to regulate the excretion of iron. Small amounts of iron are lost daily via the gastrointestinal tract, shed skin cells, and urine even in healthy people. Certain medications and diseases increase the losses.

Physiologic status also influences iron loss. Postmenopausal women lose 0.7 to 0.9 milligrams of iron per day, men 0.9 to 1.2 milligrams per day, whereas women of reproductive age lose an average of 1.3 to 1.4 milligrams per day because of menstrual losses averaged over the month (Gropper and Smith, 2013).

Blood contains about 0.5 milligram of iron per milliliter, so a blood donor would lose 250 milligrams per unit donated (Mast, Lee, Schlumpf, et al, 2012). Someone who donates every 2 months, then, would have to replace iron at the rate of 4 milligrams per day over and above the RDA all year long.

Dietary Reference Intakes

For DRIs see Appendix A. For food and other sources, see Table 7-10. To investigate the mineral content of a particular item, go to http://ndb.nal.usda.gov or to http://nutritiondata.self.com.

Vegetarian diets are estimated to provide iron at 10% bioavailability, partly because they lack the MPF factor, rather than the 18% from a mixed Western diet. Hence the requirement for iron is 1.8 times higher for

TABLE 7-8 ■ Factors Affecting Iron Absorption	
INCREASE	**DECREASE**
Large alcohol intake	Phytic or oxalic acids
Meat, fish, or poultry	Coffee or tea (tannins)
Vitamin C	Less gastric acid, antacids
	Calcium and zinc

TABLE 7-9 ■ **Improving Iron and Zinc Nutrition in Vegetarian Diets**

GOAL	STRATEGY	RATIONALE
Increase the total amount of iron and zinc consumed.	Select foods rich in iron and zinc at all meals. Consume cereals and pasta fortified with these nutrients.	Obtaining sufficient iron and zinc without animal products requires careful planning.
Make use of contamination iron.	Use cast iron cookware or steel woks for vegetable casseroles or curries, spaghetti sauces, or stewed fruits.	Moist, acidic foods have increased iron content when thus cooked for a long period. Even 20 minutes has shown an effect (Fairweather-Tait, Fox, and Mallilin, 1995).
Expand the intake of absorption enhancers.	Consume fermented foods such as yogurt and oriental soy products (tempeh, miso, natto, and soy sauce). Include a good source of vitamin C at every meal.	Certain organic acids (citric, lactic, malic, and tartaric) prevent the formation of insoluble iron and zinc phytates. The addition of milk and yogurt to a plant-based diet high in phytate increases zinc bioavailability without affecting iron bioavailability (Rosado, Díaz, and González, et al, 2005). Ascorbic acid is the most effective enhancer of nonheme iron absorption when consumed with the nonheme iron. It reduces ferric to ferrous iron that is more soluble at the pH of the duodenum and small intestine.
Reduce the intake of absorption antagonists.	Consumption of both sprouted whole-grain cereals and legumes and yeast-leavened baked products can potentially reduce the phytic acid content of a meal. Soak legumes before cooking. Delay drinking coffee and tea until at least 2 hours after meals.	Microbial fermentation can enhance bioavailability of iron and zinc via hydrolysis induced by microbial phytase enzymes derived from microflora on the surface of cereal grains or from yeast. Because phytic acid is relatively water soluble, soaking reduces the phytic acid of most legumes These beverages reduce nonheme iron absorption 40%–60%.
Avoid taking high doses of mineral supplements.	Dietary sources alone are unlikely to compromise iron and zinc status.	Antagonistic interactions between copper and zinc and between nonheme iron and zinc are most likely when high doses of supplemental zinc and nonheme iron are ingested without food.

SOURCE: Adapted from Gibson, Donovan, and Heath (1997).

TABLE 7-10 ■ **Trace Minerals**

MINERAL	ADULT RDA/AI AND FOOD PORTION CONTAINING IT*	FUNCTIONS	SIGNS AND SYMPTOMS OF DEFICIENCY	SIGNS AND SYMPTOMS OF EXCESS	BEST SOURCES
Iron	8–18 mg (female) 8 mg (male) 2.6–5.8 oz Braunschweiger	Component of hemoglobin	Fatigue, lightheadedness Shortness of breath Hypochromic, microcytic anemia	Hemosiderosis Hemochromatosis	Liver, other red meats Clams Oysters Lima and navy beans Dark green leafy cooked vegetables Dried fruit
Iodine	150 mcg 3/8 tsp iodized salt	Component of thyroid hormones	Goiter Cretinism Myxedema	Acnelike lesions Goiter	Iodized salt Saltwater seafood
Fluoride	3–4 mg 4.3–5.7 L fluoridated water	Hardens teeth	Dental caries	Mottled teeth Increased caries	Fluoridated water Seafood Brewed tea
Zinc	8–11 mg 3.6–5 oz beef chuck roast, lean only	Component of 70 enzymes Involved in DNA and RNA synthesis Necessary for collagen formation Serves role in immunity	Growth failure Hypogonadism Delayed wound healing Impaired night vision Impaired taste Delayed sexual maturation	Copper deficiency Suppressed immune response	Red meat, especially organ meat Seafood, especially oysters Poultry Pork Dairy products Whole grains
Copper	900 mcg 1.8 oz lobster	Cofactor for enzymes involved in hemoglobin synthesis and cell respiration Necessary for melanin formation	Menkes disease Anemia Demineralization of skeleton Depigmentation of skin and hair Impaired immune function	Wilson disease Copper deposits in liver, kidneys, brain, spleen, and cornea	Organ meats Shellfish Nuts Seeds Legumes Dried fruit

(continued)

TABLE 7-10 ■ Trace Minerals (Continued)

MINERAL	ADULT RDA/AI AND FOOD PORTION CONTAINING IT*	FUNCTIONS	SIGNS AND SYMPTOMS OF DEFICIENCY	SIGNS AND SYMPTOMS OF EXCESS	BEST SOURCES
Selenium	55 mcg 3.6 large hard-cooked eggs	Part of many enzymes Necessary for iodine metabolism Protects against the toxicity from mercury, cadmium, and silver	Keshan cardiomyopathy	Sour milk or garlic breath odor Fatigue Nail and hair loss	Brazil nuts Meats Seafood Dairy products Eggs
Chromium	20–35 mcg 0.5–0.9 oz American cheese	Thought to potentiate action of insulin	Weight loss Impaired glucose utilization Elevated blood lipids Peripheral neuropathy	Rarely related to food Metallic taste	Meats, especially organ meats Fish Poultry Cheese Peanuts Whole grains
Manganese	1.8–2.3 mg 1.1–1.4 cups cooked spinach	Involved in amino acid and carbohydrate metabolism Required for bone formation	Dermatitis Decreased growth of hair and nails Skeletal defects Changes in hair and beard color	Accumulated mineral in brain In miners: liver damage and Parkinson-like syndrome Central nervous system impairment	Whole grains Dried fruits Nuts Cooked green, leafy vegetables
Cobalt	Not established	Component of vitamin B_{12}	Not reported		Meat Poultry Fish Eggs Milk, cheese
Molybdenum	45 mcg ¼ cup cooked navy beans†	Cofactor for enzymes involved in catabolism of sulfur-containing amino acids and purines	Parenteral nutrition clients only: tachycardia, headache, mental disturbances, coma	Hyperuricemia Gout	Meat Fish Poultry Legumes Whole grains

*Examples only; not suggested for sole source of a day's intake.
†Mineral omitted from many nutrient databases.

vegetarians than for other Americans. Very strict vegetarians' iron availability may be as low as 5% (Institute of Medicine, 2001).

Sources

The Western diet contains an estimated 5 to 7 milligrams of iron per 1000 kilocalories. In the United States, one-third of dietary iron is supplied by grains, one-third by meats, and one-third by other sources. Absorption also varies among the sources of iron. Ten to 30% of iron is absorbed from liver and other meats; less than 10% is absorbed from eggs; and less than 5% is absorbed from grains and most vegetables.

Many foods are fortified with iron, but its bioavailability depends on the compounds used. Iron from spinach, iron supplements, and contamination iron are absorbed at a 2% rate. Clinical Application 7-6 describes one way iron becomes available from nonfood sources.

Deficiency

Perhaps the most significant worldwide nutritional problem, iron deficiency affects more than 2 billion people, including half the women and children in developing

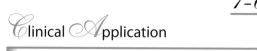

7-6
$\mathscr{C}$linical $\mathscr{A}$pplication

Contamination Iron

Cooking in iron pots can increase the iron content of foods. This source of dietary iron is called **contamination iron.** Significant transfer occurs during simmering of acidic foods, especially tomatoes. For instance, 3½ ounces of spaghetti sauce cooked for 3 hours in a cast iron pot contains almost 90 milligrams of iron, compared to less than 5 milligrams of iron when cooked in a glass container (Zhou and Brittin, 1994). The East Indian practice of cooking curries in cast iron woks also was shown to increase iron content 4- to 12-fold (Fairweather-Tait, Fox, and Mallillin, 1995). The absorption rate of contamination iron is the same as that of supplements—2%.

countries (Wessling-Resnick, 2014). Iron deficiency **anemia** occurs in 2% to 5% of adult men and postmenopausal women in the developed world often caused by gastrointestinal blood loss. The most important causes of such blood loss are colonic or gastric cancers that need to be ruled out (Goddard, James, McIntyre, and Scott, 2011).

Iron deficiency can be determined by laboratory tests such as plasma ferritin and transferrin saturation before a person's hemoglobin value drops sufficiently to diagnose anemia, in which iron stores are severely depleted (Gropper and Smith, 2013). The anemic client often complains of lightheadedness, shortness of breath on exertion, and possibly soreness of mouth and tongue, and physical examination reveals pallor and probably an increased pulse rate.

The effects of low iron status on infants and young children included impaired growth (short stature) and low intelligence quotient scores (Wessling-Resnick, 2014). Iron-deficient children given supplements showed substantially improved school performance in 3 months. Iron deficiency also leads to defective information processing in adult women whose verbal learning and memory improve with iron administration (Chitambar and Asok, 2014). Mutations in iron loading genes are associated with Alzheimer disease, prompting investigations into clinical applications of chelation therapy for the illness (Wessling-Resnick, 2014).

A person who is anemic has insufficient hemoglobin to provide oxygen to the cells of the body. The features of the red blood cells are characteristic of various anemias. In iron-deficiency anemia, the red blood cells are microcytic (smaller than normal) and hypochromic (contain less hemoglobin, giving the cell less color than normal).

RISK OF DEFICIENCY

In the United States, population groups that frequently have inadequate iron intake are as follows:

- Infants and young children
- Adolescents in their early growth spurts
- Women of childbearing years
- Pregnant women (Gropper and Smith, 2013)

Iron deficiency is estimated to occur in 30% to 50% of clients following **bariatric** surgical procedures that bypass the duodenum and jejunum related to low intakes of iron-rich foods and interference with absorption (Tymitz, Magnuson, and Schwitzer, 2014). Other illnesses or treatments that increase gastrointestinal blood loss such as long-term use of nonsteroidal anti-inflammatory medications should be considered when assessing iron nutriture. More information on iron deficiency in pregnant women is included in Chapter 10. Iron deficiency in children appears in Chapter 11.

ASSESSMENT DATA

Although no single test is diagnostic for iron deficiency, a common test to determine the hemoglobin level of the blood delivers valuable assessment data. The normal level for men is 14 to 18 grams per 100 milliliters of blood; for women it is 12 to 16 grams. Another common laboratory test is the **hematocrit,** which measures the percentage of red blood cells in a volume of blood. Normal hematocrit levels are 40% to 54% for men and 36% to 46% for women. Persons living above 4000 feet in altitude will have higher normal values. Low hemoglobin and hematocrit levels are late indicators of iron deficiency.

In early iron deficiency, before hemoglobin and hematocrit readings drop, serum ferritin is a good indicator of iron stores under most conditions but can be falsely high due to infection and inflammation (Gropper and Smith, 2013). As the deficiency progresses, **serum transferrin** levels will rise if the body, in attempting to compensate, manufactures more transferrin to increase iron-carrying capacity (Lichtin, 2013).

TREATMENT

Supplemental iron is best absorbed when taken on an empty stomach, but gastrointestinal side effects often provoke noncompliance. Even taking the supplement with food or close to mealtime is better than not taking it at all. Accompanying the supplement with meat or vitamin C–rich foods and avoiding coffee, tea, milk, and cereals with it should increase absorption. Also, beginning at a lower dosage and then increasing it as tolerance develops is sometimes a useful strategy. Enteric-coated preparations are available but may not dissolve until beyond the duodenum, where absorption is most effective.

Hemoglobin levels can be used to monitor the effectiveness of treatment. After rising slowly for 2 weeks, hemoglobin typically increases by 0.7 to 1 gram per week so that supplementation should correct anemia in 2 months (Lichtin, 2013). Iron therapy should be continued for several months after hemoglobin and hematocrit levels return to normal to enable the body to rebuild iron stores.

In developing countries with high levels of infectious diseases, iron administration for anemia has been followed by increased morbidity from infections. Because bacteria also require iron, when the body's supply increases, they thrive. In 2006, the World Health Organization and the United Nations Children's Fund released a joint statement advising that, in regions where the prevalence of malaria and other infectious diseases is high, iron and folic acid supplementation should be limited to those who are identified as iron-deficient. When target groups have already been identified as being iron-deficient, iron supplementation is the intervention of choice for the treatment of anemia and other manifestations of iron deficiency. For prevention of iron deficiency, however, supplements are probably the least desirable of the available interventions, particularly for infants and children (Raiten, Namasté, and Brabin, 2011).

Toxicity

For basic information on mineral toxicity, see Table 7-4. Iron absorption is effectively controlled in healthy people even when meat intake is high and foods are fortified.

Surplus iron is stored in the liver as **hemosiderin.** When large amounts of hemosiderin are deposited in the liver and spleen without tissue damage, a condition called **hemosiderosis** results. If prolonged, it can lead to **hemochromatosis,** a disease of iron metabolism affecting 1 million Americans (Johnson, 2008b), in which iron accumulates in and damages tissues (see Genomic Gem 7-2).

Clients with alcoholism, although often lacking many other nutrients, sometimes suffer from iron overload. Some alcoholic beverages themselves contain a significant amount of iron. For example, inexpensive red wines contain 10 to 350 milligrams of iron per liter.

Dietary iron overload is common in parts of sub-Saharan Africa. It results from the consumption of large volumes of beer home-brewed in iron pots or ungalvanized steel drums from which it acquires a high iron content. Prevention involves fermenting the home-brewed beer in iron-free containers (Kew, 2010).

Toxicity from supplemental iron tablets is a major threat to children. The body's absorptive controls for dietary iron are circumvented by the large amounts of soluble iron in pharmaceutical preparations. In the United States, iron is the most common cause of accidental pediatric poisoning deaths in children younger than the age of 6 years (see Clinical Application 7-7).

Prenatal multivitamins are the source of iron in most lethal ingestions among children. Doses of 20 to 60 milligrams of elemental iron per kilogram of body weight are mildly to moderately toxic and more than 60 milligrams per kilogram can cause severe symptoms and morbidity (O'Malley, 2009). Ferrous sulfate, the most commonly prescribed iron supplement, consists of 20% to 30% elemental iron so that the minimal toxic dose could result from six and one-half 195-milligram over-the-counter tablets taken by a 28-pound child. Signs and symptoms begin with acute gastroenteritis within 6 hours of iron ingestion, followed by a latent period of up to 24 hours, then shock, seizures, and liver failure (O'Malley, 2009).

The Consumer Product Safety Commission requires child-resistant packaging for iron preparations

---

Genomic Gem 7-2
Hereditary Hemochromatosis

This **autosomal recessive** disease is associated with mutations in genes with resultant diminished hepcidin synthesis and increased absorption of iron. The disorder has a **homozygous** frequency of 1:200 and a **heterozygous** frequency of 1:8 in people of northern European ancestry. It is uncommon among blacks and rare among people of Asian ancestry. Of clients with clinical hemochromatosis, 83% are homozygous. For unknown reasons, however, clinical disease is much less common than predicted by the frequency of the gene occurrence. Therefore, many homozygous people do not manifest the disorder (Frankel, 2009) indicating that additional genetic and environmental factors modify the severity and clinical penetrance of disease (Weiss, 2010). Nevertheless, first-degree relatives of clients with hereditary hemochromatosis should be screened to locate other cases early.

The hemochromatosis gene, abbreviated HFE, is located on chromosome 6. It instructs cells in the liver and intestine to produce the HFE protein that

- interacts with other proteins on the cell surface to detect the amount of iron in the body and
- regulates the production of hepcidin, the master iron regulatory hormone.

More than 20 mutations in the HFE gene have been identified as causing the most common type of hemochromatosis. Two particular mutations are responsible for most cases, each substituting one amino acid for another used to make the HFE protein:

- Tyrosine for cysteine at position 282
- Aspartic acid for histidine at position 63 (U.S. National Library of Medicine, 2012)

Signs and symptoms are caused by deposits of iron in various organs and may include hyperpigmentation of the skin, diabetes, joint symptoms, and erectile dysfunction (Frankel, 2009). In affected clients, early treatment by phlebotomy can prevent organ damage. Treatment involves regular removal of blood (200–250 milligrams of iron per unit) through **phlebotomy** until a satisfactory serum ferritin level is achieved (Gropper and Smith, 2013). In addition, the drug *deferoxamine* may be administered to bind with iron, forming a water-soluble complex that is excreted in the urine (Vallerand, Sanoski, and Deglin, 2013). Dietary interventions can also be therapeutic:

- Avoid iron and vitamin C supplements, including multivitamin–multimineral preparations.
- Consume red or organ meats in moderation.
- Avoid alcohol.
- Do not consume raw shellfish lest it contain an organism (*Vibrio vulnificus*) that can cause fatal infections in persons with iron overload and cirrhosis (Chung, Misdraji, and Sahani, 2006).

Untreated, hemochromatosis leads to organ failure and death. Possible new treatments might include hepcidin-enhancing agents (Weiss, 2010).

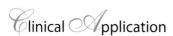

Clinical Application

Precautions to Prevent Medication Poisoning in Children

Health-care providers should impress upon parents the enormous threat medications and supplements pose for small children. The products should be stored:

■ Out of reach
■ Out of sight
■ With child-resistant caps intact

Adults should take medicines out of the child's view to avoid modeling a behavior that could harm the child.

If a child ingests any medication or supplement, a poison control center should be consulted *immediately* without waiting for signs and symptoms to appear.

in certain forms and specified strengths, and the FDA requires a warning label on solid dosage forms of iron (U.S. FDA, July 18, 2011).

Iodine

In the human body, iodine is usually found and functions in its ionic form, iodide. The body of the average adult contains about 15 to 20 milligrams of iodide. The thyroid gland in the neck contains 70% to 80% of the total body iodide and takes up approximately 120 micrograms of iodide per day (Gropper and Smith, 2013).

Function and Control of the Thyroid Gland

The main function of iodine is its participation in the synthesis of thyroid hormones, which are essential for proper maturation of the nervous system, particularly in utero and for the first few years after birth. Devastating consequences result from deficiency of iodine during those years (see Deficiency later in this section).

The thyroid gland secretes **thyroxine (T_4)** and **tri-iodothyronine (T_3)** in response to **thyroid-stimulating hormone (TSH)** from the anterior pituitary gland. Both T_3 and T_4 increase the rate of oxidation in cells, thereby increasing the rate of metabolism. When serum levels of T_3 and T_4 are adequate, secretion of TSH ceases. This is called a **negative feedback cycle:** TSH stimulates T_4 and T_3 production until a sufficient level of those hormones stops the secretion of TSH; when T_4 and T_3 levels drop, more TSH is secreted.

Absorption and Excretion

Iodine is rapidly absorbed, mostly from the stomach but also from the duodenum, and excreted by the kidneys, which have no mechanism to conserve iodine. After performing their functions, T_4 and T_3 are degraded by the liver, and the iodine content is excreted in bile. Some iodine is lost in sweat, which may be important in hot climates if intake is low (Gropper and Smith, 2013).

Dietary Reference Intakes and Sources

For DRIs see Appendix A. For food and other sources, see Table 7-10.

Iodine can come from foods, either naturally present or fortified, or from incidental sources.

IN FOODS AND WATER

Foods that are naturally high in iodine include saltwater fish, shellfish, and seaweed. The iodine content in plants varies with the mineral content of the soil in which they are grown. Table salt fortified with iodine (100 micrograms of iodine in 1/4 teaspoon of salt) has been available in the United States since 1924. It and dairy products are important sources of iodine in the United States (Perrine, Herrick, Serdula, and Sullivan, 2010).

Iodine has antibacterial properties and is sometimes used to purify drinking water. If the region is also iodine deficient, the mineral in the water can serve both purposes.

INCIDENTAL

Sometimes iodine is present as a side effect of processing. For example, iodine solutions can be used to sterilize milk pasteurization vats; some iodine may remain on the vat and be mixed into the next batch of milk to be processed. Iodine is also used to improve the texture of bread dough. In reproductive-age American women, dairy products were found to make important contributions to iodine status whether or not pregnant or lactating (Perrine, Herrick, Serdula, and Sullivan, 2010).

Deficiency

Iodine deficiency is the leading cause of preventable mental retardation worldwide (Ronald, 2011). Since the introduction of iodized salt, overt deficiency has rarely been encountered in North America even though processed foods typically do not contain iodized salt (Gropper and Smith, 2013). Deficiencies have occurred in individuals who avoid iodized salt and seafood and vegans who consume sea salt, which contains virtually no iodine.

An infant of a vegan mother was diagnosed with goiter (discussed subsequently) at 10 days of age. Notably, the mother also had a goiter. Both improved with treatment. The infant's goiter disappeared by 2 months of age (Shaikh, Anderson, Hall, and Jackson, 2003).

Two lifelong residents of the United States developed iodine deficiency because they avoided iodized salt and seafood. The only prescribed treatment was to alter their diets. These cases illustrate the necessity of individual assessment. Even though iodized salt and seafood are available in a region, some people, for reasons of their own, will choose not to partake (Nyenwe and Dagogo-Jack, 2009).

Diagnosis of thyroid malfunction can be readily evaluated by measuring protein-bound iodine and the serum levels of T_4 and T_3. The clients just described responded to increased iodine in their diets, confirming the diagnosis of iodine deficiency. A definitive diagnosis can be made with a 24-hour urine iodine excretion test (Nyenwe and Dagogo-Jack, 2009).

LOCAL EFFECTS

When the thyroid gland does not receive sufficient iodine, it increases in size, from a normal adult organ weighing 10 to 25 grams, growing to 500 to 700 grams (1 to 1.5 pounds) in its attempt to increase production of thyroid hormones. This enlargement of the thyroid is called **goiter** (Fig. 7-9). Sometimes the gland may attain sufficient size to impede breathing or swallowing. Unfortunately, in rare cases, replacement of iodine does not reduce the goiter, especially after long-standing deficiency, so that surgery or radiotherapy may be needed.

In some cases, prolonged iodine deficiency can short-circuit the negative feedback control system, resulting in autonomous thyroid nodules that produce T_3 and T_4 in response to dietary iodine rather than to

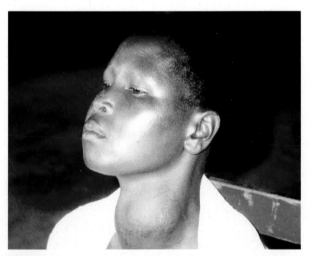

FIGURE 7-9 Woman with a goiter. (Reprinted from Kenya Medical Mission Web site, with permission.)

TSH. Iodine given to these people may cause **hyperthyroidism** (Laurberg, 2014).

Because of iodine-poor soil, the Great Lakes States and the Rocky Mountain States once were considered the "goiter belt." Now that food is distributed nationally and internationally and iodized salt is readily available, goiter is less common in the United States. Other countries continue to have significant effects of iodine deficiency (Box 7-1).

SYSTEMIC EFFECTS

Severe **hypothyroidism** during pregnancy results in **cretinism** in the newborn. As a consequence of the mother's thyroid deficiency, the infant exhibits mental and physical retardation. Cretinism is a congenital condition (present at birth). Prevention focuses on diagnosing and treating iodine deficiency in pregnant women.

Hypothyroidism due to iodine deficiency occurring in older children and adults is called **myxedema.** In areas where salt fortification is difficult to implement, treatment may consist of iodized oil, potassium iodide, or iodine (Gropper and Smith, 2013). Hypothyroidism can also be a side effect of medications, including the mood stabilizer *lithium* (Vallerand, Sanoski, and Deglin, 2013).

Interfering Factors

Substances called **goitrogens** may block the body's utilization of iodine. Goitrogens found in vegetables belonging to the cabbage family, including cauliflower, broccoli, Brussels sprouts, rutabaga, and turnips, are unlikely to

---

Box 7-1 ■ *Worldwide Iodine Deficiency*

About 200 to 300 million people worldwide are iodine-deficient (Gropper and Smith, 2013), and 2 billion people are at risk for iodine deficiency (Zimmermann and Andersson, 2011). Fifty-four countries are iodine-deficient (World Health Organization, 2012), particularly in mountainous areas or places with eroded soil. Insufficient iodine intake principally affects people in South Asia and sub-Saharan Africa. A singular case of goiter in Sudan yielded a 4.7-kilogram specimen (10.4 pounds) after surgical excision (Nada, Ahmed, Vilallonga, et al, 2011).

Even in developed Western countries, iodine deficiency exists. About 50% of Europe remains mildly iodine deficient (Zimmerman, 2009), probably because fewer than 50% of the households there use iodized salt compared with 90% of households in North and South America that use it (Gropper and Smith, 2013). In areas with a high prevalence of goiter because of lack of iodine in the food and water, the condition is termed **endemic** goiter.

Progress has been made with the universal iodization of salt since the World Health Organization increased efforts to promote national salt fortification programs. The cost amounts to five U.S. cents per person per year (World Health Organization, 2012).

cause goiter because of the relatively small amounts consumed and because cooking destroys the goitrogens. The only food linked to goiter is cassava, a starchy root eaten in developing countries (recall **konzo** and cyanide in Chapter 4). A metabolite of cassava prevents uptake of iodine by the thyroid (Gropper and Smith, 2013).

Toxicity

For basic information on mineral toxicity, see Table 7-4. Chronic toxicity may develop with an intake greater than 1.1 milligrams per day. Clients exposed to frequent large amounts of radiographic contrast dyes or the drug *amiodarone* also need to have their thyroid function monitored (Johnson, 2008a).

Fluoride

In body fluids, fluorine exists as fluoride, a salt of hydrofluoric acid, or as an **ion.** About 99% of the body's fluoride accumulates as fluorapatite in bones and teeth. Fluoride seems to make bone mineral less soluble and hence less likely to be reabsorbed.

Nearly 100% of soluble fluoride found in fluoridated water and toothpaste is rapidly absorbed from the stomach and small intestine, but absorption diminishes to 50% to 80% when fluoride is consumed as foods. Calcium and magnesium are thought to form insoluble complexes with fluoride, decreasing its absorption. Approximately 90% of excess fluoride is rapidly excreted in urine, most of the remainder in feces, and only minor amounts in sweat (Gropper and Smith, 2013).

Functions

Fluoride stimulates osteoblast production and mineral deposition in children's bones. In adults, however, new bone stimulated by fluoride may lack normal structure and strength (Gropper and Smith, 2013). Fluoride supplementation, either in short- or long-acting forms, is not approved by the U.S. FDA for the prevention or treatment of osteoporosis (Tucker and Rosen, 2014).

Fluoride's major contribution to human health relates to its role in preventing dental caries. In **plaque** and saliva, fluoride inhibits demineralization and enhances remineralization of early carious lesions. Whether in water or toothpaste, fluoride works in two main ways:

■ by slowing the activity of bacteria that cause decay and
■ by combining with the enamel on the surface of the teeth to make it stronger and more resistant to decay.

Fluoride in drinking water, although at a lower concentration than in toothpaste, maintains a constant low level of fluoride in the dental plaque and saliva all day.

Toothpaste provides a high level of fluoride, but only for 1 or 2 hours after brushing, so the two sources complement one another (Centers for Disease Control, December 16, 2011).

Dietary Reference Intakes and Sources

For DRIs see Appendix A. For food and other sources, see Table 7-10.

Food and beverages prepared with fluoridated water contain increased fluoride. Tea accumulates fluoride in the leaves so that brewed tea contains 1 to 6 milligrams per liter with decaffeinated varieties containing the larger quantities (Gropper and Smith, 2013).

Previous recommendations for fluoride in drinking water (0.7–1.2 milligrams per liter) were based on geographic areas considering variations in water intake in warm climates. Over the past several decades, many factors, including the advent of air-conditioning, have reduced geographic differences in water intake. The new recommendation of 0.7 milligrams of fluoride per liter of water is intended to prevent tooth decay while minimizing the risk for dental **fluorosis.** Besides the environmental changes, the new recommendation acknowledges that more sources of fluoride besides water (over-the-counter dental products, professional dental treatments, and supplements) are available than when water fluoridation was first introduced in the United States (Centers for Disease Control, December 16, 2011).

The U.S. Environmental Protection Agency, which is responsible for the safety and quality of drinking water in the United States, sets a maximum allowable limit for fluoride in community drinking water at 4 milligrams per liter (Centers for Disease Control, December 16, 2011).

The oral health of Americans over the past 50 years has improved significantly, mostly because of effective prevention and treatment efforts. One major success is community water fluoridation, which now benefits about 70% of Americans who receive water through public water systems. Information on county and community water systems can be obtained at http://apps.nccd.cdc.gov/mwf/index.asp. Unfortunately, dental caries (tooth decay) in children aged 2 to 5 have increased (Healthy People 2020, 2012).

Concern has been raised that children consuming conditioned water or bottled water instead of fluoridated tap water would receive suboptimal amounts of fluoride. Neither boiling nor charcoal-based water filtration systems remove fluoride from water; however, distillation and reverse osmosis treatments are effective in decreasing fluoride in water (Centers for Disease Control, December 16, 2011).

The FDA does not require bottled water manufacturers participating in interstate commerce to list the fluoride content on the label, but it does require that fluoride additives be listed. Intrastate commerce regulation is left to the individual states. If the label lacks the desired information, consumers should contact the bottled water's manufacturer to ask about the fluoride content of a particular brand (Centers for Disease Control, January 7, 2011).

Toxicity

For basic information on mineral toxicity, see Table 7-4.

Dental fluorosis can result when children regularly consume higher-than-recommended amounts of fluoride during the teeth-forming years, age 8 and younger. Most dental fluorosis in the United States, about 92%, appears as white spots on the tooth surface that often only a dental professional would notice. Moderate and severe forms of dental fluorosis cause more extensive enamel changes. The severe form in which pits may form in the teeth rarely occurs where the level of fluoride in water is less than 2 milligrams per liter (Centers for Disease Control, December 16, 2011).

Excessive consumption of fluoride over a lifetime may result in skeletal fluorosis affecting millions worldwide (Kurland, Schulman, Zerwekh et al, 2007), leading to pain and tenderness. It also may increase the likelihood of bone fractures. Severe skeletal fluorosis is rare in the United States (Centers for Disease Control, December 16, 2011) but has occurred with

- Habitual consumption of large volumes of instant tea (Whyte, Totty, Lim, and Whitford, 2008)
- Presumed secretive ingestion of toothpaste (Kurland et al, 2007).

After the FDA approved a health claim for fluoridated bottled water containing 0.6 to 1.0 milligrams of fluoride per liter to read "Drinking fluoridated water may reduce the risk of dental caries or tooth decay," another concern regarding possible excessive intake arose. Infant formulas as manufactured contain low fluoride levels. To avoid the possibility of excessive fluoride ingestion by infants from preparing powdered or concentrated formulas with fluoridated water, parents can use low-fluoride bottled water to mix infant formula. The infant's health-care provider should be asked about the proportion of the baby's feedings that should be prepared with low-fluoride bottled water products. These waters are labeled as deionized, purified, demineralized, or distilled, unless they specifically list fluoride as an added ingredient (Centers for Disease Control, April 27, 2012).

Acute toxicity has followed accidental ingestion of supplements or of excessive amounts of toothpaste. Death has been reported with intake as low as 5 milligrams of fluoride per kilogram of body weight (Gropper and Smith, 2013).

Package labeling directs caregivers to limit the amount of fluoridated toothpaste for children younger than 6 years of age to "a pea-sized amount," which should not be swallowed. Parents should consult a dentist or physician before using such toothpaste for a child younger than 2 years of age.

Zinc

The bodies of adult humans contain 1.5 to 2.5 grams of zinc, found in all organs, tissues, and body fluids, but 86% is contained in skeletal muscle and bone; it is also abundant in the central nervous system, however, where it affects transmission of impulses (King and Cousins, 2014). Zinc is incorporated into the structure of at least 70 and perhaps more than 200 enzymes (Gropper and Smith, 2013).

One essential zinc-containing respiratory enzyme, *carbonic anhydrase*, catalyzes carbon dioxide and water into carbonic acid to allow rapid disposal of carbon dioxide. Zinc is essential for the growth and repair of tissues because it is involved in the synthesis of DNA and RNA. Zinc is associated with insulin and is a component of a protein, *gustin*, concerned with taste acuity. The production of active vitamin A for the visual pigment rhodopsin requires zinc. It is integral to collagen formation for wound healing, participates in alcohol metabolism, and plays a role in providing immunity (Gropper and Smith, 2013). Its effect on the common cold is a matter of debate (see Clinical Application 7-8).

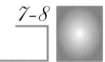

$\mathcal{C}$linical $\mathcal{A}$pplication *7-8*

Zinc for the Common Cold?

Whether zinc should be recommended to ward off or minimize symptoms of the common cold has been studied since at least 1993. Two meta-analyses found that zinc shortened the duration of the common cold when started within 24 hours of onset of symptoms. One analyzed 13 studies totaling 966 subjects (Singh and Das, 2011); the other analyzed 17 studies totaling 2121 people. The latter also determined that zinc shortened the duration of cold symptoms in adults but not in children (Science, Johnstone, Roth, et al, 2012). Both analyses showed side effects of bad taste and nausea were common in people taking zinc and neither offered firm recommendations because of the variety of research designs they analyzed. Another physician declined to recommend zinc for the common cold based on a conglomeration of varied studies but also allowed that for clients who want to take *something*, a zinc preparation would be a wiser choice than an antibiotic (Auwaerter, 2011). Taking zinc lozenges according to the package directions would deliver twice the UL for zinc, but the directions also refer the customer to a physician if symptoms persist beyond 7 days, so the excessive intake should be short term if the instructions are followed.

The FDA advised consumers not to use certain zinc-containing nasal products marketed as cold remedies (which were not proven to be effective) after receiving more than 130 reports of users having lost their sense of smell. In some people, the loss was long-lasting or permanent, posing a safety risk if they could not detect noxious odors in the environment such as smoke, a gas leak, or spoiled food (U.S. FDA, 2009).

Absorption, Control, and Excretion

Zinc is released from foods in the acid environment of the stomach and absorbed from the small intestine, mainly the duodenum and upper jejunum through some of the same absorption sites as iron. Control of zinc levels is achieved through limitations on absorption that varies from 10% to 80% but typically amounts to 20% to 30% of the zinc in the U.S. diet. Greater percentages of zinc are absorbed when the diet contains lesser amounts of it (Gropper and Smith, 2013).

Up to 80% of zinc excretion occurs via feces. Small amounts are lost in urine, in exfoliated skin cells, in sweat, in semen, and in menstrual flow. Because hair contains about 0.1 to 0.2 milligrams of zinc per gram, hair loss is also a route for zinc depletion (Gropper and Smith, 2013).

Dietary Reference Intakes and Sources

For DRIs see Appendix A. For food and other sources, see Table 7-10. To investigate the mineral content of a particular item, go to http://ndb.nal.usda.gov or to http://nutritiondata.self.com.

In the body, zinc is recovered from pancreatic and biliary secretions in the gastrointestinal tract for reuse (Gropper and Smith, 2013).

The requirement for dietary zinc may be as much as 50% greater for vegetarians, particularly vegans, as for persons consuming a mixed diet (Amit, 2010; Institute of Medicine, 2001).

Interfering Factors

Less zinc is absorbed from plant foods than from animal foods. Phytates, especially in cereals and legumes, irreversibly bind with zinc in the intestinal lumen except when the plant foods are fermented, a process that releases the zinc (King and Cousins, 2014). Conditions or medications that decrease gastric acidity impede zinc absorption. Iron and zinc compete for the same absorption sites. Zinc and nonheme iron interact when ingested together in solution and when 20 milligrams or more of iron is consumed. The effect is not always apparent when taken with a meal and varies with the form of the nutrients. For maximum absorption, separating zinc and nonheme iron supplement doses is advised (Gropper and Smith, 2013). In a similar reaction, zinc and calcium or copper may interact. In addition, phytates, oxalates, and tannins, all reduce the absorption of zinc.

Deficiency

Zinc intake correlates directly with protein consumption. Groups at risk because of limited meat intake include the poor, the elderly, and vegetarians. Zinc deficiency in adults can also occur as a result of diseases that either hinder zinc absorption or cause excessive amounts of zinc to be excreted in urine. Zinc deficiency effects are as follows:

- In children
  - Growth retardation
  - Skeletal abnormalities
  - Delayed sexual maturation
- In adults
  - Alopecia
  - Loss of taste sensation
  - Poor wound healing
  - Impaired immunity (Gropper and Smith, 2013)

The World Health Organization and United Nations Children's Fund recommend the routine use of zinc supplementation to help reduce the duration and severity of diarrhea and to prevent subsequent episodes (World Health Organization, 2011). A review of trials found preventive zinc supplementation in children is associated with a reduction in diarrhea mortality of 13% and pneumonia mortality of 15% but has no effect on malaria mortality (Yakoob, Theodoratou, Jabeen, et al, 2011).

A rare **autosomal recessive** disease, **acrodermatitis enteropathica,** causes zinc deficiency that can be fatal if untreated. A mutation in a zinc transport protein causes poor absorption. Among the signs and symptoms are impaired growth, diarrhea, and skin lesions. High doses of zinc are given to compensate for the defective absorptive mechanism (Gropper and Smith, 2013).

Toxicity

For basic information on mineral toxicity, see Table 7-4. Because zinc can be toxic if consumed in excessive amounts, it should be obtained from foods, not from routine or long-term supplementation (see Clinical Application 7-8).

Cases related to zinc excess were attributed to

- swallowed coins that released zinc into the body (Hassan, Netchvolodoff, and Raufman, 2000; Pawa, Khalifa, Ehrinpreis, et al, 2008), including one fatality (Kumar and Jazieh, 2001), and
- overuse of zinc-containing denture adhesive (Doherty, Connor, and Cruickshank, 2011; Trocello, Hinfray, Sanda, et al, 2011) including one fatality (Afrin, 2010).

Copper

The healthy adult body contains about 50 to 150 milligrams of copper, found in all body tissues and most secretions. The organs with the most copper per gram are the kidneys, liver (the main storage site that controls copper balance), and brain (Gropper and Smith, 2013). Copper is a cofactor for enzymes involved in hemoglobin synthesis and cell respiration and is required for melanin pigment formation. A mutation in a copper-dependent enzyme causes albinism (Gropper and Smith, 2013), the partial or total absence of pigment in the hair, skin, and eyes. It is usually transmitted as an autosomal recessive trait.

Gastric secretions aid in the release of bound copper in foods. Although some absorption is possible in the stomach, most copper is absorbed from the small intestine, chiefly the duodenum. Typically, 50% to 80% of ingested copper is absorbed with higher percentages occurring at low intake levels. The major route of excretion is via bile into the feces, through which the liver maintains copper balance, but molybdenum can increase urinary excretion of copper (Gropper and Smith, 2013).

Dietary Reference Intakes and Sources

For DRIs, see Appendix A. For food and other sources, see Table 7-10. To investigate the mineral content of a particular item, go to http://ndb.nal.usda.gov or to http://nutritiondata.self.com.

In the United States, adult intake averages 1 to 1.6 milligrams. The body may also recycle copper from digestive secretions (Gropper and Smith, 2013).

Interfering Factors and Deficiency

High intakes of iron and zinc interfere with copper metabolism. Phytates hinder copper absorption, but most people in the United States do not consume enough phytates to affect copper status.

Individuals at increased risk of copper deficiency are those:

- Taking medications that make the stomach less acid
- Consuming zinc supplements, typically 40 milligrams or more per day
- With gastrointestinal diseases permitting malabsorption
- With kidney diseases that increase losses (Gropper and Smith, 2013)

Copper deficiency is a commonly reported long-term complication of **bariatric surgery** (Btaiche, Yeh, Wu, and Khalidi, 2011). Deficiency has been documented in malnourished and premature infants and as a result of the prolonged administration of parenteral nutrition (see Chapter 14) solutions deficient in copper (Chitambar and Asok, 2014). Other cases occurred after prolonged jejunostomy feeding which were corrected by a daily cocoa powder supplement (Nishiwaki, Iwashita, Goto, et al, 2011).

Because of copper's link with iron utilization, copper deficiency produces a hypochromic, microcytic anemia that requires treatment with copper, not iron. Other manifestations of copper deficiency are:

- Bone abnormalities
- Impaired immune function
- Depigmentation of the skin and hair (Gropper and Smith, 2013)

A hereditary abnormality causing defective copper elimination from cells is the cause of **Menkes disease.** Most tissues accumulate excess copper but not to toxic levels because the absorption of copper from the gastrointestinal tract is subsequently blocked. The lack of copper in other tissues produces signs and symptoms of copper deficiency (Collins, 2014). The disease is inherited as an **X-linked** recessive trait. Standard treatment involves parenteral administration of *copper-histidine.* If treatment is initiated before 2 months of age, neurodegeneration can be prevented, while delayed treatment is ineffective (Kodama, Fujisawa, and Bhadhprasit, 2012).

Toxicity

For basic information on mineral toxicity, see Table 7-4.
A genetic mutation causes **Wilson disease,** which is inherited as an autosomal recessive trait affecting copper absorption and transport into the central nervous system and into various enzymes (Aldenhoven, Klomp, van Hasselt, et al, 2007). Because of defective biliary excretion, copper accumulates in the liver, brain, kidneys, and eyes (Gropper and Smith, 2013). Clinical manifestations are highly variable and comprise acute liver failure, chronic hepatitis and cirrhosis, as well as neurological or psychiatric symptoms (Hiroz, Antonino, Doerig, et al, 2011).

A dietary prescription to avoid foods high in copper can augment chelation therapy. Zinc supplements may be given to counter copper uptake and molybdenum supplements to enhance urinary excretion (Gropper and Smith, 2013). Treatment will be required for a lifetime.

Selenium

The total body selenium is about 20 milligrams. The highest concentrations of this mineral occur in the thyroid gland, kidneys, liver, heart, pancreas, and muscle. Because of their similar chemistry, selenium can often substitute for sulfur (Gropper and Smith, 2013). An analogue of the amino acid methionine called selenomethionine can be incorporated into body proteins in place of methionine (NIH Office of Dietary Supplements, 2011).

Selenium is integral to more than 25 enzymes that primarily function as **antioxidants.** Selenium is necessary for iodine metabolism and may regulate thyroid hormone production (Gropper and Smith, 2013). It also protects against the toxicity of mercury, cadmium, and silver (Sunde, 2014).

Selenium does not require digestion, and absorption throughout the small intestine does not appear to be regulated. Homeostasis of the mineral is thought to be maintained by urinary excretion that represents 50% to 60% of selenium losses. Up to 50% of the mineral is lost in feces, but some is also lost through the lungs and skin (Gropper and Smith, 2013).

Dietary Reference Intakes and Sources

For DRIs, see Appendix A. For food and other sources, see Table 7-10. To investigate the mineral content of a particular item, go to http://ndb.nal.usda.gov or to http://nutritiondata.self.com.

The amount of selenium present in plant foods depends on the selenium content of the soil and water where the foods are grown. Areas noted for low concentrations affecting local foodstuffs are New Zealand, Finland, and Denmark as well as portions of China and Russia. Selenium in fish, especially if contaminated with mercury (see Chapter 10), may have lower bioavailability because of unabsorbable mercury–selenium complexes (Gropper and Smith, 2013).

In contrast, the soil of northern Nebraska and the Dakotas has very high levels of selenium. Brazil nuts may contain as much as 544 micrograms per ounce, although they may contain much less. Because of the possibility of high selenium content, it is wise to consume Brazil nuts only occasionally (NIH Office of Dietary Supplements, 2011). Additionally, some plants, such as wheat, broccoli, and garlic, hyperaccumulate selenium from the soil (Gropper and Smith, 2013).

Deficiency and Toxicity

Selenium deficiencies have been produced in animals but are unlikely in humans who eat meat on a regular basis. Nevertheless, some exceptions exist, notably clients receiving long-term restricted intake, for example, those:

- Taking phenylketonuria formulas
- Receiving parenteral nutrition as sole source of nutrients
- Consuming ketogenic diets (see Chapter 15)

Several parenterally fed clients developed heart disease that responded to selenium treatment. Inclusion of selenium in the infusion is now routine (NIH Office of Dietary Supplements, 2011). After two children on ketogenic diets for intractable epilepsy died suddenly, their post mortem examinations revealed selenium-deficiency cardiomyopathy (Bank, Shemie, Rosenblatt, et al, 2008).

Approximately 20% of the population of China is affected by selenium deficiency (Yang, Chen, and Feng, 2007). A deterioration of the heart due to selenium deficiency has occurred in residents of China's Keshan province. Early diagnosis and treatment is essential because selenium supplementation may reverse the potentially fatal outcome (Saliba, El Fakih, and Shaheen, 2010); however, selenium cannot reverse the cardiac failure once it occurs (Sunde, 2014). Coxsackie virus appears to be a cofactor in the development of Keshan disease. Without adequate selenium, benign strains of the virus mutate into virulent strains to which some of the symptoms of Keshan disease are attributed.

Signs and symptoms of selenium deficiency include:

- Poor growth
- Muscle pain and weakness
- Depigmentation of hair and skin
- Whitening of nail beds (Gropper and Smith, 2013)

For basic information on mineral toxicity, see Table 7-4. Selenosis, toxicity from selenium, has occurred in miners and people overdosing with supplements. See Chapter 15 for information regarding a manufacturing error causing selenosis. The most common sign of selenosis is loss of hair and nails (Sunde, 2014). Acute poisoning from gram amounts of selenium is lethal with damage to most organ systems (Gropper and Smith, 2013).

Chromium

The adult body contains approximately 4 to 6 milligrams of chromium. High concentrations are found in the kidney, liver, muscle, spleen, heart, pancreas, and bone. Only about 0.4% to 2.5% of dietary chromium is absorbed depending on intake, with the greater absorption taking place at lower intake levels. Chromium is absorbed throughout the small intestine, especially the jejunum. Ninety-five percent of excretion is via the urine, the content of which reflects current intake, not chromium status. Small amounts are lost as skin cells are shed. Fecal content reflects unabsorbed, not excreted, mineral (Gropper and Smith, 2013).

Chromium is thought to potentiate the action of insulin but the mechanism of action is uncertain. The results of chromium supplementation on insulin sensitivity have been conflicting, and its use for type 2 diabetes is controversial. No support has been found for chromium supplementation to increase strength or muscle or to decrease fat tissue (Gropper and Smith, 2013), and the Federal Trade Commission ordered the discontinuation of such claims for the supplement chromium picolinate for 20 years (U.S. Federal Trade Commission, 1997).

For DRIs see Appendix A. For food and other sources, see Table 7-10.

Vitamin C may enhance absorption, but antacids and phytates decrease absorption of chromium.

Individuals receiving parenteral nutrition (see Chapter 14) without chromium have shown these signs of deficiency:

- Weight loss
- Peripheral neuropathy
- Impaired glucose utilization
- High plasma levels of free fatty acids (Gropper and Smith, 2013).

For basic information on mineral toxicity, see Table 7-4. Chromium toxicity usually occurs from direct contact or inhalation in industry. For a long time, prolonged exposure to chromium has been known or suspected to adversely affect the skin and respiratory tract (Urbano, Ferreira, and Alpoim, 2012). The mineral has widespread industrial uses as a pigment, in the production of stainless steel, and in chrome plating.

Recently questions have surfaced regarding the long-term biological effects of wear debris from artificial hips. The physiological effects of systemic exposure to chromium, cobalt, nickel, and aluminium alloy nano-particles that are released both from metal-on-metal and polyethylene-on-metal prostheses are poorly understood and are cause for concern (Polyzois, Nikolopoulos, Michos, et al, 2012).

However, the effects of the misuse of supplemental chromium are clear. To enhance weight loss, a 33-year-old White woman (who had been diagnosed with schizophrenia and depression within the year) ingested chromium picolinate, 1200 to 2400 micrograms daily. After 4 to 5 months, she did achieve weight loss but also acquired anemia, liver dysfunction, and kidney failure which required blood transfusions and hemodialysis to resolve the toxic effects of this over-the-counter supplement (Cerulli, Grabe, Gauthier, et al, 1998). See Chapter 15 more for information on dietary supplements.

Manganese

The body contains only 10 to 20 milligrams of manganese, which is found in highest concentrations in the bones, liver, pancreas, and kidneys. Manganese is involved in the formation of bone and cartilage. Enzymes from nearly every class can be activated by manganese but, with few exceptions, are not manganese-specific. Thus manganese's role can frequently be taken by magnesium or other divalent **cations** (Gropper and Smith, 2013).

Absorption throughout the small intestine typically is less than 5% with higher rates of absorption occurring with low intakes and females absorbing greater amounts than males for unknown reasons. Absorption is inhibited by nonheme iron, copper, oxalates, phytates, and fiber. When ingested in amounts about 4 to 8 times the recommended intake, manganese decreases iron absorption up to 40%. More than 90% of manganese excretion is accomplished by the liver via bile, with small losses through sweat and skin desquamation (Gropper and Smith, 2013).

For DRIs, see Appendix A. For food and other sources, see Table 7-10. To investigate the mineral content of a particular item, go to http://ndb.nal.usda.gov or to http://nutritiondata.self.com.

Deficiency is unlikely except when manganese is deliberately eliminated from the diet. Among other signs and symptoms, the client displays:

- Dermatitis
- Decreased growth of hair and nails
- Changes in hair color (Gropper and Smith, 2013)

For basic information on mineral toxicity, see Table 7-4. Manganese toxicity most often results from inhalation exposure in occupational settings, characteristically causing Parkinsonian-like symptoms and psychological changes. A 3-month course of parenteral nutrition (see Chapter 14) with manganese, thereby bypassing the regulatory mechanism of the gut and liver, caused hypermanganesemia with seizures in one 10-year-old female (Hsieh, Liang, Peng, and Lee, 2007). Complicating the diagnostic process, whole-blood manganese levels do not necessarily correlate with intake or status (Gropper and Smith, 2013).

Illustrating the overlapping metabolism of manganese and iron and in one case, cobalt, magnesium toxicity affected two 5- and 6-year old girls. Each presented with **pica,** emotional lability, neurological gait disorders, iron deficiency, and **polycythemia.** In both cases, well water was identified as a potential source of manganese, commonly higher than guidelines recommend in wells in the Maritime Provinces of Canada where each lived. In both cases, however, the precise reason for their particular neurotoxic susceptibility was not identified (Brna, Gordon, Dooley, and Price, 2011; Sahni, Léger, Panaro, et al, 2007).

Cobalt

For food and other sources of cobalt, see Table 7-10. DRIs for cobalt have not been established.

As an essential component of the vitamin B_{12} molecule, cobalt is necessary for red blood cell formation, but a nutritional role for the ionic form of cobalt has not been demonstrated (Gropper and Smith, 2013). Cobalt deficiency has caused anemia in ruminants but has not been reported in humans.

Occupational cobalt exposure in cobalt processing plants and hard-metal industry has produced adverse reactions in heart and lung function. The use of cobalt-chromium hard-metal alloys in orthopedic joint replacements, in particular, in metal-on-metal bearings in hip joint arthroplasty, has created an entirely new source of internal cobalt exposure. The metal nanoparticles have been demonstrated to be clearly more toxic than larger, micrometer-sized particles, thus making the concept of nanotoxicology a crucial new discipline (Simonsen, Harbak, and Bennekou, 2012). Case reports include the following:

■ A 56-year-old man with acute cobalt poisoning following revision of a hip prosthesis (Pelclova, Sklensky, Janicek, and Lach, 2012)
■ Delayed cobalt hypersensitivity developing several years after use of cobalt in the opposite hip (Perumal, Alkire, and Swank, 2010)
■ A 41-year-old woman with bilateral metal-on-metal hip arthroplasties of 3- and 5-year durations presented with extremely high chromium and cobalt blood levels at 12 gestational weeks. A healthy male infant was delivered at 38 weeks with elevated chromium and cobalt blood levels, but by 14 weeks of age, the infant's development seemed uneventful without signs of toxicity (Fritzsche, Borisch, and Schaefer, 2012)

Molybdenum

The body contains about 2 milligrams of molybdenum, a cofactor for enzymes involved in the metabolism of sulfur-containing amino acids and **purines.** Both in absolute amounts and in concentration, molybdenum is found primarily in the liver, kidneys, and bone. About 50% to 85% of molybdenum in foods is absorbed without digestion from the proximal small intestine. Because it binds to copper in the intestinal tract, *tetrathiomolybdate*, a pharmaceutical preparation of molybdenum, is used in the treatment of copper toxicity, including Wilson disease, and some cancers. Molybdenum is mainly excreted by the kidneys, which are thought to promote homeostasis, but small amounts are lost via bile in feces and in sweat and hair (Gropper and Smith, 2013).

For DRIs, see Appendix A. For food and other sources, see Table 7-10.

An inherited recessive deficiency of sulfite oxidase that requires molybdenum produces severe neurological damage and death in childhood. Deficiency has also been reported in a client receiving prolonged parenteral nutrition (see Chapter 14) who displayed tachycardia, headache, mental disturbances, and coma (Sardesai, 1993).

For basic information on mineral toxicity, see Table 7-4. At intakes of up to 1500 micrograms per day, molybdenum seems to be relatively nontoxic (Gropper and Smith, 2013).

Figure 7-10 illustrates the food groups contributing to the intake of major and trace minerals.

Ultratrace Minerals

For DRIs for boron, nickel, and vanadium, see ULs in Appendix A.

Arsenic, a colorless, odorless mineral, is found mostly in skin, nails, and hair, which can be analyzed to determine long-term exposure. Because arsenic is excreted primarily by the kidney, urinary excretion is used to identify short-term exposure (Gropper and Smith, 2013).

Arsenic occurs naturally in rocks, soil, and water, but agricultural and industrial contamination of those resources is the major contributor to the amount of arsenic in the United States. Residues of arsenic in pesticides remain in the soil for decades to be taken into crops used for foods. Arsenic has no known biological function in plants, which have some defensive mechanisms to detoxify arsenic, but when they are overwhelmed, the plants show growth inhibition, chlorophyll degradation, nutrient depletion, and oxidative stress (Moreno-Jiménez, Esteban, and Peñalosa, 2012).

Although some foods contain arsenic in a less toxic organic form, the form in drinking water is the more toxic inorganic form. Inorganic arsenic may be found in foods because it is present in the environment, both as a naturally occurring mineral and because of activity such as past use of arsenic-containing pesticides. Long-term exposure to high levels of arsenic is associated with higher rates of skin, bladder, and lung cancers as well as heart disease (U.S. FDA, September 21, 2012). The FDA has set an allowable level for arsenic in bottled drinking water of 10 micrograms per liter (U.S. Food and Drug Administration, August 24, 2011), the same value used for public water systems (U.S. Environmental Protection Agency, March 6, 2012) and has proposed the same level for inorganic arsenic in apple juice (U.S. Food and Drug Administration, July 12, 2013).

Rice is different from most other grains in that it more readily accumulates arsenic. The U.S. Food and Drug Administration has been collecting data on arsenic in foods, including rice and juices since 1991 but does not have an adequate scientific basis to recommend changes in rice consumption (September 21, 2012). Of particular concern to some researchers is the consumption of rice in infant foods that contain predominantly inorganic arsenic. If an infant's body weight is factored into the equation, even low concentrations of arsenic would exceed the comparable amount that an adult would receive from drinking 1 liter of water at the maximum permitted level of arsenic (Jackson,

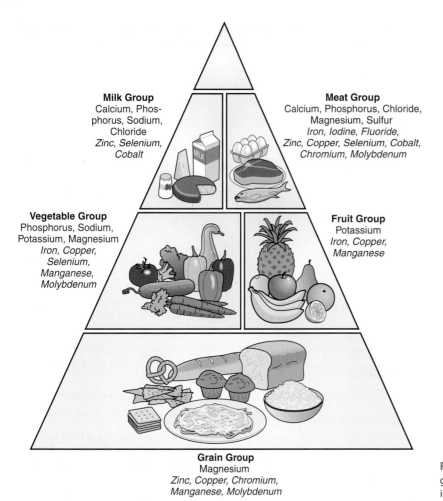

Milk Group
Calcium, Phos-
phorus, Sodium,
Chloride
*Zinc, Selenium,
Cobalt*

Meat Group
Calcium, Phosphorus, Chloride,
Magnesium, Sulfur
*Iron, Iodine, Fluoride,
Zinc, Copper, Selenium, Cobalt,
Chromium, Molybdenum*

Vegetable Group
Phosphorus, Sodium,
Potassium, Magnesium
*Iron, Copper,
Selenium,
Manganese,
Molybdenum*

Fruit Group
Potassium
*Iron, Copper,
Manganese*

Grain Group
Magnesium
*Zinc, Copper, Chromium,
Manganese, Molybdenum*

FIGURE 7-10 This pyramid illustrates the food groups supplying the various minerals. Italics indicate trace minerals.

Taylor, Punshon, and Cottingham, 2012). Based on its analyses of fruit juices and rice products, Consumers Union asked the FDA to set limits for arsenic in rice products and fruit juices as a starting point. In the meantime, to limit exposure to arsenic in rice:

■ Babies should have no more than one serving of infant rice cereal per day.

■ Children under 5 years of age should not have rice drinks as part of a daily diet.

■ Rice should be rinsed, then cooked in 6 cups of water per 1 cup of rice, and drained before serving. About 30% of the inorganic arsenic in the rice is removed by this procedure (Arsenic in your food, 2012).

It may be hard to believe that arsenic has medical uses. It has a place in the treatment of a specific form of leukemia but comes with risk of life-threatening cardiovascular and hematologic side effects (Vallerand, Sanoski, and Deglin, 2013).

Boron is found mainly in bone, teeth, nails, and hair, the body's content totaling between 3 and 20 milligrams. More than 70% of excretion is in urine as boric acid with smaller amounts of boron lost in feces and sweat. Clear biochemical functions in humans

have not been demonstrated, but beneficial effects on bones, cell membranes, and the immune system have been observed. Plant foods are particularly rich in boron (Gropper and Smith, 2013).

Nickel is found in highest concentrations in the thyroid and adrenal glands. It is also found in hair, bone, lung, heart, kidney, and liver but the total amount in the body is thought to be about 10 milligrams. No specific biological role in humans has been identified. Nickel is released into the environment with the combustion of nickel-containing products and is found in higher levels in foods of plant rather than animal origin. Most absorbed nickel is excreted in urine, but sweat concentrations can be fairly high and small amounts are lost via bile. Chronic toxicity, usually from occupational inhalation, causes respiratory and other systemic disorders including cancer (Gropper and Smith, 2013).

Silicon is involved in the normal formation, growth, and development of bones, connective tissues, and cartilage. Intake mostly comes from plant foods, with whole cereal grains and root vegetables especially rich sources. The kidney is considered the major organ of excretion; urinary silicon is significantly correlated with intake. Long-term use of silicon-containing antacids appears to contribute to particular types of kidney stones. *Silicosis* is a progressive fibrosis of the lungs caused by inhalation of silica dust (Gropper and Smith, 2013).

Vanadium, totaling about 100 to 200 micrograms in the body, is found mainly in bone, teeth, lung, and thyroid gland. No specific biological function has been identified. Absorption is less than 10%. Excretion is mainly in urine with small amounts in bile. Rich food sources include shellfish, black pepper, parsley, and dill seed. Vanadium toxicity from intakes above 10 milligrams produces:

■ A green tongue (due to vanadium deposits)
■ Gastrointestinal disturbances.
  Miners with chronic toxicity exhibit:
■ Hypertension
■ Neurological disorders

■ Liver, heart, and kidney damage (Gropper and Smith, 2013)

Other Minerals that have an Impact on Health

Aluminum, lead, and mercury are found in the body not because of nutritional needs but as the result of environmental contamination. See Chapter 10 for recommendations regarding mercury avoidance for pregnant women and Clinical Application 7-9 for more information on lead poisoning.

Aluminum, a metal frequently found in the environment, puts clients especially at risk when it contaminates pharmaceutical products used for hemodialysis or parenteral nutrition (see Chapter 14) because such

7-9

Clinical Application

Lead Poisoning (Plumbism)

Lead is a contaminant in the human body derived from inhalation, ingestion, or skin contact. The effects of lead toxicity, including neurological damage and retardation, can be devastating and permanent in fetuses and children because of the immature blood–brain barrier and either direct blood vessel transfer to the fetus or increased gastrointestinal absorption in children that is further enhanced if iron deficiency is present (Brown and Margolis, 2012). Black and Hispanic children are at greater risk of lead poisoning than white children, as are all low-income children. In Minnesota, 22% of refugee children had blood lead levels (BLLs) above 10 micrograms per deciliter (mcg/dL) compared to 1.6% of U.S. children (Centers for Disease Control, March 29, 2012).

No blood lead level (BLL) has been declared safe. The *level of concern* has been renamed *reference value* (based on the 97.5th percentile of the BLL distribution in U.S. children aged 1 to 5 years) and lowered from 10 mcg/dL to the current value of 5 mcg/dL (Centers for Disease Control, May 25, 2012a). A BLL of 70 mcg/dL or higher is a medical emergency (Meyer, Pivetz, Dignam, et al, 2003), whereas one of 100 mcg/dL or higher is life-threatening (Centers for Disease Control, March 31, 2006).

Not food, but lead-based paint in older homes is the primary source of poisoning in inner-city children, as was the case of a 2-year-old child who died from acute lead poisoning (Centers for Disease Control, 2001). Children may eat paint chips that have an appealing sweet taste but a principal mode of ingestion is lead dust on hands, toys, and household objects that young children are prone to put into their mouths. Lead paint in homes built before 1977 when residential lead-based paint was discontinued in the United States pose a particular risk to children and fetuses whose nervous systems are still being developed.

About 90% of total body lead in adults is accumulated in the bones, where it remains for decades and may be released during pregnancy as a side effect of mobilizing calcium for tissue building. BLLs reflect only recent or continued lead exposure, not accumulated bone lead levels that can be measured in the tibia and patella with special techniques (Rosin, 2009).

Because lead freely crosses the placenta, lead poisoning during pregnancy harms the woman and invariably produces congenital lead poisoning at BLLs higher than those of the mother. Details of a sample of cases suggest areas to be assessed.

■ Among 15 severely lead-poisoned pregnant women, 70% were Hispanic, all of whom ingested soil, clay, or pottery as the source of lead (Shannon, 2003; see **pica** in Chapter 10).
■ In New York City, six cases of lead poisoning in pregnant women were linked to folk remedies from India (Centers for Disease Control, August 24, 2012). See Chapter 15 for additional information on products sold as dietary supplements.
■ In the United Kingdom, a veterinarian treating severely lead-poisoned cats living amid housing renovations referred their pregnant owner for medical follow-up (Doumouchtsis, Martin, and Robins, 2006).

Other sources of lead are solder in metal food and beverage cans and lead that leaches out of glazes on serving utensils and containers, especially those containing acidic juices and wine (Hackley and Katz-Jacobson, 2003; Valadez-Vega, Zúñiga-Pérez, Quintanar-Gómez, et al, 2011). In the 1980s, lead was eliminated from solder in food cans in the United States but is still used in other countries (Olympio, Goncalves, Günther, and Bechara, 2009). Reports of ingestion of lead from dishware or foreign packaging materials still appear sporadically. Imported products, some privately obtained, have recently been implicated. Cases of lead poisoning in children have been discovered by astute clinicians attributed to:

■ Candy packaged in lead-containing wrappers from Mexico (Centers for Disease Control, 2002)
■ A product called Sindoor used for food coloring by Asian parents led to diagnoses of lead poisoning in both parents after their mainly breastfed 13-month-old son's routine test showed a BLL of 57 mcg/dL (Vassilev, Marcus, Ayyanathan, et al, 2005)

(Continued)

Clinical Application—cont'd

- A cosmetic powder from Nigeria applied to the eyelids of a 6-month-old male infant (Centers for Disease Control, August 3, 2012)
- An amulet from Cambodia with beads of 45% lead, worn about the neck and accessible to the mouth of a 15-month-old male since the age of 3 months (Centers for Disease Control, January 28, 2011)

In addition to lead-based paint, older homes also may have plumbing that could contaminate drinking water. Ten infants were poisoned from formula reconstituted with lead-contaminated water (Shannon and Graef, 1992). Because boiling increases the concentration of lead in water, the need to boil water for infant formula needs individual evaluation. To decrease the chance of lead leaching into drinking or cooking water:

1. Run water for 2 minutes in the morning before drawing water to drink.
2. Use cold water for cooking and drinking.

Local health departments are able to direct people to appropriate laboratories if they wish to have their water tested.

Although fetuses and children are the most susceptible to damage from lead poisoning, adults can be affected also.

- Fourteen days after ingesting of a "handful" of lead shot, a 15-year-old boy was admitted for elevated lead level. X-ray examination showed pellets in the appendix. After laparoscopic appendectomy, 50 pellets were recovered from the appendix (Banner, Schaeffer, Badillo, et al, 2012).

- A 34-year-old man displayed symptoms of lead toxicity 14 years after sustaining a gunshot-associated femoral fracture with retention of lead bullet fragments. Two large lead bullet fragments were found in a fluid-filled cyst in surgery (Eward, Darcey, Dodd, and Zura, 2011).

Long-term consequences of lead exposure include associations with:

- Intellectual impairment even at BLLs below 10 mcg/dL
- Delinquency and crime rates (Olympio, et al, 2009)
- Hypertension, kidney disease, cardiovascular disease, and cognitive decline in the elderly (a possible source of the lead is bone that is resorbed as a result of osteoporosis; Rosin, 2009)

Foremost is the avoidance of further exposure through environmental control. Nutritional tactics can be used as well:

- Iron and calcium supplementation to compete with lead for absorption
- A reduced-fat diet and frequent meals to decrease gastrointestinal absorption of lead

Use of chelating agents that will bind with lead are recommended if the BLL is greater than 45 mcg/10 dL; however, experts should be consulted because fatal hypocalcemia has occurred following inappropriate prescribing (Centers for Disease Control, March 3, 2006).

intake bypasses any possible defense by the gastrointestinal system. Aluminum toxicity can cause serious central nervous system and bone effects.

In 2004, the U.S. FDA mandated labeling requirements for aluminum content in all parenteral solution components and set maximum exposure values.

- One study determined that meeting the FDA exposure recommendation of <5 mcg/kg/day was possible only in clients weighing more than 50 kilograms (110 pounds), whereas almost half the exposure to aluminum occurred in babies weighing less than 3 kilograms or 6.6 pounds (Poole, Hintz, Mackenzie, and Kerner, 2008).
- Comparison of all products for parenteral nutrition solutions available in the United States revealed that although measured aluminum concentrations were less than the labeled values, large lot-to-lot variations existed. In addition, manufacturer-to-manufacturer differences were significant (Poole, Pieroni, Gaskari, et al, 2011).

Neonates are at an increased risk of aluminum toxicity because of large doses for their size, immature kidneys, and bypassed gastrointestinal absorption. Compared with preterm infants given specially formulated low aluminum parenteral nutrition, those receiving standard infusions had reduced developmental scores at age 18 months and lower lumbar spine bone mineral content at 13 to 15 years (Fewtrell, Bishop, Edmonds, et al, 2009).

Although the pharmacist can strive to decrease aluminum toxicity in **neonates,** it remains difficult to reach the mandated threshold for exposure (Wier and Kuhn, 2012); however, pharmacists can choose products with the least aluminum when compounding parenteral nutrition solutions. Additionally, changes are needed in manufacturing processes for parenteral nutrition components and in labeling requirements. Current labels indicate estimated aluminum content at the product's expiration date that universally exceeded the measured amounts, whereas labeling the actual value at the time of product release would allow health professionals to more accurately assess aluminum exposure of their clients (Poole et al, 2011).

On a positive note, routine testing of hemodialysis clients' serum aluminum levels led to elimination of pumps that presumably contaminated the dialysate. The clients displayed no symptoms, and their blood levels of aluminum decreased after the pumps were removed from service (Centers for Disease Control, 2008).

Mineral Supplementation

Excessive intake of nutrients can be as harmful as insufficient intake. For most healthy people, foods are the preferred source of minerals. For reasons that will be clarified in Chapter 15, mineral supplements produced by a pharmaceutical manufacturer are the best choices.

People who take supplements are advised not to take more than the RDAs or AIs for each mineral without consulting their health-care providers, who should always be informed of supplements their clients take. In the case of some minerals, toxicity is possible at levels slightly above the recommended intake amounts. In addition, an excess of one mineral may cause a deficiency of another. Consideration should also be given to regular intake of fortified foods and beverages when advising use of mineral supplements.

Supplements of iron are often prescribed for pregnant women and of calcium for older women at risk for osteoporosis. Most multimineral supplements contain small amounts of calcium and magnesium relative to their RDAs, so individual supplements of those minerals may be suggested for individuals who need them (NIH Office of Dietary Supplements, January 12, 2012).

Because iron deficiency is uncommon among adult men and postmenopausal women, those persons should only take iron supplements when prescribed by a physician because of their greater risk of iron overload (NIH Office of Dietary Supplements, 2007).

Keystones

- Minerals are inorganic substances that help regulate body functions without providing energy, but unlike vitamins, minerals become part of the body's structure and enzymes.

- Major minerals are present in the body in amounts of 5 grams (1 teaspoonful) or more; the daily recommended intake is 100 milligrams or more. Trace minerals are those with lesser amounts. Calcium, sodium, and potassium are major minerals. Iron, iodine, and zinc are trace minerals.

- Calcium is essential to the structure of bones and teeth and to nerve conduction, muscle contraction, and blood clotting. Milk, seafood with bones, and fortified orange juice are good sources of calcium.

- Iron is an essential component of hemoglobin that transports oxygen throughout the body. Red meat; cooked dark green, leafy vegetables; and fortified cereals are good sources of iron.

- Calcium, sodium, and potassium are essential to normal nerve and muscle function.

- Deficiency of iodine can result in goiter; of selenium, in cardiomyopathy; and of fluoride, in dental caries.

- Iron deficiency is one type of anemia; cretinism and goiter are caused by iodine deficiency. Keshan disease is a cardiomyopathy caused by selenium deficiency. Menkes and Wilson diseases are inherited inabilities to metabolize copper producing deficiency and toxicity respectively.

- Assuming no related diseases, individuals who should be assessed for potential mineral imbalances are those who shun whole categories of foods, vegetarians, dairy avoiders, and consumers of supplemental minerals in excess of the RDA/AIs.

- Persons fed artificially in which normal gastrointestinal absorptive processes are bypassed or whose intake consists of compounded formulas or of foods particularly rich in single nutrients should be carefully monitored. Additionally, storage vessels made of copper or containing lead have caused toxicities, as have medical devices that released aluminum into treatment solutions.

- Teaching clients to safeguard iron-containing supplements from children and to seek immediate medical attention should ingestion occur is of prime importance in preventing those poisoning deaths. Careful assessment of the swallowing or overuse of nonfood items could identify potentially hazardous practices that have led to zinc and fluoride poisoning deaths.

CASE STUDY *7–1*

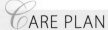

Mrs. B is a 34-year-old woman who has related her fear of osteoporosis to the nurse. A recent visit to a 75-year-old aunt crystallized this fear. The aunt has become stooped and recently broke her hip. Mrs. B is especially concerned because she has often been told she resembles this aunt. Mrs. B asks, "Is there anything I can do to prevent this from happening to me?"

A 24-hour recall of dietary intake revealed a total of 1 cup of milk and no other dairy products. Mrs. B did consume two 3-oz servings of meat. Mrs. B has three small children and stated that they are exercise enough for her. She sits outside and watches them play on every nice day.

Mrs. B is 5 feet, 3 inches tall and weighs 110 lb. She is white with fair skin.

CARE PLAN

Subjective Data

Fear of osteoporosis ■ Family history positive for osteoporosis ■ Less than RDA for calcium previous 24 hours ■ Met MyPlate guideline for meat group previous 24 hours ■ No planned exercise program

Objective Data

Height: 5 ft 3 in. ■ Weight: 110 lb (BMI 19.5) ■ White, fair, slight build

Analysis

Self-identified need regarding prevention of osteoporosis related to aunt's history of disease.

Plan

DESIRED OUTCOMES EVALUATION CRITERIA	ACTIONS/INTERVENTIONS	RATIONALE
Client will list appropriate actions to maintain a strong skeleton after teaching session	Teach client how to consume 1000 mg of calcium daily: 3 cups of milk or equivalent	One cup of milk contains approximately 300 mg of calcium +100 mg from other sources
	Teach client factors favoring calcium absorption: vitamin D	If client chooses unfortified dairy products for calcium content, vitamin D may become insufficient depending on available sun exposure
	Teach client role of exercise in strengthening bones	Weight-bearing exercise stimulates the osteoblasts to build bone

At a follow-up visit, Mrs. B indicated she had increased her consumption of dairy products but had not begun a planned exercise program. The nurse referred Mrs. B to a local Women's Health Center.

 7-1

Director of Women's Health Center's Notes

The following Director of Women's Health Center's Notes are representative of teamwork documentation.

Subjective: Interested in strengthening bones due to fear of familial osteoporosis

States no activity impediments

Objective: BMI = 19.5

Passed intake activity screen

Analysis: Increased risk of osteoporosis based on family history and physical characteristics

Plan: Suggest ultrasound heel bone mineral density for baseline value

Beginning-level walking program with group 3 times weekly, solo 3 times weekly.

Critical Thinking Questions

1. What additional dietary information would you need before recommending good sources of calcium for Mrs. B?

2. What other assessment data would be helpful to broaden the scope of preventing osteoporosis?

3. Is the problem described in the Case Study a significant one for a 34-year-old woman? Why or why not?

Chapter Review

1. Like vitamins, minerals give no energy to the body. Unlike vitamins, minerals:
   a. Are completely absorbed from the intestinal tract
   b. Become part of the structure of the body
   c. Cause few clinical problems because of their widespread abundance in foods
   d. Cannot accumulate to the extent that they cause problems

2. Which of the following foods is the best source of iron?
   a. Eggs
   b. Baked beans
   c. Beef
   d. Spinach

3. Which of the following individuals would be at greatest risk for a mineral deficiency?
   a. Someone who consumes no dairy products
   b. Someone who consumes no shellfish
   c. Someone who consumes no red meat
   d. Someone who drinks tea or coffee with every meal

4. Cretinism and goiter are caused by deficiency of _____.
   a. Copper
   b. Selenium
   c. Iodine
   d. Zinc

5. Calcium is necessary for strong bones and teeth. It is also necessary for:
   a. Assisting with the production of insulin
   b. Maintaining stomach acidity
   c. Preventing blood clots
   d. Enabling muscle contraction

Clinical Analysis

Mrs. H is a 30-year-old mother of three children, all younger than 5 years of age. On her 6-week postpartum visit, her hemoglobin level was 10 grams per 100 milliliters of blood. She is given a prescription for ferrous sulfate and referred to the office nurse for nutrition counseling regarding her iron intake.

Mrs. H tells the nurse that she eats what the children eat: cold cereal and milk for breakfast, peanut butter and jelly sandwiches and maybe a banana for lunch, and casseroles of tuna or hamburger for dinner. Mrs. H is a heavy coffee drinker, consuming 10 cups per day, two with each meal and a total of four others during "coffee breaks."

The H family is lower-middle class. Mr. H is a long-distance truck driver and is away from home for long intervals. Mrs. H has some knowledge of iron needs and sources because of her three pregnancies. She is reluctant to continue the ferrous sulfate she has been

Clinical Analysis—cont'd

taking throughout her pregnancy. "It binds me up," she tells the nurse. Also, Mrs. H maintains she cannot eat liver: "It gags me."

1. Which of the following statements by Mrs. H would indicate she understood the nurse's instructions correctly?
   a. "I should eat a little meat, fish, or poultry with every meal containing grain, fruit and vegetable sources of iron."
   b. "I should increase the fiber in my diet because it will increase the absorption of iron."
   c. "If I want an alcoholic beverage, beer contains the most iron in a readily absorbable form."
   d. "Since I am taking an iron supplement, it is not important how I eat."

2. To meet the safety needs of the H children, the nurse instructs Mrs. H to keep her ferrous sulfate in a locked cupboard. The reason for this is:
   a. Interactions of iron tablets with vitamin supplements intended for children can cause deficiencies of water-soluble vitamins.
   b. The human body has no effective means of excreting an overload of iron.
   c. Iron poisoning, although rare, can occur if a child ingests more than 30 tablets of ferrous sulfate.
   d. Because iron binds with calcium, an overdose of iron would cause rickets.

3. Based on her current habits, which of the following changes to her lifestyle would be likely to increase Mrs. H's iron absorption from food?
   a. Changing her meal times to allow 5 hours to elapse between them.
   b. Avoiding citrus fruits and juices with meals.
   c. Trying alternate forms of liver such as in sausage.
   d. Delaying coffee and tea drinking to 2 hours after a meal.

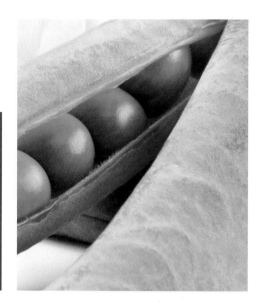

8

Water

LEARNING OBJECTIVES

After completing this chapter, the student should be able to:

■ List the functions of water in the body.

■ Relate locations of the water by age and gender to the potential for harm caused by imbalances.

■ Describe the initial stimulus and the end results of the hormonal control mechanism of water balance in the body.

■ Connect the concept of osmolality to choices for providing the body's nutrient needs.

■ Recognize the roles of the two major organs that maintain acid–base balance.

■ Categorize average gains and losses of fluid in a healthy adult over a 24-hour period.

■ Contrast the regulation, costs, and benefits of tap versus bottled water.

■ Identify methods of assessing water balance in the body.

■ Distinguish between heat exhaustion and heatstroke as to signs and symptoms and first-aid treatment.

■ Outline situations in which water deficit or excess may become lethal.

Water in Human Nutrition

*W*ater is the largest single constituent of the human body, and the need for water is more urgent than the need for any other nutrient. Humans can live a month without food but only 6 days without water.

More than half of body weight is water, which is found in and around the cells, within the blood and lymph vessels, and in various body cavities. Some tissues have significantly more water than others:

■ Muscle tissue is 70% water.
■ Fat tissue is 30% water.
■ Bone tissue is 10% water.

A man's body is 60% to 65% water, whereas a woman's body is just 50% to 54% water. Men have higher water content than women because of their greater muscle mass. Women and obese persons, who have higher body fat content, tend to have less water

for any given weight (Bailey, Sands, and Franch, 2014). The body of a 70-kg (154-lb) man would contain about 42 liters of water.

Age also affects the proportion of water in a body. Compared with the 50% to 65% for women and men, an infant's body is 75% water. Premature infants may be 80% water by weight. Infants, especially premature infants, are at high risk of fluid imbalances because of the proportion and distribution of water in their bodies. The adult proportion of water to body weight is reached at about 3 years of age (Gropper and Smith, 2013).

Fluid Compartments

Body fluids are contained in intracellular and extracellular compartments (Fig. 8-1). These compartments are separated by semipermeable membranes, which allow some substances to pass through and prevent

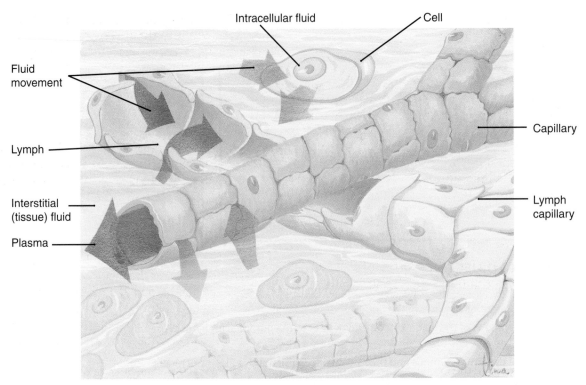

FIGURE 8-1 Water compartments, showing the names water is given in its different locations and the ways in which water moves between compartments. (Reprinted from Scanlon, VC, and Sanders, T: *Essentials of anatomy and physiology*, 6th ed. FA Davis, Philadelphia, 2011, p. 30, with permission.)

the passage of other substances. Water passes freely through the membranes.

Thirteen water transport proteins, called aquaporins (AQP), have been identified in humans. Thirteen is the final number because the human genome project is complete (Ishibashi, Hara, and Kondo, 2009). Aquaporins are membrane proteins that function as water-selective channels in the plasma membranes of many cells and help to explain the speed at which water moves across cell membranes, including the selective absorption found in different areas of the kidney. Seven aquaporin water channels are expressed in human kidneys, where they have key roles in maintaining body water **homeostasis.** Mutations in AQP2 can result in **diabetes insipidus** (Holmes, 2012).

Three aquaporins are expressed in the brain, playing important roles in the homeostasis of its fluids, a critical function given the rigid skull that restrains expansion of its contents. Aquaporin1 (AQP1) is involved in cerebrospinal fluid formation, whereas Aquaporin4 (AQP4), the predominant brain water channel, is implicated in brain edema formation and resolution (Zelenina, 2010). In the future, treating brain edema by modulating AQP4 expression or function may be possible (Xu, Su, and Xu, 2010). An autoantibody to AQP4 has been described as a marker of a unique form of multiple sclerosis involving the optic nerve and spinal cord for which alternative tests are not available (Verkman, 2009).

Both eyes and ears have functions involving fluids. AQP0 not only functions as a water channel in the eye but also plays a structural role in maintaining the transparency and accommodation of the ocular lens. Mutations in the AQP0 gene result in genetic cataracts (Chepelinsky, 2009). Eight AQP subtypes have been identified in the membranous labyrinth of the inner ear. Disturbed AQP function may have pathophysiological relevance and may turn AQPs into therapeutic targets for the treatment of inner ear diseases (Eckhard, Gleiser, Arnold, et al, 2012).

The importance of aquaporins in the rapid passage of water across plasma membranes in the gastrointestinal tract should be self-evident. The aquaporins most abundantly expressed in the whole gut are AQP1, 3, 7, 10, and 11 (Laforenza, 2012). In both cancer and brain edema, current therapies are limited, and new pharmacological approaches focused on AQPs offer exciting potential for clinical advances (Yool, Brown, and Flynn, 2010). Although no specific inhibitors of aquaporins are available yet, the search for drugs to modulate the expression and functions of aquaporins is the focus of ongoing research efforts (Ishibashi, Kondo, Hara, and Morishita, 2011).

Intracellular Fluid

The fluid inside the cells is called intracellular. In adults, intracellular water constitutes about 65% of body water. In infants, approximately 46% of the body water is intracellular.

Extracellular Fluid

All fluid outside cells is extracellular. In adults, about 35% of the body's water is extracellular, whereas in infants, the approximate proportion is 54%. Figure 8-2 illustrates those relationships. The difference is important because extracellular fluid is more easily and rapidly excreted than is intracellular fluid. **Extracellular fluid** includes interstitial, intravascular, lymph, and transcellular fluids.

INTERSTITIAL FLUID

Located between the cells or surrounding the cells, interstitial fluid assists in transporting substances between the cells and the blood and lymph vessels.

INTRAVASCULAR FLUID

Intravascular fluid is found within the blood vessels, arteries, arterioles, capillaries, venules, and veins. The liquid part of the blood is called **plasma;** the liquid part of the blood without the clotting elements is called **serum.** As is illustrated in Figure 8-3, 91.5% of plasma is water.

LYMPHATIC FLUID

The venous system cannot collect and return all the fluid from the tissues to the heart. **Lymph,** via the lymphatic vessels, assists in returning the fluid part of blood to the heart.

TRANSCELLULAR FLUID

Transcellular fluids include cerebrospinal fluid, pericardial fluid, pleural fluid, synovial fluid, intraocular fluids, and gastrointestinal secretions. Transcellular fluids are constantly being secreted into their spaces and reabsorbed into the vascular system. Figure 8-4 shows the approximate distribution of water in the four compartments.

Usage

No storage tanks for water exist in the body; water continually moves from one body compartment to another and is often reused by the body to perform different tasks.

Functions

As a component of cells, water helps give the body shape and form, and as the major constituent of blood, it helps to maintain blood volume and blood pressure. It is part of the structure of many of the body's large molecules, such as protein and glycogen. Some body water also serves as a lubricant, as in mucus secretions and joint fluid.

Water helps to regulate body temperature by absorbing the heat produced by fever and the heat resulting from metabolic processes. On average, tissue metabolism generates 100 kilocalories per hour. The blood carries excess heat to the skin, where it is dissipated by perspiration or radiation.

Water is a **solvent** for minerals, vitamins, glucose, and other small molecules. (The substance that is dissolved in a solvent is called a **solute.**) See Box 8-1 for a list of the functions of water in the body.

Absorption

A small amount of water can be absorbed into the bloodstream from the stomach, but a liter of water can be absorbed from the small intestine in an hour. The daily absorption of water by the small intestine is up to

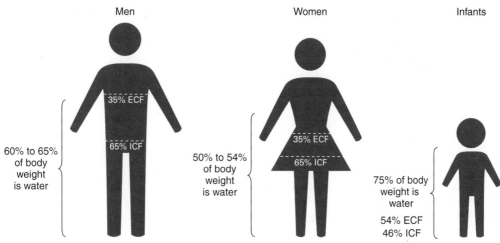

Men

35% ECF

65% ICF

60% to 65% of body weight is water

Women

35% ECF

65% ICF

50% to 54% of body weight is water

Infants

75% of body weight is water

54% ECF
46% ICF

FIGURE 8-2 The relative amounts of body weight that are intracellular and extracellular water in men, women, and infants.

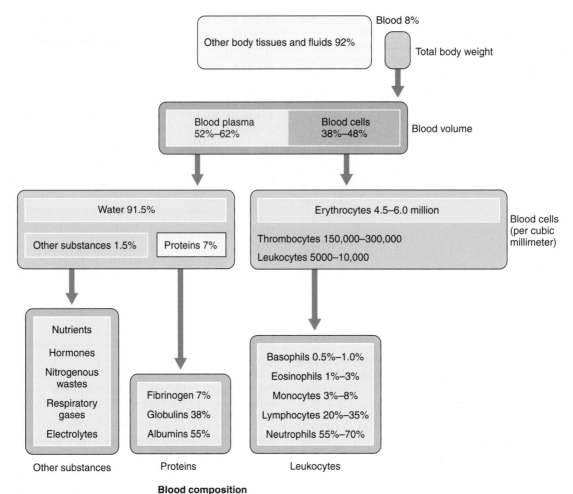

Blood composition

Components of blood and relationship of blood to other body tissues

FIGURE 8-3 Blood constitutes 8% of body weight. The largest single component of the blood is water. (Reprinted from Venes, D [Ed.]: *Taber's cyclopedic medical dictionary*, 21st ed. FA Davis, Philadelphia, 2009, p. 283, with permission.)

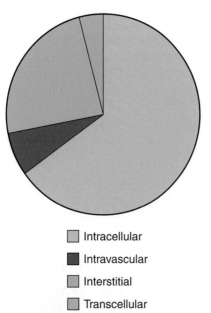

- Intracellular
- Intravascular
- Interstitial
- Transcellular

FIGURE 8-4 Proportionate amounts of water in the four fluid compartments in the body. (Reprinted from Williams, L, and Hopper, P: *Understanding medical surgical nursing*, 4th ed. FA Davis, Philadelphia, 2011, p. 70, with permission.)

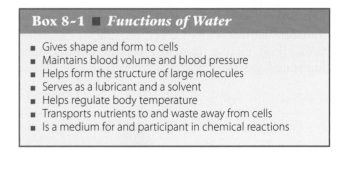

Box 8-1 ■ *Functions of Water*

- Gives shape and form to cells
- Maintains blood volume and blood pressure
- Helps form the structure of large molecules
- Serves as a lubricant and a solvent
- Helps regulate body temperature
- Transports nutrients to and waste away from cells
- Is a medium for and participant in chemical reactions

15 liters per day and by the colon 5 liters per day (Popkin, D'Anci, and Rosenberg, 2010).

Under conditions that disrupt an individual's automatic adaptive mechanisms, water may be retained. The accumulation of excessive amounts of fluid between the cells (in the interstitial spaces) is called **edema.** Conditions that may cause such water retention include:

- Venous or lymphatic blockage
- Heart failure
- Severe protein deficiency (see Chapter 4)

- Sodium retention
- Some kidney conditions

When finger pressure displaces excess fluid over a bony area the sign is termed **pitting edema.** Although the fluid remains inside the body, it is lost to circulation (Fig. 8-5).

As a result of injury or trauma, the capillaries become more permeable so that more fluid and cells can travel to the site of the injury to begin repairs, or healing. This process also causes swelling, or edema, at the site of an injury—blisters at the site of burns, for example, where fluid leaves the vessels and accumulates in the skin. As is noted in Chapter 22, correct fluid replacement is a high priority for severely burned clients.

In most cases, localized edema is not deadly; however, accumulation of fluid in the brain (cerebral edema) or in lung tissue (pulmonary edema) is life-threatening. Cerebral edema may result from tumors, toxic chemicals, or infection. Pulmonary edema can be a consequence of a failing heart or irritation of the lung, as seen in a client who inhales toxic gases.

Excessive water also can be dispersed throughout the body. This condition is called **water intoxication,** which can be caused by excessive water intake (either by the intravenous or gastrointestinal route), cerebral concussion, or hormonal disorders. Many of the symptoms are caused by diluting the concentration of the minerals in the body's fluid compartments.

Dietary Reference Intakes

*Dietary Reference Intakes (DRIs) have been established for total water from food and beverages; see Appendix A. For all ages and physiological conditions, the level of certainty is an Adequate Intake (**AI**), not a Recommended Dietary Allowance (RDA).*

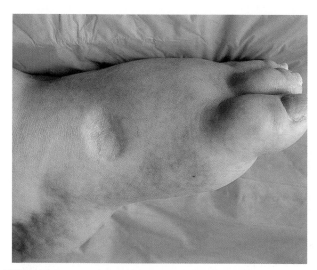

FIGURE 8-5 Finger or thumb pressure over a bony area displaces edematous fluid; shown here as pitting edema of the foot. (Reprinted from Williams, L, and Hopper, P: *Understanding medical surgical nursing,* 4th ed. FA Davis, Philadelphia, 2011, p. 397, with permission.)

Approximately 80% of water needs are expected to come from fluids and 20% from foods. Larger intakes are required by physically active people or those in hot environments.

The previously publicized negative effects of caffeine and alcohol on water balance have been refuted by evidence showing the diuretic effects of those substances to be transient. Appropriately responding to thirst sensation and mealtime beverages are usually adequate to maintain hydration. Acute water toxicity is a hazard in individuals rapidly consuming much more than the kidneys' maximal excretion rate of 0.7 to 1.0 liter per hour (Institute of Medicine, 2004).

Ordinarily, breast milk alone can supply an infant's needed water even in a desert. At the opposite end of the age spectrum, older adults often have a blunted sense of thirst, and their water needs may be affected by disease and medication.

Physiology of Body Fluids

To help with understanding the information in this section, see Box 8-2 on elementary chemistry.

Box 8-2 ■ *Elementary Chemistry*

An element is a primary, simple substance that cannot be broken down by ordinary chemical methods into any other substance. Oxygen is an element, as are sodium, chlorine, and the other minerals considered earlier.

Atoms

Elements are composed of smaller parts called atoms. In the center of an atom is the nucleus, which contains protons and neutrons and gives an atom its weight and mass. Circling around the nucleus like satellites are electrons. These electrons are arranged in a consistent manner: a maximum of two in the orbit or shell closest to the nucleus, and a maximum of eight in each of the outer shells. The ability of an atom to react chemically depends on the number of "empty slots" in the outermost electron shell.

Chemical Bonding

A compound is a substance created by the chemical bonding (joining) of two or more kinds of atoms (elements). A chemical bond is the force that binds atoms together. A compound is formed when atoms share electrons or when one atom donates one or more electrons to another atom. For example, water (a liquid) is formed when two atoms of hydrogen (a colorless, odorless gas) are joined with one atom of oxygen (another colorless, odorless gas), hence the abbreviation H_2O.

A sodium atom has only one electron in its outer shell; a chlorine atom has seven. In close proximity, the sodium atom donates the electron in its outer shell to the outer shell of the chlorine atom. With the loss of its electron, the sodium now has an electrical charge of +1 and is called a sodium **ion** (Na^+). Ions with positive charges are referred to as **cations.** The chlorine atom, which gained an electron, now has a charge of −1

(continued)

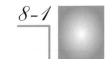

Box 8-2 ■ *Elementary Chemistry—cont'd*

and is called a chloride ion (Cl⁻). Ions with negative charges are referred to as **anions.**

Because these ions have opposite charges (+ and −), they are attracted to one another and unite, forming sodium chloride (NaCl). The chemical bond that holds the sodium and chloride ions together is called an **ionic bond.** Sodium can donate its single electron to other elements beside chlorine, and other elements can form ionic bonds as well (see Fig. 8-6).

Electrolytes

An **electrolyte** is an element or compound that, when dissolved in water, separates (dissociates) into ions capable of conducting an electrical current. These electrically charged particles are then available to take part in other chemical reactions. The properties of electrolytes permit some diagnostic tests as well as offer potential hazards (see Clinical Application 8-1).

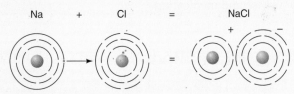

FIGURE 8-6 Formation of an ionic bond. An atom of sodium loses an electron to an atom of chlorine. The two ions formed have unlike charges, are attracted to one another, and form a molecule of sodium chloride. (Reprinted from Scanlon, VC, and Sanders, T: *Essentials of anatomy and physiology*, 6th ed. FA Davis, Philadelphia, 2011, p. 26, with permission.)

The Effect of Electrolytes on Water Balance

Each fluid compartment has an electrolyte composition that serves its needs and has automatic mechanisms designed to keep it electrically neutral, or balanced. The positive ions within a compartment must equal the negative ones. When shifts and losses occur, compensating shifts and gains reestablish electroneutrality.

Important Body Electrolytes

Mineral ions strongly influence not only water balance but also osmotic pressure, blood pressure, and acid–base balance. See Table 8-1 for a summary of the major body electrolytes.

Because electrical activity is determined by the concentration of electrolytes in a given solution, electrolytes are measured by the total number of particles in solution rather than their total weight. The unit of measure in the United States is the **milliequivalent (mEq),** expressed as mEq/liter. The concentration of a pharmaceutical solution is also measured in milliequivalents. Clinical Calculation 8-1 shows the conversion of milligrams of sodium chloride to milliequivalents.

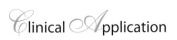

8-1

Clinical Application

Diagnostic Uses and Potential Hazards of Electrolytes

Skin sensors attached to an electrocardiograph can trace the electrical activity of the heart. The resulting graphic record is called an **electrocardiogram (ECG).** The machine's sensors on the skin can detect the electric current because blood is an electrolyte solution and thus capable of conducting electricity. The same principle applies to the use of an electroencephalograph, a device that traces brainwave activity. The record obtained from this machine is called an **electroencephalogram (EEG).**

The characteristics of electrolyte solutions that allow these machines to sense electrical activity can also be hazardous. A fluid-filled tube, such as a nasogastric tube or catheter, can conduct stray electricity from faulty electrical devices to the client's heart and could result in dysrhythmias. The electricity in the shock may be minuscule but enough to be fatal if it happens at the wrong time in the cardiac cycle. The health-care worker should be vigilant for defective electrical equipment, tagging it for repair and replacing it immediately.

TABLE 8-1 ■ Major Body Electrolytes

ELECTROLYTE	FLUID COMPARTMENT*	FUNCTIONS
Cations		
Sodium (Na⁺)	Extracellular	Major cation in extracellular fluid. Na⁺ concentration in fluids determines the distribution of H_2O by osmosis. The kidney uses Na⁺ with H⁺ and HCO_3^- to regulate acid–base balance.
Potassium (K⁺)	Intracellular	Major cation in intracellular fluid. K⁺ with Na⁺ maintains water balance. The kidney uses K⁺ with Na⁺ and HCO_3^-, to regulate acid–base balance.
Calcium (Ca²⁺)	Extracellular†	Participates in permeability of cell membranes, transmission of nerve impulses, muscle action.
Magnesium (Mg²⁺)	Intracellular	Regulates nerve stimulation and normal muscle action.
Anions		
Chloride (Cl⁻)	Extracellular	Major anion in extracellular fluid. With Na⁺, helps maintain water balance and acid–base balance.
Bicarbonate (HCO_3^-)	Extracellular	Most important extracellular fluid buffer.
Phosphate (HPO_4^{2-})	Intracellular	Within the intracellular fluid, phosphates and proteins buffer 95% of the body's carbonic acid and 50% of other acids.

*Extracellular fluid and intracellular fluid both contain all the cations and anions listed in this table but are labeled as either extracellular fluid or intracellular fluid according to the concentration. For example, sodium ions make up 142 of the total 155 milliequivalents per liter (of the cations) in the extracellular fluid.
†Of the cations, 3% in extracellular fluid and 1% in intracellular fluid.

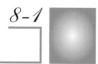 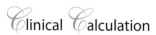

8-1

Clinical Calculation

Converting Milligrams to Milliequivalents

Milligram is a measure of weight. Milliequivalent is a measure of the concentration of electrolytes (number of particles) per volume of solution. The concentration of electrolytes in any given solution determines its chemical activity.

Electrolytes are expressed as milliequivalents per liter of solution whether referring to blood values or intravenous solutions.

To convert milligrams to milliequivalents, it is necessary to know

- the number of milligrams per liter,
- the molecular weight of the substance, and
- its valence, a number indicating the combining power of an atom, found in many dictionaries.

A teaspoonful of table salt in 1 liter of water will produce a 0.5% solution. A teaspoonful is roughly 5 grams. Because table salt is 40% sodium and 60% chloride, the liter of 0.5% salt water would contain 2 grams (2000 mg) of sodium and 3 grams (3000 mg) of chloride.

Two other values are needed: atomic or molecular weights and valences. The atomic weight for sodium is 22.9898. Sodium has a valence of 1. The formula for converting milligrams to milliequivalents is:

$$mEq/L = \frac{(mg/L) \times valence}{molecular\ weight} = \frac{2000 \times 1}{22.9898} = 87\ mEq/L\ of\ sodium$$

Continuing, we can use the same formula with different values to calculate the milliequivalents of chloride. The atomic weight for chlorine is 35.453. Chlorine has a valence of 1.

Filling in the values for chloride, we have:

$$mEq/L = \frac{(mg/L) \times valence}{molecular\ weight} = \frac{3000 \times 1}{35.453} = 85\ mEq/L\ of\ chloride$$

Then, adding the sodium and chloride, we have:

$$87 + 85 = 172\ mEq/L\ in\ the\ 0.5\%\ solution.$$

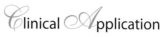 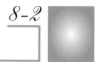

8-2

Clinical Application

Osmosis in the Kitchen

To make sauerkraut, cabbage is sliced finely and placed in the bottom of a crock. Salt is added to the dry cabbage in layers that are tamped down until the crock is full. At this point, liquid will have gathered, pulled from the cabbage pieces by the concentrated salt. A heavy plate topped with bags of water is placed atop the cabbage to continue squeezing the water from the cabbage as it ferments. The crock is covered with a cloth. After 5 or 6 weeks, the crock is full of juice, and the cabbage has become sauerkraut.

To make a small batch of sauerkraut, use 2 teaspoons of canning salt per pound of cabbage.

Osmotic Pressure

Osmosis is the movement of water (or another solvent) across a semipermeable membrane from an area with fewer particles to one with more particles. The result, as long as the difference is reasonable, is an equalization of concentration on either side of the membrane. Clinical Application 8-2 describes an experiment to demonstrate osmosis.

The size of the molecule and its ability to ionize determines the number of particles in a given concentration. Electrolytes readily ionize in solution. Disaccharides and monosaccharides do not ionize.

Osmosis is a passive process. The movement of some substances, however, is active. Some substances require active transport mechanisms to push them through a membrane. Two such transport mechanisms are the sodium pump and the potassium pump. Located

in cell membranes, these pumps are actually proteins that move ions.

Sodium pumps move sodium ions out of cells (and water follows).
Potassium pumps move potassium ions into cells.

In this manner, the body maintains electrolyte concentrations of the intracellular and extracellular fluid compartments. Active transport requires energy to operate.

DETERMINATION OF OSMOTIC PRESSURE

When two solutions on either side of a semipermeable membrane have different concentrations, pressure develops. This pressure, which is exerted on the semipermeable membrane, is called **osmotic pressure.** Osmotic pressure causes a solvent such as water to cross the membrane, but the solutes (particles) that are outside the membrane cannot go through.

OSMOLALITY AND NUTRITION

The measure of the osmotic pressure exerted by the number of particles per volume of liquid is referred to as its **osmolarity.** The unit of measure for osmotic activity is the **milliosmole.** Clinically, osmolarity is usually reported in milliosmoles per *liter*. **Osmolality,** in contrast, is the measure of the osmotic pressure exerted by the number of particles per weight of solvent, usually reported in milliosmoles per *kilogram*. The normal value for osmolality of human blood serum is about 275 to 295 milliosmoles per kilogram.

In dilute aqueous solutions such as those in the body, only a small numerical difference is found between osmolarity and osmolality, and the terms and values are often used interchangeably (Gropper and Smith, 2013). The primary determinant of osmolality in the extracellular fluid is sodium.

Fluids are designated **isotonic** if they approximate the osmolality of blood plasma. Two commonly administered isotonic intravenous fluids are 5% glucose in water and 0.9% sodium chloride. Fluids exerting less osmotic pressure than plasma are labeled **hypotonic.** Those exerting greater osmotic pressure than plasma are called **hypertonic.**

Achieving the correct osmolality of fluids administered intravenously (by needle or tube into the vein) is crucial. A solution that is too concentrated pulls water out of the red blood cells, and the cells shrivel and die. A solution that is too weak allows water to be pulled into the red blood cells until the cells burst. For these reasons, isotonic solutions are given with red blood cell products.

Intravenous solutions containing sufficient nutrients to provide all a person's known needs are so hypertonic that they must be infused into a very large vein so that they are diluted quickly by the substantial volume of blood flowing past the infusion port or catheter. This procedure is called parenteral nutrition and is described in Chapter 14.

Oral fluids also can be categorized by osmotic pressure. Plain water is hypotonic. Whole milk at 275 milliosmoles per liter is close to isotonic but is not recommended for infants for another reason related to its metabolism (see Chapter 11). Ginger ale, with 510 milliosmoles per liter, and 7-Up®, with 640, are both hypertonic. The significance of these differences will become apparent in the section on treatment of fluid volume abnormalities.

SERUM ELECTROLYTES

The electrolyte content of blood can also be reported in milliequivalents per liter. The normal serum sodium level is 135 to 145 milliequivalents per liter. In most cases, because sodium is the most influential extracellular ion, osmolarity of the extracellular fluid can be estimated clinically by doubling the serum sodium value. Normal serum sodium doubled would be 270 to 296 milliosmoles per liter. Normal osmolality of the serum is about 300 milliosmoles per kilogram. This simple method gives a close approximation.

The other ion that health-care providers monitor carefully in clients with potential fluid and electrolyte imbalances is potassium. Most of the potassium in the body is inside the cells, at a concentration of 150 milliequivalents per liter. By contrast, potassium concentration in the blood is only 3.5 to 5.0 milliequivalents per liter. Even slight variations above or below these values can produce severe consequences. The heart muscle is particularly sensitive to high or low levels of potassium; abnormal levels can produce cardiac arrest.

Although proteins play a role in fluid balance (discussed subsequently), they normally remain in the cell or extracellular fluid. Therefore, sodium, potassium, and chloride ions provide the most movement across cell membranes to maintain osmotic pressure and fluid balance (Gropper and Smith, 2013).

The Effect of Plasma Proteins on Water Balance

The body has highly developed mechanisms that maintain a constant flow of water and:

- Nutrients to cells
- Waste materials from cells

Adequate blood pressure is necessary for this transport system to function. Blood pressure is the force exerted against the walls of the arteries by the beating heart. It is reported in two numbers, for example, 120/80 (measured in millimeters of mercury, mm Hg). The top number is the pressure when the heart beats, called **systolic pressure.** The bottom number is the pressure between beats, called the **diastolic pressure.** One of the factors necessary to maintain blood pressure is a sufficient volume of blood in the arteries and veins.

Water and nutrients in the blood are pushed out through the thin walls of the capillaries into the interstitial fluid by **hydrostatic pressure** (blood pressure) supplied by the heart. From the interstitial compartment, the water and nutrients cross cell membranes to bathe and nourish the cell. Plasma proteins, including **albumin,** remain in the capillaries because they are too large to squeeze through the capillary wall.

Inside the capillaries, the remaining plasma proteins exert **colloidal osmotic pressure (COP).** At this point, the COP is greater than the hydrostatic pressure, thereby pulling water and waste materials from the interstitial fluid into the capillaries to maintain blood volume. Clinical Application 8-3 describes a condition in which a low serum protein is the cause of water imbalance.

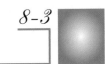

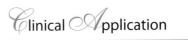

8-3

Clinical Application

Protein–Energy Malnutrition and Water Balance

Starving children often look plump (see Fig. 4-4) because they are edematous. Such children are victims of **kwashiorkor,** a disease of protein-energy malnutrition, which commonly occurs in children just after weaning when their diets do not have as much protein as found in their mothers' milk.

Protein plays a crucial role in maintaining fluid volume in blood vessels. Children with kwashiorkor develop edema because they do not have enough plasma proteins remaining in the capillaries to pull water back into the circulatory system. Thus, water accumulates in the interstitial spaces. After treatment begins, plasma proteins will pull the retained water into the blood, and the children will appear emaciated.

Regulation of Water Intake and Excretion

The body has mechanisms regulating both the intake and the excretion of water. To achieve homeostasis, the body's automatic monitoring and regulating mechanisms are activated by deficits or excesses of water amounting to only a few hundred milliliters (Popkin et al, 2010).

Normally, thirst governs water intake. Excretion is controlled mainly by two hormones:

1. Antidiuretic hormone causes the body to reabsorb (retain) water
2. Aldosterone causes the body to retain sodium

Thirst Mechanism

Thirst is the desire for fluids, especially water. Thirst normally occurs when 10% of the intravascular volume is lost or when cellular volume is reduced by 1% to 2%. When blood contains too little water, its osmotic pressure increases. Special sensors in the **hypothalamus** monitor the osmotic pressure as the blood circulates in the brain. When the hypothalamus detects an increase in osmotic pressure, the gland triggers a desire to drink.

Antidiuretic Hormone

If thirst is not alleviated, the hypothalamus increases production of **antidiuretic hormone (ADH),** which is then secreted from the posterior pituitary gland. ADH, also named **vasopressin,** causes the kidneys to return more water to the bloodstream rather than spill it into the urine. A rise in osmolality by 2% to 3% stimulates enough ADH to maximally concentrate the urine. The opposite is also true: a decline in osmolality by 2% to 3% produces maximally dilute urine (Bailey et al, 2014).

ADH also constricts arteries to increase blood pressure. A similar situation occurs by putting a finger over the end of a garden hose, narrowing its diameter, thus increasing pressure of the flowing water.

In **diabetes insipidus,** the hypothalamus does not secrete ADH or the kidneys do not respond appropriately. If the hypothalamus is not secreting ADH, a pharmaceutical preparation can be given. Clinical Application 8-4 provides information about a condition called syndrome of inappropriate antidiuresis (SIAD).

Aldosterone

The release of **aldosterone,** a hormone secreted by the adrenal glands, is another water-balancing mechanism in the body. Aldosterone causes sodium ions to be

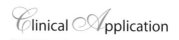 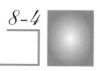

Clinical Application 8-4

Syndrome of Inappropriate Antidiuresis

The syndrome of inappropriate antidiuresis (SIAD), formerly called the syndrome of inappropriate secretion of antidiuretic hormone (SIADH), is the most frequent cause of hyponatremia (Frouget, 2012). In 10% of clients, however, antidiuretic hormone (ADH or vasopressin) is undetectable, leading to the new name for the condition (Vantyghem, Balavoine, Wémeau, and Douillard, 2011). Normally, increased blood osmolality stimulates the posterior pituitary gland to release ADH. When enough water is returned to the bloodstream by the kidney, ADH secretion stops. Several diverse situations cause syndrome of inappropriate antidiuresis (SIAD). Examples of causes include the following:

- Central nervous system disorders (infections, hemorrhage, multiple sclerosis)
- Lung disease (pneumonia, tuberculosis, cystic fibrosis)
- Some tumors (oat cell of lung, carcinoma of pancreas, lymphoma, leukemia)
- Certain drugs (selective serotonin reuptake inhibitors or SSRIs, chemotherapeutic agents, antidepressants)
- Surgery-induced severe nausea, pain (Esposito, Piotti, Bianzina, et al, 2011)

The signs and symptoms of SIAD are those of hyponatremia (see Table 7-6). Familiarity with the client's usual personality is crucial. In one case, a grandson successfully advocated for his grandmother. Her uncharacteristic sleepiness for days after surgery alarmed him enough to say, "This is not grandma." His persistent efforts culminated in a diagnosis of SIAD with transfer to the intensive care unit.

Hyponatremic patients without serious signs or symptoms of cerebral edema do not require urgent therapy to raise the serum sodium, but the underlying causes should be treated. Chronic or mild hyponatremia has been linked to falls, impaired gait and attention, and fractures. Depending on their extracellular fluid volume status, management of their fluid and sodium intakes may be part of the therapeutic plan (Vaidya, Ho, and Freda, 2010).

In stark contrast, hyponatremia with cerebral symptoms is a medical emergency in which treatment delay may prove fatal. The emerging consensus calls for prompt bolus treatment of symptomatic hyponatremia with hypertonic saline (Overgaard-Steensen, 2010) or saline infusions (Esposito et al, 2011). Saline therapy requires careful and frequent monitoring of the effects on blood values to avoid complications associated with too rapid correction of the hyponatremia, such as **osmotic demyelinating disease** (Sterns, Hix, and Silver, 2010; see Chapter 7). During treatment of hypernatremia, serum electrolytes should be monitored every 2 hours and infusion rates adjusted to avoid too rapid a correction (Bailey et al, 2014).

returned to the bloodstream by the kidneys rather than to be spilled into urine. Sodium, the most influential extracellular ion, pulls water along with it.

The stimulus for the release of aldosterone is decreased pressure of the blood supplying kidney tissue. In response, the kidneys produce **renin** that acts with secretions from the liver and the lungs to produce **angiotensin II.** The cascade continues as shown in Figure 8-7.

The other side of sodium retention is potassium loss. Within fluid compartments, positively charged particles must equal negatively charged ones. When sodium is retained, to maintain electroneutrality, the kidney excretes more potassium under the influence of aldosterone.

Acid–Base Balance

The body is well equipped to digest and metabolize acidic and basic foods without jeopardizing its acid–base balance, assuming normal amounts are ingested. The use of substances such as baking soda to treat an upset stomach should be discouraged, however, because the baking soda can be absorbed into the blood, thereby affecting the whole body. Nonabsorbable antacids designed to treat stomach upsets and used according to directions are a better choice than baking soda.

Acids are compounds that yield hydrogen ions when dissociated in solution. The more hydrogen ions a solution contains, the more concentrated the acid. Bases, or alkalis, are substances that accept hydrogen ions. Acidity or alkalinity is measured by a scale called **pH** for *potential of hydrogen.*

The pH scale ranges from 0 to 14: acids are rated 0 to 6.999; 7.0 is neutral; bases (alkalis) are greater than 7. On the scale, 1 would indicate a strong acid, and 14 a strong base. Figure 8-8 illustrates the pH scale, showing placement of acid, neutral, and alkaline fluids. The difference between units is 10-fold. Thus, lemon juice at a pH of 2 is 10 times as acidic as orange juice with a pH of 3.

Physiologically, a substance is an acid or base depending on whether it will donate or accept a hydrogen ion after metabolism in the body. For example, both citric acid in fruit sodas and phosphoric acid in colas are classified as acids chemically, but citric acid becomes a base after metabolism in the liver, whereas phosphoric acid is unchanged (Bailey et al, 2014). See Chapter 7 for the effects of phosphorus on calcium intake and phosphoric acid on bone.

The action of the lungs, kidneys, and buffer systems of the body maintains the balance between too much and too little acid in body fluids. These buffer systems minimize significant changes in the pH of body fluids by controlling the hydrogen ion (H+) concentration.

Buffers are substances that can neutralize both acids and bases. Proteins (hemoglobin) and the **bicarbonate** (HCO_3^-)–carbonic acid (H_2CO_3) system are the most important buffers in the extracellular fluid. Phosphate (HPO_4^{2-}) and proteins are two important buffers in the intracellular fluid.

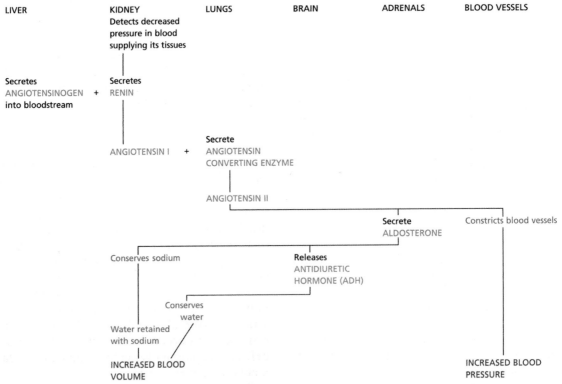

FIGURE 8-7 Hormonal control of water balance. Although the kidneys do most of the work, the complex process also involves the liver, lungs, brain, adrenal glands, and blood vessels.

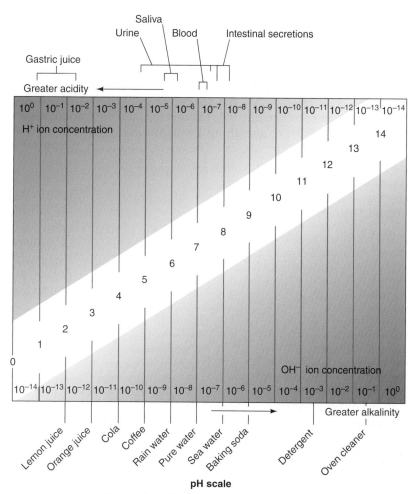

FIGURE 8-8 Representation of the pH scale with usual readings for body fluids, beverages, and household products. (Reprinted from Venes, D [Ed.]: *Taber's cyclopedic medical dictionary*, 21st ed. FA Davis, Philadelphia, 2009, p. 1764, with permission.)

Extracellular Fluid

The normal pH of the extracellular fluid is 7.35 to 7.45. The body is continually working to maintain the pH within this narrow range, which is slightly alkaline despite the acidity of the waste products of metabolism. A blood pH below 6.8 or above 7.8 is usually fatal (Fournier, 2009). A pH of 6.8 produces shock, coma, and respiratory failure. The symptoms of severe alkalemia are those of hypocalcemia because at a pH greater than 7.75, not enough ionized calcium is available for cardiac contractility, leading to death if uncorrected (Bailey et al, 2014).

Extracellular fluid contains both positive sodium ions (Na^+) and negative bicarbonate ions (HCO_3^-). When a strong acid is introduced into the fluid, a chemical reaction takes place yielding sodium chloride (a salt), which is neutral, and carbonic acid (a weak acid). **Carbonic acid** breaks down to carbon dioxide and water, which are excreted by the lungs (exhaled) and kidneys respectively.

When a strong base (alkali) enters the system, carbon dioxide and water (the two main waste products of cellular metabolism) react to form carbonic acid to counteract the alkaline effect of the base. The end products of this reaction are water and a weak base that does not drastically affect the pH.

RESPIRATORY SYSTEM

The lungs help maintain pH by varying the amount of carbon dioxide (CO_2) exhaled. Retained carbon dioxide makes the body fluids more acidic because it reacts to form carbonic acid, a source of hydrogen ions. Too much carbonic acid, or too much of any acid, results in **acidosis,** a condition that causes the lungs to automatically increase the rate and depth of breathing, eliminating more carbon dioxide and water.

This respiratory response to acidosis begins within minutes of an increase in acidity. Respiratory compensation for acidosis is 50% to 75% effective and is an extremely important component in the regulation of pH. The respiratory system acts quickly but can eliminate only carbonic acid.

The homeostatic system can be subverted by rapid breathing caused by anxiety which triggers paresthesias (peripheral and perioral), peripheral tetany (eg, stiffness of fingers or arms), fainting, and sometimes all of these findings. Tetany occurs because respiratory **alkalosis** causes both hypophosphatemia and hypocalcemia (Lechtzin, 2012). See hypocalcemia in Chapter 7.

The first aid recommended for hyperventilation resulting from anxiety is breathing through only one nostril with the mouth closed. The previous technique, breathing into a paper bag, can lead to hypoxia (Venes, 2013).

RENAL SYSTEM

Metabolic acids, usually derived from the diet, as well as excess carbonic acid, must be eliminated in urine. The main metabolic acid is sulfuric acid obtained from the metabolism of the sulfur-containing amino acids methionine and cysteine. Inorganic phosphates used as food additives (e.g., colas) may also increase the acid content of the diet (Bailey et al, 2014).

The kidney spills or retains hydrogen, sodium, and bicarbonate ions as necessary to maintain an acceptable pH in blood. For example, in response to acidosis, the kidneys excrete hydrogen ions and reabsorb sodium and bicarbonate ions. Conversely, in response to **alkalosis,** the kidneys conserve hydrogen ions and excrete sodium and bicarbonate ions. The kidneys initiate these actions within 24 hours but require 3 to 4 days to compensate for changes in blood pH.

Similarly, when aldosterone stimulates the kidney to retain sodium, potassium is excreted to maintain electrolyte balance. Neither the respiratory nor the renal systems will overcompensate to send the individual into the opposite state (Fournier, 2009).

Intracellular Fluid

The normal pH of the intracellular fluid is 6.8 to 7.0, slightly acid to neutral. Within the intracellular fluid, organic phosphates and proteins are the most important buffers. These substances buffer 95% of the body's carbonic acid and 50% of other acids. Protein is the most powerful and plentiful buffer system in the body.

Of the body's proteins, hemoglobin has the largest buffering capacity. Thus, red blood cells have 70% of the buffering power of the blood. This buffering capacity allows large quantities of carbon dioxide to be transported from the tissues to the lungs, with only a small change in venous pH compared with arterial pH.

When blood contains excessive hydrogen ions, the ions move into the cells to be buffered. Then, to maintain electroneutrality, potassium moves from the intracellular to the intravascular compartment, raising serum potassium levels.

Water Balance and Imbalances

For optimum health, water intake must equal water output. Contrary to popular advice, little support is found for the notion that additional water in adequately hydrated individuals confers any benefit (Popkin et al, 2010).

Muckelbauer, Libuda, Clausen, et al (2009) attempted to demonstrate a link between water consumption and risk of obesity. In this study, socially deprived second and third graders in Germany were provided drinking water and information throughout the school year. The children increased their water intake without significantly affecting juice or soft drink consumption. The program resulted in a 31% reduction in the risk of overweight. However, because hydration status was not measured, the results are not conclusive.

Sources of Water

Plain water from the tap or bottled water are obvious sources, but much of our water is consumed in other beverages. Skim milk is 91% water, and whole milk is 88% water. Water itself may contain other nutrients in varying amounts. Hard water has calcium, magnesium, and often iron. Water conditioners used to soften water replace those minerals with sodium. Drinking softened water increases some people's sodium intake excessively. For this reason, most experts recommend that the cold water in the kitchen be unsoftened.

We obtain about 4 cups of water per day in foods. Some foods that are solids also have high water content: head lettuce is 96% water, celery is 95% water, and raw carrots are 88% water. *To investigate the water content of a particular item, scroll down to "other" at http://nutritiondata.self.com. If you select a 100-gram portion, the grams of water listed is also the percentage.*

Water is also a product of metabolism, which yields about 1 cup of water per day in the average person. Each energy nutrient produces a different amount of metabolic water:

- 1 gram of carbohydrate produces 0.60 gram of water.
- 1 gram of fat produces 1.07 grams of water.
- 1 gram of protein produces 0.41 gram of water.
- *But* 1 ounce of pure alcohol *requires* 8 ounces of water for its metabolism.

Consumers can choose from multiple sources of drinking water. U.S. water utilities supply more than 1 billion gallons of tap water an hour, every hour of the day (Fishman 2012). Yet many city water supplies are questionable because of aging distribution systems and a deteriorating regulatory climate. The Natural Resources Defense Council graded water quality in 19 cities, concluding that drinking water purity improved slightly during the previous 15 years in most cities but that overall tap water quality varies widely from city to city. Only six cities received a grade of good or excellent (2000). See Box 8-3 for a new concern about water supplies.

Bottled water is not automatically safer than tap water in the United States. Ironically, 49% or more of bottled water actually *is* tap water (Consumer Reports, 2011). Often the label reveals little about the contents: 18% of bottled water brands do not reveal their water's geographic source, and 32% omit information on treatment methods and purity testing (Leiba, Gray, and Houlihan, 2011). The Natural Resources Defense Council found approximately 22% of bottled water tested contained, in at least one sample, contaminant levels that exceeded strict state health limits (2008).

See Table 8-2 for a brief comparison of these two main sources of drinking water, Figure 8-9 for a serving suggestion, Dollars & Sense 8-1 for the environmental cost of bottled water, Dollars & Sense 8-2 for cultural influences of water choices, and Dollars & Sense 8-3 for a compromise choice.

Losses of Water

We lose water in obvious ways, called **sensible water losses,** as in perspiration and urine. We also lose water in less obvious ways, called **insensible water losses,** as through breathing.

Sensible Water Losses

Sensible water losses include losses of the major extra-cellular ions, sodium and chloride. Three important routes commonly account for sensible water losses:

1. Through the skin as perspiration
2. Through the kidney as urine
3. Through the gastrointestinal tract in the feces

PERSPIRATION

Evaporation of sweat is the main means of dissipating the body's heat produced by exercise. In extreme cases, a person may perspire at the rate of 2 liters per hour. For example, during a marathon race, runners may lose 6% to 8% of their body weight, primarily as

---

Box 8-3 ■ *Pharmaceuticals in Drinking Water*

A relatively recent concern is that of contamination of water supplies with pharmaceuticals excreted by the body or discarded into the sanitary system. Current federal standards do not regulate pharmaceuticals in drinking water, although the Environmental Protection Agency has the authority to determine if pharmaceuticals are hazardous waste (Anderko, Chalupka, Gray, and Kesten, 2013).

Several studies have demonstrated adverse effects from long-standing, low-dose exposures in both aquatic and terrestrial wildlife, although human toxicity related to trace levels of pharmaceuticals in the water supply remains unknown (Strauch, 2011). At the least, the technique of flushing all unused or outdated

medications down the toilet is outmoded. The U.S. Food and Drug Administration (July 15, 2013) continuously updates a list of drugs that *should be flushed* along with instructions for disposing of other medications in household trash such that their theft or misuse is unlikely. Some communities have take-back programs to redistribute or correctly destroy unwanted drugs.

A combination of conventional and various advanced water treatments have been explored to reduce the pharmaceuticals in drinking water. Long term, it may be that providing millions of gallons of **potable** tap water for industrial and sanitary uses is unsustainable and that nonpotable water in toilets may portend a trend eastward from the western states.

TABLE 8-2 ■ Comparison of Bottled Water and Municipal Water Regulations

	BOTTLED WATER	PUBLIC WATER
Regulatory Agency	Food and Drug Administration (FDA)	Environmental Protection Agency (EPA)
Subject to Regulation	Only that sold state-to-state, = 30%–40% of bottled water	All systems with >14 service connections or serving >24 people
Number of States Regulating Intrastate Bottlers	40	
Testing for Bacteria	Once a week	20 times/month for small systems 100+ times/month for large systems
Chemical Testing	Annually	Quarterly
Allowable Lead Level	5 parts per billion	15 parts per billion*
Allowable Arsenic Level	10 parts per billion	10 parts per billion
Certified Labs to Test	No	Yes
Required Reporting to State or Federal Governments	No	Yes

*Requires treatment to reduce level. Level set considering aging pipes.
Sources: Chalupka (2005), National Resources Defense Council (2000), Sharfstein (2011), U.S. Environmental Protection Agency (2012).

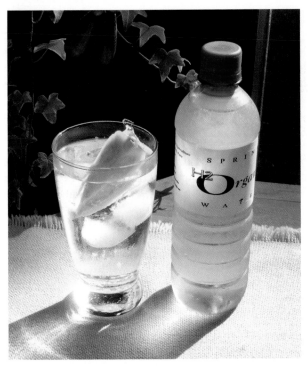

FIGURE 8-9 Either choice will hydrate a person. Although cost is not the only factor to consider, it is significantly less for a glass of tap water (even with ice and a lemon wedge) than a bottle of water.

perspiration. A 150-pound person could then lose 9 to 10½ pounds, or 4.3 to 5 liters, of fluid.

Sweat is not pure water. It is salty to the taste, hypotonic, and its composition varies from person to person. On average, one liter of perspiration contains, with wide ranges for each, approximately:

- 40 to 45 milliequivalents of sodium
- 3.9 milliequivalents of potassium
- 3.3 milliequivalents of magnesium
- 39 milliequivalents of chloride

Consequently, even a sweat loss of 5 or 6 liters entails small amounts of electrolytes so that rehydration with water should be adequate (Gropper and Smith, 2013). An unconditioned person's sweat may contain 100 milliequivalents of sodium per liter whereas the sweat of a well-conditioned individual may contain just 30 mEq/L (Bailey et al, 2014).

See Clinical Application 8-5 for information on heat-related illnesses.

URINE

In the normal, healthy person with average exertion throughout the day, urine output is roughly equal to

$ Dollars & Sense 8-1

Bottled Water: Use and Costs

Americans spent $21.7 billion on bottled water in 2011 for 9.1 billion gallons of water. This amounts to 29.2 gallons of bottled water per person compared with 18.2 gallons per person in 2001. In 2011, 222 bottles of water were sold for every person in the country (Fishman, 2012).

Refilling one's own reusable water bottle in New York City every day would cost 48 cents per year compared with buying a $1 daily bottle of water that would cost $346 for the year. That figure assumes redemption of all the deposits by returning 365 empty bottles (Giorgianni, 2011).

Labels are as likely to confuse as clarify. Artesian, distilled, mineral, PWS (public water source, or tap water), purified, spring, and sparkling (not soda water and seltzer that are soft drinks) have recognized definitions. In contrast, "glacier water" and "mountain water" have no standard definitions (Consumer Reports, 2012).

The price an individual pays for bottled water tells just part of the story. Environmental costs in dollars and in diverted resources add up:

- Manufacturing the plastic for the bottles uses 17 million barrels of crude oil annually, enough to fuel 1 million vehicles on the road for 12 months.

- Recycling is the destiny for only about 13% of the bottles, with the remainder (2 million tons in 2005) consigned to U.S. landfills. Plastic bottles take centuries to decompose, and if they are incinerated, toxic byproducts, such as chlorine gas and heavy metals, are released into the atmosphere.
- Pumping, processing, transporting, and refrigerating bottled water requires the energy of more than 50 million barrels of oil annually (Didier, undated).

More than a dozen colleges and universities have banned the sale of bottled water on campus, often under pressure from student organizing campaigns that encourage students to drink tap water. The cities of New York, Seattle, San Francisco, and Chicago's Cook County have banned use of government funds to purchase bottled water (Fishman, 2012).

Still, the United States remains the largest market for bottled water. The next two, in order, are China and Mexico, both countries in which tap water is either unavailable or typically not considered safe to drink (Fishman, 2012). See Dollars & Sense 8-2.

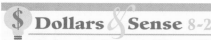

$ Dollars & Sense 8-2

Culture Influences Water Choices

Both economic and health issues regarding choices of drinking water have an effect on minority families. Of 216 parents (four-fifths Latino), 34% of Latino parents never drank tap water, and 44% never gave it to their children, typically because they thought it caused illness, which may have been true in their native countries. Of the lowest-income families (<$15,000 per year), 65% always gave bottled or filtered water to their children. In addition, approximately 40% of children who never drank tap water did not receive fluoride supplements (Hobson, Knochel, and Byington, et al, 2007).

Of 632 respondents evenly divided by ethnicity, African American and Latino parents were more likely than White parents to give their children mostly bottled water. Minority children were given bottled water exclusively three times more often than non-Latino white children (Gorelick, Gould, Nimmer, et al, 2011).

Of a group of mainly African American children and adolescents, 38% drank only bottled water. In addition, 24% were not aware of fluoride content of tap water (Huerta-Saenz, Irigoyen, Benavides, and Mendoza, 2012).

Without question, bottled water's cost is exorbitant compared with tap water. Municipal tap water costs $0.0015 per gallon, whereas bottled water can cost up to $10 a gallon or 7 cents per ounce (Discover Chiropractic, 2012). See Dollars & Sense 8-3 for a compromise solution.

Not only is bottled more expensive than tap water, the quantity of fluoride in bottled water is uncertain. Moreover, a lack of fluoride may increase the risk for dental caries (see Chapter 7).

$ Dollars & Sense 8-3

Filtered Tap Water

If the taste of tap water is disagreeable, simple water filters may improve it significantly. Filters can improve taste, odor, and clarity and remove some contaminants (Consumer Reports, May 2010). A basic pitcher can be had for about $10 with additional costs of $90 annually for the filters that would filter 2.6 quarts of water per day. For increased output, the filter may be changed more frequently. An added advantage is that the pitcher can be stored in the refrigerator for easy access to cold water.

Carrying a reusable aluminum bottle filled with filtered tap water instead of single-use plastic bottles can save dollars for the individual and the environment for everyone. Just remember to wash the bottle regularly.

8-5

Clinical Application

Heat-Related Illnesses

From 1991 to 2009, 7233 heat-related deaths occurred in the United States, an average of 658 per year (Centers for Disease Control, June 7, 2013). Heatstroke, the most serious and potentially life-threatening heat-related illness, is a medical emergency (Becker and Stewart, 2011). Causes can be high ambient temperatures over a period of days (classic heatstroke) or vigorous exercising in warm or hot environments that affects the person quickly (exertional heatstroke). Delayed access to cooling is the leading cause of morbidity and mortality in persons with heatstroke. Cold water immersion is the treatment of choice when available. It is associated with the lowest morbidity and mortality rates, and clients with exertional heatstroke treated with cold water immersion have a survival rate of almost 100% (Becker and Stewart, 2011).

Untreated heat illness can progress quickly to serious, potentially fatal illness (Centers for Disease Control, July 29, 2011). The body temperature of someone with heatstroke can rise to 106°F or higher within 10 to 15 minutes (Centers for Disease Control, May 18, 2012). See Table 8-3 for a summary comparison of heat exhaustion and heatstroke.

CLASSIC HEATSTROKE

Once core temperature (best measured rectally) reaches 104°F, cellular damage occurs, initiating a cascade of events that may lead to organ failure and death (Becker and Stewart, 2011). In France, mortality rate from heatstroke in the intensive care unit (ICU) was 63.6% (due to multiple organ failure if death occurred within 7 days of ICU stay or due to neurological disability if occurring later). Classic heatstroke may prove fatal even though cooling procedures and intensive care management are started promptly (Pease, Bouadma, Kermarrec, et al, 2009). About 20% of survivors of heatstroke have residual brain damage, regardless of intervention (Knochel, 2010).

Persons at greatest risk of classic heat-related illness are:

■ Young children
■ Older adults
■ Individuals with chronic medical (especially heart and lung or mental) disorders
■ Clients taking medications that interfere with salt and water balance (Becker and Stewart, 2011)

(Continued)

Clinical Application—cont'd

Heat-Related Illnesses

EXERTIONAL HEATSTROKE

Heat-related injuries occur quickly in physically active individuals in warm or hot environments. Between 2001 and 2009, an estimated 5946 persons were treated in U.S. emergency departments each year for a heat illness sustained while participating in a sport or recreational activity. Incidence was highest among males (72.5%) and those aged 15 to 19 years (35.6%), requiring hospitalization for 7.1% (Centers for Disease Control, May 18, 2012).

Since 1995, 42 football players have died from heatstroke (31 high school, 8 college, 2 professional, 1 sandlot). In 2009, 3 high school and 1 college football players died of heatstroke (Mueller and Colgate, 2010). Among high school athletes, heat-related illnesses resulting in time lost from athletics were related to body mass index categories. The majority of athletes so affected were either overweight (37.1%) or obese (27.6%). Fat, because of its insulating property, decreases heat loss, thereby increasing the risk for heat illness (Centers for Disease Control, August 20, 2010).

Sixty percent of exertional heat illnesses among high school athletes occurred in August and of those reported during practice, 32% occurred more than 2 hours into the practice session. The exertional heat illness rate in football athletes was 11.4 times that in all other sports combined (Kerr, Casa, Marshall, and Comstock, 2013).

All heat illnesses in high school athletes are preventable (Centers for Disease Control, August 20, 2010), leaving no excuse for football players dying of heatstroke (Mueller and Colgate, 2010). Guidelines from the National Athletic Trainers' Association specify acclimatization (gradual progression of duration and intensity of exercise) over 14 days and fluid replacement in amounts equaling sweat and urine losses to limit weight loss to a maximum of 2% per day (Centers for Disease Control, August 20, 2010).

TABLE 8-3 ■ Serious Heat-Related Illnesses

	HEAT EXHAUSTION	HEATSTROKE—MEDICAL EMERGENCY
Pathophysiology	Loss of water and salt in sweat	Loss of body temperature regulation Progresses to multiple organ dysfunctions
Symptoms	Headache Weakness, fatigue Dizziness, fainting Muscle cramps	Lethargy Throbbing headache Disorientation
Signs	Coherent	Delirium Convulsions Coma
Temperature	Usually <102.2°F	>104°F
Pulse	Weak, thready, rapid	Full, bounding, rapid
Respirations	Shallow, rapid, quiet	Difficult, loud
Skin	Cool, clammy, sweaty	Flushed, hot, dry (unless from exertion or just progressed from heat exhaustion)
First-aid treatment	Move to cool location Lie down Elevate feet Loosen clothing Monitor temperature If able to drink: ½ tsp salt in ½ glass of water orally every 15 min until medical help arrives	Move to cool location Lie down Elevate head Remove clothing Ice bags to neck, axillae, groin Spray with water while fanning Monitor airway, breathing, circulation until medical help arrives

liquid intake. A well-hydrated individual produces light yellow or straw-colored urine. A minimum amount of urine must be excreted each day to carry away the waste products resulting from metabolic processes. This function, called obligatory excretion, eliminates 400 to 600 milliliters per day. The kidneys function more efficiently when they receive an abundant water supply because economizing on water while producing more concentrated urine takes more energy and increases wear on the kidney tissues. Strong evidence supports reduced risk of kidney stones in individuals with good hydration (Popkin et al, 2010).

The hourly urine output of seriously ill clients is monitored but the amounts must be interpreted in relation to the client's situation. Even if a person is losing massive amounts of fluid through the gastrointestinal tract, such losses do not rid the body of metabolic wastes as efficiently as the kidney does. Adults should excrete 40 to 80 milliliters of urine per hour, although the amount varies throughout the day and night. Children's urine output should be at least 1 mL/kg body weight/hour (see Clinical Calculation 8-2).

GASTROINTESTINAL SECRETIONS

Regarding water balance, normally the gastrointestinal tract's net activity down to the level of the jejunum is secretion of water and electrolytes. Beyond that point, the net activity is resorption of water and electrolytes (Bailey et al, 2014).

Abnormal gastrointestinal function can cause extensive fluid loss. Location of the loss determines signs and symptoms. Gastric juice is acid, whereas intestinal juices are alkaline. Therefore, conceptually, gastrointestinal losses are divided into those lost above the outlet of the stomach, the **pyloric sphincter,** and those lost below it.

Above the Pylorus

The common causes of losses above the pylorus are vomiting or stomach suctioning. Two organs secrete digestive juices above the pylorus: the salivary glands in the mouth and the gastric glands in the stomach. The ions lost in secretions above the pylorus are:

- Sodium
- Potassium
- Chloride
- Hydrogen

About 1 liter of saliva per day is mixed with food or just swallowed. The stomach secretes about 1.5 to 2.5 liters of gastric juice per day. If gastric juices are lost, hydrogen ions in the hydrochloric acid are also lost, putting the person at risk for alkalosis.

Below the Pylorus

The usual causes of losses below the pylorus are diarrhea and intestinal suctioning. Gastrointestinal secretions below the pylorus contain:

- Sodium
- Potassium
- Bicarbonate

Two to three liters of intestinal secretions per day flow into the bowel to digest food. Normally, bile is released from the gallbladder into the small intestine at the rate of 1 liter per day. The total gastrointestinal secretions amount to 6.5 to 8.5 liters per day. Yet because water is absorbed back into the blood from the large intestine, normal feces from an adult contain only 100 to 200 milliliters of water.

Insensible Water Losses

An invisible amount of water is lost through the lungs and the skin. These are insensible losses amounting to between 800 and 1000 milliliters of water daily. Breath is visible only in cold weather. Even in warmer weather and indoors, people lose 400 milliliters of water per day in exhaled air. Deep respirations or a dry climate increase the amount of water lost.

The insensible loss of water through the skin is evaporative. It is almost pure water and nearly electrolyte-free. This insensible water loss amounts to 6 milliliters per kilogram of body weight in 24 hours, which is a baseline amount.

Environmental conditions influence the amount of water lost. Greater losses occur:

- At high temperatures
- At high altitudes
- In low humidity

Clinical Calculation 8-3 shows how to estimate insensible water loss. Burns, phototherapy, radiant warmers, or fever will increase the amount of insensible water loss. Fever increases evaporative losses by about 12% per degree Celsius of temperature elevation.

Clinical Calculation 8-4 shows how fever affects **evaporative water losses.** Table 8-4 lists average fluid gains and losses for 24 hours.

Assessment of Water Balance

Gathering data on water losses is straightforward: daily weight or documenting intake and output.

Weight

Daily weight is the single most important indicator of fluid status. An easy way to relate volume to weight is

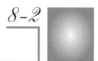

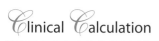 **Clinical Calculation**   *8-2*

Hourly Urine Output in Children

Children should excrete 1 milliliter of urine per kilogram of body weight per hour. What would be a normal hourly urine output for a child who weighs 50 pounds?

First, convert pounds to kilograms. There are 2.2 pounds per kilogram.

$$\frac{50\ lb}{2.2\ lb/kg} = 22.7\ kg$$

Then multiply weight in kg × 1 mL/hour

$$22.7 \times 1 = 22.7\ mL/h$$

Thus, a 50-lb child normally should excrete 22.7 mL/h of urine per hour.

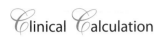

8-3

Clinical Calculation

Insensible Water Loss Through the Skin

The rule of thumb for insensible water loss through the skin is 6 mL/kg per 24 hours. How much insensible water loss would be expected for a 154-lb client?

First, convert pounds to kilograms:

$$\frac{154\ lb}{2.2\ lb/kg} = 70\ kg$$

Then multiply the client's weight in kilograms by the estimated standard:

$$70\ kg \times 6\ mL/kg = 420\ mL$$

Thus, this client's insensible water loss in a 24-hour period is expected to be 420 mL.

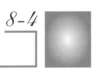

8-4

Clinical Calculation

Evaporative Water Loss in Fever

Fever increases the amount of evaporative loss by 12% for every degree Celsius of fever. If the 154-lb client in Clinical Calculation 8-3 had a fever of 102.2°F, how much additional evaporative loss would he or she sustain?

Temperatures can be reported in Fahrenheit or Celsius degrees, and the conversion formulas account for the fact that the Celsius scale sets freezing at zero and the Fahrenheit sets it at 32°.

To convert Fahrenheit to Celsius, subtract 32 and multiply by 5/9.

$$102.2 - 32 = 70.2 \times 5/9 = 39°C$$

This client's temperature would be 39°C.
Likewise, a normal temperature of 98.6°F would be converted as

$$98.6 - 32 = 66.6 \times 5/9 = 37°C$$

The client had insensible losses of 420 mL.
The client has an elevation of 2°C, which would increase evaporative loss by 24%.

$$420\ mL \times 0.24 = 100.8\ mL \text{ additional evaporative water loss}$$
$$420\ mL + 100.8\ mL = 520.8 \text{ total insensible water loss through the skin}$$

To convert from Celsius to Fahrenheit, the formula is: °C × 9/5 + 32.

to remember "a pint is a pound the world around." One liter is 1 kilogram or 2.2 pounds.

Acute weight loss in adults is rated as follows:

Mild volume deficit, 2% to 5% loss
Moderate volume deficit, 5% to 10% loss
Severe volume deficit, >10% loss

TABLE 8-4 ■ Average Fluid Gains and Losses in Adults in 24 Hours			
FLUID GAINS		**FLUID LOSSES***	
Energy metabolism	300 mL	Kidneys	1200–1500 mL
		Skin	500–600 mL
Oral fluids	1100–1400 mL	Lungs	400 mL
Solid foods	800–1000 mL	Intestines	100–200 mL
Total Gains	2200–2700 mL	**Total Losses**	2200–2700 mL

*Includes sensible and insensible losses.

Fluid balance in an infant is much more precarious than in an adult. Because a greater proportion of the infant's body water is in the extracellular space, infants can lose water more rapidly than adults. Therefore, a loss of 5% of body weight (or other findings in Table 8-5) in an infant merits medical attention. Proportionate concern is justified for children up to the age of 3 years when adult proportions of fluid distribution normally occurs and the child usually can verbalize thirst.

Weight changes can be caused by metabolic events as well as by fluid shifts. If a client receives no oral, enteral, or parenteral nutrition, the loss of body tissue may amount to 0.3 to 0.5 kilogram per day.

Similarly, the loss of effective circulatory volume is not always an external loss. Weight gain may accompany circulatory loss. See Clinical Application 8-6 for insight into internal fluid losses.

Intake and Output

In a healthy person, liquid intake and output should be approximately equal. Measuring intake is easier than measuring output, but it still is frequently inaccurate. Most institutions post the amounts that food and beverage containers hold. Amounts remaining should be measured and subtracted from the total liquid served.

Rather than assume that clients have consumed everything missing from the pitcher or tray, the nurse should ask if they drank the fluid (as opposed to, for instance, giving it to a visitor). Updating the intake form throughout the day rather than at the end of a shift is likely to produce a more complete record. Record the amount of water from ice chips as one-half of their volume. One cup of ice chips yields only ½ cup of water.

Fluid lost into a dressing or a diaper can be estimated by weighing it. Subtract the dry material's weight from the total. One gram of weight equals 1 milliliter of water. **Specific gravity** is the weight of a substance compared with that of distilled water. Normal specific gravity of urine is 1.010 to 1.025, but a lower value is common in newborns. So although the weight of a diaper wet with urine is not exactly the same as if it were wet with water, this method of recording incontinent urine is adequate in most situations.

TABLE 8-5 ■ Signs and Symptoms of Abnormal Fluid Volume

	INSUFFICIENT FLUID VOLUME	EXCESSIVE FLUID VOLUME
Symptoms		
Gastrointestinal	Thirst Loss of appetite (decreased blood to intestines)	Nausea Loss of appetite (edema of the bowel)
Signs		
General	Weight loss Depressed fontanel (infant) Sunken eyes (infant) Lack of tears when crying (infant)	Weight gain Edema
Skin and mucous membranes	Dry mucous membranes Decreased skin **turgor** (not reliable in elderly)	Skin stretched and shiny
Cardiovascular system	**Orthostatic hypotension** (pressure decrease of 15 mm Hg in systolic or diastolic) Increased pulse rate upon standing Increased hematocrit values (unless red blood cells also lost) Narrowing **pulse pressure** Filling of dependent hand veins takes longer than 5 seconds	Decreased hematocrit values Increasing **pulse pressure** Emptying of elevated hand veins takes longer than 5 seconds
Urinary	Decreased urine output Concentrated, dark urine	**Polyuria** Dilute, light urine
Gastrointestinal	Vomiting (decreased blood to intestines) Longitudinal furrows on tongue	Vomiting (edema of intestines)
Central nervous system	Confusion, disorientation	Deteriorating consciousness

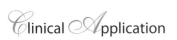 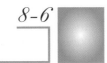

Clinical Application 8-6

Identifying Third-Space Losses

Large amounts of fluid can accumulate in several places in the body outside the circulatory system. These losses are called **third-space losses.** Certain diseases cause **ascites,** the accumulation of fluid (often amounting to several liters), not within the bowel but around it in the abdominal cavity. Other third-space losses involve internal bleeding or the collection of fluid in the chest cavity. An alert nurse can spot an early clue to third-space losses: decreasing urine output despite seemingly adequate fluid intake.

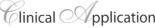

Clinical Application 8-7

Avoiding Misinterpretation

One client was told to "drink a lot of fluid" when he was discharged from the hospital. He interpreted this to be 3 to 4 gallons per day! His kidneys did their best, but kidneys cannot excrete plain water. In a few days, the client was back in the hospital for correction of electrolyte imbalance.

- Be specific when teaching clients.
- Document both the teaching content and the client's response to the information.

In a sick person, intake and output totals may not balance every day. The client's intake and output should be assessed over a period of several days because a single-day evaluation can lead to missing the big picture. See Clinical Application 8-7 for teaching and documentation tips regarding fluid intake and Box 8-4 for a practical assessment tip regarding output.

Water Imbalances

Fluid volume is unbalanced if it is insufficient or excessive. Signs and symptoms of both are shown in Table 8-5. To assess fluid volume through observation of hand veins, raise the client's hand above the heart. Normally, the veins will collapse in 3 to 5 seconds. Then lower the hand below the heart. The veins should refill in 3 to

5 seconds. The veins of a person with insufficient fluid volume require more than 5 seconds to refill. Reverse the procedure to assess excessive fluid volume in which the veins will take more than 5 seconds to empty.

Fluid compartments do not operate in isolation: if one is out of balance, the other compartments eventually will be affected as the body attempts to equalize osmotic pressure across the compartments.

Box 8-4 ■ *Visual Assessment of Fluid Balance*

In persons with normal organ function, a good day-to-day measure of hydration status is the color of urine. Urine of light yellow color usually reflects normal fluid balance, whereas concentrated urine of a deeper color may indicate dehydration.

Insufficient Fluid Volume

Treating insufficient fluid volume with appropriate fluids is essential, as is correcting the cause. Hypotonic fluids are given to replace fluid volume and correct electrolyte imbalances orally if possible but by nasogastric tube or intravenously if necessary (Clinical Application 8-8). Although hypotonic, plain water orally is not advised for treating insufficient fluid volume because it is likely to inhibit thirst and to increase urine output.

Parents should be informed of the desired treatment outcomes for a child with diarrhea. Oral electrolyte solutions, although clearly life-saving and effective in maintaining hydration, do not necessarily reduce stool volume or the duration of diarrhea. Rapid oral rehydration with the appropriate solution has been shown to be as effective as intravenous fluid therapy in the treatment of dehydrated clients. Sodium and glucose in the correct proportions can be passively cotransported with fluid from the gut lumen into the circulation to restore intravascular volume. All of the commercial rehydration fluids are acceptable for oral rehydration therapy (ORT). They contain the following:

- 2 to 3 g/dL of glucose
- 45 to 90 mEq/L of sodium
- 30 mEq/L of base
- 20 to 25 mEq/L of potassium
- Osmolality of 200 to 310 mOsm/L (Huang, Anchala, Ellsbury, and George, 2012)

If hypertonic solutions are given orally to correct fluid loss, the concentrated solution would remain in the stomach longer than water, providing satiety and restraining water intake. In addition, hypertonic solutions draw fluid from the bowel wall into the lumen, resulting in osmotic diarrhea. Some commercial laxatives and enemas are hypertonic solutions.

In addition to causing osmotic diarrhea, hypertonic solutions allow less sodium and water to be absorbed than from the ORT solutions. Ginger ale (565 milliosmoles per liter [mOsm/L]) and apple juice (700 mOsm/L) are poor choices for rehydration in prolonged diarrhea, owing to their high glucose and low electrolyte concentrations. Another popular choice, chicken broth, is also not advised. It contains no carbohydrate, just 2 mEq of sodium, with an osmolality of 330 mOsm/L (Huang, Anchala, Ellsbury, and George, 2012).

Thickened hydration solutions are also available for clients who have difficulty swallowing thin liquids. A dietitian should be consulted before using food thickeners, inasmuch as some of them bind with water, making water less available for absorption.

An alternative to intravenous rehydration in selected clients is the use of hypodermoclysis. In this technique, fluid is introduced into the subcutaneous tissue, in the thighs or abdomen, for instance, usually by means of a pair of long needles. A drug may be used to aid in dispersal of the solution.

Excessive Fluid Volume

When a person becomes ill and the control mechanisms stop working, the individual can retain fluid intracellularly or extracellularly. In addition, a person can overwhelm his or her own homeostatic mechanisms with voluntary water consumption. Such cases were reported in 17 military trainees who were hospitalized to treat overhydration (O'Brien, Montain, Corr, et al, 2001) and in hyponatremic Boston Marathon runners (Almond, Shin, Fortescue, et al, 2005). Analysis of military cases involving three deaths indicated the clients had consumed more than 5 liters, usually 10 to 20 liters, of water within a few hours although guidelines provide safety by limiting fluid intake during times of heavy sweating to 1 to 1.5 L per hour (Gardner, 2002). Another preventive measure used by long-distance runners is the ingestion of high-sodium gels, which can counter hyponatremia if used appropriately (Peate, 2005).

As with insufficient fluid volume, the remedy for excessive fluid volume is to treat the cause. Osmotic diuretic drugs such as *mannitol* remain in the extracellular

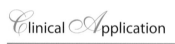

Clinical Application *8-8*

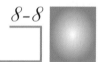

Oral Electrolyte Solutions

Originally, oral electrolyte solutions were designed to combat diarrheal diseases in developing countries. They proved so useful that they have since been modified for use in Western nations. One commonly used oral electrolyte solution is Pedialyte®, available over-the-counter without a prescription. One liter of Pedialyte contains sodium chloride and potassium citrate yielding the following electrolytes:

45 mEq sodium (Na⁺)	35 mEq chloride (Cl⁻)
20 mEq potassium (K⁺)	30 mEq citrate, a base (⁻)
65 mEq cations	65 mEq anions

Pedialyte® is mildly hypotonic, about 250 milliosmoles per liter. It also contains a concentration of glucose that promotes sodium and water absorption, 25 g/L, which also contributes 100 kilocalories per liter.

Pedialyte® is designed for hydration maintenance of an infant or child experiencing vomiting or diarrhea. If the client becomes dehydrated, as evidenced by loss of 5% of body weight, medical attention is needed. Intravenous fluids or an oral rehydration solution of different composition from Pedialyte® may be prescribed for the dehydrated child.

space. By increasing the osmotic pressure there, these drugs pull excess fluid from the cells to be excreted by the kidney.

Nutritionally, the client may be on a restricted fluid regimen. The physician may prescribe an intake of no more than 1000 milliliters in 24 hours. This amount compensates for insensible losses through the skin and lungs. It is essential to supply fluid as prescribed and to teach the client the reason for the restriction. Over a period of several days, the obligatory urine output and any diuretic therapy will help the client's body excrete the excess fluid.

Keystones

- Water transports nutrients to cells and heat and waste from cells; provides the volume needed to maintain blood pressure; becomes a structural component of cells and large molecules; and serves as a lubricant, solvent, and medium for chemical reactions.

- Of an adult's body weight, 50% to 65% is water, 35% of it extracellular. Of an infant's body weight, 75% is water, 54% of this extracellular, which can be lost quickly under adverse conditions.

- When the kidneys detect decreased blood pressure supplying its tissues, it begins a complex sequence of hormonal release involving the lungs, the adrenals, and the brain. The result is constricted blood vessels that increase blood pressure and conservation of sodium and water by the kidney that increases blood volume.

- Osmolality measures the osmotic pressure of fluids in the body or administered to it. Fluids are isotonic, hypotonic, or hypertonic compared with the osmolality of human serum. Hypertonic intravenous solutions require large vessels to quickly dilute the solution, and hypertonic oral solutions may counteract efforts to rehydrate an individual with diarrhea.

- Within minutes of detected acidosis, the lungs help to maintain acid–base balance by varying the amount of carbon dioxide exhaled; however, these organs are limited to eliminating carbonic acid. The kidneys eliminate excess carbonic acid and other acids but react slowly, within 24 hours, and may take 4 days to correct acid–base imbalances.

- The average adult gains fluids from oral fluids (1250 mL), solid foods (900 mL), and metabolism (300 mL), which total 2450 mL in 24 hours. During the same time, fluid would be lost through the kidneys (1350 mL), skin (550 mL), lungs (400 mL), and intestines (150 mL) to again total 2450 mL.

- The Environmental Protection Agency requires that all but the smallest public water systems be tested by certified laboratories more frequently than bottled water manufacturers, with results reported to governmental bodies. The Food and Drug Administration regulates bottled water as a food, exempting intrastate sales and labeling for naturally occurring fluoride but mandating a lower allowable lead level than in tap water, although at a cost of up to 10,000 times the cost of tap water.

- Daily weight is the single most important indicator of fluid status, but consideration must be given to the complete clinical situation when interpreting results. The second major technique to assess water balance in the body is an accurate intake and output record, including visual inspection of urine color.

- Heat exhaustion, resulting from loss of water and salt in sweat, is differentiated from heatstroke by mental clarity; a temperature below 102.2°F; weak, thready pulse; shallow, quiet respirations; and a cool, clammy skin. Heatstroke presents with the opposite signs, results from a loss of body temperature regulation, and can progress to multiple organ failure. First aid while awaiting emergency medical technicians involves salt water orally for heat exhaustion if possible and rapid cooling of the body with water, ice packs, and fanning for heatstroke.

- Dehydration from fluid losses can be lethal, with infants at high risk. Hyponatremia from dysregulation of hormonal water balance or from voluntary overhydration has proved fatal.

CASE STUDY *8-1*

Mr. N, a 75-year-old retired office worker, recently arrived from his summer home in the north to his winter home in Florida. After leaving temperatures in the 40s, he had looked forward to enjoying the 85°F weather. Although Mr. N had hired someone to care for his small yard while he was away from Florida, he still had to do a number of chores, which he tackled with a vengeance.

After 1½ hours, Mr. N began to get a headache. He felt a bit weak and dizzy but continued his work. He was nearly finished with the outside tasks.

Half an hour later, Ms. N found her husband lying on the ground and called to their neighbor, a retired nurse.

The nurse noted that Mr. N's skin was pale and cool but that he was perspiring profusely. He was conscious and coherent but said he felt weak. The nurse took Mr. N's pulse. It was 90 beats per minute, regular but weak. His respirations were 12 per minute and shallow.

The nurse provided the emergency care described in the following care plan. (Of course, she did not write it all out before helping Mr. N.)

CARE PLAN

Subjective Data

Had worked outside in 85°F heat for 2 hours ■ Headache, weakness, dizziness ■ Recently arrived from colder climate

Objective Data

Conscious, coherent ■ Skin pale, cool, wet with perspiration ■ Pulse 90, regular and weak ■ Respirations 24 and shallow

Analysis

Heat stress related to excessive loss of hypotonic fluid (sweat) as evidenced by wet, pale skin and weak, rapid pulse.

Plan

DESIRED OUTCOMES EVALUATION CRITERIA	ACTIONS/INTERVENTIONS	RATIONALE
Client will remain conscious and oriented, with a pulse rate no greater than 90 beats/min, until the emergency team arrives.	Instruct Ms. N to call emergency medical services and return to help.	In an emergency situation, the nurse stays with the client. Potential electrolyte imbalance requires medical care.
	Loosen Mr. N's clothing.	Loosening the clothing will allow maximum air exchange and permit relaxation.
	With Ms. N, move client to shade or provide shade where he lies.	Mr. N must get out of the sun. Depending on the situation, he might be moved indoors, but perhaps the two women could not manage to move him.
	Keep client lying down with legs elevated slightly.	Lying down permits maximum blood circulation to the brain. Raising the legs increases the return of blood to the heart. The head should not be lowered because this causes venous congestion in the brain.
	Ask Ms. N to prepare a half glass of water with ½ teaspoonful of salt in it. Administer salty water to Mr. N.	Although this is a hypertonic solution, sodium is readily absorbed by the intestine, so it is unlikely to cause osmotic diarrhea. Only 5% of consumed sodium remains in the feces. The kidneys control sodium levels in the blood. This client has lost water and sodium chloride in perspiration.

8-1

Emergency Medical Technician's Notes

The following emergency medical technician's notes are representative of teamwork documentation.

Chief Complaint: Collapsed while performing yard work

Subjective: Oriented to person, place, time

Hesitant in answers

Wife reports 75 years old, no chronic illnesses, baby aspirin daily for cardiovascular prevention

Objective: Temperature 101.0°F axillary

Pulse 108, weak, thready

Respirations 22, shallow

B/P 105/70

Skin cool, clammy

Analysis: Heat exhaustion

Plan: Rehydrate with 0.9% sodium chloride at 250 mL/hour

Monitor vital signs every 5 minutes

Transport to emergency department

Critical Thinking Questions

1. Reread the narrative. At what points in the narrative or in your expansion of the story could you envision Mr. N avoiding this incident?

2. The case study narrative does not discuss Mr. N's usual dietary intake. What dietary modifications can you think of that would make Mr. N's situation of overworking in the heat more critical?

3. What would you include in a presentation on preventing heat-related illnesses for an audience of elderly residents such as Mr. N, who follow the sun for the winter?

Chapter Review

1. Which of the following people has the greatest percentage of body weight as water?
   a. A 154-pound man
   b. A 120-pound woman
   c. An 18-pound boy, 14 months old
   d. An 8-pound girl, 4 days old

2. Which of the following areas of regulation is stricter for bottled water than for tap water?
   a. Allowable lead level
   b. Frequency of testing for bacteria and chemicals
   c. Number of customers affected
   d. Requirements to report to authorities

3. Which of the following amounts is correct for average gains from oral fluids in adults for 24 hours?
   a. 500 to 600 mL
   b. 800 to 1000 mL
   c. 1100 to 1400 mL
   d. 2200 to 2700 mL

4. The single most important indicator of fluid status in the body is
   a. Collapsing of hand veins
   b. Daily weight
   c. Intake and output records
   d. Pulse pressure changes

5. Heat exhaustion is caused by:
   a. Insufficient secretion of antidiuretic hormone (ADH)
   b. Loss of water and salt in sweat
   c. Inability to perspire
   d. Retention of excessive water

Clinical Analysis

Baby I, a 4-month-old boy, is being seen at a neighborhood clinic because he has developed diarrheal stools within the past 2 days. At birth, he weighed 7 pounds, 8 ounces. Since then he has gained steadily. Three days ago, he weighed 12 pounds, 8 ounces. Baby I's present weight is 12 pounds, 2 ounces.

Mrs. I has been feeding the baby his usual formula. He drinks eagerly but then has an explosive bowel movement with loud crying. Baby I has had six bowel movements per day instead of his usual two.

1. With this history, what physical assessment measures would the nurse include initially?
   a. Condition of hair, strength of grasp, presence of sucking reflex
   b. Heart sounds, lung sounds, blood pressure
   c. Skin turgor, fontanel fullness, moisture of mucous membranes
   d. Urine specific gravity, observation of diaper rash

2. Which of the following recommendations by the nurse would show understanding of supportive care of this client?
   a. Give Baby I whole milk to maintain nutrition.
   b. Continue, as Mrs. I has been doing, to allow the bowel to empty itself.
   c. Substitute orange juice for the formula for 3 days.
   d. Start Baby I on an oral electrolyte solution.

3. The nurse instructs Mrs. I to return for additional care for Baby I if one of the following events occurs. Which one would indicate the need to reassess Baby I?
   a. The baby sleeps soundly and has to be awakened for a night feeding.
   b. The baby has three loose bowel movements the day after beginning treatment.
   c. The baby continues to lose weight or passes blood in the stool.
   d. The baby gains more than two ounces per day.

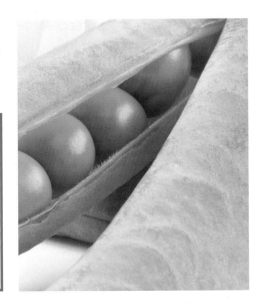

Digestion, Absorption, Metabolism, and Excretion

LEARNING OBJECTIVES

After completing this chapter, the student should be able to:

- List the anatomic structures that make up the gastrointestinal tract.
- Describe the processes of digestion, absorption, metabolism, and excretion.
- Discuss how cells use nutrients.
- Describe appropriate dietary treatments for lactose intolerance, lipid malabsorption, food allergies, and gluten-sensitive enteropathy.
- List the ways the body eliminates waste.

Every part of the human body requires nutrients from food for energy, maintenance, and growth. Food is composed of complex substances that must be broken down to simpler forms for cell use.

The **cell** is the ultimate destination for food's nutrients. Digestion, absorption, and metabolism are the three interrelated processes that act on food to prepare it for use. A fourth process, excretion, is the elimination of undigestible or unusable substances. This chapter discusses all the bodily activities, organs, and systems involved in these major processes.

Overview of the Major Processes

The first step in preparing food for use is digestion. During **digestion,** food is broken down mechanically and chemically in the gastrointestinal tract into forms small enough for **absorption** into the blood or lymphatic system.

After absorption, the nutrients usually are transported to the liver, where they may be adjusted to suit the body's needs. **Metabolism,** the sum of all physical and chemical changes that take place in the body, determines the final use of individual nutrients as well as

medications. What the cells cannot use becomes waste that is eliminated through **excretion.**

Digestion

Digestion takes place in the alimentary canal with the aid of its accessory organs.

Alimentary Canal

The **alimentary canal** is a long, muscular tube that extends through the body from the mouth to the anus. It includes:

- The oral cavity
- Pharynx
- Esophagus
- Stomach
- Small intestine
- Large intestine

Muscle rings, called **sphincters,** separate segments of the alimentary canal. The sphincters act as valves to control the passage of food. When the muscles contract, the passageway closes; when the muscles relax, the passageway opens.

The **mucosa** lines the alimentary canal and secretes **mucus,** which lubricates the canal and helps facilitate the smooth passage of food. The mucosa secretes the digestive enzymes of the stomach and small intestine.

Accessory Organs

Three **organs** located outside of the alimentary canal are considered part of the digestive system—the liver, gallbladder, and pancreas. They make important contributions to the digestive process.

LIVER

The **liver** is the second largest single organ in the body (skin is the largest). The liver performs many functions, but its primary digestive function is the production of **bile,** which breaks down dietary fats. Bile exits the liver via the hepatic **duct** (a narrow tube that permits the movement of fluid from one organ to another).

GALLBLADDER

The **gallbladder** is a 3- to 4-inch sac that concentrates and stores bile until it is needed in the small intestine. Bile is delivered to the small intestine through the common bile duct. About 2 to 3 cups of bile are secreted each day into the alimentary canal.

PANCREAS

The **pancreas** secretes enzymes that are involved in the digestion of all the energy nutrients. These secretions are collectively known as pancreatic juice. Pancreatic juice is carried to the small intestine via the pancreatic and common bile ducts.

Digestive Action

Mechanical and chemical digestion occur simultaneously throughout the alimentary canal. **Mechanical digestion** is the physical breaking down of food into smaller pieces. **Chemical digestion** involves the splitting of complex molecules into simpler forms.

Mechanical Digestion

Examples of mechanical digestion include chewing, or **mastication,** and swallowing, peristalsis, and emulsification. **Peristalsis** is a wavelike movement that propels food through the entire length of the alimentary canal. This one-way movement is caused by the alternate contraction and relaxation of the circular and longitudinal muscles that make up the external muscle layer of the alimentary canal. Other muscular activity churns the food, reducing it to successively smaller particles and mixing it with digestive secretions. All of these muscular actions are regulated by a network of nerves within the wall of the alimentary canal.

Chemical Digestion

Many **chemical reactions** are involved in digestion. **Hydrolysis** is a chemical reaction in which a substance is split into two smaller and simpler substances by the addition or the taking up of the elements of water. When the substance is split one hydrogen (H) attaches to one of the products and the hydroxyl (OH) attaches to the other product. For example, the conversion of starch to maltose, of fat to glycerol and fatty acids, and of protein to amino acids all involve hydrolysis. The hydrolysis of nutrients is achieved mostly through the action of digestive enzymes, which are present in:

- Saliva
- Gastric juice
- Pancreatic juice
- Intestinal juice

Each enzyme is specific in its action, and it acts only on a particular substance. Enzymes sometimes require the presence of additional substances, such as activators, coenzymes, or hormones, for activation. More than 500 enzymes are involved in the digestive process; this chapter discusses a few of the major ones.

In addition to enzymes, other secretions and chemicals are used in digestion. For example, mucus lubricates passages and facilitates the movement of food. It also protects the inside walls of the alimentary canal from acidic solutions. Another example is **electrolytes,** which are substances that conduct an electric current in solution. **Hydrochloric acid (HCl)** is an electrolyte and performs many functions necessary to the digestive process. A third example is bicarbonate, which is a basic solution that enters the small intestine and assists in digestion. Bicarbonate is defined in Chapter 8.

SECRETIONS

The quantity of mucus, electrolytes, water, and enzymes released during the digestive process depends on several factors.

Hormones frequently initiate a given secretion. For example, the presence of food in the stomach stimulates the cells to release a hormone called gastrin. Gastrin stimulates the release of hydrochloric acid. When the stomach's content is sufficiently acidic, it turns off further release of gastrin. When gastrin is no longer being released, hydrochloric acid is no longer released.

Emotions and conditioned responses can affect the amount of a secretion released. For example, the smell of a roasting turkey on Thanksgiving causes the release of hydrochloric acid in the stomach. Stress and tension can also produce this effect, sometimes with deleterious results.

The food in the gastrointestinal tract can influence the release of alimentary canal secretions. Drinking coffee, for instance, causes a hormone to be released into the stomach that in turn causes the secretion of hydrochloric acid. Another trigger for the release of bile from the gallbladder is the presence of fat in the small intestine. A chain of reactions in which one event causes another, and then another, is common in all biological **systems.**

END PRODUCTS

Four to 6 hours after a meal, the body has broken down the food into some trillion molecules. Each of the energy nutrients is broken down into simpler molecules.

- Carbohydrates are digested into monosaccharides.
- Fats are broken down into molecules of glycerol, fatty acids, and monoglycerides.
- The end products of protein digestion are amino acids and small peptides.

Researchers think that as much as one-third of dietary protein is absorbed into mucosal cells as dipeptides and tripeptides. Vitamins, minerals, and water are also released during digestion.

The Food Pathway

Food passes through the mouth into the oral cavity, where it is chewed and exposed to chemicals in the saliva. The tongue voluntarily forces the mass of food, called a **bolus,** into the pharynx, which is responsible for the reflex action of swallowing. The bolus then enters the esophagus, a muscular, mucus-lined tube, and is propelled downward by peristalsis to the stomach.

Both mechanical and chemical digestion occur in the stomach, reducing the food to a semifluid mass that is released into the small intestine. Further digestion takes place in the small intestine, and most of the absorption of nutrients occurs there as well. Any food remaining after digestion and absorption passes into the large intestine and is excreted as fecal matter.

Oral Cavity

The **oral cavity,** the hollow space in the skull directly behind the mouth, includes the roof of the mouth, the cheeks, and the floor of the mouth. Within the oral cavity are the teeth, tongue, and openings of the ducts of the salivary glands.

DIGESTIVE ACTION

Food entering the oral cavity is chewed and broken down into smaller particles. This mechanical action increases the surface area of the food for exposure to saliva, a digestive secretion produced by the **salivary glands.** Saliva moistens and softens the food for swallowing and contains the digestive enzyme known as **salivary amylase,** which converts starch to maltose (a disaccharide) or to the shorter chains of glucose. Because simple sugars (monosaccharides) require no digestion, some absorption may occur in the mouth. The chemical digestion of more complex carbohydrates (starch) continues until the hydrochloric acid in the stomach halts the action of the salivary amylase. Box 9-1 discusses the dietary treatment of dysphagia.

Box 9-1 ■ *Dietary Treatment for Dysphagia*

It is estimated that as many as 22% of Americans older than age 50, have a swallowing disorder called dysphagia, literally meaning difficulty swallowing. There are two types of dysphagia:

- Oropharyngeal—difficulty in safe transfer of a liquid or food bolus from the mouth to the esophagus
- Esophageal—difficulty in passing food down the esophagus

A swallowing disorder may cause coughing, but not always. As a result, food particles may pass into the lungs (aspiration), allowing bacteria to multiply, which may cause aspiration pneumonia. Dysphagia may be seen after some surgeries and radiation treatment to the head, neck, and/or esophagus, especially for cancer treatment. Premature infants may have difficulty with their suck, swallow and breathing coordination. Individuals with cognitive decline or **traumatic brain injury (TBI)** may also have difficulty swallowing. Dysphagia is commonly seen in clients with neurologic disorders such as stroke, Parkinson's disease, multiple sclerosis, and amyotrophic lateral sclerosis. Studies have cited incidences of individuals who have strokes with dysphagia anywhere from 25% to 70%, with a resulting high prevalence of pneumonia (Garcia, 2010; National Institutes of Health, 2010). It is estimated that in adults admitted to a health-care institution, dysphagia may be present in (Castrogiovanni, 2008):

- 61%—acute trauma centers
- 41%—rehabilitation centers
- 30%–75%—nursing homes
- 25%–30%—hospitals

Diets for dysphagia that safely meet nutrient needs range from nothing by mouth (NPO) to total oral feedings. Candidates for oral feedings should demonstrate the ability to perform a safe swallow by a bedside evaluation or a modified **barium swallow,** be alert and able to follow directions, and be oriented to self and the task of eating.

(continued)

Box 9-1 ■ *Dietary Treatment for Dysphagia—cont'd*

Dysphagia diets provide graduated steps from the most easily managed food to the ones most difficult to manage:

- Liquids range from thick to thin.
- Solids range from pureed to regular.
- The most conservative starting point is thickened liquids and pureed textures.
- Liquids and solids may be progressed independently.
- High-protein, high-calorie between-meal feedings as necessary.

Precise diet orders specify both the texture of solid foods and the consistency of liquids as well as other therapeutic modifications. To address the multiplicity of dysphagia diet terminology and practices, a multidisciplinary task force developed the National Dysphagia Diet (NDD) based on existing scientific evidence (Garcia, 2010; McCallum, 2003). The NDD has four levels:

Level 1: Dysphagia Pureed

- Homogenous, cohesive, puddinglike
- Requires minimum chewing

Level 2: Dysphagia Mechanically Altered

- Cohesive, moist, semisolid
- Requires some chewing ability

Level 3: Dysphagia Advanced

- Nearly all textures except hard, sticky, or crunchy foods
- Requires some chewing ability, foods still need to be moist and bite-sized

Level 4: Regular

- Any solid texture

Hydration is also a challenge for clients with dysphagia; as a result, thickening agents are commonly used to increase a client's fluid intake. Using thickening agents to modify beverages, soups, and pureed foods is both an art and a science. Commercial thickening agents, instant potato flakes, unflavored gelatin, and dehydrated baby foods and cereals can all be used. The nurse should recognize that thickeners may:

- become thicker with time.
- add significant carbohydrate kilocalories to clients' diets.
- react differently in various foods.
- affect palatability of the thickened item.

In addition, being aware that some foods, such as ice cream and gelatin, change their consistency at body temperature is important, and so is following recipes and mixing complementary flavors. For example, tomato juice can be used to thin spaghetti sauce. Another important thing to note is that each client needs his or her diet highly individualized. For instance, foods with mixed consistency such as vegetable soups with chunks and cereal with milk may not be appropriate for an individual who cannot swallow such foods. For individuals who have problems forming a food bolus, foods such as rice, scrambled eggs, corn, peas, and legumes may cause problems because these foods do not form a cohesive bolus. For other clients, foods that crumble, such as crackers, cornbread, and unmoistened ground meats, may not be appropriate.

A preprinted sheet of dos and don'ts is of limited usefulness for many clients. A nurse, speech therapist, occupational therapist, and registered dietitian may collectively devote many sessions to the developing individualized diet plans and determining the best positions for clients during feeding times.

The nurse is an essential part of the team because he or she is in constant contact with the client. The nurse can monitor the diet's implementation and identify any issues or problems that may occur (Garcia, 2010).

Signs and symptoms of dysphagia include the following:

- "Gurgly" voice
- Coughing or choking with food and fluid intake
- Nasal regurgitation
- Pocketing of food in cheeks
- Drooling
- Difficulty in initiating a swallow
- Excessive chewing
- Poor tongue control
- Poor lip closure
- Lack of body position control
- Slurred speech
- Refusal to eat
- Absence of gag reflux
- Excessive time spent eating
- Multiple swallows required to clear a single bolus of food
- Pain on swallowing
- Verbal complaints of food stuck in the throat
- Lack of attention to eating

On observation, these clients may have a documented weight loss, edema, poor skin turgor, and open wounds. These are all signs of poor nutrition.

For the client, safe swallowing includes the following tips:

- Eat slowly.
- Avoid distractions while eating.
- Do not talk while eating.
- Remove loose dentures.
- Sit up while eating.
- Position head correctly.
- Use a teaspoon and take only one-half teaspoon of food or liquids at a time.
- Swallow completely between bites or sips.
- Select foods and fluids of appropriate consistency.

Pharynx

The **pharynx** is a muscular passage between the oral cavity and the esophagus. No digestive action occurs there. The pharynx continues the movement of the bolus by the reflexive action of swallowing. The bolus then enters the esophagus.

Esophagus

The **esophagus** is a muscular tube about 10 inches long that takes food from the pharynx to the stomach. No digestive action occurs there. Peristalsis forces the bolus into the stomach with the help of mucous secretions. Between the esophagus and the stomach is the cardiac sphincter (the first portion of the stomach is called the cardia), which opens to permit passage of food. The sphincter then closes to prevent the backup of stomach contents.

Stomach

The **stomach** is a J-shaped sac that extends from the esophagus to the small intestine. Folds in the mucous membrane, called **rugae,** allow the stomach to expand and to smooth out when full. There is no need to eat constantly, partly because the stomach serves as a reservoir for food—it takes 4 to 6 hours for food to pass completely through to the small intestine. The stomach influences appetite by signaling to decrease intake when distended and to increase intake when empty and contracting (Colaizzo-Anas, 2007). Stomach size also influences the amount of food eaten, and its size is related to the amount of food habitually eaten.

Gastric juice, the collective secretions of the stomach, consists of hydrochloric acid, mucus, and the enzymes pepsin, **rennin,** and **gastric lipase.** Many factors influence the rate of gastric emptying, including the amount of gastric juice, meal composition (percent of fat, carbohydrate [CHO], or protein), meal particle size, and some hormones. Liquids empty in less time than solids do. The primary hormone that influences gastric emptying is **cholecystokinin (CCK),** which inhibits gastric emptying. Another hormone, leptin, which is secreted in the gastric mucosa in addition to fat cells, enhances the action of CCK (Colaizzo-Anas, 2007).

DIGESTIVE ACTION

In the stomach, the chemical digestion of protein begins, and further mechanical digestion takes place. Some water and minerals, certain drugs, and alcohol are absorbed in the stomach. Even before food enters the mouth, the sight or smell of it can cause the gastric mucosa to excrete the hormone **gastrin.** This hormone stimulates the secretion of gastric juice so that there is some present in the stomach when the food arrives. Mucus partially protects the stomach's lining from the corrosive effects of gastric juice.

The hydrolysis of protein begins when hydrochloric acid activates and then converts **pepsinogen** to its active form, **pepsin.** A protein molecule consists of hundreds of amino acids joined by **peptide bonds.** Such chains of amino acids linked by peptide bonds are called **polypeptides.** Pepsin breaks down large polypeptides into smaller ones. In infants, the milk protein casein is broken down by the enzyme rennin, which coagulates (curdles) the milk. In addition to activating pepsin, hydrochloric acid destroys harmful bacteria, makes certain minerals such as iron and calcium more absorbable, and maintains the pH (1–2) of the gastric juice.

Another enzyme, gastric lipase, breaks down some milk butterfat molecules into smaller ones. This enzyme is most active in infants; the more alkaline environment of an infant's stomach enables gastric lipase to work more effectively than it does in adults.

The mechanical digestion occurring in the stomach comes from the churning action of the stomach's muscular walls. This activity agitates the contents of the stomach, thoroughly mixing the food with gastric juice. In this way, the food is reduced to a semifluid mass of partially digested material called **chyme.** Peristaltic waves push the chyme toward the **pyloric sphincter,** the valve separating the stomach from the small intestine. With each peristaltic wave, a small amount of **chyme** is forced through the pyloric sphincter into the small intestine.

Gastroparesis, delayed gastric emptying, can be caused by a variety of pathologies including diabetes mellitus, neuropathic disorders, connective tissue diseases, infiltrating diseases, and postsurgical complications. Symptoms of gastroparesis include:

- Nausea
- Vomiting
- Early satiety
- Bloating or fullness
- Abdominal discomfort

Many clients are asymptomatic (no symptoms). Complications of gastroparesis include:

- Fluid and electrolyte abnormalities
- Inadequate nutritional intake
- Weight loss
- Difficult blood glucose control

Dietary treatment includes small feedings, low-fat foods, low-residue foods, and frequent feedings. Gastric motor and sensory function is complex, and the care of clients with gastroparesis is a challenge.

Ileus, a temporary loss of peristalsis, is another common pathology of gastrointestinal motility. Dietary treatment for ileus is nothing by mouth, or NPO, until the problem is resolved medically.

Small Intestine

The **small intestine** is the longest portion of the alimentary canal, approximately 20 feet (610 cm) in length. It extends from the pyloric sphincter of the stomach to the large intestine. The small intestine is looped and coiled in the central part of the abdominal cavity, surrounded by the large intestine. It consists of three parts: the **duodenum** is the first 10 inches, the **jejunum** is the middle 8 feet, and the **ileum** is the last 11 feet. Ninety percent of the digestive action in the alimentary canal and nearly all end-product absorption of digestion occur in the small intestine.

The entry of chyme into the duodenum stimulates the secretion of two hormones, secretin and CCK. Collectively, these hormones are responsible for the secretion and release of bile and the secretion of pancreatic juice.

Secretin stimulates the production of bile by the liver and the secretion of sodium bicarbonate juice by the pancreas. The bile salts in bile emulsify fats, and sodium bicarbonate juice (which is alkaline) neutralizes the gastric juice that enters the duodenum. This neutralization is necessary to prevent damage to the lining of the duodenum. Mucus secreted by intestinal glands also provides some measure of protection against such damage.

CCK stimulates the contraction of the gallbladder, an action that forces stored bile into the duodenum. It also stimulates the secretion of pancreatic enzymes, which are essential for the breakdown of carbohydrates, fats, and proteins.

Intestinal juice is also secreted in response to the presence of chyme in the duodenum. The peristaltic action of the small intestine mixes the bile, the pancreatic juice, and the intestinal juice with the chyme as it moves toward the colon. The collective action of these juices yields the final products of digestion.

DIGESTION OF CARBOHYDRATES

The action of pancreatic and intestinal enzymes completes carbohydrate digestion. Pancreatic **amylase** breaks down any remaining starch into maltose. And the action of three enzymes (maltase, sucrose, and lactase) located in the walls of the small intestine reduces the disaccharides maltose, sucrose, and lactose to monosaccharides. Each of these enzymes is specific for a given disaccharide:

> **Maltase** breaks down maltose to glucose and glucose.
> **Sucrase** breaks down sucrose to glucose and fructose.
> **Lactase** breaks down lactose to glucose and galactose.

Often, low levels of these intestinal enzymes leads to intolerances for the respective disaccharides.

In fact, approximately 70% of the world's population has some degree of lactose intolerance from a lack of the intestinal enzyme lactase. Clinical Application 9-1 discusses carbohydrate intolerances, including lactose intolerance. Table 9-1 lists food items that are lactose-free, low in lactose, and high in lactose. Table 9-2 contains a lactose-restricted diet with a sample menu.

DIGESTION OF FATS

Fats are emulsified by bile salts in the small intestine before they are digested further. **Emulsification** is the physical breaking up of fats into tiny droplets. In this way, more surface area of the fat is exposed to the chemical action of the enzyme pancreatic lipase. Pancreatic lipase completes the digestion of fats by reducing

---

9-1

Clinical Application

Intolerances

Some individuals are deficient in the enzyme lactase and are unable to digest lactose into glucose and galactose. The resulting condition is called lactose intolerance.

Lactose intolerance, the most common of these conditions, may occur in 60% to 100% of Hispanics, Blacks, and Southeast Asians. The condition can be hereditary or secondary to other disease processes involving the small intestine. After eating or drinking milk products, the client commonly experiences these symptoms of lactose intolerance:

- Abdominal cramping and pain
- Loose stools
- Flatulence (gas)

Dietary treatment of lactose intolerance involves three steps:

1. Identifying food items that contain lactose.
2. Eliminating all sources of lactose from the diet.
3. Establishing an individual tolerance level on a trial-and-error basis. The tolerance levels for lactose vary widely.

TABLE 9-1 ■ Lactose in Foods

Lactose-Free Foods

Broth-based soups unless made with added whey

Plain meat, fish, poultry, peanut butter

Breads that do not contain milk, dry milk solids, or whey

Cereal, crackers

Fruit, plain vegetables

Desserts made without milk, dry milk solids, or whey

Tofu and tofu products, such as tofu-based ice cream substitute

Nondairy creamers

Low-Lactose Foods (0–2 grams/serving)

Milk treated with lactase enzyme, ½ cup

Sherbet, ½ cup

Aged cheese, 1–2 oz

Processed cheese, 1 oz

Butter or margarine

Commercially prepared foods containing dry milk solids or whey

Some medications and vitamin preparations may contain a small amount of lactose. Generally, the amount is minimal and is tolerated well.

High-Lactose Foods (5–8 grams/serving)

Milk (whole, skim, 1%, 2%, buttermilk, sweet acidophilus), ½ cup

Powdered dry milk (whole, nonfat, buttermilk—before reconstituting), ⅛ cup

Evaporated milk, ¼ cup

Sweetened condensed milk, 3 tbsp

Party chip dip or potato topping, ½ cup

White sauce, ½ cup

Creamed or low-fat cottage cheese, ¾ cup

Dry cottage cheese, 1 cup

Ricotta cheese, ¾ cup

TABLE 9-1 ■ Lactose in Foods (Continued)
Cheese food or cheese spread, 2 oz*
Sour cream, ½ cup
Heavy cream, ¾ cup
Ice cream or ice milk, ¾ cup
Half and half, ½ cup
Yogurt, ½ cup†

*Lactose content is higher than that of aged cheese and of processed cheese because of the addition of whey powder and dry milk solids.

†Yogurt may be tolerated better than foods with similar lactose content because of hydrolysis of lactose by bacterial lactase found in the culture. Tolerance may vary with the brand and processing method.

triglycerides to diglycerides and monoglycerides, fatty acids, and glycerol.

Lactose in Cheeses

The lactose content of cheeses varies. One gallon of milk is required to produce 1 lb of cheese. During cheese making, liquid **whey** is separated from the solid curd (similar to the curd in cottage cheese). Most of the lactose in cheese is contained in the whey. In

TABLE 9-2 ■ Lactose-Restricted Diet

Description

This diet restricts foods that contain lactose. Soy-milk substitutes are used as a milk replacement. Individual tolerances should be taken into consideration because some clients may tolerate foods low in lactose (see Table 9-1).
Note: All labels should be read carefully for the addition of milk, lactose, or whey.

Indications

This diet is used for the management of clients exhibiting the signs and symptoms of lactose intolerance, Crohn disease, short bowel syndrome, or colitis. Persistent diarrhea and excessive amounts of gas may be lessened by decreasing lactose intake.

Nutritional Adequacy

This diet is low in calcium, riboflavin, and vitamin D. Supplementation is recommended.

FOOD GROUP	ALLOWED	AVOIDED
Milk	Hard, ripened cheese Ensure® Boost® Ensure Plus® Soy milk Lactaid-treated milk Coffee Rich®	Unripened cheese Fluid milk Powdered milk Milk chocolate Cream Most chocolate drink mixes Most coffee creamers
Breads and Cereals	Most water-based bread (French, Italian, Jewish, Graham crackers) Ritz crackers without cheese	Bread to which milk or lactose has been added (check label)
Fruits	Any	None
Vegetables	Fresh, frozen or canned without milk	Creamed, buttered, or breaded vegetables
Meat	Those not listed under "Avoided" Kosher prepared meat and/or milk products	Breaded or creamed meats, fish, or poultry Most luncheon meats Sausage Frankfurters
Desserts and Miscellaneous Items	Angel food cake Gelatin desserts Milk-free cookies Popcorn made with milk-free margarine Pretzels Mustard, catsup, pickles	Most commercially made desserts Sherbet Ice cream Toffee Cream candies Most chewing gums

SAMPLE MENU

Breakfast	Lunch/Dinner	
1/2 cup orange juice	3 oz baked chicken	1 slice milk-free bread
1/2 cup cream of wheat	Baked potato	2 tsp milk-free margarine
2 slices whole grain milk-free bread	1/2 cup carrots	Angel food cake with fresh fruit topping
2 tsp milk-free margarine	Sliced tomato	Coffee
Jelly		
Coffee		
1/2 cup nondairy "creamer"		

ripened cheese, the small amount of lactose entrapped in the curd is transformed into lactic acid, which does not require lactase for absorption.

Generally, cheese must age for more than 90 days to be lactose free. These cheeses are considered hard-ripened (low in lactose):

- Blue
- Brick
- Brie
- Camembert
- Cheddar
- Colby
- Edam
- Gouda
- Monterey
- Muenster
- Parmesan
- Provolone
- Swiss

These cheeses are considered soft cheeses and thus contain more lactose:

- Cream cheese
- Neufchatel
- Ricotta
- Mozzarella
- Cottage cheese

Products

Clients on a lactose-free diet should read all labels carefully to see if milk or milk solids, lactose, or whey have been added to the products. Many toothpastes and over-the-counter medications contain a small amount of lactose. Generally, the amount is very small and is tolerated well.

Lactaid is an over-the-counter product specially designed for individuals with lactose intolerance. Lactaid is a natural enzyme that is available in a tablet form. Some grocery stores also sell milk that has been pre-treated with the lactase enzyme. This product will digest 70% of the lactose in milk into glucose and galactose. As a result, most lactose-intolerant persons can drink Lactaid-treated milk or, after consuming the tablets, eat foods that contain lactose and digest the lactose comfortably. Milk treated with Lactaid is slightly sweeter than regular milk. The sweeter taste results naturally when lactose is broken into glucose and galactose.

A lactose-restricted diet may be low in calcium, riboflavin, and vitamin D. Clients should be instructed in alternative sources of these nutrients or advised to take supplements.

Lingual lipase is an important enzyme in infants but not in adults.

DIGESTION OF PROTEIN

Although hundreds of enzymes are involved in protein digestion, this text reviews only a few of the major ones. The shorter polypeptides, resulting from the stomach's digestive action, are broken down further by pancreatic and intestinal enzymes. Two of the major pancreatic enzymes are **trypsin** and **chymotrypsin,** which have inactive precursors that are activated by other enzymes.

The intestinal wall also secretes a group of enzymes known as **peptidases,** which act on the smaller molecules produced by the pancreatic enzymes, reducing them to single amino acids and small peptides, the final products of protein digestion.

Table 9-3 summarizes the digestion of carbohydrates, fats, and proteins by body organ (mouth, stomach, and small intestine) and identifies action as mechanical or chemical.

Absorption

The end products of digestion move from the gastrointestinal tract into the blood or lymphatic system in a process called **absorption.** The **lymphatic system** transports **lymph** from the tissues to the bloodstream, which is technically part of the circulatory or cardiovascular system. All fluid in the lymphatic system enters the blood after it collects in the thoracic duct, which opens into the subclavian vein. Lymph enters the bloodstream through the subclavian vein. Only after nutrients have been absorbed into either the blood or lymphatic system can the body's cells use them.

The end products of digestion include monosaccharides from carbohydrate digestion, fatty acids and glycerol (and often monoglycerides) from fats, and small peptides and amino acids from protein digestion. Absorption occurs primarily in the small intestine.

Small Intestine

The inner surface of the small intestine has mucosal folds, villi, and microvilli to increase the surface area for maximum absorption (Fig. 9-1). The mucosal folds are like pleats in fabric. On each fold (pleat) are millions of fingerlike projections, called **villi.** Each villus has hundreds of microscopic, hairlike projections (resembling bristles on a brush), called **microvilli,** on its surface. The large surface area resulting from this arrangement fosters the movement of nutrients into the blood or lymphatic system. The structure of the mucosa serves as a unit that accomplishes the absorption of nutrients.

Within each villus is a network of blood capillaries and a central lymph vessel called a **lacteal.** The villi absorb nutrients from the chyme by way of these blood and lymph vessels. Monosaccharides, amino acids, glycerol (which is water soluble), minerals, and water-soluble

TABLE 9-3 ■ Summary of Digestion			
NUTRIENT	**MOUTH AND ESOPHAGUS**	**STOMACH**	**SMALL INTESTINE**
Carbohydrates Yield	Mechanical	Mechanical	Mechanical
	Mastication	Peristalsis	Peristalsis
	Swallowing	Mucus	Mucus
	Peristalsis	Chemical	Chemical
	Mucus	None	Pancreatic enzymes: Pancreatic amylase
	Chemical		Intestine enzymes:
	Salivary amylase		Maltase
			Sucrase
			Lactase
Monosaccharides			
Fats Yield	Mechanical	Mechanical	Mechanical
	Mastication	Peristalsis	Peristalsis
	Swallowing	Mucus	Mucus
	Peristalsis	Chemical	Gallbladder: bile*
	Mucus	Gastric lipase†	Chemical
	Chemical		Pancreatic enzymes: Pancreatic lipase
	None		
	Lingual lipase in infants		
Glycerol, fatty acids, and monoglycerides			
Proteins Yield	Mechanical	Mechanical	Mechanical
	Mastication	Peristalsis	Peristalsis
	Swallowing	Mucus	Mucus
	Peristalsis	Chemical	Chemical
	Mucus	Rennin	Pancreatic enzymes: Trypsin, chymotrypsin
	Chemical	Pepsin	Intestinal enzymes: Peptidases
	None	Hydrochloric acid	
Amino acids and small peptides			

*Emulsifies fat.
†Digests butterfat only.

vitamins are absorbed into the blood in the **capillary** network. Because short- and medium-chain fatty acids have fewer carbons in their chain length, they are more water soluble than long-chain fatty acids. Thus, they are absorbed directly into the blood as well.

These water-soluble nutrients, including short- and medium-chain fatty acids, eventually enter into hepatic portal circulation (via the portal vein) and travel to the liver. **Hepatic portal circulation** is a subdivision of the vascular system by which blood from the digestive organs and spleen circulates through the liver before returning to the heart. In the liver, the nutrients are modified according to the body's needs.

Because long-chain fats are not soluble in water and blood is chiefly water, fat-soluble nutrients cannot be absorbed directly into the blood. Instead, fat-soluble nutrients—including long-chain fatty acids, any monoglycerides remaining from fat digestion, and fat-soluble vitamins—are first combined with bile salts as a carrier. This complex of fat-soluble materials is then absorbed into the cells lining the intestinal wall.

After the fat is absorbed, the bile separates from it and returns to recirculate. Within the intestinal cells, an enzyme reduces any remaining monoglycerides to fatty acids and glycerol. In a process called triglyceride synthesis, the fatty acids, glycerol, and absorbed long-chain fatty acids recombine (within the intestinal cells) to form human triglycerides.

Next, special proteins cover the newly formed triglycerides and any other fat present (such as cholesterol) to form lipoproteins called **chylomicrons,** which are released into the lymphatic system via the lacteals. Remember that the lymphatic system is connected to the blood system. The protein wrapping these packages of fat enables the chylomicrons to move into the blood via the **thoracic** lymphatic duct (and hence into portal blood). In the liver, lipids are also modified to suit the needs of the body before distribution to body cells. Table 9-4 describes some of the nutrient modifications made in the liver.

The **ileocecal valve,** which relaxes and closes with each peristaltic wave controls further passage of undigested food. This valve prevents backflow and ensures that chyme remains in the small intestine long enough for sufficient digestion and absorption.

The small intestine's structure decreases in size, or wastes away, during starvation, stress, medically indicated bowel rest, and whenever the small bowel is not used. After 1 week of a protein-deficient diet, the microvilli shorten (Colaizzo-Anas, 2007). Even an individual who is ill with a flulike virus and does not eat for several days may need several additional days to regain

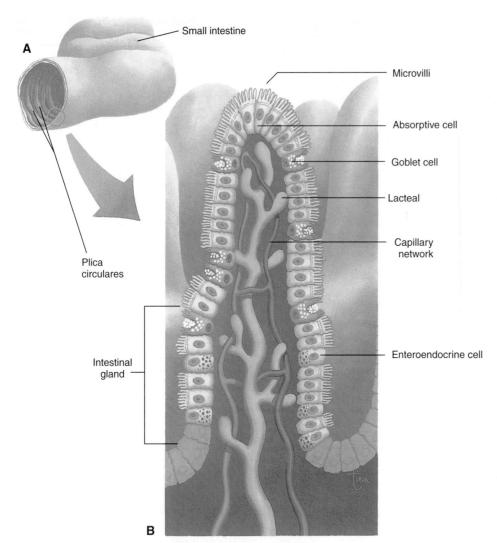

A

Small intestine

Microvilli

Absorptive cell

Goblet cell

Lacteal

Capillary network

Plica circulares

Intestinal gland

Enteroendocrine cell

B

FIGURE 9-1 Cross-section of the small intestine. The multiple folds greatly increase the surface area of the small intestine. (Reprinted from Scanlon, VC, and Sanders, T: *Essentials of anatomy and physiology.* FA Davis, Philadelphia, 2003, with permission.)

TABLE 9-4 ■ Metabolic Modifications in the Liver	
ENERGY NUTRIENT	**MODIFICATION**
Carbohydrates	Fructose and galactose changed to glucose, excess glucose converted to glycogen
Lipids	Lipoproteins formed, cholesterol synthesized, triglycerides broken down and built
Amino Acids	Nonessential amino acids manufactured, excess amino acids deaminated and then changed to carbohydrates or fats, ammonia removed from the blood, plasma proteins made
Other	Alcohol, drugs, and poisons detoxified

his appetite after recovery from the illness. Eating six small low-fat meals daily assists in appetite recovery. See Dollars & Sense 9-1.

Large Intestine

The **large intestine,** also called the **colon,** extends from the ileum (last part of the small intestine) to the anus. When chyme leaves the small intestine, it enters

the first portion of the large intestine, the **cecum** (the appendix, an organ with no known function, is attached to the cecum). It then travels slowly through the remaining parts of the large intestine: the ascending colon, the transverse colon, the descending colon, the sigmoid colon, the **rectum,** and the anal canal.

Water is the main substance absorbed by the large intestine. However, the absorption of some minerals and vitamins also occurs in the colon. Up to 80% of the water is extracted in the cecum and the ascending colon and returned to the bloodstream. Vitamins synthesized by intestinal bacteria, including vitamin K and some of the B complexes, are absorbed from the colon. After absorption and digestion have taken place, the remaining waste products are eliminated in the feces through the rectum.

Elimination

Absorption of water into the bloodstream slowly reduces the water content of the material left inside the large intestine, and the waste product (feces) has a solid

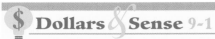

Dollars & Sense 9-1

Reintroducing Food After an Illness

Dehydration can be costly if it involves a trip to the emergency department. The cells of the gastrointestinal tract turn over every few days; therefore, if one cannot or will not eat for just a few days, gastrointestinal cell replacement ceases. Among the reasons for not eating are the stomach flu, common cold, a major dental procedure, or childhood illnesses such as measles.

In all these situations, the client will experience some discomfort when food is reintroduced. Symptoms may include abdominal cramping and diarrhea. To prevent a costly trip to the emergency department because of dehydration, everyone should consume liquids if at all possible when ill. If emeses (vomiting) prevent intake, introduce liquids first during recovery, not spicy or solid foods. Good liquid choices include the following:

- Popsicles
- Apple juice
- Grape juice
- Cranberry juice
- Broth
- Tea
- Gelatin

TABLE 9-5 ■ Factors Decreasing Absorption	
Medications	Antacids
	Laxatives
	Birth control pills
	Anticonvulsants
	Antibiotics
Parasites	Tapeworm
	Hookworm
Surgical Procedures	Gastric resections
	Any surgery on the small intestine
	Some surgical procedures on the large intestine
Disease States	Infection
	Tropical sprue
	Gluten-sensitive enteropathy
	Hepatic disease
	Pancreatic insufficiency
	Lactase deficiency
	Sucrase deficiency
	Maltase deficiency
	Circulatory disorders
	Cancers involving the alimentary canal
Medical Complications	Effects of radiation therapy
	Chemotherapy

Note: Most of these conditions are discussed in later chapters.

consistency. Mucus, the only secretion of the large intestine, provides lubrication for the smooth passage of the feces. By the time feces reach the rectum, it consists of 75% water and 25% solids. The solids include cellular wastes, undigested dietary fiber, undigested food, bile salts, cholesterol, mucus, and bacteria.

Indigestible Carbohydrates

The body cannot digest some forms of carbohydrates because it lacks the necessary enzyme to split the appropriate molecule. Some vegetables and legumes contain these indigestible sugars and fibers. Intestinal gas is formed partly in the colon by the decomposition of undigested materials. Foods that may cause intestinal gas in one person may not in another because each person has slightly different bacterial colonies in the colon.

Factors Interfering With Absorption

Malabsorption is the inadequate movement of digested food from the small intestine into the blood or lymphatic system. Malabsorption can cause malnutrition. Table 9-5 lists factors that interfere with the absorption of nutrients. Note in the table that many diseases, medications, and some medical treatments have a negative impact on the absorption of nutrients. Clinical Application 9-2 discusses surgical removal of all or part of the alimentary canal and the effect on absorption. Clinical Application 9-3 discusses inadequate absorption.

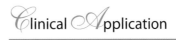

Clinical Application 9-2

Surgical Removal of All or Part of the Alimentary Canal

Clients may need to have a portion of the small intestine surgically removed for a variety of reasons. These clients are frequently at a nutritional risk because they are either permanently or temporarily unable to absorb essential nutrients. In such cases, a nutritional assessment is indicated. In the past, some clients elected to have a portion of the alimentary canal removed to lose weight. This procedure is discussed in Chapter 16.

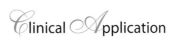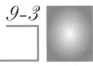

Clinical Application 9-3

Inadequate Absorption

Visually inspecting a client's feces can confirm a suspicion of poor digestion or absorption. Large chunks of food indicate a problem with digestion. A large amount of liquid or near-liquid stools suggests poor absorption. A simple question directed to the client, such as "Are your stools formed?" can provide some information. Sometimes, however, a client's concept of normal may be different from the health-care provider's.

The cells lining the inside layer of the small intestine have a very short life. The smallest structures are replaced every 2 to 3 days. Although this rapid cell turnover helps to promote healing after injury, it also allows vulnerability to any nutritional deficiency or process that might interfere with cell reproduction. Genomic Gem 9-1 describes celiac disease, in which ingestion of gluten causes an autoimmune response that damages the lining of the small intestine.

Gut failure describes a situation in which the small intestine fails to absorb nutrients properly. Symptoms of gut failure include:

- Diarrhea
- Malabsorption
- Poor response to oral feedings

A vicious cycle starts when the cells lining the small intestine fail to reproduce because they

---

Genomic Gem 9-1
Celiac Disease

Celiac disease is also known as celiac sprue, nontropical sprue, and **gluten-sensitive enteropathy.** It is an immune response to gluten, a protein found in wheat, rye, and barley. Oats may also be problematic if they were grown in soil previously planted with wheat, rye, or barley. In the United States, crop rotation is a common practice. Individuals with celiac disease suffer from a wide variety of nutritional problems.

Gluten is mainly found in foods but may also be found in medicines, vitamins, and lip balms. It is a digestive disease, affecting 1 in 141 people in the United States, which damages the small intestine and interferes with absorption of nutrients from food. Celiac disease is a genetically determined condition. Some grain proteins cause an autoimmune response that damages the lining of the small intestine, causing damage to or destroying of the villi and malabsorption of nutrients (National Institutes of Health, 2012a, 2012b). This effect may be related to an allergic reaction and can be either severe or mild. In the severe form, the loss of intestinal mucosa causes malnutrition by impairing the intestine's ability to absorb nutrients, including carbohydrates, proteins, fats, and fat-soluble vitamins.

Lactose intolerance is common in clients with celiac disease. Because the mucosa of the small intestine is damaged, there is a resulting decrease in lactase, an intestinal enzyme that helps digest lactose from milk.

Treatment of celiac combined with lactose intolerance involves using a lactose-free, gluten-free diet. This is a complex diet for a dietitian to plan and for the client to follow. Clients benefit from being kept on the lactose-free restriction only until intestinal cell regeneration occurs, often between 6 months to a year but can take up to 2 years (Ojetti, et al, 2007).

Because untreated celiac disease results in intestinal villous damage and malabsorption, nutritional assessment to prevent and treat malnutrition and iron deficiency anemia is imperative (The Academy 2013). See Table 9-6 for lists of foods containing gluten, including several prepared foods containing thickened sauces. For a positive outcome, the client on a gluten-restricted diet must have extensive teaching. Table 9-7 lists products that can be substituted for flour in many recipes.

TABLE 9-6 ■ Gluten-Restricted Diet

Description
This diet is free of cereals that contain gluten: wheat, oats, rye, and barley. Oats may be included in the diet if the oats are guaranteed to be gluten free.

Indications
This diet is used to treat the primary intestinal malabsorption found in celiac disease.

Adequacy
Kilocalorie (energy) intake may be inadequate to replace previous weight loss. This diet may not meet the recommended dietary allowances for B-complex vitamins, especially thiamin. Iron intake may be inadequate for the premenopausal woman.

FOOD GROUPS	FOODS THAT CONTAIN GLUTEN	FOODS THAT MAY CONTAIN GLUTEN	FOODS THAT DO NOT CONTAIN GLUTEN
Beverage	Cereal beverages (e.g., Postum®), malt, Ovaltine®, beer and ale	Commercial* chocolate milk, cocoa mixes, other beverage mixes, dietary supplements	Coffee, tea, decaffeinated coffee, carbonated beverages, chocolate drinks made with pure cocoa powder, wine, distilled liquor
Meat and Meat Substitutes		Meat loaf and patties, cold cuts and prepared meats, stuffing, breaded meats, cheese foods and spreads; commercial soufflés, omelets, and fondue; soy protein meat substitutes	Pure meat, fish, fowl, egg, cottage cheese, peanut butter
Fat and Oils		Commercial salad dressing and mayo, gravy, white and cream sauces, nondairy creamer	Butter, margarine, vegetable oil
Milk	Milk beverages that contain malt	Commercial chocolate milk	Whole, low-fat, and skim milk; buttermilk

TABLE 9-6 ■ Gluten-Restricted Diet (Continued)			
FOOD GROUPS	**FOODS THAT CONTAIN GLUTEN**	**FOODS THAT MAY CONTAIN GLUTEN**	**FOODS THAT DO NOT CONTAIN GLUTEN**
Grains and Grain Products	Bread, crackers, cereal, and pasta that contain wheat, oats (if not gluten free), rye, malt, malt flavoring, graham flour, Durham flour, pastry flour, bran, or wheat germ; barley; millet; pretzels; communion wafers	Commercial seasoned rice and potato mixes	Specially prepared breads made with wheat starch,[†] rice, potato, or soybean flour or cornmeal; pure corn or rice cereals; hominy grits; white, brown, and wild rice; popcorn; low-protein pasta made from wheat starch
Vegetables		Commercially seasoned vegetable mixes; commercial vegetables with cream or cheese sauce; canned baked beans	All fresh vegetables; plain commercially frozen or canned vegetables
Fruits		Commercial pie fillings	All plain or sweetened fruits; fruit thickened with tapioca or cornstarch
Soup	Soup that contains wheat pasta; soup thickened with wheat flour or other gluten-containing grains	Commercial soup, broth, and soup mixes	Soup thickened with cornstarch, potato rice or soybean flour; pure broth
Desserts	Commercial cakes, cookies, and pastries	Commercial ice cream and sherbet	Gelatin; custard; fruit ice; specially prepared cakes, cookies, and pastries made with gluten-free flour or starch; pudding and fruit filling thickened with tapioca, cornstarch, or arrowroot flour
Sweets		Commercial candies, especially chocolates	
Miscellaneous		Ketchup, prepared mustard, soy sauce, commercially prepared meat sauces and pickles, vinegar, flavoring syrups (syrups for pancakes or ice cream)	Monosodium glutamate, salt, pepper, pure spices and herbs, yeast, pure baking chocolate or cocoa powder, carob, flavoring extracts, artificial flavoring
SAMPLE MENU			
Breakfast	**Lunch/Dinner**		
½ cup orange juice Cocoa Puffs®, Sugar Pops®, Puffed Rice® 2 slices gluten-free bread 1 poached egg 1 cup milk 2 tsp margarine Jelly	Chicken breast Baked potato ½ cup broccoli Lettuce/tomato salad French dressing Sour cream ½ cup milk Cornstarch pudding		

*The terms *commercially prepared* and *commercial* are used to refer to partially prepared foods purchased from a grocery or food market and to prepared foods purchased from a restaurant.
†Wheat starch may contain trace amounts of gluten. Avoid if not tolerated.
Note: Medications may contain trace amounts of gluten. A pharmacist may be able to provide information on the gluten content of medications.

TABLE 9-7 ■ Gluten-Free Substitutions for 2 Tablespoons of Wheat Flour
3 tsp cornstarch
3 tsp potato starch
3 tsp arrowroot starch
3 tsp quick-cooking tapioca
3 tbsp white or brown rice flour

do not have the necessary nutrients for cell replacement. The result is chronic diarrhea caused by malabsorption. In turn, the malabsorption leads to malnutrition, which prevents cell reproduction (see Fig. 9-2).

STEATORRHEA

Some diseases and medications result in the malabsorption of fat. In these conditions, clients have **steatorrhea,** or fat in the stools. In many cases, the inhibition of pancreatic lipase, an enzyme necessary for the digestion of fats, causes the condition. Treatment typically involves using medications and decreasing dietary fat.

Food Allergies

A food **allergy** is sensitivity to a food that does not cause a negative reaction in most people. Clients commonly use the term **food allergy** as a generic term that encompasses a broad range of symptoms triggered by

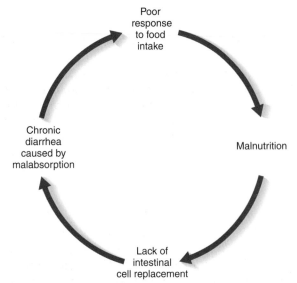

FIGURE 9-2 "Gut failure." Gut failure is a self-perpetuating cycle. Poor response to food intake leads to poor intestinal cell regeneration, which leads to chronic diarrhea caused by malabsorption.

certain foods. The medical community reserves the term to immunologically mediated abnormal reactions to foods that are life-threatening.

A true allergy requires meticulous avoidance of the implicated food to minimize the risk of potentially life-threatening reactions. Avoidance includes:

■ No eating
■ No touching
■ No smelling

Individuals may be genetically predisposed to a food allergy.

Some food allergies may be due to an alteration in absorption. The susceptible person absorbs a part of a food before it has been completely digested. The incomplete digestion of protein in particular is responsible for many allergic reactions. Box 9-2 provides a list of food allergy triggers.

Box 9-2 ■ *Food Allergy Triggers*

Common triggers for food allergies include:

■ Eggs
■ Fish
■ Gluten
■ Milk
■ Peanuts
■ Shellfish
■ Soy
■ Tree nuts

Less common triggers include:

■ Fruits
■ Vegetables

Metabolism

After digestion and absorption, nutrients are carried by the blood (usually after being modified in the liver cells) to all cells of the body. After entry into the cells, the nutrients from food undergo many chemical changes, which result in either the release of energy or the use of energy.

Metabolism is the sum of all chemical and physical processes continuously going on in living organisms, comprising both anabolism and catabolism. Catabolic reactions usually result in the release of energy. Anabolic reactions require energy.

Catabolic Reactions

In the cells, glucose, glycerol, fatty acids, and amino acids can be broken down even further. These nutrients are held together by bonds that require energy to form and that, when broken, release energy. The breakdown of the fuel-producing nutrients yields carbon dioxide, water, heat, and other forms of energy. Eventually, the carbon dioxide is exhaled, and the water becomes part of the body fluids or is eliminated in urine. Fifty percent or more of the total potential energy usually is lost as heat. The remaining available energy is temporarily stored in the cells as adenosine triphosphate (ATP).

ATP, a high-energy compound that has three phosphate groups in its structure, is available in all cells. Practically speaking, ATP is the storage form of energy for the cells because each cell has enzymes that can initiate the hydrolysis (breakdown through the addition of water) of ATP. In this reaction, one or more phosphate groups split off and subsequently release energy. If one phosphate group is removed, the result is ADP (adenosine diphosphate) plus phosphate.

Many steps are involved in the catabolic process responsible for the release of this energy. These steps require one or more of the following agents: enzymes, coenzymes, or hormones. Some vitamins and minerals act as coenzymes. Oxygen is also necessary for the full release of any potential energy. The addition of oxygen to the reaction is called **oxidation.** During the many steps that occur, energy is released little by little and stored as ATP.

The breakdown process includes the formation of intermediate chemical compounds such as **pyruvate** (pyruvic acid) and **acetyl CoA.** Acetyl CoA can be broken down further by entering a series of chemical reactions known as the **Krebs cycle** or the TCA (tricarboxylic acid) cycle. Figure 9-3 is a simplified schematic of the steps involved in the release of energy by the cells.

STORAGE OF EXCESS NUTRIENTS

If the cells do not have immediate energy needs, the excess nutrients are stored. Glucose is stored as glycogen in liver and muscle tissue; surplus amounts are

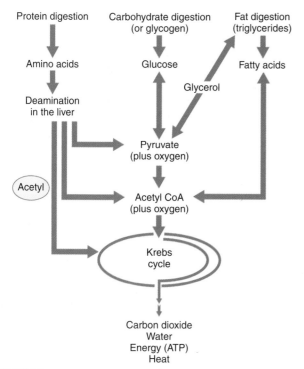

FIGURE 9-3 Energy production in the cells. Energy is released bit by bit during the further breakdown of amino acids, glucose, glycerol, and fatty acids.

converted to fat. Glycerol and fatty acids are reassembled into triglycerides and stored in adipose tissue. Amino acids are used to make body proteins; any excess is deaminated (stripped of nitrogen) and ultimately used for glucose formation or stored as fat. If energy is not available from food, the cells will seek energy in those body stores. Fat cannot be used to meet the body's need for glucose; however, protein can be converted into glucose. If CHO intake is inadequate, the body will break down lean body mass (protein stores) to meet its glucose need.

Anabolic Reactions

Once immediate energy needs have been met, cells utilize nutrients as needed for growth and repair of body tissue. The cellular supply of ATP is used first. When this instant energy source is exhausted, glycogen and fat stores are used. In addition to building up body protein, other anabolic reactions include the recombination of glycerol and fatty acids to form triglycerides and the formation of glycogen from glucose.

Excretion of Waste

Materials of no use to the cells become waste that is eliminated through excretion. Solid waste and some liquid is disposed of in the feces. The digestive system needs assistance from other body systems in the disposal of nonsolid waste. The lungs dispose of gaseous waste. Most liquid waste is sent first to the kidneys and then to the **bladder** to be eliminated in the urine. Some liquid waste is disposed of by the skin through perspiration.

Carbon dioxide (CO_2) is a gas that is eliminated through the lungs each time one exhales. The amount of carbon dioxide exhaled depends on the type of fuel (lipid, protein, or carbohydrate) or the source of fuel that the body is currently burning for energy. For example, more CO_2 is produced when carbohydrates are utilized than when protein or fat are used.

The skin removes some of the liquid waste in the form of perspiration or water, and some is excreted in the feces. The kidneys eliminate most of the excess water, sodium, hydrogen, and urea. **Urea** is synthesized in the liver from the nitrogen resulting from the breakdown of amino acids. Some water is also removed from the body each time one exhales.

Keystones

- The cell is the ultimate destination for the nutrients in food.
- Digestion is the process through which food is broken down for use by cells: carbohydrates are broken down to monosaccharides, fats are reduced to glycerol and fatty acids, and proteins are split to yield amino acids.
- Secretions from the salivary glands, stomach, small intestine, liver, and pancreas assist in chemical digestion.
- Absorption refers to the movement of food from the gastrointestinal tract into the blood and lymphatic systems.
- Metabolism involves anabolism and catabolism. The liver plays a major role in metabolism.

(Continued)

Keystones—cont'd

■ Energy is released little by little from the end products of digestion in a series of chemical reactions.

■ Energy nutrients not needed immediately by the cells are stored as glycogen and adipose tissue.

■ The human body cannot convert fat into glucose, but it can convert protein into glucose.

■ The metabolism of food produces waste. Waste products are released from the body in feces, urine, perspiration, and exhaled air.

■ Many ailments and diseases, including malabsorption, disaccharide intolerances, allergies, and gluten-sensitive enteropathy, are related to the structure and function of the gastrointestinal system.

CASE STUDY *9–1*

Mr. H is 25 years old, 6 feet tall, and weighs 170 lb (dressed without shoes). He has a medium frame, as determined by measuring his wrist circumference. Mr. H has been admitted to the hospital for an elective arthroscopic (surgical procedure) on his right knee. During the nursing admission process, Mr. H complained of gas pains and frequent loose stools. He stated that he does not avoid any particular foods and has a healthy appetite. He claims to drink about 3 cups of milk each day. The client complains of losing 5 lb during the previous month. Mr. H uses the restroom twice during the interview to "move his bowels." The second time you inspect the stool. The client's stool is loose and unformed.

The next day you note that a diagnosis of lactose intolerance has been made. A lactose-restricted diet is ordered.

The following nursing care plan originates on the day the client is admitted. The physician uses the information collected from the nurse in making his or her diagnosis. Please note that the client has already met the first desired outcome and part of the second; the outcomes have been charted. The client has not met the third desired outcome.

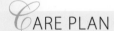ARE PLAN

Subjective Data

Client complains of gas pains and loose stools. Client states that he does not avoid any particular foods. He drinks milk.

Objective Data

Client observed to use the restroom twice in 9 minutes to defecate. Visual inspection shows loose and unformed stool.

Analysis

Diarrhea related to client's complaints of loose unformed stools as evidenced by the client's need to use the restroom twice in a 9-minute period and by direct observation of one loose and unformed stool.

Plan

DESIRED OUTCOMES EVALUATION CRITERIA	ACTIONS/INTERVENTIONS	RATIONALE
The client will assist in ruling out causes for his loose stools and report his signs and symptoms to the nurse.	Teach the client to observe and record the pattern, onset, frequency, characteristics, amount, time of day, and precipitating events related to occurrence of diarrhea. Refer client to the dietitian to determine usual food intake and nutritional status.	Observation and documentation of the client's response to these factors will assist in determining the cause of his loose stools.

CASE STUDY *(Continued)*

DESIRED OUTCOMES EVALUATION CRITERIA	ACTIONS/INTERVENTIONS	RATIONALE
	Determine exposure to recent environmental contaminants, such as drinking water, food-handling practices, and proximity to others who are ill.	
	Review drug intake for medications affecting absorption (see Table 9-5).	
The client will eliminate causative factors at once after these factors have been determined.	Follow through with the elimination of causative factors, restrict intake if necessary, note change in drug therapy, if any.	Elimination of the causative factors should decrease the frequency of loose, unformed stools. The client needs to be instructed on the relationship of his diarrhea to causative factors.
The client will have formed stools within 24 hours after the causative factors have been eliminated.	Document stool consistency.	Whenever possible, an objective measure should be used to evaluate the success of any client intervention. Stool consistency is an objective measure for treatment response to diarrhea and malabsorption.
If he or she is willing, refer the client to the registered dietitian.		

9-1

Dietitian's Note

The following Dietitian's Notes are representative of the documentation found in a client's medical record. The SOAP acronym refers to subjective and objective information, assessment, and plan. Subjective is what the client reports. Objective is what has been previously documented, such as doctor's diagnosis, laboratory information, results of diagnostic procedures and measurements. Assessment is the interviewer's interpretation of the subjective and objective information combined. Dietitians may chart the nutrition diagnosis here. Plan is action or actions the provider intends to do as a result of the assessment.

SOAP: Client states he has no previous knowledge of food- and nutrition-related recommendations. States he feels much better after milk restriction. Client expressed interest in learning more about diet. Formerly client drank three glasses of milk per day. He is concerned about calcium and vitamin D deficiencies. He misses eating soft and fresh cheese. Client claims a recent 5-pound weight loss that he attributes to frequent loose stools.

Objective: Prescribed diet (Rx) = lactose-restricted diet; medical diagnosis (Dx) = lactose intolerance

Assessment: Food- and nutrition-related knowledge deficit related to weight loss and loose stools as evidenced by client statements that he has no prior exposure to lactose-restricted diet and cessation of loose stools 24 hours after the diet was started. Oral and written instructions were provided. Special emphasis was placed on food sources of calcium and vitamin D that are low in lactose. Client demonstrated an understanding of the diet by verbally planning a lactose-free menu for one diet without error.

Plan: Recommend a calcium and vitamin D supplement. Client instructed to call the outpatient dietitian with questions. The phone number was provided. Follow-up visit in 1 week.

Critical Thinking Questions

1. The client asks you how long he will need to follow this diet and whether he will ever be able to reintroduce milk to his diet. What do you tell him?

2. What would you tell the client if the diet were only partially effective in controlling the diarrhea?

Chapter Review

1. An appropriate snack for a child on a gluten-free diet would be:
   a. Crackers and peanut butter
   b. Half of a cheese sandwich
   c. Potato chips and an oatmeal cookie
   d. Rice cakes and a banana

2. Solid body waste is stored in the:
   a. Large intestine
   b. Gallbladder
   c. Small intestine
   d. Stomach

3. Gaseous waste is expelled:
   a. In the urine
   b. In the feces
   c. Through the lungs
   d. Through the skin

4. The end products of protein digestion are:
   a. Glycerol and fatty acids
   b. Amino acids
   c. Fatty acids
   d. Monosaccharides

5. A food commonly responsible for an allergic reaction is:
   a. Chicken
   b. Peanuts
   c. Rice
   d. Carrots

Clinical Analysis

1. The nurse is visiting Mr. D, who is receiving home health care. His caregiver is concerned that Mr. D chokes on liquids but swallows semisolid food well. Which of the following actions by the nurse would be the most appropriate?
   a. Recommend a soft diet.
   b. Recommend a fluid restriction.
   c. Refer Mr. D to a speech therapist.
   d. First, advise client to drink thickened liquids and then refer to both a speech therapist and then a registered dietitian.

2. Brenda, a 3-year-old, has been admitted to the pediatric unit with a diagnosis of celiac disease. The doctor ordered a gluten-free diet. Which of the following meals would be compatible with the diet order?
   a. Goulash, green beans, and milk
   b. Hamburger on bun, French fries, and a chocolate shake
   c. Tomato soup, grilled cheese, applesauce, and a cookie
   d. Baked chicken, baked potato, sour cream, green beans, peaches, and milk

3. Mr. P is on a low-fat diet (20 grams) to control his steatorrhea. An appropriate snack would be:
   a. Fruit
   b. Nuts
   c. Cheese
   d. Cookies

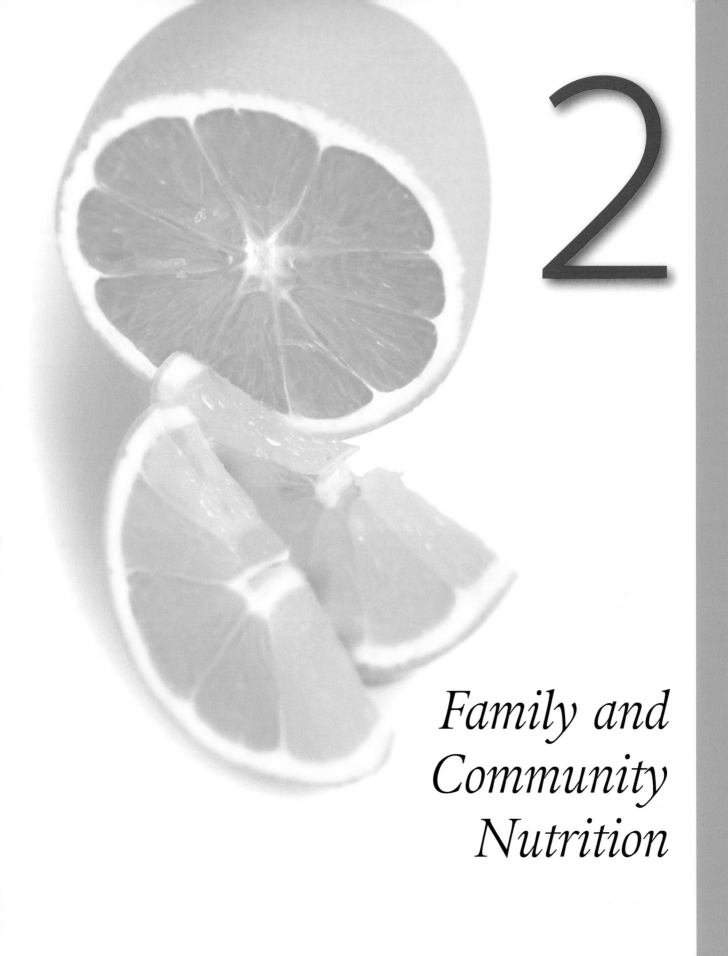

2

Family and Community Nutrition

10

Life Cycle Nutrition: Pregnancy and Lactation

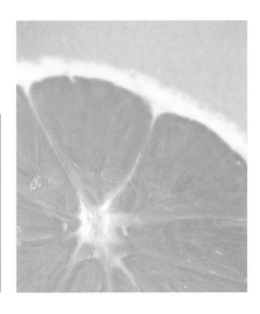

LEARNING OBJECTIVES

After completing this chapter, the student should be able to:

■ Compare the nutritional needs of a pregnant woman with those of a nonpregnant woman of the same age.

■ Contrast the nutritional needs of a pregnant adolescent with those of a pregnant adult.

■ Explain why folic acid intake is critical for women of childbearing age.

■ Identify substances to be avoided by pregnant and breastfeeding women.

■ Discuss the dietary treatment of common problems of pregnancy.

■ List three advantages that breastfeeding confers on the mother.

The needs for many nutrients change at different stages of life. Human beings are most vulnerable to the impact of poor nutrition during periods of rapid growth. This chapter focuses on the period of most rapid growth, that of the unborn child. If the essential nutrients are not present to support growth during that critical time, permanent damage to tissues and organs can occur.

Nutrition During Pregnancy

An expectant mother's nutritional status can affect the outcome of pregnancy. For example, during the first month of **gestation,** the mother must be well nourished so that the **placenta** that forms will be healthy. Because the entire **embryo** and **fetus's** major body organs form within 2 to 3 months of conception, nutrition during this time is critical to the health of the child. Required nutrients come from the mother's diet or body stores.

The placenta is not just a passive conduit for nutrients, however. The placenta performs multiple functions that are essential for fetal survival, growth, and development. These functions include transport of gases, nutrients, and waste products (Kim, Zhao, Jiang, et al, 2012). The placenta also provides a barrier to the transfer of some substances such as maternal red blood cells and bacteria.

After the birth and weaning of a child, the mother needs time to rebuild her nutrient stores. Research has demonstrated that infants that are spaced at least 2 years apart are less likely to be born premature, of **low-birth-weight (LBW),** or malnourished (Dibaba, 2010). Whether related to birth spacing or not, these complications are not evenly distributed throughout the population. A significant association has been demonstrated for women who are African American to be at a higher risk for having an infant who is delivered preterm or of LBW (Janevic, Stein, Savitz, et al, 2010). The best action an expectant mother can take for her unborn child is to enter the pregnancy with good nutrient stores and to consume a well-balanced diet while pregnant. She must also avoid harmful substances, such as alcohol and contraindicated drugs, including over-the-counter and prescription preparations.

From **implantation** to birth, the fertilized **ovum** (which weighs less than 100 mcg) develops into an infant who weighs about 3.4 kilograms (7.5 pounds) on average. During this period of rapid growth and development, the mother needs additional nutrients, including kilocalories, protein, and certain vitamins and minerals.

Energy Needs

For dietary reference intakes (DRIs) for macronutrients, see Appendix A. For digestible carbohydrate and protein DRIs, see Table 10-1.

Increased energy is needed to sustain the mother and for the development of the fetus and the placenta. From the fourth through the sixth month, the second trimester, much of this energy supports the growth of the uterus (womb) and other maternal tissues. During the seventh through ninth months, the third trimester, much of the energy supports the fetus and the placenta. To meet this increased metabolic workload and to spare protein for tissue building, a pregnant woman needs an extra:

- 340 kilocalories per day in the second trimester
- 452 kilocalories per day in the third trimester

On average the pregnant woman will need to increase daily caloric intake by approximately 300 kilocalories per day. The increase in calories should be from high nutrient density foods (Ural, 2010).

Fat Needs

For DRIs for fat, see Appendix A.

Long-chain polyunsaturated fatty acids (LC-PUFAs) have demonstrated crucial importance in the development of the fetal retina and brain (Schwartz, Drossard, Dube, et al, 2009). LC-PUFAs, docosahexaenoic acid (DHA), and arachidonic acid (AA) accumulate in the fetal brain rapidly during the third trimester of gestation and during the early postnatal period (Rioux, Belanger-Plourde, LeBlanc, and Vigneau, 2011). These essential fatty acids can be supplied directly from the diet or synthesized from the omega-6 fatty acids and omega-3 fatty acid families. Because of the importance of DHA to fetal brain development, it is recommended that pregnant women consume 300 mg each day (Rioux et al, 2011). See Chapter 18 for more information on omega-3 fatty acids.

The adequate intakes (AIs) for omega-6 fatty acids (linoleic acid) and omega-3 fatty acids (alpha-linolenic acid) are increased during pregnancy and lactation compared to amounts designated for other women.

Food sources of linoleic acid are the following oils:

- Corn
- Safflower
- Sunflower

Alpha-linolenic acid is found in these oils:

- Canola
- Flaxseed
- Soybean
- Walnut (see Chapter 18)

Important sources of DHA are fish and shellfish, because conversion by the body is not required. Consequently, a pregnant woman's diet should contain oils as well as seafood within the limits described in the section Certain Species and Amounts of Fish.

Protein Needs

For DRIs for protein, see Appendix A and Table 10-1.

Protein is required to build fetal **tissue.** The mother also needs adequate protein for growth of her tissues. Her blood volume increases in anticipation of blood loss at delivery. Her breasts develop in preparation for lactation. Her uterus enlarges and contains a sac filled with **amniotic fluid.** For those reasons, the recommended dietary allowance (RDA) for protein for pregnant women is 54% more than for nonpregnant women. Translating this need to the exchange system, 2 extra

TABLE 10-1 ■ RDAs and AIs for Selected Minerals and Energy Nutrients							
LIFE STAGE GROUP	CALCIUM (MG/DAY)	FLUORIDE* (MG/DAY)	IODINE (MCG/DAY)	IRON (MG/DAY)	ZINC (MG/DAY)	CARBOHYDRATE (G/DAY)†	PROTEIN (G/DAY)
Pregnancy							
<19 years	**1300**	3	220	27	12	175	71
19–50 years	**1000**	3	220	27	11	175	71
Lactation							
<19 years	**1300**	3	290	10	13	210	71
19–50 years	**1000**	3	290	9	12	210	71

AI, adequate intake; RDA, recommended dietary allowance.
*AI.
†Based on its role as primary energy source for the brain.
Values in boldface indicate RDA; AIs are in light face.
Source: www.iom.edu/Activities/Nutrition/SummaryDRIs/~/media/Files/Activity%20Files/Nutrition/DRIs/5_Summary%20Table%20Tables%201-4.pdf

cups of milk (16 grams of protein) and 1.5 additional ounces of meat (10.5 grams of protein) each day would more than meet the increased protein requirement.

Protein intake becomes a hazard to the fetus when the mother has phenylketonuria and is eating inappropriately. The goal of treatment with phenylketonuria is to maintain phenylalanine levels within safe limits. The limit in pregnant women is 120 to 240 umol/L to ensure normal growth and prevent mental retardation in the fetus (Giovannini, Verduci, Salvaticit, Pacit, and Riva, 2010). All women should be asked directly if they have ever had a special diet prescription. The healthcare provider should investigate further when a woman cites a history of troubled pregnancies, congenital abnormalities, a mentally retarded infant, spontaneous abortion, or stillbirth. See Clinical Application 4-2 and Genomic Gem 4-1 in Chapter 4.

Vitamin Needs

Pregnant women have an increased need for some vitamins. They must avoid taking excessive amounts of others because of potential hazard to the fetus.

Water-Soluble Vitamins

For DRIs for vitamins during pregnancy and lactation, see Appendix A. For selected vitamins during pregnancy and lactation, see Table 10-2.

A pregnant woman's RDA for vitamin C is 13% higher than that of a nonpregnant woman. Vitamin C is necessary for collagen formation and tissue building.

The RDAs for all the B vitamins except biotin are modestly increased for pregnancy. The increased requirements are understandable—particularly for thiamin, niacin, and vitamin B_6, which are coenzymes involved in energy metabolism. See the section on hyperemesis gravidarum for information specific to thiamin deficiency. Two other B vitamins are of special concern in pregnancy: vitamin B_{12} and folic acid.

VITAMIN B_{12}

For DRIs for vitamins during pregnancy and lactation, see Appendix A. For selected vitamins during pregnancy and lactation, see Table 10-2.

The vitamin B_{12} RDA is only slightly increased for pregnant and lactating women. The placenta appears to concentrate vitamin B_{12} because serum levels in the newborn are about twice the maternal levels. Vitamin B_{12} is concentrated and stored in the fetal liver during pregnancy and provides the infant with stores to sustain them for the first several months of life.

Strict vegetarians are at high risk of nutritional Vitamin B_{12} deficiencies, which can have a greater effect on the infant than on the mother (Guez, Chiarelli, Menni, et al, 2012). Vegetarians need to ensure adequate intake of Vitamin B_{12} from fortified foods or supplements. Fortified food and supplements made from cobalamin provide a physiologically active form of the vitamin, whereas products that list only vitamin B_{12} might include nonbioavailable sources. Vitamin B_{12} deficiencies have shown to result in neurological insult to the infant.

FOLIC ACID

For DRIs for vitamins during pregnancy and lactation, see Appendix A. For selected vitamins during pregnancy and lactation, see Table 10-2.

The RDA for folic acid for all women of childbearing potential specifies synthetic folic acid from fortified foods or supplements. In addition, food folate from a varied diet is expected to be consumed.

These recommendations are based on clinical studies that showed that 4 mg of folic acid daily prevented 72% of **neural tube defects (NTDs)** in infants of women who have already delivered a child afflicted with the defect (Simpson, Shulman, Brown, and Holzgreve, 2010; see Box 10-1). The Centers for Disease Control and Prevention (CDC) quickly recommended the treatment for such high-risk women beginning folic acid 1 month before conception and continuing until

TABLE 10-2 ■ RDAs for Selected Vitamins for Pregnancy and Lactation									
LIFE STAGE GROUP	VITAMIN A (MCG/DAY)	VITAMIN C* (MG/DAY)	VITAMIN D (MCG/DAY)	VITAMIN E (MG/DAY)	THIAMIN (MG/DAY)	NIACIN (MG/DAY)	VITAMIN B_6 (MG/DAY)	FOLATE† (MCG/DAY)	VITAMIN B_{12} (MCG/DAY)
Pregnancy									
<19 years	750	80	15	15	1.4	18	1.9	600	2.6
19–50 years	770	85	15	15	1.4	18	1.9	600	2.6
Lactation									
<19 years	1200	115	15	19	1.4	17	2.0	500	2.8
19–50 years	1300	120	15	19	1.4	17	2.0	500	2.8

RDA, recommended dietary allowance.
*Smokers require an additional 35 mg/day of vitamin C.
†Women able to become pregnant should consume 400 micrograms of synthetic folic acid from fortified foods/supplements besides food folate.
Source: www.iom.edu/Activities/Nutrition/SummaryDRIs/~/media/Files/Activity%20Files/Nutrition/DRIs/5_Summary%20Table%20Tables%201-4.pdf

---

Box 10-1 ■ *Neural Tube Defects: Occurrence, Pathophysiology, and Side Effects of Supplementation*

Neural tube defects (NTDs) are the most common preventable type of birth defect in the world, and affect approximately 1 in 1000 children worldwide (Fehr, Fehr, Penner Protudjer, 2011).

The neural tube is embryonic tissue that develops into the brain and spinal cord. A critical time in the development of this structure is from conception through the fourth week of pregnancy. Interference with normal development at that time produces major congenital defects, including **anencephaly, meningoencephalocele, spina bifida,** and **meningocele.** Unfortunately, the neural tube develops before many women are aware they are pregnant.

As a multifactorial condition, the exact connection of NTDs to folic acid is unclear, but folate is directly or indirectly essential for cell function, division, and differentiation. The exact mechanism through which consumption of folate reduces the risk of NTD remains unclear and is still being researched (Agarwal and Phadke, 2012).

In addition to preventing NTDs, folic acid seems to reduce the risk of other birth defects, especially cardiac anomalies, urinary tract anomalies, and orofacial clefts and its relationship to other conditions is under investigation (Simpson, Shulman, Brown, et al, 2010).

---

3 months of pregnancy. Studies have demonstrated that periconceptional consumption of adequate folic acid, of 4 mg daily, can prevent 50% to 70% of NTDs (CDC, 2010).

Despite recommendations for women of childbearing age to increase folic acid intake, most women have not done so. Consequently, folic acid has been added to the enrichment protocol for cereal-grain products in the United States since January 1998; 140 mcg of folic acid has been incorporated into each 100 grams of grain. Following the initiation of folate fortification, the prevalence of spina bifida decreased 31% and of anencephaly 16% (Ramirez de Arellano, 2010). Data demonstrate that Hispanic women continue to be at a significantly greater risk for having a baby affected with NTD than non-Hispanic white women and black women, who also have a lowest risk (CDC, 2010). See Genomic Gem 10-1 for more information on risk factors for NTDs.

Although there is strong data that conclusively confirms a decreased incidence in NTD when women consume adequate folic acid before and during pregnancy, data suggests that less than 50% of women of childbearing age are actually taking folic acid daily (Rofail, Colligs, Abetz, et al, 2012). A woman's knowledge of folic acid and its role in preventing NTDs is essential for reducing the risk of NTD. Health-care providers need to increase their efforts to promote adequate folic acid intake among fertile women. Specific target populations include the following:

- Young women
- Hispanic and black women
- Women with low incomes
- Women with less than a high school education (Fehr et al, 2011)

Fat-Soluble Vitamins

For DRIs for vitamins during pregnancy and lactation, see Appendix A. For selected vitamins during pregnancy and lactation, see Table 10-2.

Genomic Gem 10-1

The Genesis of Neural Tube Defects

Most cases of neural tube defects (NTD) occur in women without a history of the disorder, but there is evidence of a genetic component to this multifactorial condition. There is a higher recurrence risk to siblings in families with an NTD child. Because folic acid is so clearly protective, much research has focused on its metabolic pathways. Variants of several folate-related genes have been significantly associated with risk for NTDs.

Among other findings suggesting a genetic component are the following:

- There is a 10- to 20-fold higher recurrence risk to siblings in families with an NTD child (Pangilinan, Molloy, Mills, et al, 2012).
- Ethnic and racial differences in NTD prevalence— Hispanic women continue to have higher rates of NTD than non-Hispanic white women (National Center on Birth Defects and Developmental Disabilities, 2011).
- A risk still being evaluated is the paternal risk. Studies are looking at male exposure to dioxin, which can be absorbed from food products or environmental waste. Exposure can lead to mutations in spermatozoid that can lead to an increased risk of NTDs (Safi, Loyeux, and Chalouhi, 2010).

Among the environmental factors associated with NTDs, other risks that are being studied are maternal diabetes, maternal obesity, socioeconomic status, maternal hyperthermia, and use of caffeine and antiepileptic medications (Au, Ashley-Koch, Northrup, 2010). While awaiting clear understanding of causality, the ability to prevent approximately 70% of NTDs through the administration of folic acid is a remarkable advance.

The RDA for vitamin E and the AI for vitamin K are the same for pregnant women as for mature, nonpregnant women. Interfering with normal physiology can create problems, however. During normal pregnancy, the placenta transfers limited amounts of vitamin K to the fetus. Significant bleeding problems are rare, but infants are treated with vitamin K at birth (see Chapter 11). Vitamins D and A merit special mention even for normal pregnancies.

VITAMIN D

The same controversy about the adequacy of the AI for vitamin D (see Chapter 7) spills into discussions regarding the needs of pregnant women.

Vitamin D has multiple functions in the growth and development of the fetus, including immune system development, brain development, and cellular differentiation (Dorr and Allen, 2010). Attention is being brought to the effects of maternal vitamin D deficiency in relationship to the development and outcomes of the infant. If a woman is vitamin D deficient, it appears to have a greater impact on fetal than maternal bone health (Wagner, Taylor, Dawodu, et al, 2012). Severe vitamin D deficiency during gestation and early life is a primary cause of rickets in infants and children and can be accompanied by hypocalcemic seizures (Dror and Allen, 2010).

Further research is being done to investigate the current vitamin D recommendations for pregnant women.

VITAMIN A

Vitamin A excess in pregnant women has been related to birth defects. Vitamin A as retinol or retinoic acid in excess of 10,000 IU per day or treatment with **isotretinoin** during the first trimester increases the risk of **retinoic acid syndrome.** The characteristic fetal deformities include the following:

- Small or no ears
- Abnormal or missing ear canals
- Brain malformation
- Heart defects

Three ounces of beef liver may contain 27,000 IU, and 3 oz of chicken liver, 12,000 IU. A pregnant woman who eats liver regularly may consume enough vitamin A to pose a risk to her baby. A well-balanced diet should supply the RDA for pregnant women, and a supplement is generally not recommended (Ural, 2011).

Some prenatal vitamins substitute beta-carotene, which is not associated with birth defects, for preformed vitamin A or omit vitamin A entirely. Table 10-3 lists the RDAs and ULs in micrograms and International Units for vitamin A for pregnancy and lactation. Remember the conversion to IUs depends on the source (see Clinical Calculation 7-1).

Isotretinoin, a vitamin A metabolite used to treat severe acne, is hazardous to the fetus with almost a 30% risk of malformations if a woman is exposed to isotretinoin during the first trimester (Malvasi, Tinelli, Buia, De Luca, 2009). Despite a pregnancy prevention program started by the manufacturer of isotretinoin in 1988 and subsequent upgrades (one called iPLEDGE), women are still becoming pregnant while taking the drug. Requiring client registration and negative pregnancy tests before each prescription is dispensed have not eliminated the danger to fetuses.

Women of childbearing age taking isotretinoin should adhere to strict contraceptive protocols, including simultaneous use of two reliable methods. A woman who ceased taking isotretinoin 3 months before becoming pregnant still manifested teratogenic effects: conjoined twins (Malvasi et al, 2009).

In contrast, vitamin A deficiency (VAD) is a greater problem than toxicity in developing countries. VAD is a public health problem in Africa with preschool-age children and women of reproductive age being at the greatest risk (SanJoaquin and Molyneux, 2009). VAD has been associated with night blindness, severe anemia, increased maternal mortality for 1 to 2 years following delivery, and premature and/or LBW deliveries (Mulu, Kassu, Huruy, et al, 2011).

Mineral Needs

For DRIs for minerals during pregnancy and lactation, see Appendix A. For selected minerals during pregnancy and lactation, see Table 10-1.

The trace mineral iron plays a major role in the health of the mother and fetus and therefore appears first in the discussion. Other minerals of special concern in pregnancy are calcium, iodine, fluoride, and zinc.

TABLE 10-3 ■ DRIs for Vitamin A During Pregnancy and Lactation

	RDA		UL	
	MICROGRAMS AS RAEs (RAEs)	IUs	MICROGRAMS AS PREFORMED ONLY	IUs
Pregnancy				
<19 years	750	2475	2800	9240
19–50 years	770	2541	3000	9900
Lactation				
<19 years	1200	3960	2800	9240
19–50 years	1300	4290	3000	9900

DRI, dietary reference intakes; IUs, international units; RAEs, retinol activity equivalents; RDA, recommended dietary allowance.

Iron

For DRIs for minerals during pregnancy and lactation, see Appendix A. For selected minerals during pregnancy and lactation, see Table 10-1.

During pregnancy, the mother's plasma volume increases by about 45% to 50% by the 34th week of gestation, and her red cell mass increases by about 33%. Besides supporting the mother's increased blood volume, iron supports the red blood cells in the fetus, placenta, and umbilical cord. As a result, the net iron cost of a singleton (one fetus) pregnancy is estimated at 1 gram. Even moderate iron deficiency anemia (IDA) is associated with twice the risk of maternal death.

The fetus receives all iron stores from the mother, with 600 mg coming from maternal dietary intake and 400 mg coming from maternal stores (McArdle, Lang, Hayes, and Gamblind, 2011). IDA in the first trimester is associated with greater than a twofold increase in the risk of LBW or preterm delivery (Scholl, 2011). Long-term IDA during pregnancy may cause permanent damage to the brain, which negatively affects intelligence, cognitive abilities, and behavior later in life (Milman, 2012).

Fortunately, the body adjusts to limited or abundant iron sources, and iron absorption is enhanced in the second and third trimesters of pregnancy. Rates of iron absorption vary so that women who begin pregnancy:

- with adequate iron stores, absorb about 10% of ingested iron;
- with low iron stores, absorb about 20%; and
- anemic, absorb about 40%.

The RDA for iron for pregnancy assumes an absorption rate of 20%. The average maternal need for extra iron averages close to 800 mg, elemental iron daily; 300 mg is required for the fetus and the placenta, which will be delivered at the expense of the mother (Gautam, Sahg, Sekhri, and Sahal, 2008). Prophylactic iron at 60 mg per day is recommended by the World Health Organization for all pregnant women for 6 months (Picciano and McGuire, 2009). Even when she takes supplements, a woman's hemoglobin and hematocrit should be monitored regularly. Lower values are expected during the first and second trimesters because expanding blood volume dilutes the concentration of red blood cells.

Prescribed iron supplements may not be taken. Economic factors or side effects, such as nausea, cramps, gas, and constipation, may influence intake. Although oral iron preparations are best absorbed if taken 1 hour before or 2 hours after meals, individualizing the schedule is better than the client choosing to eliminate the supplement altogether. Iron supplements should be taken as directed. Clinical Application 10-1 illustrates the principle of knowing the client as well as the subject matter.

10-1

Clinical Application

Effective Teaching

The facts presented by a health-care provider are often misunderstood by the client or perceived as counter to the client's goals. The following incidents illustrate the point (Galloway and McGuire, 1996).

1. When anemic pregnant women were given iron tablets, they took the supplement until they felt better and then stopped, thinking they were cured. Prevention is a new concept to people in many countries.
2. Anemic pregnant women accepted the notion of iron supplements to correct "too little blood" but were fearful that too much iron would give them too much blood so that they would bleed more extensively at delivery.
3. Presenting the idea that iron would produce bigger babies was a disincentive for anemic pregnant women, who thought they then would face a more difficult labor.

Teaching is more than presenting facts, especially when the goal is changed behavior. Local knowledge and cultural perspective are essential to the health-care provider promoting a new health practice. For instance, it would help to know that some Puerto Rican women are likely to avoid iron as a "hot" food during pregnancy (Purnell, 2013).

Calcium

For DRIs for minerals during pregnancy and lactation, see Appendix A. For selected minerals during pregnancy and lactation, see Table 10-1.

Throughout pregnancy, approximately 30 grams of calcium are transferred to the fetus, most of it in the third trimester. Fetal calcium deposition typically peaks to 350 milligrams per day in the third trimester and maternal absorption increases to meet that demand (Hacker, Fung, and King, 2012). More calcium is absorbed by the intestine during pregnancy because of increased maternal vitamin D to meet the fetus's needs (Mahadevan, Kumaravel, and Bharath, 2012).

Maternal bone loss that occurs to support the demands of pregnancy and lactation are recovered by 1 year postpartum (Hacker et al, 2012). Chapters 7 and 8 describe the effects and interactions of calcium and vitamin D.

Transient osteoporosis is a rare, self-limiting syndrome typically characterized by hip pain in the third trimester of pregnancy accompanied by radiologic osteopenia; other joints may be affected as well. Etiology is unclear, with the left hip more often involved than the right and bilateral hips affected in 25% to 30% of pregnant women. Usual treatment is supportive during the mean duration of 6 to 8 months. The condition usually resolves in 3 to 6 months (Mahadevan et al, 2012).

One study indicates an almost twofold increase of developing postmenopausal osteoporosis in women with a history of adolescent pregnancy (Cho, Shin, Yi, et al, 2012). Some women who develop pregnancy osteoporosis may have genetically determined low peak bone mass that increases their risk for bone loss and the high bone turn over in pregnancy may cause further deterioration (Mahadevan et al, 2012).

Iodine, Fluoride, and Zinc

For DRIs for minerals during pregnancy and lactation, see Appendix A. For selected minerals during pregnancy and lactation, see Table 10-1.

As part of thyroid hormones, iodine is essential to the control of metabolism. During the second half of pregnancy, resting energy expenditure increases by as much as 23%. The RDAs for iodine are increased by 46% and 93% for pregnant and lactating women over those of other women. In the United States, a pregnant woman's usual need for iodine is met by the use of iodized salt. Severe maternal deficiency can cause cretinism in the newborn (see Chapter 8).

The fetus begins to develop teeth at the 10th to 12th week of pregnancy. Fluoride crosses the placenta so that the concentration in fetal circulation is one-fourth that of the mother; fluoride is found in fetal bones and teeth. The American Academy of Pediatric Dentistry (2012) does not support the use of prenatal fluoride supplements. The AI for pregnancy and lactation is the same as for nonpregnant women.

Zinc is not mobilized from the mother's tissues. To provide for the fetus, the mother needs regular intake. Well-balanced diets provide the RDA for women who are pregnant and lactating, and supplementation is not recommended (Ural, 2011). The RDAs for pregnant and lactating women are about 50% higher than those for other women. Lean meat from beef chuck roast, 3.5 to 4 ounces, would provide these RDAs.

Water and Weight Gain

Plasma volume during pregnancy expands by about 50%, necessitating a fluid intake of about 9 cups daily.

The recommended weight gain during pregnancy has varied over the years. Clinical Calculation 10-1 shows how to determine a goal for weight gain in pregnancy based on prepregnancy weight. On average, a woman of normal weight should gain 2 to 4 pounds during the first trimester, followed by 1 pound per week for the remainder of the pregnancy. There are charts that can be used to plot weight gain based on prepregnancy BMI. Examples charts can be found at: www.nal.usda.gov/wicworks/Sharing_Center/NY/ prenatalwt_charts.pdf. Table 10-4 shows the typical

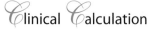 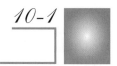

Clinical Calculation   *10-1*

Determining Recommended Weight Gain During Pregnancy

Body mass index (BMI) = Weight in kilograms/Height in meters^2
Suppose a woman is 5 ft, 4 in. tall and weighs 125 lb.

$$5 \text{ ft, 4 in.} = 64 \text{ in.}$$
$$1 \text{ m} = 39.371 \text{ in.}$$
$$\frac{64}{39.371} = 1.6 \text{ m}$$
$$\frac{125 \text{ lb}}{2.2 \text{ lb/kg}} = 56.8 \text{ kg}$$
$$\text{BMI} = \frac{56.8}{(1.6)^2} = \frac{56.8}{2.56} = 22.2$$

Looking at the following table, we see that 22.2 is in the normal category. Recommended weight gain for this woman is 25 to 35 lb.

Recommended Weight Gain for Pregnancy

BMI CATEGORY	KILOGRAMS	POUNDS
<18.5 = underweight	12.5–18	28–40
18.5–24.9 = normal	11.5–16	25–35
25–29.9 = overweight	7–11.5	15–25
>30 = obese	6.8	15

Short women and women of various racial or ethnic groups should follow the same recommendations. Teenagers who are pregnant should also use BMI as a guide to weight gain.

distribution of pounds between the baby and the mother's tissues.

Many women receive no nutritional gestational weight gain advice, and one study shows that overweight and underweight women were more likely than normal weight or obese women to receive incorrect advice (Groth and Kearney, 2009). Gaining less than recommended is associated with fetal growth retardation, low birth weight, and increased **perinatal mortality.**

TABLE 10-4 ■ Here's How It All Adds Up	
Baby	7–8 pounds
Amniotic fluid	2 pounds
Placenta	1 ¹/₂ pounds
Increased blood volume	3–4 pounds
Increase fluid volume	3–4 pounds
Increased weight of uterus	2 pounds
Breasts	2 pounds
Mother's fat stores	6–8 pounds
Total	**25–35 pounds**

Source: Adapted from Mayo Clinic Pregnancy Week by Week (2011).

Nearly half of normal weight and two-thirds of overweight women have been found to exceed weight gain guidelines, which increases the risk of childhood and adolescent obesity, weight gain, and obesity in the mother (Phelan, Phipps, Abrams, et al, 2011). Excessive weight gain during pregnancy is associated with increased risk of gestational diabetes, **caesarean deliveries,** and postpartum infections (Phillips, 2012).

Meal Pattern

Mature women who become pregnant require relatively few modifications in MyPlate recommendations for adults.

Except for iron, MyPlate recommendations should suffice for healthy women. Healthy People 2020 recommend that women who are capable of becoming pregnant choose food high in heme iron and take an iron supplement as needed. Pregnant women should eat a diet that is varied in fruits, vegetables, lean proteins, and whole grains to ensure adequate nutrient consumption.

Pregnant teenagers need nutrients to provide for their own growth as well as that of the fetus. A client, 16 years old, weighing 120 pounds who is physically active 30 to 60 minutes per day would require additional grains, vegetables, and meat/beans in the second and third trimesters. Clinical Application 10-2 relates the particular hazards of teenage pregnancy.

Women of dissimilar ages, sizes, and lifestyles would require different intakes. Individualized meal planning based on age, height, prepregnancy weight, and activity level is available at www.choosemyplate.gov/SuperTracker/myplan.aspx.

Clinical Application   *10-2*

Teenage Pregnancy

The average girl does not reach her full height or attain gynecologic maturity until age 17. When pregnant before that age, she is still growing but has a fetus to nourish as well. Infants born to still-growing adolescents, weigh an average of 155 grams (0.3 lb) less than those born to adult women. Rates of spontaneous abortion, preterm delivery, and low birth weight are higher in growing than in nongrowing adolescents.

All women of childbearing age, including adolescents, who were overweight or obese before becoming pregnant, have increased risks of **cesarean delivery,** hypertension, gestational diabetes, and stillbirth (Zera, McGirr, and Oken, 2011).

Because many pregnant adolescents have low incomes, referral to appropriate sources of assistance is a crucial part of their nutritional care.

Careful food selection is critical for all pregnant women but especially for pregnant teens who may have unbalanced diets and for women who restrict or eliminate whole categories of food such as vegetarians. Thorough nutritional assessment, ideally before pregnancy or at least very early in pregnancy, could yield huge dividends by decreasing complications and improving newborns' health. Dollars & Sense 10-1 describes some food assistance programs available to improve nutrition.

Substances to Avoid

While pregnant or nursing, women are urged to limit caffeine intake and to eliminate these items from their diets:

- Alcohol
- Soft cheeses and ready-to-eat meats
- Certain species and amounts of fish
- Undercooked meat and unwashed produce

Serious allergies to nuts and seeds affect less than 1% of the population. See Chapter 11 for information on food allergies. The American Academy of Pediatrics currently does not recommend dietary restrictions for the purpose of protecting children from allergies during pregnancy or lactation (2008).

Alcohol

A pregnant woman who drinks alcoholic beverages is endangering her baby because alcohol readily crosses the placenta, and the fetus has inadequate enzymes to detoxify it. The amniotic fluid also acts as a reservoir for alcohol, which prolongs fetal exposure (Pinto and Schub, 2012). Alcohol use during pregnancy accounts for the leading preventable cause of birth defects and developmental disabilities (CDC, July 12, 2012). The fetus is most vulnerable during the first trimester when basic structural development occurs.

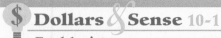

$ **Dollars** & **Sense** 10-1

Food Assistance

Supplemental food assistance is available for families in the Supplemental Nutrition Assistance Program (**SNAP**) and for women and children in the **Supplemental Feeding Program for Women, Infants, and Children (WIC).** The latter program served 9.17 million people in 2010, including 4.86 million children and 2.14 million infants. It provides supplemental foods monthly to low-income pregnant or postpartum women, infants, and children up to age 5. WIC is available in all 50 states plus 40 other territories and jurisdictions (U.S. Department of Agriculture [USDA], 2011).

First recognized in 1973, **fetal alcohol syndrome (FAS)** is most easily diagnosed between the ages of 4 and 14. FAS has specific diagnostic criteria:

■ Three characteristic facial features: smooth philtrum, thin upper lip, and short palpebral fissures (Fig. 10-1)
■ Prenatal and postnatal growth deficits
■ Central nervous system abnormalities, such as head circumference at or below the 10th percentile, neurological problems, or functional deficits

In 1996, the term *fetal alcohol spectrum disorder* was introduced to encompass several diagnostic categories covering the wider range of alcohol effects in infants and children that do not meet the criteria for FAS.

Because researchers have not been able to determine safe levels of alcohol during pregnancy, women should be encouraged to abstain. The task of protecting the unborn is formidable. One of the goals of Healthy People 2020 is to increase the percentage of pregnant women abstaining from alcohol use to 98% (CDC, July 12, 2012). Despite warnings on the effects alcohol can have on fetal development and outcomes, one of eight women in the United States continues to drink during her pregnancy (Bakhireva and Savage, 2011). One study demonstrated the prevalence of binge drinking was 15% among nonpregnant women and 1.4% among pregnant women (CDC, July 12, 2012).

Approximately 50% of pregnancies in the United States are unplanned, for women engaging in risky drinking behaviors and not using effective contraceptive methods the risk of FAS is increased. Brief interventions by health-care providers have succeeded in reducing such risks (CDC, July 12, 2012). Information on prenatal alcohol screening and intervention programs is available at:

www.cdc.gov/ncbddd/fas
www.fascenter.samhsa.gov

In addition, curricular materials for parents, educators, and juvenile justice workers are available at:

www.cdc.gov/NCBDDD/fasd/freematerials.html

Soft Cheeses and Ready-to-Eat Meats

Listeriosis is a bacterial foodborne illness caused by *Listeria monocytogenes*. For the mother, the symptoms of listeriosis tend to mild and flulike, but the bacteria can be passed via the placenta to the fetus resulting in spontaneous abortion, premature delivery, stillbirth, neonatal meningitis, and septicemia (Smith and MacLaurin, 2011). Listeriosis is rare, but has a high mortality rate of 20% to 30 % (Allerberger and Wagner, 2010).

The organism can grow at refrigeration temperatures so foods that are concerning are foods that are chilled and consumed without preheating or cooking (Amar, Little, Gillespie, et al, 2012). Outbreaks of listeriosis have been associated with raw or contaminated milk, soft cheeses, smoked seafood, sprouts, and ready-to-eat meats. Widespread outbreaks have occurred affecting:

■ 22 people in 14 states, with 2 adult deaths and 1 spontaneous abortion, traced to ricotta salata cheese from a single packing plant (CDC, 2012a) and
■ 139 people in 28 states, with 29 deaths and 1 spontaneous abortion, caused by contaminated cantaloupes from a farm in Colorado (CDC, 2012b).

The **incubation period** may be 3 to 70 days after a person has eaten the contaminated food. In addition to the general rules for safe food handling, pregnant women should:

■ Avoid soft cheeses (feta, Brie, Camembert, blue-veined, and Mexican-style cheese like queso fresco). However, hard cheeses, processed cheeses, cream cheese, cottage cheese, and yogurt may be eaten safely. Eat only cheeses that are labeled as made with pasteurized milk.
■ Cook leftover foods or ready-to-eat foods (hot dogs, sausage, deli meats) until steaming hot (165°F).
■ Not eat refrigerated meat spreads at all or refrigerated smoked seafood without cooking it.
■ Not consume unpasteurized milk or foods made from it.
■ Refrigerate foods within 2 hours and use leftovers within 3 to 4 days.
■ Use a thermometer and keep the refrigerator at 40°F or lower and the freezer at 0°F or lower.

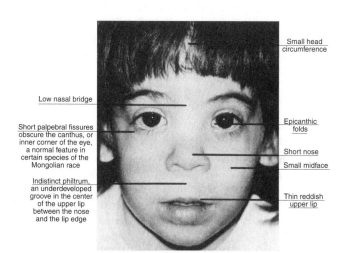

Small head circumference

Low nasal bridge

Short palpebral fissures obscure the canthus, or inner corner of the eye, a normal feature in certain species of the Mongolian race

Epicanthic folds

Short nose

Small midface

Indistinct philtrum, an underdeveloped groove in the center of the upper lip between the nose and the lip edge

Thin reddish upper lip

FIGURE 10-1 Specific facial signs of fetal alcohol syndrome include microcephaly, or small head size; small eyes and/or short eye openings; and an underdeveloped upper lip with flat upper lip ridges. (Reprinted from Feldmen, EB: *Essentials of clinical nutrition.* FA Davis, Philadelphia, 1988, p. 164, with permission.)

Certain Species and Amounts of Fish

Fish and shellfish can be a major source **of methylmercury,** a widespread environmental neurotoxin that can be harmful to fetal brain development (Mahaffey, Sunderland, Chan, et al, 2011). Because of high levels of mercury in some species of fish (those that grow larger and live longer), the Food and Drug Administration (FDA) and the Environmental Protection Agency have advised pregnant women and women who may become pregnant, nursing mothers, and young children to avoid eating:

- Shark
- Swordfish
- King mackerel
- Tilefish

If chosen as the week's seafood meals, albacore tuna or tuna steak should be limited to 6 ounces per week, whereas up to 12 ounces per week may be consumed of species of seafood with lower amounts of mercury:

- Shrimp
- Canned light tuna
- Salmon
- Pollock
- Catfish

Fish sticks and fish sandwiches at fast food restaurants generally contain species with lower amounts of mercury. Local advisories should be sought to determine the safety of recreationally caught fish. Women can find fish consumption advisories at: http://water.epa.gov/scitech/swguidance/fishshellfish/fishadvisories.

Developing nervous tissue is at particular risk, hence the warning regarding pregnant women and young children. Effects of methylmercury can include:

- Fetal abnormalities
- Microcephaly
- Severe mental and physical retardation
- Visuomotor abilities
- Memory and attention (Karagas, Choi, Oken, et al, 2012)

Over time, the body eliminates mercury, but it can accumulate in the body faster than it can be removed.

Undercooked Meat, Unwashed Produce, and Cat Litter

Health-care providers should reinforce the principles of food hygiene to pregnant women. An infection with *Toxoplasma gondii*, a harmful parasite, causes an estimated 400 to 4000 cases of congenital **toxoplasmosis** annually, producing:

- Mental retardation
- Blindness
- Epilepsy

The wide range of the estimate occurs because the disease is not nationally reportable or widely recognized as a threat by pregnant women. Only 48% of mothers of affected infants recognized risk factors of the disease, a situation that could possibly have been prevented by education.

The diagnosis is made through serological testing for *Toxoplasma* immunoglobulin (Ig)G, IgM, and IgA antibodies (Rahbari, Keshavarz, Shojaee, et al, 2012). Mothers who contract the disease are often asymptomatic, but the risk of transmitting to the fetus remains. Currently in the United States, there is not universal screening of pregnant women. Treatment of congenital toxoplasmosis has been shown to reduce the severity of symptoms and improve outcomes (Stillwaggon, Carrier, Sautter, and McLeod, 2011). The protozoan is spread via undercooked meat, unwashed fruits and vegetables, contaminated soil, and cat feces. To prevent the infection, pregnant women should:

- Cook meat, poultry, and seafood thoroughly.
- Clean items that those raw foods have contacted with hot soapy water.
- Peel or meticulously wash raw fruits and vegetables before eating.
- Keep cats indoors and feed them only cooked food or prepared cat food.
- Avoid changing cat litter or, if not possible, use mask and gloves and wash hands carefully afterward.
- Use a thermometer and keep the refrigerator at 40°F or lower and the freezer at 0°F or lower.

The FDA has compiled an extensive free educational kit on food safety for pregnant women and medical professionals. Available in English and Spanish, topics include methylmercury, *Listeria*, and *Toxoplasma*. Health educators can learn how to obtain the materials at www.fda.gov/downloads/Food/ResourcesForYou/HealthEducators/UCM094856.pdf.

Caffeine

Caffeine metabolism decreases progressively from the first to third trimester, with a doubling of the half-life of caffeine, which results in a higher concentration in the fetus (Maslova, Bhattacharya, Lin, and Michels, 2010). There have been numerous studies regarding the ingestion of caffeine and the effects on pregnancy with inconsistent results. Studies suggest that caffeine may be consumed during pregnancy but should be limited to no more than 200 mg per day (Phillips, 2012).

Overall, caffeine intake of less than 300 mg per day is unlikely to delay conception or to increase the risk of spontaneous abortion or birth defects.

Problems and Complications of Pregnancy Affecting Nutrition

The physiological changes that take place in a woman's body during pregnancy may cause a variety of conditions. Some of the common problems, such as morning sickness and leg cramps, are usually annoying but only occasionally require medical intervention. Other conditions, such as hypertensive disorders of pregnancy and gestational diabetes, can be hazardous and demand medical intervention.

Common Problems

Four of the most common problems of pregnancy are:

1. Morning sickness
2. Leg cramps
3. Constipation
4. Heartburn
5. Pica

MORNING SICKNESS

Hormonal changes, some which produce relaxed gastrointestinal muscle tone, cause the nausea and vomiting of pregnancy. About 70% to 85% of pregnant women experience nausea and vomiting during pregnancy, but only 17% actually experience the symptoms only in the morning (Summers, 2012). Compared with women without morning sickness, women who have it consumed significantly less meat and more carbohydrate in the first trimester, differences that were maintained throughout the pregnancies. In addition, the women with morning sickness delivered a half week earlier than those without it (Latva-Pukkila, Isolauri, and Laitinen, 2010).

The occurrence and duration of these events vary widely, and they are not confined to mornings. Control of the problem without medication is the goal. Eating dry crackers before getting out of bed is the classic preventive. Other suggestions are as follows:

- Avoid fatty foods.
- Eat fruits and complex carbohydrates in small, frequent meals.
- Consume cold foods rather than hot foods.
- Drink liquids between rather than with meals.
- Eat a high-protein snack at bedtime.

In most cases, morning sickness subsides after the first trimester. With the usual caution regarding herbal products (see Chapter 15), ginger can be used as a first-line therapy for nausea and vomiting (Nayeri, 2012). Vitamin B_6 can be used to reduce the severity of nausea and thiamine should be part of standard care for clients with greater than 3 weeks of vomiting (Summers, 2012).

LEG CRAMPS

Pregnant women often complain of leg cramps. One cause may be neuromuscular irritability due to low serum calcium, but the evidence that supplemental calcium reduces cramping is weak. Because of its close link to calcium metabolism, magnesium deficiency has been postulated to cause leg cramps. Magnesium salts compared with placebo may be more effective at 3 weeks at reducing leg cramps (Young, 2009).

Staying well hydrated is of primary importance, followed by maintaining adequate intakes of potassium, sodium, calcium, and magnesium. A noninvasive procedure to prevent muscle cramps is to stretch the muscles before exercise and, for nighttime cramps, before bedtime.

CONSTIPATION

Decreased gastrointestinal muscle tone, increased water absorption from the intestines, and the growing uterus pressing on the intestines cause constipation, which can affect up to 38% of pregnant women (Trottier, Erebara, and Bozzo, 2012). Adequate fluid intake, regular exercise, and a high-fiber diet should relieve this condition. Ideally, the suggested amount of fiber intake, 30 grams per day, should be achieved with food rather than pharmaceutical preparations. Foods high in fiber but relatively low in kilocalories are listed in Table 10-5. Women experiencing constipation

TABLE 10-5 ■ Nutrient-Dense Foods High in Fiber			
FOOD	QUANTITY	GRAMS OF DIETARY FIBER	KILOCALORIES
Grains			
All Bran	½ cup	9	81
Bran buds	⅓ cup	13	75
100% Bran	⅓ cup	8	83
Fruits			
Apple, raw with skin, chopped	1 cup	3	65
Orange sections, raw	1 cup	4	85
Pear, raw with skin	One small	5	86
Prunes, cooked, unsweetened	½ cup	4	133
Vegetables/Legumes			
Baked beans, in tomato sauce with pork	½ cup	5	116
Brussels sprouts, cooked from frozen	1 cup	6	65
Kidney beans, canned	½ cup	7	108
Navy beans, cooked from dry	½ cup	10	128
Green peas, cooked from frozen	½ cup	4	62

during pregnancy are also encouraged to increase daily water intake and participate in moderate amounts of activity daily.

HEARTBURN

A burning sensation beneath the breastbone is called heartburn. Hormonal changes cause relaxation of the cardiac sphincter, located between the esophagus and the stomach. That and the upward pressure on the diaphragm from the enlarging uterus can cause reflux of gastric contents into the esophagus and the burning sensation.

Avoiding spicy or acidic foods and taking small, frequent meals can control heartburn. Other helpful measures include sitting up for an hour after a meal as well as elevating the head while sleeping. Pregnant women should not self-medicate with sodium bicarbonate or antacids. The bicarbonate can be absorbed, producing alkalosis. Antacids decrease iron absorption by decreasing gastric acids, thus increasing the risk of anemia.

PICA

Pica is the compulsive ingestion of nonfood items, usually dirt, clay, laundry starch, baking soda, or ice. It is an ancient behavior and a regional practice that is mainly influenced by culture. Most notable in some regions of the southern United States, pica occurs in conjunction with inadequate diets due to poverty, but it also occurs in women at other socioeconomic levels. Many women with pica have it only during pregnancy, believing it cures the annoyances of pregnancy or ensures a beautiful baby. Others contend that the substances they ingest taste good to them.

Health concerns about pica include:

- Inadequate nutrition due to substitution of nonfood items for nutritious foods
- Iron-deficiency anemia
- Constipation
- Lead poisoning

Nutritional deficiencies that may be associated with pica are iron, calcium and zinc. Iron deficiency is most commonly seen in women who report eating clay (Cooper, 2010). Lead is also a concern for women who report eating dirt or lead-based paint. Lead poisoning can cause irreversible neurological damage (Cooper, 2010).

Women who have migrated to an area where pica is uncommon may continue the custom. A caring, nonjudgmental interviewer may encourage a woman to reveal that she has a craving for and is eating nonfood items. The interview could lead to preventive therapy and a teaching opportunity.

Complications of Pregnancy

Three complications of pregnancy with nutritional ramifications are:

- Hyperemesis gravidarum
- Hypertensive disorders of pregnancy
- Gestational diabetes

HYPEREMESIS GRAVIDARUM

Severe nausea and vomiting persisting after the 14th week of pregnancy is called **hyperemesis gravidarum.** Its incidence is reported to be higher in multiple pregnancies and other conditions associated with increased pregnancy hormone levels. The etiology and pathogenesis are unknown. It develops most often in Western countries and in first pregnancies.

Hospitalization will occur in approximately 1% to 5% of women with hyperemesis for the treatment of:

- Severe dehydration
- Electrolyte imbalance
- Weight loss greater than 5%
- Ketonuria
- Muscle wasting (Wegrzyniak, Repke, and Ural, 2012)

Major vitamin deficiencies have resulted from hyperemesis gravidarum:

- Hyponatremia can cause symptoms of headache, nausea, and vomiting.
- Deficiencies of vitamins B_6 and B_{12} can result in peripheral neuropathy.
- Deficiency of thiamine has caused Wernicke encephalopathy in pregnant clients (Summers, 2012).

See Chapters 7 and 20 for information on Wernicke encephalopathy. Sometimes this disease has resulted in fatal outcomes in the mother or the fetus (Nayeri, 2012). Prophylactic thiamine supplementation should be considered in the care of hyperemesis (Wegrzyniak et al, 2012).

Hyperemesis gravidarum requires treatment for the health of the woman and the fetus. Studies show that women with hyperemesis gravidarum were more likely to deliver babies who were small for gestational age or delivered before 37 weeks compared with women without hyperemesis (Wegrzyniak et al, 2012). Many approaches have been used to treat hyperemesis gravidarum:

- Pyridoxine
- Ginger
- Rehydration
- Enteral and parenteral nutritional support
- Antiemetics (without teratogenic effects)
- Corticosteroid therapy

HYPERTENSIVE DISORDERS OF PREGNANCY

Hypertensive disorders affect 7% to 9% of pregnancies (Magee, Abalos, von Dadelszen, et al, 2011) and include:

- Chronic hypertension
- Gestational hypertension
- Preeclampsia
- Eclampsia

Hypertension is blood pressure greater than 140 mm Hg systolic or greater than 90 mm Hg diastolic. Fetal complications include growth restriction, prematurity, and stillbirth. Distinctions among the categories and a summary of risks, pathophysiology, and treatments follow.

- *Chronic hypertension* existed before pregnancy—or is diagnosed in retrospect when gestational hypertension or the hypertension of preeclampsia does not resolve after delivery. Complications that can develop associated with chronic hypertension are preterm birth and LBW babies (Shennan and Vousden, 2010).
- *Gestational hypertension* occurs after 20 weeks of gestation without proteinuria. Approximately 14% to 45% of these women will develop preeclampsia (Mustafa, Ahmed, Gupta, and Venuto, 2012).
- **Preeclampsia** occurs after 20 weeks of pregnancy with proteinuria. It affects 3% to 8% of pregnant women in the United States (Uzan, Carbonnel, Piconee, et al, 2011). Risk factors for preeclampsia include:
  - First pregnancy
  - Multiple fetuses
  - Mother older than 35 years
  - African American race
  - Obesity
  - History of preeclampsia
  - Chronic hypertension.
- **Eclampsia** is the occurrence in preeclamptic women of seizures not attributable to another cause. It is an obstetrical emergency. The woman requires intensive care because she is at high risk for cerebral hemorrhage, circulatory collapse, and kidney failure. The fetus, too, is in grave danger.

All forms of hypertension in pregnancy are related to inflammation, **oxidative stress,** and endothelium dysfunction, which results in Hemolysis, Elevated Liver enzymes and Low Platelet count syndrome (HELLP; Uzan et al, 2011). A review of some genetic factors related to preeclampsia appears as Genomic Gem 10-2.

Definitive treatment of preeclampsia, aside from delivery of the fetus and placenta, awaits elucidation of its cause. Without question, careful monitoring of pregnant women and early intervention is crucial.

Although delivery is the only treatment for preeclampsia, risk for complications continues after delivery. For both prophylaxis against and treatment of eclampsia,

Genomic Gem 10-2
Susceptibility to Preeclampsia

Transmission of genetic risk factors for preeclampsia can occur through the mother or the father. The risk of fathering a preeclamptic pregnancy is increased in men who fathered a preeclamptic pregnancy with a different partner and also men who are born from a preeclamptic pregnancy (Mustafa et al, 2012). There is a twofold to fivefold higher risk of preeclampsia in pregnant women with a history of the disorder (Uzan et al, 2011).

A contributor to the development of preeclampsia is poor placental development. As the pregnancy continues, maternal endothelial dysfunction occurs. Genetic explanations are still being proposed. Although preeclampsia is thought to originate in the placenta, the maternal endothelium is most affected (Mustafa et al, 2012). An exaggerated inflammatory response to pregnancy may occur in genetically susceptible women. Those who were homozygous for a particular allele had the greatest risk for preeclampsia. Black women with preeclampsia were more than three times as likely as normotensive black women to have certain combinations of alleles; white women were twice as likely. Other inflammatory factors such as bacterial and viral infections may exaggerate the normal inflammatory response to pregnancy.

magnesium sulfate has been used for decades and the reduction of maternal and neonatal complications are well established (Uzan et al, 2011).

Long-term health effects have emerged after hypertensive disorders of pregnancy. Preeclampsia can continue to affect women 20 to 30 years after the delivery, when these women have increased cardiovascular mortality rates. Women with a history of preeclampsia are at a significantly increase risk to develop hypertension, ischemic heart disease, stroke, type 2 diabetes, and venous thromboembolism compared with women without history of the disease (Mustafa et al, 2012).

GESTATIONAL DIABETES

The emergence of diabetes in pregnancy, **gestational diabetes,** is considered to be a form of type 2 diabetes (see Chapter 17) that usually appears between weeks 24 and 28 of gestation when an increase in insulin resistance occurs (Cheung, 2009). It affects 5% of pregnancies, and its incidence is increasing with the global increase in obesity and type 2 diabetes (Rice, Illanes, and Mitchell, 2012).

Among these changes is the production of hormones by the placenta that decrease insulin sensitivity and increase insulin resistance in the mother to ensure a constant, optimum level of glucose for the fetus. When the mother's insulin supply is inadequate or ineffective, her high blood glucose is transferred to the fetus, who secretes his own insulin to lower the glucose content of his blood by converting it to fat, hence the hallmark result of diabetes in pregnant women: large newborns.

Risk factors for gestational diabetes are:

- Occurrence of gestational diabetes in a previous pregnancy
- Previous delivery of an infant weighing more than 9 pounds
- Family history of diabetes
- Maternal obesity (greater than 120% of ideal body weight)

Most women return to normal glucose levels after delivery; however, these same women are at a greater risk of developing type 2 diabetes in 15 to 20 years. Lifestyle modifications, aiming for a 5% to 7% reduction in body weight and participating in exercise regimes are two interventions that can be effective in the prevention of developing type 2 diabetes (Cheung, 2009).

Treatment of gestational diabetes, requiring an aggressive team approach, is included in Chapter 17. The cornerstone of treatment is diet therapy and women should be referred for dietary therapy. Because insulin does not cross the placenta, insulin is the recommended method of controlling blood glucose during pregnancy when dietary approaches alone have failed (Cheung, 2009).

The Breastfeeding Mother

The goals of Healthy People 2020 is to increase breastfeeding rates to:

- 82% of mothers who ever breastfeed
- 60% of those who breastfeed until the infant is 6 months old
- 34% of those who breastfeed until the infant is 1 year old

Initiation of breastfeeding rates in the United States continue to rise going from 74.6% in 2008 to 76.9% in 2009, exceeding the Healthy People 2010 goal. Mexican American and non-Hispanic whites exceeded the goal, but just 65% of non-Hispanic black infants were ever breastfed, still a significant increase from 36% in 1993–1994.

Breastfeeding rates varied greatly within the Mexican American community. When *immigrant* is defined as born outside of the United States, 59% of Mexican immigrant mothers breastfed for at least 6 months compared with 24% of Mexican nonimmigrants. Hispanic women who are more acculturated are two times less likely to breastfeed than less-acculturated women (Faraz, 2010). Figure 10-2 shows the percentage of 6-month-old infants by race/ethnicity being breastfed in the United States from 2000 through 2008. Chapter 11 covers the advantages of breast milk for the infant.

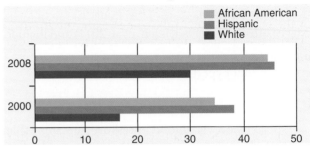

Breastfeeding Rates

FIGURE 10-2 U.S. breastfeeding rates, 2000–2008: percentage of infants who were still breastfed at 6 months of age by race/ethnicity group. (*Source:* Centers for Disease Control, February 8, 2013; *MMWR*, Progress in increasing breastfeeding and reducing racial/ethnic differences—United States, 2000–2008. Available at: www.cdc.gov/mmwr/preview/mmwrhtml/mm6205a1.htm?s_cid=mm6205a1_w.)

Nutritional Needs

For DRIs during pregnancy and lactation, see Appendix A. For selected energy nutrients and minerals, see Table 10-1.

MyPlate recommendations are for the mother to enter a "Daily Food Plan for Moms" to individualize an eating plan while following the general MyPlate recommendations. The site can be found at: www.choosemyplate.gov/supertracker-tools/daily-food-plans/moms.html.

A common recommendation for the breastfeeding woman is to drink a glass of fluid with meals and to limit caffeinated beverages to two to three cups per day.

Calcium

The primary source of calcium in human milk is calcium resorbed from the mother's bones, a process that is not prevented by increased calcium intake from foods or supplements. Moreover, the lost skeletal calcium is rapidly replaced after weaning with complete recovery occurring in most women even with closely spaced pregnancies and long periods of lactation. Bone formation occurs rapidly and density normalizes within 2 to 6 months of weaning (Mahadevan et al, 2012).

Mobilization of calcium from the mother's bones also frees sequestered lead. Release of maternal bone lead stores into the circulation can lead to lead transfer to the fetus (Ettinger et al, 2009). Meeting daily calcium requirement can decrease maternal lead levels in both circulation and breast milk (Ettinger, Lamadrid-Figueroa, Tellez-Rojo, et al, 2009).

Energy

The average lactating woman produces 26 ounces of milk daily, but the amount varies greatly. Emptying the breast stimulates more milk production. Breast milk contains about 20 kilocalories per ounce, now the standard for term infant formulas (see Chapter 11). Some of the energy for the milk comes from the mother's dietary intake, some from fat stores accumulated during pregnancy.

Effect of Maternal Deficiencies

The mammary gland can extract most nutrients from the circulation so that breast milk may contain adequate levels of nutrients even when the mother's intake is inadequate. Levels of water-soluble vitamins in human milk depend on maternal intake, and evidence suggests that the mammary gland may take priority in folate use over the mother's own blood-forming needs. Persistent maternal vitamin deficiencies, however, may result in inadequate concentrations in the milk. For instance, vitamin B_{12} deficiency in vegetarian mothers has caused neurological impairment, failure to thrive, and developmental regression in their breastfeeding infants (Linville, Ritchie, and Novak, 2012). Vitamin B_{12} deficiency can cause irreversible neurologic damage in infancy before diagnosis (CDC, 2012).

In contrast, the concentrations of the major minerals in human milk do not correspond to the mother's blood levels, but the trace mineral iodine is dependent on maternal dietary intake (Leung, Perarce, and Braverman, 2011). As recounted in Chapter 8, iodine is critical for normal neurological development and is the one mineral, along with vitamins thiamin, riboflavin, vitamins B_6 and B_{12}, and vitamin A, categorized as priority nutrients. Because low maternal intake or stores of these nutrients are reflected in human milk, supplementing the lactating mother can restore her milk to adequate levels thus providing a healthier intake for the nursing infant.

Benefits to the Mother

Several advantages to the mother are associated with breastfeeding. Breast milk is less expensive than formula (Dollars & Sense 10-2) and is always ready at the correct temperature. Contamination during formula making is usually not a concern. Nursing the infant encourages the new mother to sit down several times a day. On the other hand, without pumping her breasts and storing the milk (see Chapter 11), the task of feeding the infant is hers alone.

Breastfeeding has unique advantages:

1. Helps the uterus return to its nonpregnant state more quickly.
2. Assists in birth spacing under certain conditions.
3. May be protective against later breast cancer.

$ Dollars & Sense 10-2

Savings With Breastfeeding

Breastfeeding is less costly than bottle-feeding. The additional foods the mother consumes are less expensive than infant formula, which may cost a family $700 the first year. In addition to individual benefits, breastfeeding can help the environment by reducing costs and waste associated with formula production, marketing, and distribution.

Aids Uterine Involution

During breastfeeding, the sucking of the infant stimulates the release of **oxytocin** from the posterior pituitary gland in the brain. Oxytocin causes the uterine muscles to contract and helps return the uterus to its nonpregnant size while reducing postpartum blood loss.

Assists in Birth Spacing

The effectiveness of **lactational amenorrhea (LAM)** was found to be 98% effective in women who remained amenorrheic provided that the infant is fully breastfed and is less than 6 months old (Garad, McNamee, Bateson, and Harvey, 2012). LAM was found to be less effective if expressed milk was used routinely. Consequently, breastfeeding is not suggested as the sole means of birth spacing if other methods are available and acceptable to the client. Because estrogen inhibits lactation, means of contraception other than those containing estrogen are advised if the woman continues to breastfeed.

Lessens Risk of Cancer

Over the long term, breastfeeding has been associated with a decreased risk of breast cancer later in life, especially among premenopausal women. Studies report a 4.3% reduction in breast cancer for every 12 months of breastfeeding and a 32% reduction in risk for BRCA1 mutation carriers (Kotsopoulous, Lubinski, Salmena, et al, 2012). Less-convincing evidence suggests an association between breastfeeding duration appears to be associated with a reduction in the risk of maternal ovarian cancer (Jordan, Siskind, Green, 2010). Some of the factors in cancer's complex etiology are described in Chapter 21.

Techniques of Breastfeeding

The medical and nursing staff will assist the mother to start breastfeeding her infant. Even mothers of twins and premature babies can successfully breastfeed with additional education and support. Some general principles to aid in breastfeeding have been established.

The mother and infant should be permitted to spend as much time together as possible during the first 24 hours after birth. This practice permits bonding of infant and mother. Some areas encourage fathers to "room in" also to bond with the baby.

One correct position for breastfeeding is shown in Figure 10-3. It is "tummy-to-tummy." The infant should face the breast squarely. If the breast is very large, the mother must take care to prevent it from blocking the infant's nose lest it impede infant's breathing. When nursing, the infant should grasp the entire areola (the colored portion around the nipple) to prevent the nipples from becoming sore.

Most infants will take 80% to 90% of the milk from each breast in the first 4 minutes of nursing. Because nursing stimulates further milk production, the mother should alternate which breast she offers first to start the feeding. This technique will stimulate further milk production because a breast that baby has completely drained will produce milk at a faster rate than one that has only been partially emptied. Allowing the baby to nurse on one breast at each feeding allows the baby to receive both foremilk and hindmilk.

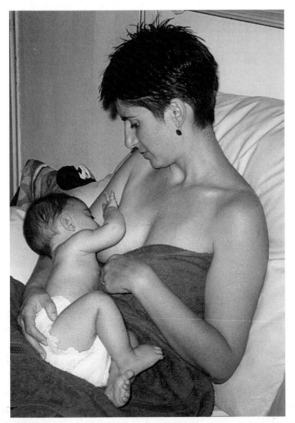

FIGURE 10-3 One correct breastfeeding position, "tummy-to-tummy." The infant takes the entire areola in its mouth. Notice how focused the mother is on the baby.

Encouraging Breastfeeding

Pediatricians are encouraged to provide information on the benefits and methods of breastfeeding so that the mother can make an informed choice. Prenatal encouragement increases breastfeeding rates and identifies potential problem areas.

Hospital and birthing center practices should focus on rooming in, early and frequent breastfeeding, skilled support, and avoidance of artificial nipples, pacifiers, and formula. Infants should be assessed while nursing at 2 to 4 days of age, with liberal use of referral, including lactation consultants (Weddig, Baker, and Auld, 2011). Box 10-2 summarizes a program to increase breastfeeding worldwide.

Knowledge of and respect for a family's cultural traditions will assist the health-care provider when promoting breastfeeding. For instance, one group of Native

---

Box 10-2 ■ *The Baby-Friendly Hospital Initiative*

The Baby-Friendly Hospital Initiative (BFHI) is a global UNICEF/World Health Organization (WHO)–sponsored effort to promote breastfeeding. As of 2012, 149 U.S. hospitals and birthing centers in 34 states are designated Baby-Friendly (Baby-Friendly, 2012). This is currently 5.8%, which is below the Healthy People 2020 goal of 8%.

WHO and UNICEF recommend implementing the following practices in every facility providing maternity services and care for newborn infants:

Ten Steps to Successful Breastfeeding

1. Have a written breastfeeding policy routinely communicated to all health-care staff.
2. Train all health-care staff in skills necessary to implement this policy.
3. Inform all pregnant women about the benefits and management of breastfeeding.
4. Help mothers initiate breastfeeding within a half hour (United States, 1 hour) of birth.
5. Show mothers how to breastfeed and how to maintain lactation even if they are separated from their infants.
6. Give infants no food or drink other than breast milk unless medically indicated.
7. Practice rooming-in: allow mothers and infants to remain together 24 hours a day.
8. Encourage unrestricted breastfeeding.
9. Give no pacifiers or artificial nipples to breastfeeding infants.
10. Foster the establishment of breastfeeding support groups and refer mothers to them on discharge from the hospital or clinic (Baby-Friendly, 2012).

In addition, Baby-Friendly institutions are expected to abide by the WHO International Code of Marketing of Breast Milk Substitutes that forbids accepting free formula or other gifts and grants from formula producers. Distributing sample packs of formula or literature bearing the name of a formula product to breastfeeding mothers is also not permitted (CDC Vital Signs, 2011).

Americans saw breastfeeding as the "natural way" or even as a moral choice calling it the "right way" to feed a baby. Decision making in this and other traditional societies involves not just the mother but also the family and the community.

Adoptive mothers have successfully breastfed their infants by using physical stimulation and breast pumps to establish a milk supply. A breastfeeding supplementary system, the Lact-Aid or Medla SNS Nursing Trainer System, are available to provide additional milk while the infant is nursing at the breast. Compelling stories of women who have breastfed adopted infants offer encouragement to others (Adoptive Breastfeeding Resource, 2008).

On the other hand, overselling of the benefits and ease of breastfeeding has resulted in starvation deaths of infants (see Chapter 11). Not only should the mother's choice be respected and supported, but also the infant's condition should be monitored appropriately regardless of the feeding method chosen.

Maternal Contraindications to Breastfeeding

Most women can feed their infants at breast. A few contraindications to breastfeeding include the mother's use of illegal drugs and certain medications, particular illnesses in the mother, and the mother's exposure to toxic chemicals. **Galactosemia,** an absolute contraindication due to a metabolic defect in the infant, is covered in Chapter 11.

Medication Use

Mothers are sometimes counseled to interrupt breastfeeding or to wean the infant, without a compelling medical reason (Jones and Breward, 2010). Although many medications the mother takes are secreted in breast milk, most do not affect the milk supply or the infant when taken in recommended doses. The great majority of antidepressants are safe during breastfeeding, but controversies remain that may cause women to stop breastfeeding prematurely (Davanzo, Copertino, De Cunto, et al, 2010).

Particularly if the medication can be administered directly to infants, the amount received in breast milk is unlikely to be harmful, but the capabilities of the livers and kidneys of premature and young infants as well as the characteristics of the medication should be considered. In rare cases, a mother's metabolism of a drug endangers a breastfeeding infant. See Genomic Gem 10-3.

Diagnostic radioactive compounds require temporary cessation of breastfeeding until the drug has left the mother's system; therapeutic doses are a contraindication. Cytoxic drugs, illegal drugs, psychotropic drugs,

Genomic Gem 10-3
Ultrarapid Metabolizers of Codeine

In 2007, the FDA issued a warning to health-care providers about a rare but potentially lethal side effect that can affect the infants of nursing mothers who are taking codeine-containing analgesics. Some people are ultrarapid metabolizers of codeine with a specific **cytochrome P450 enzyme** (CYP2D6 genotype). See Chapter 15 for a discussion of these isoenzymes.

People with a certain variation in a liver enzyme allow them to convert codeine to its active metabolite, morphine, more rapidly and completely than other people (Madadi, 2010). A breastfeeding mother with this genotype can accumulate unusually high morphine levels in her serum and breast milk, putting her nursing infant at risk for morphine overdose. One healthy, 13-day-old breastfeeding baby died of such a morphine overdose even though his mother was taking codeine at a reduced dose because she, too, had suffered side effects (FDA, 2010).

The prevalence of the ultrarapid metabolizers of codeine varies among different populations and is less than 10% for most groups. In some groups of North Africans, Ethiopians, and Saudis the prevalence may be as high as 29% (Blumenfeld, 2010). The FDA has cleared a genetic test that can determine a person's CYP2D6 genotype, thus identifying individuals who can rapidly metabolize codeine, although the test is not routinely used (Madadi, 2010).

Because codeine has been used for postpartum pain for decades and is generally considered the safest narcotic pain reliever for breastfeeding mothers, absent genotyping of every new mother, careful, informed observation of mothers and infants is critical. Breastfeeding mothers need to be prescribed the lowest effective dose of codeine and the medication should be discontinued within 4 days of use if possible (Madadi, 2010). Health-care providers should teach nursing mothers who may be taking codeine about the signs of morphine overdose in themselves (extreme sleepiness and constipation) and in infants (increased sleepiness, trouble breastfeeding, breathing difficulties, and limpness). The mother should report any of those signs to her health-care provider or seek medical attention immediately.

Newborn breastfed babies usually nurse every 2 to 3 hours and should not sleep more than 4 hours at a time. Mothers should also be aware that morphine may remain in the infant's body for up to several days after the last codeine dose.

heavy alcohol use, and women who are opioid dependent should be discouraged from breastfeeding because of the potential risk to the infant (ABM Clinical Protocol, 2009). The physician should be consulted about both prescription and nonprescription drugs the mother takes.

Substances that are commonly not thought of as drugs may also affect the breastfed infant. These include alcohol and caffeine. The American Academy of Pediatrics (APA; 2012) recommends against the use of alcohol by breastfeeding mothers except for an occasional small drink and then only if a 2-hour delay occurs until the next feeding. Alcohol is water-soluble that passes effortlessly into breast milk and the concentration of alcohol in both foremilk and hindmilk are equal or greater to that in the mother's blood (Bowen and Tumback, 2010).

Caffeine in breast milk usually contains less than 1% of the caffeine ingested by the mother. There is reduced metabolism of caffeine in the infant so the drug can accumulate (Casey, 2012). The APA recommends no more than three cups of caffeine-containing drinks a day.

Altered Physiology or Pathology

The APA states that contraindications to breastfeeding are limited and include galactosemia and mothers who are positive for human T-cell lymphotrophic virus type I or II or untreated brucellosis. Mothers with untreated tuberculosis, who have active herpes simplex lesions on their breasts or who have developed varicella 5 days before or 2 days after delivery, and those infected with H1N1 influenza should not breastfeed but may express their milk for feedings.

In the industrialized world, it is not recommended that HIV-positive mothers breastfeed. In developing countries, where alternatives to human milk are not readily available, the risk of malnutrition and infectious disease may outweigh the risk of acquiring HIV from human milk.

Exposure to Toxic Chemicals

Certain chemicals, such as DDT and PCB, have been shown to be **teratogenic,** causing congenital defects. Concern has been raised about the transmission of toxic chemicals to the infant through breast milk. Once ingested, if the body has no means of excreting the chemicals, the contaminants are stored in adipose tissue. When the lactating mother's fat stores are mobilized to produce milk, it, too, contains the chemicals.

Some experts think that the risk to the infant is minimal unless the mobilization of the mother's fat is due to inadequate intake. Others say that there is no hazard unless the woman has had occupational exposure to the chemicals or has consumed a large amount of fish from contaminated waters. Women with concerns about the issue should discuss them with their health-care providers.

Keystones

- To support her own and the fetus's growth, a pregnant woman requires increased intake of many nutrients, especially kilocalories, protein, folic acid, and iron. Vitamin B_{12} status should be assessed in vegans.

- All women capable of becoming pregnant should consume 400 mcg of folic acid from fortified foods or supplements to decrease risk of neural tube defects in the embryo.

- The pregnant woman should avoid ingesting alcohol, soft cheeses, ready-to-eat meats, certain species and amounts of fish, undercooked meats, unwashed produce, and immoderate amounts of preformed vitamin A.

- Nutritional interventions are sometimes helpful for common complaints of pregnancy: morning sickness, leg cramps, constipation, and heartburn. Tact and diplomacy may be required to counsel women who have pica.

- Medical intervention and nutritional support are indicated for clients with hyperemesis gravidarum, hypertensive disorders of pregnancy, or gestational diabetes.

- Some maternal contraindications to breastfeeding are ingestion of certain medications and drugs, some illnesses, including AIDS and untreated tuberculosis, and exposure to toxic chemicals.

CASE STUDY *10-1*

Ms. T is a 21-year-old sexually active woman who has been followed in a family planning clinic for 3 years. She has been faithful about keeping appointments and taking her oral contraceptives. She also takes the multivitamin/ multimineral supplement containing 400 mcg of folic acid about four times a week "when she remembers and eats breakfast." She is taking no other medications. She and her immediate family have no known allergies. Now she relates that she is seriously considering becoming pregnant and wonders if they can afford to start a family. Her boyfriend proposed at her 21st birthday celebration. The couple has no pets but they do enjoy outdoor sports. Ms. T denies knowledge of means to minimize fetal risk and states she drinks a beer or a glass of wine on Saturdays and Sundays. She does not smoke. She received the standard measles, mumps, and rubella (MMR) vaccination as a child.

Ms. T is 5-ft 3-in. and weighs 104 lb. She has a small frame. Her hemoglobin was 14 g/dL, and hematocrit was 42% last month.

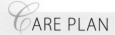 ARE PLAN

Subjective Data

Expressed interest in becoming pregnant ■ Concerned about the costs of parenthood ■ Regular moderate alcohol intake ■ History of compliance with medical regimen ■ Immunized against MMR

Objective Data

89% of healthy body weight ■ Hemoglobin 14 g/dL, within normal limits (WNL) ■ Hematocrit 42%, within normal limits (WNL)

Analysis

Increased risk to potential fetus related to current lifestyle and underweight

Plan

DESIRED OUTCOMES EVALUATION CRITERIA	ACTIONS/INTERVENTIONS	RATIONALE
Will affirm today her intention to abstain from alcohol when attempting to achieve a pregnancy and throughout gestation.	Teach Ms. T about fetal alcohol syndrome.	No amount of alcohol is presumed to be safe in pregnancy.
	Use photographs of affected children.	"A picture is worth 1000 words." Photographs introduce visual learning and have an impact on feelings.
Will take multivitamin, multimineral supplement every day beginning tomorrow.	Reiterate that vitamin preparation should contain 400 micrograms of folic acid.	This is the RDA for all women capable of becoming pregnant.
	Review the value of a varied diet and good sources of food folate.	The RDA also emphasizes the importance of food folate.
Will eat breakfast or equivalent morning nourishment every day beginning tomorrow.	Review Dietary Guidelines with Ms. T. Explore means to take nourishment in morning.	This is a good habit to acquire. Once Ms. T achieves pregnancy, supplying the embryo/fetus with a steady supply of nutrients is critical.
Will recount the limits to vitamin A intake during pregnancy by next visit.	Inform Ms. T of RDA for vitamin A in pregnancy. Alert Ms. T to the large amounts of preformed vitamin A in liver and liver products. Caution against supplements of vitamin A in addition to the multivitamin, multimineral tablet.	Teratogenic effects usually occur during the first trimester.
	Discuss the safety of beta-carotene (provitamin A) in pregnancy.	Beta-carotene has not been associated with birth defects. Supplements containing provitamin A are considered safe for pregnant women at the RDA level.
Will list actions to take to minimize exposure to *Listeria* infection by 10 weeks before attempted conception.	Provide Ms. T with a list of cheeses to avoid and those that are considered safe. Review rules for safe handling of ready-to-eat meats.	Because the incubation period of *Listeria* is up to 10 weeks, avoidance of possibly contaminated food should begin well before conception.

DESIRED OUTCOMES EVALUATION CRITERIA	ACTIONS/INTERVENTIONS	RATIONALE
	Alert her to report flulike symptoms promptly to her primary health-care provider.	Antimicrobial therapy may prevent fetal infection and the associated high mortality.
Will monitor own intake of fish to remain within recommended limits by conception.	Emphasize complete abstinence from shark, swordfish, king mackerel, and tilefish. If available, use food models showing the weekly limits of 12 ounces or 6 ounces of fish.	These advisories from the FDA and the EPA to minimize the exposure of the fetus to methylmercury show the seriousness of the threat.
Will discuss discontinuing oral contraceptive therapy and attempting conception with the primary health-care provider before changing her regimen.	Advise Ms. T about the possibility of birth defects with some oral contraceptives.	Progestins may cause birth defects if taken early in pregnancy.
Will continue planning optimal nutrition for herself and her prospective child.	Refer Ms. T to local Supplemental Feeding Program for Women, Infants, and Children.	If eligible, she could begin receiving food assistance when she becomes pregnant.

10-1

WIC Program Director's Notes

The following Supplemental Feeding Program for Women, Infants, and Children (WIC) Program Director's Notes are representative of the documentation found in a client's medical record.

Subjective: Interested in possible food assistance when she achieves pregnancy

Objective: Completed WIC application

Analysis: Meets eligibility requirements for

- Residency in state
- Household income

- Nutrition risk due to underweight—documented by family planning nurse

Does not currently meet categorical eligibility requirement:

- Is not pregnant
- Has no dependent children

Plan: Place application in pending file

Encourage client to activate application when she becomes pregnant

Critical Thinking Questions

1. If Ms. T were to achieve a pregnancy, what would her month-by-month recommended weight gain be? If she expresses concern about "gaining too much weight" when within the recommended amounts, how would you counsel her?

2. Are there other issues you believe ought to be raised with Ms. T before she attempts to become pregnant? Are they more or less important than the ones addressed in the Care Plan? Why?

3. Assuming Ms. T becomes pregnant, how would you approach anticipatory guidance regarding complications of pregnancy affected by nutrition?

Chapter Review

1. Throughout pregnancy and lactation, how many whole grains should she consume?
   a. All grains should be whole grains
   b. Half of grains consumed should be whole
   c. One serving of whole grains per day
   d. Whole grains should be avoided

2. Which of the following substances are contraindicated during pregnancy?
   a. Alcohol and swordfish
   b. Cocoa and peanut butter
   c. Coffee and well-done beef
   d. Tea and cheddar cheese

3. Which of the following principles is not recommended by the Baby-Friendly Hospital Initiative?
   a. Feeding on demand
   b. Keeping mother and infant together 24 hours a day
   c. Hydrating the infant with sterile water until the mother's milk supply is established
   d. Putting the infant to breast within 1 hour of birth

4. The RDA for folic acid specifies 400 mcg of synthetic folic acid from fortified foods or supplements for:
   a. All women capable of becoming pregnant
   b. Women taking oral contraceptive medications
   c. Women of northern European descent
   d. Breastfeeding mothers

5. If a pregnant woman complains of heartburn, she should be instructed to:
   a. Increase her intake of milk products
   b. Decrease her overall food intake
   c. Rest in bed after eating
   d. Avoid spicy or acidic foods

Clinical Analysis

Ms. S is a 15-year-old girl who thinks that she is 2 months pregnant. She has not told anyone else of the pregnancy. She is unsure if she wants to keep the baby or not. Her purpose in disclosing the information to the school nurse is to obtain assistance with weight control so she has more time to make up her mind.

1. On the basis of the above information, which one of the following interventions would be of highest priority at this time?
   a. Designing a weight-control program that is high in calcium
   b. Giving information on the desirability of breastfeeding the infant
   c. Instructing the girl regarding substances that are likely to harm the fetus
   d. Scheduling a visit with a social worker to help the girl decide on a course of action

2. Knowing that adolescents are often lacking in certain nutrients, the nurse would want to assess the girl's intake of:
   a. Cola, coffee, and tea
   b. Fruits, vegetables, milk, and red meat
   c. Fried foods and pastries
   d. Poultry, seafood, and white bread

3. Ms. S complains of morning sickness. The nurse instructs her to:
   a. Eat breakfast later in the morning
   b. Drink at least two glasses of liquid with every meal
   c. Increase her intake of whole-grain breads and cereals to 2 ounces per meal
   d. Drink a large glass of skim milk at bedtime

11

Life Cycle Nutrition: Infancy, Childhood, and Adolescence

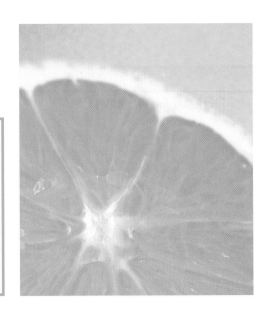

LEARNING OBJECTIVES

After completing this chapter, the student should be able to:

- Describe normal growth patterns and corresponding nutritional needs for a full-term infant, a toddler, a school-age child, and an adolescent.
- Explain why breast milk is uniquely suited to the human infant's capabilities.
- Discuss the rationale for the sequence in which semisolid foods are introduced into an infant's diet.
- List causes and treatments of five common nutritional problems of infancy.
- Summarize common nutritional problems of the preschool child.
- Relate ways in which a child can be encouraged to establish good nutritional habits.
- Identify areas of concern regarding the typical adolescent's diet.
- Devise a comprehensive plan to prevent obesity in a target population of children or adolescents.

Good nutrition is essential for infants and children. Because of public health efforts, U.S. infant mortality rates have decreased significantly. Of every 1000 infants born alive in:

- 1940, 47 died before the age of 1 year.
- 1960, approximately 26.0 died.
- 2011, 6.05 died (Hoyert & Xu, 2012).

The goal of Healthy People 2020 is to reduce the infant mortality rate (IMR) to 6.0 per 1000 live births or less for all racial/ethnic groups. Infant mortality rates in 2010 were 11.61 per 1000 live births for Black infants and 5.19 per 1000 live births for White infants, demonstrating a 2.2 times higher mortality rate for Black infants (Murphy, Zu, and Kochanek, 2012). Low birth weight and short gestational age are leading causes of IMR in the United States. In 2010, the low birth weight rate for non-Hispanic Black women was 13.53%, 7.14% for non-Hispanic White women, and 6.97% for Hispanic women (Martin, Hamilton, Ventura, et al, 2012). Of the 13 million premature infants born worldwide, 90% will survive

past infancy (Deng, 2010). Nutritional management has a major function in survival and subsequent growth and development of low birth weight infants (Dabas, Kumar, and Singh, 2010).

This chapter focuses on periods of rapid **growth** during infancy, childhood, and adolescence. In addition to nutritional needs for all periods of growth, the chapter considers the stages of physical and **psychosocial development** for these ages, noting ways in which food relates to psychosocial development. Toward the end of the chapter is a discussion of overweight and obesity, major public health issues for children and adolescents that, unless checked, do not bode well for the health of Americans.

Psychosocial Development

American psychoanalyst **Erik Erikson** divided life into eight stages, each of which involves a psychosocial developmental task to be mastered and an opposite negative trait that emerges if the task is not mastered. Even if a developmental task is successfully mastered, a new situation may arise, challenging the person to reaffirm his or her mastery. Erikson's developmental tasks through adolescence appear in Table 11-1.

Nutrition in Infancy

Infancy, the first year of life, is a critical period for growth and development.

Growth

Growth is the progressive maturation and increase in size of a living thing. The only time humans grow faster than in infancy is the 40 weeks before they are born. An infant's birth weight should:

■ Double by 4 to 6 months of age
■ Triple by 1 year

From a birth length of about 20 inches, an infant grows to about 30 inches by age 1.

An infant's *rate of growth* is more significant than absolute values. The growth charts on DavisPlus or at www.cdc.gov/growthcharts reflect growth patterns of all children in the United States.

In 2006, the World Health Organization (WHO) released new standards for growth and development. The children measured for these standards were raised in an optimal environment (breastfed, nonsmoking home) for proper growth. The standards are applicable to all children regardless of ethnicity, socioeconomic status, or type of feeding (WHO, 2006). The WHO Child Growth Standards establishes that breastfed infants are the standard for measuring healthy growth, and previous growth charts utilized a combination of breastfed and artificially fed children.

During the first few days after birth, an infant loses weight as he or she adjusts to his or her new environment and food supply. Among his or her adaptations is learning to feed compared with receiving a continuous supply of nutrients in utero. The amount of weight lost in these first few days should not exceed 7% of the birth weight (Mulder, Johnson, and Baker, 2010). The newborn (or *neonate*, as an infant is called during the first 28 days after birth) usually returns to its birth weight within 14 days.

The period most critical to brain development extends from conception into the second year of life. Brain cells increase most rapidly before birth and during the first 5 or 6 months after birth. To attain maximum brain growth, the infant needs optimal nutrition.

Development

The gradual process of changing from a simple to a more complex organism is **development.** Becoming a mature individual involves psychosocial and physical changes, not only an increase in size.

Psychosocial Development of the Infant

The psychosocial developmental task of the infant is to learn to **trust** (see Table 11-1). The parent who responds promptly and lovingly to the infant's cries is teaching the infant to trust. If the caregiver handles the infant inconsistently—gently one time and roughly the next—however, the infant learns to mistrust.

Failure to thrive (FTT) is a descriptive term used to describe inadequate growth or the inability to maintain growth (Cole and Lanham, 2011). A child may receive a diagnosis of FTT when his or her arc of growth slips by two major percentiles on a growth chart (Bates, 2010) or when weight falls below the fifth percentile on multiple occasions.

Inadequate caloric intake is the most common etiology associated with FTT and can be related to problems with feeding including poor sucking and swallowing, breastfeeding difficulties or difficulty transitioning to solid foods, insufficient breast milk or formula, excessive juice consumption, or caloric absorption problems (Cole and Lanham, 2011). It can be helpful to assess caregiver–infant interactions related to feeding practices. In situations in which physical care is provided but a tender relationship does not develop, infants may actually suffer stunted physical growth. Caregiver education regarding feeding techniques, child cues and developmental stages can be helpful in addressing nonorganic causes of FTT.

Physical Development

Development proceeds at a different pace in various tissues and organs. Proper feeding practices are based on the maturation rate of body organs (see Table 11-2).

TABLE 11-1 ■ Erikson's Theory of Psychosocial Development		
STAGE OF LIFE	**DEVELOPMENTAL TASK**	**OPPOSING NEGATIVE TRAIT**
Infancy	Trust	Distrust
Toddler	Autonomy	Doubt
Preschooler	Initiative	Guilt
School-age child	Industry	Inferiority
Adolescent	Identity	Role confusion

TABLE 11-2 ■ Physical Characteristics of Infant That Affect Nutrition

SYSTEM	INFANT'S LIMITED CAPACITY	ADAPTATIONS AND MATURATIONS	ADJUSTMENT IN FEEDING	BY 1 YEAR OF AGE
Gastrointestinal	Salivary and pancreatic amylases are inadequate to digest complex carbohydrates for several months.	Has lingual lipase to digest fat, an enzyme lacking in adults.	Delay offering complex carbohydrates.	
	Intestine permits absorption of whole proteins.		Delay offering foods likely to be allergenic until 1 year old.	
	Stomach holds about 1 oz.		Frequent feedings	Stomach holds about 8 oz.
Nervous	Suckles with up-and-down motion of the tongue for 3 to 4 months.	Rooting reflex well developed. When the infant's cheek is stroked, the head turns toward that side to nurse.	Feed breast milk or infant formula. If semisolid food is offered at this time, the natural motion of the tongue tends to spit it out.	
		After 4 months, the infant can suck using orofacial muscles. The tongue moves back and forth instead of up and down.	Semisolid food is more likely to be swallowed than spit out.	
		At 6 months has hand-to-eye coordination to put food into mouth.	Offer appropriate finger foods.	
		At 7 months can chew appropriate foods.	Increase variety of food offered.	
Urinary	Young infant's kidneys have limited capacity to filter solutes.	By end of the second month of life, kidneys can excrete the waste of semisolid foods.	Delay semisolid foods at least until 2 months of age, preferably 4 to 6 months.	Kidneys at full functional capacity.

Nutritional Needs of the Term Infant

For DRIs, see Appendix A. In general, infants' values are based on the contents of breast milk. In 2008, the American Academy of Pediatrics recommended that all infants receive a daily intake of 400 IU of vitamin D beginning in the first few days of life (Minarich and Silverstein, 2011).

A normal pregnancy is 38 to 42 weeks. An infant born after a normal pregnancy is a **term infant.** Breast milk is the species-specific food for human infants. Its characteristics are the standard for infant formulas, which replicate many of the components of breast milk but cannot supply all of its desirable qualities.

Energy and Macronutrients

Resting metabolic rates of infants are high as evidenced by:

- Normal pulse rate of 120 to 150 beats/min
- Normal respiratory rate of 30 to 50 breaths/min
- Large proportion of skin surface to body size requiring energy for temperature regulation

An activity such as crying may double the infant's energy expenditure.

Energy needs for the first 6 months of life are 108 kilocalories per kilogram of body weight per day. From 6 to 12 months of age, the energy need is 98 kilocalories per kilogram per day.

Table 11-3 lists the macronutrients of special importance for infants with comparisons of the relevant components of breast milk and cow's milk. Clinical Application 11-1 discusses a carbohydrate source that should not be given to infants. Box 11-1 identifies some research linking cognitive development to breastfeeding.

Micronutrients

The general recommendations for vitamin and mineral supplementation in infants are listed in Table 11-4. Despite the recommendation by the American Academy of Pediatrics to supplement breastfed infants with vitamin D, only 36.4% of pediatricians surveyed did so. Among parents of predominantly breastfed infants who indicated that their child's doctor recommended vitamin D, just 44.6% gave the supplement to their child (Taylor, Geyer, and Feldman, 2010).

VITAMINS

The routine administration of vitamin K to all infants is mandatory. Infants are at a higher risk for hemorrhagic disease due to lack of vitamin K transfer across the placenta, low levels in breast milk, immature liver, and low bacterial production in the colon (Gopakumar, Sivji, and Rajiv, 2010). Vitamin K deficiencies can result in Vitamin K deficiency bleeding with 50% of infants presenting with intracranial hemorrhage (Labarque, Ngo, Penders, VanDeCasseye, and Pelt, 2011).

MINERALS

Compared with cow's milk, breast milk contains:

- One-third the sodium, potassium, and chloride
- One-eighth the phosphorus of cow's milk, an amount that accommodates the limited function of the infant's kidneys

TABLE 11-3 ■ Macronutrient Needs of Term Infant				
	NUTRIENT NEEDED	**BREAST MILK**	**COW'S MILK**	**CONTRAINDICATIONS**
Carbohydrate	Galactose is necessary for brain cell formation.	Breast milk contains amylase that is 40–60 times more active than that of cow's milk.		Honey (Clinical Application 11-1)
Fat	Fat and cholesterol are necessary for rapidly growing brain and nervous system, bile, and hormones.	Provides 55% of kilocalories from fat as concentrated energy source. Contains lipase to begin digestion for the infant so about 95%–98% of the fat in human milk is absorbed.		Reduced-fat milks before age 2
	The developing nervous system needs arachidonic and docosahexaenoic (DHA) fatty acids, the main omega-6 and omega-3 fatty acids of the central nervous system.	These two fatty acids, essential for retinal and neural development are found in human milk.	Not present	
Protein		Human milk contains 70% whey (easily digested) and 30% casein. The major whey protein in breast milk is alpha-lactalbumin, with an amino acid pattern much like that of the body tissues.	18% whey, 82% casein	

Adapted from Brown (2008); Rioux, Belanger-Plourde, LeBlanc, & Vigneau (2011); Schwartz, Drossard, Dube (2010); Xavier, Rai, K., & Hedge (2011).

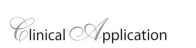

Clinical Application 11-1

Honey Is a Danger to Infants

Infants should not be given honey until after their first birthday because honey frequently contains botulism spores acquired from plants or the soil. Up to 25% of honey products have been found to contain spores. Processing the honey does not destroy these spores.

There were 112 confirmed cases of botulism in the United States in 2010. Of the 112 cases, 85 or 76% of cases were infant botulism (Centers for Disease Control, 2011).

If the spores are ingested by an infant, they become active in his or her intestinal tract and produce a neurotoxin that block the production or release of acetylcholine (Chaudhry, 2011). Symptoms include:

- Constipation
- Weakness
- Weak cry
- Poor feeding
- Poor head control (Vasquez, 2008)

The spectrum of symptoms can range from the mild end of the spectrum, in which the infant does not require hospitalization but may develop feeding difficulties and FTT, to the severe end, characterized by respiratory difficulties that result in death (Brook, 2007).

Physicians are required to report all cases of infant botulism promptly to state and local health departments.

These differences in mineral content affect the osmolality of the milk and the workload of the kidneys (see Clinical Application 11-2). *Unmodified* cow's milk is inappropriate for young infants.

Box 11-1 ■ *Research Linking Cognitive Abilities to Breastfeeding*

Early research associated breastfeeding with slightly enhanced performance on tests of cognitive development but this remains an issue of debate. Breast milk contains arachidonic (ARA) and docosahexaenoic (DHA) fatty acids, which accumulate during the brain growth spurt from the third trimester until age 2 (Morales, Bustamante, Gonzalez, et al, 2011).

- One study demonstrated that early breast milk intake promoted brain development at a structural level resulting in larger total brain volume and increase white matter (Isaacs, Fischi, Quinn, et al, 2010).
- Other studies indicate nutritional advantages for child cognition related to higher concentrations of DHA in breastfed infants (Morales et al, 2011).

Factors such as higher socioeconomic status and level of education are also demonstrating an effect on cognition. This issue is still under investigation. Adding ARA and DHA to infant formulas corresponds to other efforts to mimic breast milk. Neither supplemented formula nor breastfeeding should be viewed as a magic elixir to boost intelligence.

The daily turnover of water in the infant is approximately 15% of body weight.

The Breastfed Infant

Breast milk is designed for human infants and is the standard against which substitute milks are measured. Breastfeeding rates in the United States are at an all-time high (see Fig. 10-3), but compared with other countries, they are still low.

Benefits of breastfeeding include:

- Breastfed infants have been shown to have decreased rates of otitis media, respiratory infections, and diabetes type 1 and type 2 (Watkins and Dodgson, 2010).

Water

The infant's body is about 75% water. By 3 years of age, the body has developed so it has the adult proportion of about 60% water (Gropper, Smith, and Groff, 2009).

11-2

$\mathscr{C}$linical $\mathscr{A}$pplication

Renal Solute Loads

When selecting an infant formula, it is necessary to distinguish two measures of osmotic pressure. One is the osmotic pressure the formula presents to the gut. The other examines what remains to be excreted by the kidney after digestion, absorption, and metabolism have taken place.

These leftovers are excess electrolytes and byproducts of protein metabolism. The osmotic pressure of these leftovers presented to the kidney for disposal is called the renal solute load. Cow's milk contains higher amounts of protein, sodium, potassium, and chloride, which place the greatest burden on the infant's immature renal system. Breast milk, in contrast, provides the least burden.

When fluid intake is low or when extrarenal water losses are high, the infant may become dehydrated. The kidneys may be unable to retain enough water after excreting the renal solutes. The resulting negative water balance, if prolonged, can lead to serious dehydration. Strong epidemiological evidence shows that cow's milk or formulas with similarly high potential renal solute load increases infants' risk of hypernatremic dehydration.

MILK FORMULA	POTENTIAL RENAL SOLUTE LOAD mOsm/L	mOsm/100 kcal
Human milk	93	14
Milk-based formula	135–260	20–39
Cow milk	308	23

Data from Foman (2000).

TABLE 11-4 ■ Vitamin and Mineral Supplementation for Infants			
SUPPLEMENT	**PRESCRIBED FOR**	**SITUATION**	**RATIONALE**
Vitamin			
D	Breastfed infants Partially breastfed infants Formula-fed infants ingesting <1 L of fortified formula	Beginning in the first few days of life	
K	All infants	Single intramuscular dose of vitamin K after the first breastfeeding and within 6 hours of birth	Until the infant's intestine becomes colonized with *Escherichia coli* from the environment, he or she is at risk for bleeding problems
C	2-week-old formula-fed infants, if vitamin is not in formula	Synthetic preferable to juices (orange juice in particular may be allergen)	
B_{12} as cobalamin	Breastfed infant, if mother is strict vegetarian	See Chapter 10	Growth failure and neurological impairment due to cobalamin deficiency occurred in breastfeeding infants of vegetarian mothers
Mineral			
Calcium	Premature infants	See Clinical Application 11-5	Breast milk contains about one-sixth to one-quarter the calcium in cow's milk 67% of breast milk calcium is absorbed vs. 25% of cow's milk calcium
Phosphorus	Premature infants	See Clinical Application 11-5	
Iron	Term infant, when birth weight has doubled Formula-fed premature, from onset Fortified human milk-fed premature, when full enteral feeding established	Iron-fortified formula is recommended	Breast milk contains about 0.5 mg iron/L but 50% is absorbed Only 10% is absorbed from cow's milk or fortified formulas
Fluoride	All children >6 months of age Children >3 years of age	If drinking water contains <0.3 ppm If drinking water contains <0.6 ppm	

Sources: American Academy of Pediatrics (2012); American Academy of Pediatric Dentistry (2012); Centers for Disease Control and Prevention (2012); Gopakumar, Sivji, and Rajiv (2010); Minarich and Silverstein (2011).

■ Artificially fed infants have higher incidence of gastrointestinal infection and are more likely to develop atopic dermatitis, die from sudden infant death syndrome, and be overweight (Brodribb, 2012).

Human breast milk banks make milk available for infants whose mothers do not produce enough milk.

The goals of Healthy People 2020 are to increase breastfeeding rates to:

■ 82% of mothers who ever breastfeed
■ 25% who exclusively breastfeed until infants are 6 months old
■ 34% who breastfeed until infants are 1 year old

The American Academy of Pediatrics recommends exclusive breastfeeding (nothing but breast milk and vitamins, minerals, and medications) for the first 6 months of life.

Practices conducive to breastfeeding and lactation are covered in Chapter 10. Care of ill or frail infants must be individualized. Clinical Application 11-3 explains the procedures for storing human milk.

Composition of Breast Milk

Breast milk accommodates the infant's needs during the weeks an infant is nursing, even during the course of a single feeding. Breast milk varies from mother to mother and even in one mother with the time of day. It also varies with the lactation cycle. The variation in content also offers the infant a variety of taste experiences (see Table 11-5).

Unique Advantages of Breastfeeding

One well-documented advantage to breastfeeding that has not been duplicated by formulas is protection against infectious disease. Other advantages are limited improvement in the presentation of allergic disease and a possible negative association with obesity.

PROTECTION AGAINST DISEASE

In both developing and industrialized countries, breastfeeding reduces the incidence of gastrointestinal and respiratory diseases and otitis media (middle ear infection). Any breastfeeding is associated with a reduction in gastrointestinal tract infections, whereas the development of lower respiratory tract infections and otitis media is reduced in infants who exclusively breastfeed

TABLE 11-5 ■ Breast Milk Components			
	SECRETED	**APPEARANCE**	**COMPONENTS**
Colostrum	2–4 days after delivery	Thin, yellow, cloudy fluid	High kilocalorie High protein Antibodies White blood cells Fat-soluble vitamins Minerals
Mature	72–96 hours after delivery As long as breastfeeding continues	Milky	High lactose High vitamin E Calcium:phosphorus ratio of 2:1 (prevents calcium deficient tetany) Antibodies (decreased at 3 months) Antioxidants Foremilk (beginning of feeding): less fat Hindmilk (end of feeding): more fat to increase satiety At 3 months, fewer immunoglobulins

Sources: Brown (2008); *Merck Manual* (2010–2011).

for more than 4 months (Breastfeeding, 2012). Studies have also demonstrated any amount of formula feeding significantly increases the infant's risk of developing otitis media (McNeil, Labbok, and Abrahams, 2010).

Breast milk contains bioactive components that protect the infant from disease by:

■ Transfer of passive immunity from mother to infant (Hurley and Theil, 2011)
■ Antioxidant activity of human milk (Elisia and Kitts, 2011)

Among the infection-fighting agents in breast milk are immunoglobulin (Ig)A and leukocytes or white blood cells (WBCs).

PREVENTION OF ALLERGIES

The young infant's gastrointestinal tract can permit the passage of whole proteins into the bloodstream. These proteins can stimulate an allergic response in susceptible infants.

Breastfeeding is protective against allergies for infants with at least one first-degree relative with allergic disease. Exclusive breastfeeding for 3 to 4 months (compared with feeding formula made with intact cow's milk protein) reduces the incidence of clinical asthma, atopic dermatitis, eczema and celiac disease (Breastfeeding, 2012).

If breast milk is unavailable or insufficient, infants at high risk of **atopy** may be fed special formulas. **Hydrolysis** splits whole proteins into smaller particles that are less likely to cause allergic reactions. Extensively hydrolyzed formulas are preferable to unhydrolyzed or partially hydrolyzed formulas because they have been shown to reduce the incidence of certain atopic disease

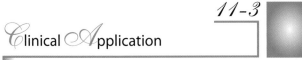

11-3

*C*linical *A*pplication

Storage of Human Milk

Careful collection and storage are necessary to preserve the sterility and quality of expressed human milk. The Centers for Disease Control and Prevention has specific guidelines for the collection and storage of human breast milk, including storage at room temperature for no longer than 6 to 8 hours, in an insulated cooler for 24 hours, in the refrigerator for 5 days, and in the freezer of the refrigerator for 3 to 6 months. Breast milk can be frozen for longer periods of time, up to 6 to 12 months, if stored in a chest or upright freezer.

The Human Milk Banking Association of North America follows strict guidelines in screening for infectious disease, criteria of pasteurization, storage and distributions of donated milk (Geraghty, Heier, and Rasmussen, 2011). The majority of donated milk is provided to premature, hospitalized infants.

(Alexander, Schmitt, Tran, et al, 2010). Parents should be encouraged to consult with their health-care provider before switching formulas because dietary changes have only been shown to be effective in children with established food allergies (Robinson, 2011).

Current evidence does not support a major role for maternal dietary restrictions during pregnancy or lactation as protective against allergies. In addition, little evidence backs the delayed introduction of complementary foods beyond 4 to 6 months of age as a strategy to prevent atopic disease.

NEGATIVE ASSOCIATION WITH OBESITY

There is strong evidence that suggests breastfed infants have a lower risk of later obesity than formula-fed infants (Whitney, 2011). There is a 15% to 30% reduction in adolescent and adult obesity rates if any breastfeeding occurs in infancy (Breastfeeding, 2012).

The mechanisms involved, although poorly understood, include aspects of the feeding process as well as the components of breast milk. Breastfed infants gain weight more slowly and are leaner than formula-fed infants. This is attributed to infant self-regulation of energy nutrients: breastfed babies follow internal cues to stop feeding when full, and bottle-fed infants can be influenced by the caretaker (Oddy, 2012). The higher protein content in formula is thought to increase the risk of obesity through effects on hormones such as insulin (Gibson-Moore, 2011).

In the United States, whereas rates of breastfeeding have risen slowly, childhood obesity rates have increased dramatically. Approximately 10% of children younger than 2 years old and 21% of children between 2 and 5 are overweight (Dolinsky, Siega-Riz, Perrin, & Armstrong, 2011). Breastfeeding is just one intervention that can be used to help achieve a normal body weight.

Genetic Abnormalities Affecting Breastfeeding

Among the conditions commonly included in newborn screening tests are two that have profound implications for the infant's nutritional intake. One affects carbohydrate metabolism and the other protein metabolism.

In **galactosemia,** the infant's lack of an enzyme to metabolize galactose is an absolute contraindication to breastfeeding. Galactosemia is inherited as an autosomal recessive trait. If untreated, the child will suffer growth failure, mental retardation, or death. Treatment involves a soy formula containing no lactose or galactose and lifelong avoidance of milk products.

The mother of an infant with phenylketonuria (see Clinical Application 5-2) often chooses to feed the child only the special formula. Breastfeeding the infant requires both limited amounts of breast milk and the special formula. To determine the amount of breast milk the infant may consume to keep his or her blood levels within the therapeutic limits requires constant monitoring and consultations, but it has been done successfully. Every state has at least one medical center for treating metabolic defects. The maternal and child health division of the state health department can assist with locating such a facility.

The Formula-Fed Infant

As good as it is, exclusive breastfeeding is not possible for all mothers and infants. Infant formula is the only food that is regulated by its own law, the Infant Formula Act of 1980, which sets minimum levels of 29 nutrients and maximal levels of 9 nutrients. Formulas for full-term infants must contain 20 kilocalories per ounce. As much as possible, commercial formulas are designed to match the qualities of human breast milk.

Formulas contain more protein than breast milk. The cow's milk proteins do not contain the optimal amino acids for human infants. Enough protein is included in the formula to provide a sufficient distribution of amino acids.

The saturated fats of cow's milk are poorly digested by the infant. In formulas, vegetable oils replace the saturated fats.

Formula Preparations

Commercial formulas come in three forms: powder (to mix with water), liquid concentrate, and ready-to-feed (see Table 11-6).

Directions for preparing the formula will be given by the health-care provider. Commonly discussed issues include:

■ Cleanliness/sterility of equipment
■ Water to use for dilution:
  ■ Sterility
  ■ Fluoride content
  ■ Possible lead contamination (see Clinical Application 8-8)
■ Safe storage
■ Use of correct strength formula (Formula too concentrated or too dilute can cause severe electrolyte imbalances. Some cases have been fatal.)

TABLE 11-6 ■ Forms of Formulas		
	ADVANTAGES	**DISADVANTAGES**
Liquid Concentrate	Relatively easy to prepare	Opened cans require refrigeration Must be used within 48 hours
Powder	Less waste Possible to prepare a small amount	Unsterile powder may be unsafe for premature infants
Ready-to-Feed	Most convenient No calculating or measuring	Most expensive (see Dollars & Sense 11-1)

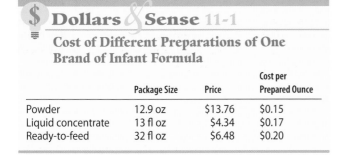

$ **Dollars & Sense** 11-1

Cost of Different Preparations of One Brand of Infant Formula

	Package Size	Price	Cost per Prepared Ounce
Powder	12.9 oz	$13.76	$0.15
Liquid concentrate	13 fl oz	$4.34	$0.17
Ready-to-feed	32 fl oz	$6.48	$0.20

- Safe heating of the formula before feeding the infant
- Discarding prepared bottles of formula unrefrigerated for 1 hour or partially consumed

Using a microwave oven for infant foods is not recommended. Heat may be unevenly distributed and continues to build even after the food has been removed from the oven.

Feeding Techniques

Approximately every 4 hours, the infant awakens for feedings. By the age of 2 to 3 months, the baby probably will have eliminated one feeding, so the schedule is five times a day. By 6 months, most infants are feeding four times a day.

The baby is positioned in the crook of the arm, almost as if breastfeeding. The parent's or caregiver's touch is important to the infant's development. Correct techniques include the following:

- The nipple holes should be large enough for milk to drip out on its own without shaking the bottle.
- The nipple should always be filled with milk to prevent the infant from swallowing air while feeding.
- Daily formula intake for an infant should be 1.5 to 2 ounces per pound of body weight, but growth is a better measure of health than the amount of formula swallowed.
- A single feeding should not exceed 8 ounces.

Propping an infant with a bottle is never acceptable because choking is a real hazard.

Special Formulas

Special formulas are available for infants who are allergic to cow's milk, those with galactosemia or lactose intolerance, and those with fat-absorption problems. See Clinical Application 11-4 for a brief description of such formulas, which are commonly soy-based.

For a formula to be considered hypoallergenic, it should be well tolerated by at least 90% of individuals who are allergic to the parent protein from which that formula has been derived. Elemental formulas derived from synthetic amino acids are well tolerated by practically all individuals, including those allergic to extensively hydrolyzed formulas (Bahna, 2008).

11-4

Clinical Application

Soy Protein Formulas

The isolated soy protein formulas marketed today are all free of cow's milk protein and lactose and are iron-fortified.

The American Academy of Pediatrics recommends using soy protein-based formulas in term infants for:

- Galactosemia and hereditary lactase deficiency
- Those whose parents desire a vegetarian diet
- Secondary lactose intolerance following acute gastroenteritis

In contrast, the Academy *does not* recommend soy protein-based formula under the following circumstances:

- Preterm infants
- Cow's milk allergy
- Routine treatment of colic
- Healthy or high-risk infants to prevent atopic disease

Adapted from Bhatia and Greer (2008).

Palatability becomes an issue as the infant develops more discerning tastes. Hydrolysis produces bitter-tasting peptides. Soy formulas and rice formula were judged to have the best tastes, followed by the whey hydrolysates. Extensively hydrolyzed protein formulas result in reduced palatability (Alexander et al, 2010).

The full-term infant's digestive, nervous, and urinary systems are immature—an even greater issue for premature infants. Clinical Application 11-5 summarizes some of the nutritional problems and appropriate interventions used for premature infants.

Hazards of Formula Feeding

On a few occasions, improperly manufactured formulas have been responsible for vitamin and mineral deficiencies in infants. This is an unacceptable, but fortunately rare, occurrence. A more common hazard, and one an individual nurse can monitor, is the improper preparation and use of formulas by the parent. Formulas can be:

- The wrong strength
- Prepared with contaminated water, equipment, or hands
- Kept at feeding temperature too long. Body temperature is "just right" for bacteria to multiply, whether in the body or in a formula bottle.

Choice of Breast or Bottle

In the United States, infants can be well nourished whether breastfed or bottle-fed. To raise a child successfully takes more than simply supplying the

Clinical Application

Premature Infants

Premature infants are born before 37 weeks' gestation. By birth weight, premature infants are categorized as:

- Low birth weight (LBW)—less than 2500 g (5.5 lb) at birth
- Very low birth weight (VLBW)—less than 1500 g (3.3 lb)
- Extremely low birth weight (ELBW)—less than 1000 g (2.2 lb).

An infant can be both premature and LBW or VLBW. Not all premature infants weigh less than 2500 grams. Nor are all LBW infants premature, but birth weight is the most powerful single predictor of an infant's future health status. LBW infants are approximately 13 times more likely to die within the first 28 days of life than heavier babies (Namiiro, Mugalu, McAdams, and Ndeezi, 2012).

Maternal factors associated with prematurity include smoking, previous premature delivery, history of chronic disease, infection, and either very low or high BMI (Nour, 2012). A genetic variant has also been implicated (see Genomic Gem 11-1).

PROVIDING NOURISHMENT

- The infant's ability to coordinate sucking, swallowing, and breathing are not developed before the 32nd or 34th week of gestation. As a result, premature infants often require enteral or intravenous feeding. Enteral tube feeding will conserve energy even in an infant who is able to suck.
- Human milk from the infant's mother is the gold standard to nourish VLBW infants (da Matta Aprile, Feferbaum, Andreassa, and Leone, 2010). Compared with term mothers' milk, preterm milk has more protein, sodium, and host defense factors but less calcium, phosphorus, and magnesium. Human milk fortifiers add protein, carbohydrate, vitamins, and minerals to the breast milk (see Fig. 11-1). Moreover, the mother's enzymes and antibodies are still available to the baby.
- Special formulas for premature infants are designed to provide for the infant's growth needs despite the immature digestive system.
  - Ready-to-feed preparations should be used rather than powdered formulas that cannot be sufficiently sterilized.

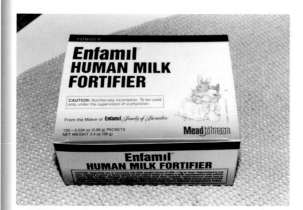

FIGURE 11-1 Human milk fortifier, when *added to human milk*, increases the amount of protein, carbohydrates, and selected vitamins and minerals available to meet the needs of rapidly growing low-birth-weight infants. These are not nutritionally complete supplements.

- Safe handling demands that prepared formula should not be at room temperature for more than 4 hours.
- Formulas with 22, 24, and 28 kcal/mL are available.
- Preterm infants lose crucial intrauterine nutrient accumulation and storage and have limited energy and reserves (Rayyan, Devlieger, Jochum, and Allegaert, 2012). Due to low vitamin reserves, premature infants require higher doses of supplemental vitamins than are term infants.
- Because of poor bone calcification and muscle development, premature infants may need calcium, phosphorus, and sodium supplements. Metabolic bone disease (MBD), including osteopenia and rickets, may develop secondary to decreased mineral stores and increased mineral demands in the postnatal period (Mitchell, Rogers, Hicks, and Hawthorne, 2009). MBD occurs in 50% to 60% of infants with 28 weeks' gestation and in those with birth weight of 1000 grams or less (Chauhan, Sarkar, and Bhimte, 2011).
- Preterm infants are at a greater risk for iron deficient anemia due to smaller iron stores at birth and a greater requirement. Iron supplementation can improve iron status and reduce the risk of anemia and associated side effects (Long, Yi, Li, et al, 2012).

TRACKING PROGRESS

Premature infants should not be evaluated against standards set for term infants.

- Premature infants should have their chronological age corrected by gestational age.
- Special growth grids for premature infants to 38-month gestational age are available.
- Premature infants will have periods of catch-up growth that will initially be seen in head circumference followed by weight and length.

NECROTIZING ENTEROCOLITIS

The most serious gastrointestinal disorder of neonates is **necrotizing enterocolitis (NEC),** an acquired injury to the bowel. This inflammatory bowel disease of neonates results in inflammation and bacterial colonization of the bowel wall (Claud, 2009). NEC causes significant morbidity and mortality in preterm infants, occurring in:

- 10% of all ELBW (<1000 g) infants
- 5% of all VLBW (<1500 g) infants

Established risk factors include:

- Preterm birth
- Low Apgar scores
- Enteral feeding
- Maternal hypertensive disease of pregnancy (Patel and Shah, 2012)

The precise etiology of this multifactorial disease process remains elusive. Consequently, treatments are symptomatic and surgical. The single most important predictor of outcome, besides gestational age, is whether the disease has progressed to a point requiring surgical intervention. Infants with NEC requiring operation have a 50% survival rate (Afrazi, Sodhi, Richardson, et al, 2011).

Breastfeeding is the most effective preventative measure for NEC. Feeding preterm infants human milk has been associated with a 58% reduction in the incidence of NEC (Breastfeeding, 2012).

Genomic Gem 11-1
Possible Contributor to Premature Delivery

About one-half the cases of premature delivery have no identified cause. There is evidence that supports genetic variants that contribute to preterm birth. The genes that are of major focus are those involved with host response to infection/inflammation and those involved in the breakdown of amniotic membranes that encase the fetus (Anum, Springel, Shriver, and Strauss, 2009). If the membranes are weak, they are more likely to rupture early and lead to preterm delivery (Bryant, Worjoloh, Caughey, and Washington, 2010).

Black women are nearly twice as likely to give birth prematurely as White women. The variant described above is present in approximately 12.4% of Black women and 4.1% of White women.

Although research is looking at genetic contributions of racial disparities in preterm birth, the complexity of the problem is appearing to be a combination of both genetic and environmental effects rather than genetic factors alone.

correct ratio of nutrients. The mother's informed decision should be supported and appropriate teaching provided.

An estimated 5% of women may be unable to produce a full milk supply for anatomic or medical reasons. Moreover, because infants' sucking stimulates milk production, difficulty with the process may result in diminished milk supply.

It is not uncommon for infants to lose weight in the first days of breastfeeding, which can lead to loss of maternal confidence in breastfeeding and then to discontinuation or formula supplementation. Although some weight loss is expected, the infant needs to be monitored closely because weight loss greater than 10% is associated with increased risk of hypernatremic dehydration and hyperbilirubinemia, which can lead to the recommendation of formula supplementation (Bokser, Flaherman, and Newman, 2010; Mulder, Johnson, and Baker, 2010).

Infants should:

- Be observed while suckling at 2 to 4 days of age by a knowledgeable health-care provider
- Have its weight monitored by the same health-care provider

All parents should be taught to expect the infant to have at least:

- Four good-sized bowel movements and
- Six saturated diapers per day

Most important, enthusiastic support for breastfeeding should never delay provision of formula when medically indicated.

Advancing the Diet

Teaching the infant to consume the foods he will receive throughout life is a gradual process. First, semisolid foods are given to complement breast milk or formula. Eventually drinking from a cup will replace suckling.

Semisolid Foods

No proof exists of the folk wisdom that the early feeding of solid food to infants promotes their sleeping through the night. At 3 months, 75% of infants sleep all night, regardless of diet. If solid foods are introduced too early, the infant may develop allergies because of the permeability of the intestine.

The American Academy of Pediatrics supports exclusive breastfeeding (nothing but breast milk and vitamins, minerals, and medications) for 6 months while recognizing that infants are often developmentally ready for complementary foods between 4 and 6 months of age.

The infant should achieve voluntary control of swallowing at 3 to 4 months. Before being offered solid food, the infant should be able to control his or her head and trunk. With this ability, the baby can turn away when satisfied. By this time, the infant is drinking 8 ounces of formula or a similar estimated amount of breast milk and yet becomes hungry in less than 4 hours.

In introducing solid food, it is best to follow the infant's lead. To avoid later feeding problems, solid foods should be started when the baby is interested. Babies ready for solid food are hungry and not fussy about tastes (Fig. 11-2). Children learn from adults; parents should avoid showing distaste for particular foods.

Waiting too long to introduce solid foods may delay the infant's acquiring the skill to manipulate the tongue

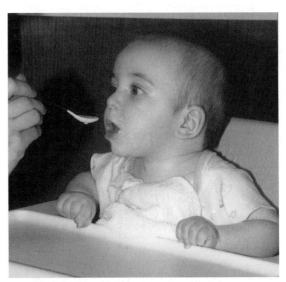

FIGURE 11-2 This 5-month-old baby is experiencing semisolid food for the first time. His readiness is clear. Notice how eager he is, how focused on the spoon.

and mouth appropriately. Early in the transition to semi-solid foods, the amount consumed is likely to be small so the main source of nutrients continues to be milk.

FEEDING

New foods should be introduced one at a time and a week apart so that if a problem develops, the responsible food can be readily identified. A food should be tried for 3 to 5 days before the infant is permitted to reject it. Only a taste or two is sufficient for the first try.

A commonly used schedule for introducing new foods appears in Table 11-7. The baby's physician may modify it to meet individual needs. No evidence supports the superiority of a particular sequence of food introduction. In particular, infants might benefit from early introduction of iron-rich foods such as iron fortified cereals and pureed meats, especially if being breastfed, to prevent the development of iron deficiency anemia. Single-ingredient food and food that the infant can chew and swallow safely should be offered (Clinical Application 11-6).

The parent should heat a small amount to serve the infant. Food that has been heated and not consumed should be discarded because of possible contamination with salivary enzymes and bacteria. Food that has been opened but not heated should be stored in the covered jar in the refrigerator and used within 3 days.

LEARNING ABOUT FLAVORS

Eating adult foods is a skill that babies must learn, but their culture affects the food choices they will be offered. The fetus will experience flavors from the mother's diet in swallowed amniotic fluid. One study found that infants whose mother drank carrot juice in the third trimester enjoyed carrot-flavored cereals more than infants whose mother did not drink carrot juice or eat carrots (Beauchamp and Mennella, 2011). Infants will later experience some of these flavors in breast milk that reflects the foods, spices, and beverages consumed by the mother that can account for culturally determined flavor preferences (Mennella, Forestell, Morgan, and Beauchamp, 2009).

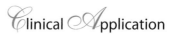

11-6

Clinical Application

Avoiding Choking Accidents

Each year, several hundred infants, as well as older children, choke on food. On average, one death every 5 days is reported in children from infancy to 9 years of age.

- Hot dogs, or frankfurters, are involved most often in infant choking. Apples, cookies, and biscuits are also frequent causes of choking in infants. Peanuts and grapes are the most dangerous for 2-year-old children, whereas 3-year-olds still face a risk from hot dogs.
- Other foods typically implicated in choking accidents appear in the following table by category. Because the child can safely eat many other foods, the prudent course is to avoid the listed foods when possible. If a choking incident occurs, any caregiver should be able to perform cardiopulmonary resuscitation (CPR) should it become necessary.
- Small children should always be supervised while they are eating, and they should be seated at a table to eat. Likewise, eating in a moving vehicle is discouraged.

HARD FOODS	STRINGY FOODS	STICKY FOODS	PLUG-SHAPED FOODS
Apples	Beans	Bread	Whole grapes
Carrots	Celery	Chewing gum	Hot dogs
Cookies		Peanut butter	
Corn			
Hard candy			
Nuts			
Peanuts			
Popcorn			
Raisins			
Other raw vegetables			
Seedy items (e.g., watermelon)			

Weaning the Infant

Teaching the infant to use a cup is a gradual process. In most cases, the baby will show interest in the cup at 4 to 6 months. For these early attempts, and if the

TABLE 11-7 ■ Suggested Progression for Offering Foods to Infant at Low Risk of Allergies		
AGE OF INFANT	**FOOD**	**RATIONALE/PRECAUTIONS**
4 Months	Infant cereal mixed with formula	Because of risk of allergies, rice offered first; wheat after age 12 months. Read labels: some mixed infant cereals contain wheat.
5–6 Months	Strained vegetables	Less sweet than fruits; thought less likely to be rejected if offered before fruit.
6–7 Months	Strained fruits	Will be well accepted; humans have strong preference for sweets.
6–8 Months	Finger foods (bananas, crackers)	Encourages self-feeding. Different textures may aid speech development.
7–8 Months	Strained meats	May be introduced earlier to add iron and zinc to the diet. Offer variety. (See Clinical Application 11-6.)
10 Months	Strained or mashed egg yolk	Start with ½ tsp. Due to possible allergy, delay egg white until 1 year old.
10 Months	Bite-sized cooked foods	Select appropriate foods. See Clinical Application 11-6.
12 Months	Foods from adult table	Select suitable foods, prepared according to baby's abilities.

infant is not exclusively breastfed, water can be offered. If the mother decides to wean the child from breast or bottle before its first birthday, the replacement should be infant formula, not unmodified cow's milk.

The bottle-fed infant may not be ready to give up the bottle until 12 to 14 months of age. If bedtime bottles have not been used, weaning will proceed more rapidly. It is best to substitute the cup for the bottle for one feeding period at a time. After using the new schedule for 5 days or so, the new method is substituted for a second feeding.

Nutritional Problems in Infancy

Common problems of nutrition in infancy are summarized in Table 11-8. The table includes some home remedies, but if an infant does not improve rapidly from a nutrition-related problem, parents should seek medical attention.

Allergies

Food allergies affect approximately 6% of children in the United States (Wang, 2010). Food allergies can be IgE-mediated, non-IgE-mediated, or a combination of both (Wang & Sampson, 2011).

IgE-MEDIATED ALLERGIES

Because true food allergies can have fatal consequences, identifying children with allergies is critical. An **allergen** is a substance that provokes an abnormal individual hypersensitivity or **allergy.** The steps in allergy production are illustrated in Figure 11-3. Proteins that are not broken down into amino acids and small peptides can enter the blood stream intact and in their most allergenic form (Smith, 2012).

The number of people with allergies is increasing rapidly both in developed and developing countries but not in underdeveloped areas. The fewer germs in the environment, the more time the immune system has to process and react to allergens. Although

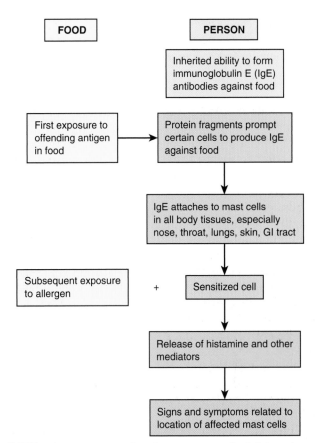

FIGURE 11-3 Development of an allergic reaction to food. (Adapted from Formanek, 2001; Taylor and Hefle, 2006.)

allergic disease is a complex condition, evidence does support a hereditary component (Kneepkens & Brand, 2010).

Common Food Allergens

The following eight protein families account for the majority of food allergies:

1. Milk
2. Egg
3. Peanut
4. Tree nuts
5. Fish

TABLE 11-8 ■ Common Nutritional Problems in Infancy		
PROBLEM	**INTERVENTION**	**COMMENTS**
Regurgitation of Milk	Handle baby gently. Burp well; sit up after feeding.	Very common for first 6 months; not serious unless vomiting is projectile or bile-tinged or baby has persistent respiratory symptoms or poor weight gain.
Constipation	Apple or pear juice after the first month of life. 1 oz per day for each month of life up to 4 oz.	Rare in breastfed infants.
Burns to Mouth	Swirl formula after heating; test well	Use water bath to heat. Formula warmed in a microwave oven continues to increase in temperature after removal.
Nursing-Bottle Syndrome	Do not use milk or juice as bedtime bottle; do not put sweetener on pacifier	See Chapter 3.

6. Crustacean shellfish
7. Soy
8. Wheat (Wang & Sampson, 2011)

In children, the most common allergenic foods are:

■ Eggs
■ Milk
■ Peanuts
■ Soybeans
■ Wheat

Children typically outgrow allergies to:

■ Eggs
■ Milk
■ Soy
■ Wheat

but not to:

■ Peanuts
■ Tree nuts
■ Fish
■ Shellfish (Burks et al, 2011)

Clinical Application 11-7 summarizes reports of fatal and near-fatal cases of **anaphylaxis** following ingestion of a food allergen. The seriousness of food allergies should never be underestimated.

Nonfood Transfers of Allergens

Allergens can be transferred by modes other than ingestion:

■ Kissing: A young woman with a severe shellfish allergy developed anaphylaxis after kissing her boyfriend who had eaten shrimp earlier in the evening (Steensma, 2003).
■ Inhalation:
   ■ An 11-year-old boy had anaphylaxis while his mother was cooking rice.
   ■ An 8-year-old girl developed anaphylaxis while white potatoes were being boiled at home.
   ■ An 8-year-old boy who had a severe milk allergy had repeated anaphylaxis after intake of dry powder inhaler, which contained trace amounts of lactose (Ramirez and Bahna, 2009).
■ Organ transplantation: pediatric client, aged 19 months, 3 years, and 16 years old, developed peanut allergies following liver transplants, according to three reports (Mavroudi, Xinias, Deligiannidis, et al, 2012).

Allergens from dissimilar sources also can evoke an allergic response. Cautions pertaining to cross-sensitivity to latex among persons allergic to various foods are listed in Clinical Application 11-8.

---

*C*linical *A*pplication   *11-7*

Anaphylactic Reactions to Food

Allergy to food can be fatal. About 30,000 cases of food allergy-related anaphylaxis are seen annually in emergency departments. The clients at the greatest risk of developing anaphylactic symptoms are those allergic to peanuts. Increased rates of peanut allergies are attributed to:

■ Increased vegetarian diets in which peanuts are seen as a good protein source
■ Increasingly common environmental exposures
■ Food preparation practices and inaccurate labeling that lead to accidental exposure

Symptoms can develop within seconds of ingestion but typically will begin within 15 minutes of exposure, and respiratory arrest can occur within 30 minutes of exposure. Symptoms include:

■ Difficulty swallowing/breathing
■ Cough and wheezing, shortness of breath
■ Hoarse voice and/or stridor
■ Edema of face and hands
■ Paleness and clamminess
■ Tachycardia
■ Loss of consciousness

Treatment and education of clients, families, health professionals, and the community need focus on the following:

■ Accidental peanut ingestion should be avoided and early signs and symptoms of allergic reaction recognized.
■ Epinephrine should be prescribed, kept available, and used for clients with IgE-mediated food allergies.
■ Children and adolescents who have an allergic reaction to food should be observed for 3 to 4 hours after the reaction at a center capable of dealing with anaphylaxis.
■ Parents of such children should be taught to ensure an emergency plan is developed and is provided to schools and other relevant institutions.
■ Schools need to have training related to identification and emergency treatment of anaphylaxis, have written emergency plans, and have labeled emergency kits.

Of clients who have experienced life-threatening symptoms on initial reaction, 71% will have similarly severe reactions in subsequent episodes. When allergy seems possible, a thorough history and a food diary may yield a list of suspected foods to test further. Skin tests and blood tests can confirm the diagnosis.

Sources: Dunbar and Luyt, 2011; Johnson and Daitch, 2011.

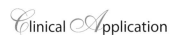
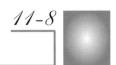

Clinical Application   11-8

Latex Allergies and Food Hypersensitivity

Individuals allergic to latex have demonstrated hypersensitivity to foods botanically unrelated to latex but that may share allergenic components. Allergies to certain fruits are described in 30% to 70% of latex-allergic clients which is referred to as latex-fruit syndrome. The fruits most commonly involved are the following:

- Avocado
- Banana
- Chestnut
- Fig (Radauer et al, 2011).

    Less commonly involved fruits are the following:

- Apricot
- Kiwi
- Mango
- Melon
- Plum
- Tomato

    Latex allergy should be ruled out in individuals allergic to any of those foods before performing clinical procedures using latex gloves.

Diagnosis

Self- or parental-diagnosis is a common practice but prone to error. Misdiagnosis leads to elimination of the wrong food or too many foods. Unnecessary elimination of foods can lead to malnutrition (Burton-Shepherd, 2012).

For infants, the timing of new foods is well advised. The signs and symptoms of food allergies may appear as long as 5 days after exposure to an allergen. Thus, allowing at least 5 days to elapse between new foods will increase chances of identifying allergens.

Treatment of Allergies

The key to treatment is avoidance of the allergen. Reading labels is likely to take over the lives of the family.

Since the beginning of 2006, when the Food Allergen Labeling and Consumer Protection Act took effect, food labels are required to state clearly whether the food contains a major food allergen. The law identifies a major food allergen as any of the eight listed earlier and any ingredient that contains protein derived from them. So if a product contains casein or whey, for example, the label must include the word *milk*. The plain language declaration requirement also applies to flavorings, colorings, and incidental additives that are or contain a major food allergen (Food Allergy & Anaphylaxis Network [FAAN], 2011).

FAAN provides educational materials to assist in analyzing labels for ingredients with allergenic potential. Its Web site has notifications of products with ingredients not included on labels. For teachers and caregivers, the organization also has a model emergency plan in English and Spanish (FAAN, 2012).

Pharmacologic management of allergy signs and symptoms includes the following:

- Antihistamines that block histamine receptors in the tissues for mild to moderate symptoms
- Epinephrine (adrenalin) with bronchodilator and vasopressor actions for severe reactions; self-administered epinephrine can be lifesaving.

    Anaphylaxis guidelines suggest:

- Treatment with epinephrine
- Teaching about self-injectable epinephrine
- Referral to an allergist
- Sending the client home with an anaphylaxis emergency plan
- Teaching about anaphylaxis and its treatment

As shown in Clinical Application 11-7, even if prescriptions have been filled, they are not always used appropriately.

Related Food Technology

In any single day, our immune systems are exposed to thousands of proteins from the environment and the food we eat. All foods we consume are potential allergens. The discrepancy between the vast numbers of proteins we encounter and the limited number that actually become allergens led to an allergy assessment strategy for genetically modified foods. This technology enables adding or changing the genes that contribute to food allergies. Biotechnology products are extensively tested for allergic effects before commercialization, which contributes to increased safety.

COW'S MILK PROTEIN–SENSITIVE ENTEROPATHY

Cow's milk allergy is thought to affect 2% to 3% of infants (Kneepkens and Meijer, 2009). In an IgE-mediated allergy, an immune system response to a specific protein leads to inflammatory changes in the gastrointestinal tract.

Symptoms resolve within 48 to 72 hours after eliminating cow's milk protein from the diet. By age 1, 40% to 50% of children will tolerate cow's milk, and by the age of 3 this rises to 75% to 90% (Burton-Shepherd, 2012). The physician should be reminded of dietary limitations so that an appropriate time can be chosen to reintroduce the offending foods.

Colic

Infantile colic occurs in 10% to 25% of infants. Although the cause of colic is unknown, the condition is named for the presumed manifestation, spasms of the muscles of the colon. The abdomen is tense, and the infant flexes his or her legs up to the belly and may appear flushed. The infant may cry for hours, starting late in the afternoon, just when caregivers are also tired and cranky. The classic definition of colic is the "Rule of Threes," crying for more than:

- 3 hours a day
- 3 days per week
- 3 weeks (Infante, Segarra, & LeLuyer, 2011)

POSSIBLE CAUSES

Suggested causes fall into two main groups:

- Gastrointestinal (food protein hypersensitivity or allergy)
- Nongastrointestinal (parental– or maternal–child interaction problems)

The various factors act together, gastrointestinal, psychosocial, and neurodevelopmental disorders have been suggested as causes for colic (Kheir, 2012).

Physiological causes have been proposed:

- Abdominal distention resulting from swallowing air. Passage of flatus seems to relieve the pain.
  - If the infant is bottle-fed, the nipple holes may be too big or too small, increasing the amount of air swallowed.
  - The breastfed infant might be swallowing air because of incorrect nursing position.
- Carbohydrate metabolism may be immature, producing transient lactose intolerance.
  - Symptoms are relieved in 5% to 20% of infants with colic after exclusion of cow's milk protein for 5 days (Landgren, Lundqvist, & Hallstrom, 2012).
  - Thirty-seven percent of strictly breastfed infants had a reduction in symptoms when the mother followed a low-allergen diet (Infantile Colic, 2011).

TREATMENT

The following interventions have sometimes helped:

- Holding the baby upright
- Burping
- Providing warm water to drink
- Diluting the formula
- Offering cold formula
- Swaddling
- Carrying the infant
- Rocking
- Making soft repetitive sounds

For breastfed infants, a 7-day trial manipulating the mother's diet reduced the crying or fussing duration by 37%. Foods omitted by the mothers were cow's milk, eggs, tree nuts, peanuts, wheat, and fish (Infantile Colic, 2012).

Even though their baby's condition is stressful for them, the parents should try not to be overly concerned. Most infants grow and gain weight despite colic.

The one proven treatment is time: 85% of infants with colic have diminished symptoms by age 3 months (Landgren et al, 2012).

Diarrhea

WHO defines diarrhea as the passage of more than three loose, watery stools a day (WHO, 2012). In developing countries, diarrhea is a common cause of mortality among children younger than 5 years old, with an estimated 2 million deaths annually. Among children in the United States, acute diarrhea accounts for:

- More than 1.5 million outpatient visits
- 200,000 hospitalizations for children under age 5
- 300 deaths per year (Chow, Leung, & Hon, 2010)

Seventy-five percent of an infant's body weight is water, 54% of it extracellular. For this reason, an infant is at high risk of rapid dehydration from diarrhea. The degree of dehydration can be estimated from the infant's weight loss with severe dehydration being classified as a weight loss of more than 10%.

CAUSES

Infants are subject to osmotic diarrhea. Overfeeding and food intolerances are common causes of diarrhea.

The most common cause of infectious **enteritis** in human infants is **rotavirus.** Gastroenteritis caused by rotavirus results in about 20 to 60 deaths in the United States annually in children younger than 5 years old, but 500,000 deaths in the same ages worldwide (Centers for Disease Control and Prevention, 2010). Severe vomiting may accompany the diarrhea.

Children between 6 months and 2 years of age are most susceptible. By age 3, most children have antibodies against the virus. The fecal–oral route is its probable mode of transmission, but the virus survives for long periods on hard surfaces, in contaminated water, and on hands.

The only single prevention and control measure are vaccines against rotavirus gastroenteritis.

PATHOPHYSIOLOGY

As a result of diarrhea, the wall of the intestine may become inflamed. The inflammation diminishes the amount of lactase produced, so the infant may exhibit temporary lactose intolerance. Distension, cramps, and osmotic diarrhea ensue. In diarrhea caused by rotavirus, the virus disrupts the normal functioning of the gastrointestinal mucosa, which stimulates gut motility causing an uncontrolled outflux of water into the intestinal lumen resulting in profuse diarrhea (Chandran, Fitzwater, Zhen, and Santosham, 2010).

TREATMENT

Treatment should begin at home at the onset of the diarrhea. Caregivers should be instructed regarding signs and symptoms of dehydration and other parameters of treatment failure. The usual protocol is as follows:

- **Oral rehydration solutions (ORS)** should be used for rehydration, which should be accomplished in 3 to 4 hours.
- An age-appropriate, unrestricted diet should be given as soon as dehydration is corrected.
- For breastfed infants, nursing should be continued.
- For formula-fed infants, diluted formula is not recommended, and special formula is not necessary.
- Additional ORS should be administered for ongoing losses through diarrhea.
- No unnecessary laboratory tests or medications should be administered.

ORSs (see Chapter 8) are lifesaving not only in developing countries but also in North America. Most infants who are vomiting can be rehydrated with oral fluids. Providing sips of ORS by teaspoon at a rate of 15 to 25 mL/kg/hour will prevent gastric distension and vomiting (Wittenberg, 2012). Ceralyte®, Oralyte®, and Pedialyte®, as well as store brands, are available at nearly all drug stores and grocery stores.

Sports drinks are not adequate substitutes for these solutions. Large amounts of fluids containing simple sugars, such as carbonated soft drinks, juice, and gelatin desserts, should be avoided because they might increase osmotic diarrhea. Liquids at room temperature are often better tolerated than warm or cold beverages.

WHEN TO CALL THE PHYSICIAN

Parents should be instructed to call the primary healthcare provider regarding an infant's diarrhea under the following conditions:

- Young or small infant
  - <6 months of age
  - <17.6 pounds in weight
- History of premature birth, chronic medical conditions, or concurrent illness
- Fever
  - 38°C (100.4°F) for infants ages <3 months
  - >39°C (102.2°F) for children ages 3 to 36 months
- Visible blood in stool

- High output, including frequent and substantial volumes of diarrhea
- Persistent vomiting
- Signs of dehydration
  - Sunken eyes
  - Decreased tears
  - Dry mucous membranes
  - Decreased urine output
- Change in mental status (e.g., irritability, apathy, or lethargy)
- Suboptimal response to oral rehydration therapy (ORT) already administered or inability of the caregiver to administer ORT.

ORS has been shown to have several benefits compared with intravenous fluid therapy (IVT) which include:

- Convenient to administer
- No associated pain or phlebitis
- ORS has been shown to have similar effectiveness in treating acute gastroenteritis in children (Suh, Hahn, & Cho, 2010).

Risk factors for increased mortality from acute diarrhea in the United States are:

- Prematurity
- Young maternal age
- Black race
- Rural residence

The decision to hospitalize an infant should consider these factors along with degree of dehydration.

Nutrition of the Toddler (Ages 1 to 3 Years)

The child's nutritional needs become more like those of adults after the first birthday. During the toddler years, growth is slower than during infancy, and although activity increases, the proportional need for kilocalories decreases compared with infancy. Thus, the child's appetite slackens.

How and what the family eats will influence the child's habits and tastes for many years. Being forced to eat a distasteful food because "it's good for you" has imprinted permanent avoidance behaviors on some individuals. Conversely, some parents expand their repertory of menu choices to set good examples for their children.

Psychosocial Development

Autonomy or independence is the psychosocial developmental task of the toddler. Every 2-year-old knows the word *no*. One way parents can assist a toddler achieve autonomy is to encourage choices from acceptable food alternatives (Fig. 11-4). If parents insist that a child eat certain items or amounts, the child may learn to use food rejection as a means of gaining attention. Later, more serious eating problems may result from such interactions. The parent can, however, create structure in the child's day by insisting the child remain at the table during mealtime whether or not items are consumed.

Physical Growth and Development

During the toddler years, growth slows. The expected weight gain in the second year may be just 4 to 6 pounds. Height may increase by about 4 inches. By age 2, however, head circumference reaches two-thirds of its adult size. *See "Growth Charts" on DavisPlus or at www.cdc.gov/ growthcharts.*

The toddler is aptly named. One of the skills acquired during this time is walking upright. As this skill is being perfected, the child's muscles of the back, buttocks, and thighs are enlarging. The bones are becoming more mineralized, and "baby fat" is disappearing.

Along with the gross motor skill of walking, the toddler's fine motor control improves. He or she is able to

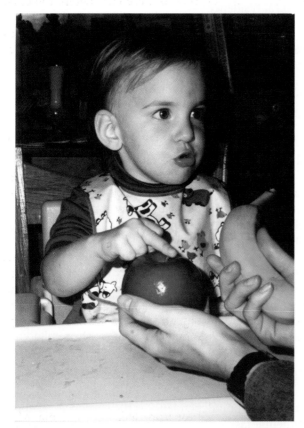

FIGURE 11-4 Autonomy is achieved in small steps. This 19-month-old girl is choosing her dessert.

use eating utensils with more finesse. The spoon is likely to reach the mouth still filled with food. The toddler's mouth is more sensitive than an adult's mouth. Foods are eaten better at lukewarm temperatures rather than hot. Thus, dawdling at the table may have a physiological basis.

Nutrient Needs and Intake

For DRIs, see Appendix A. In 2008, the American Academy of Pediatrics recommended that all children receive a daily intake of 400 IU of vitamin D (Minarich and Silverstein, 2011).

The need for many nutrients increases proportionately with body size throughout the growth years. These needs, coupled with the toddler's poorer appetite, stretch parents' ingenuity and patience. See Table 11-9 for MyPlate recommendations for 2- to 5-year-olds.

According to the American Academy of Pediatrics, despite the toddler's poorer appetite, vitamin supplements are probably unnecessary for healthy children older than 1 year (see Dollars & Sense 11-2). Special circumstances may indicate a need for supplementation.

Food Likes

Toddlers like finger foods and can learn about texture by eating them. Toddlers prefer plain foods to most mixtures such as casseroles. Familiar combinations, such as macaroni and cheese, spaghetti, and pizza, however, may be relished. Unfamiliar foods that are rejected the first time should be offered again at a later time.

Mealtimes

Toddlers are learning social skills as well as good nutritional habits. Eating is a social experience for adults most of the time; toddlers also appreciate company. Parents should be encouraged to sit down and eat with the toddler. Visiting other homes might introduce food items and experiences not encountered at home.

As with other financial decisions, families must decide on the best use of their funds. See Chapters 7 and 15 for quality issues.

Keeping to a regular schedule will help maintain the child's food intake. A 1-year-old's stomach holds just 1 cup, necessitating small servings. A serving is one-fourth to one-fifth the size of an adult's recommended serving. A good rule of thumb is to serve 1 tablespoonful for each year of age.

Eating regular meals and nutritious snacks helps to prevent fatigue and control the appetite. If high-sugar snacks are used to assuage hunger before a meal,

TABLE 11-9 ■ MyPlate Guidelines 2- to 5-Year-Olds Based on 1000 Calories/Day		
FOOD GROUP	NUMBER OF SERVINGS	SERVING SUGGESTIONS
Grains	3 ounces	Make half your grains whole. Aim for 1½ ounces of whole grains a day.
Fruit	1 cup	Eat a variety of fruit. Choose whole or cut-up fruits more often than fruit juice.
Vegetable	1 cup	Vary your veggies. Each week aim for the following: Dark green = ½ cup Red and orange = 2½ cups Beans and peas = ½ cup Starchy veggies = 2 cups Other veggies = 1½ cups
Protein Foods	2 ounces	Twice a week serve seafood. Vary proteins to include beans, peas, nuts, and seeds. Keep meat and poultry portions small and lean.
Dairy	2 cups	Drink fat-free or low fat (1%) milk. Serve fat-free or low-fat yogurt and cheese. If serving soy products make sure they are calcium-fortified.
Fats, Sugar, Sodium	3 teaspoons oil Limit fat calories and added sugar calories to 140 calories Sodium less than 2300 mg	Serve low-fat dairy. Serve lean proteins. Avoid sugary snacks and beverages. Serve fruits in natural form instead of canned fruits packed in water. Avoid processed foods.

$ Dollars & Sense 11-2

Children's Vitamins

Although the American Academy of Pediatrics does not recommend vitamin and mineral supplements for healthy children, many families provide them as insurance. If parents choose to give vitamin and mineral supplements to a child, they should be aware of the cost per year. For example:

Ages	Brand Name Product	Price/Daily Dose	Total cost
1–12 years	Children's chewable	$0.10	$36.50
12–18 years	Adult tablet	$0.07	$25.55
Total per child			$62.05

however, the more nutritious foods at the meal may be taken poorly.

New Foods

After the pureed foods of infancy, parents will be pleased to offer more attractive plates of food to the toddler. Brightly colored foods are appealing. Nevertheless, chewing may not be well developed. Tough meat or very fibrous vegetables are not for the toddler.

Foods not recommended until after the first birthday can be gradually introduced if family history of allergies is not a concern. These foods include unmodified cow's milk, egg white, wheat, citrus fruits, seafood, chocolate, and nut butters. Parents should continue to introduce foods one at a time at weekly intervals and to watch for reactions.

Even very young children make their wishes known through body movements, pushing food away, closing their mouths, and turning away from the feeder. The astute parent will respond to these cues before the child resorts to crying to communicate distress. Parents should be advised to avoid the use of external cues such as prompts, rewards, or forcing a child to clean their plate.

Daily intake should include:

- One serving of a vitamin C-rich fruit or vegetable
- One serving of a green leafy or yellow vegetable
- Limited sugar
- Grams of fiber equal to child's age +5 beginning at age 2

Parents should continue to avoid giving the toddler hazardous foods (Clinical Application 11-6). Sometimes chopping the food into tiny pieces eliminates a choking hazard. Nevertheless, a toddler should not be left alone while eating.

Because the kidneys become mature at about age 1, the toddler can tolerate salt in moderation. Preference for salty foods is an acquired taste. Because of the association between salt and high blood pressure later in life, the prudent parent will discourage the consumption of heavily salted foods.

Nutritional Concerns

Toddlers are at risk for iron-deficiency anemia. Misguided food choices may lead to inadequate intakes of nutrients and interfere with growth and development.

Iron-Deficiency Anemia

Iron deficiency affects 2.4 million children in the United States. Childhood iron-deficiency **anemia** is associated with behavioral and cognitive delays. Infants considered high risk are those of low socioeconomic status, Africans or African Americans, immigrants, those born preterm and small for gestational age, and those who did not receive an adequately supplemented formula (Aspuru, Villa, Bermejo et al, 2011). One study of 1641 toddlers investigated risk factors and racial/ethnic disparities related to iron deficiency and found the following:

- 42% were Hispanic
- 28% were White
- 25% were African American

The study also investigated the risk of obesity in relationship to iron-deficiency anemia, finding that:

- 20% of those with iron-deficiency anemia were overweight
- 8% were at risk for being overweight
- 7% were normal weight (Brotanek, Gosz, Weitzman, and Flores, 2007)

Overindulging in milk is thought to decrease the appetite for iron-rich foods, enriched cereals, meats, and some fruits and vegetables. Therefore, milk intake should be limited to 24 ounces per day for children aged 1 to 5 years. The term *milk anemia* refers to iron deficiency anemia caused by overconsumption of milk and underconsumption of iron-rich foods. Juice for toddlers should not exceed 6 ounces per day (Box 11-2).

Box 11-2 ■ *Recommendations for Juice Consumption*

For Infants

- No juice before 6 months of age
- No juice from bottles or covered cups that permit consumption throughout the day
- No juice at bedtime
- No unpasteurized juice

For Children and Adolescents

- Ages 1 to 6: Limit juice to 4 to 6 ounces per day
- Ages 7 to 18: Limit juice to 8 to 12 ounces per day
- Encourage consumption of whole fruits
- No unpasteurized juice

Assessment and Interventions

- Determine amount of juice intake for children with overnutrition or undernutrition and those with chronic diarrhea or abdominal symptoms.
- Determine the amount and means of juice intake for children with dental caries.
- Teach parents the difference between juice and juice drinks.

Source: Summarized from American Academy of Pediatrics. Policy Statement. The Use and Misuse of Fruit Juice in Pediatrics. PEDIATRICS Vol. 107 No. 5 May 2001, pp. 1210-1213. Reaffirmed August 2013.

Treatment of iron-deficiency anemia may include medication and ingestion of iron-fortified foods or foods naturally high in iron. Treatment should produce a normal hemoglobin level in 1 to 2 months, but replenishing iron stores may take 3 to 6 months (Deglin and Vallerand, 2009).

Vegetarian diets may pose a risk for iron deficiency in toddlers. The position of the Academy of Nutrition and Dietetics is that a *well-planned* vegetarian diet can provide all the nutrients needed by children at varying stages of growth. Extremely restrictive diets such as fruitarian and raw foods diets, however, have been associated with impaired growth and are not recommended for infants and children.

Milk Intake

To support brain growth and development, 1- to 2-year-old children should continue to drink whole milk. At age 2, fat intake should gradually be reduced to 30% of a child's intake and transitioning to low-fat or fat-free milk is recommended.

Nutrition of the Preschool Child (Ages 3 to 6 Years)

This is a delightful time of enthusiastic learning, including food preferences.

Psychosocial Development

Initiative is the psychosocial task to be mastered by the preschool child. Within their capabilities, children should be encouraged to set and achieve some goals of their own. Children can participate in planning and preparation of meals, and they should help in the kitchen, not just with cleanup. Preschool children can make gelatin desserts, fancy cookies, and showy relishes to foster a sense of accomplishment.

By making the meal a social time and eating slowly themselves, parents can encourage the same behavior in a child. Exemplifying good manners will be more productive than criticizing the child's manners.

Having company their own age is helpful. Children stay at the table longer and eat more in the company of their peers. Exchanging visits with a friend's child will begin to broaden the child's horizons.

Physical Growth and Development

From the third to the sixth year, a child continues to gain 4 to 5 pounds per year. A gain in height of about 2 inches per year is average so that by age 5, birth length will have doubled. Half the adult height is attained by approximately age 2 years.

Adequacy of growth should be assessed every 6 to 12 months. Growth charts remain the standard against which a given assessment is judged. *See "Growth Charts" on DavisPlus or at www.cdc.gov/growthcharts.*

Nutrient Needs and Intake

For DRIs, see Appendix A. In 2008, the American Academy of Pediatrics recommended that all children receive a daily intake of 400 IU of vitamin D (Minarich and Silverstein, 2011).

More than 30% of children in the United States take dietary supplements regularly, most often multivitamins and multiminerals. Supplement use was associated with higher family income, a smoke-free environment, not participating in the Women, Infants, and Children program (WIC), lower child body mass index (BMI), and less daily television and computer use time (Picciano, Dwyer, Radimer, et al, 2007).

Preschool children are very active. A 3-year-old may need 1300 to 1500 kilocalories per day. Serving sizes for 4- to 6-year-old children are the same as those *recommended* for adults.

Developing Good Habits

The preschool child responds best to regular mealtimes. When the adult meal will be served late, the parents have to decide if it would be better to allow the child to socialize with adults at a late meal or to feed the child early.

Preschoolers cannot eat enough in only three meals to meet their needs. By age 3, a child is able to verbalize hunger. Some nutrient-dense, low-fat choices are:

- Cottage cheese
- Low-fat yogurt
- Fresh fruit
- Raw vegetables
- Low-fat milk
- Fruit juices
- Graham crackers
- Fig bars

Concentrated sweets such as candy and soda pop should be limited.

However, too much control is undesirable. Young children naturally obey inner cues of hunger and satiety. Parents who override those cues by insisting the child eat a given amount are teaching the child to overeat. It is better to acknowledge that the child cannot consume enough at mealtime and to provide healthy snacks.

Tableware should be appropriate for the preschool child. Unbreakable dishes that are designed for stability, with deep sides to permit scooping the food onto a spoon or fork, are practical choices. Small glasses and cups, also unbreakable, with a squat design and low center of gravity, will minimize accidents and mealtime tension.

It is not too early to emphasize the importance of cleanliness. Regularly washing hands before meals and brushing teeth after meals will cultivate good health habits.

New Foods

Parents should offer new foods one at a time in small amounts. Trying something new is most acceptable at the beginning of the meal when the child is hungriest. A taste or two is sufficient if new foods are offered at regular intervals. Often 8 to 10 tries are necessary before the child develops a taste for a new food.

Parents have the advantage of being able to select the food offered. Items the parents dislike will not grace the family table regularly, if at all. Children, too, should be permitted their preferences. If an argument over food develops into a power struggle, as sometimes happens, the child will not admit to liking the food, even when it turns out to be quite tasty.

Nutritional Concerns

Preschool children should be monitored for problems. See Box 11-3 for data that can be included in pediatric nutritional screening.

Box 11-3 ■ *Nutrition Screening for Young Children*

Nutritional screening in young children is important to ensure proper growth and development and for early detection of nutritional related problems such as obesity and failure to thrive. Nutritional screening also allows time for anticipatory guidance. Various screening tools can be used that provide both subjective and objective data.

Objective data should include:

- Height/length of child and parents
- Weight
- Objective data should be plotted on growth charts at each assessment

Subjective data can include data such as:

- How many ounces of milk and juice does the child consume each day?
- How many servings of fruits and vegetables does the child eat per day?
- How many servings of whole grains does the child eat per day?
- What are main protein sources?
- How many hours of television or video watching per day?
- How many times per week does the child eat fast food meals?
- How many minutes of physical activity does the child participate in each day?

In addition, dental caries and the nutritional quality in day-care programs may be of concern.

Dental Health

The destruction of tooth enamel by dental caries (see Chapter 3) is a problem for all economic groups. The "baby" teeth, as well as the permanent teeth, deserve care and professional attention. For teeth to be correctly brushed, the parent may have to do it. Fluorosis (see Chapter 8) has occurred as a result of the overuse of supplements and the ingestion of fluoridated toothpaste. Children younger than 6 years are likely to swallow rather than to expectorate toothpaste. A pea-sized portion of toothpaste is sufficient. Regular dental checkups should be a part of the preschool child's routine.

Adequate dentition and good nutrition are mutually supportive. Nutritional counseling for parents is an important intervention for the prevention of dental carries in children. A study showed that preschool children from ages 1 to 5 years who consumed sugar-containing drinks, especially at night, and daily sugar intake were independent risk factors in the development of early childhood caries (Tinanoff, 2009).

Childcare Programs

It is estimated that approximately three-quarters of children aged 3 to 6 years old in the United States spend time in organized child care. The American Dietetic Association has addressed meeting children's nutrition and nutrition education needs while in child care. Some pertinent recommendations are:

- Children in care for 8 hours or less should be offered at least one meal and two snacks or two snacks and one meal.
- Children in the program for 8 or more hours per day should be offered two meals and two snacks or three snacks and one meal.
- Children should be served fruits and vegetables high in vitamin C daily and high in vitamin A at least three times a week.
- Caregivers should not add extra salt or sugar to food.
- Good institutional food management practices should be implemented, including good hand washing, adequate refrigeration, and proper storage of supplies.

Nutrition of the School-Age Child (Ages 6 to 12 Years)

A balanced diet suitable for healthy adults will also be good for a school-age child.

Diets should not be restricted because of the energy (kilocalorie), fat, or sugar content of any one food, nor should foods be labeled *good* or *bad*. In the first case, food may be regarded as medicine, and in the second, as "forbidden fruit." Neither viewpoint fosters positive attitudes.

Psychosocial Development

According to Erikson, the developmental task of the school-age child is **industry.** The school years are the years to build competence in many different skills. Making and keeping commitments is part of developing industry.

School-age children can participate in planning menus, shopping for food, preparing the meals, as well as cleaning up afterward (Fig. 11-5). Limiting the child's role to washing the dishes or taking out the garbage will be more likely to foster a sense of inferiority than habits of industry.

Physical Growth and Development

The average yearly growth during the school years is 7 pounds and 2.5 inches. The growth is not evenly distributed throughout the year, reflected in an inconsistent appetite. A child's progress should be tracked on the CDC growth charts to determine if growth is within the normal range. *See "Growth Charts" on Davis Plus or at www.cdc.gov/growthcharts.*

Exercise can help the school-age child's growth and development by stimulating osteoblasts and expending energy to control weight. Activities that are likely to become lifetime interests should be especially encouraged. Unlike sports such as football that are played by few adults, tennis or similar skill sports may provide an outlet for a lifetime.

By school age, the effects of good or poor nutrition will begin to be apparent. The well-nourished child will display most of the qualities listed in Table 11-10.

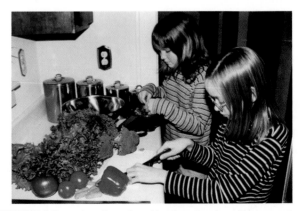

FIGURE 11-5 Preparing dinner for a friend can involve culinary practice.

TABLE 11-10 ■ Indications of Good Nutrition in the School-Age Child

General Appearance	Alert, energetic Normal height and weight
Skin and Mucous Membranes	Skin smooth, slightly moist; mucous membranes pink, no bleeding
Hair	Shiny, evenly distributed
Scalp	No sores
Eyes	Bright, clear, no fatigue circles
Teeth	Straight, clean, no discoloration or caries
Tongue	Pink, papillae present, no sores
Gastrointestinal System	Good appetite, regular elimination
Musculoskeletal System	Well-developed, firm muscles; erect posture, bones straight without deformities
Neurological System	Good attention span for age; not restless, irritable, or weepy

Nutritional Needs and Concerns

For DRIs, see Appendix A. In 2008, the American Academy of Pediatrics recommended that all children receive a daily intake of 400 IU of vitamin D (Minarich and Silverstein, 2011).

See Table 11-11 for MyPlate guidelines for 6- to 8-year-olds.

Meal Patterns and Behaviors

A school-age child cannot consume all the needed nutrients in three child-sized meals. Healthy snacks are necessary to complement the main meals. Likewise,

breakfast is essential and should contain one-fourth to one-third of the day's nutrients. Skipping breakfast has been shown to lead to consumption of higher-fat snacks later in the day, resulting in higher BMI (Corder, van Sluijs, Steele, et al, 2011).

School-age children are generally so active that they may have trouble sitting still. Requiring them to spend 15 to 20 minutes at the table for meals will increase the likelihood that they will eat a complete meal.

Concerning attention-deficit/hyperactivity disorder, studies are showing that a balanced diet high in omega-3 fatty acids and free of potential allergens, food preservatives, and high amounts of processed sugars may be a beneficial strategy used in the treatment of the disorder (Duca, 2010). Further research is being conducted.

One study showed that eating five to seven family dinners per week resulted in significantly higher frequency of breakfast consumption and higher daily servings of fruits, and those who did not report eating family dinners were three times more likely to be overweight and six times more likely to be food insecure (Fulkerson, Kubik, Sotry et al, 2009). Another study showed that females aged 9 to 14 years who ate family dinner most days of the week were less likely to initiate purging, binge eating, and frequent dieting (Haines, Gillman, Rifas-Shiman et al, 2010).

Nutrition at School

Nutrition education continues in school, focusing on foods, not nutrients. Interactions with other children

TABLE 11-11 ■ MyPlate Guidelines 6- to 8-Year-Olds Based on 1800 Calories/Day

FOOD GROUP	NUMBER OF SERVINGS	SERVING SUGGESTIONS
Grains	6 ounces	Make half your grains whole. Aim for 3 ounces of whole grains a day.
Fruit	1½ cups	Eat a variety of fruit Choose whole or cut-up fruits more often than fruit juice
Vegetable	2½ cups	Vary your veggies. Each week aim for the following: Dark green = 1½ cups Red and orange = 5½ cups Beans and peas = 1½ cups Starchy veggies = 5 cups Other veggies = 4 cups
Protein Foods	5 ounces	Twice a week, serve seafood. Vary proteins to include beans, peas, nuts, and seeds. Keep meat and poultry portions small and lean.
Dairy	2½ cups	Drink fat-free or low fat (1%) milk. Serve fat-free or low-fat yogurt and cheese. If serving soy products make sure they are calcium-fortified.
Fats, Sugar, Sodium	5 teaspoons oil Limit fat calories and added sugar calories to 160 calories Sodium less than 2300 mg	Serve low-fat dairy. Serve lean proteins. Avoid sugary snacks and beverages. Serve fruits in natural form instead of canned fruits packed in water. Avoid processed foods.

and school experiences expose a child to new foods and different cultures.

One study looked at the use of the Nutrition Detective program, which educates students on the selection of healthful foods that are minimally processed, low in added sugars and trans-fats, and rich in desirable constituents, such as fiber. The study showed that the program enhanced the ability of both students and their parents to distinguish more healthful from less healthful options (Katz, Katz, Treu, et al, 2011).

Because children need nourishment to learn and many come to school hungry, food assistance is available at school. Federally reimbursable school meals programs require participating schools to offer meals free or at reduced prices to eligible children. In 2011, 12.1 million children participated in the School Breakfast Program, and 10.1 million received their meals free or at a reduced price. See Box 11-4 and Table 11-12 for requirements.

Box 11-4 ■ *School Foods*

Federally funded school meals began in 1946 and specify nutritional content to be served (see Table 11-13).

Competitive foods are primary sources of low-nutrient, energy-dense foods that students consume that include items such as candy; chips; noncarbonated, high-sugar drinks; and soda. Federal regulations prohibit access to foods of minimal nutritional value in food-service areas during mealtimes, but schools can sell these foods at other locations during the school day. In the last decade, 39 states have passed law or policy addressing competitive foods and beverages (School, 2011).

The Institute of Medicine (2010) released standards for items available on school campuses but not part of the federally reimbursable school meals. The purpose of these stricter standards is to promote healthful eating habits. If followed, the standards would make à la carte cafeteria offerings, vending machine products, and fundraising items nearly conform to the Dietary Guidelines for Americans.

Nutrition in Adolescence

Adolescence is the period that extends from the onset of **puberty** until full growth is reached. For most individuals, adolescence occurs between the ages of 12 and 20. Adolescence is second only to infancy in the nutritional requirements necessary for growth and development. Unfortunately, most adolescents do not meet the daily recommendation for fruits, vegetables, and whole grains; they exceed the daily recommended amount of sodium; and they drink more full-calorie soda per day than milk (CDC, 2013). See Box 11-5 for information regarding energy drinks and the adolescent.

Psychosocial Development

Achieving their own **identity** is the developmental task Erikson identified for adolescents, including accepting their capabilities. In this process, teenagers "try on" various identities. Adolescents pick up fads instantly and drop them just as suddenly. Food and eating fads are part of the same pattern.

Physical Growth and Development

The term *growth spurt* is accurate. Boys and girls differ in the timing and completion of the growth spurt (see Table 11-13). To track an adolescent's growth, BMI-for-age percentile charts (2- to 20-year-old boys and girls) are available on *DavisPlus or at www.cdc.gov/ growthcharts*.

Approximately 90% or more of adult mass is obtained during childhood and puberty (Moretto, Silva, Kurokawa, et al, 2011). The peak growth spurt is

---

TABLE 11-12 ■ Federally Reimbursable School Meal Programs

	OPERATING SINCE	STUDENTS SERVED, 2011	FOOD	CURRENT REQUIREMENT
School Breakfast	1975	12.1 million	Grains and Meat/Meat Alternate	1 cup with vegetable substitution allowed. Grades K–6 have 1 oz daily minimum (7–10 oz weekly); Grades 6–8 have 2 oz minimum (10–12 oz weekly); Grades 9–12 have 1 oz minimum daily (9–10 oz weekly).
			Whole Grains	Encouraged
			Milk	All by July 1, 2014
				1 cup
				Must be fat-free (unflavored/flavored) or 1% low-fat (unflavored)
National School Lunch	1946	30.5 million	Fruit/Vegetables	¾ – 1 cup of vegetables plus ½ – 1 cup fruit per day. With weekly requirements for dark greens, red/orange, legumes, starchy
			Meat/Meat Alternate	Grades K-8 have 1 oz daily minimum (8–10 oz weekly); Grades 9–12 have 2 oz minimum (10–12 oz weekly).
			Grains	Grades K-5: 1 oz minimum (8–9 oz weekly); Grade 6–8: 1 oz minimum (8–10 oz weekly); Grades 9–12 2 oz minimum (10–12 oz weekly)
				All grains must be whole by July 1, 2014.
				1 cup
			Milk	Must be fat-free (unflavored/flavored) or 1% low-fat (unflavored).

Adapted from U.S. Department of Agriculture (2012).

Box 11-5 ■ *Energy Drink Use in Adolescents*

Energy drinks are beverages that contain higher levels of caffeine than soda and also can contain herbal supplements and vitamins. Energy drinks market the effects of improved energy, reaction time, and improved concentration, which are attractive benefits to some adolescents. There is an increase in energy drink consumption among adolescents in recent years. One study demonstrated that 31% of 12- to 17-year olds reported regular consumption of energy drinks (Burrows, Pursey, Neve, and Stanwell, 2013). Adolescents may not be educated on the differences between sports drinks and energy drinks, and use of energy drinks before and during exercise can contribute to dehydration, tremors, heat stroke, and heart attacks (Rath, 2012). Adolescents with preexisting conditions or undiagnosed conditions such as heart disease are at increased risk when consuming energy drinks. Education needs to be provided to adolescents while further research is conducted to determine the safety of energy drinks in adolescents.

TABLE 11-13 ■ Adolescent Growth Spurts

STATUS	AGE IN YEARS	
	Boys	Girls
Age in Years	12–17	9.5–14.5
Height Gain in Year of Peak Velocity	>10 cm (3.9 in.)	Possibly 9 cm (3.5 in.)
Age at Peak Growth Velocity	13–15	11–13.5
At Age 18	2.54 cm growth remains	Slightly less remaining growth than boys Growth 99% complete

TABLE 11-14 ■ MyPlate Guidelines 9- to 17-Year-Olds Based on 1800 Calories/Day

FOOD GROUP	NUMBER OF SERVINGS	SERVING SUGGESTIONS
Grains	6 ounces	Make half your grains whole. Aim for 3 ounces of whole grains a day.
Fruit	1½ cups	Eat a variety of fruit. Choose whole or cut-up fruits more often than fruit juice.
Vegetable	2½ cups	Vary your veggies. Each week aim for the following: Dark green = 1½ cups Red and orange = 5½ cups Beans and peas = 1½ cups Starchy veggies = 5 cups Other veggies = 4 cups
Protein Foods	5 ounces	Twice a week serve seafood. Vary proteins to include beans, peas, nuts, and seeds. Keep meat and poultry portions small and lean.
Dairy	3 cups	Drink fat-free or low-fat (1%) milk. Serve fat-free or low-fat yogurt and cheese. If serving soy products make sure they are calcium-fortified.
Fats, Sugar, Sodium	5 teaspoons oil Limit fat calories and added sugar calories to 160 calories Sodium less than 2300 mg	Serve low-fat dairy. Serve lean proteins. Avoid sugary snacks and beverages. Serve fruits in natural form instead of canned fruits packed in water. Avoid processed foods.

Box 11-6 ■ *Macronutrients for Children and Adolescents (4 to 18 years)*

Carbohydrates: 45% to 65% of daily calories
Protein: 10% to 30% of daily calories
Fat: 25% to 35% of daily calories

known to take place between 10 and 14 years in 95% of girls and between 12 and 16 years in 95% of boys (Busscher, Wapstra, and Veldhuizen, 2010). During the peak of the adolescent growth spurt, the mineral and protein content of the body is increased.

Nutritional Needs and Concerns

For DRIs, see Appendix A. In 2008, the American Academy of Pediatrics recommended that all adolescents receive a daily intake of 400 IU of vitamin D (Minarich and Silverstein, 2011).

See Table 11-14 for MyPlate recommendations for adolescents ages 9 to 17 year olds. Current guidelines for distribution of macronutrients can be found in Box 11-6.

Calcium and Iron

Regarding nutrients, adolescent diets are lacking in calcium and iron. Long term, deficiencies of those minerals may be manifested in osteoporosis or anemia.

Short term, evidence suggests an influence of dietary factors on fracture occurrence. Although rates of fracture vary considerably with age, sex, and maturation, they peak in early puberty. At that time, rates of bone turnover are high, but bone mineral accrual lags behind gains in height and weight. Among the factors impacting pediatric fracture incidence are the following:

■ Bone mass and bone mineral density
■ Low calcium intake
■ High body mass index
■ Excessive consumption of carbonated beverages
■ Lack of weight-bearing physical activity

- Use of corticosteroids
- Fracture sustained at young age (Valerio, Galler, Mancusi, et al, 2010)

For all children and adolescents, breakfast, or lack thereof, has an impact on overall dietary intake significantly (see Box 11-7). Teens should strive to consume three to four servings of iron-rich foods and four to five servings of calcium-rich foods daily.

Overenthusiastic Weight Control

Because of the cultural value placed on thinness, adolescents, especially girls, may restrict their dietary intake to achieve a desired slim body. Some use unhealthy practices such as fasting, diet pills, laxatives, and vomiting to remain slim. **Anorexia nervosa** affects 0.5% to 1% of 14- to 18-year-old girls and is covered in Chapter 16. Eating disorders can last for years, with consequences related to growth and development (Ayton, 2011). Participating in sports that value slimness is a risk factor for both girls and boys (see Box 11-8). One study demonstrated a total of 10% to 15% of boys who participated in weight-sensitive sports, such as wrestling, practice unhealthy weight loss behaviors (Turocy, Galler, Mancusi, et al, 2011).

Some adolescents may adopt vegetarianism as a means to control weight and body shape rather than for ecological or spiritual reasons. Regardless of the reason they have become vegetarians, these adolescents should have their nutritional status and dietary intake monitored.

Acne and Diet

Acne afflicts more than 17 million Americans with approximately 80% to 90% of adolescents affected. Acne is triggered by sex hormones stimulating the sebaceous

Box 11-7 ■ *Breakfast versus No Breakfast Effects*

Among children and adolescents, breakfast or lack of breakfast has an appreciable impact on the day's nutritive intake. One significant predictor of adolescent breakfast eating was parental breakfast eating. Skipping breakfast is more prevalent in girls and children from lower socioeconomic backgrounds (Basch, 2011).

On average, children who skipped breakfast did not make up the nutrient deficits during the remainder of the day. Breakfast skipping has also been associated with the development of unhealthy eating habits, weight gain, and obesity. It has been found that adolescents who skip breakfast are more likely to consume unhealthy beverages including soft drinks and food high in saturated fats, calories, and sugar (Leidy and Racki, 2010).

Children who eat breakfast on most days have improved attention spans, concentration, and memory as well has higher intakes of micronutrients. For benefits such as lower weight and greater satiety breakfast should be consumed daily and consist of low-glycemic, high-fiber carbohydrates and healthy proteins (Zanteson, 2012).

Box 11-8 ■ *The Female Athlete Triad*

Female athletes, who desire athletic success as well as thinness, are at risk for developing a medical condition commonly referred to as the "female athlete triad." The disorder can have a negative impact on athletes' health and performance and is characterized by low energy availability, menstrual dysfunction, and low bone mineral density.

- Low energy availability—occurs from high energy expenditure, inadequate energy intake, or a combination of both (Ducher, Turner, Kukuljan, et al, 2011).
- Menstrual dysfunction—the prevalence of menstrual dysfunction in athletes ranges from 6% to 79% (Hoch, Pajewski, Moraski, et al, 2009).
- Low bone mineral density—the prevalence of reduced bone mineral density in athletes ranges from 10% to 22% (Ducher et al, 2011). The combination of amenorrhea and low energy availability predisposes athletes for stress fractures and osteoporotic fractures later in life (Ducher et al, 2011).

All girls and women should be encouraged to participate in sports and physical activities because the benefits outweigh the risks (Hoch et al, 2009). Female athletes should be screened for the triad before participating in sports and educated about the body's need for nutrients (Warr & Woolf, 2011).

glands. The skin becomes oilier and the ducts to the glands sometimes plug up, permitting the accumulation of harmful bacteria that produce inflammation. The sebaceous glands' production of sebum may be influenced by androgens and hormonal mediators that, in turn, may be stimulated by foods.

Dietary components that have recently been revisited regarding acne are dairy products, high glycemic index foods, fat intake, and fatty acid composition (Droppelmann, Navarrete-Dechent, Nicklas, et al, 2012). On the one hand, some experts conclude that no clear proof exists as to whether culprit foods such as dairy products, chocolate, and fatty foods affect acne. Others are convinced that dairy products and high glycemic index foods influence hormonal and inflammatory factors thus increasing acne prevalence and severity (Ismail, Manaf, and Azizan, 2012). The suggested link to dairy foods speculates that milk contains hormones and bioactive molecules.

Another theory is that hyperinsulinemia initiates an endocrine sequence, resulting in increased androgens and an altered retinoid signaling pathway related to acne (Droppelman et al, 2012). Recent trials have demonstrated decreased acne after 12 weeks on a low glycemic load diet. (See **glycemic index** in Glossary.) Foods with a high glycemic load, such as white bread or potatoes, cause a rapid rise in blood glucose. Foods with a low glycemic index, such as high-fiber cereals or beans, cause a more gradual change in blood glucose.

Recent evidence has identified that reactive oxygen species, free radicals, and oxidative stress play a role in initiating acne, and antioxidant vitamins like A and E are lower in clients who have acne (Jesitus, 2012).

Omega-3 fatty acids have also been shown to suppress inflammation and appear to be beneficial in acne (Jesitus, 2012).

Overweight in Children and Adolescents

Obesity in children and adolescents has become a national epidemic and is projected to worsen over time (Stevens, 2010) Childhood overweight and obesity rates have doubled in the past three decades, whereas the overweight and obesity rates of adolescents have tripled (Garver, 2011). Box 11-9 describes the diagnosis and prevalence of overweight and obesity in children and adolescents in the United States. Table 11-15 demonstrates the percentage of children at or above the 95% for weight based on ethnicity.

Those who are overweight or obese have a higher risk of developing:

■ Type 2 diabetes
■ Hypertension
■ Negative self-image associated with psychosocial issues

More than 60% of children who are overweight before puberty will be overweight in adulthood (Rabitt and Coyne, 2012).

Some of the factors contributing to overweight and obesity in children are:

■ Unwise food choices
■ Inactivity, with television and computer games replacing active play
■ Decreased ability to self-regulate energy intake related to overcontrolling parents
■ Inability of parents to see child as overweight
■ Failure of health professionals to prioritize the diagnosis of obesity compared to other health risks (Hopkins, DeCristofaro, and Elliott, 2011)
■ Genetics (see Genomic Gem 11-2)

Strategies to prevent overweight are listed in Table 11-16. These approaches cost less than treatment of established obesity and reach the greatest number of children.

Weight management is the subject of Chapter 16. Overweight children require careful supervision to maintain normal growth and development while reducing weight and adipose tissue. Treatment of obese children requires a multicomponent program encompassing diet, physical activity, nutrition counseling, and parent or caregiver participation.

The conditions permitting or encouraging overweight among youth have evolved over many years and have become embedded in the dominant culture that involves the food industry and marketing. No single change is going to reverse the trend. Multiple interventions and strategies are needed at all levels: individuals, families, schools, communities, and the nation.

Box 11-9 ■ *Overweight in Childhood and Adolescence*

Technically, obesity refers to fatness, often measured by skinfold thickness, not weight. However, BMI is used as a surrogate measure of obesity because its components, height and weight, are readily available data and the growth charts for comparison are easily obtained. *See "Growth Charts" on DavisPlus or at www.cdc.gov/growthcharts.*

A BMI between the 5th and the 85th percentile is considered normal for children and adolescents. Values over the 95th percentile have been variously defined in this population as overweight or obese. By late adolescence, the 95th percentile is about equal to an adult BMI of 30, signifying obesity.

Figure 11-6 illustrates the increasing prevalence of overweight since 1976 in both genders and in all age groups. Table 11-15 shows **NHANES survey** results by gender, age, and ethnic group. Clearly, the distribution varies by ethnicity, but overall the percentage of children and adolescents with BMIs above the 95th percentile continued to increase.

**Obesity among children and adolescents
2–19 years of age**

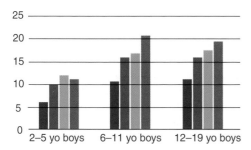
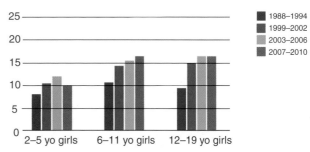

FIGURE 11-6 Statistics demonstrate there was an increase in the incidence of children, both male and female, at or above the 95th percentile of BMI from 1988 to 2010. (Source: National Center for Health Statistics. Health, United States, 2011: With Special Feature on Socioeconomic Status and Health. Hyattsville, MD. 2012. Accessed on October 22, 2013 at: www.cdc.gov/nchs/data/hus/hus11.pdf.)

TABLE 11-15 ■ Percentages of Children at or Above the 95th Percentile, NHANES 2007–2010

Ethnic Group	MALES			FEMALES		
	2–5 Years	6–11 Years	12–19 Years	2–5 Years	6–11 Years	12–19 Years
Non-Hispanic White	8.8	18.6	17.1	9.2	14.0	14.6
Non-Hispanic Black	15.7	23.3	21.2	14.2	24.5	27.1
Mexican American	19.1	24.3	27.9	9.9	22.4	18.0

Source: Health, United States, 2011: With Special Feature on Socioeconomic Status and Health. National Center for Health Statistics (US). Hyattsville (MD): National Center for Health Statistics (US): 2012 May.

Genomic Gem 11-2

It's in My Genes—Up to a Point

Up to 40% of variation in BMI is estimated to be genetic. Multiple genes are likely involved, including many affecting energy balance. Although obese parents produce the highest proportion of obese children, separating heredity from environment is problematic.

Evidence has emerged from family studies. A familial risk was shown to increase with the severity of obesity. An adult with a father, mother, brother, or sister with a BMI of 40 is at a 5 times higher risk of being obese than individuals who have only normal-weight first-degree relatives (Bouchard, 2009). Another study looking at male fraternal twins who were overfed demonstrated variance between pairs, but resemblance of weight gain within pairs, indicating some individuals are more at risk than others to gain fat when there is an energy intake surplus (Bouchard, 2009).

The 40% of BMI variance that is genetic may be treatable in the future. The 60% that is environmental can be modified with current information.

TABLE 11-16 ■ Strategies to Prevent Childhood Overweight

AGE GROUP	STRATEGY	BARRIERS	RATIONALE
Infant	Promote and support breastfeeding	Cultural norms about breastfeeding in general or in public or the workplace	Many health benefits May allow infant to control amount consumed better than with formula feeding
Toddler and Preschooler	Implement MyPlate at home and in day care/preschool Limit sweetened drinks Begin 1% or fat-free dairy Encourage daily physical activity	Parents/caregivers may be reluctant to change	Need for full-fat dairy ceases at age 2
School-Age and Adolescent	Health curriculum Active, appealing physical education for all Offering healthy food and beverages in school	Ingrained curricular models Tendency to emphasize sports that for most youth are spectator events Advertising less healthy foods to youth	Include high-intensity activities such as endurance training and popular dance Limit screen time Limit carbonated beverages
All Ages	Limit TV/computer game time to 2 hours/day Encourage at least 1 hour of physical activity daily Encourage 5 servings of fruits and vegetables daily Eat a healthy breakfast daily Encourage family meals Serve recommended portion sizes Calculate and plot BMIs yearly Advocate for healthful food choices in restaurants Discourage consumption of empty kilocalories Expand access to supermarkets with reasonably priced produce Provide safe environments for physical activity		

Adapted from American Academy of Pediatrics, 2011; Hopkins, DeCristofaro, and Elliott, 2011; Karnick and Kanekar, 2012.

Keystones

- Breast milk is especially suited to the human infant because the protein, fat, and carbohydrate in breast milk are tailored to the infant's digestive capabilities.
- After the age of 4 to 6 months, semisolid and then solid foods are added to the diet gradually, using carefully selected foods to avoid choking accidents.
- Nutritional problems in infancy include allergies, colic, and diarrhea, with the latter having the best documented treatment: oral rehydration therapy.
- Toddlers not only learn to accept new foods but also learn their culture's traditions surrounding food. Common nutritional problems for toddlers are iron deficiency and iron-deficiency anemia.
- Preschool and school-age children need healthy meals and snacks to sustain growth at a time when parents have less control over the child's eating while away from home.
- Most adolescents do not consume enough calcium to optimize their growth and development, and most girls lack iron in their diets. Self-prescribed reduction diets and poor choices of food are problems.
- Pediatric obesity is a major childhood health problem in the United States and the industrialized world, with the potential to spread in developing countries. Consequences are adult pathologies presenting decades early: hypertension, high blood cholesterol, and type 2 diabetes.

CASE STUDY *11–1*

Ms. S is a school nurse in an inner-city high school. The principal asked for Ms. S's assistance in improving the students' nutritional and fitness states. A committee was formed that included students, teachers (classroom, home economics, and physical education), cafeteria and kitchen staff, parents, and a dietitian from a nearby hospital. The following plan reflects the program they devised after many meetings.

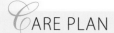 ARE PLAN

Subjective Data

Focus groups with students revealed their opinions of food and physical activity. ■ A schoolwide survey solicited suggestions for classroom content, menu items, and physical activities.

Objective Data

Analysis of school lunch menus revealed an average fat content of 38% of kilocalories. ■ Vending machines in and around school offered only high-fat snacks or those with empty kilocalories. ■ Inspection of building usage identified 2 days after school when the gym was empty but other parts of the building were in use.

Analysis

Opportunity to improve students' nutrition and fitness

Plan

DESIRED OUTCOMES EVALUATION CRITERIA	ACTIONS/INTERVENTIONS	RATIONALE
Students will have increased opportunities to choose healthful foods in and around school.	Analyze sample lunch menus monthly to select areas to improve and to note progress.	Prioritizing changes is important to budget resources. Feedback to cafeteria staff will help maintain their interest and effort to improve.

(Continued on the following page)

DESIRED OUTCOMES EVALUATION CRITERIA	ACTIONS/INTERVENTIONS	RATIONALE
	Include fresh fruit and vegetables on every lunch menu.	Fresh fruits and vegetables can offer vitamins, minerals, and fiber as well as decrease the dominance of high-fat items on the menu.
	Use student tasters to develop low-fat versions of popular dishes.	Palatability is critical in devising dishes the students will eat.
	Diversify contents of vending machines to include dairy products, fruit juices, cereal- and- dried-fruit snacks.	Items must be available to give students the opportunity to choose.
	Collaborate with biology teacher on fruit or vegetable growing as student projects.	Producing food items can stimulate interest in eating their own produce.
Students will demonstrate higher goals for their physical fitness.	Evaluate the place of physical education in the curriculum and campaign for needed changes.	To effectively prepare students for life requires offering skill development for an active life.
	Institute fitness testing in physical education classes.	Feedback to students allows them to track their progress.
	Ensure that 75% of time in physical education class is active.	Inactivity is a major contributor to overweight. Physical education class should not add to the problem.
	Institute activities students suggest, such as ethnic dances and games other than major U.S. sports.	Capitalizing on students' interests will recognize the value of their ideas. Later activities might broaden the scope to activities from other cultures.
	Arrange for supervised activities in the gym after school on the days the building would be open for other events. Vary the activities.	If community or volunteer leaders could be recruited, the cost would be minimized for the school and the students. A variety of activities would attract students other than the usual athletes who are active anyway.
Students will increase knowledge of healthful eating practices within time and budgetary constraints.	Design and promote a practical course in skills of modern life for both genders.	Practical courses will attract a different student than strictly academic courses do.
	Devise short instructional units on planning, purchasing, and preparing healthful food for classroom or after-school activity sessions.	Short units would give immediate feedback on the value of the information. Consuming the day's lesson is a bonus.
	Incorporate field trips to grocery stores as appropriate.	Expanding the students' perception of the choices open to them would offer the opportunity to increase variety in their diets.

11-1

Community Committee Work

A committee was formed to improve the area surrounding the high school to permit opportunities for daily exercise for the students. Members included YMCA staff, neighborhood business owners, and city officials.

Subjective: Parents described traffic congestion, lack of sidewalks and bike paths, and suspected undesirable activities occurring around the school.

Objective: Police reports of auto-pedestrian accidents, assaults, thefts, and drug arrests indicated increased incidence compared with the district's other high schools.

Analysis: School's environment a disincentive to walking or bicycling to and from school.

Plan:
Establish a Neighborhood Watch Program using business owners and nearby families.
Increase numbers of crossing guards and recruit volunteer monitors when students are coming and leaving school.
Improve traffic flow around the school.
Long term, construct bike paths and sidewalks to and from the surrounding neighborhoods.

Critical Thinking Questions

1. What additional interventions might be used to improve nutritional intake and increase physical activity in these students?

2. Identify possible barriers to implementing the outlined program. Suggest strategies to overcome them.

3. It is possible that the committee's goals are not compatible with those of many of the students in this high school. How could the students be persuaded to value a more healthful lifestyle?

Chapter Review

1. A nurse in a clinic would identify which of the following infants as needing additional assessment of growth?
   a. Baby girl A, 4 months old, birth weight 7 lb 6 oz, present weight 14 lb 14 oz
   b. Baby boy B, 2 weeks old, birth weight 6 lb 10 oz, present weight 6 lb 11 oz
   c. Baby boy C, 6 months old, birth weight 8 lb 8 oz, present weight 14 lb 8 oz
   d. Baby girl D, 2 months old, birth weight 7 lb 2 oz, present weight 9 lb 10 oz

2. Which of the following are advantages of breast milk that formula does not provide?
   a. Less fat and cholesterol
   b. More antibodies and digestive enzymes
   c. More fluoride and iron
   d. More vitamin C and vitamin D

3. Which of the following foods would be appropriate for a 6-month-old infant?
   a. Cocoa-flavored wheat cereal, orange juice, and strained chicken
   b. Graham crackers, strained prunes, and stewed tomatoes
   c. Infant rice cereal, mashed banana, and strained squash
   d. Mashed potatoes, strained beets, and chopped hard-cooked egg

4. Families should be encouraged to provide fortified whole milk for children until the age of
   a. 18 months
   b. 2 years
   c. 36 months
   d. 4 years

5. Which of the following individuals is at greatest nutritional risk?
   a. 3-month-old infant being fed commercial formula
   b. 3-year-old child who drinks 3 cups of milk a day
   c. 8-year-old child who eats four chocolate chip cookies and drinks two glasses of milk after school
   d. 16-year-old girl who is pregnant and attempting weight loss

Clinical Analysis

1. Mrs. T is having her 2-month-old son checked in the well-baby clinic. She tells the nurse that the baby is not sleeping through the night yet. Mrs. T's mother advised her to start the infant on cereal to "fill him up" at bedtime. Which of the following statements by the mother would indicate to the nurse the need for further teaching?
   a. "My baby can have solids at 6 months."
   b. "Most babies sleep through the night by age 3 months."
   c. "I will put the infant cereal into a bottle and enlarging the nipple hole."
   d. "I understand that early introduction of foods may increase the risk for allergies."

2. Ms. C has given a 24-hour dietary recall for her 18-month-old son. The nurse is alert to identify common causes of choking. To avoid choking accidents, which of the following groups of foods would be considered safest for a toddler?
   a. Apple quarters, green beans, and chicken noodle casserole
   b. Grapes, carrot strips, and macaroni and cheese
   c. Diced peaches, mashed potatoes, and spaghetti
   d. Watermelon chunks, cheese-stuffed celery, and sliced frankfurters

3. Ms. K has delivered a 3-lb 8-oz premature infant. She had planned to breastfeed. On which of the following statements should the nurse base her teaching?
   a. Human breast milk can be specially fortified for premature infants to increase its nutritive value.
   b. Because of their larger proportion of body weight as water, premature infants need supplemental water after every feeding.
   c. Formula feeding is advisable because room temperature feedings are better absorbed than those at body temperature.
   d. Breastfeeding a premature infant offers no advantage to the infant and is difficult for the mother because of the necessary supplements.

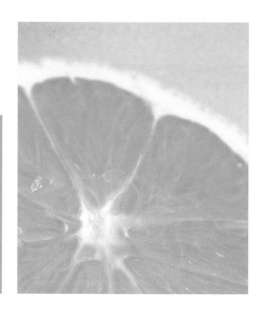

12

Life Cycle Nutrition: The Mature Adult

LEARNING OBJECTIVES

After completing this chapter, the student should be able to:

- Identify the foods and food groups most likely to be lacking or excessive in the diets of adults.
- Describe the changes in the older adult's body that affect nutritional status.
- Explain how a nutritional assessment of an older adult differs from that of a younger one.
- Illustrate ways in which food can be used to aid in the developmental tasks of adulthood.
- List several suggestions to improve food intake for older people in a variety of living situations.

The life cycle of human growth and development continues throughout the adult years. Both psychosocial and physical developments continue as a person matures. This chapter considers the impact on nutrition of the physiological and psychosocial changes that occur during young, middle, and older adult years. Because much of this book emphasizes the nutritional needs of young and middle-aged adults, the main focus of this chapter is the older adult. One major threat to health in adulthood is inactivity (Box 12-1), which can lead to overweight and obesity, the subject of Chapter 16.

Young Adulthood

Young adulthood spans ages 18 through 39. Not all 18-year-olds are adults, developmentally speaking, nor are all 40-year-olds middle-aged in thought or behavior.

Psychosocial Development

During the early years of young adulthood, the individual may be completing the adolescent task of identity. According to Erik Erikson, the developmental task of young adulthood is **intimacy** (Table 12-1). For example, people who delay commitment to a life partner until their 30s and 40s will probably be working at achieving intimacy; other 40-year-olds may be tackling the next task of generativity.

Nutrition in the Young Adult

Table 12-2 shows *MyPlate* recommendations for the adult aged 19 to 30 years.

Middle Adulthood

For this section, middle adult years are defined as those between ages 40 and 70 to match the dietary reference intakes (DRI) tables.

Psychosocial Development

Erikson's task of **generativity** involves serving as a mentor to the next generation. Teaching family members to

---

Box 12-1 ■ *The Prevalence of Inactivity in Adults*

The Healthy People 2020 initiative set a target of 32.6% of adults who report no leisure time physical activity. In 2008, 36.2% of adults in the United States reported no leisure-time physical activity, a prevalence that steadily increases with age:

- Ages 18 to 24—19%
- Ages 25 to 35—22%
- Ages 36 to 44—24%

- Ages 45 to 64—27%
- Ages 65 and older—32%

A state-by-state report card showed the prevalence of inactivity for those aged 65 years or older ranged from 19.4% in Hawaii to 54.3% in Puerto Rico (Centers for Disease Control and Prevention, 2010).

TABLE 12-1 ■ Erikson's Theory of Psychosocial Development in Maturity

STAGE OF LIFE	DEVELOPMENTAL TASK	OPPOSING NEGATIVE TRAIT	USE OF FOOD TO ACHIEVE TASK
Adult	Intimacy	Isolation	Arranging candlelight dinner
Middle Adult	Generativity	Stagnation	Teaching someone to prepare family favorite or ethnic dishes
Older Adult	Integrity	Despair	Using food fragrances or memories of food to reminisce

---

TABLE 12-2 ■ MyPlate Daily Recommendations for Adults Aged 19 to 30 Years*

FOOD GROUP	WOMEN	MEN
Fruit	2 cups	2 cups
Veggies	2½ cups	3 cups
Grain	6 oz (3 oz whole grain)	8 oz (4 oz whole grain)
Protein	5½ oz	6½ oz
Dairy	3 cups	3 cups
Oil	6 teaspoons	7 teaspoons

*Servings for those who get less than 30 minutes of moderate exercise each day.
Adapted from U.S. Department of Agriculture, ChooseMyPlate.gov (2013).

TABLE 12-3 ■ MyPlate Daily Recommendations for Adults Aged 31 to 50 years*

FOOD GROUP	WOMEN	MEN
Fruit	1½ cups	2 cups
Veggies	2½ cups	3 cups
Grain	6 oz (3 oz whole grain)	7 oz (3½ oz whole grain)
Protein	5 oz	6 oz
Dairy	3 cups	3 cups
Oil	5 teaspoons	6 teaspoons

*Servings for those who get less than 30 minutes of moderate exercise each day.
Adapted from U.S. Department of Agriculture, ChooseMyPlate.gov (2013).

prepare traditional foods, for example, may help a person achieve generativity.

Nutrition in Middle Adulthood

Table 12-3 shows MyPlate recommendations for the adult aged 31 to 50 years.

Older Adulthood

Changes in **life expectancy** and physiology affect the nutrition of older Americans.

Demographics of Aging

People are living longer. Older people constitute a larger proportion of the population. These trends are expected to continue, thus increasing the numbers of frail and dependent elderly.

Life Expectancy

In 1900, life expectancy at birth was 47 years. By 2009, however, life expectancy at birth was 78.5 years. By ethnic group, all values were record highs:

- 81.2 years for white females
- 77.6 years for black females
- 83.5 years for Hispanic females
- 76.4 years for white males
- 71.1 years for black males
- 78.7 years for Hispanic males (National Center for Health Statistics, 2011).

Proportion of Population

Steady growth is seen in the proportion of the U.S. population older than the age of 65 years. It was:

- 4.1% in 1900
- 6.8% in 1940 (5 years after Social Security was enacted)
- 9.8% in 1970 (5 years after Medicare took effect)

- 12.8% in 2011 (U.S. Census Bureau, 2011)
- Estimated to be 20% by 2030 (Gebhardt, Sims, and Bates, 2009)

The increase in the aged population is evidence of successful public health efforts: improved sanitation, an increased concern for safety, and control of communicable diseases. In 2011, two major causes of death in adults were heart disease and cancer (Centers for Disease Control and Prevention [CDC], 2013). Both causes are linked to lifestyle, including diet.

Nursing Home Residency

In 2009, 3.3 million people, with the average age of 85 years, received care in nearly 16,000 U.S. nursing homes (Toles, Young, and Ouslander, 2012–2013).

Psychosocial Development

Erikson's developmental task for older adults is **integrity,** in the sense of being whole or complete. Those who accomplish this task will look back on their lives as being worthwhile.

A technique to help the older person achieve integrity is reminiscence. Asking an older person to recall special foods can stimulate reminiscence. Familiar food odors often evoke memories.

Socially, older adults must often adapt to the loss of friends and relatives. The death of a spouse demands a tremendous adjustment. The accompanying depression and new responsibility for tasks the spouse performed may significantly affect an older person's food intake.

Physical Changes of Aging

Even without frank disease, the physical abilities of older adults diminish. "Middle-age spread" often gives way to dwindling bulk and waning strength.

The clinical guidelines on overweight and obesity in adults set a body mass index (BMI) of 25 as the upper limit of ideal weight for all adults regardless of age. Among men and women 65 years of age and older, however, a BMI in the overweight and mild (Grade 1) obesity range, BMI 25.0 to 34.9, is not associated with a significantly increased risk of mortality (Kulminski, Arbeev, Kulminskaya, et al, 2008). This finding does not negate the evidence linking overweight to arthritis, diabetes, coronary heart disease, and other conditions that may have an impact on the older person's quality of life.

Integumentary System

Many changes take place in the skin as a person ages. As subcutaneous fat is lost, the skin becomes dry and wrinkled. Less elasticity is present to spring back after a pinch to the forearm, the usual site assessed for hydration status. The skin of the forehead or over the breastbone is a more reliable site in the elderly client than the forearm.

The older adult also loses some of the ability to synthesize vitamin D from sunshine, so it may take twice as much sun exposure without sunscreens as necessary in a younger person to produce a given amount of vitamin D.

Sensory System

Four senses become markedly less acute as a person ages: vision, hearing, taste, and smell. Because the sense receptors do not deteriorate equally, some of the sense loss is attributed to changes in the central nervous system. Extensive variation exists among individuals.

EYES

Vision is often impaired. The older person sees colors in the red and yellow spectrum better than blue and green spectrum (Pinheiro and Silva, 2012). Clouding of the lens of the eye—cataract formation—decreases overall vision. Older eyes do not adjust well to glare such as that found in some supermarkets.

These vision changes may make grocery shopping burdensome. The fine-print labels on food items may be illegible to the elderly. Food preparation may become not only difficult but also hazardous if the person cannot see adequately. Colorful foods with visual appeal and strong contrast might stimulate the appetite in some elderly.

EARS

The sound receptors in the inner ear deteriorate. First to be lost is the ability to perceive high tones. The older person with poor hearing typical loses the ability to distinguish higher frequencies first, which results in the ability to hear men's voices better than women's (Tun, Villiams, Small, and Hafter, 2012). Hearing aids do not fully compensate for the hearing loss. In fact, they often magnify sideline noise to the point of distracting the wearer. The result may be social isolation when it becomes too laborious to interact with others. Socializing at meals may become embarrassing or frustrating, and older people may avoid such interaction.

NOSE AND TONGUE

For the sense of taste to function well, the sense of smell must also be intact. Food tastes bland when a person has a head cold. After age 65 many people begin to lose some sense of smell (Losing your sense, 2012). Although the sense of smell is frequently more affected by aging than the sense of taste, both faculties are important to help protect the person from noxious elements in the environment, such as spoiled or burning food or gas leaks.

Chemical taste receptors are concentrated on the tongue's surface but also are located at the base of the tongue, on the soft palate, and in other areas of the nasopharynx. Saliva acts as a solvent to present the foods to the taste buds. If the mouth is dry, taste sensations are indistinct.

Taste receptors have traditionally been known to recognize sweet, sour, salty, and bitter sensations. Receptors have been identified for *umami*, a sensation described as savory or rich. It is caused by the amino acid glutamine in its free form and is associated with monosodium glutamate (MSG). Using MSG, which contains about one-third of the amount of sodium found in table salt, in foods such as soups, gravies, and sauces improves palatability without significantly increasing sodium content (Discovering umami, 2010). Concerns regarding the physical effects such as headaches or lethargy with the use of MSG have resulted in much debate, but studies have failed to consistently demonstrate symptoms of sensitivity (Discovering umami, 2010).

Reported sensory losses are uneven. Unlike sensitivity for bitter and sour that remains intact in older clients, the perceptivity for sweet and salt declines with age, so many older clients will complain their food tastes bitter. A possible physiological mechanism is suggested by discovering neurons that are sensitive to salts and acids also respond to bitter stimuli (Travers and Geran, 2009). If a person is over salting his or her food as a result of a diminished taste sensation for salt, alternate seasonings can be used to decrease sodium consumption; these are listed in Chapter 18. A technique to increase taste sensation in geriatric clients is brushing the tongue as part of oral hygiene.

Gastrointestinal System

Particularly crucial to nutrition is gastrointestinal function. Hundreds of processes are required for the proper digestion, absorption, and metabolism of foods. Many functions of the gastrointestinal system decline significantly in older people.

DENTAL HEALTH

Older individuals are not immune to dental caries. In fact, when exposed by gum disease, the tooth root, lacking enamel, is particularly vulnerable to caries, causing increased occurrence in the elderly population. Contributing factors include the following:

- Inadequate oral hygiene
- Infrequent dental examinations and cleanings
- Salivary gland dysfunction
- Frequent snacking
- Removable partial dentures
- Long-term medication use (Raghoonandan, Cobban, and Compton, 2011)

Fluoride applied to the teeth or fluoridated water prevents caries among adults of all ages. Unfortunately, only 27 states met the Healthy People 2010 goal of having 75% of their citizens on public water supplies with fluorinated water (CDC, 2011). The goal of Healthy People 2020 is for 80% of the population to have access to fluorinated water supplies.

The major cause of tooth loss in the older adult is not dental caries but **periodontal disease,** which affects the gums (gingiva) and the apparatus attaching the tooth to the jaw. Healthy People 2020 also addresses periodontal disease, with the goal of reducing the number of adults with moderate to severe periodontal disease to 11.5% and reducing the proportion of adults aged 65 to 74 years who have lost all of their permanent teeth to 21% (U.S. Department of Health and Human Services, 2013). Dentures, like hearing aids, only partially compensate, so that dentures are about 20% as efficient as natural teeth. Advanced gum disease affects 4% to 12% of adults, and one-fourth of adults in the United States aged 65 years or older have lost all of their permanent teeth, a condition called **edentulous** (CDC, 2011).

Furthermore, a denture cannot be effective if the underlying tissue is in poor condition. Persons with upper dentures that cover the palate containing taste receptors lose some taste sensation and are also subject to impaired swallowing.

The production of saliva decreases sharply in older adults, a condition called **xerostomia.** Chewing and swallowing become more difficult, and food intake may be affected. Also, with age, less mucus and smaller quantities of enzymes are secreted.

OTHER CONDITIONS

Atrophic gastritis, a chronic inflammation of the stomach lining with decreases in size of the glands and mucous membranes is typically diagnosed in association with chronic gastritis and an increased risk of gastric cancer (Frank, Muller, Weck, et al, 2011). An extreme case is **achlorhydria,** the absence of hydrochloric acid in the stomach.

Either of these conditions may interfere with protein digestion and with vitamin and mineral absorption. Vitamin B_{12} may remain locked to the food protein, and less nonheme iron will be absorbed in the more alkaline environment. Heme iron does not require stomach acid and is mainly absorbed in the duodenum and thus is unaffected by atrophic gastritis (Villarroel, Flores, Pizarro, et al, 2011).

Intestinal **motility** decreases because of lessened muscle tone. Medications may interfere with electrolyte balance, also diminishing muscle tone. Increasing age leads to a decrease in blood flow to the liver, which can reduce the ability of the aging liver to metabolize medications (Gardiner, 2013).

Urinary System

The size of the kidneys increases until age 40 or 50 years but then decreases. With aging, the kidneys become smaller and lighter, and blood flow is reduced (Nazarko, 2010). The aging kidney loses some ability to concentrate urine and to conserve sodium. Mild hyponatrenia, the commonest electrolyte imbalance in the older population, is associated with gait and attention deficits, resulting in higher frequency of falls.

This compromised kidney function makes urine samples less reliable for nutrient analyses in the elderly. Two laboratory tests frequently are used to assess renal function: **blood urea nitrogen (BUN)** and serum creatinine. An increase in the BUN level usually indicates a decrease in kidney function. It may also be elevated in dehydration or if excessive protein is presented to the liver for breakdown, as with a high-protein diet or with gastrointestinal bleeding. Because clients with even slightly elevated BUN may not be able to excrete the waste products from protein metabolism, caregivers must be judicious about giving high-protein nutritional supplements to older people with elevated BUNs.

Creatinine, an end product of creatine metabolism, is excreted efficiently by the healthy kidney. The amount of creatinine produced is proportional to the individual's skeletal muscle mass and remains fairly constant in the absence of extensive muscle damage. The serum creatinine test has the advantage over the BUN of being little affected by dehydration, malnutrition, or liver function.

Creatinine levels may not detect decreased kidney function, however, if a slow decline in renal function occurs simultaneously with a slow decrease in muscle mass, as occurs in the aging process. Consequently, both tests may be performed to obtain a more complete diagnostic picture.

Musculoskeletal System

The major loss of body mass in the older adult involves muscle mass. It is estimated that the rate of degenerative skeletal muscle loss is 3% to 8% per decade after age 30 and accelerates with advancing age (Genaro and Martini, 2010). Because muscle is a more metabolically active tissue than fat, energy needs decline with diminished muscle mass. The losses are reversible, however. Even in the elderly, skeletal muscle protein anabolism can be stimulated by increasing dietary protein above the recommended dietary allowance (RDA) of 0.8 g/kg

per day (Gaffney-Stomberg, Insogna, Rodriguez, and Kerstetter, 2009). See Box 12-2 for information regarding sarcopenia.

Nutritional deprivation and catabolic states can affect the muscles of respiration in the chest and diaphragm. Because the older person relies more on the diaphragm than the chest muscles to breathe, a full stomach may impede breathing to a greater extent than in a younger person.

Perhaps more noticeable than the loss of muscle mass in older people is the loss of height. Bones stop growing in length between ages 16 and 18, but density increases until the late 20s (Swann, 2012). After age 30, bone loss occurs at a rate of about 0.3% to 0.5% per year. A major cause of this loss of height is osteoporosis. Osteoporosis is a chronic skeletal disease that results in decreased base mass and increases the risk of fracture (Curtis and Stafford, 2012).

Older joint surfaces are roughened by arthritis. By age 50, half of all adults have some osteoarthritis. The resulting pain and stiffness impairs the use of the hands for opening jars, chopping raw foods, and cutting cooked foods at the table. Arthritis also can affect the mandibular joint of the jaw used for chewing.

Nervous System

For many people, deteriorating brain function is the most feared loss of old age, one that is shared by their loved ones, who may see the person gradually fade from the present with the onslaught of dementia. By the time a person reaches old age, the brain has endured a lifetime of stressors, but some individuals

---

Box 12-2 ■ *Sarcopenia*

Sarcopenia is the reduced skeletal muscle mass and decline in muscle function that is associated with aging. The prevalence of sarcopenia is approximately 25% after age 60 years and 50% in people aged 80 years and older (Verdijk, Snijders, Beelen, et al, 2010). The effects of sarcopenia result in changes of daily activities, such as a slower pace of walking, less endurance, and increased difficulty in performing tasks such as stepping up a stair, rising from a chair, or stabilizing posture to prevent falls (Brass and Sietsema, 2011). Illness, chronic disease, low protein intake, and inactivity are all contributors to the development of sarcopenia.

A relationship has been demonstrated between the loss of lean muscle mass and an increase in body fat mass, which leads to a condition termed sarcopenic obesity. Resistance training has been shown to counteract these age-related changes by improving muscle mass and strength and improving balance and coordination (Ward, 2011).

Studies are currently attempting to locate a clear genetic component related to the development of sarcopenia and although the gene gremlin1 has demonstrated a pivotal role in the regulation of skeletal muscle formation further studies are required (Kasper, 2011).

weather the storms better than others. Some significant changes include:

■ Conclusive evidence exists that the adult brain shrinks with age (Gonoi, Abe, Yamasue, et al, 2010). Brain volume decreases about 0.1% to 0.2% per year between the ages of 30 and 50
■ Blood flow to the brain decreases because of narrowing of the arteries
■ Thirst sensation becomes less operative, increasing the risk of uncompensated dehydration
■ Mortality from heat stroke rises sharply in people older than 60 years

Several factors influence brain function in the elderly. More years of education, physical exercise, and cognitive stimulation are positively related to better brain function. Nutritional factors of benefit to the aging brain include:

■ Vitamins B_6, B_{12}, and folic acid
■ High intake of essential fatty acids, both linoleic acid and alpha-linoleic acid (Turner, 2011)

ALZHEIMER DISEASE

In 2013, it was estimated that Alzheimer disease affected 5.2 million Americans of all ages, with 5 million being aged 65 years or older (Alzheimer's Association, 2014). By 2025, it is estimated that 7.1 million people aged 65 or older will be living with the disease (Alzheimer's Association, 2013). Although the cause of the disease is not fully understood, a genetic predisposition is shown by the 60% to 80% hereditary risk of late-onset dementia (Casey, 2010). See Genomic Gem 12-1.

Decreased brain levels of docosahexaenoic acid (DHA) are associated with aging and have been shown to be essential for normal neurological maintenance of learning and memory (Turner, 2011). Consumption of omega-3 fatty acids (particularly DHA, for example, as obtained in one fish meal weekly) and antioxidants such as vitamin E appear to lower the risk of Alzheimer disease. Special concerns of nourishing clients with dementia are covered in Clinical Application 12-1.

PARKINSON DISEASE

Another neurological disease that is more common in older people than in younger ones is Parkinson disease (PD). In the United States, at least 500,000 people are thought to suffer from PD, and about 50,000 new cases, with an average age at onset of 60 years, are reported annually (National Institute of Neurological Disorders and Stroke, 2013). **Nutraceuticals,** foods or food products that may provide health and medical benefits, are seen as neuroprotective and thought to prevent or impede the progression of PD (Chao, Leung, Wang, and Chuen-Chung Chang, 2012). See

---

Genomic Gem 12-1

Alzheimer Disease

Although the cause of Alzheimer disease has not been fully elucidated, gene mutations may complicate the relation of nutrients to disease risk. Likewise, genetics plays a role in its onset.

One variant of the apolipoprotein E gene, the *APOE2* allele, is the clearest genetic protective factor against Alzheimer disease (Cole, Ma, and Frautschy, 2010).

The brain is highly metabolic, which makes the organ highly vulnerable to oxidative damage; this can result in protein, lipid, and DNA oxidation, which is associated with Alzheimer disease (Feng and Wang, 2012). The mixed results in studies of the antioxidant vitamin E in relation to Alzheimer disease may result from the varied genomes of the people recruited. Vitamin E from food has been associated with a modest reduction in long-term risk of Alzheimer disease among people without a polymorphism in the apolipoprotein E gene, the *APO E4* allele (Feng and Wang, 2012).

Screening tests for specific biomarkers are available for persons at high risk of the disease but not routinely utilized for clients without symptoms (New Alzheimer, 2011). Screening clients who have symptoms of cognitive impairment can assist the clients and their families prepare for the hardships of life with Alzheimer disease.

---

the section on vitamins under Nutrition in the Older Adult later in this chapter. Box 12-3 details some nutritional ramifications of the disease.

Endocrine System

The average older person is slowing down. Resting energy expenditure (REE) decreases, especially in the brain, skeletal muscle, and heart. The older adult's REE may be 10% to 12% less than that of a younger person's. Lost muscle mass is replaced, if at all, by adipose tissue that is less active metabolically than muscle.

The pancreas often secretes inadequate amounts of insulin or the body loses its ability to utilize insulin, leading to diabetes mellitus (see Chapter 17). Receptors in the kidney for antidiuretic hormone (ADH) may function poorly to produce a less effective response. Levels of aldosterone also decrease with age. Both of these changes make maintaining correct fluid volume more difficult for an older person than for a younger one.

Cardiovascular System

As the older adult continues to age, cardiac output and heart rate decrease. In response to exercise, the heart rate does not increase as effectively as in youth, nor does it return to normal as rapidly. Because of this diminishment, the elderly are at risk for diseases of the heart. Dietary modifications for heart disease are included in Chapter 18.

12-1

Clinical Application

Nutrition and Dementia

Care of clients with dementia challenges family and health-care providers because eating is fundamental to life. Clients with dementia progressively lose the ability for self-care, including feeding. A simple tool to assess the client's level of functioning is the Eating Behavior Scale, shown below. The six items assessed direct the caregivers to an appropriate strategy to assist the client without usurping a task the client still can perform.

Managing the client's environment is a major part of the care of the client with dementia.

■ Provide quiet, adequately lit dining rooms.
■ Offer clients the same seats to achieve familiarity.
■ Serve one course at a time.
■ Supply appropriate but limited utensils, large-handled if necessary.
■ Select dishes with high sides to enable the client to scoop up the food onto a spoon.
■ Serve finger foods that are within the client's capabilities.

Clients with dementia must be reminded of the steps involved in self-feeding:

■ Putting the food on the spoon
■ Directing it to the mouth
■ Swallowing

Verbal cues or guiding the client's hand can get him or her started or keep the process going. Despite the surroundings, common courtesies can be effective in reminding clients of social expectations and in maintaining their dignity. For example:

■ Introducing the client to the other people at the table
■ Providing a cup rather than a carton for milk
■ Offering foods

The effect of music in the dining room is a researched intervention for dementia clients. Selections with a slow tempo—at or below the human heart rate—tend to dampen environmental noises that might startle clients. Fewer incidents of agitated behaviors occurred during the weeks that music was played compared with weeks without music (Johnson and Taylor, 2011). Because staff members also heard the music, perhaps they also experienced some of the music's relaxing effect.

A multidisciplinary project to improve nutrition in clients with late-stage dementia not only achieved that goal but also decreased the distress of clients and nursing staff caused by the clients' swallowing problems. Among the interventions used were:

■ Thickened liquids
■ Three levels of dysphagia diets
■ Daylong snacks
■ Use of nutritional supplements

Tube feeding (see Chapter 14) has not been shown to improve the specific outcomes of survival, pressure ulcers, nutrition, and aspiration pneumonia in dementia client (American Dietetic Association [ADA], 2008).

National Institutes of Health Warren G. Magnuson Clinical Center Nursing Department

EATING BEHAVIOR SCALE (EBS)			
Patient # _____ Admit date _____ Observation date ____			
Observer initials _____ Meal start _____ Finished _____			
Patient room _____ Day room _____ Time, minutes _____			
Circle only one answer: ___ Maximum score = 18____ Total = _____			

OBSERVED BEHAVIOR	I	V	P	D
Was the patient—				
1. Able to initiate eating?	3	2	1	0
2. Able to maintain attention to meal?	3	2	1	0
3. Able to locate all food?	3	2	1	0
4. Appropriately using utensils?	3	2	1	0
5. Able to bite, chew, and swallow without choking?	3	2	1	0
6. Able to terminate meal?	3	2	1	0
Comments				

_____

_____

_____

_____

D, dependent; I, independent; P, physical assistance; V, verbal prompts.
For printing, also available on DavisPlus.

A part of the cardiovascular system, the immune system, is less effective in the older person than in the younger one. T and B cells are lymphocytes with a role in the immune system, and these cells decline in number and activity as a person ages (Ennis, 2013). In apparently healthy elderly, micronutrient supplements may enhance the immune response.

At greatest risk of immunodeficiency are persons with protein-kilocalorie malnutrition, which is associated with increased complication rates (mainly infections) and death. Table 12-4 shows some of the effects of aging on **humoral** and **cellular immunity.**

Nutrition in the Older Adult

Table 12-5 shows the MyPlate daily recommendations for people aged 51 and older. MyPlate can be used for assessing and counseling.

MyPlate

MyPlate can serve the older adult well as a guideline for healthy eating. Data has demonstrated a greater proportion of adults aged 65 or older eat five or more fruits and vegetables daily than do younger adults. In 2009, only

Box 12-3 ■ *Parkinson Disease*

It is estimated that 52% to 65% of people with PD experience weight loss, and 25% of the population are at a medium or high risk of malnutrition, with women at a greater risk than men (Walker, Davidson, and Gray, 2012). PD is a progressive neurological disorder characterized by degeneration of neurons in the area of the brain that controls movement. This degeneration causes a shortage of dopamine, a neurotransmitter or brain-signaling chemical. Among the signs of the disease are:

- Tremors
- Rigidity
- Loss of facial expression
- Gait disorders

These changes in movement can affect everyday activities such as talking, walking, swallowing, and writing (Heisters and Bains, 2012).

TABLE 12-4 ■ Some Effects of Aging on Immunity

TYPE OF IMMUNITY	LYMPHOCYTES INVOLVED	FUNCTION	EFFECT OF AGING
Humoral	B cells	Produce antibodies against foreign antigens.	Slightly fewer antibodies produced but less specific and less effective
Cellular	T cells	Protect against viruses, fungi, malignant cells, and foreign tissue grafts without using antibodies; autoimmune reactions are a dysfunction of this mechanism	Declines with age but only after age 90 in healthy people

TABLE 12-5 ■ MyPlate Daily Recommendations for Adults Aged 51 and Older*

FOOD GROUP	WOMEN	MEN
Fruit	1½ cups	2 cups
Vegetables	2 cups	2½ cups
Grains	5 oz; 3 ounces whole grains	6 oz; 3 ounces whole grains
Protein Food	5 oz	5½ oz
Dairy	3 cups	3 cups
Oil	5 teaspoons	5 teaspoons

*Servings for those who get less than 30 minutes of moderate exercise each day.

32.5% of adults consumed two or more fruits per day and 26.3% consumed three or more vegetables per day (Department of Health and Human Services and CDC, 2010). The goal of Healthy People 2020 is to increase the consumption of fruit and vegetable intake in all people greater than age two to 0.9 cups of fruit for every 1000 calories consumed and 1.1 cups of vegetables for every 1000 calories consumed.

A special Modified MyPlate for Older Adults for People Over 70 Years of Age appears as Figure 12-1. The modified MyPlate incorporates the 2010 Dietary Guidelines for Americans and highlights areas specific for the older adult including:

- Choosing spices and low sodium options
- Focus on fluid selection of water, fat-free milk, and soup
- The fork and knife are reminders to put down television remotes and cell phones and focus on the enjoyment of the meal
- Incorporate physical activity into daily life. (Tufts, 2011)

Energy Nutrients and Energy Balance

Older adults need about 5% fewer kilocalories per decade after age 40 years. Small changes have been recommended in intakes from carbohydrates, fats, and protein. As with younger people, the simplest criterion for the suitability of intake is the maintenance of a healthy body weight. Energy expenditure varies within the elderly population. Table 12-6 summarizes the estimated changes in caloric needs over the life span of the adult based on activity level.

CARBOHYDRATES AND FIBER

Older people should derive 45% to 65% of their kilocalories from carbohydrates. The RDA for carbohydrate, based on its role as primary energy source for the brain, is 130 grams per day, the same as for younger adults.

The AI for fiber is 30 grams per day for men 50 years and older and 21 grams for women in the same age

MyPlate for Older Adults

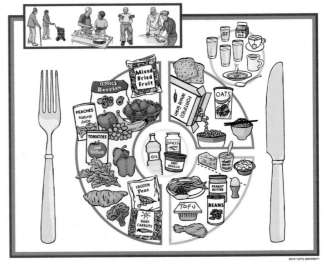

FIGURE 12-1 The Modified MyPlate for People Over 70 Years of Age. (Copyright 2011 Tufts University. For details about MyPlate for Older Adults, see www.nutrition.tufts.edu/research/myplate-older-adults.)

TABLE 12-6 ■ Estimated Calorie Needs per Day				
GENDER	AGE	SEDENTARY	MODERATELY ACTIVE	ACTIVE
Female	19–30 years old	1800–2000	2000–2200	2400
Female	31–50 years old	1800	2000	2200
Female	51+	1600	1800	2000–2200
Male	19–30 years old	2400	2600–2800	3000
Male	31–50 years old	2200–2400	2400–2600	2800–3000
Male	51+	2000–2200	2200–2400	2400–2800

Adapted from 2010 Dietary Guidelines for Americans.

group. Both of the values are less than recommended for younger adults.

FATS

Older people should derive 20% to 35% of their kilocalories from fats. Limiting fats should also increase comfort, because fat absorption is delayed in older people, leading to a feeling of fullness. Particularly among the elderly, rigid application of diet rules may be inappropriate. Restricting fat by eliminating whole milk and eggs, which are easily eaten and relatively inexpensive, could endanger nutrition in the short term for uncertain long-term benefits.

PROTEIN

Older people should derive 10% to 35% of their kilocalories from protein. The RDA for protein is 56 grams per day for adult men and 46 grams per day for adult women. Moderately increasing daily protein intake beyond 0.8 gram per kilogram of body weight may enhance muscle protein anabolism and reduce the progressive loss of muscle mass that accompanies aging. Some experts maintain that nitrogen balance studies indicate a protein intake of as high as 1.6 grams per kilogram can enhance the response of muscles to weight training, which can aid in weight loss and weight management (Li and Heber, 2011).

Although little evidence links high protein intakes to increased risk for impaired kidney function in healthy individuals, a prudent course would be to assess renal function of older individuals before embracing a higher protein intake.

Although serum albumin levels are used as a measure of body protein stores, for a given individual, serum albumin levels can indicate nutritional status, pathology, or both. It is estimated that up to 60% of older adults are malnourished on hospital admission, and nutritional status tends to decline during admission (Ross, Mudge, Young, and Banks, 2011).

Protein status is an important component in the body's defense system. In seniors with protein-energy malnutrition, decreased functions in all aspects of immunity are strongly related to protein nutritional status.

EXERCISE

Recommendations for exercise in the older adult are the same as for the younger adult; if the person is considered generally fit and has no limiting health conditions, the recommendations are as follows:

■ 2 hours and 30 minutes, 150 minutes, of moderate-intensity aerobic activity every week and
■ Muscle-strengthening activities on 2 or more days a week that work all major muscle groups (Centers for Disease Control and Prevention, 2011).

For previously sedentary persons, an exercise routine should be introduced gradually after medical clearance is received. MyPlate recommends men older than 40 years of age and women older than 50 years of age should check with their health-care providers before starting or increasing physical activity.

An objective of Healthy People 2020 is for 24% of adults to perform strength-training activities on 2 or more days per week, but only 21% achieved this goal in 2008. Strength training decreases muscle mass loss, functional decline, and fall-related injuries. The National Institute on Aging (2011) recommends that all forms of exercise be included in the older adult's exercise plan: endurance, strength, balance, and flexibility.

Vitamins

The RDAs/adequate intakes (AIs) for vitamins D is increased for older adults. The RDA for vitamin B_{12} specifies fortified foods or supplements as sources because of the possibility of malabsorption. Mean nutrient intakes from food for older adults are below the RDAs/AIs for vitamins E and K.

VITAMIN E

The RDA/AI for vitamin E is 15 mg per day for all adults. Besides functioning as a scavenger of free radicals, vitamin E has been linked to immune and cognitive functions. Oxidative stress has been shown to contribute to the etiology of dementia. Vitamin E has demonstrated the ability to decrease free-radical damage in neuronal cells, which helps to inhibit dementia progression (Feng and Wang, 2012). One study demonstrated that a daily 2000 IU supplement of vitamin E taken for 2 years delayed the placement of Alzheimer clients in residential care by 2 years due to the vitamin's effect of slowing the progression of the disease (Vitamins unlikely, 2010).

One difficulty with pinpointing effects of vitamin E is its various forms with differing functions. Tocotrienols possess powerful neuroprotective, anticancer, and cholesterol-lowering properties that are often not exhibited by tocopherols. At minute concentrations, alpha-tocotrienol, not alpha-tocopherol, prevents neurodegeneration. One study demonstrated that elderly clients with higher blood levels of all vitamin E forms had a reduced risk of developing Alzheimer compared with those who had lower levels (Turner, 2011).

Although evidence supports the effects of vitamin E on brain health, the use of supplements remains controversial. It is recommended that vitamin E be consumed in its natural form through increased consumption of fruits and vegetables.

VITAMIN K

Vitamin K can be depleted relatively more quickly than the other fat-soluble vitamins. Besides its role in blood clotting, vitamin K contributes to bone metabolism and is protective against age-related bone loss. Vitamin K deficiency has been shown to contribute to the occurrence of hip and vertebral fractures in elderly women. As with vitamin E, protective benefits of vitamin K supplements have not been confirmed for efficacy, and obtaining vitamin K from natural sources is recommended (Ahmadieh and Arabi, 2011).

Minerals

The 2010 Dietary Guidelines for sodium in the older American is an intake of less than 1500 mg per day and further reduced for those who have a chronic illness such hypertension, diabetes, or kidney disease. See Chapters 18 and 19 for more on the relationship of sodium on cardiovascular disease and renal disease.

The AI for calcium has been increased for older persons. The RDA/AI for calcium in women older than 50 years and men older than 70 years is 1200 mg per day; it is 1000 mg per day for men aged 51 to 70 years. It is reported that two groups who are deficient in daily calcium consumption are women older than age 50 and men older than the age 70 (National Institute of Health, 2013).

Calcium is best absorbed by food source, but studies have demonstrated that most postmenopausal women only consume on average 600 mg of elemental calcium per day, which leads to the recommendation of supplement usage (Spangler, Phillips, Ross, and Moores, 2011). Whether from food or supplements, calcium intake should be spread out throughout the day, with 600 mg or less being consumed at each meal.

Water

No AI for water has been established for individuals older than age 30 years. Healthy older adults need enough fluid intake to produce about 1.5 liters of light yellow urine in 24 hours.

Loss of sphincter muscle tone in women and difficulty urinating in men may prompt older people to limit their fluid intake, a practice that is not recommended. Omitting fluids in the 2 hours before bedtime, however, may help decrease the frequency of nocturia and nighttime incontinence.

One of the early signs of dehydration in the elderly is confusion, which may be difficult to ascertain in clients with dementia or altered consciousness. Signs of dehydration in the elderly are listed in Table 12-7. The increase in pulse rate on standing is an appropriate assessment technique for fluid volume status in the elderly except when heart disease and its treatments would block the physiological response.

Clients who are immobilized may need as many as 12 to 14 glasses of fluid per day. Immobility increases the calcium loss from bones. The calcium then circulates in the blood until the kidney excretes the excess. A large fluid intake dilutes the urine so that the calcium does not form stones.

Common Problems Related to Nutrition

Although arthritis, osteoporosis, and protein-kilocalorie malnutrition are not unique to the elderly, they do represent special concerns for geriatric clients. Constipation is also a frequent complaint and is covered in Chapter 20. A special food-based recipe to control the symptom of constipation that is effective in nursing home residents is given in Chapter 24.

Arthritis

This group of diseases is characterized by inflammation of various joints, often accompanied by pain, swelling, stiffness, and deformity. **Arthritis** affects an estimated 22% of the U.S. adult population (50 million persons), and 9% (21 million people) reported that arthritis limited their activities. Prevalence was high among:

- Women
- Older age groups

TABLE 12-7 ■ Signs of Dehydration in the Elderly	
BODY SYSTEM	**SIGN**
Skin and Mucous Membranes	Skin warm and dry
	Decreased turgor; pinch test may be more accurate over the sternum or on the forehead than on the hand
	Furrowed tongue
	Elevated temperature
Cardiovascular	Elevated pulse
Urinary	Increased specific gravity
	Increased urinary sodium
Musculoskeletal	Weakness
Neurological	Confusion

- Non-Hispanic Whites
- Obese or overweight individuals
- Physically inactive individuals (CDC, 2012)

OSTEOARTHRITIS

Formerly known as degenerative joint disease, **osteoarthritis** is characterized by progressive deterioration of cartilage in joints and vertebrae. Arthritis of the spine, hips, or knees is more likely to cause disability than that affecting other areas. Risk factors for osteoarthritis include:

- Aging
- Obesity
- Overuse or abuse of joints
- Trauma

Because the force exerted on the knees when walking may be up to six times the body weight, overweight people have a significantly increased risk of osteoarthritis of the knees. Thus, weight control has an important role in the prevention and treatment of osteoarthritis.

RHEUMATOID ARTHRITIS

In contrast to osteoarthritis, which is a local disease, rheumatoid arthritis is a systemic disease, affecting about 2.1 million people in the United States. Because it is a systemic disease, some have tried to modify the disease effects through diet or supplements.

Omega-3 fatty acids, in addition to blocking the formation of inflammatory compounds from omega-6 fatty acids, produce compounds that are less inflammatory and less bioactive than the ones metabolized from omega-6 fatty acids.

Osteoporosis and Fractures

Osteoporosis is covered in detail in Chapter 8. This section examines only the risks for and results of hip fracture (actually a fracture of the femur). Although half as common as reported vertebral fractures, hip fractures are much more likely to be diagnosed and treated. Clinically diagnosed vertebral fractures are estimated to represent just one-third of the total vertebral fractures. The World Health Organization has developed a fracture risk algorithm (FRAX) that can predict a person's 10-year probability of hip fracture and is based on the risk factors of age, height, weight, bone mineral density and is country-, sex-, and race-specific (Greenspan, Perera, Nace, et al, 2012). The FRAX tool can be found at: www.shef.ac.uk/FRAX/index.aspx.

INDIVIDUALS AFFECTED

It has been reported that more than 90% of hip fractures are caused by falls. Other facts about hip fractures include the following:

- About 75% of all hip fractures occur in women.
- White women are more likely to sustain hip fractures than African American or Asian women.

- Hip fracture rates increase with age. People aged 85 years or older are 10 to 15 times more likely to sustain hip fracture than those aged 60 to 65.
- Up to one in four adults who lived independently before their hip fracture remain in a nursing home for at least 1 year after their injury (CDC, 2010).

RISK FACTORS

Box 12-4 lists major risk factors for hip fractures.

PREVENTION

The most effective way to prevent fall-related injuries, including hip fractures, is to combine exercise with other fall-prevention strategies. Studies have demonstrated that exercise reduces the risk of falls in older adults (Hass, Maloney, Pausenberger, et al, 2012). Weight-bearing exercise for at least 30 minutes per day will help maintain bone strength, balance, and coordination (Swann, 2012). Examples of weight-bearing activities include activities in which the feet touch the ground walking, jogging, or dancing.

Even after sustaining a hip fracture, only a minority of elderly clients receives treatment for osteoporosis to attempt to modify the risk of future fractures. One study demonstrated that although guidelines recommend a combination of calcium, vitamin D, and antiresorptive drugs to reduce fracture by up to 50%, rates of treatment in the hospital after fracture were approximately 6% to 7% (Jennings, Auerbach, Maselli, et al, 2010).

Weight Loss and Protein-Kilocalorie Malnutrition

The older person's metabolic rate declines, primarily as a result of less lean body mass or muscle, so that loss of 5% or more of body weight requires aggressive intervention (Morley, 2006). The **anorexia of aging** is described in Box 12-5.

Treatable malnutrition has been reported to occur in 8% to 78% of hospitalized clients (Hafsteinsdottir, Mosselman, Schoneveld, et al, 2010), and up to 60% of older adults are malnourished on admission to the

---

Box 12-4 ■ *Risk Factors for Hip Fractures*

Among the risk factors for hip fractures are the following:

- Increasing age
- Female gender
- White race
- History of falls
- Insufficient exercise
- Low body mass index
- Smoking
- Long-term glucocorticoid use
- Inadequate calcium and vitamin D intake

Box 12-5 ■ *The Anorexia of Aging*

Humans and other animals of advanced age have reduced food intake. Physiological factors contributing to anorexia of aging include:

- Changes in taste and smell
- Delayed gastric emptying
- Altered digestion-related hormone secretion and hormonal responsiveness

Healthy elders have been shown to be less hungry at meal initiation and to become more rapidly satiated during a standard meal, compared with younger adults.

Nonphysiological causes include:

- Social (poverty, isolation)
- Psychological (depression, dementia)
- Medical (edentulism, dysphagia)
- Pharmacological factors

Older persons eat more in social situations than when eating alone, even when the person delivering Meals on Wheels just sits with the recipient while dining.

Decreased appetite and weight loss are commonly associated with depression (Tsai, Chou, and Chang, 2011) and studies have demonstrated an association between elderly persons who live alone with increased social isolation and diminished quality and quantity of food consumed (Callen, 2011). Older adults, who take more than 30% of all prescription drugs, are at increased risk of drug–nutrient interactions, the subject of Chapter 15.

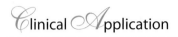 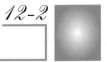

12-2

Clinical Application

Nutrition and Pressure Ulcers

The basic cause of **pressure ulcers** is impaired circulation from the weight of the body on a bony prominence or by shearing forces from pulling on the skin that damages the underlying tissue. Risk factors include:

- Immobility
- Inactivity
- Incontinence
- Impaired consciousness
- Malnutrition

Progression of the ulcer from intact skin to an open, sometimes deep sore increases the challenge to control infection, replenish nutrient losses from the wound, and promote healing.

Pressure ulcers may place clients in a hypercatabolic state, which will require an increase in calories to promote healing. Clients with pressure ulcers will require increased protein to promote a positive nitrogen balance and improve healing rates (Posthauer, 2012). Current recommendations are 1.25 to 1.5 grams of protein per kilogram of body weight if not contraindicated.

Nutritional support is only a part of the overall strategy to combat pressure ulcers. The other risk factors must be controlled and diligent nursing care provided to effectively prevent or treat this serious condition.

hospital (Ross, Mudge, Young, and Banks, 2011). Malnutrition contributes to many complications of illness, such as infections, anemia, and pressure ulcers (Clinical Application 12-2).

Food Insecurity

The main reason individuals do not consume enough protein or kilocalorie is lack of money (Box 12-6). To rectify the situation for older adults, the federal government, with an amendment to the Older Americans Act, established meal programs for senior citizens. Low-cost meals are offered at central gathering places or are delivered to the homebound and provide one-third of the RDA for elders (Fig. 12-2). The second program offered is the Senior Farmer's Market Nutrition Program (SFMNP) that offers low-income seniors coupons to exchange for fresh produce at farmer's markets and roadside stands.

Dietary Interventions

Enhancing well-consumed menu items with additional kilocalories and protein while maintaining the usual volume of food employs a "food-first" philosophy to counter weight loss. Clients may accept foods more readily than liquid supplements. Milk-based supplements that are both nutrient-dense and easy to consume might succeed for a person who is losing weight

Box 12-6 ■ *Food Insecurity*

Older adults typically are reported as having the highest rate of food security, but data demonstrate an increase in food insecurity among adults aged 65 years and older. Those who are at greatest risk are African American women, with homebound African Americans being at a 3.7 higher risk than whites to be at the highest nutritional risk (Dean, Sharkey, and Johnson, 2011). Income has also been listed as a risk factor for food insecurity.

There is emerging evidence that food insecurity can contribute to inflammation in the human body, which can contribute to increased risks of diabetes, hypertension, and cardiovascular disease. Those with food insecurity have been shown to have:

- Lower serum folate levels; folate is needed for immune system activation
- A 40% increase of having high white blood cell counts (Gowda, Handley, and Aiello, 2012).

Studies demonstrate that adults aged 60 to 90 years with food insecurity have increased risk of:

- Diminished health status
- Lower cognitive function
- Increased depression
- Obesity (Dean et al, 2011).

Some older adults are forced to make choices between purchasing food, medications, or cigarettes. One study demonstrated that although some people had inadequate food intake, they continued to allocate part of their limited resources on tobacco products (Gowda, Hadley, and Aiello, 2012).

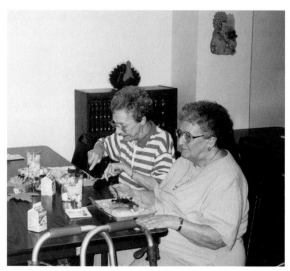

FIGURE 12-2 These women partake of an evening meal served at their residence under the auspices of the Older Americans Act and managed by a county agency.

or one who cannot chew. Studies have shown that oral liquid nutritional supplements can add calories and nutrients for older clients with inadequate dietary intake (Hines, Wilson, McCrow, et al, 2010). Another study demonstrated a reduction in falls in older frail adults who received oral nutritional supplements for 12 weeks (Neelematt, Lips, Bosmans, et al, 2012).

A more economical choice than prepared supplements may be an instant breakfast preparation. A homemade supplement recipe using ice cream is given in Dollars & Sense 12-1. To prevent dampening of appetite at mealtime, liquid caloric supplements should be given at least 1 hour before a meal.

To accommodate dentures, the person may reduce his or her intake of meats, fresh fruits, and vegetables. Assistance in selecting appropriate substitute items is in order. A recommended procedure for learning to eat and drink with dentures is explained in Clinical Application 12-3.

Nutritional Care for the Elderly

Box 12-7 lists topics to consider in a nutritional assessment.

Assessment

When assessing the elderly, special care is necessary to ensure marginal deficiencies are detected before major problems occur. Body weight and its stability are critical data in nutrition screening, yet an investigation in three large medical centers revealed that just 65.7% of clients older than 18 years reporting being weighed at admission and only 67% of those not weighed had been asked about their weight.

$ Dollars & Sense 12-1

Nutritional Supplements

Substituting Carnation Instant Breakfast® for Ensure® would save 61 cents per serving or $37 for 30 days assuming two servings per day. See calculations below.

To equal the kilocaloric content of Ensure® requires a 10-ounce serving of modified Instant Breakfast instead of eight ounces of Ensure®. The protein content of the Ensure® and Instant Breakfast made with whole milk and ice cream are equivalent. The fat, saturated fat, cholesterol, and sodium contents are higher in the homemade recipe. Whether that intake would be a major concern for the client is a clinical judgment. Other nutrients have not been compared.

To implement the Instant Breakfast® recipe also requires a refrigerator and freezer and a blender or shaker to mix the one package of instant breakfast, one cup of whole milk, and one-quarter cup of ice cream.

	Ensure	Carnation Instant Breakfast	Whole Milk	Ice Cream
Price	$7.99	$5.29	$2.99	$3.49
Package	8-oz bottles	10 packages of powder	1 gallon	1 qt
Serving size	1 bottle	1 package	1 cup	½ cup
Cost/serving	$1.33	$0.53	$0.19	$0.22
Kilocalories	250	130	150	150
Protein	9 g	5 g	8 g	2 g
Total fat	6 g	0.5 g	8 g	8 g
Saturated fat	1 g	0 g	5 g	5 g
Cholesterol	<5 mg	<5 mg	33 mg	30 mg
Sodium	190 mg	90 mg	120 mg	40 mg

12-3

Clinical Application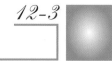

Learning to Eat With Dentures

Clients should learn to use dentures one step at a time:

1. Practice swallowing liquids with the dentures in place.
2. Practice chewing soft foods.
3. Learn and practice to bite regular foods.

Splitting the process into manageable units decreases frustration.

MINI NUTRITIONAL ASSESSMENT

The Mini Nutritional Assessment (MNA; Fig. 12-3) tool for use with older adults features two parts. The first 6 items provide a screening score and the last 12 items an assessment score that determines if further action is needed. The screening portion has the advantage of incorporating alternative measures for height if the person cannot stand and compensatory calculations for clients with missing limbs. The entire tool is available in 16 languages. Both a guide to its use and an online scoring program are available. Go to http://mna-elderly.com for more information regarding the tool and for updated resources.

The MNA has been established as a nutritional screening tool for use in a variety of care settings and allows for early detection of malnutrition risk and enables immediate intervention (Kaiser, Bauer, Ramsch, et al, 2010).

NUTRITION SCREENING INITIATIVE TOOLS

Nutritional assessment tools for use with older adults were developed by the Nutrition Screening Initiative. The following is a description of the tools.

- Determine Your Nutritional Health is a self-administered checklist with scoring directions to evaluate risk.
- Level I Screening Tool is to be administered by professionals in health or social service programs and includes directions for appropriate referrals.
- Level II Screening Tool is for use in physicians' offices and health-care institutions and includes a clinical examination, skinfold measurements, and laboratory tests.

Implementation

Some interventions are appropriate regardless of a client's living situation. Others are more focused on institutionalized elderly.

INDEPENDENTLY LIVING ELDERLY

Suggestions to increase the nourishment of elderly clients living in their own homes appear in Box 12-8.

Increasing physical activity according to the client's ability offers benefits beyond weight control. Physical activity helps to:

- Prevent heart disease and hypertension
- Improve bone mineral density
- Enhance balance and strength for activities of daily living
- Promote restful sleep

Many individuals, however, report never having been advised to exercise by their health-care providers. An intervention to enable the client to see improvement (or the need for improvement) is the keeping of an activity log.

HOSPITALIZED ELDERLY

The nurse's role in nourishing hospitalized older clients undergoing diagnostic tests is discussed in Clinical Application 12-4. Obtaining adequate food for such a client may tax the nurse's ingenuity because of timing and the need to entice a fatigued and perhaps fearful client to eat.

INSTITUTIONALIZED ELDERLY

Suggestions to increase the nourishment of institutionalized elderly appear in Box 12-9.

Providing nourishment for frail and ill elderly is a monumental task. The nurse must be aware of the client populations who are at greatest risk of undernourishment and those at that greatest need for feeding assistance.

- 86% of clients with dementia will develop difficulty with feeding (Hanson, Carey, Caprio, et al, 2011)
- Eating difficulties will occur in 40% to 80% of hospitalized stroke clients (Carlsson, Ehnfors, and Ehrenberg, 2010).

One study demonstrated that the average time it takes to assist a client with eating a meal averaged 35 to 40 minutes (Green, Martin, Roberts, and Sayer, 2011). This can become overwhelming in a high-paced health-care environment, but the nurse must remain vigilant in ensuring assistance with eating when required.

When asked, nursing home residents recalled that food tasted really good when eating with family and friends, especially in childhood. One study showed that eating with others can increase energy intake up to 76% compared with eating alone (Shepherd, 2011). When staff learn about residents' previously enjoyed foods and occasionally provide those favorites as special treats, residents maintain individuality within their peer group and among staff. Other suggestions to make mealtimes more homelike include:

- Buffet service
- Item selection that permits portion control
- Choice of accompaniments with open seating in the dining room

Mini Nutritional Assessment
MNA®

**Nestlé
NutritionInstitute**

Last name:			First name:	
Sex:	Age:	Weight, kg:	Height, cm:	Date:

Complete the screen by filling in the boxes with the appropriate numbers. Total the numbers for the final screening score.

Screening

A Has food intake declined over the past 3 months due to loss of appetite, digestive problems, chewing or swallowing difficulties?
0 = severe decrease in food intake
1 = moderate decrease in food intake
2 = no decrease in food intake   ☐

B Weight loss during the last 3 months
0 = weight loss greater than 3 kg (6.6 lbs)
1 = does not know
2 = weight loss between 1 and 3 kg (2.2 and 6.6 lbs)
3 = no weight loss   ☐

C Mobility
0 = bed or chair bound
1 = able to get out of bed / chair but does not go out
2 = goes out   ☐

D Has suffered psychological stress or acute disease in the past 3 months?
0 = yes   2 = no   ☐

E Neuropsychological problems
0 = severe dementia or depression
1 = mild dementia
2 = no psychological problems   ☐

F1 Body Mass Index (BMI) (weight in kg) / (height in m²)
0 = BMI less than 19
1 = BMI 19 to less than 21
2 = BMI 21 to less than 23
3 = BMI 23 or greater   ☐

IF BMI IS NOT AVAILABLE, REPLACE QUESTION F1 WITH QUESTION F2.
DO NOT ANSWER QUESTION F2 IF QUESTION F1 IS ALREADY COMPLETED.

F2 Calf circumference (CC) in cm
0 = CC less than 31
3 = CC 31 or greater   ☐

Screening score (max. 14 points)

12 - 14 points: Normal nutritional status
8 - 11 points: At risk of malnutrition
0 - 7 points: Malnourished   ☐☐

References
1. Vellas B, Villars H, Abellan G, et al. Overview of the MNA® - Its History and Challenges. J Nutr Health Aging. 2006;**10**:456-465.
2. Rubenstein LZ, Harker JO, Salva A, Guigoz Y, Vellas B. Screening for Undernutrition in Geriatric Practice: Developing the Short-Form Mini Nutritional Assessment (MNA-SF). J. Geront. 2001; **56A**: M366-377
3. Guigoz Y. The Mini-Nutritional Assessment (MNA®) Review of the Literature - What does it tell us? J Nutr Health Aging. 2006; **10**:466-487.
4. Kaiser MJ, Bauer JM, Ramsch C, et al. Validation of the Mini Nutritional Assessment Short-Form (MNA®-SF): A practical tool for identification of nutritional status. J Nutr Health Aging. 2009; **13**:782-788.
® Société des Produits Nestlé, S.A., Vevey, Switzerland, Trademark Owners © Nestlé, 1994, Revision 2009. N67200 12/99 10M
For more information: www.mna-elderly.com

FIGURE 12-3 Geriatric Mini Nutrition Assessment. (©Nestlé, 1994, Revision 2009, with permission. For further information, go to the MNA® Web site: www.mna-elderly.com.)

Box 12-8 ■ *Increasing Food Intake in Independently Living Elderly*

Prepare for Mealtime
- Suggest oral hygiene before meals to freshen and moisten mouth.
- Suggest smokers refrain for 1 hour before a meal to increase appetite.

Promote Social Interaction
- Encourage potluck meals with friends for those who live alone.
- Combine meals at the senior center with activities of interest.

Serve Food Attractively
- Suggest varying textures, colors, flavors.
- Suggest raw, crisp-cooked, or marinated vegetables to increase vegetable intake.
- Suggest using attractive dishes and flatware, centerpieces, tablecloths, or placemats.

Provide Nutrient-Dense Foods
- Help the client to select satisfactory meal-replacer supplements, whether commercial canned products or instant-breakfast powders.
- If additional kilocalories are needed, recommend whole milk for beverages and cooking instead of reduced-fat varieties.

Outside Help
- Obtain a home health aide to shop, do basic fix-ahead preparations.
- Provide Meals-on-Wheels for homebound.
- Refer to the social worker for food stamps, surplus commodity programs for those eligible.
- Recommend instructional materials on food purchasing, storage, cooking from county extension services.

Box 12-9 ■ *Increasing Food Intake in Institutionalized Elderly*

Prepare for Mealtime
- Provide oral hygiene before meals to freshen and moisten mouth.
- Suggest smokers refrain for 1 hour before a meal to increase appetite.
- Manage the environment by removing unsightly supplies or noxious waste.
- Allow 60 minutes to elapse after a significant amount of supplement before serving the next meal.

Promote Social Interaction
- Encourage alert nursing home residents to choose compatible mealtime companions.
- Control the noise in the dining room to avoid overstimulating those with hearing aids.

Serve Food Attractively
- Vary textures, colors, flavors.
- To increase vegetable intake, offer raw, crisp-cooked, or marinated vegetables as appetizers.
- Provide enough nonglaring light so food can be seen clearly.
- Schedule special events such as musical entertainment to enhance interest in eating.

Provide Nutrient-Dense Foods
- Add powdered milk, margarine, sugar, or ice cream to appropriate beverages and foods.
- Increase the eggs, milk, or cheese in recipes.
- When appropriate, offer 1 ounce of a nutritionally complete supplement every hour and use as "chaser" when administering medications.
- Choose milk-based beverages or beverages with sugar instead of water.
- Avoid use of low-fat or low-sugar foods.

- Using linen napkins and cups and saucers
- Allow residents to visit at their table after meals (Quiring, 2012)

Bolstering fluid intake in institutionalized elders takes planning. Frequent small drinks may be more acceptable to the client than trying to swallow large amounts with meals. See Box 12-10 for strategies to increase fluid consumption.

Box 12-10 ■ *Increasing Fluid Intake in Elderly*

- Offer clients sips of fluids frequently and with every contact.
- Leave drinks within the client's reach.
- Provide frequent mouth care.
- Offer preferred beverages.
- Establish client's normal drinking patterns.
- Position the client to a position that facilitates swallowing.
- Develop "happy hour," which can encourage socialization and fluid consumption.

Adapted from Campbell, N. (2012). Dehydration: Best practice in the care home. *Nursing & Residential Care.* 14(1): 21–25.

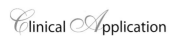 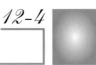

12-4

Hospitalization of the Elderly

Except in obstetrical and pediatric practices, elderly clients dominate as consumers of health care. Eighty percent of the elderly, compared with 40% of individuals younger than age 65 years, have one or more chronic diseases. In many cases, elderly clients are admitted to the hospital undernourished, and their nutritive status worsens during hospitalization.

Serving no food to a client because of diagnostic tests is starvation. The conscientious nurse obtains meals or feedings for a client who is *nil per os*, or NPO (i.e., nothing by mouth) for breakfast and lunch. There is nothing magical about the times of 8 a.m., 12 p.m., and 6 p.m. for meals. The committed nurse will arrange for adequate nourishment for clients when their tests are completed and they are permitted to eat. Dietary personnel have no idea when an individual client is finished with tests for the day until notified by the nurse.

Keystones

- Aging has an impact on almost all body systems, affecting food procurement, preparation, consumption, digestion, and metabolism.
- Supplements and fortified foods as sources of calcium and vitamins D and B_{12} are recommended for middle-aged and older adults in recognition of impaired absorption, metabolism, and synthesis as people age.
- Involuntary weight loss in the elderly should stimulate a broad search for causes: physical, environmental, financial, and social.
- Overweight increases the risk for certain diseases such as osteoarthritis and diabetes mellitus, but a body mass index in the overweight and mild obesity range is not associated with a significantly increased risk of mortality in individuals older than the age of 65 years.
- The most nutritionally vulnerable adults are nursing home residents who are unable to eat without assistance.

CASE STUDY *12-1*

Mr. E is a 70-year-old widower who relies on public transportation. His home is two blocks from the bus route and eight blocks from the nearest supermarket. Mr. E has moderately painful knees from arthritis. He has been taking the bus to the supermarket every other day so that he could manage one package on the way home. He has confided to the nurse in his doctor's office that he is ready to "just give up. It's too much trouble to eat anymore." Mr. E's weight today is 160 lb, 5 lb less than last month.

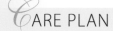

CARE PLAN

Subjective Data

Dependent on public transportation ■ Painful knees ■ Verbalized discouragement with procuring food

Objective Data

Weight loss of 5 lb in past month

Analysis

Lack of information concerning resources available to maintain senior citizens in their homes

Plan

DESIRED OUTCOMES EVALUATION CRITERIA	ACTIONS/INTERVENTIONS	RATIONALE
Mr. E will acknowledge need for assistance with meals by end of visit today.	Discuss Mr. E's weight change with him. Determine what kind of assistance he would accept.	Clients are likely to change behaviors only if the new behavior is acceptable to them.
Given several options of community support, Mr. E will select one and begin to implement the change within 3 days.	Describe Senior Citizen Nutrition Program, Meals on Wheels, home health aide shopping service, and door-to-door Care-a-Van service.	Clients may know about these programs but prefer to remain independent. Allowing the client some time to choose makes the choice more his own.
	Explore social support available from family and less-restricted friends.	Following up with a telephone call shows the nurse is committed to working through this problem with Mr. E.
	Nurse to follow up with telephone call in 3 days.	During the follow-up telephone call, Mr. E said he would like information on the Senior Nutrition Program and the Care-a-Van Service.

12-1

Senior Center Nutrition Coordinator's Notes

The following Senior Center Nutrition Coordinator's Notes are representative of the documentation found in a client's medical record.

The Nutrition Coordinator at the Senior Center interviewed Mr. E and introduced him to several "regulars" at his first noon meal at the Senior Center. On his card, she noted:

- Regular diet, no allergies
- Enjoyed woodworking and card games in past

- Major difficulty—obtaining groceries
- Will try Care-a-Van instead of bus

Follow up with alternate grocery suggestions if plan is unsatisfactory. Encourage socialization.

Critical Thinking Questions

1. What additional data could be sought in a more comprehensive assessment?

2. What other areas could be investigated to help balance to Mr. E's need for assistance with his desire for independence?

3. As you read this case, how would you define the underlying problem?

Chapter Review

1. The RDA/AI for which of the following nutrients is increased for older adults compared with younger ones?
   a. Sodium
   b. Calcium
   c. Vitamin C
   d. Vitamin K

2. The decrease in gastric acid that accompanies aging causes concern for the absorption of which of the following nutrients?
   a. Carbohydrate and water
   b. Fat and cholesterol
   c. Vitamins A and E
   d. Vitamin B_{12} and iron

3. A nurse making a home visit routinely screens for dehydration in elderly clients. Which of the following would the nurse assess?
   a. Body temperature and urine-specific gravity
   b. Tongue condition, pulse rate, and muscle strength
   c. Skin turgor and heart and lung sounds
   d. Client's intake and output records

4. Which of the following conditions is likely to contribute to vitamin D deficiency in older adults?
   a. Atrophied skin, dislike for milk, and indoor life
   b. Lack of exercise, failing hearing and vision
   c. Slowed peristalsis, diminished secretion of intrinsic factor
   d. Achlorhydria and inability to chew meats

5. Ms. P is a 58-year-old retired cook who tells the clinic nurse she regrets not having had children and grandchildren. Which of the following activities might assist Ms. P to attain generativity?
   a. Editing a cookbook for her church group
   b. Taking a class in ethnic cooking in preparation for her next trip
   c. Serving on the Meals-on-Wheels advisory board
   d. Volunteering to teach a special recipe at a local school

Clinical Analysis

Ms. O is a 76-year-old retired schoolteacher who has been admitted to a long-term care facility after surgical repair of a fractured hip.

1. While performing the Geriatric Mini Nutrition Assessment for Ms. O, to calculate the most accurate BMI, the nurse would use the client's height
   a. Listed on her driver's license
   b. At age 50
   c. As determined in the supine position with a tape measure
   d. Using the alternative knee to toe calculation

2. Ms. O reports a weight loss of 4 lb in the 3 months before her injury. Her present weight is 125 lb. Which of the following nursing actions is appropriate at this point?
   a. Asking the physician to order an appetite stimulant
   b. Ordering balanced nutritional supplements three times a day
   c. Deferring action until the team conference next week
   d. Instructing the nursing assistants to feed Ms. O

3. Because Ms. O will have limited mobility, providing adequate fluid intake is necessary to prevent complications in the _____ system.
   a. Cardiovascular
   b. Endocrine
   c. Urinary
   d. Integumentary

13

Food Management

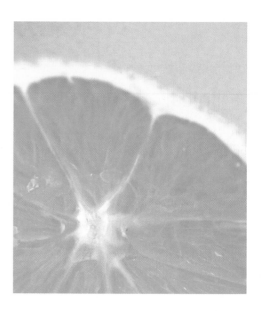

LEARNING OBJECTIVES

After completing this chapter, the student should be able to:

■ Describe the conditions under which microbiologic food illnesses can occur.

■ Identify foods that are likely to harbor disease-producing microorganisms.

■ Teach clients how to prevent foodborne illnesses.

■ Discuss the information on food labels.

*E*ffective meal management requires knowledge about food safety, including microbiological hazards, environmental pollutants, and natural food toxins. Reading food labels can help prevent nutritional hazards. How food is handled between the time it leaves the farm and the time it reaches the table affects our health and well-being. How food crops are grown and animals are raised influences health as well. As health care moves from institutions to home care, health-care workers need to understand the vital importance of safe and nutritious food (see Box 13-1).

The Centers for Disease Control and Prevention (CDC) estimates that each year, 1 in 6 Americans (48 million people) get foodborne diseases, 128,000 are hospitalized for them, and 3000 die of them (CDC 2013a). Considering the number of people involved in the growth, distribution, preparation, and service of food, our food safety record is excellent. The food supply in the United States is as safe, wholesome, and nutritious as any in the world.

Foodborne illnesses are caused by bacteria, viruses, parasites, mold, toxins, contaminants, and allergens. New strains of pathogens, or disease-producing organisms, are continually evolving; in some cases, these organisms have proven resistant to antibiotics. The development of these resistant foodborne pathogens has been attributed to increased use of antibiotics in hospitals, outpatient facilities, and veterinary applications as well as the home use of antimicrobial products (American Dietetic Association, 2009; www.foodsafety.gov).

Food contamination can happen at any point in the food supply process. The goal of the Healthy People 2020 program, a government initiative, is to improve food safety and reduce foodborne illnesses. Education is a key component of the program because proper handling, preparation, and storage of food are critical to ensure food safety (U.S. Department of Health and Human Services [USDA], 2012).

The following is recommended to reduce the risk of foodborne illness (CDC, 2013a; USDA, 2011):

■ CLEAN—Wash hands, surfaces, food
■ SEPARATE—Don't mix raw and cooked foods or use the same cutting board/utensils
■ COOK—Cook foods to safe temperatures, utilizing a thermometer; don't hold foods at temperatures <140°F.
■ CHILL—Refrigerate foods quickly after purchasing prepared foods or when storing leftovers. Keep refrigerated at ≤40°F.

Box 13-1 ■ *YOPI*

Those most at risk:
Young, **o**ld, **p**regnant, and **i**mmunocompromised clients (YOPI)—25% of the U.S. population—are at the greatest risk for foodborne illness.

Food Irradiation

Food irradiation has been used since 1905 when scientists received patents for food preservation using radiation to kill bacteria in food (Environmental Protection Agency [EPA], 2012a). It's used to kill parasites, insects, and bacteria in foods such as meat, poultry, flour, vegetables, and eggs. It also is used to delay sprouting (e.g., potatoes) and ripening (e.g., fruit) in foods (U.S. Food and Drug Administration [FDA], 2012; EPA, 2012a). When a food has been irradiated, the FDA requires the use of a label that states either "Treated With Radiation" or "Treated by Irradiation." The irradiation logo, the Radura, must also be displayed (Fig. 13-1). Foods that are not entirely irradiated but only have ingredients that are subjected to radiation, need not have a label. Also, there is no requirement for labeling of irradiated food served in restaurants (EPA, 2012b).

Microbiological Hazards

More than 250 foodborne diseases have been identified (CDC, 2012). The CDC (2013a) defines foodborne illnesses being caused by bacteria, viruses, parasites, toxins, or chemicals. Most foodborne diseases infect the tissues of the digestive tract and cause gastric distress; symptoms range from mild to severe (see Box 13-2). Microorganisms may be carried from one host to another by animals; humans; inanimate objects including food; and environmental factors, such as air, water, and soil. Many microorganisms cause disease. Under certain conditions, food becomes a vehicle for disease transmission.

It is estimated that in 2011, the top pathogens contributing to domestically acquired foodborne illnesses

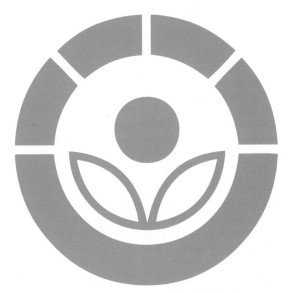

FIGURE 13-1 The Radura symbol for irradiated food labels.

> **Box 13-2** ■ *Mild and Severe Symptoms of Foodborne Disease*
>
> Mild symptoms include gastric and intestinal distress with:
>
> - Abdominal pain
> - Nausea
> - Vomiting
> - Diarrhea
> - Cramps
>
> Severe symptoms include:
>
> - Dehydration
> - Bloody stools
> - Neurological disorders
> - Death

were the Norovirus virus causing 58%, followed by the following bacteria:

- *Salmonella nontyphoida*, 11%
- *Clostridium perfringens*, 10%
- *Campylobacter*, 9%
- *Staphylococcus aureus*, 3%

Of particular concern to pregnant women is the bacterium *Listeria monocytogenes* and parasite *Toxoplasma gondii,* which can cause miscarriage, serious birth defects, and even death of a newborn (U.S. Department of Health and Human Services, 2011).

Norovirus

Norovirus is normally spread from one person to another through contaminated food, water, or environmental surfaces. Infected kitchen workers can contaminate foods they prepare if they have the virus on their hands. Sewage discharge in coastal growing waters has contaminated oysters before they are harvested (CDC, 2013a).

To prevent norovirus, the CDC (2013b) recommends:

- Washing hands frequently
- Kitchen workers wearing gloves when working with food
- Cleaning and disinfecting food preparation surfaces and equipment
- No food preparation by individuals who are ill
- Washing fruits and vegetables thoroughly before preparation or consumption
- Cooking shellfish thoroughly
- Washing clothing and table linens thoroughly

Bacterial Foodborne Disease

Bacteria are everywhere: doorknobs, countertops, hands, eyelashes, mouths, some water supplies, and food are a few of the many places where bacteria can be found.

Animal and human fluids and waste harbor bacteria and cause many foodborne illnesses. The CDC (2013a) reported that the following raw foods contribute to the majority of foodborne illnesses in the United States: foods of animal origin (meats, poultry, eggs, shellfish, and unpasteurized milk), fruits, and vegetables. The following contributes to bacterial contamination of foods:

- Bare-handed food contact by handler/worker/preparer
- Raw product/ingredient contaminates from animal or environment
- Allowing food to remain at room or outdoor temperature for several hours
- Insufficient time and/or temperature during the initial cooking/heat processing

Conditions for Growth

Bacterial growth refers to an increase in the number of organisms. Under ideal conditions, cell numbers can double every half hour: one cell becomes two, two become four, and four become eight (in an hour and a half). A single bacterium can multiply to 33 million after 12 hours. Although bacteria cannot be eradicated from our environment, bacterial growth can be controlled. For this reason, understanding the following conditions necessary for bacterial growth and microbiological food illness to occur is important:

- Source of bacteria—the bacteria must come in contact with the food.
- Food—the food must permit the bacteria to grow (increase in number) or produce a poisonous toxin. Bacteria grow in foods only within a certain pH range. This is why vinegar and lemon juice are frequently used to preserve food, such as cucumbers (pickles) and cabbage (sauerkraut). These ingredients lower the pH so bacteria cannot grow.
- Temperature—the temperature must be favorable for bacterial growth. The temperature range in which most bacteria multiply rapidly is 40°F to 140°F, the range that includes room and body temperature (Fig. 13-2).
- Time—enough time must elapse for bacteria to grow, produce a toxin, or both.
- Moisture—bacteria need water to dissolve and digest food. Foods that contain water support bacterial growth better than do dehydrated foods. This is the reason dehydration is a food preservation method.
- Ingestion—an unsuspecting person must eat the food or drink the beverage that contains the toxin or bacteria.

Bacteria are frequently odorless, tasteless, and colorless; therefore, laboratory analysis is the only way to tell whether a food will cause illness. Table 13-1 lists pathogens, common food vehicles, and symptoms.

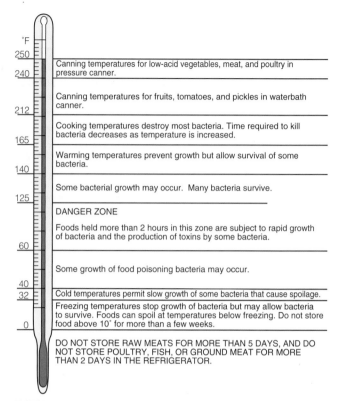

FIGURE 13-2 A temperature guide to food safety.

Food Infections

A **food infection** is caused by eating a food containing a large number of disease-producing bacteria.

SALMONELLA

Salmonella is a bacterium that can cause an illness called **salmonellosis.** It is transmitted by the consumption of contaminated foods or contact with an infected person. Some foods support the growth of *Salmonella* better than others. Common food vehicles include raw eggs, unpasteurized milk, and poultry (see Dollars & Sense 13-1).

CAMPYLOBACTER

Another type of bacteria causing food infections is *Campylobacter jejuni,* which is carried in the intestinal tracts of cows, hogs, sheep, and poultry. The most frequent source of infection is eating undercooked poultry, or foods that have been contaminated with the drippings from the raw chicken. It is the most commonly identified bacterial cause of diarrheal illness in the world (CDC, 2013a). Contaminated water or raw manure can spread the organism. For example, an animal can defecate in a vegetable garden and contaminate the produce.

Foods found to be contaminated with *Campylobacter jejuni* include raw milk, fresh mushrooms, and raw

TABLE 13-1 ■ Pathogens, Common Food Vehicles, and Symptoms (Centers for Disease Control and Prevention, 2011; www.cdc.gov)

PATHOGEN	COMMON FOOD VEHICLES (HAZARDOUS FOOD ITEMS)	SYMPTOMS
Salmonella	Raw or undercooked eggs, poultry, or meat; unpasteurized milk or juice; cheese; seafood; fresh fruits and vegetables	May lead to sudden onset of headache, fever, chills, abdominal pain, diarrhea, nausea, and vomiting. Dehydration may be severe, and fever is usually present. May develop into septicemia. Symptoms begin suddenly and last for 12–24 hours (up to 2 weeks in the elderly). See Clinical Application 13-1.
Listeria	Soft cheeses, deli meats, pâté, burritos, ice cream, unpasteurized milk, smoked seafood, deli salads, raw vegetables	Fever, chills, headache, backache, upset stomach, abdominal pain, and diarrhea. May lead to meningoencephalitis and/or septicemia in newborns and adults and miscarriage in pregnant women. Symptoms may appear within a few hours to 3 days. It may take up to 2 months to become ill.
Escherichia coli 0157:H7	Undercooked ground beef, other beef, unpasteurized milk and apple juice, contaminated raw fruits and vegetables, and water	May lead to acute hemorrhagic colitis (cramps, bloody diarrhea, nausea, vomiting, and fever). May result in hemolytic uremic failure or kidney failure. Symptoms can begin 1–9 days after contaminated food is eaten and last 2–9 days.
Campylobacter jejuni	Raw or undercooked poultry, meat, or shellfish, unpasteurized milk, water	May lead to an acute gastroenteritis of variable severity characterized by diarrhea, abdominal pain, malaise, fever, nausea, and vomiting. Guillain-Barré syndrome or meningitis have been seen in severe cases. Symptoms appear 2–5 days after eating and may last 2–10 days.
Norovirus	Produce, raw shellfish, and any other ingredient contaminated by an infected person	May lead to nausea, vomiting, diarrhea, abdominal pain, headache, malaise, and low-grade fever. Symptoms appear in 12–48 hours and usually last 1–3 days but can last 4–6.
Staphylococcus aureus	Poultry, processed meats, milk, cheeses, ice cream, mixed dishes such as potato salad, spaghetti	May cause nausea, vomiting, stomach cramps and diarrhea. Symptoms appear in 30 minutes to 6 hours and last 1–3 days.
Clostridium botulinum	Improperly processed canned food; large masses of food with air-free center	May lead to acute bilateral cranial nerve impairment and descending weakness or paralysis. Double vision, dysphasia, and dry mouth may be present. Vomiting, diarrhea, or constipation may be present initially. Symptoms appear in 18–36 hours but can occur as late as 6 hours to 10 days. Symptoms may last for weeks or months, and some residual problems can last for years. A small percentage (3%–5%), of infected people die.
Clostridium perfringens	Meats, poultry, gravies, and stews in large masses of food such as steam tables or left at room temperature	Abdominal cramping, diarrhea, vomiting, and fever are common. Incubation time is 8–16 hours. Symptoms occur within 16 hours and last for 12–24 hours (up to 1–2 weeks in the elderly).

13-1

Clinical Application

Food Safety and Immunosuppressed Clients

All clients receiving an immunosuppressive agent need counseling on food safety and sanitation. These clients have an inability to fight infections, so a relatively small number of bacteria could cause illness. **Immunosuppressive agents** are medications that interfere with the body's ability to fight infections. These drugs are used in tissue and organ transplantation procedures, such as a kidney transplant. These are also used as part of the treatment of certain diseases such as cancer. The neutrophil (white blood cell) count in the blood becomes abnormally low, a condition referred to as neutropenia, making clients susceptible to life-threatening infection. For many years a low-microbial, also known as a neutropenic, diet has been taught to immunosuppressed individuals and is still ordered by many health-care providers. The diet emphasizes the avoidance of pathogens that may be present on or in foods. Unpasteurized, undercooked, and unwashed foods as well as most cheeses, deli-counter foods, honey, and well water (unless tested and found to be free of coliforms) are to be avoided in this type of diet (The Academy of Nutrition and Dietetics, 2012). The practice has been questioned, and adherence to the diet was found to be poor. Recommendations are to teach basic food safety guidelines to clients who are immunosuppressed (The Academy 2012, Fox and Freifeld 2012, Jubelirer 2011, and Trifilio 2012). More study in this area is needed and evidence-based guidelines should be developed to provide clear information to health-care providers and clients.

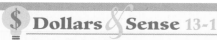

$ Dollars & Sense 13-1

Preventing Illness

Prevention of foodborne illness is one of the most effective and simple ways to stretch the health-care budget. The CDC (2011) estimates that 1 in 6 Americans get sick annually, 128,000 are hospitalized, and 3000 die from foodborne disease. It is estimated that the cost per case is $1626, with a total annual cost of $77.7 billion (Scharff, 2012).

hamburger. *Campylobacter* can be controlled by keeping food below 40°F or above 140°F and by maintaining good food-handling practices.

LISTERIA

Another pathogen is *Listeria.* This organism is problematic because the bacteria can grow slowly at refrigerated temperatures (32°F to 34°F) and on moist surfaces. Cooking facilities must be kept clean and dry to prevent the growth of this organism. Chlorine (bleach), one tablespoon per gallon of water, is also effective in inhibiting *Listeria*.

According to the CDC, every year 2500 Americans become ill with listeriosis with one of five cases resulting in death. Pregnant women become susceptible to foodborne illnesses because of changes in their immune system. Approximately one-third of listeriosis cases happen during pregnancy. Listeriosis can be transmitted to the fetus through the placenta, leading to premature delivery, miscarriage, stillbirth, or other serious health problems for the newborn. The USDA Food Safety and Inspection Service (FSIS) and the U.S. FDA provide guidelines for pregnant women (see Box 13-3).

Food Intoxication

Food intoxication is caused by the consumption of a food in which bacteria have produced a poisonous toxin.

STAPHYLOCOCCUS AUREUS

One of the most common bacteria producing a poisonous toxin is *Staphylococcus aureus,* commonly referred to as staph. Staph is reportedly in the nasal passages of 30% to 50% of healthy people and on the hands of 20% of healthy people. Infected cuts, boils, and burns harbor this organism.

Heat destroys the bacteria but not the toxins the bacteria have already produced. Because heat does not destroy the toxin, control of temperature alone will not provide protection. Prevention of staph poisoning must include good personal hygiene and keeping foods below 40°F or above 140°F.

Box 13-3 ■ *Food-Safety Guidelines for Pregnant Women (CDC, 2011)*

Pregnant women should follow these safe-eating suggestions:

- Do not eat hot dogs, luncheon meats, or deli meats unless they are reheated until steaming hot, ≥ 165°F.
- Do not eat soft cheeses such as feta, brie, camembert, blue-veined cheeses, and Mexican-style cheeses such as queso blanco fresco. Hard cheeses, such as mozzarella, pasteurized processed cheese slices, and spreads, cream cheese, and cottage cheese may be safely consumed.
- Do not eat refrigerated pâté or meat spreads. Canned or shelf-stable pâté and meat spreads may be eaten.
- Do not eat refrigerated smoked seafood unless it is an ingredient in a cooked dish such as a casserole. Canned fish such as salmon and dark tuna or shelf-stable smoked seafood may be eaten.
- Do not drink raw (unpasteurized) milk or eat foods that contain unpasteurized milk.
- Do not eat raw or undercooked eggs. This includes avoiding foods that may contain these, such as eggnog, raw cookie dough, or Caesar salad dressing.
- Do not eat raw, unwashed vegetables and sprouts (alfalfa, bean, or any other variety).

CLOSTRIDIUM BOTULINUM

Another bacterium producing a toxin is *Clostridium botulinum* and the resulting disease is **botulism.** The organism is found worldwide in soils and the intestinal tracts of domestic animals. Vegetables grown in contaminated soil harbor this organism. Botulin, the toxin produced by *C. botulinum,* is so poisonous that a single ounce is enough to kill the world's population. The spores of *C. botulinum* grow under anaerobic (without oxygen) conditions. Canned foods are processed to be anaerobic, providing an ideal medium for this bacterium's growth. Home-canned, nonacid fruits and vegetables, faultily processed commercially canned tuna, and improperly packaged smoked fish have all transmitted botulism.

Outbreaks of botulism can be avoided by the proper processing and preparation of susceptible foods. For each food, home canners should consult a reliable home-canning food guide regarding proper time, pressure, and temperature required to kill spores. As an additional precaution, all home-canned foods should be boiled for at least 10 minutes before serving to destroy botulinal toxins.

Complicating Factors

The following complicate the risk of foodborne illness:

- The worldwide overuse of antibiotics. Antibiotics kill not only pathogens but also normal flora, which help keep the disease-producing organisms in balance. Pathogens can mutate and become resistant to antibiotics.

- In the United States, the average age of the population continues to increase as life expectancy increases. Older people are more susceptible to pathogenic bacteria than younger people; fewer organisms are needed to produce symptoms in older people.
- Food production has become more centralized, an effect that has both good and bad ramifications. Food inspectors can more closely monitor the sanitation at food-processing plants, but a foodborne illness outbreak affects more people in wider geographical areas.
- As the population becomes highly educated about food safety, illnesses that in the past might have been dismissed as "stomach flu" are increasingly being identified as foodborne illnesses.
- Many foods are imported from countries whose regulatory procedures are not as stringent as those in the United States.
- Consumers are eating more meals away from home and using more convenience foods. Both behaviors increase the number of individuals involved in food handling and the time food is held in the danger zones. For example, a frozen convenience food is held in the temperature danger zone (between 40°F and 140°F) twice, once during assembly in the food-processing factory and a second time when the consumer is reheating it.
- Consumers are eating more raw food and more lightly grilled and sautéed foods, which are sometimes not cooked to proper temperatures.

Box 13-4 discusses how the simple behavior of frequent hand washing minimizes the risk of foodborne disease. Figure 13-3 pictures the correct amount of soap lather needed to cleanse hands.

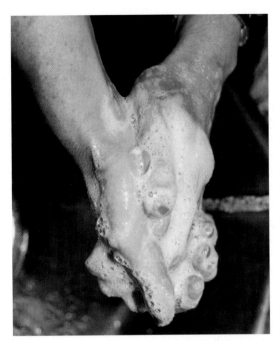

FIGURE 13-3 Amount of soap lather necessary to thoroughly cleanse the hands.

Infectious Agents

Mad cow disease, also known as **bovine spongiform encephalopathy (BSE),** is related to a disease in humans called Creutzfeldt-Jakob disease (variant CJD). Humans acquire this disease by eating beef that contains an infective agent (called a prion). A **prion** is a small protein that is resistant to most traditional methods that destroy a protein. BSE has been found in infected brain, spinal cord tissue, retina, dorsal root ganglia (nervous tissue near the backbone), distal ileum, and bone marrow in cattle experimentally infected by the oral route. Cattle acquire the infection when fed ground-up carcasses of animals, both sheep and other cattle, which contain the infected prion. Both the United States and Canada banned this feed practice for cattle in 1997, but the practice was not banned for poultry and hogs. In 2007, Canada enacted an enhanced BSE-related feed ban, which prohibited most proteins, from all animal feeds, pet foods, and fertilizers. The United States adopted similar guidelines in 2009 (CDC, 2013c).

Variant CJD has been seen primarily in young adults and is characterized initially by psychiatric and sensory problems, followed by ataxia (defective muscular coordination), dementia, and myoclonus (caused by fungus). This disease is considered a brain wasting disease (American Dietetic Association, 2009).

Parasitic Infections

A **parasite** is an organism that lives within, on, or at the expense of a living host without providing any

---

Box 13-4 ■ *Hand Washing*

The best defense against foodborne disease is hand washing and keeping the hands away from the mouth. Figure 13-2 demonstrates proper hand washing. Hands should always be washed:

- Before food preparation
- After food preparation
- After using the restroom
- Between touching another person's body, including the hands, and touching the mouth or eating
- After smoking
- Before smoking
- Between touching one person and then another person
- After covering the mouth when coughing or sneezing
- When visibly dirty
- After touching any surface area around any person who is visibly ill
- After changing an infant's diapers or touching any bodily secretion of another person

benefit to the host. Several parasites can live in animals that humans use for food. When a person eats an infected animal, he or she also consumes the parasite, and the result is illness. Common parasites are *Trichinella spiralis, Toxoplasma gondii,* and tapeworms.

TRICHINELLA SPIRALIS

Although the prevalence of this infection is low in the United States, it is significantly higher in people living in parts of Europe, Asia, and Southeast Asia.

Trichinella spiralis is a worm that becomes embedded in the muscle tissue of pigs. Pigs acquire the worm when fed meat from an animal harboring the worm in its muscle. The worm produces larvae that are protected from animal (including human) digestion. The larvae mature in the animal's stomach in 5 to 7 days. Adult worms then invade the lining of the small intestine, where they reproduce. The larvae enter the bloodstream of the animal and are carried to all parts of the body. They then penetrate the muscles, form cysts, and remain alive and infective for months. The cycle is completed when another animal eats the muscle containing the live *Trichinella spiralis* larvae.

When a human eats the larvae, usually in undercooked pork, he or she develops **trichinosis.** The symptoms of trichinosis usually appear 9 days after the ingestion of infected meat, but the time can vary from 2 to 28 days. This period of time is called the **incubation period**—the length of time it takes to show disease symptoms after exposure to the offending organism. The first symptoms, which mimic food poisoning, are nausea, vomiting, and diarrhea. When the larvae migrate into muscles, including the heart, systemic symptoms develop that include fever, swelling of the eyelids, sweating, weakness, and muscular pain. Death due to heart failure may occur.

TOXOPLASMA GONDII

This is a parasite found in food sources, such as raw or undercooked meat, as well as cat feces. Symptoms can be flulike and appear 10 to 13 days after eating, and may last months. Toxoplasmosis can cause miscarriage and birth defects including hearing loss, mental retardation, and blindness (U.S. Department of Health and Human Services 2011).

TAPEWORMS

Humans acquire tapeworms through the ingestion of raw seafood or undercooked beef and pork. Hogs and steers become intermediate hosts when they graze on sewage-polluted pastures. Tapeworm infestation can occur when human wastes contaminate freshwater streams and lakes, animal pasture, or feed.

Symptoms of a tapeworm infection may be trivial or absent. In some people, the worms attach to the jejunum

and hosts develop vitamin B_{12} deficiency, anemia, and massive infections with diarrhea. Obstruction of the bile duct or intestine can be another complication.

Viral Infections

A **virus** is a microscopic parasite that is entirely dependent on the nutrients inside host cells for its metabolic and reproductive needs. Viruses may invade the cells of people, animals, plants, and bacteria to survive and thereby cause disease. Food frequently serves as a vehicle for some viruses, including those that cause influenza and infectious hepatitis.

Food can become contaminated in its growing environment or during processing, storage, distribution, or preparation. Partly for this reason, the federal government requires all food-service workers to wear plastic gloves when handling food.

Some viruses are found in the intestinal tract of infected humans. If an infected person neglects to wash his or her hands after defecation and then handles food, the virus can contaminate the food and be passed on to unsuspecting consumers. The disease varies from a mild illness lasting 1 to 2 weeks to a severely disabling disease lasting several months.

HEPATITIS A VIRUS

The hepatitis A virus causes infectious hepatitis, a liver disease. This virus can be found in water that has been contaminated with raw sewage and in shellfish harvested from fecally contaminated water. During food processing, hepatitis A can be transmitted when polluted water is used or by fecal contamination from insects or rodents. Infected workers can transmit the virus through food they handle. The onset of viral hepatitis A is abrupt, with fever, malaise, anorexia, nausea, and abdominal discomfort. A few days later, the client may develop jaundice.

HEPATITIS E VIRUS

Every year there are 20 million hepatitis E infections and 70,000 hepatitis related deaths. Hepatitis E is a virus that causes acute sporadic and epidemic viral hepatitis. It can result in acute liver failure. The highest rates of disease are seen in regions with the lowest sanitation standards. It is transmitted through:

- Fecal contamination of water
- Foodborne transmission from ingestion of products from infected animals
- Transfusion of infected blood products
- Vertical transmission from a pregnant woman to her fetus

The onset of symptoms, which include jaundice, anorexia, enlarged liver, abdominal pain, nausea, vomiting, and fever occurs from 3 to 8 weeks after exposure to the virus (World Health Organization, 2012).

Substances Made Poisonous by Other Organisms

The consumption of toxic fish and plants can cause illness. Some molds can also produce disease (others are beneficial).

TOXIC SEAFOOD

The tissue of fish and shellfish can be naturally toxic to humans, even when the fish is fresh. The fish may not show any outward signs of illness, and there is usually no way to tell whether the fish is toxic. Because most fish toxins are stable to heat, cooking does not destroy them. **Paralytic shellfish poisoning** outbreaks have been reported involving the consumption of poisonous clams, oysters, mussels, and scallops.

Ciguatera poisoning is the most frequently reported seafood-toxin illness in the world. It is difficult to prevent because ciguatera is odorless, tasteless, and heat-stable and therefore cannot be killed by cooking or freezing. Occurrences are not due to inadequate food handling, storage, preparation or procurement methods (Friedman, Fleming, Fernandez, et al 2008). This intoxication results from eating certain fish that have consumed marine bacteria and algae associated with coastal reefs and nearby waterways. Fish eating the algae become toxic, and the effect is magnified through the food chain so that large predatory fish become the most toxic; this occurs worldwide in tropical areas. Coastal waters are routinely monitored for the presence of the organism that produces ciguatera. If excessive numbers of the organism are found, a "red tide" alert is made. The best prevention is to avoid eating fish caught during a red tide.

Scombroid fish poisoning is caused by the presence of undesirable bacteria. This poisoning occurs in fish such as tuna, mackerel, bonito, and skipjack. The bacteria produce a toxin on the flesh of fish after the fish have been caught. Scombroid fish poisoning can be prevented by the adequate refrigeration of freshly caught fish and the purchase of fish from reputable sources.

MOLDS

Molds are the most widely encountered microorganism and are spread by air currents, insects, and rodents. Some molds are beneficial, such as those used to make some cheese and soy sauce. Like bacteria, molds are often involved in food spoilage. A number of molds grow well in cold storage but are easily destroyed by heating to 140°F or higher.

Molds grow on bread, cheese, fruits, vegetables, preserves, grains, and a wide variety of other products.

Aspergillus molds produce a series of **mycotoxins** called **aflatoxins** that may be present in peanuts or peanut products, corn, wheat, and oil seeds such as cottonseed (National Institutes of Health, 2013). Many experts believe aflatoxins to be the most potent liver toxin known.

The best advice is to discard moldy bread because mold may have penetrated the entire item. Mold on natural cheese can be safely removed and the remainder of the cheese eaten, because the mold is not likely to have penetrated deeply.

Environmental Pollutants

Although environmental pollution is widespread, situations that pose a severe and immediate health danger are uncommon. The EPA regulates the use of **pesticides** and sets tolerance levels to provide a high margin of safety in food.

Chemical Poisoning

Chemical poisoning occurs when people eat toxic substances that may be intentionally or accidentally added to foods during growing, harvesting, processing, transporting, storing, or preparing foods. Two general types of chemical poisoning can occur. They are heavy metal and chemical-product contamination pesticides.

Heavy Metals

Several metals can be toxic. Metals in the soil come from rocks and minerals weathered by water erosion, metals as added ingredients or impurities in fertilizers, pesticides, manure and sludge, and airborne dust. Airborne dust comes from industrial and mining waste, fossil fuel combustion products, radioactive fallout, pollen, sea spray, and meteoric and volcanic material. This dust eventually settles to the ground and becomes part of the soil. Plants may grow normally but contain levels of selenium, cadmium, molybdenum, or lead that are toxic to humans.

The toxic action of metals is thought to be important in enzyme poisoning. For example, mercury, lead, copper, beryllium, cadmium, and silver have been found to inhibit the enzyme **alkaline phosphatase.** One function of alkaline phosphatase is in the mineralization of bone. Some diseases associated with the consumption of toxic minerals include rickets and bone tumors. Lead ingestion with a subsequent elevation of blood lead levels has been linked to toxic effects, including adverse neurologic, neurobehavioral, and developmental conditions.

Mercury is extremely toxic. It was once an occupational disease of hat manufacturers because mercury was used in the curing of animal pelts used to make hats. Inhalation of the mercury fumes led to mental deterioration, which is the origin of the term "mad hatter." Episodes of serious poisoning include those in Minamata, Japan, in which large chemical plants poured industrial waste containing mercury into nearby bays. Area residents who ate fish from the bays complained of numbness of the extremities, slurred speech, unsteady gait, deafness, and visual disturbances. Mental confusion and muscular incoordination were apparent in all the clients (Dolan, Matulka, and Burdock, 2010). Because mercury can damage the fetal nervous system, the FDA has issued a consumer alert for young children, pregnant and nursing women, and women of childbearing age not to eat large fish types in which mercury may accumulate: shark, swordfish, king mackerel, albacore tuna, and tilefish (American Dietetic Association, 2009).

Chemical Products

Chemical foodborne illness is also associated with products such as detergents, sanitizers, pesticides, and other chemicals that may enter the food supply. After such toxins have been ingested, symptoms of chemical poisoning appear in a few minutes to a few hours but usually in less than 1 hour. Nausea, vomiting, abdominal pain, diarrhea, and a metallic taste are common complaints with chemical foodborne illnesses, and death is possible (see Box 13-5).

Pesticides are chemicals used to kill insects or rodents; when accidentally mixed with food, they have caused poisonings in people. In addition, using pesticide-containing aerosols around foods and packaging materials and in food preparation areas can be dangerous. According to the EPA, studies have linked pesticides to problems such as cancer, nerve damage, and birth defects.

Pesticide residues are of great concern to consumers. **Residues** are trace amounts of any substance remaining in a product at the time of sale. Three governmental agencies regulate products that enter the U.S. food supply:

The Environmental Protection Agency (EPA)
The Food and Drug Administration (FDA)
The United States Department of Agriculture (USDA)
Food Safety and Inspection Service (FSIS)

The EPA regulates the use of potentially harmful pesticides in food production. Included among the duties of the EPA is the establishment of tolerance levels for pesticides.

The FDA regulates animal drugs, including food additives, herbicides, and environmental contaminants. The FSIS sets tolerance levels for these chemical residues in edible foods. In setting a **tolerance level,** the FSIS determines the highest dose at which a residue causes no ill effects in laboratory animals. The tolerance level is then divided by a factor ranging from 100 to 1000 to account for possible differences between animals and humans.

The numbers used assume that humans are 10 times more sensitive than the most sensitive animal species tested. In addition, a further assumption is made that children and the elderly are 10 times more sensitive than others. This is the 100-fold safety factor (multiplying 10 times 10). Thus, a large margin of safety is built into residue limits for compounds involved in the production of human food.

The FSIS enforces the residue limits in meat and poultry. The FDA is responsible for foods other than meat and poultry. When an illegal residue is found, the FDA can conduct an investigation and the FSIS can detain future shipments from the violating producer.

Natural Food Toxins

Many foods (unprocessed or uncooked) contain natural components that can harm health. Toxins in foods can be separated into five main categories, environmental, naturally occurring in the food, formed dues to mishandling of food during growing or storage, substances formed as the result of processing, and substances passed from animals to humans (Dolan et al, 2010).

Some common environmental toxins are presented in Table 13-2.

There are other naturally occurring substances in foods, which, for some individuals, necessitate the prohibition of the foods. These can be because of an autoimmune disease, inborn error of metabolism, or allergy to a food product. Table 13-3 gives some of the more commonly seen foods that must be avoided by certain individuals (Dolan et al, 2010).

Healthy people in this country who eat well-balanced diets should not worry about natural food intoxicants. However, if an individual eats large amounts of a single

---

Box 13-5 ■ *Chemical Poisoning*

Chemical poisoning can be prevented by:

■ Using each product for its intended use and in the amounts recommended
■ Reading product labels before use
■ Keeping chemicals in their original containers
■ Never storing or transporting chemicals in containers used to store food; they may be mistaken (especially by children) for food or beverages

TABLE 13-2 ■ Common Environmental Toxins

TOXIN	FOOD SOURCE	NONFOOD SOURCE	SYMPTOMS
Selenium	Plants	Microorganism conversion, soil	Hair loss, deformity and loss of nails, diarrhea, fatigue
Methyl mercury	Seafood	Bacterial action in aquatic environment, burning of coal, discharge of methyl mercury into the environment	Neurological symptoms, hearing defects, and death Developmental delays in children borne to mothers exposed
Naturally formed substances:			
Prussic acid (cyanide)	Leaves; cherry, apple and peach pits		Cellular necrosis, tissue damage, rapid breathing, trembling, incoordination
Hypericin	St. John's wort		Photosensitization, liver damage
Oxalic acid (oxalate)	Rhubarb, tea, spinach, parsley, asparagus, broccoli, Brussels sprouts, collards, lettuce, celery, cabbage, cauliflower, turnips, beans, other vegetables, and berries		Binds calcium and other minerals, making them insoluble causing decreased bone growth, kidney stones, renal toxicity, vomiting, diarrhea, convulsions, coma, impaired blood clotting
Phytic acid (phytate)	Bran and germ of many plant seeds, grains, legumes and nuts		Binds with minerals reducing bioavailability, may create mineral deficiencies or decreased protein and starch digestibility because of inhibition of digestive enzymes
Substance formed due to mishandling of food (growing and storage conditions):			
Glycoalkaloids (natural pesticides)	Potatoes, eggplant, apples, bell peppers, cherries, beets, tomatoes		Drowsiness, itchy neck, increased sensitivity (hyperesthesia), labored breathing, gastrointestinal symptoms (abdominal pain, nausea, vomiting, diarrhea)
Substances formed as the result of processing:			
Heterocyclic aromatic amines (HAAs)	Meats, poultry, fish, gravy	High heat causes reaction to form HAAs in protein foods	Carcinogenic
Trans fatty acids	Meats, milk and butter, hydrogenated liquid oils (margarines, spreads, shortenings, frying oil)		Raises low-density lipoprotein cholesterol, decreases high-density lipoprotein cholesterol, increases risk of coronary heart disease
Nitrosamines	Cheese, soybean oil, canned fruit, meat products, cured or smoked meats, fish and fish products, spices used for meat curing, beer and other alcoholic beverages	Formed from a bacterial reduction of nitrate; promoted through drying, kilning, salting, smoking or curing	Gastric cancer
Substances passed from animals to humans:			
Grayanotoxins	Honey——(from bees collecting nectar) or milk (from animals grazing) on rhododendrons, azaleas, oleander, and mountain laurel		Gastrointestinal distress

TABLE 13-3 ■ Common Foods Avoided by Specific Individuals

FOOD	REASON	CAUSE
Wheat, barley, gluten-containing foods	Gluten intolerance	Autoimmune disease
Dairy products	Lactose intolerance	Inborn error of metabolism (low or no lactase enzyme in intestine)
Milk, egg, fish, shellfish, tree nuts, wheat, peanuts, soybeans	Food allergies	Immune-mediated response to protein in foods

food at one time, he or she may experience the effects of natural intoxicants. The best protection, therefore, against the effects of natural intoxicants is to eat a wide variety of foods.

Food Additives

Additives may be introduced into food deliberately or accidentally. An **additive** is a substance added to food to increase its flavor, shelf life, or characteristics, such as texture, color, and aroma, and other qualities. In the United States, the FDA regulates food additives under the authority of the Food, Drug, and Cosmetic Act of 1938 and amendments in 1958 and 1960. These amendments include the Delaney Clause, which bans the approval of an additive if it is shown to cause cancer in humans or animals. Before using a new food additive, a manufacturer must petition the FDA for approval. The manufacturer must prove the additive is not harmful to humans at expected consumption.

Two categories of food additives are not subject to the testing and approval procedure: *prior sanctioned* and *GRAS* substances. The FDA before the 1958 Food Additives Amendment approved substances appointed as prior sanctioned. GRAS (generally recognized as safe) additives are those that have been used extensively in the past with no known harmful effects and are thought to be safe. Substances on the GRAS list have been under review since 1969. Substances on the GRAS list include sugar, salt, and vinegar.

Intentional Use

Additives are intentionally added directly to food during processing for four reasons:

1. To maintain or enhance a food's nutritional value. Vitamins, minerals, and fiber are examples.
2. To maintain a food's quality. Many additives are used to prevent the growth of microorganisms and extend a product's shelf-life. Some additives, called antioxidants, are used to prevent fats in food from deteriorating. Selected antioxidants may be effective in delaying proliferation of some cancers—mainly those related to fat metabolism, such as breast and prostate cancer.
3. To assist in processing, transporting, or holding a food. One additive that helps facilitate the processing of food is an **emulsifier,** to evenly distribute the molecules of two liquids that normally do not mix. Mayonnaise is an example of an emulsified product. Baking soda and baking powder are other commonly used additives. These substances cause such products as cakes to rise and improve their texture and volume.
4. To improve the way a food tastes, looks, or smells. Artificial colors, flavors, and sweeteners all fall into this category.

Types of common food additives are listed in Table 13-4.

Accidental Use

Some additives enter the food supply accidentally. For example, chemicals may enter food through contact with surfaces that have been cleaned with chemical solutions.

TABLE 13-4 ■ **Common Food Additives**

ADDITIVE	PURPOSE	INGREDIENT
Acidity Control Agents	Influence flavor, texture, and shelf life	Sodium bicarbonate Citric acid Hydrogen chloride Sodium hydroxide Acetic acid Phosphoric acid Calcium oxide
Antioxidants	Prevent discoloration Protect fats from rancidity	Vitamin C Vitamin E Butylated hydroxytoluene (BHT) and Butylated hydroxyanisole (BHA)
Flavors	Food enhancers	Hydrolyzed vegetable protein Black pepper Mustard Monosodium glutamate
Leavening Agents	To make dough rise	Sodium acid phosphate Sodium aluminum phosphate Monocalcium phosphate Yeast
Preservatives	To extend shelf-life	Sulfur oxide Benzoic acid Propionic acid Ethylenediaminetetraacetate (EDTA) Sodium caseinate
Stabilizers and Thickeners	To enhance texture	Gum arabic Modified starch Pectin

The Food Label

The FDA requires food labeling under the Federal Food, Drug and Cosmetic Act and its amendments. Most prepared foods, such as breads, cereals, canned fruits and vegetables, snacks, desserts, and drinks, require a food label. Nutrition labeling for raw produce (fruits and vegetables) is voluntary. Farm raised seafood must be labeled with the country of origin (www.USDA.gov). In 2006, labeling of products containing common allergens, milk, egg, fish, shellfish, tree nuts, wheat, peanuts, and soybeans was mandated by the USDA (Dolan et al, 2010). Figure 13-4 provides information on using the Nutrition Facts panel. The following list describes a food label's contents.

1. *Standardized Format:* Every label has the same layout and design; the nutrition information is titled "Nutrition Facts." Some small packages may use a simplified format.
2. *Serving Sizes:* All serving sizes listed on similar products are stated in consistently used household and metric measures to allow comparison shopping.
3. *Daily Values:* The bottom half of the Nutrition Facts panel shows either the minimum or maximum levels

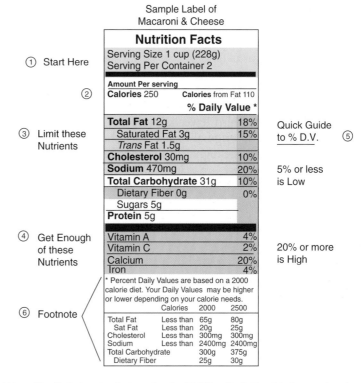

Sample Label of
Macaroni & Cheese

① Start Here

②

③ Limit these
Nutrients

④ Get Enough
of these
Nutrients

⑥ Footnote

Quick Guide
to % D.V. ⑤

5% or less
is Low

20% or more
is High

1. Start Here: The first place to start reading the Nutrition Facts Panel is the serving size and the number of servings in the package. Note how much you actually eat.

2. Calories: Displays the number of calories in the given serving size. The label also tells you how many calories are derived from fat.

3. Limit these nutrients: Eating too many of these nutrients may increase your risk of certain chronic diseases, such as heart disease, some cancers, and hypertension. Americans generally eat these nutrients in adequate amounts or too much.

4. Get enough of these nutrients: Americans often don't get enough of these nutrients.

5. Quick guide to % D.V.: % D.V. is based on 2000- and 2500-calorie diets.

6. Footnote: The D.V. are based on expert advice about some key nutrients that should be eaten daily.

FIGURE 13-4 Using the Nutrition Facts Panel on food labels. (*Source*: www.dietaryguidelines.gov.)

of nutrients people should consume each day for a healthful diet. For example, the value listed for carbohydrates refers to the minimum level, whereas the value for fat refers to the maximum level.

4. *% Daily Values:* The figures for percentage of daily values are based on a 2000-kilocalorie diet; this schema makes it easier for consumers to judge the nutritional quality of a food.

5. *Health Claims:* A **health claim** describes the relationship between a food or food component and a disease or health-related condition. Food manufacturers are allowed to write health claims on food labels that show only a preliminary promise of disease prevention. The FDA tried at one time to enforce more stringent regulations for health claims, but the court ruled that this was a violation of free speech. The FDA has only limited control on a health claim printed on a food product.

6. *A Structure/Function Claim:* A **structure/function claim** describes the role of a nutrient or dietary ingredient intended to affect the structure or function in humans or characterizes the documented mechanism by which a nutrient or dietary ingredient acts to maintain such structure or function, for example, "helps promote a healthy heart" or "helps support the immune system." Structure/function claims can be made without any scientific evidence to support the claim. The FDA has no regulatory control over a structure/function claim.

7. *Descriptors:* Terms such as *low, high,* and *free* used on food labels must meet legal definitions: For example:
   Free means less than 0.5 gram of fat per serving and tiny or insignificant amounts of cholesterol, sodium, and sugar.
   Low indicates 3 grams of fat or less per serving; also low in saturated fat, cholesterol, and/or kilocalories.

Lean signifies less than 10 grams of fat, 4 grams of saturated fat, and 95 milligrams of cholesterol per serving. (*Lean* is higher in fat than *Low*.)

Extra Lean means 5 grams of fat, 2 grams of saturated fat, and 95 milligrams of cholesterol per serving. (*Extra Lean* is lower in fat than *Lean* but not as low in fat as *Low*.)

Light (Lite) denotes one-third fewer kilocalories or one-half the fat of the original or no more than one-half the sodium of the higher-sodium version.

Cholesterol Free means the item has less than 2 milligrams of cholesterol and 2 grams (or less) of saturated fat per serving.

High in a nutrient means the food must contain 20% or more of the Daily Value for that nutrient.

Good Source Of denotes that one serving of a food is considered to be a good source of a vitamin, mineral, or fiber, containing 10% to 19% of the Daily Value for that particular vitamin, mineral, or fiber.

8. Ingredients are listed in descending order by weight. The ingredients list is required on almost all foods, even some standardized ones such as ice cream, mayonnaise, and bread.

Keystones

- The U.S. food supply is as safe, wholesome, and nutritious as any in the world, but there are no guarantees that all food purchased and eaten in the country is safe.

- Thousands of substances besides nutrients are present in foods. Most of these substances are harmless in the amounts typically eaten if the food item is selected, stored, and prepared under recommended conditions.

- Many foods contain toxic substances naturally. Only in recent years have we been able to detect and measure these toxic substances. The human body appears able to safely handle small amounts of some toxic substances without injury.

- The CDC ranks the Norovirus as causing the most foodborne illness, follow by pathogenic (disease-causing) bacterial microorganisms.

- Good food-handling methods can control most viral and microbiologic hazards.

- Selecting a wide variety of foods, storing the foods appropriately, and preparing foods correctly all help prevent illness.

- Health-care workers should teach their clients about the use of food labels and the risks of microbiologic and residual chemical hazards of foods.

CASE STUDY *13-1*

Ms. N is a 95-year-old woman who is 5 ft tall and weighs 122 lb (dressed without shoes). She has just been admitted to the nursing home. During the routine nursing admission process, Ms. N requested eggnog every night at 8:00 p.m. She stated she dislikes packaged mixes and would prefer her eggnog made with whole milk, ice cream, and a raw egg. Ms. N's physician has ordered eggnog at HS (Latin for hour of sleep, or just before bedtime) every day. Ms. N stated she has had a homemade eggnog every night for the past 50 years. The client's daughter has stated she makes her mother eggnog from raw eggs.

CARE PLAN

Subjective Data

Client stated she drinks eggnog made with a raw egg each day. ■ Client's daughter stated she makes her mother such a beverage.

CASE STUDY *(Continued)*

Objective Data
 Height: 5 ft, 0 in. ■ Weight: admitting 122 lb ■ Age: 95

Analysis
 Increased risk of infection related to consumption of raw eggs and client's advanced age.

Plan

DESIRED OUTCOMES EVALUATION CRITERIA	ACTIONS/INTERVENTIONS	RATIONALE
The client will state that raw eggs can make one ill.	Provide verbal and written information to the client and the client's daughter on the relationship between food illness and *Salmonella* infections.	Elderly clients are particularly at risk for salmonellosis.
	Have the client and the client's daughter state that raw eggs are hazardous.	Verbal recognition of a hazard is the first step in behavioral change.
The client will accept and eat another item for her evening snack.	Request the dietitian provide client with a list of other alternatives for her evening snack and evaluate whether client needs the snack.	Do not offer client an item that is not available from the Food and Nutrition Department. The client may need the nutrients in the evening snack.
	Chart acceptance or rejection of the snack.	Refusal to eat substitute snack defeats the purpose of sending the snack.

13-1

Dietitian's Note

The following Dietitian's Notes are representative of the documentation found in a client's medical record.

Subjective: Spoke with client and her daughter. The risk of *Salmonella* foodborne disease with the consumption of raw eggs in an older adult was explained to client and her daughter. A 24-hour dietary recall cross-checked with a food frequency was completed. Client has been eating three times per day, accepts all major food groups, and denies food allergies. Usual intake consists of: 6 medium-fat meats, 5 starches (3 whole grain), 3 vegetables (including a source of vitamin A), 3 fruits (including a source of vitamin C), and 6 fats. Claims good dentition, denies nausea and vomiting (N/V), constipation, diarrhea.

Objective: Albumin 3.7 mg/dL; body mass index 23; height 5 ft, 0 in.; weight 122 lb

Analysis: Usual intake about 1400 to 1450 kcal with 67 grams of protein. No laboratory, diet history, and anthropometric evidence of nutritional risk.

Estimated kilocalorie needs based on maximum ideal body weight (IBW) of 110 lb or 50 kg and 25–35 kcal/kg max equals 1250–1750 kcal.

Estimated protein need based on 50 kg and 0.8–1.2 g/kg equals 40–60 grams of protein per day.

Estimated kilocalories in homemade eggnog equals 275 kcal.

After explaining risk with the consumption of raw eggs, client agreed to have one cup of hot cocoa and a banana for her evening snack because she would need the kilocalorie from these items to meet her estimated kilocalorie needs. Client's protein intake more than exceeds estimated requirements.

Plan:
 1. Follow-up in 3 days.
 2. Order evening snack as described above.

Critical Thinking Questions

1. What other areas of the home might you inspect to minimize the risk of a foodborne illness?

2. What clients need to take extra precautions to prevent a foodborne illness?

3. Do you think it is within the scope of practice for a nurse when making a home visit to discuss unsafe food practices?

Chapter Review

1. Cold foods should be stored:
   a. At less than 50°F
   b. At less than 0°F
   c. At less than 40°F
   d. For no more than 6 hours outside the recommended temperature range.

2. The term *low* on a food label means the product contains:
   a. Less than 3 grams of fat per serving; also low in saturated fat, cholesterol, or kilocalories
   b. _____ the fat of the original
   c. Less than 10 grams of fat, 4 grams of saturated fat, and 95 milligrams of cholesterol per serving
   d. More fat than a product labeled *extra lean*.

3. Foods commonly contaminated with *Campylobacter* are:
   a. Hard-cooked scrambled eggs
   b. Raw vegetables
   c. Canned foods
   d. Raw poultry

4. The best method to control the spread of foodborne illness is by:
   a. Wearing gloves when handling food
   b. Proper hand washing
   c. Taking food supplements
   d. Avoiding certain foods

5. Farm-raised seafood must be labeled with
   a. Country of origin
   b. Grams of mercury
   c. Kilocalories in one serving
   d. Grams of protein

Clinical Analysis

1. Mr. P has brought his 35-year-old male companion who has a history of AIDS to the ambulatory care clinic for treatment for a sudden onset of headache, abdominal pain, diarrhea, nausea, and vomiting. The nurse should:
   a. Document all food consumed during the past 7 days.
   b. Inquire about food practices in the home.
   c. Inspect Mr. P's passport for foreign travel in the past month.
   d. Document the client's immunization status.

2. You are on a committee to help plan the annual hospital picnic. One employee volunteers to make Texas-style chili at home and serve it at the picnic. You have a responsibility to:
   a. Inquire how the chili will be made, transported, and held at recommended temperatures
   b. Taste the chili on arrival at the picnic for safety
   c. Check the temperature of the chili on arrival at the picnic
   d. Review the recipe for the potential use of unsafe ingredients

𝒞linical 𝒜nalysis—cont'd

3. Mr. J is an 85-year-old man recently discharged from the hospital for a partial bowel obstruction that he had surgically repaired. His wife is getting ready to serve him eggnog made with raw eggs. What would be the most effective way to determine if the client consumed any contaminated food?
   a. Ignore the situation because that is not the purpose of the visit.
   b. Inquire about any gastrointestinal pain Mr. J may have had.
   c. Instruct the wife about the safe preparation of eggs.
   d. Assess the amount of sugar used in the beverage.

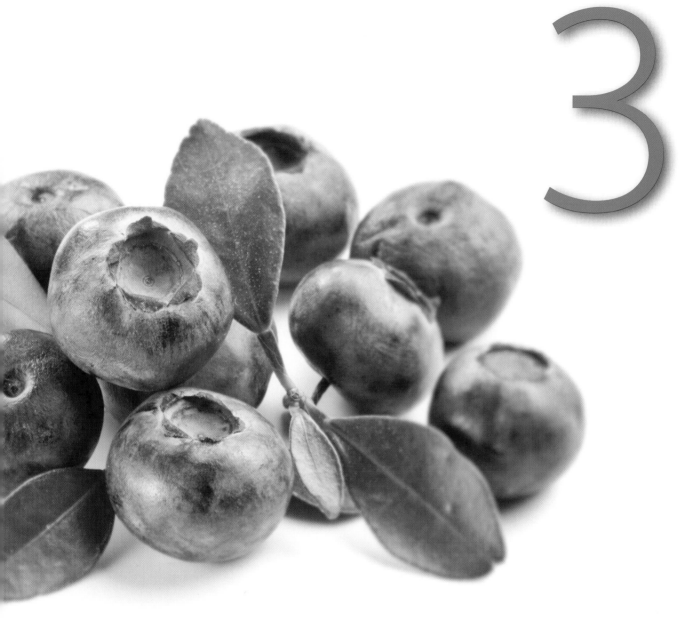

3

Clinical Nutrition

14

Nutrient Delivery

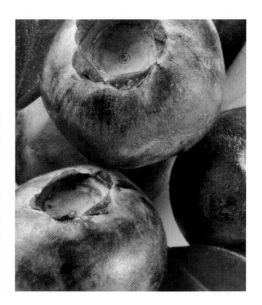

LEARNING OBJECTIVES

After completing this chapter, the student should be able to:

■ Identify three routes used to deliver nutrients to clients and potential complications with two of these routes.

■ Discuss the kinds of commercial formulas available for oral and enteral feedings.

■ Discuss why it is important to carefully control the rate of delivery and volume of enteral formula delivered to a client.

■ List the reasons for the high incidence of malnutrition in institutionalized clients and the interventions nurses can perform to combat malnutrition.

■ Describe suggested procedures for administering medications through feeding tubes.

This chapter introduces the methods commonly used to deliver nutrients to clients: oral, enteral nutrition via feeding tube, and parenteral nutrition. The major functions of dietetic services in health-care facilities are the preparation and delivery of nutrients via food and supplements and the clinical nutritional care of clients. The nutritional care of clients includes four areas:

1. Assessing the client's need for nutrients
2. Determining the best method for delivering nutrients to the client
3. Monitoring the client's nutrient intake
4. Counseling the client about nutritional needs

High-quality nutritional care helps prevent illness and disease and saves the client's and society's health-care dollars.

Food Service in Institutions

All members of the health-care team need to become familiar with some aspects of the food service in their place of employment. The scheduling of diagnostic procedures, blood work, surgery, and administration of medications is dependent on when the client last consumed food.

Meal Service Patterns

Many institutions serve three meals to clients each day as well as several between-meal feedings. Feedings between meals are available for clients in need of extra nutrients, those who desire extra food, or those who are unable to consume sufficient kilocalories at regular mealtimes. Some institutions offer a room service system, and clients may order food whenever they desire. Specific procedures are necessary to ensure that the provision of medical care is coordinated with meal delivery.

Nutritional Care Services

Institutions vary in the types of nutritional services they offer clients. A large teaching hospital or medical center frequently has nutrition professionals on staff

307

who specialize in treating particular types of clients. A critical care dietitian, for example, has special training to assess, plan, implement, and counsel clients in high-risk stages of trauma, disease, and conditions that affect nutritional support. In such settings, other health-care workers can rely on the critical care dietitian to provide technical support.

At the other end of the spectrum, in a small community hospital or a long-term care facility, a dietitian may be present only part time or as a consultant. In such circumstances, other health-care workers must plan to make the best use of the dietitian's services when he or she is available. In this situation, the nursing staff assumes more responsibility for the nutritional care of clients.

Home- and community-based programs also provide nutritional care services. For example, hospice, home-care programs, and some governmental agencies deliver nutritional care services. Frequently, a dietitian is available through any of these programs for consultation. Third-party payers increasingly cover medical nutritional care, referred to as *medical nutrition therapy* (MNT).

Screening, Assessment, Monitoring, and Counseling

Nutritional care is a responsibility of many health-care team members. The nurse is usually the first team member to interview and assess the client, often before the physician visits the client. The physician and/or physician assistant complete a physical examination of the client, order necessary treatments and diagnostic procedures, and provide either a diagnosis or tentative diagnosis. The diagnosis may change after the diagnostic tests are completed. The nurse, physician, or the physician assistant usually makes referrals to other team members. Institutions frequently require specific team members to assess each client. Figure 14-1 presents an overview of a nutrient-delivery decision-making tree.

Screening

The Joint Commission on Accreditation of Healthcare Organizations requires that a nutritional screening is completed within 24 hours of admission to an acute care facility. A health technician or nurse may utilize a series of questions, often in the form of a predetermined screening tool, which rates a client's potential nutritional risk. Changes in weight, appetite, or presence of nausea, vomiting, **dysphagia** (difficulty swallowing), and/or disease state (such as diabetes, obesity, hypertension, cancer, etc.) are reviewed. If a client has a positive screen in these areas or there are changes noted, a client may be determined to be at risk nutritionally.

Assessment

Clients found to be at a nutritional risk need to have a complete nutritional assessment by a registered dietitian (RD), which may include the following items:

- Height, weight, body mass index (BMI), and weight history
- Laboratory test values
- Food intake information
- Potential food–drug interactions
- Mastication and swallowing ability
- Client's ability to feed himself or herself
- Bowel and bladder function
- Evaluation for the presence of **pressure ulcers**
- Food allergies and intolerances
- Any other factors affecting nutritional status, such as food preferences and cultural and religious beliefs about food
- Determination of body composition
- Presence of severe burns, trauma, infection, or other physiological stressors that increase nutrient needs and are likely to prolong hospital stay
- Learning barriers such as hearing, mobility, language, need for interpreter, vision, speech, reading/writing skills, inability to follow instructions, cultural and religious barriers, learning disability, learning readiness (requests, accepts, or avoids information), and preferred learning style

The American Society for Parenteral and Enteral Nutrition (A.S.P.E.N.) Clinical Guidelines for Nutrition Screening, Assessment, and Intervention in Adults (Mueller, Compher, Druyan, et al, 2011), has defined nutrition assessment as a comprehensive approach to defining nutritional status that uses medical, nutrition, and medication histories; physical examination; anthropometric measurements; and laboratory data. In addition, A.S.P.E.N. defines any "acute, subacute or chronic state of nutrition, in which varying degrees of overnutrition or undernutrition with or without inflammatory activity have led to a change in body composition and diminished function" as Malnutrition (Mueller et al, 2011). In this context, nutrition assessment is much more than an initial client screening, as completed by nursing personnel. A comprehensive nutritional assessment requires data from physical examinations, tests, lab work, and client intake information to be analyzed by the dietitian to determine a nutritional diagnosis and plan of care.

Computer technology has greatly facilitated the client assessment process. Information may group clients such as all those with low blood albumins, on specific medications, with low weight for height, and on NPO (nothing by mouth) or on inadequate diets for longer than 3 days, for example. The consolidation of this information allows for a greater number of clients

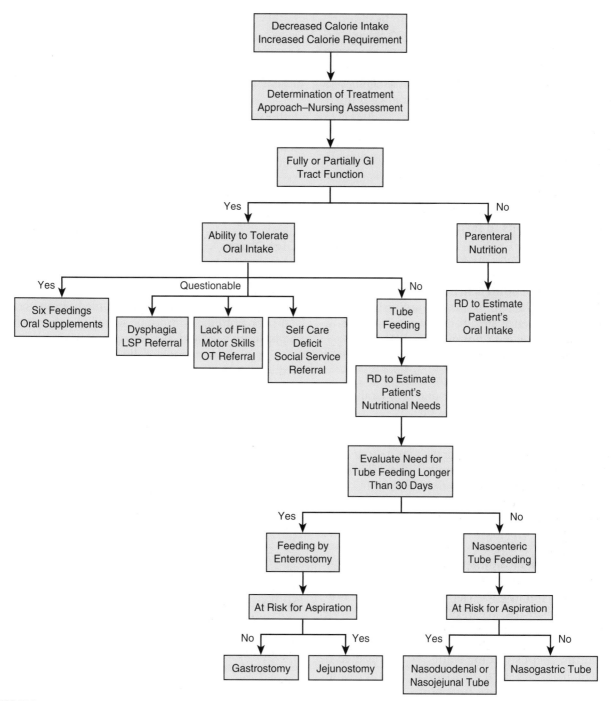

FIGURE 14-1 Nutrient delivery decision-making tree. OT, occupational therapist; RD, registered dietitian; LSP, licensed speech pathologist. (From Abbott Nutrition Pocket Guide, 2010. © 2011 Abbott Laboratories. Used with permission.)

to be identified and targeted for in-depth nutritional assessment and care.

Client care has also become standardized as a result of computer technology and the development of standards of practice. For example, a health-care organization may require clients with a blood albumin level of less than 3 mg/dL be evaluated by a registered dietitian within 24 hours of admission. A licensed speech pathologist may be required to evaluate all clients with dysphasia before the client is given any food or fluids. A registered nurse may be required to phone a physician immediately on receipt of data showing a potassium level greater than 5.0 mEq/L and document the phone call. The occupational therapist may be required to evaluate clients who are unable to feed themselves.

Regulatory agencies of long-term care facilities require that clients have a nutritional assessment performed by a registered dietitian shortly after admission. An initial assessment or screening identifies clients at nutritional risk. An in-depth assessment as defined by A.S.P.E.N. requires a care plan by several team members who coordinate services (Mueller et al, 2011).

Monitoring

All clients should be reassessed or monitored at appropriate intervals. Most organizations include the required frequency of client monitoring in their standards of practice. Some clients in hospital intensive care units require continuous monitoring. Other clients require daily, weekly, monthly, or quarterly reassessment as determined by preset guidelines.

The **client care conference** (interdisciplinary conference) is a productive means of monitoring clients. Before the conference, health-care workers gather information on the client's nutritional care including:

■ Initial nutritional screen and/or assessment
■ Present body weight and weight history
■ A record of recent food intake and/or tolerance
■ Any changes in medical condition
■ Diet order
■ Family support (or lack of)

With this information, health-care workers can more readily determine the reason for most changes in the client's nutritional status. If weight loss is identified, a review of the client's **food acceptance record,** if available, may verify whether such a weight loss is likely a result of poor food intake.

Clients whom health-care providers have determined to be at nutritional risk because of poor food intake should be treated; treatment may include a nutritional supplement, between-meal feedings, a change in the diet prescription, or a change in feeding status. If, for example, a client can no longer feed himself or herself, the client's feeding status would need to be changed from self-feed to assisted feeding. Many clients require aggressive nutritional treatment that may include enteral nutrition through a feeding tube, inserted either surgically or nasally, and/or parenteral nutrition. Monitoring the client's weight, laboratory values, and food intake is an important part of delivering high-quality nutritional care.

Counseling

All clients should be evaluated for nutritional counseling. The assumption that a client is not expected to be discharged and therefore is not entitled to education is unjustifiable. Educating the client about nutritional concerns helps the client assume responsibility for his or her own care, thus promoting self-esteem and a sense of worth.

Diet Manuals

Current accreditation standards (both long-term and acute care) require all health-care institutions to have a diet manual available to all team members. Electronic manuals are often used and may be available on an organization's computer system. The diet manual defines and describes all diets used as part of nutritional therapy for clients.

Diet Orders

The physician or designee is responsible for prescribing a diet for the client. Just as a medication cannot be administered to a client without a medication prescription, food or fluids cannot be served to a client without a physician's written diet order.

One of the functions of the diet manual is to define a diet. The diet manual is the first place to look when clients request food items not being served. The diet manual may state, for example, that the food item is restricted or not allowed on the client's prescribed diet.

Special Diets

The purpose of a special or modified diet is to restore or maintain a client's nutritional status by manipulating one or more of the following dietary aspects:

■ Nutrients such as protein, calcium, iron, sodium, potassium, and vitamin K may be increased, decreased, or held at a consistent level.
■ Kilocalories may be either restricted or increased.
■ Texture or consistency of foods may be considered. For example, if a client has dysphagia a diced diet with prethickened liquids may be ordered.
■ Fiber may be restricted or increased depending on a client's gastrointestinal (GI) function.
■ Fluid may be pushed in the case of dehydration or limited for renal or cardiac diseases.

All modified diets are variations of the general diet; the client nonetheless needs all the essential nutrients. For this reason, each modified diet must be carefully planned to provide each of the essential nutrients or a documented reason for not providing one or more essential nutrients. Physicians determine when a specific diet order is medically indicated for a client.

Common Diet Orders

Some common diet orders are for *clear liquid, full liquid, soft,* and *general* or *regular.* A clear-liquid diet is any transparent liquid that can be poured at room temperature. Gelatin, some juices, broth, tea, frozen ices, and coffee are clear liquids. A clear-liquid diet is nutritionally inadequate and normally limited in duration. Clear-liquid nutritional supplements, however, are available.

A full-liquid diet is any liquid that can be poured at room temperature. Milk, custard, all fruit juices, ice cream, strained soups, and all items allowed on the clear-liquid diet are allowed on most full-liquid diets. The major difference between a clear-liquid and a full-liquid diet is that the latter contains milk and milk products (Table 14-1 and Boxes 14-1 and 14-2).

Soft diets vary greatly from one facility to another. For example, a mechanical soft diet is ordered when the client has only a few or no teeth (edentulous). A soft diet is ordered following surgery when easily digested foods are required. A facility that specializes in treating clients with eye, ear, nose, and throat disorders may have many types of soft diets. A pureed diet usually consists of foods that have been run through a blender or food processor to meet the consistency needs of the client. Table 14-2 lists recommended foods on a pureed, mechanical soft, and soft diet.

A general or regular diet means that the client is on an unrestricted diet. Frequently, an *as tolerated* or *progressive* diet may be prescribed, which means that a clear-liquid diet is to be served initially and the diet advanced (full-liquid to soft to general) as the client is able to tolerate. The nurse may be responsible for determining the client's tolerance for food just before tray delivery. This last-minute determination of client tolerance is necessary for many clients because of fluctuating medical status.

Diets for Diagnostic Procedures

Many diagnostic procedures requiring dietary preparation are performed in hospitals.

Poor Client Preparation

Poor dietary preparation can force a client to have an expensive procedure repeated or postponed (Fig. 14-2). Figure 14-2A is an x-ray film from a poorly prepared client. Feces in the colon block the view of structures within the colon. Figure 14-2B shows the colon of a well-prepared client. In the absence of fecal material, the entire length of the colon can be visualized.

Box 14-1 ■ *Clear-Liquid Diet*

Description

The clear-liquid diet provides energy and fluid in a form that requires minimal digestive action.

Indications

The clear-liquid diet is prescribed when it is necessary to limit undigested food in the GI tract and before bowel surgery, diagnostic imaging procedures, and colonoscopic examination. A clear-liquid diet is also used during acute stages of illness to assist with fluid and electrolyte replacement and as a first step in oral alimentation after intravenous feeding, surgery, and GI disturbances.

Adequacy

This diet is inadequate in all nutrients and should be used only in the short term.

Food Allowed	Foods to Avoid
Coffee and tea	All other food and beverages
Carbonated beverages such as 7UP® and ginger ale	
Fruit-flavored gelatin, Italian ices, and popsicles	
Apple, grape, or cranberry juice	
Clear fat-free broth and bouillon	
Sugar	

Recommended to Enhance Nutrition

Nutritional supplement such as Ensure Clear® (Abbott)*
High-protein broth and gelatin desserts are also available.

Sample Breakfast, Lunch, and Dinner Menu

Clear apple, grape, or cranberry juice
Broth
Flavored gelatin
Coffee or tea
Sugar

*Clear-liquid nutritional supplement if client is on this diet for longer than two meals.

TABLE 14-1 ■ Composition of Liquid Diets						
DIET	PROTEIN (GRAMS)	FAT (GRAMS)	CARBOHYDRATE (GRAMS)	SODIUM (MEQ)	POTASSIUM (MEQ)	KILOCALORIES
Clear Liquid	5	Trace	70–95	65	20	375
Clear Liquid With Three 10-oz Servings of Ensure Clear®	32	Trace	175–200	215	23.46	915
Full Liquid	50	55	205	110	65	1500

Box 14-2 ■ *Full-Liquid Diet*

Description

The full-liquid diet provides foods and beverages that are liquid or may become liquid at body temperature.

Indications

This diet is used as a progression between clear liquids and a soft diet and after oral surgery. Acutely ill clients with a chewing or swallowing dysfunction and clients with oral, esophageal, or stomach disorders who are unable to tolerate solid foods because of strictures or other anatomical disorders find this diet useful.

Adequacy

This diet can be adequate in all nutrients according to the Recommended Dietary Allowances. Special care needs to be taken to meet folacin, iron, thiamin, niacin, vitamin A, fiber, and kilocalorie allowances.

Foods Allowed	Foods Not Allowed
Beverages	
Any beverage that pours at room temperature	All others
Breads, cereals, and grains	
None	
Fruits	
All fruit juices	All others
Vegetables	
Any vegetable juice	All others
Meats	
None	
Milk	
Any	
Fats	
Butter, margarine, cream, and oils	All others
Other	
Custard, ice cream, flavored with gelatin, sherbet, sugar, and popsicles	All others and any made coconut, nuts, or whole fruit

Special Notes

The use of a complete nutritional liquid supplement is often necessary to meet nutrient allowances for clients who follow this diet for longer than 3 days.

An oral supplement that contains fiber minimizes the potential for problems with constipation and abdominal cramping. However, liquid supplements with fiber are not indicated for all clients on full-liquid diets.

Sample Menu

Breakfast	Lunch and Dinner	Snacks
½ cup fruit juice	½ cup fruit juice	A complete nutritional supplement as needed to meet protein and kilocalorie allowances
	½ cup vegetable juice	
1 cup pasteurized eggnog	1 cup strained cream soup	
Coffee, cream, and sugar	½ cup custard	
	8-oz Ensure® or Boost® or similar product	
	Coffee as desired	

TABLE 14-2 ■ Consistency Modifications—Recommended Foods			
FOOD GROUP	PUREED DIET	MECHANICAL SOFT DIET	SOFT DIET
Soups	Broth, bouillon, strained or blenderized cream soup	Broth, bouillon, strained or blenderized cream soup	Broth, bouillon, cream soup
Beverages	All	All	All
Meat	Strained or pureed meat or poultry, cheese used in cooking	Ground, moist meats, or poultry, flaked fish, eggs, cottage cheese, cheese, creamy peanut butter, soft casseroles	Moist, tender meat, fish, or poultry, eggs, cottage cheese, mild flavored cheese, creamy peanut butter, soft casseroles
Fat	Butter, margarine, cream, oil, gravy	Butter, margarine, cream, oil, gravy, salad dressing	Butter, margarine, cream, oil, gravy, crisp bacon, avocado, salad dressing
Milk	Milk, milk beverages, yogurt without fruit, nuts, or seeds, cocoa	Milk, milk beverages, yogurt without seeds or nuts, cocoa	Milk, milk beverages, yogurt without seeds or nuts, cocoa
Starch	Cooked, refined cereal, mashed potatoes	Cooked or refined ready-to-eat cereal, potatoes, rice, pasta, white, refined wheat, light rye bread or rolls, graham crackers as tolerated	Cooked or ready-to-eat cereal, potatoes, rice, pasta, white, refined wheat, light rye or graham bread, rolls, or crackers
Vegetables	Strained or pureed, juice	Soft, cooked, without hulls or tough skin as in peas and corn, juice	Soft, cooked, vegetables, limit strongly flavored vegetables and whole-kernel corn, lettuce and tomatoes
Fruit	Strained or pureed, juice	Cooked or canned fruit without seeds or skins, banana, juice	Cooked or canned fruit, banana, citrus fruit without membrane, melon, juice
Desserts	Gelatin, sherbet, ice cream without nuts or fruit, custard, pudding, fruit ice, popsicle	Gelatin, sherbet, ice cream without nuts or fruit, custard, pudding, fruit ice, popsicle	Gelatin, sherbet, ice cream without nuts, custard, pudding, cake, cookies without nuts or coconut, fruit ice, popsicle
Sweets	Sugar, honey, jelly, candy, flavorings	Sugar, honey, jelly, candy, flavorings	Sugar, honey, jelly, candy, flavorings
Miscellaneous	Seasonings, condiments	Seasonings, condiments	Seasonings, condiments

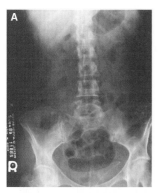
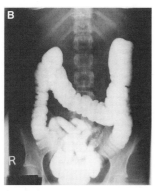

FIGURE 14-2 *A*, Image of a client who was poorly prepared for a barium enema. *B*, Image of a client who was adequately prepared for a barium enema. (Courtesy of Dr. Russell Tobe.)

Some x-ray procedures are not only expensive but also uncomfortable. The client must have the procedure repeated if necessary bodily structures cannot be visualized. Although the specific dietary preparation for x-ray studies of the colon may vary from one facility to another, dietary preparation is usually somewhat similar. The client may be instructed not to eat or drink anything after midnight on the day of the imaging study. In addition, the client may need to follow a clear-liquid diet for 12 to 48 hours before the x-ray procedure.

Many clients undergo x-ray studies as outpatients. The nurse or medical assistant working in a physician's office is usually responsible for dietary instruction before these procedures.

Misdiagnosis

Poor dietary preparation can lead to a misdiagnosis. For example, a blood sample for a fasting blood glucose (FBS) test should be drawn on a **fasting** individual; that is, one who has not had any food or beverages (with the exception of sips of water) by mouth for at least 8 hours before the blood draw. If the client eats before the procedure, his or her blood glucose level may be elevated, and this elevation may cause a misdiagnosis of diabetes. A misdiagnosis may cause a client unnecessary anxiety, medical treatment, and expense.

Importance of Nutritional Care

Malnutrition associated with acute and chronic disease is common in hospital settings. **Acute** means that the illness has a rapid onset, severe symptoms, and a short course. **Chronic** means that the illness has a long duration.

The presence and importance of malnutrition has been increasingly recognized throughout the world.

Malnutrition is one of the most common conditions affecting the care of hospitalized clients. The prevalence of adult malnutrition is estimated from 15% to 60% of patients have moderate to severe malnutrition. Many patients come into hospitals malnourished, and their acute illnesses further worsen their malnutrition and increase their length of stay (LOS) in the facility therefore increasing health-care costs (Barker, Gout, and Crowe, 2011; White, Guenter, Jensen, et al, 2012).

Malnutrition is associated with a 25% morbidity and a 5% mortality. **Morbidity** is defined as the rate of being diseased. **Mortality** is defined as the death rate. A malnourished client is more likely to be sicker and run a higher risk of death than a well-nourished client with the same diagnosis. Because malnutrition affects morbidity and mortality, it is also associated with a prolonged hospital stay.

Iatrogenic Malnutrition

The term **iatrogenic malnutrition** was first used in 1974 and refers to physician- or institution-induced malnutrition (Butterworth and Blackburn, 1975). Routine hospital practices such as extended periods of food or nutrient deprivation because of treatments, as well as diagnostic tests that interfere with the client's meal schedule or that cause a lack of appetite, are related to the high prevalence of malnutrition. Drug therapy may also affect a client's appetite. Some drugs cause drowsiness, lethargy, nausea, and anorexia. Problems related directly to an illness, such as pain, unconsciousness, paralysis, vomiting, and diarrhea, can also interfere with eating.

Today many institutions have written policies and procedures for clinicians to follow to minimize the likelihood of iatrogenic malnutrition. The tasks that clinical team members should perform to combat institutional malnutrition are discussed in Clinical Application 14-1.

Methods of Nutrient Delivery

Nutrients can be delivered to the client orally in foods or supplements, enterally by feeding tube, or parenterally through veins. **Enteral nutrition (EN)** means the feeding of an appropriate formula or liquid via a tube to a client's GI tract. **Parenteral nutrition (PN)** designates that nutrients are being provided via an intravenous route.

Figure 14-3 shows two feeding pumps. The feeding pumps are set to deliver a given rate, volume, and amount of both enteral and parenteral feedings to a client. The importance of connecting the enteral feeding to the tube that leads to the client's GI tract and

14-1
Clinical Application

Methods for Team Members to Combat Iatrogenic Malnutrition

Nursing actions can affect the nutritional health of institutionalized clients. The following behaviors minimize the likelihood of malnutrition:

- Recording height and weight
- Regular communication among nurses, physicians, dietitians, and other health-care workers
- Food-tray viewing/monitoring and documentation of client's food intake
- Careful food handling and sanitation practices for oral and enteral feedings
- Knowledge of the importance of good nutrition, nutritional supplements, and the composition of vitamin mixtures
- Monitoring the length of time clients are NPO, on liquid diets, and on intravenous feedings of only glucose
- Appreciation of the role of nutrition in the prevention and recovery from infection
- Recognition of the increased nutritional needs due to injury or illness
- Monitoring of stool frequency, urinary losses, losses by suction tubes, drainage, etc.
- Recording of weight at regular intervals
- Monitoring of behavior patterns, vomiting, and any unusual comments clients make about food
- Monitoring of client fluid intake and output

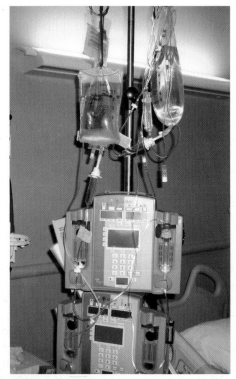

FIGURE 14-3 These two feeding pumps are set to deliver both a tube feeding and PN simultaneously. The client also has lines running for medications. Note how confusing it is to place the lines.

connecting the intravenous solution to the tube that leads directly into the blood stream cannot be overemphasized. Although this is primarily a nursing responsibility, all trained team members should make a habit of checking tube connections every time a client with two feeding routes is visited. The placement of a feeding tube into the wrong lead is called a misconnection.

Oral Delivery

Most institutionalized clients are fed orally. Whenever possible, the client should be encouraged to eat foods, because this is an optimal way for the client not only to obtain nutrients but also to experience the normal psychological and physical pleasure associated with eating.

The Menu

An institution's menu can be selective or nonselective. A selective menu is similar to a restaurant menu; clients can choose the specific menu items that appeal to them. Clients eat best when they fill out their own menus or a significant other does so for them. Marking the menu is one way in which a client can participate daily in care planning.

When an institution does not have a selective menu, one kind of meal is prepared and served to all clients. Food and labor required for providing a selective menu is more expensive than for institutions providing a nonselective menu. However, many clients may fail to eat the food from a nonselective menu because they dislike the menu item provided.

Eating Environment

Health-care workers need to create as pleasant an environment as possible immediately before and during mealtime. The room should be checked for objectionable odors, sounds, and sights. Obviously, a full bedside commode or an emesis basin nearby discourages eating. In addition, the client should be prepared to eat when the tray arrives. Cleaning the client's hands and face helps the client become more enthusiastic about eating. The client's bedside table should be cleared of all miscellaneous items, and unnecessary delays in serving the tray should be avoided. The client should be properly positioned to eat. This includes elevating the head of the bed (if his or her condition permits) and positioning the bedside table to the correct height. Assistance with opening food packages or cartons may be required.

Some clients may find the odor of food offensive. For these clients, it is best for the nurse not to uncover the food items directly in front of them, minimizing the risk of nausea. For these individuals, often oncology clients, open food trays in the hallway, or away from the client, to help dissipate the intense odors of hot foods.

Assisted Feeding Versus Self-Feeding

Some clients must be fed. Food should be offered in bite-sized portions and in the order that the client prefers. Clients should not be rushed. Talking with clients while feeding makes mealtime pleasant and signals that they are not being rushed. Personnel are encouraged to sit while feeding clients because this indicates a willingness to spend time with them and encourages relaxation.

Some nursing personnel have found they can enhance a client's food intake by mimicking normal eating behavior:

■ Sit behind the client.
■ Place your right arm over the client's arm (if you and the client are right-handed).
■ Place a fork or spoon with food in either the client's hand or your own hand (depending on the client's ability to do this maneuver).
■ Guide the client's hand to his or her mouth.

In a long-term care facility, a client's ability to feed himself or herself should be reevaluated at regular intervals. Safe feeding temperatures of hot foods should be determined in conjunction with kitchen staff by conducting timed temperature studies of test plates and trays of food, never by touching the food directly.

Assisting the Disabled Client

A client with a disability may require either total or partial assistance with eating. Partial assistance may include opening milk cartons and plastic bags containing condiments and eating utensils, buttering bread, and cutting meat. Visually impaired clients may be able to feed themselves when they know where the food is on the plate. The usual technique is to describe food placement in terms of hours on a clock face.

Some clients can feed themselves but may be slow, clumsy, and messy. A large napkin under the chin may assist in cleanup. Offering hot beverages in small amounts may minimize the likelihood of an accident.

Sometimes the consistency or form of a food may influence whether clients can feed themselves. A thin liquid, for example, may cause some clients to choke. A thicker substance such as yogurt may be better tolerated. Some disabled people are able to manage finger foods such as french fries or hard-cooked eggs.

Health-care personnel can learn the food tolerances and preferences of disabled clients by asking or observing. The physician should be notified if a client appears to be choking or coughing while being fed. A licensed speech pathologist (LSP) can be invaluable in determining the optimal solid food and liquid consistency to minimize the risk of aspiration.

Health-care workers should evaluate clients who cannot feed themselves and encourage them to remain as independent as possible in all the activities of daily living, including eating. Some clients' inability to feed themselves may be related to neuromuscular disabilities. The occupational therapist (OT) has special training in the selection and fitting of eating devices to assist such clients.

Supplemental Feedings

Many clients are unable to consume sufficient kilocalories or nutrients because of anorexia, altered GI function, an inability to eat, or an increased need for nutrients. The first step is to offer these clients additional food at or between meals. Any between-meal feedings must adhere to the client's diet order. Closely monitoring a client's food intake including supplemental feedings is important. If the client will not accept supplemental feedings, another treatment approach may be needed.

Many clients accept liquid supplementation better than solids. Many debilitated clients seem to feel less full after drinking a beverage than after eating a comparable number of kilocalories and nutrients in foods. Liquid supplements can include:

■ Milk
■ Milk shakes
■ Instant breakfast drinks
■ Commercially prepared beverages

Many commercially prepared liquid formulas are available. Increasingly, potentially beneficial nutrients that may enhance immune function such as arginine, glutamine, nucleotides, antioxidants, and fish oils are added to the various formulas and are shown to reduce infection complications and hospital LOS (Academy of Nutrition and Dietetics Critical Illness Update Evidence-Based Nutrition Practice Guidelines, 2012). Enteral formulas are classified by the U.S. Food and Drug Administration (FDA) as **medical foods,** which means they are not regulated as either a food or a drug. Although their manufacture must follow safe practices, formulas are exempt from regulations on labeling, including nutrition facts and health claims. The veracity of adult enteral formula labeling and product claims is dependent on formula vendors. Infant formula labeling and claims are regulated by the FDA (Bankhead, Boullata, Brantley, et al, 2009).

Four types of supplements are used for oral and/or enteral feedings:

1. Modular supplements
2. Standard or "polymeric" formulas
3. Elemental and semielemental formulas
4. Disease-specific formulas

MODULAR SUPPLEMENTS

A **modular supplement** contains a limited number of nutrients. Polycose, for example, contains only carbohydrate. Microlipid is an example of a lipid supplement. Modular supplements for protein include Resource Beneprotein® and Pro-Mod Liquid Protein®.

Modular supplements are available in a liquid or powder form and can be added to foods, other types of oral supplements, or tube feedings. Sometimes modular supplements are readily accepted if mixed with food. For example, Resource Beneprotein® mixed with hot cereal and mashed potatoes does not change the taste of these foods and adds a significant amount of protein to a client's diet.

Some modular products available contain two nutrients. Resource Arginine® contains both the amino acid arginine and carbohydrate. The manufacturers list these products as modular feedings because they do not contain all the essential nutrients.

STANDARD OR POLYMERIC FORMULAS

A standard or **polymeric formula** is a complete formula used when the GI tract is functional and the client needs all the essential nutrients in a specified volume. Dozens of such products are on the market. A complete supplement, such as Ensure®, Boost®, Jevity®, and Nutren Replete® should always be used when the formula is the sole source of nutrition.

Some complete nutritional supplements are also designed for tube feedings; the consistency and flavor of a feeding designed to be tube-fed may not be acceptable to the client if fed orally.

Commercial supplements should be used only after the client's requirements for nutrients have been assessed. Excess nutrients are rarely beneficial, and consuming too much of a feeding may be medically harmful. Many organs in the human body are in a stress situation in the poorly nourished client. The client's kidneys or liver may be subjected to unnecessary stress or harm if the nutrients cannot be used efficiently due to illness or disease state (see Clinical Calculation 14-1).

14-1

𝒞linical 𝒞alculation

Calculating an Oral Supplement

1. Place the client on a kilocalorie count.
2. Estimate the client's kilocalorie requirement.
   - Calculate the client's ideal body weight (IBW). Females = 100 pounds for the first 5 feet and 5 pounds for each additional inch ± 10%; males = 106 pounds for the first 5 feet and 6 pounds for each additional inch ± 10%
   - Use maximum IBW for all further calculations except those (1) who are underweight then use their actual body weight (ABW) to prevent overfeeding. (2) Use ABW for clients within their IBW range.
   - Divide the weight calculated above to obtain the client's weight in kilograms.
   - Estimated energy needs for noncritical care clients are 25 to 35 kcal/kg; energy needs for critical care clients are 20 to 30 kcal/kg.
   - Protein needs for noncritical care clients are 0.8 to 1.2 grams/kg; protein needs for critical care clients are 1.2 to 1.5 grams/kg.
   - Fluid needs are 1 mL/kg or 30 mL/kg or as tolerated to maintain fluid status.
3. Select an appropriate oral supplement for the client. Some hospitals allow clients to taste several supplements and choose the one most palatable to them.
4. Determine the difference between the client's recorded food intake and kilocalorie allowance.
5. Determine the kilocalorie concentration of the formula. This can be done by referring to either the appropriate table in the diet manual or the supplement's label. Usually formulas are between 1.0 and 2.0 kcal/mL.
6. Determine how many milliliters of formula are needed to meet the client's kilocalorie allowance.
7. Divide the total milliliters needed by the number of feedings to be offered.
8. Check to make sure the client's protein and fluid needs are within the desired range. If not, select a different supplement.

EXAMPLE

1. Assume that the client ate 550 kcal.
2. Assume that the client is a woman who weighs 132 lb and is 5 ft 2 in. tall. Client's IBW would be 100 lb + 10 lb for her additional 2 in. = 110; ± 10% = 100 to 120. She weighs more than her IBW, so use her maximum IBW of 120 to compute kilocalorie needs. 120 divided by 2.2 = 54.5 kg.
3. Client's estimated need for kilocalories is 25 to 35 kcal/kg × 54.5 kg = 1363 to 1908 kcal.
4. Assume that the client has tasted several supplements and prefers Boost Shake® 1.0.
5. The client's estimated range for kilocalories is 1363 to 1908. The client ate 300 kcal. The difference is a deficit of 1063 to 1608 kcal.

14-1

𝒞linical 𝒞alculation—cont'd

Calculating an Oral Supplement

6. Boost Shake® contains 280 kcal and 8 grams of protein in 240 mL.
7. The client stated she would prefer to drink this feeding five times per day, some on each tray, and during two between-meal feedings.
8. Assume from the client's recorded food intake that her diet contains about 10 grams of protein per day. A woman weighing 54.5 kg has an estimated protein allowance of 0.8 to 1.2 grams/kg.

    54.5 kg × 0.8 gram/kg = 43.6 g of protein to 54.5 × 1.2 grams/kg = 65.4 grams
    Subtract the 10 grams eaten from trays
    43.6 grams – 10 grams = 33.6 grams

    The supplement should provide at least 33.6 grams of protein and no more than 65.4 grams of protein (0.8 to 1.2 grams/kg of maximum IBW).

9. Five cans of Boost Shake® contain 1400 kcal and 40 grams of protein for a total of 1200 mL.
10. Eight grams of protein × 5 cans (240 mL each) = 40 grams of protein from oral supplement + 10 g of protein from food = 50 grams.
11. Double check: food intake of 300 kcal + 10 grams of protein + 1400 kcal from Boost Shake® + 40 grams of protein from Boost Shake® = 50 grams of protein total + 1700 kcal total + 1200 mL fluid total from supplement (client should be encouraged to drink at least 300 mL of water extra per day to meet her fluid needs). This information should be documented and verbally given to the nurse assigned to the client.

ELEMENTAL AND SEMIELEMENTAL FORMULAS

Another group of oral supplements includes **elemental and semielemental.** Examples of such formulas include Peptamen®, Vital®, and Vivonex®. The nutrients in these formulas are easier to absorb because they are in their simplest form, small molecules, which require little digestion. For example, maltodextrins, corn syrup solids, oligosaccharides, and glucose polymers are rapidly hydrolyzed by maltase and oligosaccharidases, which are apt to be present in the small intestine in higher concentrations than lactase.

Protein is either partially or totally hydrolyzed. Partially hydrolyzed protein (small peptides) offer an advantage over totally hydrolyzed protein (single amino acids). Peptides and free amino acids do not inhibit each other's transport across the gastrointestinal tract, and absorption of nitrogen is actually improved by the inclusion of small peptides. Easier-to-digest fats include medium-chain triglycerides. Partially hydrolyzed fats include monoglycerides and diglycerides.

Elemental and semielemental formulas contain little lactose and residue and may be given orally or enterally through a tube. These formulas are expensive and for use with clients who have limited GI function or metabolic disorders. Because elemental and semielemental formulas are less palatable than **standard feedings,** client acceptance of these as oral feedings is often a problem.

DISEASE-SPECIFIC FORMULAS

The last group of oral supplements includes special formulas designed for clients with specific metabolic problems such as diabetes, kidney, and liver disorders. These formulas are discussed in subsequent chapters.

Oral supplements are also used both in addition to or as a transition from enteral and parenteral feedings. When a client has ceased to consume foods orally for a time, a transition period is always necessary to reacclimate to oral feedings. This process can sometimes take a couple of days to months.

Enteral Tube Feeding

Tube feedings are the second way nutrients can be delivered to clients. EN is the delivery of a formula (which includes breast milk for infants) into a functioning GI tract through a tube. This feeding route should only be considered if the functioning GI tract is sufficient in length for adequate absorption and there is an inability for the client to consume nutrients, either totally or in part, orally. With some medical conditions, oral feeding is impossible, insufficient, or impractical. Several common conditions in which a tube feeding is indicated are listed in Table 14-3.

Tube feeding formulas are commercially prepared to reduce the incidence of contamination. Many medical centers use closed systems for tube feedings in which commercially prepared bags or containers of formula are ready to be hung and fed to clients. Open systems of feeding, if prepared in an aseptic manner, may be done safely in medical centers or at home by clients. Open systems require the filling of a bag or container with liquid formula. This allows the addition of modular components a client may require, such as additional fiber or protein. Many of the commercial products described in the previous section can be used for tube feeding.

TABLE 14-3 ■ Conditions Indicating a Tube Feeding

CONDITION	EXAMPLES
Client has mechanical difficulties that make chewing and/or swallowing impossible or difficult.	Obstruction of the esophagus, weakness or nausea, mouth sores, throat inflammation
Client has an intestinal disease and cannot digest or absorb food adequately.	Malabsorption syndromes
Client refuses to eat or cannot eat.	Anorexia nervosa, esophageal cancer
Client is unable to consume a sufficient amount of food because of a clinical condition.	Coma, serious infections, trauma victims, clients with large kilocalorie requirements

The medical literature addresses different opinions regarding the benefits of tube feedings for clients with dementia (Buff, 2006; Candy, Sampson, and Jones, 2009; Delegge, 2009). There has been much discussion about the practice of using feeding tubes in dementia clients because of their lack of interest or ability to eat, as well as worry about the risk of aspiration due to dysphagia. Some articles advocate ending the use of stomach tubes to feed people with advanced Alzheimer disease and other types of dementia. Clients with these conditions frequently pull the tubes out, leading nursing home and hospital staff to place the clients under close observation and, in extreme cases, restraints. An argument can be made that tube feedings deprive clients of the enjoyment that can be derived from eating and the social satisfaction that accompanies eating by hand. For this reason, most institutions have strict guidelines that all team members must follow before inserting a feeding tube into any client. For these clients, surgically inserted feeding tubes placed directly into the stomach or small intestines are frequently used rather than a nasogastric feeding tube, which is more easily pulled out.

Gastrointestinal Function

The GI tract should always be used to the extent possible. Oral supplements should be considered before tube feeding; tube feeding should always be considered before PN. There is less septic morbidity, fewer infectious complications, and significant cost savings in critically ill adults who receive EN versus PN (The Academy, 2012). Tube feeding is safer, less expensive, and more closely mimics normal feeding conditions than PN. Nutrients should be supplied intact rather than elemental or semielemental if the client has a normally functioning GI tract. **Intact nutrients** are nutrients that are not hydrolyzed, so the body must keep producing the secretions and enzymes necessary for digestion, thereby forcing the GI tract to function.

Tube Placement

Feeding tubes can enter the body through the nose or through a surgically made opening. A **nasogastric (NG) tube** runs from the nose to the stomach. A **nasoduodenal (ND) tube** runs from the nose to the duodenum. A **nasojejunal (NJ)** tube runs from the nose to the jejunum. These types of tubes are for short-term use because of client discomfort and tissue irritation.

Long-term feeding devices should be considered when the need for enteral feeding is at least 4 weeks' duration in adults, children, and infants after term age; in clients with dementia; or when a tube cannot be inserted through the nose (as in throat cancer), an **ostomy** (a surgically created opening) is created. An **esophagostomy** is a surgical opening into the esophagus through which a feeding tube is passed. A **gastrostomy** (called percutaneous endoscopic gastrostomy, or PEG) is a surgical opening in the stomach through which a feeding tube is passed; this is the most common tube insertion method.

A PEG tube can be placed **percutaneously** with the aid of an **endoscope** or surgically if the client is already undergoing abdominal surgery or has a condition that makes working with an endoscope difficult. A PEG tube may be used for feedings within 2 hours of placement in adults and 6 hours in infants and children. Percutaneous endoscopic jejunostomy (PEJ) tube placement is generally reserved for clients who are not candidates for a PEG. For example, a client who has had a gastrectomy (stomach removal) procedure requires a PEJ tube placement. A PEJ tube is also indicated for clients prone to aspiration. A.S.P.E.N. recommends that EN feedings should be started postoperatively in surgical clients within 24 to 48 hours without waiting for flatus or a bowel movement.

A critical responsibility of team members is assessment of feeding tube placement, especially with tubes inserted nasally. Radiographic confirmation must be obtained before using a feeding tube (Bankhead et al, 2009). Tubes have been mispositioned in such dangerous locations as the lungs and even the brain (Metheny and Titler, 2001). Unfortunately, feeding tubes migrate (after x-ray examination) and may move out of the stomach or jejunum. Tube migration places the client at risk for aspiration because the tube may move into the trachea. The client is also at risk if he or she regurgitates the feeding. **Regurgitation** means to cause to flow backward. If the feeding backs up into the client's lungs, a lung infection can develop.

When a client has inhaled fluids regurgitated from the stomach, he or she may develop aspiration pneumonia. **Aspiration** is the state in which a substance has been drawn up into the nose, throat, or lungs. Pulmonary aspiration is a common occurrence in hospitalized clients. Nonsurgically inserted enteral tube feeding increases the risk of aspiration and is associated with the development of nosocomial pneumonia, which significantly increases morbidity and mortality in critically ill clients.

In the past, nurses were taught and institutions recommended tinting of enteral feedings with blue dye to promote early detection of aspiration. Every time the client was suctioned, the specimen was inspected against a white background for the presence of dye. Blue dye was the favored color because blue is not found in secretions. It is now widely recognized that blue dye has toxic effects, including lactic acidosis, altered mental status, hypotension, hyperthermia, and rapid death (Super, 2003). Another problem associated with the use of blue dye is bacterial contamination. The Academy of Nutrition and Dietetics evidence-based library states that blue dyes should not be added to enteral nutrition for detection of aspiration. The risk of using the dye outweighs perceived benefits (www.adaevidencelibrary.com, 2012).

Contamination

All tube feedings provide an excellent environment for growth of microorganisms. When a client's tube feeding becomes contaminated with bacteria, the client receiving the feeding may become ill and suffer from nausea, vomiting, or diarrhea. For this reason, hospitals and nursing homes use only commercially prepared tube feedings that are packaged under sterile conditions. However, commercially prepared formulas can become contaminated if they are not handled properly after opening.

To prevent contamination, first check the can for the correct product, expiration date, and any signs of contamination, such as swelling. If the can is swollen, notify your supervisor. Do not administer a feeding from a damaged can. Other cans in the same shipment should be checked for contamination.

Good personal hygiene is essential. EN formulas must be prepared for client use in a clean environment using aseptic techniques. Sterile, liquid EN formulas should be used in preference to powdered, reconstituted formulas whenever possible. The following recommendations help reduce contamination (McCalve, Martindale, Vanek, et al, 2009):

■ Always properly wash hands and use disposable gloves.
■ Shake the container well and wipe down the lid with isopropyl alcohol, allowing it to dry before opening it.
■ Transfer the formula into a new administration bag or container.
■ Label the administration bag or container and any remaining formula carefully with the client's name, room number, the date and time the formula was opened, the amount in the container, the name of the product, administration route and rate, and other pertinent information. Other information may include whether the formula contains vitamins or other additives.
■ Reconstituted formulas made in advance should be refrigerated immediately and, if not used, discarded within 24 hours of preparation; they should be exposed to room temperature for no more than 4 hours when hung for administration.
■ Sterile, decanted formula has an 8-hour hang time.
■ Sterile, decanted formula or HBM (human breast milk) used for neonates has a limited hang time of 4 hours with administration sets changed at that time.
■ Store the formula in the refrigerator in a covered container. When a new supply of formula is received, place it in the rear of the storage area so that the older formula is used first. Check expiration dates carefully to ensure that expired product is not used for tube feedings.
■ Administration sets for open system enteral feedings must be changed at least every 24 hours.
■ A closed system bag or container is preferable for administering EN and may be hung for 24 to 48 hours per manufacturer guidelines.

Administration

Tube feedings can be administered continuously, intermittently, or by **bolus.** Clogging of the tube occurs significantly more often with continuous rather than intermittent feedings. A.S.P.E.N. guidelines (McCalve et al, 2009) recommend the following for when administering EN:

1. Evaluate all clients for risk of aspiration.
2. Ensure that the feeding tube is in the proper position before initiating feeding.
3. Client's head should be elevated at a minimum of 30° to 45°.
4. Check gastric residual volume (GRV) every 4 hours during the first 48 hours for gastrically fed clients. In adults, if the GRV is 250 mL or greater after a second gastric residual check, a promotility agent should be considered. If the GRV is 500 mL or greater, EN should be held and consideration given to a feeding tube placed in the small bowel (McCalve et al, 2009).
5. Flush tubes according to guidelines given for the type of feeding.

CONTINUOUS FEEDING

Many professionals believe that **continuous feeding** is preferable to other methods. A continuous feeding is always recommended for formulas delivered directly into the small intestine. One recommended rate is 30 to 50 mL/hour, increasing daily by 25 mL/hour to the rate necessary to meet energy needs. This gradual increase in the formula's volume gives the client's GI tract a chance to adjust to the formula and helps prevent many complications that occur in tube-fed clients. Children should be started at 1 to 2 mL/kg/hour and advanced by .5-1 mL/kg/hour every 6 to 24 hours until the goal rate is achieved. For critically ill clients, a conservative recommendation of 10 to 40 mL/hour with advancement to the goal rate in increments of 10 to 20 mL/hour every 8 to 12 hours is recommended by A.S.P.E.N. guidelines (McClave et al, 2009). Safety precautions for continuous feedings include the following:

1. Flush the tube with 30 mL of water every 4 hours in continuously fed adults and after GRV checks and medication administration; flush with as little water as possible in infants and children. Sterile water should be used with medication administration, in immuno-compromised, or in critically ill clients.
2. Allow no more than a 4-hour hang time for each bag of formula (when an open system is used) unless the formula is packaged in a sterilized delivery system (closed system).

These procedures help prevent contamination and bacterial growth. An infusion pump is necessary for precise control of a continuous feeding.

INTERMITTENT FEEDING

An **intermittent feeding** means giving a volume of feeding solution from a feeding container or bag over 30 to 40 minutes with or without a feeding pump. Clients tolerate intermittent feedings much better than bolus feedings because these feedings more closely approximate normal eating behavior. The tube needs to be flushed after each feeding to minimize bacterial growth and prevent contamination. Many mobile clients prefer intermittent feedings because they are not continuously attached to the feeding pump. Children may be started with 25% of the goal volume divided by the desired number of feedings. The volume may be increased by 25% per day as tolerated, divided by the number of feedings.

BOLUS FEEDING

Bolus feeding means giving a volume of feeding solution by gravity via syringe over approximately 15 minutes. A client is fed only four to six times per day. Feedings given by this method are frequently poorly tolerated, and clients complain of abdominal discomfort, nausea, fullness, and cramping. Some clients, however, can tolerate bolus feedings after a period of adjustment in which the volume is slowly increased. Bolus feedings entering the intestines are usually poorly tolerated. Children's bolus feedings should be initiated and advanced the same as outlined earlier in the Intermittent Feeding section.

Clients on bolus feedings should not recline for at least 2 hours after the feeding. Tubes should be irrigated (flushed with water) after each feeding to prevent contamination. The client with normal gastric function can usually tolerate 500 mL of formula at each feeding (Blouch and Mueller, 2004; McCalve et al, 2009).

Potential Complications

Complications fall into three categories:

1. Mechanical
2. Gastrointestinal
3. Metabolic

Table 14-4 reviews these complications and lists system-specific prevention strategies.

TABLE 14-4 ■ Feeding Complications and Prevention Strategies	
COMPLICATION	**PREVENTION STRATEGY**
Mechanical	
Tube irritation	Consider using a smaller or softer tube. Lubricate the tube before insertion.
Tube obstruction	Flush tube after use. Do not mix medications with the formula. Use liquid medications if available. Crush other medications thoroughly. Use an infusion pump to maintain a constant flow. Feeding should not be started until tube placement is radiographically confirmed.
Aspiration and regurgitation	Elevate head of client's bed 30 to 45 degrees at all times. Discontinue feedings at least 30 to 60 minutes before treatments where head must be lowered (e.g., chest percussion). If the client has an endotracheal tube in place, keep the cuff inflated during feedings. Gasteric Residual Volume (GRV) should be checked every 4 hours during the first 48 hours for gastrically fed clients. If ≥250 mL after a second gastric residual check, a promotility agent should be used. If the GRV is ≥250, EN should be held and consideration given to a feeding tube placed in the small bowel.

TABLE 14-4 ■ Feeding Complications and Prevention Strategies (Continued)	
COMPLICATION	**PREVENTION STRATEGY**
Tube displacement	Place a black mark at the point where the tube, once properly placed, exits the nostril. Replace tube and obtain physician's order to confirm with x-ray imaging.
Gastrointestinal	
Cramping, distention, bloating, gas pains, nausea, vomiting, diarrhea*	Initiate and increase amount of formula gradually. Bring formula to room temperature before feeding. Change to a lactose-free formula. Decrease fat context of formula. Administer drug therapy as ordered, e.g., Lactinex®, *kaolin-pectin*, Lomotil®. Change to a formula with a lower osmolality. Change to a formula with a different fiber content, including soluble fiber and excluding insoluble fiber. Practice good personal hygiene when handling any feeding product. Evaluate diarrhea-causing medications the client may be receiving (e.g., antibiotics, digitalis).
Metabolic	
Dehydration	Assess the client's fluid requirements before treatment. Monitor the client's hydration status.
Overhydration	Assess the client's fluid requirements before treatment. Monitor the client's hydration status.
Hyperglycemia	Initiate feedings at a low rate. Monitor blood glucose levels. Use hyperglycemic medication if necessary. Select a low-carbohydrate formula. Evaluate total kilocalories provided; overfeeding in a critically ill client exacerbates hyperglycemia.
Hypernatremia	Assess the client's fluid and electrolyte status before treatment. Provide adequate fluids.
Hyponatremia	Assess the client's fluid and electrolyte status before treatment. Restrict fluids. Supplement feeding with rehydration solution and saline. Diuretic therapy may be beneficial.
Hypophosphatemia	Monitor serum levels. Replenish phosphorus levels before refeeding.
Hypercapnia	Select low-carbohydrate high-fat formula.
Hypokalemia	Monitor serum levels. Supplement feeding with potassium if necessary.
Hyperkalemia	Reduce potassium intake. Monitor potassium levels.

*The most commonly cited complication of tube feeding is diarrhea.

Osmolality

The osmolality of a solution is based on the number of dissolved particles in the solution. The greater the number of particles, the higher the osmolality. At a given concentration, the smaller the particle size, the greater the number of particles present.

Oral supplements and tube feedings with a high osmolality draw body fluid into the bowel, resulting in a fluid imbalance. The symptoms are diarrhea, nausea, and flushing. The osmolality of normal body fluids is approximately 300 mOsm/kg. Hydrolyzed nutrients have a higher osmolality than intact nutrients. An **isotonic** feeding has an osmolality of 300 mOsm, the same as body fluids. A high-osmolality feeding can provide a more concentrated source of nutrients than a feeding of lower osmolality.

Sensitivity to the osmolality of oral supplements and tube feedings varies from one individual to another. All

clients need a period of adjustment to a high-osmolality formula. Most clients are able to eventually develop a tolerance to a high-osmolality formula; some clients, however, are more likely to develop symptoms of intolerance. Such clients include those who:

- Are debilitated
- Have gastrointestinal disorders
- Are preoperative and postoperative
- Have a gastrointestinal tract that has not been challenged by food for a significant period
- Have newly inserted surgically placed tubes (PEG and PEJ)

Administration of Medications

A pharmacist should always be consulted before administration of medications via a feeding tube. To minimize or prevent complications, all health-care workers should be aware of potential drug–food interactions (see Chapter 15). Clinical Application 14-2 discusses suggested procedures for administering medications through feeding tubes. Medications should *never* be added to the tube feeding formula because they can be physically incompatible with the product because of changes in the feeding's viscosity (thickness) or flow characteristics. Some medications may also cause the feeding to separate, granulate, or coagulate (McCalve et al, 2009).

Monitoring

Nutritional status, fluid balance, and GI tolerance should be monitored in tube-fed clients. Whether the

14-2

Clinical Application

Procedures for Administering Medications Through Feeding Tubes

Procedures for the administration of medications through feeding tubes may vary slightly from one institution to another. The following procedures, however, are common:

- Do not add medication directly to an enteral feeding formula.
- If possible, administer drugs in liquid form.
- If the drug is not available in liquid form, consult with the pharmacist; he or she may be able to procure a liquid form or similar drug provided by the American Society of Hospital Pharmacists in Pediatric Extemporaneous Formulation List of the manufacturer's suggestions.
- Exercise caution when calculating equivalent liquid doses. Many liquid dosage forms are intended for pediatric use, and the dose must be adjusted appropriately for adults.
- Administer crushed tablets only when no other alternatives are available.
- If administering crushed tablets, crush the tablet to a fine powder and mix with sterile water. Do not crush any tablet on the list of oral drugs that should not be crushed. Do not crush drugs with a sustained-release action or an enteric coating. If in doubt, consult the pharmacist.
- Administer each drug separately. Do not mix all the medications for one dosing time. Flush with at least 15 mL of sterile water between each medication.
- Flush the tube with at least 30 mL of sterile water before giving the medication and before restarting the tube feeding.
- To avoid causing gastric irritation and diarrhea, dilute drugs that are hypertonic or irritating to the cells that line the gastrointestinal tract, such as potassium chloride, in at least 30 mL of sterile water before administration.
- Dilute drugs, such as indomethacin—which are usually administered with meals to avoid gastric irritation—with sterile water before administration.
- Divide dosing schedules—if necessary—of sustained- or slow-release formulations of drugs used for once-daily dosing when administering in liquid form.

client requires daily or weekly monitoring depends on client acuity, duration of feeding, and the practice in the facility.

Nutritional status monitoring begins with a comparison of the client's kilocalorie and protein allowances to the volume and composition of the nutritional product used. Initially the client's kilocalorie and protein allowances are not met because a tube feeding is usually started at a low volume to increase gastrointestinal tolerance. Changes in the client's medical status and treatment, physical activity, and tolerance to the tube feeding may continually alter the volume and kind of feeding the client requires. Therefore, the caloric and protein content of the tube feeding requires reassessment.

In stable clients, serum levels of sodium, blood urea nitrogen, hemoglobin, and albumin are indicators of fluid status. Urine osmolality can be used to monitor hydration status. Urine osmolality is normally 50 to 1400 mOsm, with a usual range 300 to 900 mOsm and an average of 850 mOsm. Decreased osmolality indicates overhydration, and increased osmolality indicates dehydration.

Fluid intake and output need to be recorded daily. Fluid intake should be at least 500 mL greater than output in clients who are neither overhydrated nor underhydrated. This 500-mL surplus is needed to cover insensible losses in feces and from the skin and lungs. Clinical signs of hydration status include skin turgor, presence of axillary sweat, condition of the mucous membranes, and the presence or absence of edema. Constipation is another possible sign of dehydration.

Gastrointestinal tolerance can be assessed by the absence or presence of diarrhea, bowel sounds, nausea, distension, and vomiting. The type of feeding delivered, the volume given, or the delivery rate can cause diarrhea. Diarrhea is frequently caused by medications. Antibiotics, laxatives, H_2 receptor blockers, and antacids with magnesium can cause stools to become watery. Medications that contain sorbitol can also have a laxative effect.

Gastric residuals are usually measured several times daily or about every 4 hours in clients at risk with tubes leading into the stomach. Because elevated residuals indicate delayed gastric emptying and a potentially increased risk for aspiration, feedings are advanced only when gastric residuals are less than 250 mL (www.adaevidencelibrary.com, 2008; McClave et al, 2009).

Measurement of gastric residuals in a stable alert client who has a well-established tolerance to the tube feeding is usually not necessary. Feedings continuously dripped into the intestines do not normally produce a gastric residue because there is no place for the fluid to collect. Gastric residue measurement is most relevant in critically ill clients and others at risk for gastroparesis (Blouch and Mueller, 2004) and with other issues such as vomiting, sepsis, and sedation (McClave et al, 2009).

Home Enteral Nutrition

With the increase in home-based health-care agencies, hospitals and nursing homes discharge many clients on enteral nutrition and follow the clients closely as outpatients.

Parenteral Nutrition

PN, in which nutrients are delivered to the client through the veins (intravenously), is the third means of feeding. PN is normally used in acute care settings in the following circumstances (McCalve et al, 2009):

■ In a previously healthy individual admitted to an intensive care unit after 7 days of hospitalization when EN is not feasible.
■ There is evidence of protein-calorie malnutrition and it is not possible to feed enterally.
■ An individual is going to undergo major GI surgery, and it is not possible to feed enterally, PN should be initiated 5 to 7 days before surgery and continued after the surgery.
■ An individual undergoes major GI surgery and is not able to be fed enterally for 7 or more days.
■ If an individual is unable to meet energy requirements after 7 to 10 days by enteral route alone, PN supplementation may be considered.

Peripheral parenteral nutrition (PPN) means to feed the client via a vein away from the center of the body in a line terminating in a peripheral site (Fig. 14-4). In **central parenteral nutrition (CPN),** the client is fed via a central vein. Clients are also fed via a central line that has been inserted peripherally and threaded into the subclavian or jugular veins. This is called a peripherally inserted central catheter, or **PICC line.**

The terminology is confusing. Therefore, note whether the line terminates peripherally or centrally. CPN, PICC lines, and PPN can be used to provide partial or total daily nutritional requirements. Clients who cannot or should not be fed through the gastrointestinal tract are candidates for CPN, PICC lines, and PPN. See Box 14-3 for appropriate indications for the use of PN.

Peripheral Parenteral Nutrition

Intravenous (IV) feeding (PPN) is routine in some health-care institutions. IV solutions, usually containing water, dextrose, electrolytes, and occasionally other nutrients, are used to maintain fluid, electrolyte, and acid–base balance. Intravenous solutions do contain kilocalories. The calculation of the kilocalorie content of an intravenous solution is demonstrated in Clinical Calculation 14-2.

Amino acids and fat can be supplied peripherally. To prevent ketosis, intravenous lipid emulsions should contribute no more than 60% of the total kilocalories provided. Dextrose concentrations are limited to approximately 10%, because peripheral veins cannot withstand concentrations greater than 900 mOsmol/kg. Thus, PPN has often failed to provide

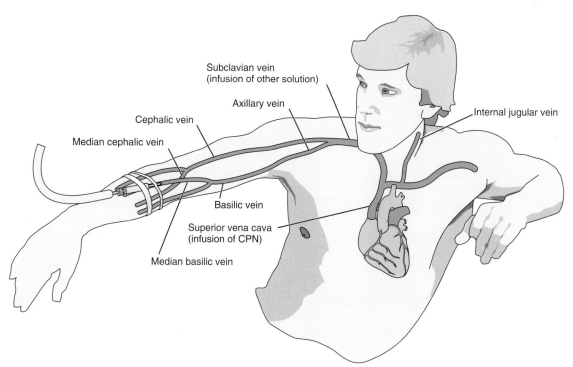

FIGURE 14-4 Correct placement of a peripherally placed central catheter (PICC).

Box 14–3 ■ *Indications for Parenteral Nutrition*

PN

PN is an effective method of nutritional support in the following situations:

- For clients who were healthy before admission to the intensive care unit and for whom no standard nutrition therapy has been provided for 7 days or longer
- If there is evidence of protein-calorie malnutrition and it is not possible to feed orally or enterally
- For individuals who will undergo major GI surgery and it is not possible to feed orally or enterally; initiate 5 to 7 days preoperatively and continue postoperatively
- For clients who have inadequate GI function.

Peripheral Parenteral Nutrition

PPN is delivered into a peripheral vein, normally the hand or forearm.

Central Parenteral Nutrition/Peripherally Inserted Central Catheter

PN delivered into a large-diameter vein, usually the superior vena cava adjacent to the right atrium. CPN is used when long-term or home PN is required.

Clinical Calculation 14–2

Calculating Kilocalories in IV Solutions

D_5W means 5% dextrose in water. The subscript following the D tells you the % of dextrose in the solution. Other common concentrations of sugar and water are $D_{10}W$ and $D_{50}W$.

A 5% concentration of dextrose means 100 mL of water contains 5 grams of dextrose. A 10% concentration of dextrose means 100 mL of water contains 10 grams of dextrose. A 50% concentration of dextrose means 100 mL of water contains 50 grams of dextrose. A simple proportion should be used to calculate the number of kilocalories in any given volume of a solution.

The formula is:

percent of concentration/100 mL = x grams of dextrose/volume of solution client received

For example, a client has received 1000 mL of D_5W:

5% of dextrose/100 mL = x grams of dextrose/1000 = 50 grams of dextrose

Proportions are solved by cross-multiplication and division: (5 grams × 1000 mL) divided by 100 mL = 50 grams of dextrose. One gram of carbohydrate given intravenously provides 3.4 kcal; thus, 50 grams multiplied by 3.4 kcal/grams = 170 kcal.

---

adequate kilocalories and other nutrients for repair and replacement of losses. PPN has been used to supplement a partially successful oral or enteral nutrition program.

A system for PPN (called all-in-one or three-in-one) has been developed that allows a higher osmotic load (1200 to 1350 mOsmol/L) to be delivered peripherally. Lipids, amino acids, dextrose, electrolytes, trace elements, and vitamins are all incorporated into one container. Tolerance of this higher osmotic mixture in peripheral veins might be attributed to the buffering and dilution effects of intravenous fats in combination with the higher pH of the amino acid solutions and the addition of heparin to the mixture.

The use of glutamine in PN therapy has been shown to reduce infectious complications in critically ill clients (Academy of Nutrition and Dietetics, 2012). It is the position of A.S.P.E.N. that specific, critically ill client populations, including postoperative or ventilator-dependent clients, can benefit from the use of glutamine in PN. A.S.P.E.N. specifies that glutamine solutions should be available for clinical use based on professional judgment of prescribers (A.S.P.E.N., 2011).

CPN and PICC Lines

When nutrients are infused into a terminal central vein, parenteral nutrition is often referred to as CPN. The **superior vena cava,** one of the largest-diameter veins in the human body, is commonly used for CPN, and CPN can deliver greater nutrient loads because the blood flow in the superior vena cava rapidly dilutes these solutions 1000-fold. Concentrations for both dextrose and amino acids are determined by the client's needs. See Clinical Calculation 14-3 for an explanation and demonstration of the calculation of a sample CPN solution. A line inserted peripherally but threaded into a central vein is CPN.

INSERTION AND CARE OF A CPN LINE

A physician or certified registered nurse inserts the PICC line, usually to the subclavian vein and into the superior vena cava. The line can be inserted at the client's bedside using strict aseptic technique. CPN solutions and PICC lines need to be sterile. The sterile mixtures consist of dextrose, amino acids, lipid emulsion, electrolytes, vitamins, trace elements, and other additives. The pharmacist usually prepares them in a sterile environment. Careful attention is required to provide vitamins and minerals to clients maintained on CPN/PICC lines to prevent problems such as Wernicke-Korsakoff syndrome (see Chapter 8, Clinical Application 20-8).

CPN requires close monitoring, and the therapy is costly. The high cost is directly related to the number

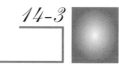

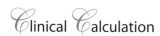

Clinical Calculation

Calculating CPN Solution/CPN Energy Nutrient Content (or PICC line)

CPN/PICC solutions are usually packed in 500-mL bags. Pharmacists prefer to use dextrose and amino acids in 500-mL bags and vary the concentration of the nutrients to achieve the appropriate nutritional parameters. For example, a 500-mL bag of dextrose mixed with a 500-mL bag of amino acids equals 1000 mL. Lipids are usually provided as 250 mL of 20% lipid (1/2 bag) or 500 mL (one bag) of 10% lipid.

The client's needs for kilocalories, protein, and fat can be accommodated by individualizing the concentration of each energy nutrient. For example, dextrose can be ordered from 5% to 70%, noted as D_5, D_{40}, D_{50}, etc. Commonly used concentrations of amino acids are 5%, 8.5%, and 10%.

NUTRITIONAL VALUES USED IN COMPUTATIONS OF CPN SOLUTIONS

Dextrose = 3.4 kcal/g
20% lipid = 2.0 kcal/mL
10% lipid = 1.1 kcal/mL
Protein = 4.0 kcal/gram
1 gram of nitrogen = 6.25 grams of protein

Calculate the total kilocalories, nonprotein kilocalories, grams of nitrogen, calorie/nitrogen ratio, and % kilocalories from fat in 500 mL of D_{50}, 500 mL of 10% amino acids, and 250 mL of 10% lipid.

Dextrose	Percent concentration × volume = grams of dextrose	0.50 × 500 = 250 gram dextrose
	Grams of dextrose × 3.4 kcal/gram = kcal of solution	250 grams dextrose × 3.4 kcal/gram = 850 kcal
Amino acids	Percent concentration × volume = grams of protein	0.10 × 500 mL = 50 grams of protein
	Grams of protein × kcal/gram = protein kcal	50 grams of protein × 4 kcal/gram = 200 kcal
Lipids	kcal/mL × volume in mL = fat kcal	1.1 × 250 mL = 275 kcal
Total kilocalories	Add kilocalories from dextrose, protein, and lipid	850 + 200 + 275 = 1325 kcal
Percent kilocalories from fat	Kilocalories from fat divided by total kcal = % fat kilocalories	275 divided by 1325 = 21% fat

calculating formula needs with the physician. The initials CNS (certified nutrition support) indicates the nurse, pharmacist, or dietitian has had advanced training in the delivery of nutrition orally, enterally, and parenterally.

MONITORING

Careful administration of the central line solution is important. Most institutions have a strict protocol that must be followed by all health-care professionals. A **protocol** is a description of the steps for performing a procedure. Protocols vary widely from one institution to another.

Most CPN protocols include the following:

■ A slow start
■ A strict schedule
■ Close monitoring
■ Instructions for increasing the volume
■ Maintenance of a constant rate
■ Instructions for a slow withdrawal

The solution may require adjustment, which can be made by increasing or decreasing any or all of the nutrients. All long-term CPN/PICC line clients should receive ongoing monitoring by a home-care clinician, including an assessment of micronutrient status, to ensure adequacy of the nutrition support regimen (Falk, 2002; McCalve et al, 2009). Careful monitoring of the client's response to central line nutrition and taking corrective measures when needed are essential for safe administration of these solutions.

Many metabolic complications are possible with CPN. Rapid shifts of potassium, phosphorus, and magnesium from the intercellular compartment to the intracellular compartment result in a lowering of nutrient concentrations in the serum. As a result, initial laboratory tests rapidly fluctuate during the course of treatment. Immediate replacement of potassium, phosphorus, and magnesium is indicated if the corresponding laboratory values of these nutrients fall below normal.

Providing glucose in excess of kilocaloric needs can result in several problems, including carbon dioxide retention with respiratory difficulty. Too high a glucose content in solutions also leads to hyperglycemia. Therefore, glucose levels should be assessed regularly and insulin may be necessary. Liver function test results may become abnormal after an excess glucose load. Excess glucose may also lead to hyperlipidemia and fatty deposits in the liver. Elevated triglyceride levels may indicate too much glucose is being infused.

The avoidance of metabolic complications directly related to a glucose overload is one reason CPN clients need to be monitored closely. Such complications can be avoided by providing only an appropriate, not an

of highly trained health-care team members required to monitor the client, the laboratory work required for monitoring, and the cost of the solution. A nurse and a dietitian are typically responsible for assessing, monitoring, and educating clients destined for home parental nutrition. The clinical dietitian on the team usually has an advanced degree and special training. The dietitian is responsible for constant nutrition assessment, monitoring, interpretation of data, and excessive, amount of kilocalories. In addition, an initial slow infusion at low concentrations prevents complications. Box 14-4 lists general recommendations for CPN monitoring.

Box 14-4 ■ *Monitoring Parenteral Nutrition*

Initial Assessment
- Vital signs (respiration, pulse, temperature)
- Body weight and height
- Serum electrolytes, glucose, creatinine, blood urea nitrogen levels
- Serum magnesium, calcium, phosphorus levels
- Serum triglycerides and cholesterol levels
- Liver function tests
- Serum albumin and prealbumin
- Complete blood count
- Energy (estimated or measured), protein, fluid, and micronutrient needs

Routine Every 4 to 8 Hours
- Vital signs

Every 24 Hours
- Weight
- Fluid intake and output
- Serum electrolytes, glucose, creatinine, blood urea nitrogen levels; daily for 5 days or until stable, then twice a week

Weekly
- Serum ammonia, SGOT,* serum calcium, phosphorus, magnesium, total protein, and albumin
- Complete blood count
- Reassessment of actual oral, enteral, and PN intake

Other monitors may be indicated depending on the client's clinical condition.

*SGOT (serum glutamic oxaloacetic transaminase) is a liver enzyme that reflects liver cellular damage when elevated (as opposed to liver obstructive disease).

TRANSITION AND COMBINATION FEEDINGS

Clients need a transition period from CPN to oral feedings. Some physicians prefer to wean clients from CPN by using a tube feeding. This is the situation shown in Figure 14-3. The client has both an enteral feeding line and CPN. Other physicians prefer to avoid the tube and wean clients orally. In the latter case, as the client's oral intake increases, the CPN solution is gradually withdrawn. Expect clients who have been on CPN for a significant time to experience some difficulty with oral feedings. They may need much encouragement to eat.

One of the problems with CPN is that the GI tract does not have to work during CPN administration. Consequently, the GI tract will have undergone some atrophy. Oral foods should be offered slowly during the weaning process. Some physicians avoid this problem by allowing some clients to consume a clear-liquid or light diet while on CPN, if their condition permits.

HOME PARENTERAL NUTRITION

Increasingly, clients are discharged on CPN. These clients need adequate follow-up by either the hospital or a community home-health agency. The pharmacist is responsible for the storage of PN solutions in most institutions. Nurses involved in home parenteral nutrition need to be aware that vitamin degradation during the storage of PN mixtures is significant and affects clinical outcome (Dupertuis, 2002; Mirtallo, Canada, Johnson, et al, 2004). Factors affecting vitamin degradation include PN bag material, temperature, and length of time between PN compounding and end of infusion into the client. The home-care nurse needs to work closely with the pharmacist and client to minimize nutrient losses in PN solutions.

Keystones

- The nutritional care of clients is a joint responsibility of all team members.
- How meals are distributed to clients and meal-service schedules are important for team members to know because they affect the administration of medications and the scheduling of clients for tests and procedures.
- Nutrition screening is an important function of nurses and may determine that a client is at nutritional risk, requiring a nutritional assessment by a dietitian.
- Nutritional care includes four areas: assessing the client's need for nutrients, determining the best method for delivering nutrients, monitoring nutrient intake, and counseling clients about nutritional needs.
- Nutrients can be delivered to clients orally, enterally via a feeding tube, or parenterally.

Keystones—cont'd

- One principle is followed when selecting a feeding route: If the gastrointestinal tract works, use it to maximum capability.
- Oral feedings should be considered before EN.
- EN should be considered before PN.
- PN can be delivered peripherally or centrally.
- Clients on either EN or PN need to be closely monitored.

CASE STUDY *14–1*

P was brought to the emergency room by ambulance; his mother accompanied him. The mother stated her son had been hit by a car while riding his bike. P is 11 years old, 4 ft 11 in. tall, and weighs 89 lb. The client's mother stated that her son was well before the accident. In the emergency room, it was observed that both his eyes were surrounded by contusions, and his throat and the left side of his face were swollen. Communication with the client was at first minimal because it was painful for him to speak. An intravenous solution of 0.9% normal saline was started in the ambulance. He was also shown to have a fractured mandible. Surgery was required, and his jaw was wired. After surgery, the boy was found to have dysphagia, thought to be caused by tissue swelling.

The physician has ordered a nasogastric feeding tube with Nutren 1.0 Fiber®. The order reads:

Day 1 Continuous drip 40 mL/h
Day 2 Continuous drip 60 mL/h
Day 3 Continuous drip 80 mL/h

Nutren 1.0 Fiber® contains 1.0 kcal/mL and 40 g of protein per 1000 mL. The physician states, "The client will remain on a tube feeding until he can consume his kilocalorie requirement orally. This client requires adequate nutrition to enable the mandible to heal properly." P is expected to be discharged on a home enteral tube feeding. His prognosis is good, and he is expected to make a full recovery.

A resident physician inserts the nasogastric tube. The nurse assists at the client's bedside. The client holds the nurse's hand tightly as the tube is inserted. He has a worried look on his face, increased facial perspiration, and increased pulse/respirations during the procedure.

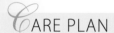

CARE PLAN

Subjective Data
Client held hand tightly during nasogastric tube insertion and appeared worried, apprehensive, and jittery.

Objective Data
Client is a trauma victim who showed increased perspiration and increased pulse/respirations during the tube insertion procedure.

Analysis
Child is showing signs and symptoms of anxiety related to feeding tube placement.

Plan

DESIRED OUTCOMES EVALUATION CRITERIA	ACTIONS/INTERVENTIONS	RATIONALE
The client's mother will state that he needs the tube feeding to heal his mandible until his jaw is unwired and he is eating to meet his total caloric needs.	Explain enteral nutrition therapy procedures as performed.	A tube feeding is unfamiliar to most clients. Knowledge about the procedure may relax the client and his mother.

(Continued on the following page)

DESIRED OUTCOMES EVALUATION CRITERIA	ACTIONS/INTERVENTIONS	RATIONALE
	As the client's condition permits, be available for "listening." Give the client a pad of paper and pencil to facilitate communication.	The client needs to vent his feelings about both the tube feeding and the situational crisis (the accident).
Teach client's mother how to safely administer enteral feeding via tube, including the rate, residual check, and proper client placement.	Review home enteral tube feeding instruction sheet, give to client's mother, and have her watch the process of starting the feeding, and if possible practice under the nurse's supervision.	It is important that the individual responsible for the safe handling of the enteral tube feeding understand, see, and, if feasible, practice the process.

TEAM WORK 14-1

Dietitian's Notes

The following Dietitian's Notes are representative of the documentation found in a client's medical record.

Subjective: Client not able to provide verbal information. Per client's mother, client was well nourished before accident. No food allergies, intolerances, or food dislikes. Client did not avoid any of the major food groups and ate at least four times a day.

Objective: 11-year-old child 4 ft 11 in. tall, weight 89 lb (40.4 kg). Client now being fed 80 mL of Nutren 1.0 Fiber® per day every hour times 24 hours. No complaints of nausea, vomiting; last bowel movement this a.m.

Analysis: Kilocalorie intake from tube feeding as ordered equals 1920 per day with 76.8 grams of protein. Client's estimated kilocalorie needs at 30 to 35 kcal/kg and 40.4 kg equals a maximum of 1414 kcal. Client's estimated protein needs are 1.0 to 1.5 g/kg actual body weight or 40.4 to 60.6. BMI = 17.9. Pt is just above the 50th percentile for BMI-for-age percentile. Laboratory values are all within normal limits.

Client is consuming no food; the tube feeding is the sole source of nutrition.

Plan: Recommend decreasing the continuous drip rate to 60 mL/hour. This would provide 1440 kcal, 1440 mL of fluid, and 57.6 grams of protein. Flush the feeding tube with 78 mL of water 6 times per day to provide fluid requirements. Will closely follow prealbumin levels and reevaluate protein content of tube feeding (adding a protein supplement) if prealbumin below normal.

Critical Thinking Questions

1. What would you do if the client pulled out the tube after insertion?

2. After he starts eating, how would you reassess the client's continued need for a tube feeding?

3. How should this client be monitored while on the tube feeding?

Chapter Review

1. Parenteral nutrition is usually indicated in the following situation:
   a. Rectal abscess
   b. Cancer esophagus
   c. Bowel obstruction
   d. Malnutrition

2. 1000 mL of a D_5W solution provides ____ grams of CHO and ____ kcal.
   a. 50 and 170
   b. 5 and 20
   c. 50 and 200
   d. 5 and 17

3. Careful administration of central parenteral nutrition includes all of the following except:
   a. A slow start
   b. Close monitoring
   c. Abrupt withdrawal
   d. A strict schedule

4. Among the following, diarrhea in a tube-fed client is most likely related to:
   a. Continuous-infusion feeding
   b. Contamination
   c. Fluid deficiency
   d. Insufficient kilocalories

5. Which of the following is not a recommended procedure for administering medications through a tube feeding?
   a. Mix all of the medications together, crush thoroughly, mix with water, and add to the formula.
   b. If at all possible, use medications in the liquid form.
   c. Flush the tube with at least 30 mL of water before giving the medication and before resuming the tube-feeding formula.

Clinical Analysis

1. Mr. J, 58 years old, visits his physician with a complaint of abdominal pain. He is scheduled for a diagnostic work-up, which will include a **barium enema** (x-ray study of his colon). Before this procedure, the nurse should instruct the client to:
   a. Eat a large breakfast on the day of the examination, such as orange juice, cereal, toast, scrambled eggs, and milk.
   b. Drink ample fluids on the morning of the examination, including at least 12 ounces of juice, 1 cup of gelatin, and broth.
   c. Take nothing orally after midnight on the day of the examination and consume only gelatin; clear broth; tea; coffee; and grape, apple, or cranberry juice on the day before the examination.
   d. Drink milk, juices, and coffee and eat only strained cream soups, ice cream, and gelatin on the day before the examination and take nothing orally after midnight.

2. Ms. L has a jejunostomy. She was discharged from the hospital last week after receiving instructions on home care from the nutrition support service. The local pharmacy is out of the Vivonex formula she has been instructed to use. As the nurse, you recommend that:
   a. She substitute Ensure®
   b. She substitute Polycose®
   c. She contact the Nutrition Support Service for instructions
   d. She substitute a standard or polymeric formula

3. Mr. W has been receiving a tube feeding of Ensure® via nasogastric tube for 3 weeks via a bolus infusion. He has just started to have loose stools (300 mL each—6 today). You should first suspect the following to be responsible for the diarrhea:
   a. A new medication added to his treatment plan
   b. Bacterial contamination
   c. Intolerance to the bolus delivery method
   d. Lactose intolerance

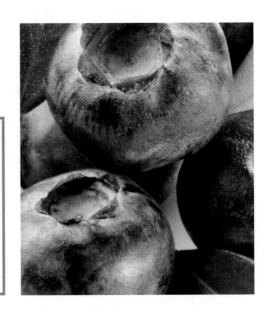

15

Interactions: Food and Nutrients Versus Medications and Supplements

LEARNING OBJECTIVES

After completing this chapter, the student should be able to:

■ Identify four groups of clients likely to experience food–drug interactions and indicate possible consequences of improper administration or management.

■ Describe four ways in which foods, nutrients, drugs, and dietary supplements can interact and give an example of each.

■ Explain why separating grapefruit juice ingestion from oral doses of affected drugs is not an effective strategy for preventing interactions.

■ Name the most common food, drug, and dietary supplement to be involved in drug–nutrient interactions.

■ List four drugs that should be administered separately from foods and supplements containing calcium, iron, magnesium, and zinc.

■ Discuss the tyramine-restricted diet and relate it to the pathophysiology involving monoamine oxidase inhibitors (MAOIs).

■ Compare and contrast the regulatory processes for products sold in the United States as dietary supplements with those for products marketed as drugs.

■ Relate the mechanism by which *warfarin* achieves anticoagulation to the diet required for therapeutic success.

■ Suggest precautions to be utilized by individuals who wish to use dietary supplements.

■ Review principles pertinent to optimizing an athlete's nutrition.

$\mathcal{D}$rug–nutrient–supplement interactions encompass any alteration in the effect of one caused by the interplay with one of the others. Drugs, whether prescription or over-the-counter (OTC), are substances intended for use in the diagnosis, cure, mitigation, treatment, or prevention of disease. OTC drugs are defined as safe and effective for use by the general public without a doctor's prescription (American College of Preventive Medicine, 2011). The complex definition of dietary supplements is explained in a later section of this chapter.

The body does not have separate pathways for food, dietary supplements, and medications. They all share the same organs and systems and may compete for carriers, enzymes, substrates, and energy (American

Dietetic Association, 2010). Inevitably those competitions produce winners and losers, the latter often the clients in whose bodies the competitions play out.

Extent of Use

Use of prescribed medications, OTC drugs, and dietary supplements is widespread in the United States. The following figures are derived from various sources.

■ Prescription drugs accounted for costs of $325.8 billion in 2012, the first time in 58 years that such spending declined (CBS News, 2013).

- OTC drug sales in all U.S. outlets amounted to $29.3 billion in 2012 (Consumer Healthcare Products Association, 2014).
- Dietary supplements reportedly sold for $11.5 billion in 2012 (Schultz, 2013).

With all those substances in play, the chances of interactions abound. In a nationally representative sample of 57- to 85-year-old Americans:

- 81% were taking prescription drugs
- 42% were using OTCs
- 49% were taking dietary supplements (Qato, Alexander, Conti, et al, 2008).

Some drugs interact with other drugs, foods, nutrients, and supplements in ways that can be beneficial or detrimental, enhancing or inhibiting the action of the other. In no sense is the information in this chapter exhaustive. Emphasis is placed on interactions that illustrate the range of known mechanisms and those that increase the risk of malnutrition or therapeutic failure. Pharmacists and dietitians use computerized databases to elicit possible problem areas. In all cases, pharmaceutical resources should be consulted when administering medications.

As used in this text, the term *drug* includes alcohol and both prescription and OTC medications. As is the usual practice in medical literature, **generic names** are given for drugs.

Some common dietary supplements that may also interact with drugs and nutrients are included later in the chapter. Because of the lack of premarketing regulation and ongoing inspections of manufacturing processes, these substances invite special scrutiny when used by clients.

Because athletes may be tempted to try to gain a competitive edge by using supplements, information on safety and effectiveness of some performance-enhancing supplements as well as food-based interventions for the athlete round out the chapter.

Mechanisms of Interactions

Interactions can be antagonistic or additive thus *warfarin's* effect is impeded by vitamin K and enhanced by vitamin E (Boullata and Hudson, 2012). Both pharmacokinetics and pharmacodynamics can be involved in interactions with nutrients or supplements.

Pharmacokinetics is the study of the action of a drug, emphasizing absorption time, duration of effect, distribution in the body, and method of excretion. Among the considerations pertinent to pharmacokinetics are:

- **Half-life**—time for a drug's concentration, usually in plasma, to be reduced by one-half.

- **Bioavailability**—proportion of the drug that reaches the systemic circulation. By definition, intravenous drugs and nutrients administered via parenteral nutrition (PN) are 100% bioavailable.
- **Presystemic clearance**—metabolism of orally ingested compounds before they reach the systemic circulation (formerly known as the **first-pass effect**).

Pharmacodynamics is the study of drugs and their actions on living organisms, as well as their physiologic or clinical effects. Pharmacodynamic effects of interactions that result in toxicities or treatment failures are major concerns of health-care providers.

For instance, *phenytoin*, a drug used to control epileptic seizures, is a folic acid antagonist that competes with the vitamin for binding sites. Its effects can be:

- pharmacokinetic, resulting in lower serum levels of *phenytoin* or
- pharmacodynamic, if seizure activity increases.

The interaction works both ways, so that long-term *phenytoin* therapy also can cause folic acid deficiency. Consequently, a folic acid supplement may be instituted with a phenytoin prescription (Pronsky and Crowe, 2012; see Table 15-1).

Starting at the pharmacy and ending with excretion of the drug or its components, interactions are classified into one of four types (see Table 15-2).

Type I Interactions

Type I interactions usually occur outside the body:

- In the intravenous or PN solution
- In the syringe where substances are admixed
- In tube feeding reservoirs
- In the respective tubings

In Europe, seven infants suffered adverse cardiopulmonary events and six of them died after intravenous administration of *ceftriaxone* and calcium-containing solutions. Contributing factors may have been the use of *ceftriaxone* at dosages higher than those approved by the U.S. Food and Drug Administration (FDA), intravenous "push" administration, and administration of the total daily dosage as a single infusion (Bradley, Wassel, Lee, and Nambiar, 2009). Subsequently, the FDA lifted its ban on coadministering *ceftriaxone* and calcium solutions for clients older than 28 days but maintained the prohibition for neonates (U.S. FDA, June 11, 2009).

No one should rely on visual inspection to identify precipitates that may be

- Too small to be seen with the naked eye or
- Invisible in opaque solutions

TABLE 15-1 ■ Nutrient–Drug Interactions

NUTRIENT	DRUG(S)	INTERACTION	INTERVENTION
Calcium	ciprofloxacin norfloxacin ofloxacin tetracycline	Combines with drugs, yielding insoluble compounds	Separate drug doses from calcium-containing foods
Folic Acid	Oral contraceptives phenytoin aspirin	Decreased absorption (Roman, 2014) Competition for binding sites Competition for binding sites	Supplementation as needed Monitor blood levels of vitamin and drugs in long-term therapy Monitor blood levels of vitamin in long-term therapy
Iron	ciprofloxacin norfloxacin ofloxacin tetracycline	Combines with drugs yielding insoluble compounds	Separate drug doses from iron-containing foods
Magnesium	ciprofloxacin norfloxacin ofloxacin tetracycline	Combines with drugs, yielding insoluble compounds	Separate drug doses from magnesium-containing foods
Niacin	isoniazid phenytoin	Drug is structurally similar to niacin Unknown mechanism	Observe for pellagra with long-term therapy Observe for pellagra with long-term therapy
Vitamin B_6	isoniazid levodopa penicillamine	Formation of a complex that makes vitamin unavailable (Type IIC interaction)	Monitor vitamin status with long-term therapy
Vitamin B_{12}	antacids nitrous oxide anesthesia nitrous oxide aerosols	Drugs neutralize gastric acid that normally facilitates separation of vitamin B_{12} from the foods containing it Nitrous oxide oxidizes the cobalt atom in cobalamin to an inactive state Same mechanism	Monitor vitamin status with long-term therapy Take thorough dietary history. Occurred in clients on restrictive vegetarian diets or their breastfed infants Check for abusive use
Vitamin D	carbamazepine corticosteroids phenobarbital phenytoin rifampin	All interfere with vitamin D metabolism in Type III interaction	All: Monitor vitamin status with long-term therapy
Zinc	ciprofloxacin norfloxacin ofloxacin tetracycline	Combines with drugs, yielding insoluble compounds	Separate drug doses from zinc-containing foods

TABLE 15-2 ■ Classification of Interactions

	CHARACTERISTICS	POSSIBLE EFFECT	EXAMPLE	INTERVENTION
Type I	Usually occur when substances are in direct physical contact, e.g., in delivery device	Physical, biochemical reactions, e.g., oxidation, precipitation	Calcium phosphate precipitates in PN solution	Follow recommendations in the literature Do not rely on visual inspection
Type II	Limited to substances taken orally or administered enterally	Increased or decreased bioavailability	Fatty meal dramatically increases bioavailability of griseofulvin	Check if client limits dietary fat Advise to take with fatty meal
A		Modified enzyme activity	Grapefruit juice inhibits intestinal isoenzyme CYP3A4, raising blood levels of many drugs	Advise client not to consume grapefruit juice when taking these drugs orally (see Table 15-3)
B		Modified transport mechanism	Water-soluble formulations of vitamin E inhibit the transfer protein, P-glycoprotein, increasing blood levels of cyclosporine and digoxin	Do not use water-soluble formulations of vitamin E with cyclosporine Monitor blood levels regularly if vitamin E is used with digoxin
C		Complexing or binding of substances	Calcium, iron, magnesium, and zinc bind with tetracycline, yielding insoluble compounds	Separate drug doses from foods and tube feedings containing these minerals by 1–3 hours

	CHARACTERISTICS	POSSIBLE EFFECT	EXAMPLE	INTERVENTION
TABLE 15-2 ■ Classification of Interactions (Continued)				
Type III	Occur after the substances have reached the systemic circulation	Changed cellular or tissue distribution	*Warfarin* interferes with synthesis of clotting factors	Equalize amounts of vitamin K-rich foods eaten day-by-day
Type IV	Affect disposition of substances by liver and kidney	Promoted or impaired clearance or elimination of substances	*Lithium* is excreted in tandem with sodium and water	Encourage stable amounts of sodium and water intake. Monitor therapeutic effect and urine specific gravity

Adapted from Chan, 2014; Mayo Clinic, 2013.

Neither should one ever inject solutions with precipitates into a client. Up-to-date references regarding compatibility should always be consulted. Calcium and phosphorus solubility limits have been published for pharmacists' use. The principal variables governing calcium and phosphorus precipitation in PN solutions are calcium, phosphorus, amino acid concentrations, temperature, and pH (MacKay, Jackson, Eggert, et al, 2011).

Clinical Application 15-1 offers some insight into the knowledge and skill necessary to administer PN safely. Some of the considerations involved with appropriate administration of tube feedings in conjunction with oral medications appear in Chapter 14.

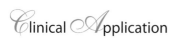
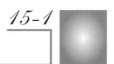

Clinical Application 15-1

Preventing Drug Interactions With Parenteral Nutrition (PN)

PN is a complex formulation of glucose, amino acids, fat emulsion, electrolytes, vitamins, and trace elements. Up to 38 additives may be included, each having individual characteristics that might contribute to interactions.

Drugs that can or should be administered as continuous infusions and that are compatible with PN are the best choices, especially in the critical care setting where fluid intake may be regulated. Alternatively, the drugs can be separated from the PN by using multiple-lumen catheters, alternating the PN infusion with medication infusion, or, if possible, oral administration of medications. The clinical pharmacist's input is critical to providing safe, effective care to clients with these complex needs.

Multivitamins should be admixed immediately before infusion. Thiamin and vitamin A are known to have a short stability in PN. For example, night blindness caused by vitamin A deficiency developed in a client whose PN was admixed in the pharmacy and later delivered to the home. Now dual-chambered bags are available to delay admixing until just before administration.

Interactions may be obvious if changes are noted in the solution or if the catheter becomes plugged, but loss of effectiveness of the drug or the PN can also occur without outward clues.

Sources: Brown, Minard, and Ziegler, 2014; Chan, 2014; Mirtallo, 2004.

Type II Interactions

In general, food stimulates gastrointestinal secretions that assist in dissolving solid forms of medication but other drugs are enteric coated with an acid-resistant shell to protect the active ingredient from gastric acid and delay dissolution until the medication reaches the alkaline intestine. Strict adherence to the package administration directions is necessary to maintain the effectiveness of the enteric coating. See Figure 15-1.

Type II interactions occur with oral or enteral intake, producing increased or decreased bioavailability of either the drug or nutrient. Each interaction can impact administration schedules. See Box 15-1 to distinguish delayed from decreased absorption. Factors influencing Type II bioavailability include:

■ Food intake
■ Modification of enzyme activity or transport mechanisms
■ Complexing or binding of drugs or nutrients so one or both are unavailable for absorption.

See Type IIC interaction and Tables 15-1 and 15-3.

Food Intake

Some drugs should be ingested into an empty stomach, some should be taken with foods, even specific foods to achieve therapeutic results.

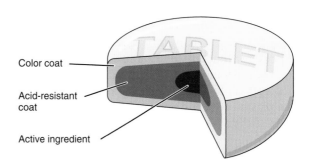

FIGURE 15-1 Enteric-coated tablet. Substances that penetrate the acid-resistant coating defeat the purpose of this type of tablet. (Reprinted from Clayton, BD, and Stock, YN: *Basic pharmacology for nurses,* 9th ed. Mosby, St. Louis, 1989, p. 56, with permission.)

Box 15-1 ■ *Delayed Versus Decreased Absorption*

Some drugs take longer to be absorbed if ingested with food, but the total amount absorbed is unchanged. This delay is the case with *verapamil,* a vasodilator. Therefore, emphasis can be placed on consistency in drug administration in relation to food intake.

However, spacing of doses in relation to food and beverage intake becomes important when a smaller amount of the drug is absorbed in the presence of food than in an empty stomach. In such a situation, correct timing of medication and other intake is necessary. This decreased absorption is the case with *captopril,* an antihypertensive agent.

Also complicating the picture, not all drugs in a given class are equally affected by interactions with food. The total amount absorbed of the quinolones *ciprofloxacin* and *ofloxacin* is reduced if taken with food, but absorption of *levofloxacin* is not reduced by food (Chan, 2014).

DRUGS TAKEN ON AN EMPTY STOMACH

Some drugs must be taken on an empty stomach. A strict protocol is used for *alendronate,* a bone resorption inhibitor given for osteoporosis. *Alendronate* must be taken first thing in the morning with plain water 30 minutes before any other medications, food, or beverages. Any intake other than water significantly decreases absorption. Moreover, the person must remain upright for 30 minutes to facilitate passage through the pylorus and minimize risk of esophageal irritation.

The antihypertensive *captopril* should be taken with only water, and food intake should be delayed for 1 hour after dosing because food decreases absorption by 30% to 50% (Gropper and Smith, 2013). An **antineoplastic** drug, *melphalan,* should be taken without food because it significantly reduces the drug's bioavailability (Pronsky and Crowe, 2012).

The following two antituberculosis drugs have significant pharmacokinetic effects if taken with food and should be taken on an empty stomach. Correct administration is particularly important with tuberculosis because of the lengthy treatment regimen.

■ Foods decrease the absorption of *rifampin* by as much as 26% and increase the time required for the drug to reach maximum concentration, while also decreasing that concentration.
■ Foods, particularly carbohydrates, can decrease the absorption of *isoniazid (INH)* by as much as 57% and the plasma concentration of the drug by as much as 30% (Arbex, Varella, Siqueira, and Mello, 2010).

DRUGS TAKEN WITH FOOD

Food increases absorption or bioavailability of several drugs of various classes. The instructions for some drugs specify that they must be taken with food and

others that a particular macronutrient is recommended to maximize absorption.

Taking with food increases the absorption of:

■ *cefuroxime,* a second-generation cephalosporin.
■ *ketoconazole,* an antifungal agent that requires a pH of <5 to dissolve (Pronsky and Crowe, 2012).
■ lovastatin, an antihyperlipidemic agent.

Taking with food increases the bioavailability of:

■ *atazanavir,* an antiretroviral drug that *must* be taken with food (Pronsky and Crowe, 2012).
■ *ganciclovir,* an antiretroviral agent for which food increases both absorption and bioavailability (Pronsky and Crowe, 2012).
■ *lopinavir,* an antiretroviral drug.
■ *nelfinavir,* an antiretroviral agent for which food intake increases blood levels 2 or 3 times (Pronsky and Crowe, 2012).

Meals containing fat favor absorption of certain drugs that require bile salts for optimal absorption. Fat also stimulates the release of cholecystokinin, which slows gastrointestinal motility, thus permitting the drug to remain in contact with the intestinal tissues for a longer time than otherwise. The extra intestinal exposure to the drug enhances its absorption.

Fatty meals are specifically recommended to accompany:

■ *griseofulvin,* an antifungal agent given infections of the skin such as athlete's foot
■ *atovaquone,* an anti-infective drug given for *Pneumocystis jiroveci* pneumonia.

All of the illustrative drugs with specific food instructions appear in Table 15-3. An example of a special intervention involving a high-fat diet to control epileptic seizures in children appears in Clinical Application 15-2. The ethics of concealing medications in food, which is a separate issue, is briefly discussed in Clinical Application 15-3.

Changes in Enzyme Activity (Type IIA Interactions)

Cytochrome P450 (CYP450) is a superfamily of more than 50 enzymes found mainly in the liver but also in the gastrointestinal tract, lungs, placenta, and kidneys. Among their functions are the production of cholesterol, the detoxification of foreign chemicals, and the metabolism of drugs. Six of the enzymes metabolize 90% of drugs, with the two most significant enzymes being CYP3A4 and CYP2D6 (Lynch and Price, 2007). That function may have evolved to protect the body from toxins.

After uptake by the intestinal epithelial cells (enterocytes), many substances are metabolized by CYP3A4

TABLE 15-3 ■ **Drug–Nutrient Interactions**

DRUG	CLASSIFICATION	INTERACTION
alendronate	Bone resorption inhibitor	Any intake but water decreases absorption
ampicillin	Anti-infective	Food, acidic juices, or carbonated beverages increase gastric degradation of drug
atazanavir	Antiretroviral	Must be taken with food to increase bioavailability
atorvastatin	Lipid-lowering agent	Grapefruit juice increases bioavailability for several days in Type IIA interaction
atovaquone	Antiprotozoal	Fatty meal increases absorption
azithromycin*	Anti-infective	Food, acidic juices, or carbonated beverages increase gastric degradation of the drug
captopril	Antihypertensive	Food decreases absorption 30%–50% by unknown mechanism; take with water and do not eat for 1 hour Potassium-containing salt substitutes increase risk for hyperkalemia in Type IV interaction
carbamazepine	Antiepileptic	Serum plasma level monitoring recommended with grapefruit juice (Pronsky and Crowe, 2012)
ceftriaxone	Anti-infective	Calcium-containing IV products, including PN, combine with the drug in a Type I interaction
cefuroxime	Anti-infective	Taking with food increases absorption
ciprofloxacin	Anti-infective	Take 2 hours before or 6 hours after calcium-containing foods, supplements (Pronsky and Crowe, 2012) Calcium, iron, magnesium, and zinc combine with the drug to form insoluble compounds in Type IIC interaction
clobazam	Anxiolytic, anticonvulsant	Grapefruit juice increases bioavailability over several days in Type IIA interaction
cyclosporine	Immunosuppressant	Grapefruit juice increases bioavailability for several days in Type IIA interaction Water-soluble formulations of vitamin E have increased blood levels of drug in Type IIB interaction
diazepam	Anxiolytic, anticonvulsant	Grapefruit juice increases bioavailability for several days in type IIA interaction
dicloxacillin	Anti-infective	Food, acidic juices, or carbonated beverages increase gastric degradation of the drug
digoxin	Antiarrhythmic	Water-soluble formulations of vitamin E have increased blood levels of drug in Type IIB interaction
enalapril	Antihypertensive	Potassium-containing salt substitutes increase risk for hyperkalemia in Type IV interaction
felodipine	Antianginal, antihypertensive	Grapefruit juice increases bioavailability for several days in Type IIA interaction
fexofenadein	Antihistamine	Fruit juice (apple, grapefruit, orange) decreases bioavailability >70% (Pronsky and Crowe, 2012)
furazolidone	Anti-infective	Tyramine-containing foods may provoke hypertensive crisis in Type III interaction
ganciclovir	Antiretroviral	Food increases absorption and bioavailability
griseofulvin	Antifungal	Fatty meal taken with drug stimulates bile secretion and increases bioavailability of the drug
indinavir*	Antiretroviral	Food precipitates the drug Bioavailability decreased with grapefruit juice (Pronsky and Crowe, 2012)
isocarboxazid	MAOI antidepressant	Tyramine-containing foods may provoke hypertensive crisis in Type III interaction
isoniazid*	Antitubercular	Food, acidic juices, or carbonated beverages increase gastric degradation of the drug Foods, particularly carbohydrates, can decrease absorption and plasma concentration of the drug Vitamin B_6 complexes with the drug in Type IIC interaction: useful in drug overdoses and in minimizing drug side effects Tyramine-containing foods may provoke hypertensive crisis in Type III interaction
ketoconazole	Antifungal	Food increases absorption Take calcium or magnesium supplement 2 hours after dose (Pronsky and Crowe, 2012) Needs pH <5 to dissolve
levodopa	Antiparkinson agent	Amino acids in dietary proteins may compete with the drug for intestinal absorption and transport across the blood–brain barrier. Control protein intake and its distribution throughout the day
levothyroxine	Thyroid preparation	Large amounts of vitamin B_6 may decrease drug effect Large amounts of calcium, iron, magnesium, or zinc may bind levothyroxine and prevent complete absorption in a Type IIC interaction Food, dietary fiber, and espresso coffee interfere with absorption (Liwanpo and Hershman, 2009)
linezolid	Anti-infective	Tyramine-containing foods may provoke a hypertensive crisis in Type III interaction
lisinopril	Antihypertensive	Potassium-containing salt substitutes increase the risk for hyperkalemia in Type IV interaction
lithium	Mood stabilizer	Increased sodium and water intake increases renal excretion of the drug, decreasing its effect Decreased sodium and water intake increases the drug's effect (Type IV interaction)
lopinavir	Antiretroviral	Food increases bioavailability
lovastatin	Lipid-lowering agent	Food increases absorption Grapefruit juice greatly increases bioavailability for several days in Type IIA interaction
melphalan*	Antineoplastic	Food significantly decreases bioavailability
mercaptopurine*	Antineoplastic	Oxidized by food into inactive metabolites
nelfinavir	Antiretroviral	Food increases blood levels by 2 or 3 times
nicardipine	Antianginal, antihypertensive	Grapefruit juice increases bioavailability over several days in Type IIA interaction

(continued)

TABLE 15-3 ■ Drug–Nutrient Interactions (Continued)

DRUG	CLASSIFICATION	INTERACTION
nifedipine	Antianginal, antihypertensive	Grapefruit juice increases bioavailability over several days in Type IIA interaction
nisoldipine	Antianginal, antihypertensive	Grapefruit juice increases bioavailability over several days in Type IIA interaction
norfloxacin	Anti-infective	Calcium, iron, magnesium, and zinc combine with drug to form insoluble compounds in Type IIC interaction
ofloxacin	Anti-infective	Calcium, iron, magnesium, and zinc combine with the drug to form insoluble compounds in Type IIC interaction
phenelzine	MAOI antidepressant	Tyramine-containing foods may provoke hypertensive crisis in Type III interaction
phenytoin	Antiepileptic	Folic acid antagonist that competes with the vitamin for binding sites Tube feedings decrease serum levels of the drugs
procarbazine	Antineoplastic	Tyramine-containing foods may provoke hypertensive crisis in Type III interaction
rasagiline	Antiparkinson agent	Tyramine-containing foods may provoke hypertensive crisis in Type III interaction
rifampin	Antitubercular	Foods decrease absorption and increase the time to reach maximum concentration, which is also decreased
selegiline†	Antiparkinson agent	Tyramine-containing foods may provoke hypertensive crisis in Type III interaction
simvastatin	Lipid-lowering agent	Grapefruit juice greatly increases bioavailability for several days in Type IIA interaction
tetracycline*	Anti-infective	Calcium, iron, magnesium, and zinc combine with drug to form insoluble compounds in a Type IIC interaction
tranylcypromine	MAOI antidepressant	Tyramine-containing foods may provoke hypertensive crisis in Type III interaction
triazolam	Anxiolytic, anticonvulsant	Grapefruit juice increases bioavailability for several days in Type IIA interaction
verapamil	vasodilator	Food delays but does not decrease absorption; consistency in drug administration in relation to food is advised
warfarin	Anticoagulant	In genetically susceptible persons, cranberry juice interferes with drug metabolism in Type IIA interaction Large amounts of vitamin K–rich foods and beverages reduce anticoagulant effect in Type III interaction High doses of vitamin E increase risk of hemorrhage (Pronsky and Crowe, 2012) Concomitant enteral feeding interferes with *warfarin* absorption, possibly through protein-binding in a Type IIC interaction

*Risk of treatment failure if taken with food (Schmidt and Dalhoff, 2002).
†Transdermal preparation does not require severe dietary restrictions at certain doses (Cohen and Sclar, 2012; Pronsky and Crowe, 2012).
Sources: Arbex, Varella, Siqueira, and Mello, 2010; Cereda, Barichella, and Pezzoli, 2010; Chan, 2014; Gropper and Smith, 2013; Pronsky and Crowe, 2012.

15-2

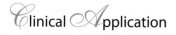

Clinical Application

The Ketogenic Diet for Seizure Control

About one-third of clients with epilepsy are pharmacoresistant. For a subgroup of this population, both children and adults, the ketogenic diet can be highly efficacious and should be considered early (Dhamija, Eckert, and Wirrell, 2013).

Originally used to treat children with **epilepsy** that is poorly controlled with medication, the ketogenic diet (high-fat, low-carbohydrate) limits kilocalories and fluid to less than the Recommended Dietary Allowance. The diet is also inadequate in micronutrients so that supplementation and close monitoring of the child's growth are essential (Papandreou, Pavlou, Kalimeri, and Mavromichalis, 2006).

The diet's mechanism of action is unknown, and ketosis alone does not explain the anticonvulsant effect, indicating that several mechanisms may exist for its effect (Lutas and Yellen, 2013). Normally, the brain derives most of its energy from glucose. When deprived of its preferred fuel, the brain uses ketone bodies for energy, a process shown to be more effective in young animals than in old ones. In humans, the ketogenic diet is more successful in children younger than 8 years than in older children, although the diet is not universally helpful (Papandreou et al, 2006).

Although the mechanisms underlying the broad clinical efficacy of the ketogenic diet remain unclear, there is growing evidence that the ketogenic diet alters the fundamental biochemistry of neurons in a manner that not only inhibits neuronal hyperexcitability but also induces a protective effect. Thus, the ketogenic diet may ultimately be useful in the treatment of a variety of neurological disorders (Kim and Rho, 2008).

About one-third of children with intractable seizures become seizure-free on the ketogenic diet, one-third have seizures significantly less frequently, and one-third do not benefit. Some children in the study continued to receive medications for their epilepsy but in reduced amounts. Nonetheless any reduction in medication improves the child's quality of life (Papandreou et al, 2006).

Analysis of four randomized controlled trials suggest that in children, the ketogenic diet results in short- to medium-term benefits in seizure control, the effects of which are comparable to modern antiepileptic drugs. However, one study of long-term outcome reports a high attrition rate for the diet. For those with medically intractable epilepsy or those in whom surgery is unsuitable, a ketogenic diet could improve seizure control, but tolerability is poor (Levy, Cooper, and Giri, 2012).

Unfortunately, the diet has several known complications: kidney stones, gallstones, anemia, and cardiac abnormalities. Nevertheless, the ketogenic diet provides an option for families with a child suffering from difficult-to-control seizures.

The ketogenic diet was also used in two cases of a rare disorder of the urea cycle, which leads to a deficiency of arginine and excessive blood ammonia. Both clients displayed refractory epilepsy, one of whom had reduced seizure frequency on the diet; the other did not (Peuscher, Dijsselhof, Abeling, et al, 2012).

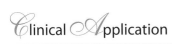

15-3

Clinical Application

The Ethics of Hiding Medications in Food

Nurses' deception of their clients, however well intentioned, when revealed may cause mistrust of that particular nurse or the health-care system in general. In addition, food universally symbolizes caring. Hiding medications in food is not an action to be taken lightly.

Clients have the right to decline treatment *unless* they are unable to discern the consequences of their decisions. The appropriate assessment of the client's mental fitness is necessary before that right is denied.

If, after deliberation with the client's advocate, colleagues, and the institution's ethics committee, deception is deemed justified, the nurse and pharmacist should ensure that the particular medication, after being crushed and mixed with food, would remain safe and effective.

No one should unilaterally decide to deceive a client just to pass medications on time (Olsen, 2012).

or returned to the intestinal lumen by a transporter protein, **P-glycoprotein (P-gp).** This process limits the amount of the substance available for absorption and provides repeated opportunities for CYP3A4 enzymes to metabolize the drug (Chan, 2014). Individuals show a wide variation in the amount of CYP3A4 in the liver and the intestine due to genetic, physiological, and environmental factors with resulting differences in the severity of interactions.

GRAPEFRUIT JUICE

An accidental discovery in 1989 that grapefruit juice, used to mask the taste of alcohol in a study, enhanced the absorption of *felodipine* has spurred research into the underlying mechanism. It appears that grapefruit juice's major effect is through the inhibition of intestinal CYP3A4 so that the oral bioavailability of affected drugs is increased dramatically, in some cases as much as fivefold, sufficient to cause drug toxicity and increased side effects or treatment failure. The interaction occurs with the first glass of grapefruit juice consumed, increases in severity with continued consumption of juice, and continues for 3 to 5 days after cessation of juice intake until the intestine can manufacture more of the enzyme (Chan, 2014).

The components of grapefruit juice vary considerably depending on the variety, maturity and origin of the fruit, local climatic conditions, and the manufacturing process. No single component accounts for all observed interactions (Grapefruit, 2012); however, no evidence suggests that eating grapefruit in moderation causes detectable inhibition of CYP3A4 enzymes (Chan, 2014). Other grapefruit products such as preserves, powdered whole grapefruit, grapefruit seed extract, and zest have been implicated occasionally (Grapefruit, 2012).

Applying this knowledge to clinical practice is complicated by the fact that even within a given class of drugs, not all agents are metabolized by CYP3A4, so some medications in the class are affected by grapefruit juice and others are not. Here are some examples.

Of calcium channel blockers, given to manage hypertension and angina pectoris, grapefruit juice:

- increases bioavailability of *felodipine, nicardipine, nifedipine,* and *nisoldipine* (see Table 15-3) but
- shows little interaction with *amlodipine* (Pronsky and Crowe, 2012).

Similarly, grapefruit juice increases the bioavailability of the benzodiazepines:

- *clobazam, diazepam,* and *triazolam* (see Table 15-3) but
- not *alprazolam* (Pronsky and Crowe, 2012).

Likewise, differing effects with grapefruit juice are seen with statin drugs, given to lower cholesterol and prevent ischemic heart disease:

- *simvastatin* and *lovastatin* had greatly increased blood levels when given with grapefruit juice,
- *atorvastatin* showed a lesser effect than with the previous two drugs (see Table 15-3), but
- *pravastatin* exhibited no effect (Pronsky and Crowe, 2012).

An immunosuppressive agent used to prevent rejection of transplanted organs, *cyclosporine,* is metabolized by intestinal CYP3A4, and elevated blood levels have occurred when administered with grapefruit juice.

In short, avoiding grapefruit juice during oral therapy with affected drugs is well advised. This is particularly true with drugs with a narrow **therapeutic index** and serious side effects that high levels of the drug may evoke (see Table 15-3).

CRANBERRY JUICE

A similar mechanism but a different isoenzyme is proposed to explain an interaction between the anticoagulant *warfarin* and cranberry juice. *Warfarin* is metabolized by the cytochrome P450 isoenzyme CYP2C9, and cranberry juice contains flavonoids known to inhibit P450 enzymes.

Examples of pharmacokinetic cranberry–*warfarin* interactions include:

- A woman with two episodes of elevated **international normalized ratios (INRs)** 3 months apart after consuming 1.5 and 2 quarts of cranberry juice cocktail daily for 2 to 4 days (Hamann, Campbell, and George, 2011)
- An 85-year-old woman on chronic *warfarin* therapy for atrial fibrillation whose INRs increased two- to

threefold after two separate ingestions of cranberry sauce (Haber, Cauthon, and Raney, 2012)

■ A man with an INR of 6.45 (therapeutic range of 2 to 3) without abnormal bleeding after drinking a half gallon of cranberry-apple juice in the week before the elevated INR (Paeng, Sprague, and Jackevicius, 2007)

The following cases exemplify pharmacodynamics interactions:

■ After a chest infection, a client subsisted almost solely on cranberry juice for 2 weeks while taking his prescribed medications, *digoxin, phenytoin,* and *warfarin*. He died of gastrointestinal and pericardial hemorrhage (Suvarna, Pimohamed, and Henderson, 2003).

■ A client with a prosthetic mitral valve developed a persistently elevated INR 2 weeks after starting to drink cranberry juice. Subsequent symptoms included postoperative bleeding problems (Grant, 2004).

■ A client taking stable doses of *warfarin* who developed major bleeding and high INR values soon after starting daily cranberry juice had no other identifiable reasons for the high INR. Fortunately, discontinuation of the juice consumption resolved the problem (Rindone and Murphy, 2006).

■ An elderly man who consumed only cranberry juice for 2 weeks while maintaining his usual dosage of *warfarin* died from internal hemorrhage (Griffiths, Beddall, and Pegler, 2008). See Table 15-3.

In some of the cases cited above, the clients ingested unusually large amounts of cranberry juice. Small controlled trials failed to link moderate ingestion of cranberry juice to *warfarin* effects:

■ Giving 240 mL of cranberry juice twice daily for 1 week to 10 clients stabilized on *warfarin* did not statistically change their prothrombin times (Mellen, Ford, and Rindone, 2010).

■ Compared with a matching placebo, 240 mL of cranberry juice daily for 2 weeks did not produce significantly different INRs in 30 clients on stable *warfarin* anticoagulation (Ansell, McDonough, Zhao, et al, 2009).

The last-mentioned two controlled studies used a total of 40 subjects who likely did not encompass the range of genetic possibilities for metabolizing the juice and the drug (see Genomic Gem 15-1). Especially in situations with clear genetic influences, investigations that genotype subjects likely would yield more conclusive findings than do general population studies.

LICORICE

Clinical Application 15-4 describes interference with cortisol metabolism caused by licorice consumption.

Changes in Transport Mechanism (Type IIB Interactions)

A nutrient can also inhibit P-glycoprotein as is the case with water-soluble formulations of vitamin E. Administration of this form of vitamin E to liver transplant recipients and healthy volunteers increased *cyclosporine* bioavailability by up to 80%. By the same mechanism, this form of vitamin E increased oral bioavailability of *digoxin* but showed no pharmacodynamic effects, probably because the volunteer subjects were young and healthy. Rather than the vitamin E itself, the interaction is likely caused by a substance added in the manufacturing process (Chan, 2014). See Table 15-3.

Hence, a client taking *cyclosporine* could be in major trouble if he concurrently consumes grapefruit juice

---

𝒢enomic 𝒢em 15-1

Genetic Factors in *Warfarin* Response

Genetic factors explain a higher proportion of variability in *warfarin* response than age, body size, race, concurrent disease, and medications. The identified genes chiefly responsible for the genetic effect are:

■ CYP2C9 that codes for an enzyme that metabolizes *warfarin*
■ VKORC1 that codes for *warfarin's* target enzyme (Kim, Ko, Lee, et al, 2012).

Clients with mutated CYP2C9 are very sensitive to *warfarin*, displaying over-anticoagulation with standard doses. CYP2C9 enzyme, mainly expressed in the liver, is involved in the metabolism of about 10% of all drugs. A large variation among individuals exists in CYP2C9 activity, which accounts for differences in drug response and in adverse effects. Approximately 5% to 14% of Caucasians, 0% to 5% of Africans, and 0% to 1% of Asians lack CYP2D6 activity, and these individuals are known as poor metabolizers (Zhou, Liu, and Chowbay, 2009).

Warfarin also affects the ability of VKORC1 to mediate vitamin K activation. Polymorphisms of this gene also vary by nationality and have been linked to differences in effective maintenance doses of *warfarin* (Kim, Ko, Lee, et al, 2012). In fact, initial variability in the INR response to *warfarin* was more strongly associated with genetic variability in the pharmacologic target of *warfarin*, VKORC1, than with CYP2C9 (Schwarz, Ritchie, Bradford, et al, 2008).

Whether sufficient evidence exists to justify genotype-based *warfarin* dosing is a matter of debate. A major contributing factor is lack of third-party reimbursement for the relatively expensive testing (Stack for Education Committee, 2011).

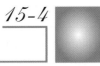

Clinical Application

Licorice Affects Cortisol Metabolism

Natural licorice, a flavoring agent, contains glycyrrhizic acid, which when metabolized inhibits an enzyme that controls the conversion of cortisol to cortisone in the kidney. The result is the enhanced mineralocorticoid effect of cortisol, leading to hypokalemic hypertension (Bailey, Sands, and Franch, 2014). When eaten in excess, licorice can cause sodium and water retention, hypertension, hypokalemia, and alkalosis as shown in the following cases.

■ Life-threatening hypokalemic paralysis occurred as a result of consuming licorice as a tea sweetener (a common custom among the Arab population) superimposed on long-term consumption of licorice candy (Elinav and Chajek-Shaul, 2003).
■ Muscle weakness progressed to paralysis in an elderly Asian man with hypertension, hypokalemia, and metabolic alkalosis, attributed to a 3-year daily ingestion of tea flavored with natural licorice root (Lin, Yang, Chau, and Halperin, 2003).
■ Hypertension and hyperkalemia in a 52-year-old man with lower-extremity edema caused by daily consumption of more than 0.5 L of licorice-based aperitif over the holidays (Brasseur and Ducobu, 2008).
■ Peripheral edema and weight gain in a 49-year-old woman who consumed 4 to 7 licorice candy cigars to prevent constipation during a 2-week trip (Johns, 2009).

These clients did not realize the risks of their habits. Besides these deliberate ingestions, however, a person may consume natural licorice unknowingly because it is used to flavor many foods, some chewing tobacco, chewing gum, alcoholic beverages, some laxatives, and herbal medicines (see later section in this chapter). Herbal medicines containing licorice or its active ingredient, glycyrrhizic acid, caused paralysis in two elderly individuals that discontinuation and appropriate electrolyte replacement therapy corrected (Cheng, Chen, Chau, and Lin, 2004; Yasue, Itoh, Mizuno, and Harada, 2007).

Because most licorice candy consumed in North America is artificially flavored, this interaction of natural licorice with an endogenous hormone is easily overlooked.

and water-soluble vitamin E, both of which are readily available and for most people, innocuous. Such a situation demands vigorous and effective client education.

Complexing or Binding of Substances (Type IIC Interactions)

Well documented interactions involve minerals and mineral-fortified foods, vitamin B$_6$, and enteral feedings.

MINERALS AND MINERAL-FORTIFIED FOODS

Tetracycline, an anti-infective agent, combines with calcium, iron, magnesium, and zinc to form insoluble compounds. The drug and the nutrient thus bound are both less available for absorption. For this reason,

tetracycline should be administered 1 hour before or 3 hours after:

■ Taking iron supplements
■ Eating iron-containing foods (red meat, egg yolks)
■ Consuming milk, other dairy products or, calcium-fortified juices
■ Taking antacids or multivitamins containing magnesium, aluminum, calcium, or zinc

Tetracycline should be taken without food or milk to avoid a high risk of treatment failure. Bioavailability of *tetracycline* is reduced

■ Up to 57% when taken with food
■ 65% with dairy products
■ 81% with iron supplements

Even a small amount of milk in coffee or tea can reduce the drug's bioavailability by 49% (Schmidt and Dalhoff, 2002). See Tables 15-1 and 15-3.

Some *fluoroquinolones* react with metal cations in the same manner as does *tetracycline.* See *ciprofloxacin, norfloxacin,* and *ofloxacin* in Table 15-3 and the nutrients in Table 15-1. Impaired absorption has been found with enteral feeding so that withholding tube feedings for 1 hour before and after the dose of medication is usually suggested.

Foods or supplements containing large amounts of calcium, iron, magnesium, or zinc also may bind *levothyroxine* and prevent complete absorption (Vallerand, Sanoski, and Deglin, 2013).

DRUGS INTERACTING WITH VITAMIN B$_6$

Both *penicillamine* and *isoniazid (INH)* combine with pyridoxol phosphate to inactivate it, causing distal, progressive symmetric neuropathy in clients on long-term *INH* therapy for tuberculosis. Treatment involves discontinuation of *INH* or pyridoxine supplementation (Roman, 2014).

The anti-Parkinson agent *levodopa* forms a complex with vitamin B$_6$. The kidney then excretes this complex in the urine rather than returning it to the bloodstream. This interaction can be used therapeutically.

■ With *levodopa,* supplemental *pyridoxine:*
  ■ Should be limited to <5 mg per day to avoid decreased drug effect.
  ■ May be added to a levodopa regimen to prevent vitamin B$_6$ deficiency, while also decreasing the effectiveness of levodopa.
■ With *isoniazid, pyridoxine* can:
  ■ Be used as a supplement to limit the extent of the polyneuropathy that is a common side effect of *isoniazid* (van der Watt, Harrison, Benatar, and Heckmann, 2011).
  ■ Be given intravenously to treat *isoniazid* toxicity which is among the most common causes of

drug-induced seizures in the United States, including the case of a 10-month-old found with his parent's *INH* (Minns, Ghafouri, and Clark, 2010). In one case of attempted suicide, regional efforts were required to obtain sufficient supplies of IV pyridoxine (Morrow, Wear, Schuller, and Malesker, 2006). See Tables 15-1 and 15-3.

ENTERAL FEEDING

Although the exact mechanism is unknown but bearing characteristics of a type IIC interaction, decreased serum levels of the antiepileptic drug *phenytoin* when administered with nasogastric feedings are well documented. Serum levels of the drug rebound when the feedings are discontinued. Initiating enteral feedings on clients previously stabilized on *phenytoin* resulted in a 70% reduction in serum *phenytoin* concentrations. Monitoring of serum *phenytoin* levels two or three times a week if administered with tube feedings is recommended (Chan, 2014). See Table 15-3.

A significant difference in INR values has been demonstrated in intensive care clients receiving *warfarin* and enteral nutrition either continuously or paused for *warfarin* administration. Therefore, continuous enteral nutrition should be withheld for 1 hour before and after *warfarin* administration (Dickerson, Garmon, Kuhl, et al, 2008). See Table 15-3.

Type III Interactions

Type III interactions occur after the nutrient or drug has reached the systemic circulation that delivers nutrients and drugs throughout the body to be metabolized by multiple organs. Two interactions with pharmacodynamic effects involve *warfarin* and *monoamine oxidase inhibitors* (MAOIs).

Vitamin K and *Warfarin*

The most commonly prescribed anticoagulant, *warfarin,* is given to prevent blood clot formation in clients with that history, other clotting disorders, and those with mechanical devices in the cardiovascular system.

MECHANISM OF INTERACTION

Warfarin works by competing with vitamin K at its binding sites, thus inhibiting the synthesis of vitamin K–dependent clotting Factors II, VII, IX, and X, prolonging clotting time, and "thinning" the blood.

Eating large amounts of foods high in vitamin K during anticoagulant therapy with *warfarin* decreases or may even negate the desired effect of the drug. Clients should not stop eating foods containing vitamin K, but they should avoid large variations in the amounts eaten.

A problem might arise if they eat mounds of green leafy vegetables one day and then none for the following several days (see Table 15-4).

An experiment using diets that decreased vitamin K intake by 80% or increased it by 500% during a 4-day in-hospital stay demonstrated significant changes in the clients' INRs, thus supporting the relevance of diet to therapeutic anticoagulation (Franco, Polanczyk, Clausell, and Rohde, et al, 2004). Analysis of dietary records estimated that for each increase in 100 micrograms of vitamin K intake, the INR would be reduced by 0.2 points. Additionally, OTC multivitamin supplements contain enough vitamin K_1 to significantly alter coagulation parameters (Rohde, de Assis, and Rabelo, 2007).

In Brazilian clients with vascular disease, fluctuations in phylloquinone (vitamin K_1) intake, particularly from kidney beans were associated with variations in prothrombin times and INRs (Custódio das Dôres, Booth, Martini, et al, 2007).

Even beverages that are significant sources of vitamin K can interfere with therapeutic anticoagulation efforts. The following cases illustrate the need

TABLE 15-4 ■ **Basic Vitamin K-Controlled Diet**

FOODS HIGH IN VITAMIN K (NO MORE THAN 1 SERVING/DAY)*	SERVING SIZE	MCG VITAMIN K
Kale, cooked	½ cup	531
Spinach, cooked	½ cup	441
Collards, cooked	½ cup	418
Swiss chard, raw	1 cup	299
Swiss chard, cooked	½ cup	287
Mustard greens, raw	1 cup	279
Turnip greens, cooked	½ cup	265
Parsley, raw	¼ cup	246
Broccoli, cooked	1 cup	220
Mustard greens, cooked	½ cup	210
FOODS MODERATELY HIGH IN VITAMIN K (NO MORE THAN 3 SERVINGS/DAY)*		
Collards, raw	1 cup	184
Spinach, raw	1 cup	145
Turnip greens, raw	1 cup	138
Endive lettuce, raw	1 cup	116
Brussels sprouts, cooked	½ cup	110
Broccoli, raw	1 cup	89
Cabbage, cooked	½ cup	82
Green leaf lettuce	1 cup	71
Soybeans, mature, cooked	1 cup	66
Romaine lettuce	1 cup	57
Asparagus	4 spears	48

*Research protocol; client's RD will individualize. *Consistency is key.*
Sources: Academy of Nutrition and Dietetics, 2012; National Institutes of Health, 2003; http://nutritiondata.self.com.

to regularly monitor clients taking *warfarin* not only for effective anticoagulation but also for changes in dietary intake.

- A 44-year-old man who had been stabilized on the drug but who later consumed one-half to one gallon of green tea per day dropped his INR out of therapeutic range within 1 week of starting the tea intake (Taylor and Wilt, 1999).
- A 64-year-old woman who had been stabilized on *warfarin* while drinking pomegranate juice 2 to 3 times weekly discontinued the juice intake and her INR became subtherapeutic (Komperda, 2009).

Table 15-4 shows a basic diet for *warfarin* therapy. Many health systems have developed protocols for anticoagulation diets. Note that "green leafy vegetables" are not universally interchangeable and that the mode of preparation has an impact on vitamin K content:

- Cooked spinach has 4 times the vitamin K of cooked Brussels sprouts.
- Cooked broccoli has 2.5 times the vitamin K of raw broccoli.

The client's dietitian will individualize the diet prescription to accommodate food preferences. It is important that the food pattern used when the *warfarin* dose is stabilized be continued on subsequent days and weeks. The key to effective *warfarin* therapy is consistent intake of foods containing substantial vitamin K.

Despite its efficacy, *warfarin* remains underused in clinical practice because of its variable dose response, diet and medication interactions, and need for frequent monitoring. New classes of targeted anticoagulants are being developed that avoid the many pitfalls of the vitamin K antagonists (Hylek, 2013).

OTHER FACTORS AFFECTING WARFARIN

Abnormal intestinal function and pharmacokinetics of the drug also affect the effectiveness of *warfarin*.

Intestinal Conditions
Even a short-term change in physical health can affect *warfarin*'s pharmacodynamics, as has been reported in cases of diarrhea that may interfere with the absorption of dietary and **endogenous** vitamin K. Excessive anticoagulation has occurred in clients with:

- Protracted diarrhea (Roberge, Rao, Miske, and Riley, 2000)
- Relapsing Crohn disease symptoms partly attributed to chronic malabsorption of vitamin K (Fugate and Ramsey, 2004)

Clients with inflammatory bowel disease have a greater incidence of vitamin K deficiency and malabsorption. Such clients may not absorb oral vitamin K,

given to reverse elevated INRs but may require parenteral products (Fugate and Ramsey, 2004).

Clients taking *warfarin* experiencing diarrhea or decreased food intake should have their INRs monitored more frequently than usual and *warfarin* dosages adjusted accordingly. Note: Drugs other than *warfarin* may interfere with endogenous vitamin K; see Clinical Application 15-5.

Protein Binding
Warfarin is 99% bound to plasma proteins (Vallerand et al, 2013). A client with low levels of serum albumin as a result of malnutrition or disease is at risk for drug toxicity with drugs that are usually highly bound to albumin. The drug that is bound to protein is inactive, whereas the unbound drug circulating in the blood is active and able to exert its intended therapeutic effect. Figure 15-2 sketches two consequences of the competition between drugs and foods or nutrients for protein binding sites.

Tyramine and Monoamine Oxidase Inhibitors

The usual abbreviation for this group of drugs is **MAOI (monoamine oxidase inhibitor).** Several antidepressants are MAOIs, and some other drugs produce similar reactions with tyramine (see Table 15-5).

MECHANISM OF DRUG ACTION

MAOIs prevent the breakdown of **dopamine** and **tyramine,** chemicals necessary for proper functioning of the nervous system. The drugs' therapeutic effects are to increase the concentration of epinephrine, norepinephrine, serotonin, and dopamine in the central nervous system, thus counteracting depression.

In the peripheral nervous system, MAOIs also prevent the release of the norepinephrine that builds up in the nerves. The stores of norepinephrine become especially high in the nerves that regulate the size of blood vessels. The result is a decreased ability to constrict peripheral blood vessels. The vasodilation thus produced leads to hypotension.

To compound the situation, the drugs also inhibit the body's normal response to a low blood pressure,

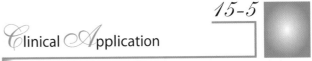

15-5

𝒞linical 𝒜pplication

Vitamin K Deficiency in an Infant

Anti-infective drugs, besides fighting pathogens, destroy beneficial intestinal bacteria that synthesize vitamin K. Cerebral hemorrhage in a 4-month-old infant was attributed to isoniazid and rifampin therapy for congenital tuberculosis and immaturity of vitamin K absorption or metabolism processes (Kobayashi, Haruta, Maeda, et al, 2002).

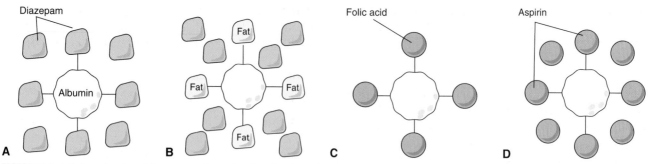

FIGURE 15-2 *A,* Four molecules of diazepam are bound to the albumin molecule, leaving the other four molecules of diazepam free to leave the bloodstream for the central nervous system. *B,* Fat displaces the diazepam from the albumin molecule so that all eight molecules of diazepam are immediately free to exert sedative effects on the central nervous system. *C,* Four molecules of folic acid are attached to the albumin molecule and able to circulate through the kidney intact. *D,* Aspirin displaces the folic acid from the albumin molecule, and the separate molecules of folic acid are likely to be excreted in the urine.

TABLE 15-5 ■ Tyramine-Restricted Diet		
DESCRIPTION	**INDICATION**	**ADEQUACY**
Restricts food with naturally high levels of tyramine	Used when clients receive drugs classified as monoamine oxidase inhibitors (MAOIs) and those with MAOI activity. Antidepressants: *isocarboxazid phenelzine tranylcypromine* Anti-infectives: *isoniazid linezolid* Antineoplastics: *procarbazine* Antiparkinson: *rasagiline selegiline*	Adequate in all nutrients according to the current Recommended Dietary Allowances if the individual makes appropriate food choices
FOOD GROUP	**TO AVOID**	**TO USE MODERATELY**
Breads and cereals	None	None
Fruits and vegetables	Avocados Bananas Figs Broad (fava) beans Chinese pea pods Eggplant Fermented soy products Italian flat beans Mixed Chinese vegetables Raspberries Sauerkraut	None
Dairy	Aged cheese (brick, blue, brie, cheddar, camembert, Swiss, romano, Roquefort, mozzarella, parmesan, provolone) Sour cream Yogurt	Gouda cheese, processed American cheese
Meat and fish	Any canned meat Anchovies Beef or chicken liver Sausage (bologna, salami, pepperoni, summer) Fish (caviar, dried fish, salt herring)	
Beverages	Ale, beer, sherry, red and white wines	Coffee, colas, hot chocolate (1–3 cups per day)
Other	Chocolate, bouillon and other protein extracts, protein supplements, meat tenderizer, soy sauce, yeast concentrates	

that is, an increased heart rate. Thus, the individual taking MAOIs displays the unusual combination of hypotension and bradycardia.

EFFECT OF FOOD ON MAOIS

Some foods contain **tyramine,** a metabolic intermediate product in the conversion of the amino acid tyrosine to epinephrine. Foods that contain degraded protein, such as aged cheese, are high in tyramine. When a client taking MAOIs consumes foods or beverages high in tyramine, the drugs prevent the normal breakdown of tyramine. The tyramine oversupply consequently leads to excessive epinephrine, producing hypertension. Sometimes the blood pressure is severely elevated, which can cause intracranial hemorrhage.

As with many substances, individuals' responses to tyramine vary. Four factors interact to determine the severity of reaction:

1. The amount of tyramine ingested
2. The type and dose of the MAOI
3. Client susceptibility
4. The time between the drug dose and a tyramine-containing meal

TYRAMINE-RICH FOODS

Many foods contain enough tyramine to create problems for clients receiving MAOIs. The amount of tyramine varies even in different samples of a particular food. Table 15-5 describes the tyramine-restricted diet. Because this interaction can be life-threatening, the best advice to give a client is to avoid all foods capable of causing problems, even though a small amount of the food, or a given batch of a product, might be safe. The effects of MAOIs and interactions with foods may persist for 2 weeks after they have been discontinued (Pronsky and Crowe, 2012).

MAOIs, despite proven efficacy for depression, are underprescribed due, in part, to concerns about required dietary and drug restrictions. A transdermal MAOI delivery system (*selegiline*) lessens or avoids the need for dietary restrictions (Cohen and Sclar, 2012) but only at lower doses (Pronsky and Crowe, 2012).

Protein Intake and Levodopa

Levodopa is given for Parkinson disease. The amino acids in dietary proteins may compete with the drug for transport across the **blood–brain barrier.** Low-protein diets with protein intake shifted to the evening have proved helpful in stabilizing drug effects (Pronsky and Crowe, 2012). In addition, low-protein products designed for chronic renal failure are safe, tasty, well tolerated, and useful in improving both levodopa fluctuations and client adherence to low-protein dietary regimens (Cereda, Barichella, and Pezzoli, 2010). See Table 15-3.

Vitamin D: Multiple Interactions

Corticosteroids increase the **catabolism** of the matrix of the bone, inhibit the osteoblasts from building new bone, and prevent the liver from processing vitamin D. When this lack of vitamin D results in insufficient calcium absorption by the intestine, parathyroid hormone causes withdrawal of calcium from the bones and osteoporosis results. Because of the seriousness of this adverse effect, monitoring of the client's vitamin D status should be ongoing during long-term corticosteroid therapy (see Table 15-1).

Phenytoin, in addition to previously detailed interactions, also affects bone metabolism, reducing bone mineral density and increasing the risk of fractures. The mechanism is presumed to entail an upregulation of enzymes, resulting in an imbalanced conversion of vitamin D into inactive metabolites (Meier and Kraenzlin, 2011). By nature a long-term therapy for seizure prevention, *phenytoin* requires conscientious monitoring of the client's bone health and institution of osteoporosis preventive measures.

Two other enzyme-inducing antiepileptics that increase the metabolism of vitamin D in a similar manner are *carbamazepine* and *phenobarbital* (Meier and Kraenzlin, 2011). The antituberculosis drug *rifampin* also creates a risk of vitamin D deficiency (Pronsky and Crowe, 2012). The Endocrine Society Clinical Practice Guideline suggests that clients taking glucocoids and anticonvulsant medications be given at least two to three times more vitamin D than the Recommended Dietary Allowance (RDA) for their age group to satisfy their need for the vitamin (Holick, Binkley, Bischoff-Ferrari, et al, 2011). See Table 15-1.

B Vitamins: Multiple Interactions

Water-soluble vitamins are particularly susceptible to drug interactions during long-term therapy. Folic

acid's absorption is decreased by oral contraceptives (Roman, 2014). Documented cases of interactions include the following with niacin and vitamin B_{12}.

NIACIN

Phenytoin has been related to pellagra:

■ A client with cerebral palsy receiving *phenytoin, valproic acid,* and *diazepam* for years was treated with multiple therapies from numerous physicians before the diagnosis of pellagra was reached. Symptoms resolved in 2 months with niacin and multivitamin supplementation, and the cause was attributed to the anticonvulsants (Lyon and Fairley, 2002).

■ Three weeks of *phenytoin* therapy was credited with causing pellagrous dermatitis in a 3-year-old child that resolved within 3 weeks of niacin supplementation and within 2 weeks of replacing *phenytoin* with *carbamazepine* (Kaur, Goraya, Thami, and Kanwar, 2002).

The mechanism producing pellagra in those cases is unknown, possibly an alteration in absorption of vitamins or interference with synthesis of niacin from tryptophan.

Pellagra is also a well-known complication of *isoniazid (INH)* therapy for tuberculosis. Because *INH* is structurally similar to niacin, the body recognizes it as niacin and reduces its production of the vitamin from tryptophan (Das, Parajuli, and Gupta, 2006). In Turkey, a 7-year-old boy's case of *INH*-induced pellagra was resolved with niacin therapy (Bilgili, Karadag, Calka, and Altun, 2011).

VITAMIN B_{12}

An oral antidiabetic agent, *metformin,* is a known pharmacological cause of vitamin B_{12} deficiency, but the responsible mechanisms are not established (Mazokopakis and Starakis, 2012). Long-term treatment with *metformin* can potentially lead to neuropathy, which is also a complication of diabetes. Annual monitoring of vitamin B_{12} status is recommended (Pierce, Chung, and Black, 2012). The RDA for vitamin B_{12} and the amount available in general multivitamins may not be enough to correct this deficiency among clients with diabetes (Reinstatler, Qi, Williamson, et al, 2012).

Long-term, recurrent exposure to *nitrous oxide,* commonly used in anesthesia, irreversibly oxidizes the cobalt atom in cobalamin, thus destroying the cobalamin-dependent enzyme methionine synthase (Carmel, 2014). Undiagnosed vitamin B_{12} deficiency often contributes to the untoward result in cases involving *nitrous oxide* anesthesia, but substance abuse is an additional cause. Examples of case reports follow.

■ One woman so affected had been a vegetarian for 10 years and for 5 years had restricted her intake to apples, nuts, and raw vegetables while avoiding legumes. (See Chapters 6 and 10 regarding vegetarianism and vitamin B$_{12}$ deficiency.) *Nitrous oxide* was one component of the anesthesia this client received to repair a traumatic hip fracture. Six weeks later, she was unable to walk and was diagnosed with degeneration of the spinal cord. The client improved with cobalamin injections but still had some residual effects 1 year after anesthesia (Rosener and Dichgans, 1996).

■ Severe neurological impairment occurred in two infants following *nitrous oxide* anesthesia. A 6-month-old female, breastfed by a mother who avoided dairy and meat products without vitamin supplements, was diagnosed as severely vitamin B$_{12}$-deficient after anesthesia with *nitrous oxide* and after suffering diffuse cerebral atrophy (McNeely, Buczulinski, and Rosner, 2000). The case of the second infant had an additional contributing factor (see Genomic Gem 15-2).

■ Young adults have been affected with ataxia and progressive ascending numbness in the extremities resulting from inhaling *nitrous oxide* from whipped cream containers over several months. One individual recovered, and the other two were lost to follow-up (Lin, Chan, Chang, and Su, 2011). A fourth client who fell from a 6-foot-high wall was initially thought to have traumatic injuries but later was diagnosed with myelopathy from *nitrous oxide* abuse that resolved with treatment (Ghobrial, Dalyai, Flanders, and Harrop, 2012).

It is thus prudent for vegetarians to take preventive cobalamin supplements especially during pregnancy and while breastfeeding and to avoid *nitrous oxide* anesthesia. Treatment of *nitrous oxide* toxicity must be started early and administered parenterally because reversal of the toxicity can be incomplete (Carmel, 2014).

Type IV Interactions

Interactions between drugs and nutrients can continue as the kidneys excrete waste products of metabolism.

Sodium, Fluids, and Lithium

Both sodium intake and increased fluid intake affect the mood stabilizer *lithium*, which is one of several drug options for the long-term treatment of bipolar (formerly manic-depressive) disorder. This drug is absorbed, distributed, and excreted with sodium and may result in the following scenarios.

■ Decreased sodium intake with decreased fluid intake may lead to *lithium* retention manifested by slurred speech, decreased coordination, drowsiness, and muscle weakness or twitching.

■ Increased sodium intake and increased fluid intake increase the excretion of *lithium*, thus worsening signs and symptoms of mania.

Use of loop diuretics or angiotensin-converting enzyme (ACE) inhibitors significantly increases the risk of hospitalization for lithium toxicity in the elderly (Juurlink, Mamdai, Kopp, et al, 2004). Because of the interaction with salt and water intake, clients who take *lithium* may be taught to monitor the concentration or specific gravity of their urine (see Table 15-3).

Salt Substitutes and ACE Inhibitors

The ACE inhibitors lower blood pressure by preventing conversion of angiotensin I to angiotensin II, thereby decreasing aldosterone secretion and increasing excretion of sodium and water (see Fig. 8-7) and increasing retention of potassium. Clients receiving ACE inhibitors such as *captopril, enalapril,* and *lisinopril* should be monitored for **hyperkalemia** (see Table 15-3).

Hyperkalemia has been reported in two clients using salt substitutes containing potassium while receiving

---

Genomic Gem 15-2

Inherited Defect in Nitrous Oxide-Cobalamin Interaction

A 3-month-old male was anesthetized twice with *nitrous oxide* for biopsy and removal of a mass on his left leg. Seventeen days after the resection, he suffered seizures and apnea. Computed tomography scan revealed generalized atrophy of the brain. The infant died 46 days after the second surgery (Selzer, Rosenblatt, Laxova, and Hogan, 2003).

He was determined to have an inherited defect of the *MTHFR* gene that provides instructions for making an enzyme used to process amino acids, culminating in the conversion of the amino acid homocysteine to another amino acid, methionine. At least 40 mutations in the *MTHFR* gene have been identified in people with homocystinuria (U.S. National Library of Medicine, 2011).

Eventually, investigation revealed that the infant's father and one of his uncles had elevated serum homocysteine levels. In addition, the infant's sibling with a low homocysteine level was receiving long-term high-dose vitamin B therapy. Neither the father nor the sibling had received *nitrous oxide* (Selzer et al, 2003).

In another case, a man with diabetes, history of stroke, and hyperhomocystinemia developed new sensorimotor symptoms and urinary incontinence 4 weeks after prolonged exposure to *nitrous oxide* anesthesia during amputation (Ahn and Brown, 2005). These cases illustrate the critical importance of a thorough history to ascertain vitamin B$_{12}$ deficiency before administering *nitrous oxide* anesthesia.

ACE inhibitors. In each case, serum potassium returned to normal after cessation of the salt substitute. One client had to be resuscitated after cardiac arrest before the contribution of a salt substitute to his hyperkalemia became apparent (Ray, Dorman, and Watson, 1999).

Folic Acid Displaced by Aspirin

Plasma proteins can bind with nutrients as well as drugs. When there are insufficient binding sites on the plasma proteins for all of the drug or nutrient, the excess accumulates in the bloodstream as free, small particles. The kidney is likely to excrete these small particles rather than to restore them to the bloodstream.

One common drug that interferes in this manner with a nutrient is *acetylsalicylic acid,* or *aspirin.* It displaces folic acid from its plasma protein. The kidney then excretes the folic acid in the urine (see Fig. 15-2). Increased consumption of foods high in folic acid is recommended with long term high dose aspirin therapy (Pronsky and Crowe, 2012).

Dietary Supplements

In 2009, consumers spent $26.7 billion on supplements that have been taken by more than half of American adults (Consumer Reports, 2011). Only 23% of products were used based on recommendations of a health-care provider (Bailey, Gahche, Miller, et al, 2013). Compared with nonusers of dietary supplements, users tend to be:

- Older
- Female
- White
- Living in a food-secure household (Kennedy, Luo, and Houser, 2013)
- More physically active
- Less likely to smoke
- Slimmer with a lower BMI
- Higher in educational attainment (Consumer Reports, 2011)
- Insured for health-related expenses
- Moderate users of alcohol
- Higher in socioeconomic status (Bailey, Gahche, Miller, et al, 2013)

Consequently, attributing effects to dietary supplements apart from lifestyle is problematic.

A 2007 survey found that 17.7% of American adults had used "natural products" (i.e., dietary supplements other than vitamins and minerals) in the previous 12 months (National Institutes of Health,

March 2010). About 25% of persons taking prescription medications also take a dietary supplement and two-thirds of them do not tell their physicians about their dietary supplement use, perhaps because they do not consider supplements to be legitimate drugs or to carry risks (Gardiner, Phillips, and Shaughnessy, 2008). As this section details, neither of those assumptions is justified.

Compared with the number of possible interactions between supplements and medications, only a small proportion have been examined or reported. The occurrence and clinical significance of many drug–nutrient interactions remains unclear. Those likely to be those of clinical significance, however, are interactions involving drugs with a narrow **therapeutic index** such as *cyclosporin, digoxin, indinavir,* and *warfarin* (Chen, Serag, Sneed, et al, 2011; Shi and Klotz, 2012).

Special Rules

The rules for labeling the nutrient content of foods and drugs in the United States are much more stringent than those applied to dietary supplements.

Before receiving permission to market a new drug, the pharmaceutical company must conduct rigorous tests on animals and on people in randomized, double-blind clinical trials. Randomization requires that participants be assigned by coin toss or equivalent unbiased method to receive the investigative drug or not. **Double-blind** trials are experiments in which neither the subject nor the investigator knows whether a subject is receiving the treatment or a **placebo.**

For foods, label information must be supported by research or scientific agreement, which is not the case with dietary supplements.

Because it is not required by law, research into the effectiveness and adverse effects of dietary supplements is limited. Most dietary supplements, because the evidence is inadequate to permit health or nutrient content claims, must use structure–function claims (Institute of Medicine, 2005). The standard for the structure–function claim for dietary supplements is simply that it be truthful and not misleading (see Box 15-2).

An additional problem pertains to overlapping areas of regulatory responsibility. Food labeling is regulated by the FDA and the U.S. Department of Agriculture, whereas advertising is regulated by the Federal Trade Commission (FTC). The standards and methods used by these agencies differ (Heimbach, 2008). The FTC, along with the FDA, has been cracking down on food and beverage makers for allegedly overselling the health benefits of their products (Klein, 2010).

Box 15-2 ■ *Regulation of Dietary Supplements*

The Dietary Supplement Health Education Act of 1994, referred to as DSHEA, created the first regulatory structure for this class of products. The FDA provides primary oversight of dietary supplements along with drugs and most foods (Swanson, Thomas, and Coates, 2014).

Under the provisions of DSHEA, dietary supplements can be sold unless shown by the FDA to be unsafe, adulterated, or labeled in a misleading manner. The burden of proof in this case rests with the FDA, not with the manufacturer, and no prior notice from the manufacturer of intent to sell is required unless the product contains a new dietary ingredient. The Bioterrorism Act does require manufacturers to register with FDA before producing or selling supplements and in 2007, the FDA published comprehensive regulations for Current Good Manufacturing Practices for those who manufacture, package or hold dietary supplement products (U.S. FDA, December, 2010).

Under DSHEA, a dietary supplement is defined as a product taken by mouth that

1. contains a dietary ingredient: vitamin, mineral, herb; botanical, amino acid, enzyme, tissue; or a concentrate, metabolite, or constituent extract from the ingredients previously mentioned.
2. is in the form of a supplement (meaning tablet, capsule, soft gel, gelcap, liquid, or powder).
3. is not represented as a food or sole item of a meal or of the human diet (U.S. Food and Drug Administration, May 20, 2009).

DSHEA does not limit the serving size or the amount of nutrients in any form of dietary supplement, but its regulations spell out the nature of the claims that can be made for a product on the label and its format. The following types of statements are allowed:

1. Health claims that have substantial scientific support or, if limited support, the claim must contain qualifying statements

2. Nutrient content claims that describe the level of the nutrient or dietary ingredient in a product compared with an established daily value
3. Structure/function claims that describe the product's effect on structure or function of the body or on general well-being. These claims must also include the following information displayed prominently on the label:
"This statement has not been evaluated by the Food and Drug Administration. This product is not intended to diagnose, treat, cure or prevent any disease."

Manufacturers of dietary supplements that make structure/function claims on labels or in labeling must submit a notification to the FDA that includes the text of the structure/function claim no later than 30 days after marketing the dietary supplement (U.S. FDA, May 20, 2009).

For instance, a structure/function claim could state the product "helps to maintain bone health." If the label said the product is used to treat arthritis, it would be disallowed as a medical claim. Monitoring the system is incomprehensible. In the 10 years after the passage of DSHEA, the number of dietary supplement products on the market ballooned from an estimated 4000 to more than 29,000 (Atwater, Montgomery-Salguero, and Roll, 2005).

The FDA maintains a MedWatch program to receive information about possible adverse effects of dietary supplements. Health-care providers and consumers can report these events online at www.fda.gov/Safety/MedWatch/HowToReport/default.htm or by calling 1-800-FDA-1088. The identity of the client is kept confidential.

DSHEA has supporters of the status quo as well as those calling for regulation of dietary supplements in the same manner as pharmaceuticals. Health-care providers should know the current system and be aware of changes to provide wise counsel to clients.

Areas of Concern

With botanical products, nature keeps some of the ingredients secret. Not all the constituents of these products have been identified, and they may exert more than one physiological effect in the human body. Therefore, when ingesting one of them, a person takes not only the active ingredient that is purported to have the desired medicinal effect but also other substances in the plant tissue as well.

Among those other substances may be defensive chemicals the plant has evolved to protect itself from predators. Despite a long history of use, little is known about the toxicity of botanical products. Most such knowledge comes from acute cases of toxicity sporadically reported, but recently some scientific studies have been conducted.

Manufacturers and distributors of dietary supplements must record, investigate, and forward to the FDA any reports they receive of serious adverse events associated with the use of their products that are reported to them directly (U.S. FDA, March 14, 2013). Because the FDA's responsibility begins only after the products have been packaged and marketed,

the maintenance of quality is the responsibility of the manufacturer.

In May 2008, the FDA reported 201 individuals with adverse reactions to liquid nutritional supplements containing excess selenium and chromium resulting in the largest epidemic of selenosis in the history of the United States (Aldosary, Sutter, Schwartz, and Morgan, 2012). The affected products, distributed to 15 states, were voluntarily recalled (U.S. FDA, May 1, 2008).

Besides the dearth of information and questionable manufacturing practices, issues of standardization, contamination, and interaction with other substances are major concerns. ConsumerLab.com, in testing more than 2400 dietary supplements over 11 years, found 25% with a quality problem, primarily because of an inadequate amount or substandard ingredients followed by contamination with heavy metals (Swanson, Thomas, and Coates, 2014).

Lack of Standardization

The potency of herbal products varies with the:

- Climate and soil conditions
- Life cycle of the plants from which they come

Great differences in the quantities of active ingredients have been found, depending on:

- The source
- The species and part of the plant used
- Storage conditions
- Time of harvest
- Method of processing
- Country of origin
- Inclusion of look-a-like plants

Without consistent products, research cannot be generalized as a basis for evidence-based practice.

Botanical products can come to market not containing the ingredients on the label. For example, analysis of:

- Echinacea preparations determined that labeled species content was correct in only 52% of the samples and 10% contained no echinacea at all (Gilroy, Steiner, Byers, et al, 2003).
- 54 samples of St. John's wort determined that just 2 of them (3.7%) contained active ingredients within 10% of the amounts stated on the label (Draves and Walker, 2003).

Discerning the species of a plant product by visual inspection is not always possible:

- Chinese star anise (*Illicium verum*) when used as a spice is on the **Generally Recognized As Safe (GRAS) List** but
- Japanese star anise (*Illicium anisatum*) causes neurological and gastrointestinal toxicities.

Seven infants, ages 2 to 12 weeks, were treated at Miami Children's Hospital for star anise poisoning. Symptoms included irritability, hyperexcitability, vomiting, abnormal eye movements, and seizures (Ize-Ludlow, Ragone, Bruck, et al, 2004). After approximately 40 individuals, including about 15 infants, became ill following ingestion of star anise teas, the FDA issued an advisory to not drink such beverages because the particular variety of star anise involved in these illnesses could not be identified (U.S. FDA, September 10, 2003). Additional cases have been reported in a 3-month-old in Virginia (Madden, Schmitz, and Fullerton, 2012) and a 2-month-old in France (Perret, Tabin, Marcoz, et al, 2011).

New technology offers assistance in distinguishing Chinese from Japanese star anise through nondestructive testing (Vermaak, Viljoen, and Lindström, 2013).

Contamination With Dangerous Substances

Botanical products have been contaminated with toxic substances. Heavy metals and prescription medications are frequently cited as contaminants.

HEAVY METALS

The FDA Tolerable Daily Diet Lead Intake is:

- 6 mcg for children <6 years of age
- 25 mcg for pregnant women
- 25 mcg for adults (Liva, 2007)

The U.S. Pharmacopoeia (see Box 15-3) limits the presence of heavy metals in nutritional supplements to:

- 3 ppm for arsenic, cadmium, and mercury
- 10 parts per million (ppm) for lead

Additionally, the FDA limits lead to 0.1 ppm in candy likely to be consumed frequently by small children (Liva, 2007).

Ayurvedic medicine, a system of traditional medicine native to India, stresses natural plant-based medicines, often with the addition of sulfur, arsenic, lead, copper, and gold to the more than 600 formulations (Gunturu, Nagarajan, McPhedran, et al, 2011). In August through October 2005, one-fifth of both U.S.-manufactured and Indian-manufactured Ayurvedic medicines purchased via the Internet contained detectable lead, mercury, or arsenic. Among the metal-containing products, 95% were sold by U.S. Web sites and 75% claimed to use good manufacturing practices. All metal-containing products exceeded one or more standards for acceptable daily intake of toxic metals (Saper, Phillips, Sehgal, et al, 2008).

From 1966 to 2007, 76 cases of lead **encephalopathy** potentially associated with traditional medicine were located as follows:

- 5% in adults, at least one of whom had residual neurological impairment and

---

Box 15-3 ■ *Standards for Health-care Products*

The U.S. Pharmacopeial Convention (USP), a nongovernment, nonprofit organization, sets standards for drugs, dietary supplements, biologics, and other articles used in health care. Substances listed as USP meet standards of purity and strength as determined by chemical analysis or animal responses to specified doses. A zero tolerance policy for pesticides applies to food and botanicals.

A voluntary verification program for dietary supplements is available to assure consumers of the safety of the products they buy. Certain supplements with known safety concerns are excluded from the program:

- Ephedra
- Kava
- Comfrey
- Chaparral
- Aristolochia

The USP mark on a product verifies the accuracy of the label, the strength and quantity of the contents, the lack of contaminants according to federal standards, and the use of good manufacturing practices (Srinivasan, 2006; USP Convention, 2013).

- 95% in infants and young children of which 8 cases were fatal and at least 15 had residual neurological deficits (Karri, Saper, and Kales, 2008).

Those are only the cases in which the lead poisoning proceeded to encephalopathy. Young children and fetuses of pregnant women are at special risk for the toxic effects of lead because these Ayurvedic products are used to treat infertility in women (Centers for Disease Control and Prevention, July 9, 2004).

Additional cases of lead poisoning continue to be reported, such as in:

- A 58-year-old woman in Connecticut seen twice in the emergency department, hospitalized, endoscoped extensively, before a blood test for anemia triggered analysis of blood lead levels. She had been taking Ayurvedic medicine to assist with diabetes control (Gunturu, Nagarajan, McPhedran, et al, 2011).
- A 12-month-old child of Thai parents in Massachusetts, attributed to an Asian tongue powder given to absorb toxins. Case–finding located one additional poisoned infant (Woolf, Hussain, McCullough, et al, 2008).

DRUGS

Dietary supplements have also been contaminated with prescription medications. Because of the special rules governing the dietary supplement industry, discovery of the contaminants frequently occurs long after the products are first marketed.

While studying natural anti-inflammatory substances in human placental blood, investigators detected an unknown substance. It was subsequently identified as the drug *colchicine,* which is used to treat gout, traced to five women who consumed ginkgo biloba during pregnancy. Further searching located the drug in samples of ginkgo biloba distributed commercially in the area. *Colchicine* has the potential to be **teratogenic** (Petty, Fernando, Kindzelskii, et al, 2001).

In 2007 and 2008, two voluntary recalls of three dietary supplements involved contamination with the prescription drug *sildenafil.* The danger is a possible interaction with nitrates, found in some prescription drugs such as *nitroglycerin,* would lower blood pressure to dangerous levels. The contamination was discovered by the FDA, not the manufacturer or distributor (U.S. FDA, June 18, 2009; December 14, 2010).

Analysis of 20 samples of dietary supplements marketed for weight control revealed:

- 2 were strictly herbal
- 4 corresponded to the ingredients on the label
- 14 were adulterated (Vaysse, Balyssac, Gilard, et al, 2010)

These are not isolated instances. A search on the FDA Web site in 2013 for "sildenafil" and "undeclared ingredient" yielded 59 entries, excluding the FDA archives.

Difficulty Obtaining Reliable Information

Supplement labels are often lacking needed information. For example:

- Experienced pharmacists could not discern ingredient information from some of the labels in one survey (Atwater, Montgomery-Salguero, and Roll, 2005).
- Analysis of labels on St. John's wort showed the vast majority did not adequately address clinically relevant safety issues. At best, 8% included information on pertinent drug interactions (Clauson, Santamarina, and Rutledge, 2008).

Often a consumer's source of information about a dietary supplement is the seller of the product. Analysis of 443 Web sites identified 55% that contained claims to treat, prevent, diagnose, or cure specific diseases despite the prohibition of such statements (Morris and Avorn, 2003).

Reliable information on the quality of dietary supplements is available from:

- FDA at www.fda.gov/Food/DietarySupplements/default.htm
- NIH National Library of Medicine at www.nlm.nih.gov/medlineplus/druginfo/herb_All.html
- NIH Office of Dietary Supplements, at http://ods.od.nih.gov/Research/PubMed_Dietary_Supplement_Subset.aspx
- NIH National Center for Complementary and Alternative Medicine (NCCAM) at http://nccam.nih.gov

Easy to Underestimate Potential Harm

Both the name "dietary supplements" and the ease of procurement can mislead consumers about their possible impact on medications. For those reasons or others, many clients do not inform their health-care providers about their use of dietary supplements.

- Of 458 outpatient veterans, 43% were taking at least one dietary supplement with prescription medications, of which 45% had a potential for a significant drug–dietary supplement interaction (Peng, Glassman, Trilli, et al, 2004).
- Forty-five percent of children seen in one emergency department over a 3-month period had been given an herbal product by their caregivers, of whom just 45% had discussed the herbal therapy with the child's primary health-care provider (Lanski, Greenwald, Perkins, and Simon, 2003).

So many botanical products have the potential to increase bleeding times that the American Society of

Anesthesiologists recommends all herbal medications be discontinued 2 to 3 weeks before elective surgery (Frost, 2006).

Supplements Reported to Interact With Drugs

Knowledge and caution are necessary to weigh the risks and benefits of dietary supplements (see Fig. 15-3). Although statistics do not predict individual responses, St. John's wort and ginkgo as well as magnesium, calcium, and iron had the greatest number of documented interactions with medications (Tsai, Lin, Simon Pickard, et al, 2012). Examples of purported mechanisms of action, case reports, and experts' advice follow.

St. John's wort

St. John's wort has been favorably compared to pharmaceutical antidepressants in some studies, but significant interactions with medications have been discovered. Clinical trials indicate that St. John's wort, via CYP3A4 and/or P-glycoprotein induction, reduces the plasma concentrations (and/or increases the clearance) of *atorvastatin, cyclosporin, digoxin, fexofenadine, indinavir, nifedipine, simvastatin, verapamil,* and *warfarin,* among others (Izzo and Ernst, 2009). Caution is indicated when St. John's wort and medications metabolized by CYP3A4 and/or P-glycoprotein are used together (see Table 15-6).

Altered clinical status resulted from adding St. John's wort to an antipsychotic drug in the following case. A woman with schizophrenia, stable on *clozapine,* deteriorated after she started self-medicating with St. John's wort. Her psychiatric condition and plasma *clozapine* level improved after withdrawal of St. John's wort (Van Strater and Bogers, 2012).

Because the bioavailability of oral contraceptives is reduced when administered concurrently with

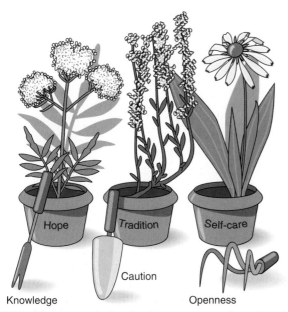

FIGURE 15-3 Because of cultural traditions, many people use botanical products as they seek a measure of self-care and hope. Those who use botanical products, however, need to cultivate knowledge and caution in their choices. They also should practice openness with their health-care providers.

TABLE 15-6 ■ Documented Dietary Supplement–Drug Interactions			
DIETARY SUPPLEMENT	**DRUG**	**DRUG CLASS**	**EFFECT**
Garlic	*indinavir*	Antiretroviral	Decreased drug effect
	nelfinavir	Antiretroviral	Decreased drug effect
	ritonavir	Antiretroviral	Reduced plasma level of drug
	saquinavir	Antiretroviral	Reduced plasma level of drug
	warfarin	Anticoagulant	Reduced plasma level of drug Increased drug effect
Ginkgo Biloba	*aspirin*	Antiplatelet agent	Increased bleeding
	clopidogrel	Antiplatelet agent	Increased bleeding
	ibuprofen	Nonsteroidal anti-inflammatory agent (**NSAID**)	Increased bleeding
	nifedipine	Antihypertensive	Increased drug effects
	omeprazole	Antiulcer agent	Increased drug effects
	trazodone	Antidepressant	Increased drug effects
Ginseng	*imatinib*	Antineoplastic	Drug-induced hepatotoxicity
	phenelzine	Antidepressant	Increased drug effect
	warfarin	Anticoagulant	Decreased drug effect
Glucosamine	*warfarin*	Anticoagulant	Increased drug effect Caution if shellfish allergy
St. John's wort	*alprazolam*	Anxiolytic	Increased drug clearance and decreased drug effect
	atorvastatin	Lipid lowering agent	Decreased drug effect
	clozapine	Antipsychotic	Decreased drug effect
	cyclosporine	Immunosuppressant	Rejection of transplanted organs
	digoxin	Antiarrhythmic	Decreased drug level and effect
	fexofenadine	Antihistamine	Decreased drug effect
	indinavir	Antiretroviral	Decreased drug level and effect
	nifedipine	Antihypertensive	Decreased drug level
	Oral contraceptives	Hormones	Reduced bioavailability and contraceptive failure
	simvastatin	Lipid-lowering agent	Decreased drug effect
	verapamil	Vasodilator	Decreased drug effect
	warfarin	Anticoagulant	Increased drug clearance and decreased drug effect

Sources: Bilgi, Bell, Ananthakrishnan, and Atallah, 2010; Boullata, 2005; Knudsen and Sokol 2008; Izzo and Ernst, 2009; Pronsky and Crowe, 2012; Van Strater and Bogers, 2012.

St. John's wort, women should use additional methods to avoid unintended pregnancy (Rahimi and Abdollahi, 2012). However, only 50% of community pharmacists and 11% of health food store clerks identified the interaction when asked directly (Sarino, Dang, Dianat, et al, 2007).

Ginkgo Biloba

Ginkgo biloba is promoted to enhance mental functioning through improved cerebral circulation. The evidence that ginkgo biloba has predictable and clinically significant benefits for people with dementia or cognitive impairment is inconsistent and unreliable (Birks and Grimley Evans, 2009). Neither does convincing evidence support ginkgo's effectiveness for acute ischemic stroke, intermittent claudication, or tinnitus and evidence for ginkgo's effect on age-related macular degeneration is inconclusive (Roland and Nergård, 2012).

Individuals have experienced spontaneous bleeding while taking ginkgo as in a reported case of post-laparoscopic cholecystectomy bleeding in a client taking ginkgo biloba (Fessenden, Wittenborn, and Clarke, 2001). Fifteen published case reports described a temporal association between using ginkgo and a bleeding event, but in 13 of the cases, the clients had other risk factors for bleeding. In six cases, however, it was clear that when ginkgo was stopped, the bleeding did not recur (Bent, Goldberg, Padula, and Avins, 2005).

Ginkgo does not interact with *warfarin* or *aspirin* directly but does have antiplatelet activity. Cumulative effects become apparent when ginkgo is combined with other drugs affecting coagulation. In combination with nonsteroidal anti-inflammatory drugs, especially aspirin, ginkgo reportedly caused severe bleeding, including intracranial bleeding (Gardiner, Phillips, and Shaughnessy, 2008). In one case, the addition of *ibuprofen* to a 2-year intake of ginkgo biloba extract concluded after 4 weeks with a fatal cerebral hemorrhage (Meisel, Johne, and Roots, 2003). Not surprisingly, ginkgo is listed as increasing bleeding risk with *warfarin* (Vallerand, et al, 2013). See Table 15-6.

Ginseng

Three varieties of ginseng, Asian, American, and Siberian, have different properties and interactions. Persons taking American ginseng and *warfarin* should be monitored when changing herbal products or even using a new bottle of the same product (Gardiner, Phillips, and Shaughnessy, 2008).

A 26-year-old man with chronic myelogenous leukemia who had taken *imatinib* for 7 years with no complications presented with right upper quadrant pain. His only lifestyle modification prior to the diagnosis of hepatotoxicity was daily ingestion of Panax ginseng via energy drinks for the previous 3 months. Ginseng is known to inhibit CYP3A4, the primary enzyme involved in the metabolism of *imatinib*. The result of their interaction was hepatotoxicity (Bilgi, Bell, Ananthakrishnan, and Atallah, 2010).

Panax ginseng also increases bleeding risk with *warfarin* (Vallerand, et al, 2013).

Garlic

Garlic is promoted for cardiovascular health. Whereas several trials have suggested that garlic has possible blood pressure-lowering effects, a larger number of published studies have reported virtually no effect. It is notable that all positive studies were performed using subjects with elevated **blood pressure** and that, by contrast, almost all negative studies used subjects with normal blood pressure. Compared to placebo, a Japanese traditional preparation of crushed garlic and egg yolk significantly reduced **systolic blood pressure** in mildly hypertensive subjects but not in those with lower blood pressure readings (Nakasone, Nakamura, Yamamoto, and Yamaguchi, 2013).

In a test of the pharmacokinetic effect of garlic on antiretroviral medicines, 21 days of garlic powder supplementation reduced plasma *saquinavir* concentrations in healthy volunteers. Likewise, 4 days of garlic extract supplementation reduced *ritonavir* concentration but less dramatically (Gurley, Fifer, and Gardner, 2012).

In addition, garlic also increases bleeding risk with *warfarin* (Vallerand, et al, 2013). See Table 15-6.

Glucosamine–Chondroitin

Glucosamine and chondroitin are substances found in the human body in and around cells of cartilage. Consumers sometimes take one or both supplements for osteoarthritis. The American Academy of Orthopaedic Surgeons recommended against the supplements (Richmond, Hunter, Irrgang, et al, 2009). A later meta-analysis showed that after 2 to 3 years of daily consumption, glucosamine and chondroitin sulfate may delay radiological progression (joint space narrowing) in clients with osteoarthritis of the knee (Lee, Woo, Choi, et al, 2010).

Although not an endorsement from the American Academy of Family Physicians, and noting the evidence was mixed, an article in the organization's journal listed the option of the supplementation by citing a double-blind randomized controlled trial. It showed little benefit from the use of glucosamine combined with chondroitin in participants with mild knee osteoarthritis, but a greater benefit was noted in persons with moderate to severe pain (Ringdahl and Pandit, 2011).

Untoward reactions that have occurred with glucosamine use:

- One case of liver toxicity was reported in a 55-year-old woman taking glucosamine. Several of her liver enzymes were elevated to 10 times the upper limit of normal. One week after discontinuing glucosamine, serum transaminases fell dramatically, with some returning to normal limits. Four weeks after glucosamine was discontinued, all her liver tests were normal (Ebrahim, Albeldawi, and Chiang, 2012).
- A 71-year-old man had received *warfarin* 7.5 mg/day for 5 years for atrial fibrillation, while treating himself with the supplement glucosamine hydrochloride and chondroitin sulfate for arthritis. After tripling his dose of the supplements, the client's INR was out of therapeutic range within 3 weeks. Modifying the doses and finally discontinuing the supplements restored the *warfarin* to therapeutic levels in another 32 days (Knudsen and Sokol, 2008).

A search of the FDA MedWatch database revealed 20 reports of glucosamine or glucosamine-chondroitin use with *warfarin* to be associated with increased INRs or increased bleeding or bruising. One report described an intraventricular bleed and subdural hematoma, which resulted in a persistent vegetative state (Knudsen and Sokol, 2008).

The World Health Organization adverse drug reactions database documented 21 spontaneous reports of increased INR associated with glucosamine use, 17 of which resolved when glucosamine was stopped. A single published case report was located of concomitant use of glucosamine-chondroitin sulfate potentiating the effect of *warfarin*. In aggregate, available information suggests that the use of *warfarin* and glucosamine may lead to an increased INR (Knudsen and Sokol, 2008).

Caution is urged in clients with shellfish allergies who wish to take glucosamine (Pronsky and Crowe, 2012). See Table 15-6.

Hepatotoxicity From Dietary Supplements

Untoward effects have occurred with dietary supplements even without drug interactions such as the spontaneous bleeding cited earlier for ginkgo. Exact estimates on the frequency of adverse hepatic reactions resulting from dietary supplements are unknown (Stickel, Kessebohm, Weimann, and Seitz, 2011). A few examples are recounted in this section.

Over 22 months, supplement use alone accounted for the most cases of fulminant liver failure referred to one transplant service, exceeding *acetaminophen* toxicity and viral hepatitis. Ten clients were recent or active users of potentially hepatotoxic supplements; seven of them had no other identified cause for hepatic failure (Estes, Stolpman, and Olyaei, et al, 2003).

A previously healthy 28-year-old female bodybuilder had been taking two dietary supplements for 1 month before becoming jaundiced and unable to exercise. Her acute liver failure was caused by a dietary supplement and "fat burner" containing usnic acid, green tea, and guggul tree extracts. She developed encephalopathy but survived after liver transplantation. Of all the ingredients, usnic acid may have been predominantly responsible for the hepatoxicity (Krishna, Mittal, Grewal, et al, 2011).

Two females, aged 33 and 40 years, experienced severe acute hepatitis in the setting of documented Hydroxycut exposure, an herbal weight loss supplement. It may contain as many as 11 ingredients, of which 3 have prior data suggesting liver toxicity. An alternative cause for the toxicity was not found in these two women (Dara, Hewett, and Lim, 2008).

A Prudent Course

Clients at greatest risk from drug–dietary supplement interactions are:

- Children
- The elderly
- People with chronic diseases or impaired organ function
- People taking many medications over a long period of time
- People taking medicines with high risk of interactions (anticoagulants, antiepileptics, antimicrobials)
- Individuals with genetic variants in drug metabolism

The fact that many botanical products have been used for centuries does not negate their dangers. Clearly, "let the buyer beware" holds true. To protect clients, thorough assessment is vital. Often the use of dietary supplements does not come to light until late in the treatment cycle. Did health-care providers ask the clients about use of dietary supplements? If so, was it done in a manner that permitted them to reveal their practices without feeling ridiculed or condemned? Some items to consider when assessing diet supplement use are listed in Clinical Application 15-6.

Education is essential. Without disparaging a client's background, the health-care provider must counter the concept that "everything natural is safe." Substances

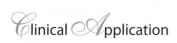
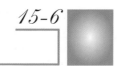

Clinical Application 15-6

Assessment for Dietary Supplement Use

Questions the nurse might ask to determine supplement use:

■ What kinds of herbal products, dietary supplements, or other natural remedies do you take?
■ Do you give any of them to children?
■ Do you find the recommended dose satisfactory?
■ Have you changed doses recently?
■ Are you taking any prescription or over-the-counter medications for the same purpose? Or for opposite purposes?
■ Have you used this product before? For how long?
■ Where do you obtain these products?
■ Is anyone else in your household taking botanical products?
■ Are you allergic to any plant products?
■ Are you pregnant, planning to become pregnant, or breastfeeding?

strong enough to produce the effects attributed to dietary supplements are medicines, no matter what the law currently allows for distribution. Such substances should be treated with respect, including the use of childproof containers.

Enhancing Athletic Performance

Physical training and proper nutrition are vital for success in sports. In general, the diet that is optimal for good health is also optimal for most athletes. Energy and macronutrient needs, especially carbohydrate and protein, must be met during times of high physical activity to maintain body weight, replenish glycogen stores, and provide adequate protein to build and repair tissue. Sports nutrition has several objectives:

■ To foster good health
■ To promote adaptations to training
■ To help athletes recover quickly after each training session
■ To foster optimal performance during competition (Williams, 2014)

Nutrition for Athletes

As long as competitive sports have existed, athletes have attempted to improve their performance by ingesting a variety of substances. This practice has given rise to a multi-billion-dollar industry that aggressively markets its products as performance enhancing, often without objective, scientific evidence to support such claims (Bishop, 2010).

Ergogenic aids are substances, devices, or practices that enhance an individual's energy use, production, or recovery. They encompass equipment, clothing, training exercises, psychological preparation, and dietary supplements, the topic of this section. For athletes the aid is any means of enhancing energy utilization, including energy production, control, and efficiency.

Many athletic organizations prohibit the use of certain pharmacological, physiological, and nutritional aids. The World Anti-Doping Agency (2013) lists prohibited substances on its Web site. The National Collegiate Athletic Association (NCAA) Web site lists banned substances as well as rules governing testing (2012).

Several surveys of supplements available through the Internet and at retail have confirmed that many are contaminated with steroids and stimulants that are prohibited for use in elite sports. To help ensure that the risks of censure to an athlete are minimal, many reputable manufacturers have their products rigorously tested by sports antidoping laboratories (Judkins and Prock, 2012).

Some ergogenic aids clearly fall into the classes of nutrients included in Chapters 2, 3, 4, 6, 7, and 8, whereas others do not, although they may be substances with physiological functions. The ergogenic aids included in this chapter are categorized either as nutrients corresponding to those in the above listed chapters or as nonnutrients.

Nutrients

The Acceptable Macronutrient Distribution Ranges (AMDRs) are broad enough to cover the macronutrient needs of most active individuals, but alternate formulas based on body weight have been developed for athletes (see Clinical Calculation 15-1). These requirements can generally be met by dietary management without the need for supplements.

CARBOHYDRATE

Carbohydrate is the body's main dietary energy source for:

■ **Anaerobic** (1 to 2 minutes) and
■ **Aerobic** (more than 3 minutes) exercise

It is the only fuel that can be used anaerobically (Rosenbloom, 2012).

Suggested daily intakes of carbohydrate per kilogram of body weight are:

■ 6 to 10 grams for the average athlete in training
■ 10 to 12 grams for 2 to 3 days before prolonged endurance events (Williams, 2014)

These amounts exceed the AMDR, which is designed for 97% to 98% of individuals of a given age,

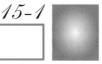

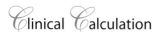 *15-1*

Clinical Calculation

Individualizing Macronutrient Recommendations for the Athlete

Depending on kilocalorie needs and the sport, athletes may need these adjustments in diet.

	GRAMS/KILOGRAM BODY WEIGHT	SUGGESTED DISTRIBUTION RANGE
CHO	7–11	50%–70% of kcal
Protein	1.2–1.7	12%–20% of kcal
Fat	0.8–2	20%–30% of kcal

If an athlete, 70 kg (154 lb), 5 ft 9 in., runs an average of 10 miles per day, lifts weights 3 or 4 times a week, and needs 3600 kcal/day, his suggested intake would be:

CHO

7 grams × 70 kg = 490 grams; 11 grams × 70 kg = 770 grams
490 grams × 4 kcal/gram = 1960 kcal; 770 grams
× 4 kcal/gram = 3080 kcal

$$\frac{1960}{3600} = 54\% \qquad \frac{3080}{3600} = 86\%$$

CHO intake = 54% to 86% of 3600 kcal

PROTEIN

1.2 grams × 70 kg = 84 grams; 1.7 grams × 70 kg = 119 grams
84 grams × 4 kcal/gram = 336 kcal; 119 grams × 4 kcal/gram
= 476 kcal

$$\frac{336}{3600} = 9\% \qquad \frac{476}{3600} = 13\%$$

Protein intake = 9% to 13% of 3600 kcal

FAT

0.8 grams × 70 kg = 56 grams; 2 grams × 70 kg = 140 grams
56 grams × 9 kcal/gram = 504 kcal; 140 grams × 9 kcal/
grams = 1260 kcal

$$\frac{504}{3600} = 14\% \qquad \frac{1260}{3600} = 35\%$$

Fat intake = 14% to 35% of 3600 kcal

Adapted from Carlson (2008) and Rodriguez, et al, (2009).

gender, or female reproductive status. Athletes should choose healthy carbohydrates, whole grains, legumes, fruits, and vegetables as part of a balanced diet. Guidelines for carbohydrate intake during exercise are listed in Table 15-7. If an individual has no time to eat before an event, consuming 30 grams of carbohydrate in easy

to digest foods (grits, bagel, banana, or yogurt) 5 to 10 minutes before it starts may improve performance. Recreational athletes who work out 3 or 4 times a week and are eating carbohydrates with meals probably do not need to supplement with extra carbohydrate before exercising (Rosenbloom, 2012).

The maximum amount of glucose that can be oxidized is 60 grams per hour. More than that can lead to gastrointestinal discomfort. Ultraendurance athletes who exercise for 4 hours or longer can consume up to 90 grams of carbohydrate per hour if multiple sources of carbohydrate (sucrose, glucose, fructose) are used because the gut uses different transporters for each (Rosenbloom, 2012).

Carbohydrate intake also is necessary after exercise to restore glycogen stores. Ingesting 1.2 to 1.5 grams of carbohydrate per kilogram of body weight per hour appears to maximize glycogen synthesis for 4 to 5 hours after exercise (Williams, 2014).

Recommended distribution of macronutrients for athletes (see Clinical Calculation 15-1) clearly emphasizes carbohydrate intake. Elite Kenyan runners consume 75% of their kilocalories as carbohydrate (Carlson, 2008). They are also very lean, an advantage in their sport, which demands economy of motion. Weightlifters, in contrast, benefit from an increased body mass, particularly muscle mass (Williams, 2014). A perceived need to minimize body size to succeed in some sports can lead to the Female Athlete Triad (see Chapter 11).

PROTEIN AND AMINO ACIDS

Because most athletes consume adequate amounts of protein due to high kilocaloric intakes, supplemental protein is unnecessary. The use of amino acid or powdered protein supplements are not better than intact, high-quality protein foods when adequate energy is consumed (Sandon, 2011). Both resistance and endurance training exercise induce protein catabolism during exercise, but protein synthesis predominates in the postexercise recovery period (Williams, 2014). Exercise, particularly resistance exercise, has an interactive effect with ingested protein leading to positive muscle protein balance. Although the response might be slightly greater when protein is ingested immediately following exercise, the effect lasts 24 hours, so each ingestion of protein during that time results in

TABLE 15-7 ■ Advice for CHO Intake During Exercise

APPROACH	ATHLETE'S SKILL LEVEL	DURATION	CHO INTAKE	RATIONALE
Traditional	All	All	30 to 60 grams/hour	Improved performance even during short, high-intensity exercise
New	All	2–3 hours	60 grams/hour	Presumed limit of effective CHO metabolism
	Well trained and conditioned	>2.5 hours	90 grams/hour from multiple sources (i.e., glucose + fructose)	Different sources utilize different intestinal transporters

Adapted from Cermak and van Loon, 2013; Jeukendrup, 2010, 2013.

accretion of muscle protein (Tipton, 2011). Milk has repeatedly been shown to acutely increase muscle protein synthesis and to lead to lean mass gains; it may also decrease muscle damage when consumed after exercise (Sandon, 2011).

The American College of Sports Medicine, the American Dietetic Association, and Dietitians of Canada (Rodriguez, DiMarco, Langley, et al, 2009) concluded that protein requirements are higher in very active persons than in the general population, suggesting daily amounts of:

- 1.2 to 1.7 grams per kilogram of body weight in resistance athletes
- 1.2 to 1.4 grams in endurance athletes

These amounts are approximately 50% to 100% higher than the RDA, but well within the AMDR of 10% to 35% of daily energy intake given additional kilocalories the athletes require. Meeting these requirements can be achieved by consuming natural food sources (Williams, 2014). No benefit has been found for consuming more than 2 grams per kilogram per day (Sandon, 2011).

A vegetarian diet per se is not associated with detrimental effects in athletes, but an optimal protein intake should be achieved through careful planning with an emphasis on protein-rich plant foods. **Rhabdomyolysis** has occurred in a young athlete following a poorly planned vegetarian diet (Borrione, Spaccamiglio, Salvo, et al, 2009).

Individual amino acid supplements and related protein metabolites are not considered to be effective in improving exercise performance (Williams, 2014). Also, the maximum amount of protein that most adults can use per day is 0.9 grams per pound of body weight (Chicago Academy of Nutrition and Dietetics, undated).

A comparison of three sports protein supplements sold on the Internet by major retailers appears in Dollars & Sense 15-1. A fourth seller did not include the information sought for comparison. The cost for 10 grams of protein from the sampled whey protein supplements exceeds that of 60% of the food items analyzed in Dollars & Sense 4-3.

Case reports linking whey protein supplements to acne in adult males and adolescents also might give a potential user pause:

- Five adult male bodybuilders developed acne after consumption of whey protein (Simonart, 2012).
- Five male clients aged 14 to 18 years experienced onset of acne shortly after beginning supplementation with at least 6 different brands of whey protein supplements. All responded poorly to acne treatment regimens (Silverberg, 2012).

Acne vulgaris has been linked to milk ingestion, both whole and skim milk. Whey protein may be the fraction of dairy products that promotes acne formation (Silverberg, 2012).

The questionable efficacy of supplements as well as the expense and possible side effects should encourage an athlete to seek protein in food, not supplements.

WATER

Normal hydration is the goal for athletes. Dehydration degrades aerobic exercise and mental performance in warm to hot environments. Fluids should be consumed during exercise to prevent excessive dehydration (loss of more than 2% of body weight).

Sweat losses vary depending on:

- The activity
- Clothing
- Equipment
- Environmental conditions
- Individual differences in sweat rates

Serious athletes may sweat from 0.5 to 2 liters per hour. Some football players, often with large body weights, reportedly can lose 8 liters of sweat per day in hot weather. Customized plans for fluid intake can be designed based on sweat rates estimated from weight lost during exercise. Replacing only the fluids lost is the goal. Drinking at least 16 to 20 ounces of fluid, emphasizing sports drinks for the sodium content, for every pound that was lost while exercising is recommended (Rosenbloom, 2012). Skeletal muscle cramps are thought to be related to dehydration, electrolyte deficits,

$ Dollars & Sense 15-1

Comparison of Sports Powdered Whey Vanilla Supplements

Product	Price	Package	Serving Size	Protein Grams/serving	CHO Grams/serving	Cost/serving	Cost/10 Grams of Protein*
A	$19.99	2 lb	1.2 oz	25	3	$0.74	$0.296
B	$29.49	2 lb	1.1 oz	24	4	$1.01	$0.424
C	$17.99	14.1 oz	0.95 oz	15	5 (fiber)	$1.21	$0.808

*Compare to Dollars & Sense 4-3.

and muscle fatigue (American College of Sports Medicine, Sawka, Burke, et al, 2007).

Possibly refuting that theory, triathlon participants displayed no significant differences between athletes with cramps and those without in prerace–postrace serum electrolyte concentrations and body weight changes (Schwellnus, Drew, and Collins, 2011). An alternative theory, altered neuromuscular control, is suggested as the principal pathophysiological mechanism causing exercise associated muscle cramps (Schwellnus, 2009).

Hydration before, during, and after exercise is essential nonetheless. Athletes are more likely to voluntarily replace fluid losses when beverages are cold, flavored, and sweetened (Sandon, 2011). See Clinical Application 15-7 for suggestions to maintain hydration. Specially formulated sports drinks are necessary for:

- Extended exercise duration
- Hot, humid climates
- High sweat rates
- Individuals who lose salt (Sandon, 2011)

An ideal recovery beverage should not only contain carbohydrate and protein but also electrolytes, including about 0.3 to 0.7 grams sodium per liter of fluid to help restore sodium lost through sweat (Spaccarotella and Andzel, 2011). Low-fat chocolate milk consists of a 4:1 carbohydrate:protein ratio (similar to many commercial recovery beverages) and provides fluids and sodium to aid in post-workout recovery. Consuming chocolate milk immediately after exercise and again at 2 hours postexercise appears to be optimal for exercise recovery and may attenuate indices of muscle damage (Pritchett and Pritchett, 2013).

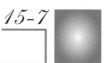

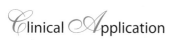

Hydration Suggestions for Athletes

In amounts:

- Day before competition, drink enough to ensure adequate hydration.
- At least 4 hours before exercise, slowly drink about 5 to 7 mL of fluid/kg body weight.
- If no urine is produced or if urine is dark 2 hours before exercise, drink another 2 to 3 mL/kg body weight.
- Do not drink excessively to avoid dilutional hyponatremia.
  In fluids chosen, carbohydrate-electrolyte solutions:
  - Containing 6% to 8% carbohydrate to help increase body stores of glucose and glycogen
  - Containing 20 to 50 mEq sodium/liter and/or salty foods or snacks to help stimulate thirst and retain fluid

Sources: Rosenbloom, 2012; Sandon, 2011; Williams, 2014.

Four hours after exercise, individuals who consumed milk or salted milk were in positive fluid balance, whereas those who consumed sports drinks or water were not (Sandon, 2011).

Consuming excessive water, however, can lead to electrolyte imbalances. During long events, an athlete's blood is shunted to the skeletal muscle with less blood flow to the kidneys. If fluids are overconsumed, the kidneys may not be able to excrete the excess fluid producing dilutional hyponatremia (American College of Sports Medicine, Sawka, Burke, et al, 2007). For examples, see Chapter 8.

Nonnutrients

Many ergogenic aids are promoted for athletes, some with little scientific evidence for efficacy and safety. Only four are included here based on availability of information in the medical literature: bicarbonate, creatine, caffeine, and glycerol. Bicarbonate, creatine, and caffeine, are supported by a strong research base (Maughan, Greenhaff, and Hespel, 2011).

BICARBONATE

Muscular activity generates lactic acid as a waste product with consequent lowering of blood pH. The ingestion of sodium bicarbonate before intense exercise may buffer lactic acid in the muscle cell, which could temper the metabolic acidosis that contributes to fatigue. Supplementation with buffer salts increases serum pH and may enhance performance in repetitive exercise tasks that maximize energy production for 1 to 6 minutes (Williams, 2014). For example, there is good evidence that sodium bicarbonate ingestion has improved multiple-sprint performance (Bishop, 2010).

Ingestion of such salts is generally considered safe but may cause acute gastrointestinal distress and diarrhea, which might be lessened by smaller doses over a longer time (Williams, 2014). The overall effect size for the influence of sodium bicarbonate on performance was moderate and was significantly lower for specifically trained as opposed to recreationally trained participants (Peart, Siegler, and Vince, 2012).

CREATINE

Creatine is a nonprotein substance synthesized in the body from the amino acids arginine, glycine, and methionine. Creatine is produced endogenously, mainly in the liver, kidneys, and to a lesser extent in the pancreas, at an amount of about 1 gram per day. Another 1 gram is obtained through an omnivorous diet predominantly derived from meats (Cooper, Naclerio, Allgrove, and Jimenez, 2012). When combined with phosphate, the resulting compound, phosphocreatine, serves as a storage form of energy that is released with anaerobic muscle contraction.

The mechanisms by which creatine acts in the human body to improve physical and cognitive performance are still not clear (Cooper, et al, 2012) but creatine has been recognized as the most effective nutritional supplement in enhancing exercise tolerance, muscle strength and lean body mass (Gualano, Roschel, Lancha-Jr, et al, 2012). Creatine supplementation has been shown to be effective on predominantly anaerobic intermittent exercise. It also can help to maintain total creatine pool after injury and to attenuate muscle damage induced by a prolonged endurance training session (Cooper, et al, 2012). Despite the general positive effects, some athletes are nonresponders (American Academy of Nutrition and Dietetics, January 2013). See Box 15-4.

The form of creatine that has been most extensively studied and commonly used in dietary supplements is creatine monohydrate. Studies have consistently indicated that creatine monohydrate supplementation increases muscle creatine and phosphocreatine concentrations by approximately 15% to 40%. Newer forms of creatine have been purported to have better physical and chemical properties, bioavailability, efficacy, and/or safety profiles than creatine monohydrate. However, there is little to no evidence that any of the newer forms of creatine are more effective and/or safer than creatine monohydrate whether ingested alone and/or in combination with other nutrients (Jäger, Purpura, Shao, et al, 2011).

Creatine supplementation has been shown to reduce the body's endogenous production of creatine; however, levels return to normal after a brief period of time when supplementation ceases. Although at present, ingesting creatine as an oral supplement is considered safe and ethical, safety cannot be guaranteed, especially when administered for a long period of time to different populations including the young and the elderly (Cooper, et al, 2012). Excess intake may cause diarrhea, and individuals with kidney or liver disease should consult their health-care provider before starting supplementation (Williams, 2014).

CAFFEINE

Caffeine mobilizes fat stores and stimulates working muscles to use fat as a fuel, which delays depletion of muscle glycogen and allows for prolonged exercise. The critical period in glycogen sparing appears to occur during the first 15 minutes of exercise, when caffeine has been shown to decrease glycogen utilization by as much as 50%. The effect on performance, which was observed in most experimental studies, was that participants were able to exercise longer before exhaustion occurred (Higgins, Tuttle, and Higgins, 2010). There is good evidence that caffeine can improve single-sprint and multiple-sprint performance (Bishop, 2010) and may enhance performance in prolonged, high-intensity, intermittent anaerobic exercise as needed for soccer and rugby (Williams, 2014). Caffeine has been shown to be an effective ergogenic aid for endurance athletes when ingested before and/or during exercise in moderate quantities, 3 to 6 milligrams per kilogram of body weight. Also, abstaining from caffeine for at least 7 days before use will optimize the effect (Higgins, et al, 2010), but larger doses do not add to the ergonomic effect (Williams, 2014).

As an ergogenic compound, caffeine raises the heart rate and blood pressure. Consequently, adverse effects, typically manifesting with ingestion of more than 200 milligrams of caffeine, include insomnia, nervousness, headache, rapid heart rate, arrhythmia, and nausea. Caffeine is also on the NCAA Banned Drugs List if concentrations in urine exceed 15 micrograms/milliliter (2013).

Caffeine is the most common stimulant in energy beverages, a relative newcomer to the market. Regulation of energy beverages, including content labeling and

---

Box 15-4 ■ *Fast- and Slow-Twitch Muscle Fibers*

Human muscles contain a genetically determined mixture of both slow and fast fiber types that seem to influence how muscles respond to training and physical activity. On average, individuals have about 50% slow-twitch and 50% fast-twitch fibers in most of the muscles used for movement (Quinn, 2012).

Slow-twitch (Type I) muscle fibers are more efficient at using oxygen to generate ATP for continuous, extended muscle contractions over a long time before becoming fatigued. They are helpful in aerobic exercise and distance or sustained events.

Fast-twitch muscle fibers (Type II) use anaerobic metabolism to create fuel and are much better at generating short bursts of strength or speed than slow-twitch muscle fibers but fatigue more quickly. Fast-twitch fibers generally produce the same amount of force per contraction as slow muscles, but they fire more rapidly. Having a greater number of fast-twitch muscle fibers is helpful for sprinters.

Genetics influences natural ability in various sports, whether they demand speed or strength. Olympic sprinters possess about 80% fast-twitch fibers, whereas marathoners have 80% slow-twitch fibers. Some research shows evidence of muscle fibers changing from one type to another, suggesting that fiber type can change with a vigorous training schedule (Cluett, 2004).

Regarding response to creatine supplementation, responders showed the greatest percentage of Type II (fast-twitch) muscle fibers followed by quasi-responders and nonresponders. Overall, responders have a lower initial level of total muscle creatine content and with a greater population of Type II fibers, thus a higher potential to improve performance in response to creatine supplementation (Cooper, et al, 2012).

health warnings, differs across countries, with some of the laxest requirements in the United States. Therefore, it should be no surprise that the United States ranks as the world's largest consumer at roughly 290 million gallons in 2007, or 3.8 quarts per person per year. Hundreds of different brands of energy beverages are now marketed, with caffeine content ranging from a modest 50 mg to an alarming 505 mg per can or bottle. By comparison, an 8-oz cup of coffee contains:

- 110 to 150 milligrams for drip
- 65 to 125 milligrams for percolated
- 40 to 80 milligrams for instant.

In addition to caffeine however, energy beverages contain an array of other ingredients, the effects of which, singly or in combination, remain unstudied (Higgins, et al, 2010). For example, an otherwise healthy 28-year-old man in Australia consumed excessive amounts of a caffeinated "energy drink" throughout a day of motocross racing and suffered a cardiac arrest the following day (Berger and Alford, 2009).

GLYCEROL

To increase tolerance for fluid loss during exercise, athletes may attempt to hyperhydrate by consuming extra fluid before exercise. Because a large fluid intake is typically accompanied by diuresis, hyperhydrating is difficult. Enter glycerol with the capacity to enhance body fluid retention. Glycerol-containing beverages create an osmotic gradient in the circulation favoring fluid retention, thereby facilitating hyperhydration and protecting against dehydration (van Rosendal, Osborne, Fassett, and Coombes, 2010).

Glycerol-induced hyperhydration has been shown to increase endurance performance that starts declining at a dehydration level (loss of >2% of body weight). Consequently, glycerol-induced hyperhydration would be required only to fill the gap when athletes anticipate that they could not consume enough fluid during exercise to prevent dehydration. A method of calculating such a requirement is available (Goulet, 2010).

Glycerol hyperhydration can increase body water by one liter or more. Side effects from glycerol ingestion are rare, but include nausea, gastrointestinal discomfort, and light-headedness (Van Rosendal, et al, 2010). Moreover, for some sports, the increase in body weight from the retained fluid could be a detriment.

Advice for Athletes

Products marketed to athletes to provide the macronutrients needed before, during, and after exercise are not superior to ordinary foods but may

have some advantages. They are portable and pre-measured, thus convenient. Trying them out in training, not during competition, is wise. Whether a recovery shake is worth the expense when low fat chocolate milk or a hard-boiled egg will serve as well needs thoughtful decision-making (Rosenbloom, 2012). Before using any supplements, the athlete, with the advice of a health-care provider, parents, and coach, should evaluate the supplement carefully. Although most of the supplements described herein appear safe when using the recommended dose, the effects of higher doses (as often taken by athletes) on indices of health remain unknown, and further research is warranted. Finally, anecdotal reports suggest that team-sport athletes often ingest more than one dietary supplement, and little is known about the potential adverse effects of ingesting multiple supplements (Bishop, 2010).

The same advice given for the general dietary supplements applies to those marketed for athletes. Just because they are available OTC does not ensure safety. For most supplements, the evidence is weak or even completely absent (Maughan, Greenhaff, and Hespel, 2011). One 24-year-old man developed acute renal failure while taking creatine and multiple other supplements for bodybuilding. Fortunately, complete recovery followed discontinuation of the supplements (Thorsteinsdottir, Grande, and Garovic, 2006).

The list of prohibited substances of the World Anti-Doping Agency classifies the administration of several steroids in sports as doping. Besides the classical steroids, more and more products appear on the market for dietary supplements containing steroids that have never been marketed as approved drugs, mostly without proper labeling of the contents (Parr and Schänzer, 2010). Of 634 samples of nonhormonal supplements from 15 countries, 14.8% contained prohibited anabolic androgenic steroids not declared on the label (Geyer, Parr, Mareck, et al, 2004).

Every attempt should be made to ascertain quality of supplements and ingredients. Several certification programs provide testing facilities for manufacturers of both raw ingredients and end products to ensure the absence of prohibited substances (Maughan, Greenhaff, and Hespel, 2011).

Athletes should seek advice from qualified nutritionists. Sports nutrition is a specialty practice for dietitians who often assist professional and college athletes maximize their performances in their chosen activity through individualized nutrition prescriptions.

Some basic suggestions for fueling the body for high-energy expenditure sports appear in Table 15-8. The timing and distribution of nutrients is intended to ensure adequate glycogen levels and to maximize protein synthesis and recovery.

TABLE 15-8 ■ Exercise Fueling Basics for Athletes*

TIME	CHO	PROTEIN	FAT	WATER	EXAMPLE	RATIONALE
3–5 Hours Before Exercise; About ⅓ of Kilocalories for Day	60% of kcal	15%–20% of kcal	20%–25% of kcal			
45–60 Minutes Before Exercise	30–50 grams	10–15 grams	5 grams or less	2 cups	2 cups 1% fat chocolate milk (52 grams CHO 16 grams protein 6 grams fat)	Tops off glycogen stores that an overnight fast depletes. Increases fluid absorption: 2.7 grams of water bound to 1 gram of glycogen
0–60 Minutes After Exercise and Every 2–3 Hours Thereafter	90–110 grams	15–30 grams	Modest	1 cup per pound of weight lost	2 cups granola, 1 cup skim milk with ¼ cup powdered milk (130 grams CHO, 30 grams protein)	Milk, containing sodium and potassium, can help restore fluid balance also.

*Depending on athlete's size, the sport, environmental conditions, etc.
Adapted from Carlson, 2008; Pritchett and Prichett, 2013; Rosenbloom, 2012; Sehnert, 2008.

Responsibilities of Health-Care Professionals

The standards for hospital accreditation and client safety by the Joint Commission address existing or potential food–drug interactions, specifically considering the reduction of harms by anticoagulant therapy (Boullata and Hudson, 2012). Preventing or modifying pharmacodynamic effects of drug–nutrient–supplement interactions is a team effort involving physicians, pharmacists, dietitians, and nurses. Health-care agencies often assign the client teaching to certain members of the team to ensure that no one will be missed. For instance, pharmacists may be responsible for teaching clients receiving *warfarin* therapy and dietitians for teaching those receiving tube feedings. Nurses often do the discharge teaching and follow-up with a telephone call to field questions after the client returns home.

Persons at highest risk for food and drug interactions are those who:

■ Take many drugs, including alcohol
■ Require long-term drug therapy
■ Have poor or marginal nutrition
■ Are critically ill
■ Receive enteral or parenteral nutrition

The main predictors of drug–nutrient interactions in a client are:

■ Increased age
■ Multiple chronic illnesses
■ Current use of multiple medications and supplements (Chan, 2014)

The most commonly cited substances in interactions from three categories are:

■ Among supplements, St. John's wort
■ Among drugs, *warfarin*
■ Among foods, grapefruit juice

Polypharmacy, the concurrent use of a large number of drugs, is a risk factor for untoward reactions, particularly if the person is treated by many prescribers. The elderly are particularly vulnerable because they take more than 30% of prescription drugs that presumably are more potent than OTC drugs.

Regardless of the age of the client, each additional drug or dietary supplement exponentially increases the potential for interactions (Chan, 2014). The elderly are likely to be on long-term regimens for chronic diseases, further increasing the risk of adverse effects, as exemplified in Figure 15-4. Other groups at risk of food and drug interactions are infants and adolescents because of high nutrient needs and immature detoxification systems. Clinical Application 15-8 reviews triggers that should prompt a further search for drug–nutrient interactions.

The consequences of improper scheduling of drugs and foods or nutrients can be:

■ Treatment failure
■ Toxicity
■ Increased expense

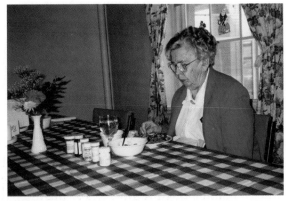

FIGURE 15-4 This woman has several risk factors for drug–nutrient interactions. She is elderly, is on a multiple-drug regimen, and takes some of her medications with a meal.

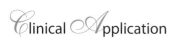 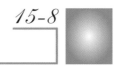

15-8

Clinical Application

Screening Clients at Risk for Drug–Nutrient Interactions

Further nutritional assessment may be in order if a client:

- Reports a recent weight change.
- Abuses alcohol.
- Consumes a modified diet, prescribed or self-imposed, including one with significant changes in protein content.
- Receives tube feedings.
- Takes many medications or dietary supplements, some with meals, some known to interfere with nutrition.
- Shows worsening of signs and symptoms of disease.
- Displays laboratory values indicating nutrient depletion.

Health-care providers should keep up with the scientific findings to counsel clients appropriately. Overbroad prohibitions should be avoided because some complementary and alternative medicine therapies may improve the client's well-being. Also, a client's autonomous choices should not be unduly skewered by unfounded concerns (Gilmour, Harrison, Asadi, et al, 2011). On the other hand, the possibility of identifying the client's inherent ability to metabolize drugs to the best advantage offers exciting opportunities to individualize treatment and minimize interactions.

Keystones

- Persons at risk for food–drug interactions are those who take many drugs, require long-term medication therapy, have immature or impaired metabolic systems, or receive enteral or parenteral nutrition, any of which can result in treatment failure, drug toxicity, or nutritional deficiency.

- Interactions can take place in the delivery device (Type I: *ceftriaxone* with calcium-containing IV solutions) or within the body by affecting absorption and bioavailability (Type II: *simvastatin* with grapefruit juice), cellular or tissue distribution (Type III: excessive cooked greens with *warfarin*), or disposition by the liver or kidneys (Type IV: irregular sodium intake with *lithium*).

- Separating grapefruit juice from drugs metabolized by CYP3A4 is an inadequate intervention because the juice and drug do not interact directly. Rather the juice inhibits intestinal CYP3A4 causing the excessive bioavailability of the drug to last several days until the intestine produces more of the enzyme.

- The most commonly cited interactions, sometimes life-threatening, involve grapefruit juice, *warfarin*, or St. John's wort interacting with each other or with another food, drug, or dietary supplement.

- To avoid the formation of insoluble compounds with calcium, iron, magnesium, and zinc, the following drugs should be separated from substances containing those metal cations: ciprofloxacin, norfloxacin, ofloxacin, and tetracycline.

- When a client taking MAOIs consumes foods or beverages high in tyramine, the drugs prevent the normal breakdown of tyramine, which leads to excessive epinephrine that produces hypertension, sometimes severe. A tyramine-restricted diet limits selected foods in every food group except grains.

- In the United States, prescription and OTC drugs are tested in randomized, double-blind clinical trials before being marketed. Food label information must be supported by research or scientific agreement. In contrast, dietary supplements can be sold unless shown by the FDA to be unsafe, adulterated, or labeled in a misleading manner.

- *Warfarin* achieves anticoagulation by competing with vitamin K at its binding sites, thus inhibiting the synthesis of vitamin K–dependent clotting factors. To attain therapeutic goals, the client should avoid large swings in the intake of foods high in vitamin K, mainly green leafy vegetables. Elimination of food is unnecessary; consistency of intake is key.

(Continued)

Keystones—cont'd

■ Persons taking dietary supplements should be aware of the risks associated with their production, not assume "natural" products are inherently safe, obtain as much credible information as possible, and always inform their health-care providers of their use.

■ Athletes should consume a healthy diet emphasizing appropriate proportions of carbohydrate and protein for their body and sport, take care to hydrate appropriately, and, if dietary supplements are desired, select those certified to contain labeled ingredients and no substances prohibited for athletes.

CASE STUDY *15-1*

Mr. K, a 48-year-old accountant, is admitted to the hospital for treatment of deep vein thrombosis (DVT) and correction of INR of 1.2 signifying almost no therapeutic effect of his prescribed *warfarin*. His treatment of DVT includes intravenous administration of the antithrombotic heparin until oral *warfarin* level becomes therapeutic between 2.0 and 3.0. (See Type III Interactions for mechanism.) His admitting nurse recorded a previous episode of thrombophlebitis 5 months ago for which he has been medicated with *warfarin* and monitored with blood work to prevent recurrence.

The factors possibly contributing to his current illness relate to a road trip Mr. K took to his 30th high school reunion. He drove 13 hours, virtually nonstop, both going to the reunion and returning. In addition, Mr. K described his food intake on his trip as significantly different from usual. He "pigged out" on Southern cooking, consuming large amounts of cooked greens at least twice a day over the 4-day reunion. "But I didn't eat any of the salads," he said. He could not recall specifics of the dietary instruction he had received during his initial bout with thrombophlebitis except that he needed to equalize intake of green, leafy vegetables.

A vitamin K–controlled diet was ordered for him and a consultation with the RD scheduled. On the basis of these data and his observations, the admitting nurse prepared a care plan. The portion of it pertinent to food and drug interactions appears below.

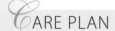

CARE PLAN

Subjective Data

Takes prescribed *warfarin* at same time each day ■ Faithful in reporting for blood work and keeping follow-up appointments ■ Significant change in vitamin K–containing foods in the past 10 days

Objective Data

Wearing *warfarin* Medic Alert bracelet
INR = 1.2 in doctor's office before admission

Analysis

Lack of correct information regarding self-care related to food–drug interaction as evidenced by described recent food intake contributing to DVT

Plan

DESIRED OUTCOMES/ EVALUATION CRITERIA	ACTIONS/INTERVENTIONS	RATIONALE
Client will understand requirements of diet related to *warfarin* therapy by discharge.	Schedule RD consultation.—Done	RD will individualize diet prescription.
	Observe food intake on actual vitamin K–restricted diet.	Current practices should clarify educational needs.

CASE STUDY *(Continued)*

DESIRED OUTCOMES/ EVALUATION CRITERIA	ACTIONS/INTERVENTIONS	RATIONALE
Client will prepare for dietitian's consultation by listing food preferences related to vitamin K content.	Provide writing materials if necessary. Prompt with questions about usual daily intake.	Review of current practices may stimulate questions to ask the dietitian.
Client will state that the key to successful *warfarin* therapy is day-to-day consistency of vitamin K intake.	Emphasize RD will individualize diet plan to accommodate preferences. Stress consistency of intake of foods high in vitamin K is essential to successful *warfarin* therapy.	Advance preparation will maximize effect of RD's instruction. Review and redundancy enhances learning.

15-1

Dietitian's Notes—next day

The following notes are representative of the documentation found in a client's medical record.

Subjective: Had been classifying any raw green vegetable as forbidden by his diet. Thought cooking destroyed vitamins, including vitamin K, and therefore cooked vegetables would be safe to eat as desired. Favorite vegetables include broccoli, Brussels sprouts, cabbage, "and greens if someone cooks them."

Objective: INR today 1.5

Nurse's note states he did not eat the tossed salad with broccoli and lettuce served for dinner, stating, "They're not on my diet." Reminded that he was served a vitamin K–controlled diet.

Analysis: Faulty understanding of diet for warfarin therapy

Plan: Client will demonstrate 100% proficiency at identifying amounts of vegetables represented by food models.

Client will demonstrate 80% proficiency at sorting preferred foods with significant vitamin K content into a quasi-exchange daily dietary pattern.

Client will report to RD by telephone the result of his first postdischarge INR and his progress regarding dietary intake.

𝒞ritical 𝒯hinking 𝒬uestions

1. What other information about meals might the RD have obtained that would bear on the ability of this client to maintain a vitamin K–restricted diet?

2. In light of the anticoagulation failure just described, do you believe this client is motivated to improve his lifestyle to avoid future occurrences of thrombophlebitis? Why or why not?

3. Would this situation be likely to have developed in the same way if the client had been a woman? Why or why not?

Chapter Review

1. Which of the following clients is at greatest risk for food–drug interaction?
   a. A 50-year-old man with no current disease who takes one baby aspirin daily to prevent heart disease
   b. A 75-year-old woman taking medication for several chronic diseases
   c. A 39-year-old man who usually consumes two cocktails before dinner
   d. A 25-year-old pregnant woman who is taking a prenatal vitamin supplement and calcium tablets

2. For which of the following items is there most agreement that athletes require increased amounts compared with more sedentary individuals?
   a. Creatine
   b. Glucosamine
   c. Glycerol
   d. Protein

3. Which of the following statements by a client prescribed simvastatin would indicate he understood the instructions?
   a. "One glass of grapefruit juice a day is as much as I can have."
   b. "I can have grapefruit juice for breakfast since I take the pill at bedtime."
   c. "I won't drink grapefruit juice while I am taking this drug."
   d. "I can start with 1 ounce of grapefruit juice and work up to 4 ounces over a month's time."

4. A client taking lithium is most likely to experience increased mania with:
   a. Decreased fluid intake and decreased sodium intake
   b. Decreased fluid intake and increased potassium intake
   c. Increased sodium intake and decreased potassium intake
   d. Increased sodium intake and increased fluid intake

5. Individuals following a vitamin K–controlled diet as outlined in the text may have three servings per day of all of the following except:
   a. Cooked collards or spinach
   b. Raw broccoli or spinach
   c. Endive or Romaine lettuce
   d. Asparagus and leaf lettuce

Clinical Analysis

Mr. A is being admitted to a long-term care facility. He is a 45-year-old posttrauma client. The motor vehicle accident in which he became paralyzed below the waist also killed his wife and daughter. The accident occurred 6 months ago. In the meantime, he has been treated at a rehabilitation center. He is depressed and freely shares his feelings of guilt and loss. The depression has interfered with his progress toward rehabilitation and also contributed to a 20-pound weight loss since the accident. After many trials of various antidepressants, he is now receiving *phenelzine*. The following questions relate to his care.

1. Close attention to Mr. A's diet is essential. Which of the following foods will he have to avoid completely?
   a. Baked beans, dates, and roast beef
   b. Sugar, molasses, and maple syrup
   c. Bologna, cheddar cheese, and wine
   d. Green beans, whole-wheat bread, and oranges

Clinical Analysis—cont'd

2. When teaching nursing assistants about the dietary restrictions needed by Mr. A, the nurse should be sure the nursing assistants understand that:
   a. The potential complication can be life-threatening.
   b. Mr. A is to be kept unaware of the seriousness of his condition.
   c. As time goes on, the forbidden foods can be added to the diet slowly, one at a time.
   d. If Mr. A does not cooperate in his dietary care, his paralysis is likely to worsen.

3. Ms. O is seeking advice at a clinic before becoming sexually active. She is leaning toward the use of oral contraceptives. She tells the nurse that she takes some herbal products "to keep my strength up and get me through the day." Which of the following products would raise the greatest concern for the nurse?
   a. Natural vitamin C from rose hips
   b. Ginger
   c. St. John's wort
   d. Protein supplement for athletes

16

Weight Management

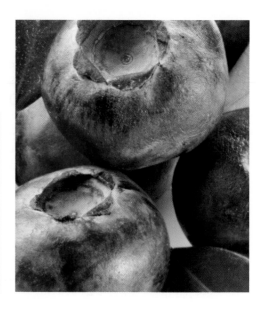

LEARNING OBJECTIVES

After completing this chapter, the student should be able to:

- List basic principles of energy imbalance.
- Discuss the effects of weight loss on the body.
- Identify the medical, psychological, and social problems associated with too much and too little body fat.
- Discuss the federal guidelines for the identification, evaluation, and treatment of overweight and obesity in adults.
- Describe the symptoms commonly exhibited by a client with anorexia nervosa and/or bulimia.
- Evaluate at least three fad diets used for weight reduction.

Weight management is a concern not only from a personal viewpoint but also from a societal perspective. Consequences of excessive body weight cause many individuals to suffer economically, socially, mentally, and physically (see Dollars & Sense 16-1).

Studies have repeatedly shown that at any one point in time, more than 40% of the population describe themselves as trying to lose weight. Approximately 85% of those who lose weight will regain their original weight within 5 years. Although this sounds dismal, it also means that 15% of all people who lose weight are successful over the long term. Weight management, although difficult, is not impossible, and the financial and health benefits of weight control, both to the individual and society, are enormous.

Terminology and Classification

Historically the classification of people as underweight, normal weight, overweight, and obese has been a challenge for practitioners. Yet how a person is classified is becoming more important. Third-party payers (insurance companies and state and federal governments) want an individual to meet specific criteria before they will grant financial approval for treatments. Percentage body fat is the true measure of how to classify clients, but there are problems with this measurement. Therefore, body mass index (BMI) and waist circumference are the most commonly used methods for classifying clients (Table 16-1).

$ Dollars & Sense 16-1

Costs of Obesity

According to a national study, costs associated with obesity demonstrated a cost of $1429 more for obese patients compared to those of normal weight and total annual health-care costs of $147 billion in associated costs related to obesity in 2008 (CDC, 2012). Approximately one-half of these costs were paid for by Medicaid and Medicare. These costs do not include the indirect costs attributed to obesity such as absenteeism and decreased productivity.

TABLE 16-1 ■ Classification of Overweight and Obesity by BMI, Waist Circumference, and Associated Disease Risks

| | BMI (kg/m²) | Obesity Class | DISEASE RISK* RELATIVE TO NORMAL WEIGHT AND WAIST CIRCUMFERENCE† | |
			Men 102 cm (40 in.) or Less Women 88 cm (35 in.) or Less	Men >102 cm (40 in.) Women >88 cm (35 in.)
Underweight	<18.5		—	—
Normal	18.5–24.9		—	—
Overweight	25.0–29.9		Increased	High
Obesity	30.0–34.9	I	High	Very high
	35.0–39.9	II	Very high	Very high
Extreme Obesity	40.0+	III	Extremely high	Extremely high

*Disease risk for type 2 diabetes, hypertension, and CVD.
†Increased waist circumference also can be a marker for increased risk, even in persons of normal weight.
Source: National Heart, Lung, and Blood Institute. Available at www.nhlbi.nih.gov/health/public/heart/obesity/lose_wt/bmi_dis.htm.

Percentage Body Fat

An individual's percentage body fat is associated with her or his health risk. The most accurate definition for obesity is a body fat content greater than 30% to 33%. The exact percentage is defined differently by various professional groups. The optimal fat content for females is 18% to 22%. The optimal fat content for males is 15% to 19%. Women tend to present with about a 10% higher body fat composition compared with men. However, percentage body fat is expensive to measure accurately.

Techniques used to measure body fat involve underwater weighing, tissue x-ray examinations, ultrasound, electrical conductivity, computed tomographic scans, and magnetic resonance imaging scans. Electrical impedance is used by some health-care workers, but this method is gaining disfavor because of a lack of consistent results. Limitations include less accuracy in extremely obese persons; overhydration and underhydration; hormone abnormalities; and the need for a qualified technician. Thus, measurement of body fat is of limited usefulness for persons trying to lose weight. The other procedures previously mentioned are expensive and not available in clinical settings.

Body Mass Index

The National Institutes of Health (NIH) recommends and encourages all health-care professionals to use BMI to classify clients as underweight, normal weight, overweight, and obese in clinical settings. The classification of an individual as underweight, normal weight, overweight, and obese is defined according to BMI:

- Underweight <18.5
- Normal 18.5 to 24.9
- Overweight 25 to 29.9

- Obese class 1 >30
- Severely obese class 2 >35
- Morbidly obese class 3 >40
- Super obese >50

Individuals can calculate their own BMI using Clinical Calculation 16-1. Or they can use a Body Mass Index Chart (Table 16-2) to determine BMI without doing any calculations. The more complex calculation for BMI is weight in kilograms divided by height in meters squared. There are also online calculators and applications that can be downloaded to mobile phones at http://nhlbisupport.com/bmi.

Although BMI correlates with the amount of body fat a person has, it does not measure body fat. Some athletes may have a BMI that identifies them as overweight, but they do not have excessive amounts of body fat. The extra pounds are lean body mass acquired from rigorous training.

Similarly, a teen with a normal BMI may have all the health-related consequences of obesity if the client has a high body fat content of greater than 33%. The teen

16-1

𝒞linical 𝒞alculation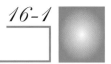

Steps in Calculating BMI

A BMI can be calculated in three easy steps.

1. Multiply weight in pounds by 703.
2. Multiply height in inches by height in inches.
3. Divide the product of step 1 by the product of step 2.

    For example, for a 166-pound person who is 5 ft 6 in. or 66 in. tall:

1. 166 × 703 = 116,698
2. 66 × 66 = 4356
3. 116,698 divided by 4356 = 26.7

TABLE 16-2 ■ Body Mass Index Chart

BMI	19	20	21	22	23	24	25	26	27	28	29	30	31	32	33	34	35	36
Height (Inches)								Body Weight (Pounds)										
58	91	96	100	105	110	115	119	124	129	134	138	143	148	153	158	162	167	172
59	94	99	104	109	114	119	124	128	133	138	143	148	153	158	163	168	173	178
60	97	102	107	112	118	123	128	133	138	143	148	153	158	163	168	174	179	184
61	100	106	111	116	122	127	132	137	143	148	153	158	164	169	174	180	185	190
62	104	109	115	120	126	131	136	142	147	153	158	164	169	175	180	186	191	196
63	107	113	118	124	130	135	141	146	152	158	163	169	175	180	186	191	197	203
64	110	116	122	128	134	140	145	151	157	163	169	174	180	186	192	197	204	209
65	114	120	126	132	138	144	150	156	162	168	174	180	186	192	198	204	210	216
66	118	124	130	136	142	148	155	161	167	173	179	186	192	198	204	210	216	223
67	121	127	134	140	146	153	159	166	172	178	185	191	198	204	211	217	223	230
68	125	131	138	144	151	158	164	171	177	184	190	197	203	210	216	223	230	236
69	128	135	142	149	155	162	169	176	182	189	196	203	209	216	223	230	236	243
70	132	139	146	153	160	167	174	181	188	195	202	209	216	222	229	236	243	250
71	136	143	150	157	165	172	179	186	193	200	208	215	222	229	236	243	250	257
72	140	147	154	162	169	177	184	191	199	206	213	221	228	235	242	250	258	265
73	144	151	159	166	174	182	189	197	204	212	219	227	235	242	250	257	265	272
74	148	155	163	171	179	186	194	202	210	218	225	233	241	249	256	264	272	280
75	152	160	168	176	184	192	200	208	216	224	232	240	248	256	264	272	279	287
76	156	164	172	180	189	197	205	213	221	230	238	246	254	263	271	279	287	295

Height (Inches)								Body Weight (Pounds)										
58	177	181	186	191	196	201	205	210	215	220	224	229	234	239	244	248	253	258
59	183	188	193	198	203	208	212	217	222	227	232	237	242	247	252	257	262	267
60	189	194	199	204	209	215	220	225	230	235	240	245	250	255	261	266	271	276
61	195	201	206	211	217	222	227	232	238	243	248	254	259	264	269	275	280	285
62	202	207	213	218	224	229	235	240	246	251	256	262	267	273	278	284	289	295
63	208	214	220	225	231	237	242	248	254	259	265	270	278	282	287	293	299	304
64	215	221	227	239	238	244	250	256	262	267	273	279	285	291	296	302	308	314
65	222	228	234	240	246	252	258	264	270	276	282	288	294	300	306	312	318	324
66	229	235	241	247	253	260	266	272	278	284	291	297	303	309	315	322	328	334
67	236	242	249	255	261	268	274	280	287	293	299	306	312	319	329	331	338	344
68	243	249	256	262	269	276	282	289	295	302	308	315	329	328	335	341	348	354
69	250	257	263	270	277	284	291	297	304	311	318	324	331	338	349	351	358	365
70	257	264	271	278	285	292	299	306	313	320	327	334	341	348	355	362	369	376
71	265	272	279	286	293	301	308	315	322	329	338	343	351	358	365	379	379	386
72	272	279	287	294	302	309	316	324	331	338	346	353	361	368	375	383	390	397
73	280	288	295	302	310	318	325	333	340	348	355	363	371	378	386	393	401	408
74	287	295	303	311	319	326	334	342	350	358	365	373	381	389	396	404	419	420
75	295	303	311	319	327	335	343	351	359	367	375	383	391	399	407	415	423	431
76	304	312	320	328	336	344	353	361	369	377	385	394	402	410	418	426	435	443
BMI	37	38	39	40	41	42	43	44	45	46	47	48	49	50	51	52	53	54

To use the table, find the appropriate height in the left-hand column. Move across to a given weight. The number at the top of the column is the BMI at that height and weight. Pounds have been rounded off.

may have a history of minimal physical activity and poor food choices. The health-care professional should carefully evaluate the results of any BMI measurement along with other nutritional assessments (laboratory data, physical examination, and diet history).

Waist Circumference

Waist circumference is also used to classify fat distribution and central obesity. Waist circumference has emerged as an independent predictor of cardiometabolic disease including insulin resistance, diabetes, and cardiovascular disease (Grossniklaus, Gary, Higgins, and Dunbar, 2010). Women with a waist circumference greater than 35 inches and men with a waist circumference greater than 40 inches are at a higher health risk than those with a lower waist circumference (NIH, 2014). The NIH recommends waist circumference measurement for both the ease of measurement and low cost.

Prevalence and Incidence of Overweight and Obesity

The prevalence of obesity in the United States has had a startling increase since the mid-1970s. Figure 16-1 illustrates these trends more dramatically than words. **Prevalence** means the total number of cases of a specific disease divided by the number of individuals in the population at a certain time.

Many experts are concerned about the incidence and prevalence of obesity in the nation's children. **Incidence** is defined as the frequency of occurrence of any event or condition over time and in relation to the population in which it occurs. Asian American children have the lowest incidence of obesity. Native American children have the highest incidence of obesity. Thus, one could conclude obesity is partially genetic in origin. Data from two National Health and Nutrition Examination Surveys comparing obesity data from 1988–1994 and 2009–2010 demonstrate the following (Centers for Disease Control and Prevention [CDC], 2012):

- For non-Hispanic White boys, the prevalence of obesity increased from 11.6% to 17.5%.
- For non-Hispanic Black boys, the prevalence increased from 10.7% to 22.6%.
- For Mexican-American boys, the prevalence increased from 14.1% to 28.9%.

- For non-Hispanic White girls, the prevalence increased from 8.9% to 14.7%.
- For non-Hispanic Black girls, the prevalence increased from 16.3% to 24.8%.
- For Mexican-American girls, the prevalence increased from 13.4% to 18.6%.

Basic Science of Energy Imbalance

To understand the science of energy imbalance, think of the human body as a machine. Tens of thousands of researchers have spent years studying how the human body reacts to a kilocalorie imbalance. It is not adequate to say people weigh too much or too little because they overeat and do not exercise enough or vice versa. We need to ask: Why does someone's body seek or not seek food or exercise, when the human machine has adequate or inadequate energy available? What is not working? First, a brief outline of the science of energy imbalance follows.

Energy Imbalance

Energy imbalance results when the number of **kilocalories** eaten does not equal the number used for energy. An individual can determine whether food intake is meeting energy needs by monitoring

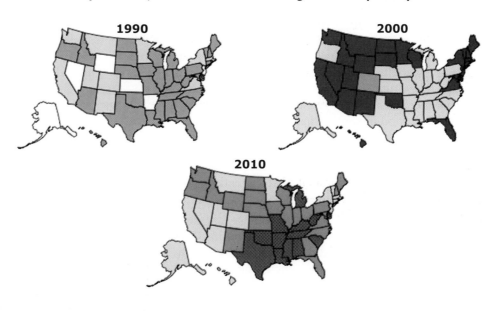

Obesity Trends* Among U.S. Adults
BRFSS, 1990, 2000, 2010
(*BMI ≥30, or about 30 lbs. overweight for 5'4" person)

1990

2000

2010

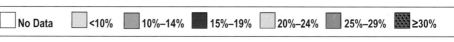

FIGURE 16-1 U.S. Obesity Trends 1990 to 2010 (www.cdc.gov/obesity/data/trends.html).

| | No Data | <10% | 10%–14% | 15%–19% | 20%–24% | 25%–29% | ≥30% |

his or her weight. If more kilocalories are eaten than are used by the body, weight gain will occur. If fewer kilocalories are eaten than are used by the body (and protein intake is adequate), weight loss will occur. (A low protein intake over an extended period will eventually lead to fluid retention and a subsequent weight gain from the fluid retained. In this situation, energy imbalance is difficult to ascertain by body weight alone.) Anyone can determine whether he or she is in energy balance by monitoring his or her weight over time. (This assumes normal hydration.)

There are two basic principles of energy imbalance. First, it takes a specific number of kilocalories to gain or lose a pound of body fat. Second, the body stores energy and uses that stored energy in a highly specific manner.

The Five-Hundred Rule

To lose 1 pound of body fat per week, an individual must eat 500 kilocalories fewer per day than his or her body *expends* for 7 days. To gain 1 pound of body fat per week, the individual must eat 500 kilocalories more per day for 7 days than his or her body expends. The gain or loss of body fat need not occur during the course of a week; the kilocalorie surplus or deficit may occur over a month or year. The principle is the same. The total number of kilocalories required to gain or lose a pound of body fat is 3500. Too many kilocalories from any source of carbohydrates, fat, and/or protein promote weight gain. The 500 rule means that weight loss is independent of diet composition.

The key term here is *expend*. As you learned in Chapter 5 on energy balance, the human body has some small subtle internal mechanisms that cause more or fewer kilocalories to be expended in some situations. The human body also has some small subtle internal mechanisms that cause the individual to eat more or less food in some situations.

Body Fat Stores

Excess kilocalories from any source (fat, carbohydrate, or protein) are stored as body fat in adipose fat tissue, which can accumulate in unlimited amounts. This accumulation can lead to overweight and, eventually, obesity. During a kilocalorie deficit, the body first seeks the energy necessary to sustain body functions in glycogen stores, which are limited. When a kilocalorie deficit occurs for longer than about 1 day, the body seeks the energy necessary to sustain its functions in both body fat stores (adipose tissue) and

protein stores (organ and muscle mass). Weight loss always includes some loss of lean body mass (LBM). How much LBM is lost depends on how the weight loss is achieved.

Energy Imbalance and Body Composition

Weight loss affects body composition, and body composition affects health. The human body's two largest components (after water) are fat and lean mass that includes protein. Protein is stored primarily in muscle tissue, organs, and certain body chemicals. Preservation of lean body mass and optimal health go hand in hand. A loss of structural body content (e.g., heart and respiratory muscles, kidney, liver, body chemicals) is undesirable. Exercise can preserve and somewhat increase lean body mass. Weight gain increases body fat content. Weight loss decreases both body fat and lean body mass. An understanding of the difference between body fat content and lean body mass content is crucial to understanding the science of energy imbalance. The health benefits of weight loss are all related to a loss of body fat and not a loss of lean body mass (see Genomic Gem 16-1).

Loss of Fat Versus Loss of Water and Protein

Most people, especially the overweight, can lose only about 2 pounds of body fat a week by eating less. Any weight loss beyond that is probably due to loss of water and/or lean muscle tissue. There is always some loss of body protein along with body fat during

---

Genomic Gem 16-1

Obesity Genetic or Environmental?

Research has demonstrated that among mothers who were obese during pregnancy, 52% of their offspring were obese during childhood, 62% at adolescence, and 44% during early adulthood (Rooney, Mathiason, & Schuberger, 2011) This does not mean that a child with a high complement of susceptibility genes will inevitably become overweight, but his or her genetic endowment gives them a stronger predisposition. Our environment gives children unprecedented opportunities to overeat and be sedentary. Therefore, nutritious food and participation in daily physical activity should be provided to counterbalance the effect of genetics and help should be given to those who are more susceptible to obesity.

weight loss. This loss occurs because lean body mass is more metabolically active and therefore burns more kilocalories than fat tissue. The loss of body protein from reduced food intake is greater than the loss of body protein from a combination of reduced food intake and regular exercise. Thus, physical activity during weight loss protects lean body mass. Also, the greater the rate of weight loss, the more LBM is lost.

Severity of Obesity and LBM

Weight loss affects body composition of lean and obese people differently. The amount of lean body mass an individual loses during weight reduction depends on the degree of severity of the obesity. Obese animals tolerate starvation better than thin ones, and the same is true of humans. *Tolerate* means that they conserve body protein during weight loss. This means overweight and mildly obese individuals are at a higher risk of becoming protein-depleted during rapid weight loss. Rapid weight loss (0.5 to 1.0 pounds per day), if sustained for many weeks, is associated with an excessive loss of lean body mass and protein depletion of the heart. Malnutrition of the heart muscle can lead to sudden death. As an individual loses more and more fat during rapid weight loss, the ability to conserve lean body mass decreases. Thus, the length of time an individual diets as well as his or her beginning total body fat content have an impact on the amount of lean body mass lost.

Consequences of Obesity

Obesity can lead to many adverse consequences. For example, the distribution of body fat affects a person's susceptibility to medical problems, and the **psychological** ramifications of obesity are significant. Clients are commonly enmeshed in a tangle of societal, cultural, prejudicial, and psychological issues. Many clients find great difficulty in breaking the cycle of behaviors that contribute to obesity. With an understanding of the issues, health-care providers can educate overweight and obese clients about the need for weight loss and encourage these clients to lose weight.

Social

The social consequences of obesity are connected to cultural expectations and the documented prejudice many obese people experience.

Cultural Expectations

Culture, in this context, refers to the convictions of a given people during a given period. Currently, many Americans perceive leanness as being attractive and desirable and fatness as being unattractive and undesirable. Some studies have demonstrated that culture can affect attitudes toward thinness. Black women often chose a larger ideal body type and are less affected by thin images, whereas white women are more dissatisfied with their weight (Baugh, Mullis, Mullis, et al, 2010). Yet what is and has been considered attractive has changed over time. Leanness has not always been the preferred body build. For example, during the 1800s, an overly fat body was considered the most attractive. Carrying excess weight meant that the person was well-to-do—that he or she could afford to overeat. Our society is slowly changing perceptions of what is attractive. For example, many perceive women with well-developed muscles as being more attractive than their lean, not-so-muscular counterparts. The increased numbers of female bodybuilders demonstrate this attitudinal shift.

In the United States, obese people have been under intense pressure to lose weight. Evidence of this pressure is the billions of dollars spent on weight-reduction programs and special foods each year. In an effort to be more attractive, many obese clients try to lose weight. Over time, however, most people regain the weight they have lost and commonly gain an additional few pounds. Thus, a self-defeating cycle begins. Clients generally need to be reminded that, although body weight is important, health and wellness are even more important.

Documented Prejudice

Research has documented health-care professionals, including both physicians and nurses, often have biases toward obese clients. Studies have demonstrated that health-care providers may view obese clients as noncompliant, lazy, and unattractive (Wolf, 2010). Health-care workers need to try to understand their own feelings about fatness, obesity, and obese persons. Sometimes, health-care workers unconsciously insult obese clients. For example, comments made in front of clients, such as "It will take three of us to move this client," are hurtful. Health-care providers should treat obese clients with respect, kindness, and patience.

Psychological

Obesity can be associated with a range of psychological problems, which may result from food restriction (Box 16-1). One important psychological consequence of obesity is body image disturbances.

> **Box 16-1** ■ *Psychological Consequences of Food Restriction*
>
> Food restriction, either voluntary or involuntary, has consequences. Xenophon in ancient Greece described a "ravenous hunger" in soldiers who had been deprived of food during a military campaign. During World War II, Keyes et al (1950) studied the effects of semistarvation on subjects. The effect of food restrictions in rats has also been studied. In many studies, the subjects responded to food deprivation with extraordinarily similar behaviors. First, restrained eaters did not necessarily have much, if any, long-term weight loss. Second, restraining one's eating made one highly susceptible to bouts of excessive eating even after restrictions were lifted. Third, study subjects exhibited **cognitive** and emotional changes when food was restricted, including heightened emotional responsiveness; cognitive disruptions, including distractibility; and a focus on food and eating (Polivy, 1996).
>
> Health-care providers need to caution clients about the consequences of restrained eating. Overweight clients need to be helped to give up their crash diets and to be advised to eat balanced healthful diets that include whole grains, fruits, vegetables, and nonfat dairy products. Abandonment of the short-term "diet mentality" and adoption of long-term lifestyle changes will enhance physical and psychological well-being.

Body Image Disturbances

Body image is the mental picture a person has of himself or herself. A disturbed body image can manifest itself in two ways. First, people with distorted body images are usually dissatisfied with their bodies. Chronic complaints, demands for extra attention, and frequent negative statements made by clients about the way they look may be signs of an underlying body image disturbance.

Second, persons with distorted body images frequently do not view their bodies realistically. For example, people may view themselves as having certain body parts larger than they actually are. A later section in this chapter discusses clients with anorexia nervosa, a mental health disorder, who frequently have body image disturbances. Very thin clients who have this condition frequently view themselves as overweight despite valid evidence to the contrary.

Medical

Obesity is considered a major health problem in the United States and is also considered a chronic medical condition. People who are overweight or obese are more likely to develop health problems such as:

- Hypertension
- Dyslipidemia (e.g., high total cholesterol or high levels of triglycerides)
- Type 2 diabetes

- Coronary heart disease
- Stroke
- Gallbladder and liver disease
- Osteoarthritis
- Sleep apnea and respiratory problems
- Gynecological problems (abnormal menses and infertility) (CDC, 2012)

The distribution of body fat affects risks. **Abdominal obesity,** in which excess weight is between the client's chest and pelvis, is more dangerous than gluteal-femoral obesity. Clients with abdominal obesity are said to be shaped like an apple and are especially vulnerable to chronic disease risks associated with excessive body weight. A man's waist should measure less than 40 inches (102 cm), and a women's waist should measure less than 35 inches (88 cm).

It is estimated that more than 50% of U.S. adults have abdominal obesity that increases their risk of developing insulin resistance, diabetes, and cardiovascular disease (Grossniklaus, Gary, Higgins, and Dunbar, 2010). In **gluteal-femoral obesity,** the excess weight is around the client's buttocks, hips, and thighs. Clients with gluteal-femoral obesity are said to be pear-shaped and are not as susceptible to chronic disease risks associated with excessive body fat.

The **waist-to-hip ratio** measures central distribution of fat. Waist-to-hip ratio is calculated by dividing waist circumference by hip circumference. A ratio of 1.0 or more in men and 0.85 or more in women indicates too much central weight compared with total body fat, which is a risk factor for obesity-related medical conditions (Swann, 2010).

Treating obesity is an important means of controlling some major chronic and degenerative diseases. For example, blood pressure levels can be reduced by a diet high in fruits and vegetables and low in fat. Up to 2½ cups of fruits and 4 cups of vegetables are recommended for a very active male 18-year-old. Up to 1½ cups of fruits and 2 cups of vegetables are recommended for a 65-year-old sedentary female.

Factors Influencing Food Intake

Lifestyle behaviors, appetite, satiety, and, questionably, macronutrient energy distribution influence food intake.

Lifestyle

These factors affect how much is eaten and influence kilocalorie consumption:

- Variety—The greater the variety of food served, the more kilocalories consumed.

- Taste—The better food tastes, the more is eaten.
- Weekend activity—Eating at regular times and planning non-food-related activities for weekends may assist in weight control.
- Skipping breakfast—People who regularly skip breakfast are more likely to be obese. Those eating four or more times daily are less likely to be obese. The fourth meal should be a small snack. Skipping meals is not a good weight-control strategy.
- Eating out—Eating meals away from home is associated with increased energy intake (Bezerra, Curioni, and Sichieri, 2012).
- Speed—The faster food is eaten, the more is consumed because it takes a little longer for satiety signals to reach the brain. The more foods need to be chewed, the fewer kilocalories are eaten because it takes time to chew the food.
- Soda intake—The consumption of sweetened soda is associated with excess energy intake (Taber, Stevens, Evenson, et al, 2011).
- Dietary fat—High dietary fat foods tend to be higher energy-dense foods.

Lifestyle behaviors that are responsible for *decreased* energy expenditure also increase body weight.

- Sedentary activities—The more hours spent on screen time, watching television, playing video games, or being on the computer, the less time is spent being physically active.
- Changes in energy expenditure—Small daily decreases in energy expenditure, such as getting up to change the channels on the television and opening the garage door manually may be significant over the course of a year.

Physiology

Numerous hormones and neuropeptides that stimulate or inhibit food intake through central and peripheral mechanisms have been identified. Molecules that affect metabolic rates and energy expenditure are also an area of current research. Figure 16-2 illustrates multiple molecules and pathways involved in the

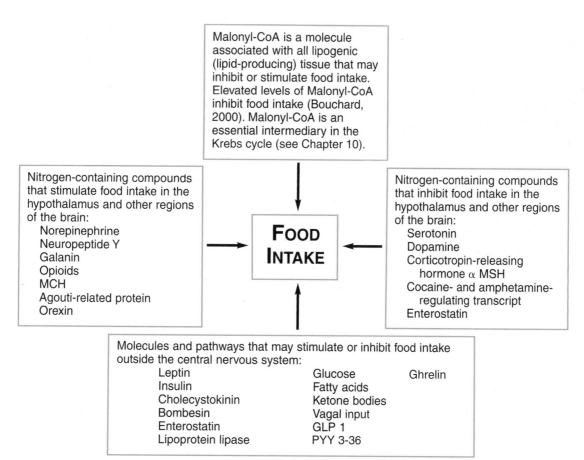

FIGURE 16-2 The hormones, molecules, and pathways that influence food intake through central or peripheral mechanisms. (Adapted from Bouchard, C: Inhibition of food intake by inhibitors of fatty acid synthase. N Engl J Med 343:25, 2000.)

internal regulation of food intake. In general, there is redundancy and counterbalance among these pathways so that, for instance, the inhibitory effect of one molecule is dampened by another. This intricate redundancy and counterbalance makes effective treatment of obesity complex. Perhaps as researchers learn more about the human energy balance system, more effective and safe treatments for imbalances may be available.

The brain, stomach, small intestine, and fat cells are all part of this complex energy balance system. The stomach, small intestines, and fat cells send messages to the brain to turn on or turn off eating. The triggers that influence food intake include satiety signals and hunger signals. When the brain, for instance, receives a satiety signal, animals stop eating.

Peptide hormones produced from the gastrointestinal tract are considered regulators of appetite and are released in response to nutritional stimuli (Moss, Dhillo, Frost, and Hickson, 2012). Ghrelin is one example of a gastric-made polypeptide that stimulates growth hormone and regulates food intake. Release of ghrelin increases food intake.

Neuropeptide Y is one example of a polypeptide in the brain that results in increased food intake. This chemical causes carbohydrate cravings, initiates eating, decreases energy expenditure, and increases fat storage. All of these actions favor positive energy balance and weight gain. Leptin, a protein made by fat cells, is a hormone that acts on the hypothalamus to decrease food intake. Leptin acts on receptors to counteract effects of feeding stimulants secreted by cells in the gut and in the hypothalamus. Interestingly, blood leptin levels are generally increased in obese individuals and are proportional to the total amount of visceral fat in the body (Klempel and Varady, 2011). This is a short summary of the many ways the body has evolved to cope and survive during repeated cycles of feast and famine. Appetite can also be influenced by gastrointestinal distention to decrease food intake and contractions of an empty stomach to increase food intake. Satiety signals are sent from this area to the brain.

Macronutrient Energy Composition

Researchers have conducted many studies on the role of macronutrient composition in energy balance. Following is a brief summary of this research. Protein has the greatest effect on satiety, followed by carbohydrate and then fat (Stubbs, Whybrow, and Lavin, 2010). The brain appears to need some carbohydrate (delivered as glucose) for an individual to achieve satiety. In addition, fiber expands the stomach to assist in counteracting the release of polypeptides that increase food intake. In summary, eating a well-balanced meal that is planned to provide the energy nutrients within the accepted macronutrient distribution range (AMDR) is the best approach to weight management.

Glycemic Index

A low glycemic diet may also help with weight management, although studies are still producing conflicting findings. Some experts believe that eating carbohydrates that have a low glycemic index (GI) may result in a spontaneous reduction in food intake. GI is a measure of how much the blood glucose level increases after consumption of a particular food that contains a given amount of carbohydrate. A slice of white bread or glucose is the reference food. All other foods' GIs are set in comparison to white bread or glucose and are ranked according to their potential to raise blood glucose compared with the reference white bread or glucose. Foods with a low GI are thought to promote satiety and decrease food intake. The glycemic index of mixed meals is not known. Following are some examples of the glycemic index of selected foods. Note: The reference food is white bread:

- White bread, 100
- Glucose, 138
- Fructose, 26
- Honey, 126
- Whole-wheat bread, 100
- Rye (whole grain, pumpernickel), 88
- Cornflakes, 121
- Banana, 84
- Baked potato, 116
- Kidney beans (canned), 74
- Ice cream, 69
- Sucrose, 83
- White rice (polished, boiled 10 to 25 minutes), 81
- Oatmeal, 85
- All-bran, 74
- Plum, 34
- Sweet potato, 70
- Lentils (green, canned), 74
- Skim milk, 46
- Orange, 59
- Orange juice, 71
- Yogurt, 52
- Soybeans (canned), 22

If the reference food is glucose, the numbers will be different, but not wrong. Many factors influence a food's GI. The rate of consumption and the time of day a food is eaten may increase or decrease a particular food's GI. Other components in a food besides carbohydrate influence a food's GI, including fat, fiber, and protein content and starch characteristics. How a food is prepared and processed influences GI. Physiological effects, including pregastric hydrolysis, gastric emptying rate, intestinal response, hydrolysis and absorption, pancreatic and gut hormone response, and colonic effects, influence a food's GI. Nondietary factors that influence a food's GI include medications taken, stress, physical activity, and overall health status.

Clinical use of GI as a guide to food selection may provide a health benefit and appears to be without adverse effects. Hints to incorporate the GI into the diet include these suggestions:

- Keep it simple—substitute whole grains and fresh fruits and beans for higher-GI foods.
- Focus on foods that contribute the most carbohydrate, such as bread, breakfast foods, and potatoes.
- Do not worry about foods that contribute 5 or fewer grams of carbohydrate in a serving. Some nutritionally dense foods, such as carrots, have a higher GI but contain a low amount of CHO in a serving.

Theories About Obesity

Theories about obesity are plentiful. Box 16-2 discusses one theory: the malfunctioning hypothalamus.

Efficient Metabolism

Some obese individuals actually require fewer kilocalories for normal body functions than do lean individuals. Some obese individuals thus use kilocalories very efficiently.

Brown Fat

Brown fat, a special type of fat cell, accounts for less than 1% of total body weight. Brown fat burns kilocalories and then releases the energy as heat. Energy released as heat is not stored as body fat. Some obese people may have defective brown fat or less brown fat than lean people.

Set Point Theory

The set point theory argues that each individual has a unique, relatively stable, adult body weight based on

---

Box 16-2 ■ *Can a Malfunctioning Hypothalamus Cause Weight Gain?*

The brain partially controls hunger and satiety. The hypothalamus, located in the brain, appears to be the center for weight control. A malfunctioning hypothalamus could cause an individual to receive incorrect hunger signals, thus stimulating continued eating and signaling weight gain. Appetite, satiety, and hunger may be incorrectly processed by a malfunctioning hypothalamus.

Various areas of the hypothalamus are sensitive to at least 13 neurochemicals, and these areas are involved in the regulation of hunger, eating, and satiety: the ventromedial nucleus and the lateral lobe in the hypothalamus are the two most significant areas.

- The ventromedial nucleus, which is activated by **serotonin** and antagonized by norepinephrine, mediates satiety.
- The lateral lobe, which is activated by norepinephrine and/or dopamine and antagonized by serotonin, mediates hunger and thirst.

Selective hypothalamic neurotransmitters are now being considered as medications to alter the brain sensation of hunger, appetite, and satiety. However, more research is necessary to understand better long-term and short-term effects of these medications.

---

biologic factors. Hence, an obese person may have a higher set point than a lean counterpart.

Number of Fat Cells

Obese individuals have many more fat cells than do their lean counterparts. A kilocalorie deficit can reduce the fat in each cell but cannot break down the cell. Once manufactured, a fat cell exists until death. Empty fat cells release a chemical messenger that travels to the brain and sends a message to the reduced obese person to fill the depleted fat cells. As a result, the reduced obese person must learn to constantly ignore internal hunger signals. Ignoring such pains can be done for a short period, but long-term adaptation to hunger is difficult.

Enzymes in the Metabolic Chain

Lipoprotein lipase is an enzyme that is involved in the uptake of fatty acids for the manufacture of fat in individual fat cells. Research has shown that the activity of this enzyme increases during weight reduction. This action makes fat cells even more efficient in synthesizing fats.

Obesogens

New research is emerging regarding **obesogens**. Obesogens are chemicals in the environment that are thought to have different mechanisms of action, some affect the number or size of fat cells and others are thought to affect appetite, satiety, food preferences, and energy metabolism (Holtcamp, 2012). Known and suspected obesogens include the following:

■ Diet: fructose and monosodium glutamate
■ Smoking: nicotine
■ Pharmaceuticals: estradiol
■ Industrial chemicals: bisphenol A (BPA)
■ Organophosphate pesticides
■ Environmental pollutants: lead, benzo[a]pyrene (Holtcamp, 2012)

Federal Guidelines

There are clear advantages to weight loss by overweight and obese clients. The primary reason should be to decrease the risk of disease. Treatment is also indicated for persons who have an obesity-related disorder. Options offered to clients should depend on their degree of overweight and obesity.

Advantages of Weight Loss

Federal clinical guidelines for identifying overweight and obesity in adults focuses on the medical benefits to be derived from weight loss. This panel recommends:

■ Weight loss to lower blood pressure in overweight and obese persons with high blood pressure
■ Weight loss to lower elevated levels of cholesterol, low-density lipoprotein cholesterol, and triglycerides and to raise low levels of high-density lipoprotein cholesterol in overweight and obese persons with dyslipidemia (see Chapter 18)
■ Some weight loss to lower elevated blood glucose levels in overweight and obese persons with type 2 diabetes

Determining Overweight and Obesity

According to U.S. federal guidelines, practitioners should use the BMI and waist circumference to classify the degree of energy imbalance in clients. Body weight alone can be used to follow weight loss and to determine efficacy of treatment (NIH, 2009).

Treatment of Energy Imbalances

Federal guidelines address goals for weight loss, how to achieve weight loss, goals for weight maintenance, how to maintain weight loss, and special treatment groups.

Goals for Weight Loss

The initial goal of weight loss should be to reduce body weight by 10% from the baseline (current weight). With success, further weight loss can be attempted, if indicated. Safe weight loss occurs at about 1 to 2 pounds per week for a period of 6 months, with the subsequent strategy based on the amount of weight lost (Shay, Shobert, Seibert, and Thomas, 2009).

Achieving Weight Loss

The approach to weight loss should depend on professional evaluation and the client's BMI, waist circumference, and other factors. These are some of the weight-loss treatment options for clients:

■ Dietary therapy (also called medical nutrition therapy)
■ Physical activity
■ Behavior therapy
■ Pharmacotherapy
■ Weight-loss surgery
■ Combined therapy (some or all of the above)

Diet Therapy

A weight-loss diet should include a reduction in total kilocalories averaging a 500 to 1000 kcalorie per day decrease while maintaining a daily consumption of 1000 to 1500 kcalories per day. Diets must maintain adequate amounts of all nutrients and should provide at least:

■ 45% of kilocalories from carbohydrate
■ 20% of kilocalories from fat
■ 10% of the kilocalories from protein or 0.8 gram/kg, whichever is higher
■ Remaining 25% of kilocalories open to negotiation with the client
■ 25 to 35 grams of fiber
■ All essential vitamins and minerals

The meal plan should be one the client can and will follow. When clients are given a standardized meal plan, weight loss is not usually successful. However, when behavior modification, nutritional counseling, and exercise recommendations support the meal plan, weight loss can be more successful.

Different clients need different types of dietary directions. A few clients want to be told what to eat and will follow through with appropriate behaviors. Some clients prefer receiving simplified instructions and do not want to learn a complicated diet. Following ChooseMyPlate Guidelines and using a Super-Tracker (US. Department of Agriculture [USDA], 2013) dietary plan may work well for the latter type of client (provided behavior modifications and the need for exercise are also discussed). Portion control must be emphasized.

A common tool used for teaching portion control and energy nutrient distribution is the Academy of Nutrition and Dietetics (AND) Exchange Lists. These lists provide detailed meal plans and clearly spell out portion sizes, making them an ideal guide for health-care workers when they serve and monitor weight-reduction diets.

Another advantage of the AND Exchange Lists is that the system teaches clients the composition of foods, such as which foods contain sugar, which fat. The disadvantage to this meal planning system is that learning it takes a relatively long time, so some clients become discouraged. See the Exchange Lists in Appendix B. Weight Watchers uses a variation of this meal planning system with some success.

There are also numerous smartphone and computer applications available for the more technologically advanced client. Certain applications allow clients the ability to track their daily intake of calories and nutrients and log exercise minutes. The program also allows the client the ability to scan bar codes on packaged food items to enter nutrient data. Online and mobile applications give clients objective, visual cues that can assist in holding the client accountable for their weight loss goals.

Sometimes clients are unable to make drastic changes in their food intake and become discouraged. In this situation, nutritional counselors should encourage clients to make major behavioral changes in their eating habits slowly. The goal in weight-reduction counseling is to help the client make permanent lifestyle changes.

Physical Activity

Population studies conducted in the United States, Great Britain, and France suggest that the rapidly increasing prevalence of obesity in recent decades may be largely due to increasing sedentary behaviors, perhaps to a greater extent than dietary excesses. Some nutrition counselors advocate a nondieting approach to weight control. Exercise and healthy eating is encouraged instead of adherence to a rigid diet plan.

Physical activity should be part of any comprehensive weight-loss and weight maintenance program because it:

■ Modestly contributes to weight loss in overweight and obese adults
■ May decrease abdominal fat
■ Increases cardiopulmonary fitness
■ Increases lean body mass

Initially, adults should participate in moderate levels of exercise for 150 minutes, or 2 hours and 30 minutes,

each week. The person who is attempting to lose weight should gradually increase the duration of their exercise with some adults having to participate in 300 minutes of exercise a week to achieve their weight loss goals (see Genomic Gem 16-2).

To identify individuals at risk for heart disease, a health-care provider should screen all clients before making exercise recommendations. Clients with known heart, lung, or metabolic disease should have a physician-supervised stress test before beginning an exercise program.

When following an exercise program, fluid intake should be adequate. Individuals should drink water before, during, and after exercise, and they should pay close attention to thirst to prevent dehydration. Four ounces of water every 15 minutes is usually sufficient, but when temperatures are high, additional fluids may be necessary. During hot weather, the thirst mechanism may not be adequate to prevent dehydration in many elderly persons and in individuals involved in heavy exercise. Such persons need to drink water even if they are not thirsty.

One method to determine if fluid intake is adequate is to weigh oneself before and after exercise. One pound of water (sweat) weighs 16 ounces or 2 cups. Therefore, for every pound of sweat lost during exercise, the person needs to drink 2 cups of water. Another indication that fluid intake is adequate is urine that is clear and has a minimal odor.

Behavior Modification

Behavior modification is a useful adjunct to weight loss and maintenance plans. It is assumed that eating and exercise are learned behaviors and with modification changes in body weight can be achieved (Burke and

---

Genomic Gem 16-2
Body Build and Propensity for Obesity

The propensity to be physically inactive may be at least partly determined by genetics. Individuals with certain body builds may be genetically predisposed to engage in less spontaneous physical activity and to have relatively low energy requirements. However, physical activity behaviors also influence whether we stay lean or become obese. For example, note these two studies:

1. One showed that overweight or obese Hispanic children were less likely to get the recommended levels of moderate physical activity and less likely to participate in team sports compared with their nonobese peers (Yand and Yang, 2011).
2. Another showed that people who had an increase in physical activity appeared to have improved eating patterns as well (Annesi and Marti, 2011).

Wang, 2011). A client's motivation to enter weight-loss therapy and his or her readiness to implement a plan require evaluation. Permanent weight loss can result only from a permanent change in eating and exercise behaviors. See Box 16-3 for common weight-reduction strategies.

Pharmacotherapy

According to federal guidelines, Food and Drug Administration–approved weight-loss medications may be used as part of a comprehensive weight-loss program, which includes diet and physical activity, for clients with a BMI equal to or greater than 30 and no concomitant obesity-related risk factors or diseases. For clients with a BMI equal to or greater than 27 and concomitant obesity-related risk factors or diseases, medications may also be indicated.

Medications should never be used without lifestyle modification. Medication therapy for obesity should be continually monitored for efficacy and safety and discontinued if the client does not lose weight. Table 16-3 lists weight-loss medications, actions, and adverse effects.

Surgery

Weight-loss surgery is an option for selected clients with clinically extreme or severe obesity (BMI >40 or >35 with comorbid conditions) when less-invasive methods of weight loss have failed and the client is at high risk for obesity-associated morbidity or mortality.

Numerous surgical procedures are used to treat obesity. The removal of fat tissue through a vacuum hose is called **liposuction. Lipectomy** is surgical removal of adipose tissue. Both of these procedures are done more for cosmetic reasons than for weight control. A **jejunoileal bypass** involves the removal of a part of the small intestine. Clients lose weight after this procedure because they cannot absorb all the food they eat, although this places these clients at a nutritional risk. The jejunoileal bypass procedure is rarely performed currently; however, health-care providers are likely to encounter clients who have had this procedure.

Two of the most commonly performed surgeries for weight management are **gastric banding** and **gastric bypass (Roux-en-Y)** with the Roux-en-Y technique being the preferred approach (Burke and Wang, 2011). Diagrams of these procedures are shown in Figure 16-3.

Gastric banding involves the placement of an adjustable band to create a small stomach pouch. When the stomach is smaller or reduced, only a limited amount of food can be consumed at one feeding. This induces weight loss from reduced kilocalorie intake. The Roux-en-Y gastric bypass procedure has been considered the "gold standard" and results in the creation of a small gastric pouch (Furtado, 2010). Before surgery, the surgeon specifies a diet, and the client must make an enormous commitment to follow the diet exactly and choose foods carefully. The following

---

Box 16-3 ■ *Behavior Modification Techniques to Share With Clients*

These behavior-change tips can help facilitate a weight-loss program.

Self-Monitoring

- Keep a food diary and record all food and fluid intake.
- Keep a weekly graph of weight change.
- Keep an exercise diary.

Stimulus Control

- At home, limit all food intake to one specific place.
- Plan food intake for each day.
- Rearrange your schedule to avoid inappropriate eating.
- Sit down at a table while eating.
- Use a smaller dinner plate.
- At a party, sit a distance from snack foods, eat before you go, and substitute lower kilocalorie drinks for alcohol.
- Decide beforehand what you will order at a restaurant.
- Have the restaurant bag half the meal to go before serving the meal.
- Save or reschedule everyday activities for times when you are hungry.
- Avoid boredom; keep a list of activities on the refrigerator.
- Remove high-fat food from the home.

Slower Eating

- Drink a glass of water before each meal. Drink sips of water between bites of food.
- Swallow food before putting more food on the utensil.
- Try to be the last one to finish eating.
- Pause for a minute during your meal and attempt to increase the number of pauses.

Reward Yourself

- Chart your progress.
- Make an agreement with yourself or a significant other for a meaningful reward.
- Do not reward yourself with food.

Cognitive Strategies

- View exercise as a means of controlling hunger.
- Practice relaxation techniques.
- Imagine yourself ordering a side salad, diet dressing, low-fat milk, and a small hamburger at a fast-food restaurant.
- Reframe negative thoughts with positive thinking.
- Enhance social support.

TABLE 16-3 ■ Weight-Loss Medications

DRUG	ACTION	ADVERSE EFFECTS
Phentermine (Adipex)	Norepinephrine, dopamine, and serotonin reuptake inhibitor	Increase in heart rate and blood pressure, heart palpitations, and vasodilation Reports worldwide of deaths
Diethylpropion (Tenuate)	Stimulates the central nervous system to decrease appetite	Increase in heart rate and blood pressure Insomnia
Orlistat (Xenical or reduced strength formula Alli)	Inhibits pancreatic lipase, decreases fat absorption	Decrease in absorption of fat-soluble vitamins Soft stools and anal leakage Possible link to breast cancer
Lorcaserin (Belviq)	Serotonin receptor agonist	Insomnia Dry mouth Constipation Fatigue
Phentermine and extended-release topiramate (Qsymia)	Norepinephrine, dopamine, and serotonin reuptake inhibitor	Increased heart rate Increase risk of birth defects Tingling of hands and feet Insomnia Dry mouth

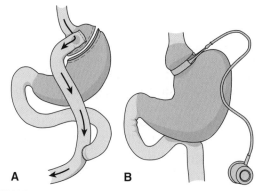

FIGURE 16-3 Surgery for weight loss. *A,* Roux-en-Y stomach bypass: large portion of stomach and duodenum are bypassed. *B,* Adjustable gastric banding: stomach opening can be tightened or loosened over time to change the size of the passage.

is a description of a typical progressive diet plan; some surgeons use a variation:

Phase 1: Clear liquids: 64 ounces per day of sugar-free and noncarbonated clear liquids consumed in small amounts immediately after the surgery; no straws. The focus of phase 1 is the prevention of dehydration of the patient.

Phase 2: Pureed: This phase begins after the patient is tolerating clear liquids and may last up to 1 month: The patient can begin introducing up to 6 small meals of 60 to 90 mL of pureed food. The patient should include high-protein foods, begin taking chewable vitamin and mineral supplements, and continue to maintain hydration with 64 ounces of liquid per day that should be consumed between meals. The patient needs to focus on foods that are low in fat and sugar.

Phase 3: Adaptive/soft food: Phase 3 will generally last 1 to 2 months. Foods can include soft foods including protein, fruits, and vegetables. The patient should attempt to eat five small meals of ⅓ to ½ cup of mechanical soft foods and progress to four meals of ½ to ¾ cup of soft food. The patient will continue to take a chewable vitamin and mineral supplement, hydrate with 64 ounces of fluid per day that is consumed between meals, but may begin to add in low-fat, low-calorie fruits and vegetables.

Phase 4: Stabilization/food of regular consistency: The patient resumes eating foods of regular consistency eating three meals of nutrient-rich foods that are low in fat and sugar (Furtado, 2010).

Food to avoid: fibrous vegetable, raw vegetables, carbonated sweetened beverages, high-calorie sweets, and snack foods such as French fries, potato chips, and nuts. Caffeine should also be limited.

Another surgical option is the **gastric sleeve** procedure. During the procedure, the surgeon removes approximately 85% of the stomach until it resembles a tube or sleeve. This newer surgical approach will also result in strict, postprocedure, dietary changes similar to those listed earlier.

Bariatric surgeons usually depend on team members to screen and monitor clients, who typically have several sessions with the team before the procedure is done. Most surgeons screen and monitor clients because the liability risk is great if clients are not screened and educated.

Clinical Application 16-1 discusses problems that clients often encounter after gastric surgery and suggests general guidelines for these clients to follow. Clients should be followed carefully postoperatively

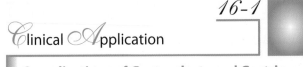

Clinical Application   16-1

Complications of Gastroplasty and Gastric Bypass

There are many potential acute complications of gastric surgery for weight reduction. These include:

- Nausea, vomiting, bloating, and/or heartburn: These signs and symptoms can be caused by overeating, not chewing food well, eating too quickly, drinking cold or carbonated beverages, using drinking straws, or eating gassy foods.
- Obstruction: An obstruction is the blockage of a structure. In this case, a blockage can occur close to the area stapled. A frequent cause of obstruction is poorly chewed food. The result is stomach pain, nausea, and vomiting.
- Dumping syndrome: Intake of concentrated sweets and large quantities of fluids causes quick dumping of food into the small intestine. Abdominal fullness, nausea, diarrhea 15 minutes after eating, warmth, weakness, fainting, racing pulse, and cold sweats are symptoms of this syndrome.
- Among the long-term risks is osteoporosis, due to decreased calcium absorption.

because of risks for deficiencies such as iron, folic acid, and vitamin B_{12}. Clients are also at risk for maladaptive eating behavior. Clinical Application 16-2 discusses surgery guidelines for these clients postsurgery.

Expected results from gastric surgery procedures should always be explained to clients. No permanent effects can be promised, and having the surgery does not mean that afterward the client can overeat without weight gain. Ninety percent of weight loss occurs in the first year, and clients typically begin to gain again in the second and third years. The client should view

the procedure as a tool to be used in conjunction with behavioral training—the small pouch helps clients learn to reduce and slow down food intake. After the first year, because of pouch stretching or intestinal adaptation, much of the effect of the surgery can be negated, and the lost weight may be regained. However, one study did demonstrate that in patients who underwent a surgical intervention as a treatment for weight loss, 94% maintained 20% of their weight loss at years 2 and 6 postprocedure (Adams et al, 2012).

Weight-Loss Maintenance

Weight regain typically occurs after weight loss. A program of dietary therapy, physical activity, and behavior therapy enhances the likelihood of weight-loss maintenance. Drug therapy can also be used according to the guidelines published by the National Institutes of Health; however, drug safety and efficacy beyond 1 year of total treatment have not been established.

Research suggests, however, that frequent contact between clients and practitioners increase the success of weight loss and maintenance therapies (Shay et al, 2009).

The National Weight Control Registry (NWCR) was founded in 1994 to investigate people who have had long-term successful weight loss and maintenance. There are currently 10,000 people registered, and they report the following behaviors as contributing to their continued weight loss success:

- Have maintained diets low in calories.
- Have maintained diets low in fat.
- 78% report eating breakfast daily.
- 75% weigh themselves at least weekly.
- 62% watch less than 10 hours of television each week.
- 90% exercise, on average, 1 hour per day (NWCR, 2013).

The Role of Nutrition Educators

Appropriate roles for nutrition educators include:

- Providing accurate information
- Assisting children to prevent unhealthy weight gain (see Box 16-4)
- Warning against dangerous practices such as self-imposed starvation diets that eliminate one or more of the major food groups and encourage the intake of only one food group (see Table 16-4)
- Guiding clients to understand the risks and benefits of weight loss and weight-loss programs, products, medicines, procedures

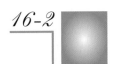

Clinical Application   16-2

Post–Gastric Surgery Nutrition Guidelines

These strategies can help clients adjust after surgery:

- Eat three to six small meals per day.
- Eat slowly.
- Chew food thoroughly.
- Eat very small quantities.
- Stop eating when full.
- Do not eat longer than 30 minutes at a time.
- Drink most fluids between meals.
- Select a balanced diet.
- Take a chewable multivitamin–multimineral supplement.
- Exercise regularly.

Box 16-4 ■ *Weight Management in Children*

These are three ways in which individuals and communities can help children enjoy the physical activities that can aid in weight management.

Develop appropriate activities—The enjoyment of physical activity should start young. Children aged 2 to 5 years should engage in active play several times a day. Examples of appropriate activities for young children include ballet lessons, tricycle or bike riding, walking daily with a family member, swimming lessons, and sledding (Fig. 16-4).

Develop play areas—Communities need to develop safe play areas for children. Local school districts should be encouraged to offer more opportunities for young people to be active in a noncompetitive environment.

Encourage noncompetitive activities—A totally sedentary child who is uncomfortable in a competitive situation will gain important health benefits from physical activity. Children aged 6 to 17 should engage in 1 hour of physical activity each day at a moderate to vigorous aerobic intensity.

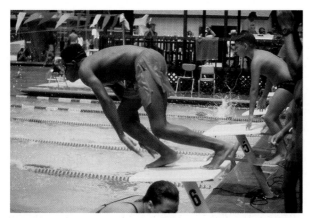

FIGURE 16-4 This boy is diving into the swimming pool, while exercising during his swim.

- Teaching clients to evaluate the risks and benefits of surgery for themselves
- Referring clients to health-care professionals, including physicians and dietitians, when appropriate
- Helping clients set realistic goals (see Box 16-5)
- In states that have regulations, assist in efforts to enforce these standards for safe weight loss

Reduced Body Mass

Clients with a reduced body mass are as difficult, if not more difficult, to treat as overly fat clients. Body fat has important roles in insulation and protection of body

---

TABLE 16-4 ■ Weight-Loss Diets in the Popular Media

Fad diets come and go. Typically, fad diets limit a person to a few specific foods or food combinations and do not provide kilocalories within the acceptable macronutrient range and the nutrient density so necessary for optimal health. For example, the brain needs sufficient carbohydrate (CHO) for optimal function. One hundred and thirty grams of CHO is the average minimum amount of glucose used by the brain, and the acceptable macronutrient range for CHO is 45% to 65% of kilocalories. The following describes three popular diets, along with the diet author's rationale. Studies have demonstrated that modified-carbohydrate diets result in greater weight loss at the 12-week follow-up compared with low-fat, low-calorie diets, but results are comparable at 12 months (Shikany, Desmond, McCubrey, and Allison, 2011). Studies have also demonstrated that the South Beach and Zone diets did not result in nutritional deficiencies if fiber-rich, whole grains are consumed, but strict CHO restriction of 50 grams of CHO or less can result in inadequate consumption of thiamine, folic acid, vitamin C, iron, and magnesium (Clifton, 2011). Studies have failed to demonstrate long-term safety of modified-carbohydrate diets. These diets are not widely endorsed by the health-care community; however, health-care professionals should know which diets their clients may be following.

NAME OF DIET	RATIONALE OF DIET'S AUTHOR	DESCRIPTION
Atkins	Claims processed CHO and insulin rather than excess kilocalories are responsible for weight gain and obesity.	Four phases: ■ Phase 1: Induction—eat protein, healthy fat, and vegetables with 20-g net CHO. ■ Phase 2: Ongoing weight loss—continue phase 1 foods and increase CHO by 5 g week until 25–45 g net CHO. ■ Phase 3: Premaintenance—eat phase 2 foods and introduce fruits, legumes, breads and grain by adding 10 g CHO each week. ■ Phase 4: Lifetime maintenance—eat phase 3 foods and increase CHO to ≥75 g.
South Beach	The faster sugars and starches are absorbed, the more weight is gained. The goal is to stabilize blood sugar and eliminate cravings. Low glycemic index meals suppress appetite and reduce food intake later in the same day in comparison to higher glycemic index meals (see below).	Three phases: ■ Severe CHO restriction for first 2 weeks. ■ Reintroduction of "good CHO" (those with a low glycemic index, such as whole grains, fruits, vegetables) during phases 2 and 3. ■ Consistent mealtimes and plentiful water.
Zone	Only through eating in the "Zone" can the body reach its physical peak. The author claims that cellular inflammation makes us gain weight by turning fat cells into "fat traps," which trap calories that can't be released to be used for energy. The kilocalorie intakes of the meal plans are between 1000 and 1700 kilocalories.	The zone is 40% CHO, 30% protein, and 30% fat. All food is measured, and only precise portion sizes are eaten. CHO serving sizes are small (⅛ cup of pasta).

Health-care and wellness professionals can assist clients in setting realistic goals for weight reduction and encourage loss of modest amounts of weight. Typically, clients have an unrealistic weight-loss goal. Despite considerable professional agreement that weight losses of 5% to 10% from baseline are successful for reducing comorbid conditions associated with obesity, obese clients often desire weight losses two to three times greater than this. For example, a weight-reduction diet may be planned to allow for a 1 pound per week weight loss. The client may expect to lose 5 pounds per week. A female client may expect to be able eventually to wear a size 5 dress as a result of dieting. This expectation is not realistic for some clients with large bones. Studies have demonstrated that an unrealistic weight loss expectation is one of the most frequently cited reasons for failing to maintain weight loss (Ohsiek and Williams, 2011). Health-care workers provide a valuable service when they teach clients, especially those who are overweight, how to set achievable goals that will allow for maintenance and prevent future weight gain.

organs. A client with a low body fat content usually has a loss of lean body mass as well, and loss of this functioning tissue concerns clinicians. Women may cease to ovulate and menstruate when the percentage of body fat falls below 15% to 17%. The client may experience cardiac abnormalities and become more prone to infections. These clients are at risk for osteoporosis in the long term.

Classification

A person with a BMI below 18.5 should be evaluated before being classified as underweight. A man with a body fat content less than 15% and a woman with a body fat content less than 18% (if known) need to be evaluated and assessed before being classified as having a reduced body mass. The only reliable method to determine if the individual is at a nutritional risk is to do a complete nutritional assessment.

Consequences

Long-term follow-up of studies indicates that excessive leanness is associated with increased mortality and decreased life expectancy. However, the causes of mortality are different from those associated with excess weight. An excessively lean person is almost twice as likely to succumb to respiratory diseases such as tuberculosis. In addition, these clients have greater difficulty maintaining body temperature during cold weather. Infections and disturbances of the gastrointestinal tract are more likely in an underweight person, as is fragile bone structure and osteoporotic changes.

Causes

A person may be underweight because of genetic factors or because of a long-term or recent weight loss. A recent weight loss can often be related to a recent new medical diagnosis (such as trauma), a psychological diagnosis, or socioeconomic issues.

Rapid Loss Increases Risk

The greater the rate of weight loss, the more the client is at a nutritional risk. **Rate** means loss per unit of time. For example, a 20-pound weight loss in 2 weeks is an excessive weight loss. Such a client has lost a large amount of lean body mass. However, a 20-pound weight loss during a 20-week period could be attributed mostly to a loss of body fat with a minimal loss of lean body mass. If the client began with surplus body fat stores, a loss of 20 pounds may not place this client at a very high nutritional risk. If the client had a reduced body mass, even a slow weight loss may place him or her at a high nutritional risk. Laboratory data are useful to determine a client's nutritional risk level.

Not all changes in body weight are caused by insufficient kilocalorie intake. For example, a client may lose several pounds of body weight over the course of a single day as a result of diuretic therapy. The weight loss in this instance would be due to water loss and not to body fat or protein loss (see Box 16-6).

Eating Disorders

There are numerous theories to the cause of the development of eating disorders, but most agree the cause is a combination of biological, social-culture, and psychological factors. Many experts are concerned about the prevalence of anorexia nervosa, bulimia, and binge-eating, which may all result in nutritional problems. In the United States, as many as 10 million females and 1 million males are fighting a life-and-death battle with an eating disorder.

One method for determining whether a client is eating enough food is to monitor his or her food intake. Kilocalorie intake is monitored by recording actual food consumption and calculating the kilocalories eaten. Utilizing programs such as the USDA's SuperTracker provides a user-friendly way to assist with calculations and developing dietary plans. The program can be found at www.supertracker.usda.gov/default.aspx.

Anorexia Nervosa

Anorexia nervosa is a medical condition that results from self-imposed starvation. Symptoms include:

- Recent unplanned weight loss of 5% or more
- Decreased resting energy expenditure (REE)
- **Amenorrhea** (cessation of menstruation)
- Constipation
- Excessive hair loss
- Abnormal sleeping patterns
- Preoccupation with food
- Body image disturbance
- Misconception about physical status
- Intake of only 500 to 800 kilocalories per day
- Slow eating
- Increased physical activity
- Social isolation
- Intense fear of becoming obese
- Poor muscle tone

The disorder appears at a rate of 80% to 85% in young women at age 12 to 25 years and the disorder occurs 10 to 20 times more frequently in females than in males (Wozniak, Rekleiti, and Roupa, 2012). The client may resort to a variety of devices to lose weight, including starvation, vomiting, and laxative use. The disorder may be life-threatening.

Bulimia

Bulimia is more common than anorexia nervosa, especially during adolescence and young adulthood. The mean age for females at diagnosis was 23 years. An estimated 1.1% to 4.2% of females have bulimia nervosa in their lifetime. The condition is rare in males.

Bulimics binge and purge. **Binging** involves the consumption of as much as 5000 to 20,000 kilocalories per day. **Purging** is the intentional clearing of food out of the system by vomiting and/or using enemas, laxatives, and diuretics. Individuals with bulimia are more apt to maintain a normal weight by restricting food and dieting before binging episodes (Hannon-Engel, 2012). Athletes such as ballerinas and gymnasts sometimes are bulimic. The female triad is a serious syndrome comprising three interrelated components (see Chapter 11):

- Disordered eating
- Amenorrhea
- Osteoporosis

Binge-Eating Disorder

Binge-eating disorder (BED) is recognized as a distinct eating disorder in the Diagnostic and Statistical Manual of Mental Disorders, Fifth Edition (DSM-5). Binge-eaters eat large amounts of high-fat and high-sugar foods in short periods of time, unlike the bulimic; binge eaters do not follow a binge with a purge. BED affects 1% to 2% of the population with a 3:2 female to male ratio. Clients with BED may be overweight or obese and often experience feelings of shame and guilt (Disordered eating, 2012). Binge-eaters can often associate eating at times of stress or emotional distress, eating "unconsciously," and eating until they are uncomfortably full (Campbell, 2012). BED can contribute to the development of obesity and obesity related conditions.

Treating Eating Disorders

The treatment of eating disorders requires a multidisciplinary approach including nutritional counseling; psychotherapy which can include behavioral therapy, family therapy, and group therapy; psychopharmacology therapy and the use of antidepressants; and medical therapy to correct complications related to the illnesses. It is important to help the client discover the reason he or she chooses to eat, not eat, binge, or purge. Some of these clients have symptoms including a fixation on food, weight, physique, or exercise (see Box 16-7).

> **Box 16-7** ■ *Treating Eating Disorders in the Hospital Setting*
>
> Some clients may be admitted to the hospital for treatment if they demonstrate severe weight loss, hypotension, electrolyte disorders, suicidal ideation or psychosis, or the failure of outpatient treatment (Wozniak, Rekleiti, and Roupa, 2012). Careful recording of kilocalories consumed and expended is indicated. Close monitoring of clients is often indicated during meals and until 2 hours after meals because these clients may attempt to hide food in their clothes, mouth, bedding, or anywhere else. It is sometimes necessary for the nurse to accompany these clients to the bathroom. Clients with eating disorders have been known to flush their food down the toilet or engage in purging activities such as self-induced vomiting after a meal. Clients will require daily weights.

Keystones

- Energy imbalance results from an inequality of energy intake and expenditure.
- The reason an individual eats more or fewer kilocalories than needed to maintain a stable body weight is only partially understood.
- Reasons a person may be in energy imbalance are both internal and external.
- Weight loss decreases both body fat and lean body mass.
- Care needs to be taken to minimize the loss of lean body mass during weight reduction.
- Exercise should be encouraged because it helps minimize the loss of lean body mass during weight reduction.
- Exercise, a well-balanced diet, and behavior modification are all essential components of a sound weight-reduction program.
- The prevention of energy imbalance is the key to decreased health-care costs nationally.
- Medications and surgical interventions may be indicated for individuals who meet the criteria set by the guidelines.
- Treating the client who has a reduced body mass is a concern for health-care workers.

CASE STUDY *16-1*

The client arrives at the physician's office for a routine blood pressure check. Her blood pressure is 150/95. Her medications include 100 mg Lopressor daily and 25 mg hydrochlorothiazide daily. The client works nights as a cashier at a service station and days at a dry cleaner. Her BMI is 28. She recently had a stress test that was considered normal. The doctor would like the client to lose weight to help lower her blood pressure.

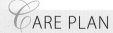 ARE PLAN

Subjective Data

Client stated, "I can barely afford my blood pressure medication, and the doctor has encouraged me to lose about 14 pounds. I know I need to eat less and exercise more. I need to spend less money on medications. I know I'm not too smart because I only completed the sixth grade in school." A food frequency record showed that this client usually eats four times each day. Her usual pattern includes 3 cups of low-fat milk, 8 starches (mostly refined), ½ cup of vegetables, 1 piece of fruit, 6 to 8 ounces of meat, 5 fats, 1 dessert, and an occasional beer. She eats fast food two nights each week and has pizza weekly for lunch. "I am desperate and will do anything to lose weight." The client has health insurance that will pay for one wellness program per year.

Objective Data

Blood pressure 150/95 ■ height 5 ft 6 in ■ BMI 28; waist circumference 36 ■ stress test was normal.

Analysis

Energy imbalance ■ kilocalorie intake greater than kilocalorie expenditure. Overweight as evidenced by BMI of 28 and waist circumference of 36, probably contributing to hypertension.

CASE STUDY *(Continued)*

Plan

DESIRED OUTCOMES EVALUATION CRITERIA	ACTIONS/INTERVENTIONS	RATIONALE
Increase physical activity.	Recommend Mrs. R monitor her exercise behaviors and try to walk at least 30 minutes three times per week and increase to 7 days per week as able.	Self-monitoring of lifestyle behaviors promotes behavioral change. Sedentary individuals receive the most health benefit from even small amounts of exercise.
Consume foods in appropriate portions following the MyPlate Guide.	Review MyPlate model with Mrs. R with emphasis on whole grains, fruits and vegetables, lean proteins, and the limiting of fats. Review portion sizes indicated on this teaching tool.	The MyPlate Guide is a good tool to use for clients with a lower reading level and promotes a high-fiber, low-fat diet.
Client will state why a weight loss of 1 to 2 pounds per week may reduce her blood pressure.	Explain to the client that the rate of weight loss is important and why.	A 1- to 2-pound per week weight loss will minimize the loss of lean body mass. Self-starvation rarely results in long-term weight loss for overweight clients.
Refer client to the local hospital's wellness center that incorporates diet, behavior modification, and exercise in the program.	Explain to the client why you are referring her to this particular program.	The best wellness programs include diet, exercise, and behavior modification.

 16-1

Follow-Up Note From Hospital's Wellness Program

Thank you for your referral to our program. Client has met with our registered dietitian, exercise physiologist, and psychologist during group sessions. She has attended most sessions and has done remarkably well. She has lost a total of 5 pounds at the rate of .1 to 5 pounds per week for the past 8 weeks. We were also able to arrange a scholarship for her to attend the program for 8 more weeks. She keeps good food and exercise records. She has made several friends in the class and says she looks forward to this night out with her new friends. Thank you again for this referral.

Cordially,

Wellness Program Director

Critical Thinking Questions

1. What foods does this client need to eat less, and what foods does she need to eat more?

2. What would you tell the client if after 1 week she gained a pound, even though she had given up her daily dessert and had increased her vegetable intake to 5 servings each day?

3. What other dietary modifications would you recommend?

Chapter Review

1. To lose 2 pounds of body fat per week, an individual must eat ____ fewer kilocalories each day for 7 days without a change in energy expenditure.
   a. 1000
   b. 1500
   c. 2000
   d. 2500

2. A very rapid rate of weight loss (1 pound per day) in an adult who is slightly overweight:
   a. Usually encourages permanent changes in behavior
   b. May lead to sudden death in some clients
   c. Will preserve lean body mass
   d. Fosters long-term weight maintenance

3. An obese client should be enrolled in a weight-management program and meet the following criteria before medications are tried:
   a. BMI of 20 and a waist circumference of 30 inches
   b. In a male, waist circumference of at least 35 inches and a BMI of 27
   c. A BMI of 27 and no concomitant obesity-related risk factors
   d. In a female, a waist circumference of at least 35 inches and a BMI of 30 or greater

4. A client with anorexia nervosa:
   a. Has an increased resting energy expenditure
   b. Frequently complains of constipation
   c. Is not likely to have a body image disturbance
   d. Typically seeks the company of others

5. An elderly overweight smoker should first be encouraged to:
   a. Lose weight
   b. Quit smoking
   c. Lose weight and quit smoking using any means possible
   d. Be evaluated to determine if weight loss is indicated and bone health is adequate

Clinical Analysis

1. Mrs. R is a 40-year-old mother of three. She has arthritis in both knees. She weighs 180 pounds, has a medium frame, and is 5 ft, 3 in. tall. Her BMI is 32. Her physician has told her to lose weight to help reduce her knee pain. According to Mrs. R, she never thought she was overweight until she was 24 years old. At this time, her weight started increasing. When she weighed 140 pounds, she started to diet. One time she lost a total of 25 pounds, which she promptly regained plus an additional 5 pounds. The client described four additional **weight cycles.** Mrs. R claims she cannot exercise because "it is too painful on my knees." She has tried every conceivable type of diet, including a comprehensive medically

supervised weight-control program. Mrs. R states that for the past year, no matter how little she eats, she cannot lose weight even on a 1200-kilocalorie diet. Mrs. R:
   a. Apparently knows a great deal about low-kilocalorie foods, because she has successfully lost weight before
   b. Knows very little about foods, because she always regained the weight she lost
   c. Lacks motivation, because she has an inability to follow through with the appropriate behavior
   d. Should be discouraged from further attempts to control her weight

Clinical Analysis—cont'd

2. Mrs. M had a slow weight gain for about 10 years. She asks for advice concerning how to best manage her weight. Mrs. M lives a sedentary lifestyle, eats three well-balanced meals each day, and enjoys going out to dinner with her husband one night each week. Her BMI is 27. Mrs. M would most likely benefit from:
   a. Decreasing her meal frequency
   b. Increasing her physical activity
   c. Taking a medication to lose weight
   d. Not going out to dinner with her husband each week

3. Mr. P wants to lose weight and has a BMI of 30 and a waist circumference of 41. Initially, the nurse should advise Mr. P to:
   a. Follow a 1200-kilocalorie diet.
   b. Ask his doctor for a medication to assist in weight reduction.
   c. Self-monitor and write down his food intake and physical activity.
   d. Refer the client to a surgeon for an evaluation.

17

Diet in Diabetes Mellitus and Hypoglycemia

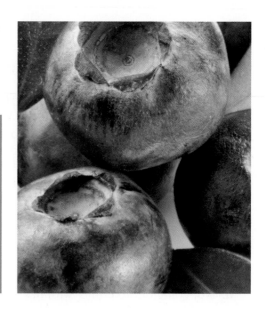

LEARNING OBJECTIVES

After completing this chapter, the student should be able to:

■ Define and classify diabetes mellitus and describe the treatment for each type of the disorder.

■ Discuss the goals of nutritional care for persons with diabetes mellitus.

■ List nutritional guidelines for people with diabetes mellitus for illness, exercise, delayed meals, alcohol, hypoglycemic episodes, vitamin and mineral supplementation, and eating out.

■ Describe the types of hypoglycemia and dietary treatment.

This chapter introduces the importance of nutrition in diabetes mellitus (simply referred to as diabetes throughout the rest of this chapter) and hypoglycemia. These two diseases are associated with insulin secretion and/or resistance to insulin accompanied by characteristic long-term complications. Diabetes mellitus is caused by the low secretion and/or utilization of insulin. Hypoglycemia is seen in suboptimal treatment of diabetes and in other causes such as gastric surgery, some medications, and hormone and enzyme deficiencies. The Centers for Disease Control and Prevention (CDC) estimates the prevalence of diagnosed and undiagnosed diabetes in the United States for all ages in 2010 to be 25.8 million or 8.3% of the population—18.8 million people diagnosed and 7 million undiagnosed. Nationally, diabetes is the seventh leading cause of death (CDC, 2011). Type 2 diabetes is frequently not diagnosed until complications occur. Approximately one-quarter of individuals who have diabetes may be undiagnosed (ADA 2013a). It is estimated that as many as 1 in 3 U.S. adults could have diabetes by 2050. The economic cost of diagnosed cases of diabetes was $245 billion dollars in 2012, which is up 41% from $174 billion in 2007 (American Diabetes Association [ADA], March 2013a). Nutrition is integral to the management of diabetes.

Definition and Classification

Diabetes can be defined as a group of disorders with measurable persistent hyperglycemia, which results from defects in insulin production, insulin action, or both. **Hyperglycemia** means an elevated level of glucose in the blood. Definitions and classifications for the various subclasses of diabetes have been standardized. Diabetes may produce symptoms of excessive urine production, thirst, excessive hunger, blurred vision, and, in some cases, weight loss (ADA, 2012a; CDC, 2011).

Diagnosis

Diabetes is diagnosed and defined by laboratory analysis of the blood. In 2010, the ADA (2013b) adopted the use of a glycosylated hemoglobin (A1C) of 6.5% or higher as a diagnosis for diabetes mellitus in adults. A1C levels indicate the level of blood glucose control an individual has had over approximately 2 to 3 months. If blood glucose is high, the excess attaches to the hemoglobin, causing the A1C level to be high.

Advantages of utilizing the A1C test include:

- Fasting is not required for the blood test
- Levels reflect an average level of blood glucose over time
- Greater preanalytical stability
- Less impact during periods of stress and illness.

Disadvantages of utilizing the A1C test include:

- Greater cost associated with the test
- Decreased availability in remote regions of the country and world
- Controversy in differences of normal levels in different race/ethnicity groups
- Uncertainty exists with the usage in children
- Unable to use in individuals with abnormal red cell turnover, such as occurs in pregnancy, with recent blood loss or transfusion, and in some forms of anemia

For individuals who cannot be diagnosed by using A1C levels, the diagnosis of diabetes must be done using blood glucose levels. This is still a valid method to diagnosis diabetes. Fasting glucose levels of at least 126 milligrams per **deciliter** (mg/dL) are required for a diagnosis of diabetes in nonpregnant adults. Fasting is defined as no kilocalorie intake for at least 8 hours. A fasting blood glucose level of 100 to 125 is diagnosed as prediabetes or **impaired fasting glucose.** Casual or random blood glucose (RBG) greater than 200 mg/dL plus classic symptoms (increased urination, increased thirst, weight loss) are also an established method for diagnosing diabetes in adults and children. A test result, which is diagnostic of diabetes, should be repeated to confirm the diagnosis. A random blood glucose between 140 and 199 mg/dL is diagnostic of prediabetes. Random means the blood sample is tested without regard to time of day, prior diet, and physical activity (ADA, 2013b). Refer to Clinical Application 17-1 for an explanation of other tests used for diabetes.

Classification

There are four clinical classes of diabetes: type 1, type 2, gestational (GDM), and other, secondary causes. The two major forms are **type 1** and **type 2.**

Prediabetes occurs in individuals with impaired glucose tolerance but who are not yet diagnosed with diabetes. This is an important group to diagnose and treat because they are more likely to be diagnosed with diabetes.

17-1

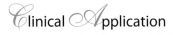 Clinical Application

Laboratory Tests for Diabetes Mellitus

Biochemical tests for diabetes include fasting blood sugar, glucose tolerance test, urine tests, and glycosylated hemoglobin.

FASTING BLOOD SUGAR

A measurement of a **fasting blood sugar (FBS)** is performed routinely on most diabetic clients. In preparation, the client should be instructed not to smoke, eat, or drink for 8 hours before the test. Water is the exception because it will not interfere with test results. The test ideally should be done after at least 3 days of unrestricted diet (150 grams of carbohydrate per day) and unlimited physical activity. The individual should remain seated throughout the test. If the client usually takes insulin or a hypoglycemic agent, the medication should not be taken or given until the blood test is done. Normal FBS should be less than 100 mg/dL. A finding of 126 mg/dL or greater is diagnostic of diabetes.

GLUCOSE TOLERANCE TEST

In the **glucose tolerance test,** 75 grams of anhydrous glucose dissolved in water is given orally or intravenously after a fasting blood sugar sample has been drawn. Blood samples are then drawn at specified intervals. The client's ability to process glucose can be evaluated by this means. A blood glucose value above or equal to 200 mg/dL at 2 hours and at least one other sample at less than 2 hours are required for the diagnosis in nonpregnant adults. A normal 2-hour blood sample would have an upper level of 140 mg/dL. Values between 140 and 199 mg/dL are indicative of impaired glucose tolerance or prediabetes. In the absence of unequivocal hyperglycemia, these criteria should be confirmed by repeat testing on a different day (ADA, 2013b).

Clients may need to discontinue certain drugs for 3 days before the test and follow a high-carbohydrate diet of 300 grams of carbohydrate per day. The client should be given written instructions explaining the pretest dietary requirements. An inadequate diet before the glucose tolerance test may diminish carbohydrate tolerance and cause high glucose levels, creating a false-positive result. During the test period, the client should be instructed not to have anything by mouth except water. Tobacco, coffee, and tea can alter the test results.

URINE TESTS

For most people, when blood glucose reaches 180 to 200 mg/100 mL, the kidneys begin to spill glucose into the urine. This point of spillage is called the **renal threshold.**

At one time, this test was assumed to reflect the glucose content of the blood, but the renal threshold varies from individual to individual. The renal threshold may also change in a given individual with decreasing kidney function. Although urine tests are used as screening tests, they are less reliable than the blood glucose tests available for home use.

URINE ACETONE

As a consequence of the body's inability to metabolize glucose, fat is partially broken down for energy. The intermediate products of fat

(Continued)

Clinical Application—cont'd

Laboratory Tests for Diabetes Mellitus

breakdown are ketone bodies. These ketone bodies build up in the blood because the quantity of fat being catabolized exceeds the body's capacity to process these intermediate products effectively. As this occurs, ketone bodies begin to spill into the urine. One of the ketone bodies is acetone, which can be measured in urine. The presence of acetone in the urine is called **ketonuria,** a sign that the diabetes is out of control. Clients may be taught to test for urinary ketones if their blood glucose level exceeds 240 mg/dL. When a client exhibits ketonuria, the physician and diabetes educator should be consulted for changes in the diet prescription and/or insulin dosage.

GLYCOSYLATED HEMOGLOBIN (A1C)

Glucose attaches to the hemoglobin molecule in a one-way reaction throughout the 120-day life of the red blood cell. In a high-glucose environment, a greater percentage of the hemoglobin is glycosylated.

This blood test is performed on a random blood sample; the client does not have to fast. The result is not influenced by exercise or diabetic drugs.

Because the **glycosylated hemoglobin** value reflects the average blood glucose level for the preceding 2 to 3 months, it is a good test of the effectiveness of long-term therapy. A client cannot follow the prescribed regimen for just a few days before a doctor's visit and claim otherwise. Glycosylated hemoglobin values between 5.7% and 6.4% is considered prediabetes. An A1C greater than 6.4% confirms a diagnosis of diabetes.

Testing for A1C is recommended at least two times a year for people in good control and quarterly in patients who are not meeting glycemic goals or whose therapy has changed (ADA, 2013b).

Prediabetes

Impaired glucose tolerance (IGT) and impaired fasting glucose (IFG) refer to a metabolic state intermediate between normal with glucose homeostasis and diabetes. The ADA encourages the use of the term *prediabetes*. Individuals who have A1C level of 5.7% to 6.4% or a fasting glucose level of greater than 100 mg/dL but less than 126 mg/dL on more than two occasions meet the criteria for IGT or IFG. IGT may represent a step in the development of types 1 and 2 diabetes, heart disease, and stroke. It is estimated that in 2010, there were approximately 79 million Americans over age 20 with prediabetes (CDC, 2011). Approximately 11% of individuals who are diagnosed with prediabetes develop type 2 diabetes each year. IGT and IFG are associated with abdominal obesity, dyslipidemia, and hypertension. Lifestyle intervention, which helps increase physical activity, a decrease in 5% to 10% body weight, and medications such as metformin have helped prevent or delay the development of diabetes (ADA, 2013b).

Type 1

Type 1 diabetes has also been called **insulin-dependent diabetes mellitus (IDDM),** juvenile-onset diabetes, and type I diabetes. This form of diabetes accounts for 5% to 10% of those with diabetes. Of those diagnosed with type 1 diabetes, 75% are individuals younger than 18 years of age. This type of diabetes normally results from a cellular-mediated autoimmune destruction of the β-cells of the pancreas, which produce insulin. The rate of the destruction is variable. Although mostly found in children and adolescents, it can occur at any age. Clients with this disorder cannot survive without daily doses of

insulin because the pancreas does not produce sufficient insulin for glucose uptake. This situation results in elevated blood glucose. After treatment starts, clients on medications that lower their blood glucose levels may have problems with too low a blood glucose level. These variations in blood glucose levels make clients prone to two conditions.

1. The first condition is **ketoacidosis.** The signs of ketoacidosis are hyperglycemia and excessive ketones. Ketoacidosis is discussed later in this chapter.
2. The second condition is **hypoglycemia,** or a low blood glucose level.

Individuals with type 1 diabetes are more prone to other autoimmune disorders such as Graves disease, Hashimoto thyroiditis, Addison disease, vitiligo, celiac sprue, autoimmune hepatitis, myasthenia gravis, and pernicious anemia. Some, but few, individuals with type 1 diabetes have no evidence of autoimmunity. It is thought their diabetes is strongly inherited, seen mostly in African or Asian ancestry. Their need for insulin replacement therapy may come and go (ADA, 2012b).

Type 2

Type 2 diabetes has also been called **non–insulin-dependent diabetes mellitus (NIDDM),** adult-onset diabetes, and type II diabetes. Most of these clients are obese, and weight reduction usually improves their ability to process glucose. These individuals have insulin resistance and may have varying degrees of insulin deficiency. Initially, and sometimes throughout the course of the disease, insulin injections are not required. However, some of them do require insulin injections because of persistent hyperglycemia. Clients with type 2 diabetes can manufacture some insulin but often do not make enough or cannot use insulin efficiently. The risk of developing type 2 diabetes increases with age, obesity, lack of physical activity, in women with previous GDM, and individuals with dyslipidemia and is associated with a strong genetic component (see Genomic Gem 17-1). Ninety percent to 95% of people with diabetes in the United States have type 2 (ADA, 2012a). Because of the increasing rate of obesity in children, 1 in 3 cases of diabetes is type 2 (National Institutes of Health, 2013). The CDC estimates that approximately 3600 children are diagnosed with type 2 diabetes annually. The ADA recommends screening in children 18 years and younger who are overweight (BMI >85th percentile for age and sex, weight for height, or weight >120% of ideal for height), who also have a maternal or family history of diabetes, signs of insulin resistance, or whose race/ethnicity make them more likely to have diabetes (ADA, 2013b). The prevalence is markedly increased among different racial/ethnic subgroups (CDC, 2011):

■ Native Americans
■ Asian Americans
■ African Americans
■ Mexican Americans
■ Alaska Natives
■ Puerto Ricans

The onset of this disorder is gradual, with the severity often not enough for individuals to notice any symptoms. However, during this undiagnosed period macrovascular and microvascular complications may occur (ADA, 2012a). Table 17-1 summarizes the differences between type 1 and type 2 diabetes.

Gestational Diabetes

Gestational diabetes (GDM) occurs in approximately 7% of all pregnancies. GDM carries risks for the mother, fetus, and neonate. Guidelines recommend that all women be assessed for their risk of GDM at

TABLE 17-1 ■ Type 1 and Type 2 Diabetes Mellitus Comparisons (ADA 2012b)

	TYPE 1	TYPE 2
Cause	Beta cells damaged	Tissues resist insulin
Most Common Age at Onset	Younger than 20 years	Older than 45 years
Medication	1. Insulin injections or pump 2. Insulin injections or pump and oral agents 3. Insulin drip during critical illness	1. None 2. Oral agents 3. Some individuals may require insulin injections to attain optimal blood glucose levels 4. Insulin drip during critical illness
Usual Body Build	Thin, underweight	Obese
Nutrition Therapy	Integration of insulin therapy, activity, and food intake. Consistent timing of insulin to food intake	Achievement of near-normal glucose, lipid, and blood pressure goals. Weight loss through diet and increased activity is desirable; bariatric surgery may be considered in extreme cases with BMI >35

their first prenatal visit. If a woman has the risk factors for diabetes such as obesity, a personal history of GDM, a family history of diabetes, or glycosuria, testing for diabetes should be done as soon as possible. Women not known to have diabetes should undergo a 75-gram oral glucose tolerance test (OGTT) at 24 to 28 weeks of gestation. The test should be done after 3 days of an unrestricted diet (carbohydrate >150 grams per day), activity, and in the morning after an overnight fast of 8 to 14 hours. The following blood levels must be met or exceeded for a diagnosis of GDM (ADA, 2013b):

■ 92 mg/dL fasting plasma glucose (FPG)
■ 180 mg/dL 1 hour after glucose load
■ 153 mg/dL 2 hours after glucose load

Clinical Application 17-2 discusses diabetes in pregnancy.

Immediately after pregnancy, 5% to 10% of women with GDM are found to have diabetes, usually type 2. Women with GDM have a 35% to 60% chance of developing diabetes in the next 10 to 20 years (ADA, 2012b; CDC, 2011).

Other/Secondary Diabetes

Most diabetes results from a primary failure of insulin production or use. Other conditions can cause diabetes such as genetic defects, surgery, medications, infections, pancreatic disease, and other illnesses. The term **secondary diabetes** is sometimes used when one of

Genomic Gem 17-1
Maturity-Onset Diabetes in the Young

Maturity-onset diabetes in the young (MODY) is a term used to describe a diabetes disorder that is found in clients younger than 25 years. This condition is genetic with a defect in the gene involved in the stimulation of the pancreatic ß cells to produce insulin. A parent with MODY has a 50% chance of passing on MODY to his or her children. Clients with MODY do not always need insulin treatment and can often be treated with oral agents and a weight-reduction diet.

17-2

*C*linical *A*pplication

Diabetes in Pregnancy

Pregnancy raises blood insulin levels in all women. It is an adaptive mechanism. Early in pregnancy, the woman's body cells store energy. Later, the woman's tissues become insulin resistant so that the fetus can draw on energy stores when the woman is fasting.

When the pregnant woman has or develops hyperglycemia, the mother's blood glucose crosses the placenta, but her insulin does not. Then the fetus produces more insulin, which increases his or her fat deposition. Women with diabetes have large babies for this reason.

Perinatal mortality of infants born to women with diabetes is higher than that of infants of women who do not have diabetes. Ketosis in early pregnancy can produce congenital malformations, central nervous system disorders, and low intelligence. With strict control of the diabetes, however, 97% of the fetuses survive, compared with 98% to 99% born to women without diabetes.

Insulin resistance is greater in the morning in pregnant women. For this reason, usually only 39 grams of carbohydrate (CHO) are planned for the breakfast meal. There is a heightened tendency for maternal ketosis during fasting, and the possible adverse effects of ketones on the fetus suggest that periods of fasting during pregnancy should be avoided. Small, frequent feedings throughout the day are recommended. A bedtime snack that contains between 15 and 45 grams of CHO is recommended to minimize an accelerated production of ketones, which has been known to occur during sleeping. Clients should be reminded not to skip meals. Following is a summary of these recommendations:

- Breakfast: 30 grams of CHO
- Lunch and dinner: 60 grams of CHO
- Snacks: between 15 and 45 grams of CHO (dependent on the client's energy allowance based on individual assessment)
- Recommend bedtime snack for all clients
- Include protein and fat at each meal (amount dependent on client's energy allowance based on individual assessment)

Nutritional regulation is central to management of diabetes in pregnant women. During pregnancy, the most commonly recommended kilocalorie distribution is 40% to 45% CHO, 20% to 25% protein, and 30% to 40% fat. The treatment goal is to prevent hypoglycemia, defined as fasting plasma concentrations of <70 mg/dL.

Hyperglycemia during early pregnancy may be teratogenic (causing abnormal development of the embryo). Oral hypoglycemic agents have been shown to cause significant risk to the fetus. In most instances, women are advised to discontinue use of hypoglycemic agents before conception. If medication is necessary to control hyperglycemia, insulin is safer for the fetus.

Early pregnancy loss and congenital malformations can be minimized by optimal medical care and client education before conception. Contraception, timing of conception, control of metabolic state, self-management techniques, assessment of diabetic complications, and other medical complications should be discussed with clients of childbearing age. The desired outcome of glycemia control in preconception is to lower glycohemoglobin to achieve maximum fertility and optimal embryo and fetal development. Preconception counseling is best accomplished by a multidisciplinary approach including an endocrinologist; internist or family practice physician; obstetrician; and diabetes educators, including nurses, registered dietitians, social workers, and other specialists as necessary. Self-management skills essential for control during pregnancy include (ADA, 2013b):

- Using an appropriate meal plan
- Timing of meals and snacks
- Planning physical activity
- Choosing time and site of insulin injections
- Using carbohydrate and glucagon for hypoglycemia
- Reducing stress, coping with denial
- Testing capillary blood glucose
- Self-adjusting insulin doses

---

these disorders is responsible for hyperglycemia. Examples include:

- Pancreatitis
- Cystic fibrosis
- Downs syndrome
- Surgical removal of the pancreas
- Cushing disease
- Maturity-onset diabetes of the young (MODY)
- Pharmacological doses of glucocorticoids (e.g., prednisone) or other hormones or drugs

The diabetes may be resolved if the cause is alleviated (such as discontinuation of drugs or resolution of pancreatitis). If the cause is not correctable, secondary diabetes is treated similarly to other forms of diabetes (ADA, 2013b).

Other types of diabetes account for 1% to 5% of individuals diagnosed with diabetes (CDC, 2011).

Functions of Insulin

Every cell in the human body depends somewhat on glucose to meet energy needs. The brain and the rest of the nervous system depend almost exclusively on glucose for energy. Normally blood glucose levels decrease and increase within a given range pre- and post-feeding. Levels are lower before eating and higher after eating. Insulin is the only hormone that lowers blood glucose. A person normally secretes insulin in response to an elevated blood glucose level. Insulin decreases blood glucose by accelerating its movement from the blood into the cells. As glucose enters the cells, it may be metabolized to yield energy, may be stored as glycogen, or may be converted to fat (Table 17-2).

The ultimate fate of glucose once it is inside the cell depends on the body's need and the amount of glucose

TABLE 17-2 ■ Metabolic Activities Promoted by Insulin	
ACTIVITY	METABOLIC PATHWAY
Movement of glucose into cells	None
Energy production from glucose	Glycolysis
Manufacture of glycogen	Glycogenesis
Fat formation from carbohydrate and protein	Lipogenesis

Note: "Genesis" means forming of.

that enters the cell. The cells' energy needs will be met first. If cells have available glucose over and above immediate energy needs, the excess glucose is stored as glycogen. Insulin stimulates the storage of glucose as glycogen. Once the glycogen stores are filled to capacity, any remaining glucose is converted to fat. The body can store about 0.4 pound of glycogen, which is equal to 800 kilocalories.

Insulin influences the metabolism of protein and fat, and stimulates entry of amino acids into cells and enhances protein formation. It also enhances fat storage in adipose tissue and indirectly inhibits the breakdown of fat for energy. If the body has ample glucose available for energy, protein and fat need not be broken down to meet energy needs. If the body does not have glucose available for energy, it will use dietary protein or break down internal body protein stores to meet its immediate need for energy.

Insulin levels fluctuate in the blood. Normally, blood insulin levels increase as the blood glucose level increases. A high level of insulin in the blood signals the cells not to break down stores for energy (Table 17-3). An anabolic, or building, state exists when metabolism is normal and glucose and insulin levels are high. Normally insulin levels decrease as the blood sugar level decreases. A low level of insulin in the blood indirectly signals the body to begin to break down body stores for glucose. Figure 17-1 illustrates glucose use by the cells.

Other Hormones

Glucagon and somatostatin assist in coordinating the storage and mobilization of the energy nutrients: carbohydrate, fat, and protein. Glucagon increases blood glucose levels and stimulates the breakdown of body protein and fat stores. Somatostatin acts locally within the Islets

TABLE 17-3 ■ Metabolic Activities Inhibited by a High Level of Insulin	
ACTIVITY	METABOLIC PATHWAY
Movement of glucose from noncarbohydrate sources, e.g., glycerol and amino acids	Gluconeogenesis
Release of glucose from glycogen	Glycogenolysis
Breakdown of fat from adipose tissue	Lipolysis

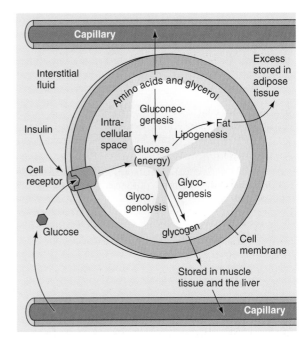

FIGURE 17-1 Insulin is necessary for glucose to gain entry into a cell. Once inside the cell, glucose can meet several fates: it can be burned as energy or stored as glycogen, or the glycerol portion of a fat molecule or some amino acids can be broken down into glucose. Some amino acids will be converted to glucose if the cell requires glucose.

of Langerhans to depress the secretion of insulin and glucagon. Evidence has shown that these hormones may not be at optimal levels in some clients with diabetes.

Cellular Sources of Glucose

Cells obtain glucose from both food that is eaten and internal glucose stores. Almost all carbohydrate eaten (except fiber), about 50% of protein eaten, and about 10% of fat eaten enter the blood as glucose. The internal body stores that can be converted to glucose are glycogen, some protein, and the glycerol portion of triglycerides. Body fat is stored as triglycerides in adipose tissue. To understand diabetes, it is necessary to know how the body coordinates all internal and external sources of glucose to maintain a normal blood glucose range.

Blood Glucose Curve

Given the vital need for every cell to have an uninterrupted supply of energy, the human body has evolved to allow an uninterrupted energy supply to reach cells without continuous eating. The blood glucose level increases after eating and decreases in the fasting state. Figure 17-2 illustrates the normal blood glucose curve.

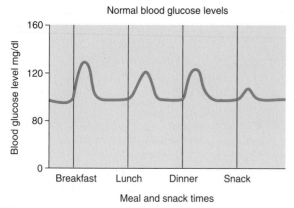

Normal blood glucose levels

FIGURE 17-2 A person's blood glucose level normally goes up after food consumption and then down between feedings.

Causes of Diabetes

When the β cells of the pancreas cannot make enough insulin, or when the body's cells are resistant to the insulin blood glucose cannot be transported into cells for their use. The result is hyperglycemia. The major causes of diabetes include genetic factors, lifestyle, autoimmune diseases, and viral infections. Some susceptibility to diabetes is genetic. However, not everyone with susceptible genes develops clinical diabetes. Before diabetes becomes apparent, this genetic susceptibility is often triggered by the individual's lifestyle or other environmental factors. A healthy lifestyle is particularly important for the *prevention* of diabetes in genetically susceptible clients. Excessive body fat, inactivity, and stress are risk factors for type 2 diabetes. A loss of body fat alone is sometimes sufficient to balance the insulin produced with a modified food intake. Sometimes emotional or physical stress is the stimulus that causes hyperglycemia. The body's stress response involves the release of epinephrine from the adrenal glands. One action of epinephrine is to raise the blood glucose level so the person has energy for the "fight or flight" response. One review found that the regular consumption of sugar sweetened and artificially sweetened beverages, but not 100% juice, appear to be a risk factor for the development of type 2 diabetes, although more study needs to be done (Fagherazzi, Viller, Saes Sartorelli et al, 2013).

Signs and Symptoms

The classic triad of signs and symptoms includes:

1. **Polyuria** (increased urination)
2. **Polydipsia** (increased thirst)
3. **Polyphagia** (increased appetite and weight loss)

The triad is most commonly seen in type 1 diabetes. The following section describes these and other signs and symptoms commonly seen in persons with diabetes.

Classic Triad

In diabetes, glucose cannot optimally move from the intravascular space across a cell membrane into the intracellular space. This is why the blood glucose level of people with diabetes remains elevated after eating. Under normal circumstances, the blood glucose level does not increase excessively because excess glucose undergoes glycolysis and is readily converted to adipose tissue or stored as glycogen inside the cell. As the glucose-rich blood circulates through the kidneys, these organs reabsorb as much glucose as they can. After this point is reached, glucose enters the urine. **Glycosuria** means an abnormally high amount of glucose in the urine. As the glucose exits the body in urine, water is pulled out also, as a result of the osmotic effect of glucose. This results in polyuria, or a large urine output. The large loss of water causes excessive thirst and polydipsia and prompts the person to drink fluids.

When glucose is not available for energy inside the cells, the body begins to break down protein and fat for energy. In untreated type 1 diabetes, the body's cells are starving. These starving cells send a message to the brain to turn on the person's appetite. The person responds by eating to satisfy the craving for food. The third most common symptom or sign of diabetes is **polyphagia,** an abnormal increase in appetite.

Other Signs and Symptoms

The abnormal carbohydrate metabolism of diabetes and its effects on the body's tissues cause other problems. Weight loss is more commonly seen in clients with type 1 diabetes than in clients with type 2. Clients with both types of diabetes may show these signs and symptoms:

- Blurred vision
- Fatigue
- Infection
- **Vaginitis** (inflammation of the vagina)
- Bladder infections
- Poor wound healing
- Impotence in men
- Kidney disorders

Complications

Both acute and chronic complications occur with diabetes mellitus. Acute complications require immediate care. Chronic complications include diseases of the eye, kidneys, heart, and nervous system. Chronic complications are responsible for the increased death rate among individuals with diabetes and the diminished quality of life that many of these clients experience.

Acute Clinical Situations

Three acute complications are seen in clients with diabetes:

1. **Diabetic ketoacidosis (DKA)**
2. Hyperglycemic hyperosmolar nonketotic syndrome
3. **Hypoglycemia**

Ketoacidosis

Individuals with type 1 diabetes who experience a profound insulin deficiency may progress to ketoacidosis. The three main precipitating factors in ketoacidosis are:

1. A decreased or missed dose of insulin
2. An illness or infection
3. Uncontrolled disease in a previously undiagnosed person

Ketoacidosis is a complex, life-threatening condition that demands emergency treatment. The predominant clinical manifestations and general principles of treatment are discussed next.

DEHYDRATION

Without insulin, glucose cannot be transferred across the cell membranes into the cells. A greatly increased number of glucose molecules (300 to 800 mg/dL) in the blood exert an osmotic effect, causing water to move from within the cells to the intravascular space and producing cellular dehydration. The body excretes the excess water, glucose, and electrolytes in urine.

ACIDOSIS

Unaware that the problem is not lack of glucose but lack of insulin, the body proceeds to increase blood glucose by mobilizing protein and fat from the tissues to be converted to glucose by the liver. Because the human body can use only the glycerol portion of the triglyceride molecule for glucose, the fatty acid portion is processed into ketones. Normally ketones are metabolized and excreted as carbon dioxide and water.

Under conditions of ketoacidosis, however, the body cannot metabolize this overload of ketones rapidly enough to maintain homeostasis. The client has excessive ketones in the blood (ketonemia) and spills ketones into the urine (ketonuria). Acetone is one of the ketone bodies for which urine is tested. The ketone bodies are acid, and thus the term ketoacidosis.

Electrolyte Imbalances

Clients with severe ketoacidosis may excrete 6.5 liters of fluid and 400 to 500 milliequivalents of sodium, potassium, and chloride in 24 hours. A fluid loss of 15% of body weight is not unusual. Most critical in the treatment of electrolyte imbalances in diabetic ketoacidosis is the body's level of potassium. As the cells are being catabolized for fuel, the intracellular potassium is transferred to the intravascular space.

Serum potassium levels can be low, normal, or elevated in the person with ketoacidosis, depending on the body's current coping mechanism. Regardless of the serum concentrations of potassium and sodium, the pathological process of diabetic ketoacidosis depletes these electrolytes. Either hypokalemia or hyperkalemia can lead to cardiac arrhythmias and must be carefully managed in clients with ketoacidosis.

Treatment

Clients with severe diabetic ketoacidosis are critically ill. Treatment includes supplemental insulin, fluid and electrolyte replacement, and medical monitoring. Serum electrolyte levels change dramatically once treatment commences. Intensive care is necessary to provide the careful monitoring and frequent adjustments in therapy required as the fluids and electrolytes are being replaced. Intravenous regular insulin will permit the use of carbohydrate for energy and will halt the body's excessive use of fat, which has produced the ketone bodies. Insulin drives glucose back into the cells. Potassium, too, moves from the intravascular space to the intracellular space, necessitating frequent measurement of the serum levels of both glucose and potassium. When the client recovers, identification of the precipitating factor for the ketoacidosis and education focused on preventing additional occurrences are essential.

Hyperglycemic Hyperosmolar Nonketotic Syndrome

The four signs of **hyperglycemic hyperosmolar nonketotic syndrome (HHNS)** are:

1. Blood glucose level >600 mg/dL
2. Absence of or slight ketosis
3. Plasma hyperosmolality
4. Profound dehydration

This life-threatening emergency is usually seen in older people with diabetes, more often in type 2 diabetics, and is normally brought on by an illness or infection. HHNS is like DKA except that the insulin deficiency is not as severe, so increased **lipolysis** (the breakdown of body lipid stores) does not occur. Because these clients do not have symptoms of vomiting, nausea, and acidosis brought on by severe ketosis, as do clients with type 1 diabetes, they often do not seek prompt medical help. Their blood sugar levels are higher and their dehydration more severe than is seen in ketoacidosis.

In these clients, prolonged osmotic diuresis and dehydration secondary to hyperglycemia lead to decreased renal blood flow and allow blood glucose to reach very high levels. Medications that cause an increase in blood glucose levels, chronic disease, and infection may contribute to this condition. Treatment includes correction of the electrolyte imbalance, hyperglycemia, and dehydration.

Hypoglycemia

In both type 1 and type 2 diabetes, an individual can develop hypoglycemia which is defined by a blood glucose level <70 mg/dL. Hypoglycemia may be caused by:

- Too much insulin (accidental or deliberate)
- Too little food intake, a delayed meal
- Excessive exercise
- Alcohol (especially in the fasting state)
- Medications such as oral hypoglycemic agents

  Symptoms may include:

- Confusion
- Headache
- Double vision
- Rapid heartbeat
- Sweating
- Hunger
- Seizure
- Coma

The treatment of hypoglycemia is discussed later in this chapter.

Chronic Complications

Clients with both type 1 and type 2 diabetes of sufficient duration are vulnerable to serious complications involving the eyes, kidneys, and nervous system.

Diabetic **retinopathy** is a disorder that involves the retina. Diabetes is a leading cause of blindness and vision loss in the adult U.S. population. The blurred vision reported by these clients is related to retinopathy. These clients are also at a higher risk for cataracts.

Diabetic **neuropathy** is a chronic complication of diabetes. Clients may complain of a lack of sensation in their extremities. They may puncture, cut, or burn their feet and not feel any pain. A wound may become infected and heal poorly. Gangrene, or tissue death, may follow. The treatment for gangrene is amputation. **Neuropathy** can affect gastric or intestinal motility, erectile function, bladder function, cardiac function, and vascular tone.

Gastroparesis (paralysis of the stomach with delayed gastric emptying) may occur and alter the absorption of meals, which makes glycemic control problematic.

Cardiovascular disease (CVD) is more common in clients with diabetes than in the nondiabetic population of the same age and gender. This is related in general to the fact that diabetes is a small-vessel disease and the critical end arteries in the heart muscle are small vessels.

Diabetic **nephropathy**, or kidney disease, is another common complication in clients with diabetes.

Tragically, some clients with diabetes do not take the threat of chronic complications seriously until much damage has occurred.

Management

The current medical goal is to *normalize* blood glucose throughout the day and to control blood pressure and blood lipids. The importance of a physician-led medical team for the management of a client's diabetes is outlined in the 2013 Standards of Medical Care in Diabetes published by the American Diabetes Association. Teams should include nurses, pharmacists, dietitians, and mental health professionals—all with proficiency in diabetes care. The goals of the treatment plan for management of the client's diabetes should be developed by the team in conjunction with the client to ensure the plan is reasonable and understandable. The client's age, work and/or school schedule, physical activity, eating habits (which include social and cultural factors) as well as other medical conditions must be taken into account when developing diabetes self-management education for clients. Clients self-monitoring of blood glucose (SMBG) is an important tool for determining the effectiveness and adherence to a treatment plan. For individuals using multiple insulin injections or an insulin pump, SMBG should be done three or more times per day. The two primary methods for health-care providers and clients to assess the effectiveness of the diabetes management plan are SMBG and A1C. Table 17-4 presents glycemic goals recommended by the American Diabetes Association (ADA, 2013b).

A landmark study known as the Diabetes Control and Complications Trial (DCCT) in individuals with type 1 diabetes demonstrated that intensive control of blood glucose levels delays the onset and slows the progression of diabetic retinopathy, nephropathy, and neuropathy (DCCT Research Group, 1993). According to this study's results, people with type 1 diabetes who followed a tightly controlled regimen, compared with those who followed a standard regimen, showed reductions of approximately:

- 76% in progression of diabetic retinopathy
- 54% in albuminuria (albumin in the urine, which may be a sign of renal impairment)

TABLE 17-4 ■ **Glycemic Goals for Diabetics**

GLYCEMIC RECOMMENDATIONS	ADULTS	CHILDREN 0–6	CHILDREN 6–12	ADOLESCENTS 13–19	GDM	GDM/PRE-EXISTING DM
Bedtime and overnight (mg/dL)	N/A	110–200	100–180	90–150	N/A	60–99*
Preprandial mg/dL	70–130	100–180	90–180	90–130	≤95	60–99*
1 hour postprandial mg/dL	<180	†	†	†	≤140	100–129
2 postprandial mg/dL	<180	†	†	†	≤120	100–129
A1C %	<7.0	<8.5	<7.0	<7.5	N/A	<6.0

*If achievable without excessive hypoglycemia.

†Postprandial blood glucose levels should be measured when there is a discrepancy between preprandial blood glucose values and A1C levels to help assess glycemia in those on basal/bolus regimens.

■ 36% in **microalbuminuria** (a more sensitive indicator of protein in the urine, which may be an early warning of renal impairment)

A tightly controlled regimen is not without problems, however. Among these is an increased incidence of insulin-induced hypoglycemic episodes. Clients undergoing intensive diabetes treatment do not face deterioration in the quality of their lives, even while the rigor of their diabetes care is increased (DCCT Research Group, 1996). Since the DCCT study was done, there have been different insulins developed with different times of onset, peak, and duration that have helped reduce the incidence of hypoglycemia. The DCCT showed that intensive insulin therapy (three or more insulin injections per day, continuous subcutaneous insulin infusion [CSII], or insulin pump therapy) improved glycemic control and improve outcomes (ADA, 2013b). This evidence has been further strengthened by a report from the United Kingdom Prospective Diabetes Study (UKPDS), which demonstrated that intensive therapy for type 2 diabetes significantly lowered the rate of diabetes-related events (UKPDS Group, 1998).

The benefits of intensive therapies has been demonstrated to continue long term for clients with type 1 with reductions in nonfatal myocardial infarction, stroke, or CVD death. Type 2 diabetics, newly diagnosed, with intensive glycemic control (<6.5%) had reductions in cardiovascular events. Studies have shown an increase in mortality due to cardiovascular events in individuals with long-standing (>9 years) type 2 diabetes. Because of the potential risks for individuals with long-standing type 2 diabetes, a history of severe hypoglycemia, advanced atherosclerosis, or an advanced age, intensive glycemic control is not recommended (ADA, 2013b).

All health-care workers should assist the general population in the early detection of diabetes and prevention of complications. As Figure 17-3 emphasizes, the three cornerstones of the management of diabetes after diagnosis are:

1. Physical activity
2. Medication
3. Nutritional management

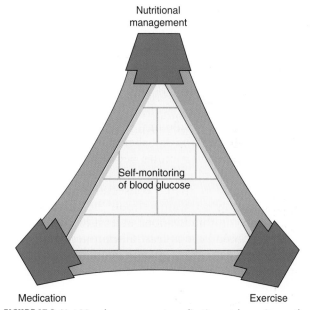

FIGURE 17-3 Nutritional management, medication, and exercise are the three components of treatment for diabetes. Each of these cornerstones has an influence on blood glucose levels. An individual can identify how each of these cornerstones affects his or her blood glucose level by self-monitoring blood glucose.

Self-monitoring of blood glucose levels enables the client to assess how each of these factors interacts.

Self-Monitoring of Blood Glucose

Many individuals monitor their own blood glucose levels with a blood glucose meter. This procedure is called **self-monitoring of blood glucose (SMBG).** Individual response to medication, diet, and exercise can be determined with SMBG and can be performed using a single drop of blood. The client obtains the drop of blood from a finger with either a lancet or a spring-loaded device. The blood sample is placed in the meter, called a glucometer, and the test results are available in less than 1 minute. The client can then adjust insulin dose and food and exercise behaviors accordingly. Many experts consider SMBG to be the most important development in diabetes management since the discovery of insulin.

SMBG has allowed clients to try to normalize their blood glucose levels throughout the day. Health-care workers need to teach clients carefully how to interpret the results of SMBG. Continual reassessment of the client's technique and blood glucose records is necessary to guide treatment decisions. SMBG helps evaluate the need for changes in diet or medications and for clients on insulin injections or pumps, monitoring should be done at least 3 times a day. Continuous glucose monitoring (CGM) devices are available to measure blood glucose and have alarms when low or high levels are measured. There are no definitive standards for SMBG for people with type 2 diabetes who are on diet control or oral medications (ADA, 2013b).

Physical Activity

Exercise plays a key role in the management of diabetes. All individuals with diabetes are encouraged to perform at least 150 minutes per week of moderate-intensity aerobic physical activity at least 3 days per week with no more than 2 consecutive days without exercise. Strength training should be performed, if there are no contraindications, at least twice per week. Children should have at least 60 minutes of physical activity every day (ADA, 2013b). People with diabetes who exercise should be encouraged to follow these guidelines:

1. Wear proper footwear and use other protective equipment if necessary.
2. Avoid exercise in extremely hot or cold environments.
3. Inspect feet daily and after exercise for open areas, blisters, punctures, swelling, and redness; report any of these signs to the physician immediately.
4. Avoid exercise during periods of poor metabolic control (blood glucose levels that are <70 or >240 mg/dL levels).
5. Wear a diabetes ID badge or bracelet.
6. Carry a source of glucose in case of a decrease in blood glucose because exercise decreases blood glucose levels.
7. Diabetics who use insulin, or insulin secretagogues, if blood glucose levels are less than 100 mg/dL before exercise, added carbohydrate should be ingested pre-exercise (ADA, 2013b).

Exercise and Type 1 Diabetes

The ADA strongly endorses an exercise program for people with type 1 diabetes because of the potential for improving cardiovascular fitness and psychological well-being. Exercise involves some risk for individuals with type 1 diabetes because it changes insulin requirements in sometimes unpredictable ways for more than 24 hours after the exercise. Retinopathy, neuropathy, and renal disease may worsen in some clients with type 1 diabetes who exercise. Blood pressure may also become elevated. For this type of client, self-monitoring of blood glucose should be incorporated into a modified exercise program tailored to individual needs and limitations. The client should demonstrate the ability to self-treat a hypoglycemic episode.

Exercise and Type 2 Diabetes

Physical activity is widely endorsed for persons with type 2 diabetes. Physical activity increases the number and binding capacity of insulin receptors, assists in lowering blood glucose levels, and reduces insulin requirements in persons who use insulin. Improved blood lipid levels occur in some clients who engage in regular exercise. This improvement helps delay or prevent the CVD complications commonly seen in these clients. Exercise also assists in weight control and improves muscle strength and flexibility.

Exercise, SMBG, and Food Intake

Clients with type 1 diabetes who exercise and all type 2 clients who engage in nonroutine exercise should monitor their blood glucose levels before, during, and after exercise. It is best to exercise 60 to 90 minutes after meals, when the blood glucose level is highest. If the blood glucose level is greater than 100 mg/dL before exercise, no additional food is usually needed if the planned exercise is of short duration and low intensity. Exercise of long duration and high intensity generally requires more kilocalories. Snacks with an additional 15 to 30 grams of carbohydrate-containing food should be ingested for every 30 to 60 minutes of exercise. Good choices for snack foods include:

■ Fruit
■ Starch
■ Milk exchanges

To prevent wide swings in blood glucose levels, care should be taken not to overeat. Too much food will cause the blood glucose level to go up too high and subsequently to drop too low.

Medications for Diabetes

Two primary types of medications are used with diabetic clients:

1. Insulin
2. Oral hypoglycemic agents

Clients with type 1 diabetes require insulin. Clients with type 2 diabetes may not require any medication, may need to have an oral hypoglycemic agent and/or insulin prescribed. Frequently, clients with type 2 diabetes are able to discontinue or reduce medications after a significant loss of body fat.

Insulin

Almost all the insulin used in the United States is human. Human insulin is manufactured by recombinant-DNA technology (biosynthetic). Human insulin (**Humulin**) produces few allergic reactions. Insulin cannot be taken orally because the gastrointestinal tract enzymes will digest it before absorption. Insulin must be administered by needle either **subcutaneously** (beneath the skin) or intravenously (IV). Only regular insulin is given IV. The substances used to delay absorption of intermediate- and long-acting insulins are not designed for IV administration. Regular insulin is usually administered IV only for the severely hyperglycemic or hospitalized client.

Insulin can also be administered with an insulin pump. These pumps are designed to provide a small inflow of insulin continuously and large inflows before eating, mimicking normal insulin secretion. Continuous subcutaneous insulin infusion (CSII) or insulin pumps have been available for nearly 25 years but have only recently been widely used.

Medications are described according to the onset, peak, and duration of action. A bolus dose of insulin is short acting and designed to cover needs for one meal. A basal dose of insulin is longer acting and usually injected once or twice a day. Table 17-5 lists the times of onset, peak, and duration of insulin. Variation in duration makes it possible to inject insulin in a pattern that is as close as possible to normal insulin activity. Ideally, the medication is planned around the diet, not vice versa. It is for the client's benefit, and long-term quality of life, to change a medication to cover food/meal ingestion for the greatest flexibility.

Oral Hypoglycemic Agents

Oral hypoglycemic agents lower blood glucose levels in type 2 diabetes. These drugs stimulate insulin release from the pancreatic beta cells, reduce glucose output from the liver, and increase the uptake of glucose in tissues. Many oral agents are being prescribed in the United States (Table 17-6). Metformin is the preferred initial oral medication given to prediabetics and diabetics, unless there is a contraindication (such as reduced kidney function or severe GI side effects). Commonly prescribed oral hypoglycemic agents include glipizide,

TABLE 17-5 ■ Times of Onset, Peak, and Duration of Action for Insulins

	TIMES IN HOURS		
	Onset	Peak	Duration
Insulin Bolus (Short Acting)			
Humalog® or lispro	15–30 minutes	30–90 minutes	3–5 hours
NovoLog® or aspart	10–20 minutes	40–50 minutes	3–5 hours
Regular	30–60 minutes	2–5 hours	5–8 hours
Apidra® or glulisine	20–30 minutes	30–90 minutes	1–2½ hours
Basal Insulin (Intermediate-Long Acting)			
Lantus**	1–1½ hours	None	20–24 hours
NPH	1–2 hours	4–12 hours	18–24 hours
Novolog 70/30*†	10–20 minutes	1–4 hours	Up to 24 hours
Lente	1–2½ hours	3–10 hours	18–24 hours
Ultralente	30 minutes–3 hours	10–20 hours	20–36 hours
Levemir®	1–2 hours	6–8 hours	Up to 24 hours

*Lantus® is a long-acting insulin that is designed to be given at HS (Latin for hour of sleep, commonly used to mean just before bedtime). Lantus® has no pronounced peaks, with a relatively constant level over 24 hours. The Food and Drug Administration approved Lantus® in early 2000 and Levemir® in 2005. †Mixture is a premixed insulin with intermediate-acting and short-acting insulin in one bottle or insulin pen.

glyburide, glimepiride, acarbose, and glitazones. Oral agents are frequently used in combinations to help get diabetics to their recommended glycemic levels without hypoglycemia. Many of the oral agents work on different cell receptor sites (ADA, 2013b).

Management of Hospitalized Clients

Increased lengths of stay and adverse outcomes are seen in hospitalized clients with hyperglycemia. In the hospitalized population with hyperglycemia, when blood glucose levels are greater than 140 to 180 mg/dL, treatment with insulin is recommended, along with checking the A1C levels so that individuals with existing diabetes can be distinguished from those with hyperglycemia triggered from acute stress. Oral diabetes medications should be discontinued during most acute hospitalizations and resumed as appropriate after discharge. Because hospitalized individuals may have a rapidly changing condition, and/or be NPO (no food by mouth) for treatment and tests, flexibility in insulin therapy is critical. A basal and bolus insulin therapy that helps prevent periods of hyper- and hypoglycemia is recommended. The three components to this type of therapy include basal insulin, which is long acting and given once per day; mealtime bolus insulin, which is fast acting and helps prevent postprandial rises in blood glucose and is given before a meal and withheld if the client is NPO; and correction insulin, which is also fast acting and given to lower hyperglycemic blood glucose levels not caused by nutritional hyperglycemia (ADA, 2013b; Magaji and Johnston, 2011).

TABLE 17-6 ■ Diabetes Oral Medications and Major Actions

CLASSIFICATION	MAJOR ACTIONS	GENERIC NAME (TRADE NAME)	COMMENTS
Sulfonylureas	Stimulate insulin release by the pancreas and may help decrease liver glucose production.	Glipizide (Glucotrol®, Glucotrol® XL) Glyburide (DiaBeta®, Micronase®, Glynase PresTabs®) Glimepiride (Amaryl®)	Glipizide must be taken on an empty stomach. Glyburide can be taken with food or on an empty stomach. Low toxicity. Use caution with elderly.
Biguanides	Decrease liver production of glucose. Increase glucose uptake into tissues.	Metformin (Glucophage®)	Given in 2–3 doses per day with meals. Not metabolized.
Meglitinide	Stimulates immediate insulin release from pancreas as needed for meals.	Repaglinide (Prandin®) Nateglinide (Starlix®)	Given in 2–4 doses per day 15–30 minutes before meals.
Alpha-Glucosidase Inhibitors	Slow the rate of digestion of starches and complex sugars.	Acarbose (Precose®)	Given in 3 doses per day with meals. 98% not absorbed. Rest excreted by kidneys.
Thiazolidinedione	Decreases insulin resistance.	Pioglitazone (Actos®) Rosiglitazone (Avandia®)	Clients need to be monitored for fluid retention and weight gain.

Medical Nutritional Management of Diabetes

Diabetes is directly related to how the body uses food. Nutrition is thus an essential component of management for all persons with diabetes. Studies have shown that clients report improved health; better control of body weight; improved control of blood glucose, blood pressure, and lipid levels; and improved use of insulin when they adhere to dietary recommendations. The goals of nutritional care for people with diabetes are the control and prevention of complications. This involves the promotion of normal nutrition and dietary modification to control blood glucose and lipid levels. Clients' nutritional goals need to be determined individually. There is no "diabetic diet" or "ADA diet," but several meal-planning approaches are widely endorsed by the ADA and the Academy of Nutrition and Dietetics (see Dollars & Sense 17-1).

Nutritional Goals

The goal of medical nutritional therapy is to educate the client with diabetes so he or she can make changes in food and exercise habits that lead to improved metabolic control. Specifically, the client needs assistance with:

1. Attaining and maintaining near-normal blood glucose levels as feasible by the coordination of food intake, **endogenous** and **exogenous** insulin and/or hypoglycemic agents, and physical activity. This goal is a challenge in some clients who have fluctuating endogenous insulin production.
2. Attaining and maintaining optimal serum lipid levels and blood pressure
3. Providing adequate kilocalories to:
   - Attain and maintain a healthy body weight for adults and normal growth and development for children
   - Recover from illnesses
   - Meet the metabolic needs of pregnancy and lactation
4. Preventing and treating the acute and chronic complications of diabetes, such as renal disease, autonomic neuropathy, hypertension, and CVD.
5. Improving overall health through good nutrition. *MyPlate, U.S. Department of Agriculture Food Guide,* and *Dietary Guidelines for Americans* illustrate and summarize nutritional guidelines for all Americans, including people with diabetes.

Goal Priority

The medications prescribed, the type of diabetes the individual has, and the client's desire to change behavior determine goal priority. A high priority for the person taking insulin is to facilitate consistency in the timing of insulin to cover meals and snacks to prevent wide swings in blood glucose. This priority requires coordination among exercise, insulin, and food intake.

A high priority for the individual with type 2 diabetes is achieving glucose, blood pressure, and lipid goals. To achieve these goals, diet is a cornerstone of treatment. Weight reduction for these clients usually improves short-term glycemic levels and long-term metabolic control. The client's motivation to lose weight needs to be carefully assessed by the health-care educator.

$ Dollars & Sense 17-1

Dietetic Foods

Clients with diabetes do not need to buy special foods labeled "dietetic." Many clients find they actually save money because they eat less food on the prescribed meal plan.

Meal Frequency

Meal spacing is more crucial in type 1 than in type 2 diabetes. Consistent timing of medication type and administration and meal size assist in stabilization of blood glucose levels in type 1 diabetes. In general, people with diabetes benefit from eating on a regular basis (every 4–5 hours), but this must be individualized based on the client's lifestyle and/or medical condition.

Client Readiness to Change

Food behaviors are difficult to change. Although some clients with diabetes do successfully change or alter food behaviors to enhance their outcomes, many clients do not, will not, or cannot change harmful food behaviors. Modification of harmful behaviors involves progression through five stages: precontemplation, contemplation, preparation, action, and maintenance. Individuals typically recycle through these stages several times before terminating negative behaviors. Following is a brief description of each stage:

1. *Precontemplation:* Individuals exhibit no intention to change behavior in the foreseeable future.
2. *Contemplation:* Individuals know they have a problem and are seriously thinking about overcoming the harmful behavior but are not ready to take action.
3. *Preparation:* Individuals plan to take action in the near future, may have taken action unsuccessfully in the past, and may report small behavioral changes.
4. *Action:* Individuals modify their behavior, experiences, and environment to overcome the harmful behavior. This stage requires considerable commitment of time and energy.
5. *Maintenance:* Individuals continue to work to prevent relapse and to consolidate gains.

Health-care workers can assist clients in the precontemplation and contemplation stages by attempting to raise clients' consciousness about the benefits of behavioral change. Stimulus control and reinforcement also help clients become more aware of the need to alter behaviors (see Weight Management). The most difficult problems posed by clients for the health educator are at the precontemplation phase (Zimmerman, Olsen, and Boswoth, 2000).

A technique called Motivational Interviewing (MI) that can be used by health-care workers helps determine what the client's interest in disease management and education is and can strengthen the client's desire to make positive changes. If the client wishes to gain better blood glucose control, the clinician working with that individual would help explore how he or she wishes to do so. Options utilizing diet, medications, and/or exercise should all be discussed and assistance with the client's goal provided. Consulting a dietitian, pharmacist, and/or physical therapist may be helpful for the client to reach and maintain his/her goal. MI has been shown to improve self-management, psychological and glycemic outcomes in type 2 diabetics (Chen, Creedy, Lin, and Willin, 2012).

The health-care educator needs to consider carefully how much information the client desires and how ready he or she is to change behaviors. For example, an educational tool that takes 3 to 4 hours to review with a client is inappropriate for someone who is willing to devote just a few minutes to learning about his or her diet. In contrast, the client who wants to learn everything he or she can about self-care will not be satisfied with an elementary meal plan.

Survival Skills

The ADA and the Academy of Nutrition and Dietetics recommend that the newly diagnosed client initially learn basic survival skills. DavisPlus contains a copy of Survival Skills, or information the client needs to know immediately. After the client has demonstrated an understanding of this basic knowledge, a firm foundation has been set for the acquisition of additional, more individualized information. Individualized food and meal plans and insulin regimens provide flexibility to accommodate lifestyle, age, and overall health status.

Meal-Planning Approaches

Several meal planning tools are available for use with the newly diagnosed client including:

- MyPlate for Diabetes
- Dietary Guidelines for Americans
- The USDA Food Guide

Any of these meal-planning approaches is considered survival-skill information. After the client understands the initial meal-planning approach, a more advanced approach should be considered. Many hospitals and private practitioners provide more comprehensive educational programs to achieve optimal blood glucose and lipid control. Different tools for meal-planning are discussed later in the chapter. Figure 17-4 illustrates a dietitian providing nutrition counseling.

Energy Nutrient Distribution

Total energy requirements for an individual with diabetes do not differ from those for individuals without diabetes. Twenty to 35 kcal/kg, depending on the client's level of physical activity, nutritional status, desire for weight loss or gain, and body weight are usually a good starting point

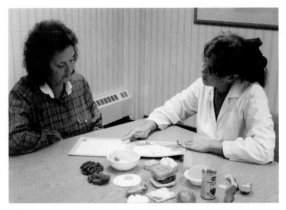

FIGURE 17-4 A diabetes educator providing nutritional counseling. The use of food models facilitates the learning process and teaches portion control.

to estimate a need for kcal. The client should eat a set amount of kcal for a few weeks and compare body weight before and after the given kcal level is consumed. Adjustments based on the treatment goals can be made, as necessary. If weight loss is desirable, the rate of loss should be 1 to 2 pounds per week. The only way to more accurately determine a client's need for energy is by indirect calorimetry and this equipment is not widely available.

The acceptable macronutrient distribution recommended for the general population is also recommended for clients with diabetes. The distribution of energy

nutrients refers to the percentage of total kilocalories that should be derived from carbohydrate, fat, and protein as well as to the division of carbohydrate, fat, and protein among the day's meals/feedings. Clinical Calculation 17-1 shows how the percentage of energy nutrients is converted to grams of carbohydrate, fat, and protein and distributed throughout the day's meals/feedings.

Macronutrient Distribution

There is no one optimal mix of carbohydrate, protein, and fat that must be followed by every diabetic. This should be individualized based upon each client's lifestyle, preference, and comorbidities. Low-fat, low-carbohydrate, and Mediterranean eating patterns have all been shown to be effective for weight loss in studies up to 2 years. Monitoring carbohydrate intake through carbohydrate counting, choices, or experienced-based estimates are recommended for achieving glycemic control (ADA, 2013b).

Dietary Guidelines for Americans recommends all people choose a variety of fiber-containing food, such as whole grains, fruits, and vegetables, because they provide vitamins, minerals, fiber, and other substances that optimize health. The contribution of carbohydrate to total kilocalorie intake should be individualized based on nutrition assessment, laboratory results, and weight and treatment goals.

17-1

𝒞linical 𝒞alculation

Distributing Energy Nutrients and Calculating a Diet

In the following example, an 1800-kcal diet is converted to 55% carbohydrate, 20% protein, and 25% fat.

$$1800 \text{ kcal} \times 0.55 = 990 \text{ kcal @ } 4 \text{ kcal/gram} = 248 \text{ grams}$$
of carbohydrate
$$1800 \text{ kcal} \times 0.20 = 360 \text{ kcal @ } 4 \text{ kcal/gram} = 90 \text{ grams of protein}$$
$$1800 \text{ kcal} \times 0.25 = 450 \text{ kcal @ } 9 \text{ kcal/gram} = 50 \text{ grams of fat}$$

In the following example, 248 grams of carbohydrate, 90 grams of protein, and 50 grams of fat are converted to a ⅕, ⅖, ⅕, and ⅕ distribution. Each fraction represents one meal; thus, ⅕ of the energy nutrients are to be provided each at breakfast, supper, and the evening snack; ⅖ of the energy nutrients are to be provided at the noon meal. Please note: ⅕ equals 20%, and ⅖ equals 40%.

$$248 \text{ grams of carbohydrate} \times 0.20 = 50 \text{ grams} \times 3 \text{ meals} = 150$$
$$248 \text{ grams of carbohydrate} \times 0.20 = 99 \text{ grams} \times 1 \text{ meals} = 99$$
$$90 \text{ grams of protein} \times 0.20 = 18 \text{ grams} \times 3 \text{ meals} = 54$$
$$90 \text{ grams of carbohydrate} \times 0.40 = 36 \text{ grams} \times 1 \text{ meal} = 36$$

Because only a small percentage of dietary fat enters the bloodstream as glucose, normally fat is not calculated into the distribution. Lunch (²/₅ distribution) would contain about 99 grams of carbohydrate

and 36 grams of protein. Each of the other meals (⅕ distribution) would contain about 50 grams of carbohydrate and 18 grams of protein.

The next step is to determine the number of exchanges to be provided from each of the six exchange groups. No exact method is used to determine this step. Usually the client is consulted to determine the amount of nonfat milk, fruits, vegetables, and so forth that he or she would be willing to consume. An effort should be made to calculate the diet with at least the recommended amount and categories of food in the MyPlate guide for diabetics (see Fig. 17-5). Many health-care workers determine the amount of nonfat milk, fruits, and vegetables to be provided first. This calculation is followed by the grams of carbohydrate to be contributed by these groups. The remaining carbohydrate is then allocated to the starch group.

Protein is determined by first calculating the amount previously provided by nonfat milk, vegetables, and starches; the remaining protein is then allocated to meat exchanges. Fat is determined by first calculating the amount previously provided by the meat exchanges; the remaining fat is then allocated to fat exchanges. The calculations and meal plan for our sample 1800 kcal with 55% carbohydrate, 20% protein, and 25% fat with a ⅕, ⅖, ⅕, and ⅕ distribution appear in Table 17-7.

TABLE 17-7 ■ Sample 1800-Kilocalorie Diabetic Diet*

DIVISION OF ENERGY NUTRIENTS AND EXCHANGES

Exchange List	Number of Daily Exchanges	Protein (90 g)	Fat (50 g)	Carbohydrate (218 g)	Breakfast	Lunch	Dinner	Bedtime
Skim milk	2	16	0	24	½	1		½
Starch	11	33	0	165	2	4	3	2
Fruit	3	0	0	45	1	1	0	1
Vegetable	3	6	0	15	0	2	1	0
Meat	5	35	25	0	1	2	1	1
Fat	5	0	25	0	1	1	2	1

MEAL PLAN AND SAMPLE MENUS

Meal Plan	Sample Menu 1	Sample Menu 2
Breakfast ½ cup skim milk 2 starch 1 fruit 1 meat 1 fat	½ cup skim milk 2 slices of toast ½ cup orange juice ¼ cup low-cholesterol egg substitute 1 tsp margarine	½ cup skim milk 1 cup of oatmeal ½ banana 1 low-fat sausage link 2 pecans
Lunch 1 skim milk 4 starch 1 fruit 2 vegetables 2 meat 1 fat	1 cup skim milk 1 cup brown rice 1 apple 1 cup green beans 2 oz stir-fried chicken 1 tsp oil	1 cup skim milk 2 slices of bread† 1 cup broth-type vegetable soup and 3 ginger snaps ½ cup pineapple juice ½ cup asparagus and 1 cup raw carrots 2 slices low-fat cheese† 1 tsp margarine†
Dinner 3 starch 1 vegetable Free vegetable 1 meat 2 fat Free	1 large baked potato ½ cup broccoli‡ Lettuce salad 1 oz ground beef 2 tbsp sour cream‡ 1 tbsp French dressing Coffee	¼ 10-in pizza, thin crust, and 2 bread sticks (4 × ½ in) Sliced tomato Lettuce salad 1 tbsp French dressing Diet soft drink
HS ½ cup skim milk 2 starch 1 fruit 1 meat 1 fat	½ cup skim milk 1½ oz pretzels 15 grapes 1 oz low-fat cheese stick 2 walnuts	½ cup skim milk 6 cups hot-air-popped popcorn 1 peach 1 tbsp Parmesan cheese 1 tbsp lite margarine

HS, hora somni (at bedtime).
*The calculations and meal plan based on 55% carbohydrate, 20% protein, and 25% fat with a ⅕, ⅖, ⅕, and ⅕ distribution.
†Cheese sandwich.
‡Potato toppings.

The ADA, in association with the American Dietetic Association (now the Academy of Nutrition and Dietetics), published general guidelines that pertain to carbohydrates and include the following (ADA, 2008):

■ A dietary pattern that includes carbohydrate (CHO) from fruits, vegetables, whole grains, legumes, and low-fat milk is encouraged for good health.
■ Monitoring CHO, whether by carbohydrate counting, exchanges, or experienced-based estimation, remains a good strategy in achieving glycemic control.

■ The use of the glycemic index and load may provide a modest benefit over that observed when total CHO is considered alone.
■ Sucrose-containing foods can be substituted for other CHO in the meal plan, if added to the meal plan, covered with insulin or other glucose-lowering medications. Care should be taken to avoid excess energy intake.
■ Like the general population, people with diabetes are encouraged to consume a variety of fiber-containing foods. However, evidence is lacking to recommend

a higher fiber intake for people with diabetes than for the population as a whole.

■ Sugar alcohols and nonnutritive sweeteners are safe when consumed within the daily levels established by the U.S. Food and Drug Administration.

Eating a diet high in refined carbohydrates is not recommended. One review found that sugar may have a long-term negative metabolic effect. It factored out obesity and inactivity. For every 150 kilocalories of sugar (equal to one 12-ounce soft drink) in a diet, there was a 1% increase in the prevalence of diabetes in a population. There was only a .1% increase seen with an additional 150 calories for other food sources (Basu, Yoffe, Hills, and Lustig, 2013). An increased intake of high-fructose corn syrup (HFCS) was associated with a 20% higher prevalence of diabetes in populations consuming HFCS (Goran, Ulijaszek, and Ventura, 2012). Conversely, a higher intake of whole grains is associated with a decreased risk of deteriorating glucose tolerance (Wirström, Hilding, Gu, et al, 2012).

Protein

The need for protein in the diabetic population is the same as for the general population if renal function is normal. Excessive dietary protein should be avoided. The concept that excessive dietary protein may have a health risk is discussed in Chapter 4. In addition, protein can increase insulin response without increasing plasma glucose concentrations. Therefore, protein should not be used to treat acute or prevent nighttime hypoglycemia (ADA, 2012c).

The primary goal regarding dietary fat in clients with diabetes is to decrease blood lipid levels. To achieve this goal, recommendations include:

■ Limit saturated fat to <7% of total kilocalories.
■ Intake of *trans*-fat should be minimized.
■ Lower dietary cholesterol to <200 mg/day.
■ Consume two or more servings of fish per week (with the exception of commercially fried fish filets) because these provide *n*-3 polyunsaturated fatty acids.

Not all clients with diabetes have these lipid abnormalities. In epidemiological studies, an increased plasma triglyceride and low high-density lipoprotein cholesterol have been associated with an increased risk for clinically apparent CVD in people with diabetes. CVD is the major cause of morbidity and mortality in individuals with diabetes (ADA, 2012b).

Carbohydrate Counting

Carbohydrate counting is another frequently used menu-planning tool. Because CHO is the energy nutrient that has the greatest influence on blood glucose levels, some clients adhere to nutritional recommendations more closely with this approach and SMBG. Clients can readily see the effect that diet has on blood glucose levels throughout the day when combined with SMBG. The advantages of the carbohydrate-counting meal plan concept include:

■ Single-nutrient focused
■ More precise matching of food and insulin
■ Flexible food choices
■ A potential for improved blood glucose, and client-controlled treatment

Challenges for the client who uses this system may include:

■ The need to weigh and measure food
■ Maintenance of extensive food records
■ Monitoring of the blood glucose before and after eating
■ The need to calculate grams of carbohydrate consumed
■ The need to maintain healthful eating and weight management

Knowledge of carbohydrate counting is often a prerequisite before consideration of insulin pump therapy. It is also a prerequisite for clients who want to learn how to calculate insulin-to-carbohydrate ratios. This type of teaching is usually done by a certified diabetes educator (CDE) and is considered advanced teaching.

The rationale for carbohydrate counting is a carbohydrate exchange (approximately 15 grams of carbohydrate) equals one starch exchange, one fruit exchange, or one milk exchange. The acceptable range is 8 to 22 grams per carbohydrate choice. Food labels, tables of food composition, and *Exchange Lists for Meal Planning* are some of the tools clients can use to determine the carbohydrate content of a particular food. Following is a typical meal plan for a client who has been taught to count carbohydrates:

Breakfast: 3 carbohydrates
Example: 1 whole bagel and 8 ounces (oz) skim milk
Lunch: 3 carbohydrates
Example: ⅔ cup plain yogurt (or sweetened w/an artificial sweetener), 1 fresh orange, and ¾ ounce whole-wheat crackers (2–5)
Dinner: 3 carbohydrates
Example: 1½ cups pasta
Snack: 1 carbohydrate (range, 8–22 grams)
Example: 8 oz skim milk

Protein and fat intake are not counted with this meal-planning system but should be given some consideration. Clients are usually counseled to eat about the same amount of protein each day and choose foods that are low in fat. For example, based on an individualized assessment, a client may be counseled to choose a food that provides approximately 3 grams or less of fat for each carbohydrate (15 grams). If a client is considering a canned entrée containing 30 grams of carbohydrate, he or she knows the food is not a good choice if it contains more than 6 grams of fat.

Exchange Lists

Exchange lists have been used for many years to teach clients portion sizes, food composition, and meal plan distribution. Many clients find this method of menu planning too complex to learn and difficult to implement. However, exchange lists are a good approach to meal planning if the client is highly motivated and the educator has sufficient time to spend with the client. Use of exchange lists are most widely taught in outpatient settings. Clinical Calculation 17-1 demonstrates how to distribute the energy nutrients and calculate a diet using the exchange system.

MyPlate for Diabetics

Figure 17-5 is the MyPlate for diabetics. This is an easy way to get started eating for diabetes. Half of the dinner plate should be filled with non-starchy vegetables such as spinach, carrots, lettuce, greens, cabbage, green beans, broccoli, cauliflower, tomatoes, cucumber, beets, mushrooms, onions, and peppers. The second half of the plate should be separated in half. One of these halves should be filled with starchy foods such as whole-grain breads, rice, pasta, tortillas, cooked beans, peas, corn, potatoes, or low-fat crackers, snack chips, pretzels, and fat-free popcorn. The last section of the plate should have low-fat proteins such as poultry without the skin, fish, seafood, lean cuts of beef and pork, tofu, eggs, or low-fat cheese. To this plate, an 8 ounce glass of non-fat or low-fat milk or 6 ounce container of low-fat, no sugar added yogurt should be added. For dessert, a small piece of fruit, or ½ cup of no sugar added fruit salad can be added for a complete meal (ADA 2013c).

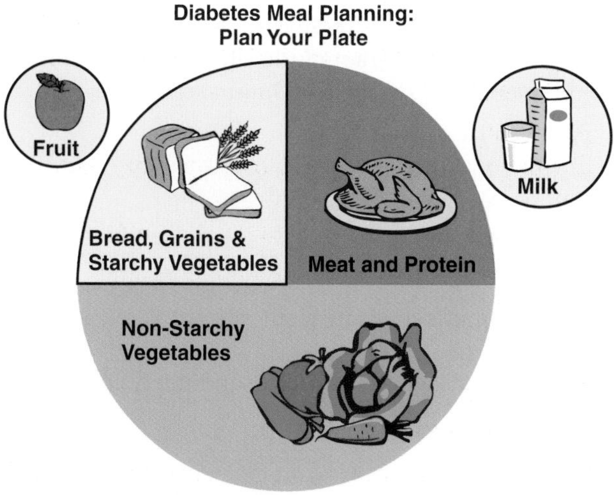

Mediterranean Diet

The Mediterranean Diet is based on the way people who live in Italy, Spain, and other countries in the Mediterranean region have eaten for centuries. The diet consists of (Dugdale and Zieve 2012):

- Plant-based meals with small amounts of meat and chicken when they are used
- Whole grains, fresh fruits and vegetables, nuts, and legumes
- Fish and seafood, limited red meat
- Olive oil as the main source of fat

The PREDIMED study (Prevencion con Dieta Mediterranea) enrolled 7447 subjects aged 55 to 80 years with either type 2 diabetes or 3 or more CVD risk factors, but no CVD at the beginning of the study. No caloric restriction or physical activity was advised or promoted in the study. A Mediterranean Diet supplemented with at least 4 tablespoons of olive oil or 30 grams of mixed nuts daily was found to reduce the incidence of myocardial infarction, stroke, and cardiovascular mortality by 30% compared with following a typical low-fat diet (Visalli, 2013).

Glycemic Index and Glycemic Load

Not all carbohydrates affect blood glucose levels in the same manner. The glycemic index (GI) was discussed in the previous chapter and can be an important tool in the improvement of diet management in diabetes. Foods with a GI less than 55 are low, 56 to 76 are moderate, and 76 to 100 are high. In general, the more processed a food is, the higher the GI. However, the determination of GI was based on the same portion of a food item and not necessarily that in a normal portion size. It is important to take the portion size into consideration when evaluating a food; in doing this, the glycemic load (GL) of the food item is calculated. GL is the GI of the food multiplied by the carbohydrate per serving, divided by 100. A food with a low GL is less than 10, medium is 11 to 19, and high is greater than

Diabetes Meal Planning: Plan Your Plate

Fruit

Bread, Grains & Starchy Vegetables

Non-Starchy Vegetables

Meat and Protein

Milk

FIGURE 17-5 MyPlate for people with diabetes shows the division of a typical plate of food, which should comprise vegetables, whole-grain starchy foods, and lean proteins.

20 (Kirpitch and Maryniuk, 2011). There can be wide variability in the calculated values of different foods. The University of Sydney, where the research on GI and GL was pioneered, lists a value for the GI of an 80-gram serving of carrots based on their state of preparation from raw, to peeled, boiled and ground, to unspecified. In this example, clients may be told to consume only raw carrots. But if the GL is calculated, based on the carbohydrate content in a serving, the GL is 1, 4, and 6, respectively (Table 17-8), all of which are considered low GL food items (www.glycemicindex.com).

When discussing the GI or GL of a food item, the following should be kept in mind as affecting the overall glycemic effect of foods (Kirpitch and Maryniuk, 2011):

■ The more processed a food, typically, the higher its GI/GL.
■ Combining foods in a mixed meal (cheese, white rice, and nonstarchy vegetables) will minimize the overall glycemic effect of one food that has a high GI/GL. In general, protein and fat have little glycemic impact, and adding the cheese to the rice will lower the overall GI/GL of the meal.
■ Fiber (insoluble) from whole grains, fruits and vegetables, and seeds provides a physical barrier slowing the breakdown of the carbohydrate and therefore have a lower GI/GL.
■ Fiber (soluble) from beans and oats is more viscous and tends to have a lower GI/GL in its more unprocessed form.

Because eating foods with a lower GI/GL lowers the glycemic response by the body, there is a lower insulin response. It has been shown that following a low GI/GL diet has the following benefits for people with diabetes (Kirpitch and Maryniuk, 2011):

■ Lower A1C by .5%
■ Decrease in hypoglycemia
■ Reduce the incidence and risk for microvascular complications
■ May be helpful in improving lipid profiles by lowering low-density lipoprotein and raising high-density lipoprotein cholesterol levels and therefore reducing the risk for cardiac disease
■ May facilitate weight loss which may improve insulin sensitivity

TABLE 17-8 ■ Glycemic Load (GL) Calculation of Carrots				
FOOD	SERVING IN GRAMS	GI	CHO GRAMS/ SERVING	GL
Carrots, raw	80	16	8	1
Carrots, peeled, boiled and ground	80	60	6	4
Carrots, unspecified	80	92	6	6

CHO, carbohydrate; GI, glycemic index.

Special Considerations

People with diabetes frequently ask questions about nutritional problems related to vitamin and mineral supplementation, alcohol, acute illness, eating out, and delayed meals.

Vitamin and Mineral Supplementation

There is no clear evidence that people with diabetes benefit from vitamin or mineral supplementation solely because they have diabetes. Routine supplementation with antioxidants, such as vitamins E and C and carotene, is not advised because of lack of evidence of efficacy and concern related to long-term safety. Benefit from chromium supplementation in individuals with diabetes or obesity has not been clearly demonstrated and are therefore not recommended (ADA, 2013b).

Dietary Supplements

It is estimated that half of all Americans use supplements and anywhere from 22% to 67% use some type of supplement on a daily basis. Individuals mistakenly believe that because something is "natural," it can't be harmful. Additionally, possible pharmacological activity of a supplement may cause interactions with other drugs and foods. Clients should always be asked what types of herbs and supplements they are taking (Shane-McWorter, 2012). These products should be assessed for interactions with other drugs. A pharmacist should be consulted with any questions. Some of the common supplements diabetics take with the likelihood of having a positive effect on their diabetes include the following (Natural Medicines Comprehensive Database, 2013):

Possibly effective:
■ Alpha lipoic acid
■ Blond psyllium
■ Caffeine
■ Chromium

Possibly ineffective supplements are:
■ Cranberry
■ Docosahexaenoic acid/eicosapentaenoic acid
■ Garlic
■ Lutein
■ Lycopene
■ Selenium
■ Vitamin C

Insufficient evidence exists for benefit to diabetes mellitus therapy for:

- Aloe
- Apple cider vinegar
- Biotin
- Bitter melon
- Branch-chain amino acids
- Buckwheat
- Calcium
- Cinnamon
- Chia
- Cocoa
- Coenzyme Q-10
- Fenugreek
- Fig
- Flaxseed oil
- Ginseng
- Stevia
- Tea (black, green, or oolong)
- Vitamin D

Alcohol

Moderate use of alcohol does not adversely affect diabetes in well-controlled clients. Recommendations are as follows (ADA, 2013b):

- If people with diabetes choose to drink, daily intake should be limited to one drink per day or less for women and two drinks or less per day for men.
- To reduce nocturnal hypoglycemia in both insulin users and insulin secretagogues, people with diabetes who choose to drink should consume alcohol with food.
- In people with diabetes, moderate alcohol consumption (when ingested alone) has no acute effect on glucose and insulin concentrations but carbohydrate coingested with alcohol (as in a mixed drink) may raise blood glucose.

Nutrition During Acute Illness

Colds and flulike symptoms can be fatal for some people with diabetes unless precautions are taken. Secretion of both glucagon and epinephrine increases during illness and contributes to an increase in blood glucose levels. This action may lead to a loss of glucose, fluid, and electrolytes. Dehydration, electrolyte depletion, and a loss of nutrients may follow. Acute illnesses can lead to DKA in type 1 and to HHNS in type 2 diabetes.

Dehydration is more rapid when electrolytes and fluids are not replaced. Vomiting, diarrhea, and fever all result in fluid loss. During acute illness, the individual should be instructed to monitor his or her blood glucose level every 2 to 4 hours until the symptoms subside. Urine ketone levels should be checked. The following guidelines are recommended by the ADA (2013c) and the National Diabetes Information Clearinghouse (NDIC):

- Ingestion of 15 to 20 grams of glucose is the preferred treatment for hypoglycemia, although any form of CHO that contains glucose may be used.
- The response to treatment of hypoglycemia should be apparent quickly. Plasma glucose should be tested again in 15 minutes because additional treatment may be necessary. This may need to be repeated several times until the blood glucose is greater than 70 mg/dL.
- Once SMBG returns to a level greater than 70 mg/dL, if the next meal is more than an hour away, a snack should be eaten.

Increased fluids reduce the risk of dehydration. Clients who are vomiting or nauseated and are unable to tolerate regular food should drink liquids that contain carbohydrate or electrolytes (Table 17-9). A general guideline is that approximately 15 grams of carbohydrate should be consumed every 1 to 2 hours. Some clients have an individually calculated sick-day menu based on the carbohydrate content of their regular diet.

Other meal-planning tips that may prove helpful during periods of acute illness include the following:

- Increase water intake, even for clients who can eat regular foods.
- Eat smaller, more frequent meals.
- Eat soft, easily digested foods.

During acute illnesses, testing plasma glucose and urinary ketones, drinking adequate amounts of fluids,

TABLE 17-9 ■ **Carbohydrate-Containing Foods for Sick Days**

FOOD	AMOUNT	GRAMS OF CARBOHYDRATE
Regular cola	½ cup	13
Ginger ale	¾ cup	16
Milk	1 cup	12
Apple juice	½ cup	15
Grape juice	⅓ cup	15
Orange juice	½ cup	15
Pineapple juice	½ cup	15
Prune juice	⅓ cup	15
Regular gelatin	½ cup	20
Sherbet	½ cup	30
Tomato juice*	½ cup	5

*High in sodium.

and ingesting carbohydrates are all important (ADA, 2008).

Eating Out and Fast Foods

The best advice for clients with diabetes who enjoy eating out is that they know their meal-planning system and order small portions.

Hypoglycemia in Diabetes

The immediate treatment goal for a glucose level of less than 70 mg/dL is to increase blood glucose to within a normal level as rapidly as possible. Take care not to overtreat hypoglycemia. If the client is monitoring his or her blood glucose level, at the first sign or symptom of hypoglycemia, he or she should measure the blood glucose level. If the blood glucose level is less than 70 mg/dL, 15 grams of glucose should be consumed, after 15 minutes, blood glucose should be measured. If blood glucose is not yet above 70 mg/dL, another 15 grams of glucose should be consumed, and blood glucose should be rechecked. This should be repeated until blood glucose is normal. The individual should then consume a snack or meal to prevent recurrence of hypoglycemia (ADA, 2013b). If glucose is not available, 15 grams of carbohydrate should be consumed, such as:

- 3 to 4 glucose tablets
- 1 serving of glucose gel
- 5 to 6 pieces of hard candies
- 4 to 6 ounces of fruit juice

- 1 cup of milk
- 1 tablespoon of sugar or honey

Clients should be advised to carry a source of carbohydrate with them at all times. A snack should be consumed if a meal or snack is delayed (preplanned or not preplanned) by a half hour or more (NDIC, 2012). The client should have at least one significant other instructed about hypoglycemia.

Teaching Self-Care

People with diabetes ultimately treat themselves. The better educated the individual is about diabetes, the greater the likelihood of his or her avoiding the acute and chronic complications of this disease. Many public health departments, hospitals, and clinics hold classes for clients with diabetes. Newly diagnosed clients with diabetes need to learn survival skills. Health-care workers often have to repeat instructions several times before the client understands the survival skills being taught.

Because of the genetic predisposition toward diabetes, many newly diagnosed clients have relatives who have suffered from the acute and chronic complications of diabetes. Hearing about such complications firsthand often creates fear in newly diagnosed clients. They need time to accept their condition. Occasionally, it may take as long as a full year before clients can grasp the principles of self-care. This is especially difficult for children (see Clinical Application 17-3). During hospitalization, it is extremely difficult to effectively educate clients. Follow-up with a certified diabetes educator (CDE) and a registered dietitian (RD) is crucial.

17-3

$\mathscr{C}$linical $\mathscr{A}$pplication

Children With Diabetes

Kilocalorie allowances are based on a person's weight. As a rough estimate, a 1-year-old child needs 1000 kcal per day. For older children, 100 kcal per year of age are added to the daily intake. For a 9-year-old child, this would equal 1900 kcal. Typically, 55% of the total kilocalories should be consumed as carbohydrate: 1900 kcal multiplied by 55% equals 1045 kcal. To convert kilocalories from carbohydrate to grams of carbohydrate, divide by 4: 1045 kcal divided by 4 kcal/gram equals 260 grams of carbohydrate.

How these grams of carbohydrate are divided among the day depends on the child's prescribed medications and lifestyle. Let's assume the child eats three meals and two snacks (at midafternoon and bedtime) and takes one dose of basal insulin in the morning and three doses of regular insulin, one before each meal.

The diet could be planned to provide 20% of the carbohydrate at each feeding. Twenty percent of 260 grams of carbohydrate equals 52 grams or 3 ½ carbohydrate choices. The child and the child's parents would be instructed to provide about 52 grams of carbohydrate at each feeding.

As long as the child eats balanced meals that provide all the essential nutrients, the source of the carbohydrate is not as important as the total carbohydrates consumed. However, nutritional teaching should emphasize the importance of complex carbohydrates and avoidance of simple sugars. A typical menu for a child might be as follows:

17-3

Clinical Application—cont'd

Children With Diabetes

Acceptable Range, 46–60 per Meal or Snack

MEAL	GRAMS OF CARBOHYDRATE	MEAL	GRAMS OF CARBOHYDRATE
Breakfast		*Midafternoon Snack*	
½ cup Honey Nut Cheerios	12 (package label)	¾ cup apple juice	23 (exchange value)
¾ cup skim milk	9 (exchange value)	13 animal crackers	25 (exchange value)
½ cup orange juice	15 (exchange value)	Total carbohydrates for snack	48
1 slice toast	15 (exchange value)	*Dinner*	
1 tsp peanut butter	0	15-in. cheese pizza	39 (table of food composition)
Total carbohydrates for meal	51	6-oz regular cola	20 (table of food composition)
Lunch		Total carbohydrates for meal	59
Ham and cheese sandwich with 2 slices of bread	30 (exchange value)	*Bedtime Snack*	
1 apple	15 (exchange value)	½ cup skim milk	6 (exchange value)
¾ cup skim milk	9 (exchange value)	Raw broccoli with dip	0 (free with this system)
Carrot sticks	0 (free with this system)	10 (1½ oz) whole-wheat crackers (no added fat)	30 (exchange value)
Total carbohydrates for meal	54	½ oz jelly beans	14 (table of food composition)
		Total carbohydrates for snack	50
		Total carbohydrates for the day	262

Hypoglycemia Not Related to Diabetes Mellitus

There are two types of hypoglycemia not related to DM, reactive and fasting. The symptoms are the same as those experienced by diabetics with hypoglycemia.

Reactive hypoglycemia is hypoglycemia that occurs within 4 hours after a meal. The causes are uncertain but may be related to an individual's sensitivity to the body's release of epinephrine or deficiency in glucagons secretion. Other causes may include gastric surgery (causing the rapid passage of food into the small intestine) and enzyme deficiencies early in life (hereditary fructose intolerance).

Fasting hypoglycemia is defined as a blood glucose level less than 70 mg/dL after an overnight fast, between meals, or after physical activity. Causes include some medications (large dose salicylates, sulfa medications, pentamidine, and quinine), alcoholic beverages (especially binge drinking), critical illnesses (affecting the liver, heart, or kidneys), hormonal deficiencies (shortages of cortisol, growth hormone, glucagons, or epinephrine), tumors (in the pancreas), and infancy and childhood conditions (hyperinsulinism, enzyme or hormonal deficiencies) (NDIC 2012).

The dietary management of reactive hypoglycemia consists of avoiding simple carbohydrates and sometimes taking small, frequent feedings. The meal plans for diabetes offer a reasonable guide to meal planning. Table 17-10 is a 1-day meal plan for this type of diet.

TABLE 17-10 ■ Sample Meal Plan for Hypoglycemic Diet	
EXCHANGE GROUP	**SAMPLE MENU**
Morning	
1 fruit	½ cup unsweetened orange juice
1 starch	¾ cup whole-grain cereal
1 meat	1 oz low-fat cheese
½ cup skim milk	½ cup skim milk
Free	Decaffeinated coffee
Mid-Morning	
1 meat	1 tbsp peanut butter
1 starch	4 whole-grain crackers
Noon	
Chef salad	
2–4 oz meat	2–4 oz lean meat
1 vegetable	Lettuce, tomatoes, and
1 fat	Dressing
1 fruit	1 small piece fresh fruit
1 cup skim milk	1 cup skim milk
1 starch	2 breadsticks (4 × ½ in.)
Midafternoon	
1 meat	1 oz low-fat cheese
1 starch	4 whole-grain crackers
Evening	
2–4 meat	2–4 oz lean meat
1 starch	½ cup potato or whole wheat pasta
1 vegetable	½ cup vegetable
1 fat	Lettuce salad with dressing
1 fruit	1 piece fresh fruit
Free	Decaffeinated coffee or tea
Bedtime	
1 starch and 1 meat	½ sandwich (1 slice whole-grain bread and 1 oz lean meat)
1 vegetable	Fresh vegetables
Free	Decaffeinated beverage

Keystones

■ Diabetes is caused by an undersecretion or underutilization of insulin and/or receptor or postreceptor defects.

■ Diabetes is actually a group of disorders with a common sign of hyperglycemia.

■ The two major types of diabetes are type 1 and type 2. Impaired glucose tolerance or impaired fasting glucose, secondary diabetes, and gestational diabetes are other categories of this disease.

■ People with diabetes suffer from acute and chronic complications.

■ Treatment involves medication, nutrition management, and exercise.

■ Nutrition is a fundamental part of treatment.

■ Hypoglycemia, a rarer condition than diabetes, is caused by over secretion of insulin and is also treated with dietary manipulation.

CASE STUDY *17–1*

Mrs. S, a 45-year-old black woman, came to your doctor's office because she had a sore that would not heal on her leg. She is 5 ft 5 in., and weighs 200 lb (body mass index [BMI] = 33.5). Vital signs are temperature 98.6°F, pulse 70 beats per minute, respirations 16 breaths per minute, and blood pressure 160/95 mm Hg.

Mrs. S reports a gradual increase in her weight since her third child was born 20 years ago. That baby weighed 12 lb. Two previous pregnancies produced infants weighing 10 and 11 lb. She has no known allergies. None of the children live at home. Mrs. S lives with her husband, who works as a construction laborer. She has been seasonally employed as a hotel maid at a nearby resort. Health insurance coverage is sporadic. They have a new insurance policy now.

Mrs. S is the oldest of six children. Her father died of a heart attack at age 60. Her mother died of a stroke at age 62. Both parents reportedly "had a little sugar." The sister who is closest to Mrs. S in age developed diabetes 3 years ago and is being treated with oral medication. Their youngest sister was diagnosed with type 1 diabetes at age 18 after an episode of mumps.

Mrs. S reports a good appetite and a fluid intake of about 3 quarts per day. Her favorite beverage is iced tea with sugar and lemon. She does most of the grocery shopping and cooking.

Mrs. S hit her left ankle with the screen door about 2 months ago. The resulting sore has not healed but has gotten worse. Mrs. S knows that a sore that does not heal is a sign of cancer, which is why she sought medical attention. The ankle now has an open lesion 5 cm in diameter over the lateral ankle bone. The entire foot is swollen to twice the size of the right foot. The bandage over the sore had greenish-yellow drainage on it. A random blood glucose test 3 hours after her last meal shows a glucose level of 400 mg/dL. Her urine glucose was negative for ketones. The physician diagnoses Mrs. S with type 2 diabetes.

The physician prescribed the following care for Mrs. S:

■ Bed rest with left leg elevated
■ Diet assessment and teaching
■ Multivitamin, 1 capsule daily
■ Culture and sensitivity of drainage from left leg
■ Cefuroxime, 250 mg, orally every 12 hours
■ Warm, moist dressing to left leg ulcer four times per day
■ Fasting blood sugar (FBS), electrolytes
■ Metformin, 500 mg with breakfast and dinner

The nurse constructed the following Care Plan for Mrs. S.

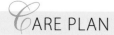ARE PLAN

Subjective Data

Family history of diabetes mellitus ■ Large appetite ■ Large fluid intake ■ Delay in seeking medical attention

Objective Data

Obesity: ht 5 ft 5 in ■ wt 200 lb ■ Newly diagnosed type 2 diabetes ■ Possible hypertension (only one reading given)
■ Open lesion 5 cm diameter over left lateral ankle ■ purulent discharge

Analysis

Lack of knowledge of disease process related to new diagnosis with type 2 diabetes. Through interviewing, client is willing to attend a diabetes class.

Plan

DESIRED OUTCOMES EVALUATION CRITERIA	ACTIONS/INTERVENTIONS	RATIONALE
Client will understand type 2 diabetes	Briefly discuss type 2 diabetes causes, effects on the body, and tools for management of the disease.	The more a client understands about the disease, the more likely she is to become part of the treatment process.
Client will verbalize self-care measures related to type 2 diabetes	SMBG will be taught using a glucometer. A blood glucose log will be given to client and asked to bring to next appointment.	Client needs to become aware of BG goals and self-management techniques to manage her diabetes.
	Refer to dietitian for nutritional assessment and education.	One of the cornerstones of treatment of type 2 is weight loss.
		Clients with diabetes essentially need to learn to treat themselves as much as possible and know when to seek medical treatment.
	Review survival skills with client (see DavisPlus for client teaching tool).	The American Diabetes Association recommends all clients with diabetes learn survival skills.
Client will verbalize willingness to continue nursing/medical regimen.	Ask the client what her interests are for her management of the diabetes, help her set achievable goals that she can work on (motivational interviewing).	The client will feel more empowered and is more likely to work towards goals she help set. This can be done over time if the client is able to return for follow-up.
	Refer to social worker for sources of food and medical attention when uninsured.	Social workers are most familiar with community resources.
	Teach principles of wound care, including effect of high blood sugar on infection.	If Mrs. S understands that high blood sugar feeds the bacteria causing the infection, she may be more willing to work hard to control the diabetes.
	Reinforce dietitian's instruction. Have Mrs. S review MyPlate for diabetes and the reason why it is important to follow.	Knowledge usually precedes behavior change.
	Have Mrs. S describe the meal plan she follows.	Short periods of instruction are most effective; frequent review of the material will help the client master it.
	Request physician's referral to diabetes class.	Insurance companies will more likely cover outpatient educational programs if ordered by a physician.

17-1

Dietitian's Notes

The following Dietitian's Notes are representative of the documentation found in a client's medical record.

Subjective: Spoke with client, who was tearful throughout our session. Client describes an uncontrollable thirst and hunger and inability to prepare food while her husband is at work. Claims her husband left her a thermos of coffee and snacks before he left for work. Snacks included bread, a jar of peanut butter, and a jar of jelly. Generally, she claims to have eaten the jars of both the peanut butter and jelly every day, along with half the loaf of bread. She didn't eat the whole loaf because she knows too much bread is bad for anyone. For dinner, her husband usually brought home fast food from the burger store (hamburgers and French fries) or pizza. Denies daily consumption of milk, fruits, and vegetables.

Objective: Diagnosis: Type 2 diabetes (newly diagnosed) with open lesion over left ankle with drainage.

Analysis: Inappropriate carbohydrate (CHO) intake related to diabetes and food and nutrition knowledge deficit as evidenced by blood glucose greater than 400 and diet history. Body mass index (BMI) 33.5. Ideal body weight based on maximum ideal body weight of 100 lb for the first 5 ft and 4 lb for each additional inch equals 120; plus or minus 10% equals 108 to 132 lb. 132 pounds divided by weight in kilograms (2.2) equals 60 kg, and this is the weight used to estimate kcal and protein needs.

Estimated kcal needs based on maximum ideal body weight and 25 to 35 kcal/kg equals 1500 to 2100. However, because weight loss is desirable for this client, would provide slightly less kcal to provide for a weight loss of about 1 lb per week. 1500 minus 500 kcal/day equals 1250 kcal/day. A 50% acceptable macronutrient distribution range was used to determine carbohydrate needs per meal: 10.5 exchanges/day or 3 per feeding and 2 for an evening snack.

Estimated kcal needs based on 1.0 kcal/kg equals 60 grams per day. Estimated protein needs on the high side to provide enough protein for wound repair.

Education: Reviewed carbohydrate counting with client. Will need much encouragement to follow through with healthful behavioral changes.

Plan:

1. Recommend to client three carbohydrate (CHO) exchanges per meal and two carbohydrate exchanges at bedtime.

2. Recommend referral to diabetes class for more education.

3. Concur that social worker would be helpful to determine eligibility for home-delivered lunch and transportation assistance to diabetes class.

17-2

Social Worker's Notes

The following Social Worker's Notes are representative of the documentation found in a client's medical record.

Arrangements have been made for the client to receive a hot lunch daily and a cold boxed dinner 5 days per week. Will contact meal delivery program.

Arrangements have also been made to provide client with transportation to and from the diabetes class.

Critical Thinking Questions

1. What symptoms in Mrs. S led to her diagnosis with type 2 diabetes?

2. Why is a home delivery of meals beneficial for Mrs. S?

3. Why is a referral to a certified diabetes educator crucial for this client?

Chapter Review

1. If a client has a history of ketoacidosis, he or she most likely has which type of diabetes:
   a. Type 1
   b. Type 2
   c. Pituitary
   d. Gestational

2. The following statement is true:
   a. Acute illness lowers blood glucose levels.
   b. Fluid and electrolyte replacement is essential during episodes of acute illness in all persons with diabetes.
   c. Persons with diabetes who have an acute illness require a vitamin and mineral supplement.
   d. Persons with diabetes should never eat forms of simple sugar.

3. Dietary guidelines for people with diabetes include:
   a. One serving of alcohol daily
   b. Consume no more than 2000 milligrams of sodium each day
   c. Restrict fat intake to less than 10% of total kilocalories
   d. Consume at least 20 to 35 grams of fiber each day

4. For most clients, the cornerstone of treatment of type 2 diabetes is:
   a. Stress management
   b. Meal planning
   c. Strict adherence to five planned meals per day
   d. Hypoglycemic drugs

5. The diet for reactive hypoglycemia includes the following features:
   a. Small, frequent meals with restricted simple sugars
   b. Three meals with ample simple sugars and high complex carbohydrate
   c. Four to six small meals that are high in fat
   d. Three high-carbohydrate meals that are moderate in fat

Clinical Analysis

1. Ms. N, a 14-year-old, was diagnosed 1 year ago with type 1 diabetes mellitus. Her blood sugar levels have been stable on intermediate-acting insulin and a 370-gram CHO diet. The teenager is now being seen in the doctor's office for routine follow-up. The nurse is reviewing Ms. N's knowledge of self-care.
   To assess knowledge, the nurse asks how the client would handle a day when the client could not eat solid foods. Which of the following answers would show understanding of the usual procedure?
   a. Skip insulin that day.
   b. Call the doctor after missing one meal.
   c. Replace the carbohydrates in the meal plan with liquids containing equal amounts of carbohydrate.
   d. Take half her usual insulin dose and double the usual fluid intake.

2. The client plays volleyball for the high school team and is moderately active during practices and games. Self-monitoring blood glucose (SMBG)

records indicate a daily glucose level of between 120 and 140 mg/dL before the time she usually plays volleyball. Which of the following behaviors are appropriate for her before playing?
   a. No additional food is indicated
   b. Increase intake by 15 grams of carbohydrate
   c. Decrease intake by 15 grams of carbohydrate
   d. Increase intake by one vegetable exchange and one fat exchange

3. The client states, "I am getting tired of pricking my finger several times a day. Why can't I manage my diabetes with urine testing like my grandmother?" Which of the following responses by the nurse would be most appropriate?
   a. "The urine test is more accurate in older people."
   b. "The point at which sugar is spilled in the urine varies even for one individual. Therefore, the blood test is more accurate."
   c. "Urine tests are more costly."
   d. "The blood test is the newest thing. Your grandmother's doctor must be old-fashioned."

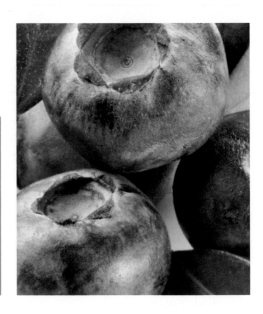

18

Diet in Cardiovascular Disease

LEARNING OBJECTIVES

After completing this chapter, the student should be able to:

■ Discuss the relationship between diet and the development of cardiovascular disease.

■ Distinguish between type II and type IV hyperlipoproteinemias as to aggravating factors and the focus of dietary modifications.

■ Identify strategies that are most likely to reduce the risk of cardiovascular disease.

■ Compare and contrast dietary modifications for clients with myocardial infarction, heart failure, and stroke.

■ Describe the DASH diet.

■ List several flavorings and seasonings that can be substituted for salt on a sodium-restricted diet.

The cardiovascular system includes not only the heart and blood vessels but the blood-forming organs as well. This chapter covers common diseases of the heart and blood vessels that can be influenced by dietary modification.

Occurrence of Cardiovascular Disease

Despite declines in recent years, heart disease and stroke remain the first and fourth leading causes of death in the United States, respectively. Of all U.S. deaths in 2011, 47% were from heart disease and stroke (National Vital Statistics Report, 2012). More than 80 million American adults suffer from cardiovascular disease (CVD) (Fang, Yang, Hong, and Loustalot, 2012). The American Heart Association developed goals for 2020 to improve the cardiovascular (CV) health of all Americans by 20% while reducing deaths from CVD and strokes by 20% through healthy diets;

exercise; decreasing dyslipidemia, blood pressure, and body weight to normal levels; and eliminating smoking (American Heart Association, 2012).

Underlying Pathology

Two major pathological conditions contribute to cardiovascular disease:

1. Atherosclerosis, the most common form of **arteriosclerosis**
2. Hypertension, included here as contributing to pathology and later in the chapter as a risk factor for cardiovascular disease

Atherosclerosis

In **atherosclerosis,** fatty deposits of cholesterol, fat, or other substances accumulate inside the artery, accompanied by inflammation. Initially, the deposited material, or plaque, is soft, but later it becomes fibrosed or hard. This disease process interferes with the pumping of blood through the artery in two ways:

■ The deposits gradually make the lumen smaller and smaller.
■ The fibrosis makes it progressively harder for the artery to constrict or dilate in response to the tissues' needs for oxygenated blood (Fig. 18-1).

When the lumen, or opening through the artery, is 70% blocked by atherosclerotic plaque, the person is likely to show symptoms of impaired circulation distal to the obstruction.

Hypertension

Blood pressure (B/P) is the force exerted against the walls of the arteries by the pumping action of the heart. Blood pressure is recorded in two numbers, for example, 120/80. The top number, **systolic pressure,** is the pressure when the heart beats. The bottom number, **diastolic pressure,** is the pressure between beats. Both pressures are reported in millimeters of mercury (mm Hg). Normal blood pressure is less than 120/80 mm Hg.

Diagnosis of Hypertension

Prehypertension increases the chance of becoming hypertensive. It is defined as:

■ A systolic reading of 120 to 139 mm Hg, or
■ A diastolic reading is 80 to 89 mm Hg.

Hypertension is defined as:

■ Blood pressure of 140/90 mm Hg or higher on at least three occasions on different dates or
■ Persons taking antihypertensive medication.

Several readings are taken on various days to eliminate the possibility of excitement or nervousness causing a transient elevation. Hypertension is classified as Stage 1 or 2 (Table 18-1). Blood pressure measurement should be part of a child's health assessment beginning at age 3 years. It is estimated that almost 75% of the cases of arterial hypertension and 90% of the cases of prehypertension in children and adolescents are currently undiagnosed (Aglony, Acevedo, and Ambrosio, 2009).

A person with hypertension may not feel sick, so blood pressure screening is often offered as a community service (Fig. 18-2). Along with temperature, pulse, and respirations, blood pressure is a vital sign that is usually taken at every health-care visit.

Types of Hypertension

Depending on the cause, hypertension is labeled primary or secondary. About 90% of hypertensive clients have primary or **essential hypertension.** There is no single, clear-cut cause for this high blood pressure.

Secondary hypertension occurs in response to another event or disease in the body. One such event is pregnancy, during which hypertension may occur (see Chapter 10). Medications also can cause secondary

Normal artery   Atherosclerotic artery

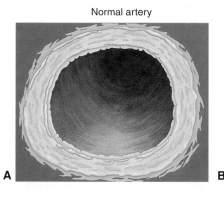
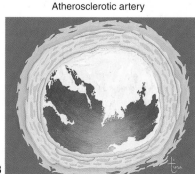

FIGURE 18-1 Cross-section of a normal coronary artery (*A*) and an atherosclerotic artery (*B*). Note both the narrowed diameter and the roughness within the lumen in the diseased artery. (Reprinted from Scanlon, VC, and Sanders, T: *Essentials of anatomy and physiology,* 5th ed. FA Davis, Philadelphia, 2007, p. 280, with permission.)

TABLE 18-1 ■ Classification of Blood Pressure for Adults and Children

CLASSIFICATION	mm Hg SYSTOLIC	mm Hg DIASTOLIC	PERCENTILE DENOTING CLASSIFICATION IN CHILDREN AND ADOLESCENTS
Normal	<120	and <80	<90th
Prehypertension	120–139	or 80–89	90th to 95th (children) >120/80 (adolescents)
Stage 1 Hypertension	140–159	or 90–99	95th to (99th + 5 mm Hg)
Stage 2 Hypertension	>159	or >99	>99th + 5 mm Hg

Source: Centers for Disease Control and Prevention, 2013; National Institutes of Health, 2007, 2013.

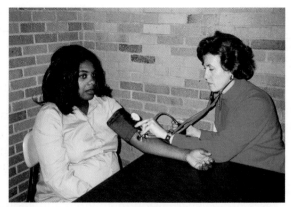

FIGURE 18-2 Hypertension is a silent killer. Blood pressure monitoring is a part of most health-system visits.

hypertension. Birth control pills that contain proges-terone stimulate the production of renin (see Fig. 8-17), which may result in an elevation in blood pressure.

As mentioned in Chapter 15, the combined intake of monoamine oxidase inhibitors (MAOIs) and tyra-mine-rich foods or beverages can cause hypertension. Secondary hypertension can also result from diseases of the kidney, adrenal glands, or nervous system.

Positive Feedback Cycle

Many cardiovascular conditions have interlocking causative factors. The interaction between atheroscle-rosis and hypertension is an example of a **positive feedback cycle.** In this situation, the presence of the second condition worsens the first. Atherosclerosis narrows the lumen of the arteries, and the smaller opening increases blood pressure. Then the higher blood pressure forces more lipids into the arterial wall, worsening the atherosclerosis, and the cycle is repeated.

End Result of Pathology

Most affected people do not have either atherosclerosis or hypertension. More commonly, they have both con-ditions. Although many organs are likely to be damaged by atherosclerosis and hypertension, the major con-cern is the effect on the heart and brain, as described in the following sections on coronary heart disease and cerebrovascular disease.

Coronary Heart Disease

When the coronary arteries that supply the heart mus-cle with blood become blocked, the result is **coronary heart disease (CHD)** or coronary artery disease (CAD). If the blockage is temporary, due to increased activity and the body's increased demand for oxygen, the person may experience **angina pectoris,** or severe pain and a sense of constriction about the heart. Rest and the administration of vasodilating medications commonly produce relief, but changes in diet and lifestyle are necessary to stave off heart damage.

However, if the vessel is blocked by atherosclerotic plaque, by a **thrombus** (blood clot), or by an **embolus** (a circulating mass of undissolved matter), the heart tissues beyond the point of obstruction receive no oxy-gen or nutrients. When this happens, the person exhibits signs and symptoms of a **coronary occlusion,** or a heart attack. When the blood supply cannot be restored quickly, myocardial cells in the affected area die. The medical diagnosis then becomes **myocardial infarction.**

Heart Failure

When the heart cannot keep up with the demands on it, **heart failure (HF)** occurs. Heart failure is any clin-ical syndrome that results from any structural or func-tional impairment of ventricular filling or ejection of blood (Yancy, Jessup, Bozkurt, et al, 2013). Causes may include the following:

- Atherosclerosis
- Hypertension
- Myocardial infarction
- Rheumatic fever
- Birth defect
- Obesity
- Diabetes

The right side of the heart normally collects the blood returning from the body and pumps it to the lungs to excrete carbon dioxide and absorb oxygen. If the right ventricle is failing, usually due to lung disease, the blood backs up into the veins that empty into the right atrium, and the client has the signs of peripheral edema. If the client has excessive fluid volume and edema of the small bowel, the client suffers from anorexia and nausea.

The left side of the heart normally receives the oxy-genated blood from the lungs and pumps it out to the body. If the left ventricle is failing, usually after a my-ocardial infarction, the blood that cannot be pumped effectively to the body backs up in the blood vessels of the lungs. Next, the fluid from the blood is forced into the lung tissue. The client will display shortness of breath and moist lung sounds and will expectorate frothy pink sputum.

In addition, if the heart cannot pump enough blood to maintain blood pressure, the body implements the renin response. Angiotensin II constricts the blood vessels, raising blood pressure. Aldosterone causes the kidneys to conserve sodium, and with it, water (see Fig. 8-17). More fluid fills the blood vessels. The higher blood pressure pushes this fluid out into the interstitial spaces, causing edema.

Obviously, one side of the heart cannot function long if the other side is failing. Therefore, the healthcare worker learns to look for early signs of heart failure in the extremities in right-sided failure or in the lungs in left-sided failure.

About 6.6 million people in the United States suffer from HF. A lifetime risk of developing HF at age 40 is estimated to be 1 in 5 with a mortality ranging from 20% to 50% (Petrone, Weir, Hanson, et al, 2012). The incidence of HF rises with age. Approximately 2% of individuals aged 65 to 69 and more than 8% of individuals over age 84 are affected. By 2050, it is estimated that 20% of the population will be aged over 65 years, and thus the incidence of HF is anticipated to rise. The mortality rate for HF is estimated to be 50% within 5 years of diagnosis. In the United States, 1 in 9 deaths are attributed, at least in part, to HF (Yancy et al, 2013).

There is a lower risk of developing HF by following these healthy lifestyle recommendations (Petrone et al, 2012):

- Regular exercise
- Moderate alcohol intake
- Consumption of fruits and vegetables
- Consumption of breakfast cereals (cereal fiber)
- Consumption of fish high in omega-3 polyunsaturated fatty acids (PUFAs)
- Supplementation with omega-3 PUFAs

The American Heart Association Guidelines (Yancy et al, 2013) recommend individuals with HF receive treatment for:

- Hypertension
- Dyslipidemia
- Obesity
- Diabetes

There are more than 1 million hospitalizations for HF annually in the United States, and 25% of those individuals are at a higher risk of all-cause related rehospitalizations within 1 month. The United States expends more than $40 billion annually for HF treatment, more than half of which is spent on hospitalizations (Yancy et al, 2013).

The American Heart Association Guidelines recommend a multidisciplinary team of clinicians, using evidence-based guidelines for the treatment of HF. Client education is critical for individuals diagnosed with HF. The transition from hospital to a community setting is especially important because of the prevalence of readmissions in HF clients. Studies have found that having intensive discharge instructions with well-coordinated follow-up care, as well as a 1-hour nurse

educator teaching session at the time of hospital discharge, improved clinical outcomes. The recommendation for treatment for individuals with HF include the following (Yancy et al, 2013):

- Pharmacological, such as omega-3 fatty acids and some hypertension medications
- Sodium restriction for those with symptomatic HF to reduce congestive symptoms (Individuals with mild HF should restrict sodium to 1500 mg/day, and those with moderate or severe HF should restrict sodium to less than 3000 mg/day).
- Exercise
- Depression screening
- Sleep disorder screening
- Weight loss in severely obese
- Fluid restriction for those with advanced HF to reduce congestive symptoms, normally in conjunction with sodium restriction (Hyponatremia in HF clients is seen due to their inability to excrete excess fluids.)

Cerebrovascular Accident

When a blood vessel in the brain becomes blocked by atherosclerosis (ischemic stroke), the tissue supplied by that artery dies. This pathology causes about 87% of strokes or **cerebrovascular accidents (CVAs)** in the United States (American Heart Association and American Stroke Association, 2012). Strokes also can be caused by an embolus or by a ruptured blood vessel. Cerebrovascular accidents are usually secondary to atherosclerosis, hypertension, or a combination of both.

Each year, approximately 795,000 strokes, 610,000 of them first attacks, occur in the United States. On average, someone has a stroke every 40 seconds (American Heart Association and American Stroke Association, 2012). Sixty percent of strokes occur in women. On average, every 4 minutes someone dies from a stroke (American Stroke Association, 2012).

Stroke is called a "brain attack" and early treatment can minimize the long-term effects of ischemic stroke, but people often ignore initial signs and symptoms or fail to react appropriately. Analysis of 56,969 persons with strokes in four states revealed that nearly 40% did not arrive at the hospital by ambulance, thereby limiting the possibility of definitive early treatment (George et al, 2009).

Individuals consuming more than five servings of fruits and vegetables daily had a 25% lower incidence of stroke than those consuming fewer than three servings (He, Nowson, and MacGregor, 2006). A diet with the following components will likely reduce the incidence of stroke (Ding and Mozaffarian, 2006):

- Low in sodium
- High in potassium

■ Rich in fruits, vegetables, whole grains, cereal fiber, and fatty fish

These are the same principles used to prevent cardiovascular conditions resulting from atherosclerosis. A heart-healthy diet may also be a head-healthy diet. The American Heart Association's 2020 goal is to improve the cardiovascular health of all Americans by 20% while reducing deaths from cardiovascular diseases and stroke by 20%. It recommends that an adult consuming 2000 calories per day should consume:

■ Fruits and vegetables: at least 4.5 cups per day
■ Fish (preferably oily fish): at least two 3.5-ounce servings/week
■ Fiber-rich whole grains: at least three 1 ounce equivalent servings/day
■ Sodium: less than 1500 mg/day
■ Sugar-sweetened beverages: no more than 450 calories/week
■ Nuts, legumes, and seeds: at least 4 servings/week
■ Processed meats: no more than 2 servings/week
■ Saturated fat: less than 7% of total energy intake

Risk Factors in Cardiovascular Disease

The occurrence of cardiovascular disease in a person cannot be predicted with certainty. Many attributes and behaviors interact to produce the illness (see Table 18-2).

Unmodifiable Risk Factors

Risk factors that cannot be changed to prevent atherosclerosis and hypertension are:

■ Age
■ Gender
■ Race
■ Family history
■ Personal medical history

TABLE 18-2 ■ Risk Factors for Cardiovascular Disease	
UNMODIFIABLE	MODIFIABLE
Age	Hypertension
Gender	High blood cholesterol
Race	Obesity
Heredity	Diabetes mellitus
Family history	Physical inactivity
Prior medical history	Alcohol intake
	Cigarette smoking

Age, Gender, and Race

Hypertension usually develops at about age 50 to 60, and coronary atherosclerosis becomes problematic more frequently in individuals older than age 40.

Risk for coronary heart disease increases in men after age 45 and women after age 55. Until menopause, women have less atherosclerosis and coronary heart disease than men, but women postmenopausal and younger diabetic women are stricken with coronary heart disease just as often as men are.

Non-Hispanic Blacks have a higher risk for hypertension and hypertension-related complications than non-Hispanic Whites and Mexican Americans (Centers for Disease Control and Prevention [CDC], 2012).

Family and Prior Medical Histories

A family history of premature coronary heart disease in a parent or sibling increases a person's risk of the disease. Premature coronary artery disease is a myocardial infarction or a coronary artery procedure before age 55 in men and 65 in women (Brunzell, 2007).

Of special concern are the inherited **hyperlipoproteinemias** (see Genomic Gem 18-1) resulting in increased lipoproteins and lipids in the bloodstream (Table 18-3). Type IV hyperlipoproteinemia is common and frequently associated with type 2 diabetes mellitus.

Genomic Gem 18-1

Type II Hyperlipoproteinemia

Type II hyperlipoproteinemia results from a single gene defect in the cell receptor that binds circulating low-density lipoproteins. It is an autosomal dominant characteristic (Jawalekar, 2012). Individuals with this defect have a rate of coronary heart disease 25 times that of the normal population. In addition, clients with the subgroup type IIA hyperlipoproteinemia generally develop heart disease 15 years earlier than the rest of the population. Some even suffer heart attacks in infancy and childhood.

Most common forms of cardiovascular disease are thought to result from many genes, acting alone or with other genes and environmental factors. The same haptoglobin phenotypes related to susceptibility to scurvy also show marked differences in susceptibility to atherosclerosis. This difference is attributable to variations in low-density lipoprotein oxidation (Delanghe, Langlois, De Buyzere, and Torck 2007). Because at least one-half the variation in serum cholesterol is genetic, determining the pathologic mechanisms could markedly improve diagnosis and treatment selection (Arnett, Baird, Barkley, et al, 2007).

Because all hyperlipoproteinemias are not the same, neither are the dietary treatments. Health-care providers should be informed about the differences and not assume that all clients with hyperlipoproteinemia receive the same diet prescription. For best results, the clinical dietitian individualizes the diet with the client.

TABLE 18-3 ■ Inherited Hyperlipoproteinemias (Fredrickson Classification)

| | | | | INCREASED PLASMA VALUES | | | | |
| | | | | Lipoprotein | | | Lipid | |
Type[+]	Frequency	Inheritance Pattern	Aggravated by/ Target of Control	Chylomicrons	VLDL	LDL	Cholesterol	Triglycerides
I	Very rare	Autosomal recessive	Fat					X
IIA	Common	Autosomal dominant	Fat			X	X	
IIB	Common	Autosomal dominant	Fat		X	X	X	X
III	Uncommon	Multifactorial	CHO	Remnants			X	X
IV	Very common	Autosomal dominant	CHO		X			X
V	Rare	Autosomal recessive	Fat and CHO	X	X		X	X

CHO, carbohydrate; LDL, low-density lipoprotein cholesterol; VLDL, very low density lipoprotein cholesterol.

[+]Type I - Familial Hyperchylomicronemia
Type IIA - Familial Hypercholesterolemia
Type IIB - Familial Combined Hypercholesterolemia
Type III - Familial Dysbetalipoproteinemia
Type IV - Familial Hyperprebetalipoproteinemia
Type V - Endogenous Hypertriglyceridemia

Source: Adapted from Dietary Management of Hyperlipoproteinemia (1980); Fauci, Braunwald, Isselbacher, et al (1998), Jawalekar (2012).

For functions and significance of the various lipoproteins, see Table 18-4.

Modifiable Risk Factors

The major modifiable risk factors for CAD are:

- Hypertension
- Elevated serum cholesterol
- Obesity
- Physical inactivity
- Diabetes mellitus
- Alcohol intake
- Cigarette smoking

Hypertension

According to the American Heart Association (Appel, Frohlich, Hall, et al, 2011), hypertension is a leading risk factor for CAD as well as the most important risk factor for stroke. People with normal blood pressure have about half the lifetime risk of stroke compared with those with high blood pressure. Hypertension affects approximately 30%, or 67 million American adults (Keenan and Rosendorf, 2011; Yoon, Burt, Louis, Carroll, 2012). Prehypertension, the precursor to hypertension, also affects another 30% of the population (CDC, 2013). For individuals who reach age 50 years, the lifetime risk of developing hypertension is 90% (Appel and Anderson, 2010). It is estimated that less than 50% of adults with hypertension control their blood pressure, and for every 10% increase in hypertension, treatment could prevent 14,000 deaths annually (Yoon et al, 2012). More than $47 billion in direct medical expenses and $3 billion in lost productivity related to hypertension are spent each year in the United States. The CDC (2013) estimated that reducing the consumption of sodium from 3300 to 2300 mg per day may reduce the incidence of hypertension by 11 million cases and save $18 billion in health care

TABLE 18-4 ■ Functions and Significance of Various Lipoproteins

LIPOPROTEIN	FUNCTION	CLINICAL SIGNIFICANCE
Chylomicrons	Transport exogenous triglycerides from intestines to blood stream	Formed in small intestine; present in blood only after a meal
VLDL	Main transporter of endogenous triglyceride	Synthesized by liver from free fatty acids, glycerol, and carbohydrate
LDL	Transports cholesterol to body cells	Evolves from VLDLs as body's cells remove triglyceride from them and attach cholesterol Carrier of about 60% of total serum cholesterol The higher the LDL level, the greater the risk of CHD Major target of cholesterol-reducing therapy
HDL	Transports cholesterol from body cells to liver to be excreted Inhibits atherosclerosis through anti-inflammatory, antioxidant and antithrombotic actions (Hausenloy and Yellon, 2008)	Synthesized by liver and intestines The higher the HDL level, the lower the risk of CHD Aerobic exercise increases HDL levels

CHD, coronary heart disease; HDL, high-density lipoprotein cholesterol; LDL, low-density lipoprotein cholesterol; VLDL, very low density lipoprotein cholesterol.

costs annually. See Table 18-1 for the classification for blood pressure levels in adults and children.

HIGH SALT INTAKE

Blood pressure values increase with age everywhere except in extremely remote areas of the world and are significantly related to salt intake. Approximately 30% to 50% of hypertensive people and smaller percentages of normotensive people are salt-sensitive, meaning their blood pressure goes up in response to ingesting sodium.

It's estimated that the average American consumes 3400 mg of sodium per day. The 2010 Dietary Guidelines for Americans recommend that everyone decrease their sodium intake. Table 18-5 lists the daily adequate intake (AI) of sodium for individuals by age group. The tolerable upper intake level (UL) was set for all individuals 14 years and older at 2300 mg of sodium per day.

Because 75% of dietary salt is found in processed foods, a public health approach to reducing salt in those items is recommended because individual educational efforts have not been successful (Appel and Anderson, 2010; Keenan et al, 2011). Frequent consumption of the following foods contribute the indicated percentage of sodium intake of Americans (2010 Dietary Guidelines for Americans):

- Yeast breads (7%)
- Chicken and chicken mixed dishes (7%)
- Pizza (6%)
- Pasta and pasta dishes (5%)

LOW POTASSIUM AND CALCIUM INTAKES

Potassium influences blood pressure because it promotes urinary excretion of sodium. However, results of studies of potassium on blood pressure have been inconsistent. High potassium intake does produce a greater reduction in blood pressure in African Americans than in Whites and in individuals with a high salt intake (Gropper, Smith, and Groff, 2009).

Calcium supplementation may result in small reductions in systolic but not diastolic blood pressure and is associated with reduced risk of hypertensive disorders of pregnancy (Gropper, Smith, and Groff, 2009). Individuals who benefit from oral calcium therapy are those who:

- Have low calcium intakes, especially less than 400 mg daily
- Have low serum calcium levels
- Are salt-sensitive (Gropper, Smith, and Groff, 2009)

Because results of calcium supplementation on blood pressure have been modest and inconsistent, calcium should not be recommended to prevent or treat hypertension (Kotchen and Kotchen, 2006). A long-term, population based study of Swedish women found that high levels of calcium supplementation (total calcium >1400 mg/day) and low calcium intake (<600 mg/day) was associated with a higher death rate from all causes, as well as CVD but not stroke (Michaelsson, Melhus H, Warensjö Lemming, et al, 2013).

A higher intake of certain foods, such as fruits, vegetables, and low-fat dairy have been correlated with a decrease in CVD occurrence. However, individual nutrients, potassium and calcium alone, have not shown an effect. The American Heart Association does not recommend taking supplements for cardiovascular health with the exception of omega-3 fatty acid fish oils for individuals with heart disease (American Heart Association, 2013b). When the benefit of an isolated nutrient alone is studied, the individual nutrient tested may have a limited effect because:

- it has a small effect alone but works in conjunction with other nutrients when present in food or
- the substance in the food causing the effect has not been identified.

See Table 18-6 for the lifestyle changes which help decrease cardiovascular disease risk.

Elevated Blood Cholesterol

Despite its categorization as a risk factor for cardiovascular disease, **cholesterol** serves vital functions in the body. Cholesterol is a component of:

- The nerve tissue of the brain and spinal cord
- The tissues of the liver, the adrenal glands, and the kidneys
- Bile

In addition, cholesterol serves as a precursor of adrenal hormones and the sex hormones.

Although some cholesterol contributes to a healthy body, blood cholesterol levels are measured to monitor risk, to promote health, and to prevent disease (see Boxes 18-1 and 18-2).

RELATIONSHIP TO DIET

About 1000 milligrams of cholesterol is processed in the body per day, but less than one-third of the body's store of cholesterol comes from the diet, exclusively

TABLE 18-5 ■ Daily Adequate Intake (AI) of Sodium for Individuals by Age Group	
AGE IN YEARS	AI/DAY (mg)
1–3	1000
4–8	1200
9–50	1500
51–70	1300
≥71	1200

TABLE 18-6 ■ Lifestyle Changes Proven to Reduce Cardiovascular Disease Risk

BEHAVIOR	GOAL	APPROXIMATE LDL-C REDUCTION	APPROXIMATE SYSTOLIC B/P REDUCTION	APPROXIMATE ATHEROSCLEROTIC CARDIOVASCULAR DISEASE RISK REDUCTION
Optimize Diet	Consume <7% kcal as saturated fat (including <1% as *trans*-fat)	8%–10%		8%–10%
	Consume <200 mg cholesterol daily	3%–5%		3%
	Consume 5–10 g soluble fiber daily	3%–5%		<1%
	Limit sodium intake to 2300 mg daily		2–8 mm Hg	3%
	Eat 5 servings fruit, vegetables daily		8–14 mm Hg	5%
	Limit alcohol to 1 (women) or 2 (men) standard drinks per day		2–4 mm Hg	10%
				3%
	Possibly consume plant sterol/stanol enriched foods, 2 g daily	6%–10%		6%
Other	10 lb weight loss	5%–8%	5–10 mm Hg	10%
	Moderate exercise 30 min daily		4–9 mm Hg	10% (some due to B/P change)
	Smoking cessation			20%

LDL-C, low-density lipoprotein cholesterol.
Adapted from American Dietetic Association (2008a, 2008b), Grundy (2006), Lichtenstein et al (2006), American Heart Association (2013a).

Box 18-1 ■ *Cholesterol Screening Goals*

A national health objective of Healthy People 2020 is to screen 82.1% of adults aged 20 years and older for blood lipid screening. Blood lipids should be screened in adults every 5 years.

Between 2005 and 2008, approximately 70.1% of U.S. adults met the goal. Of that total percentage, men were less likely than women and those without health insurance were less likely than those with health insurance to have had their cholesterol checked as recommended (CDC, 2012).

Box 18-2 ■ *Screening Children's Cholesterol*

Universal screening of children's cholesterol is recommended for all children at two time points, once between the ages of 9 and 11 and once between the ages of 17 and 21. Nonfasting total cholesterol and high-density lipoprotein cholesterol (HDL) are recommended for the initial lipid screening test. Children with elevated cholesterol or low HDL who fail at lifestyle changes of diet and exercise should be considered for pharmacological treatment at age 10 (de Ferranti and Washington, 2012; National Heart Lung and Blood Institute, 2013a). The need for screening at a younger age is determined by family history of cardiovascular disease, unknown history (i.e., adopted children), or presence of other risk factors. For these children, the first screening should take place after 2 years of age but no later than 10 years of age. Screening before 2 years of age is not recommended (Daniels and Greer, 2008; National Heart Lung and Blood Institute, 2013a).

Children who do have elevated serum cholesterol levels have to be managed carefully so that sufficient food is provided to support growth.

genetically based and seems to be caused by synthesis occurring only in the liver and not in other tissues of the body (Gropper et al, 2009).

Consumption of substances other than dietary cholesterol can also influence serum cholesterol levels. *Trans* unsaturated fatty acids in vegetable oil products are a risk factor for cardiovascular disease because they raise low-density lipoprotein cholesterol (LDL-C) levels and lower high-density lipoprotein cholesterol (HDL-C) levels. See Table 18-6 for the decrease in cardiovascular disease risk attainable by controlling fat and cholesterol intake.

MEASUREMENT OF BLOOD CHOLESTEROL

Lipids such as triglycerides (the major form of dietary fat and of stored body fat) and cholesterol (a sterol with fatlike properties) cannot dissolve in water. To travel in the bloodstream, they are bound to lipoproteins. See Table 18-4 for the functions and significance of the four main classes of lipoproteins: **chylomicrons, very low-density lipoproteins (VLDL), low-density lipoproteins (LDLs),** and **high-density lipoproteins (HDLs).**

Blood tests for serum cholesterol are reported as total cholesterol, LDL-C, or HDL-C based on cholesterol's association with the two major transport lipoproteins. Serum cholesterol itself is neither good nor bad, but the lipoproteins are associated with greater or lesser risk of CHD.

Table 18-7 shows in a simplified form how the goals for LDL-C therapy are determined based on the risks of death from myocardial infarction or CAD. A client may be prescribed pharmacological and nonpharmacological treatments. Therapeutic lifestyle changes (TLC) remain an essential modality in clinical management (Grundy, Cleeman, Merz, et al, 2004; National Heart Lung and Blood Institute [NHLBI], 2013b). Table 18-8

from foods of animal origin. Nearly all of the body's tissues can synthesize cholesterol, with the liver and the intestine producing the greatest amount. Most people can produce less cholesterol or increase its excretion in response to high levels of dietary cholesterol but others respond weakly. This is thought to be

TABLE 18-7 ■ Serum LDL-C Goals Based on Risk of Myocardial Infarction or Coronary Artery Disease Mortality

Risk factors in Columns A and B are summed. Client's risk factors are located in Column C to determine a goal for his cholesterol level (Column D).

RISK FACTOR	POSITIVE (COLUMN A)	NEGATIVE (COLUMN B)
Cigarette Smoking	+1	
BP >140/90 or Antihypertensive Drug	+1	
HDL-C <40 mg/dL	+1	
HDL-C >60 mg/dL		−1
Premature CHD in First-Degree Relative	+1	
Men >45 years; Women >55 years	+1	
Total	Add Column A	Combine Column B with Column A to determine risk factor count
	COLUMN C	COLUMN D
Classification of Risk	If These Risk Factors Present	LDL-C (mg/dL) Goal
High	CHD, other atherosclerotic disease and/or diabetes	<100
Moderate	Two or more risk factors	<130
Low	0–1 risk factors	<160

BP, blood pressure; HDL-C, high-density lipoprotein cholesterol; LDL-C, low-density lipoprotein cholesterol. The table is a simplified example. Other factors may affect clinical judgment to set goals lower.
Sources: Expert Panel on Detection, Evaluation, and Treatment of High Blood Cholesterol in Adults (2001); Goldberg (2008); Grundy et al (2004).

TABLE 18-8 ■ Cholesterol-Lowering Diets

DESCRIPTION	INDICATION	ADEQUACY
These diets limit lipids and, for some clients, sugars.	These diets are prescribed when clients have elevated serum cholesterol. Consultation with a registered dietitian is encouraged to individualize a dietary plan.	The diets are adequate in all nutrients with the possible exception of iron because of the restriction on red meat. If the client is also on a sodium-restricted diet, imitation cheese, bacon, and eggs may exceed the prescription. Clients must be encouraged to consume enough energy to maintain a healthy body weight.

Food Group	Recommended Foods
Milk	Skim milk, 1% milk, cultured buttermilk, evaporated skim or nonfat milk Nonfat or low-fat yogurt and frozen yogurt 1% or 2% fat cottage cheese Low-fat soft cheese: Farmer and pot cheese labeled no more than 2–6 g of fat/oz
Breads, Cereals, and Starches (from whole grains)	Breads (made without whole milk, eggs, or butter): whole wheat, rye, pumpernickel, pita, white, bagels, English muffins, sandwich buns, dinner rolls, rice cakes Low-fat crackers: sticks, rye crisp, saltines, zwieback Hot cereals, most dry cold cereals Pasta: noodles, macaroni, spaghetti Rice Dried peas and beans, split peas, black-eyed peas, chick peas, kidney beans, navy beans, lentils, soybeans, low-fat tofu
Fruits and Vegetables	Fresh, frozen, canned, or dried prepared without butter, cream, or cheese sauce
Meat, Poultry, Fish, Shellfish	Lean meat with fat trimmed: *Beef*—round, sirloin, chuck, loin *Lamb*—leg, arm, loin, rib *Pork*—tenderloin, leg, shoulder *Veal*—all except ground Poultry without skin Fish: Fresh or frozen cod, flounder, haddock, halibut, trout; fresh or canned-in-water tuna Shellfish: Clams, crab, lobster, scallops, shrimp
Eggs	Egg whites, egg substitute
Fats and Oils	Monounsaturated preferred (canola, olive, peanut oils) Low-fat dressings
Desserts and Snacks	Low-fat frozen desserts: Sorbet, sherbet, Italian ice, frozen yogurt, popsicles Angel food cake Low-fat cookies: fig bars, gingersnaps Low-fat candy: hard candy, jelly beans Low-fat snacks: pretzels, plain popcorn
Beverages	Nonfat beverages: carbonated drinks, juices, tea, coffee

details a cholesterol-lowering diet. Cholesterol-lowering medications are added to a healthy lifestyle, not substituted for it. LDL remains the target of therapy because a clinical trial testing the effects of an HDL-raising medication was stopped early because of adverse effects (Rader, 2007).

Obesity and Inactivity

The location of the body fat is significant: abdominal obesity is related to cardiovascular disease and diabetes mellitus more than is **gluteal-femoral obesity.** Abdominal obesity is associated with increased triglyceride levels and decreased HDL-C levels (Brunzell, 2007). The waist measurements at the umbilicus indicative of increased risk are:

■ More than 40 inches in men
■ More than 35 inches in women.

See Table 18-6 for the decrease in cardiovascular disease risk attainable by weight loss and increased physical activity. Note that weight loss contributes to improvement in both lipid level and blood pressure.

Lack of exercise contributes to many other risk factors for cardiovascular disease. For instance, activity is inversely related to blood pressure independent of being overweight in both sexes and across all ages. As well, increased physical activity has been accompanied by increased HDL-C levels with its attendant lessening of risk.

Diabetes Mellitus

Diabetic individuals have a two to three times higher risk of atherosclerosis than other people. Diabetic women lose the preventive advantages usually associated with premenopausal women regarding cardiovascular risk.

Insulin is required to maintain adequate levels of **lipoprotein lipase,** an enzyme that breaks down chylomicrons. When lipoprotein lipase is inadequate, chylomicrons and VLDL particles accumulate in the blood. After the diabetes is controlled, serum lipid levels decrease.

Lipoprotein lipase activity is greater in physically active subjects and increases with exercise, a valuable concept in the management of type 2 diabetes. Another example of altered physiology is described in Box 18-3, relating undernutrition in utero to increased risk for diabetes mellitus and cardiovascular disease in adulthood.

Metabolic Syndrome

A particular constellation of signs and symptoms labeled **metabolic syndrome** is used to designate a cluster of risk factors for cardiovascular disease. Clients

Box 18-3 ■ *Fetal Nutrition and Cardiovascular Disease in Adulthood*

Environmental influences before and shortly after birth are generally accepted as important determinants of the risk of cardiovascular disease and diabetes mellitus in adulthood (Hofman, Jackson, and Knight, 2004). Programming of the fetus may result from adaptations invoked when the materno–placental nutrient supply fails to match the fetal nutrient demand (Godfrey and Barker, 2001). One example of such shunting is the diversion of fuels to the developing brain at the expense of the muscles and pancreas (Sperling, 2004).

Studies have connected low birth weight, thinness, and short body length at birth with high death rates from cardiovascular disease and high prevalence of type 2 diabetes mellitus (Barker, 1999). The associations are seen in small-for-gestational-age babies, rather than premature infants, and are independent of social class or lifestyle. Babies who are thin at birth tend to be insulin resistant as adults and have a high prevalence of diabetes mellitus, hypertension, and hyperlipidemia as adults.

Research suggests that undernutrition during gestation alters the relationships between glucose and insulin and between growth hormone and insulin-like growth factors. In this way, the fetus adapts to its environment to permit survival, but its changed physiology makes the individual susceptible to cardiovascular disease in later life (Tompkins, 2007). See Genomic Gem 18-2.

Genomic Gem 18-2
Fetal Origins Hypothesis

Nutrient availability during fetal life can program the function of genes that lasts a lifetime by modifying which genes are expressed (can be turned on) and which remain inactive. The function of genes involved in cholesterol metabolism appear to be modified in males who weighed less than 7 lb at birth. In these men, high-density lipoprotein production decreases in response to high-fat/high-saturated-fat diets, the opposite response of that seen in men with higher birth weights (Brown, 2008).

An investigation of genes for type 2 diabetes and the metabolic syndrome attempted to relate fetal growth and genes to adult health outcomes. Small body size at birth and a particular polymorphism seemingly protected an individual against insulin resistance and type 2 diabetes in later life (Eriksson, 2008).

Metabolic syndrome is estimated to affect 35% of Americans, placing them at higher risk for cardiovascular disease, diabetes, and stroke. The American Heart Association recommends reducing the risk of metabolic syndrome through weight reduction, increasing activity, and eating a heart healthy diet (Miller, Stone, Ballantyne, et al, 2011).

with this condition display three or more of the following signs: glucose intolerance, hypertriglyceridemia, low HDL cholesterol, hypertension, and abdominal obesity (Miller et al, 2011). Specific criteria are:

■ Fasting blood glucose ≥100 mg/dL
■ Triglycerides ≥150 mg/dL

- HDL-C <40 mg/dL in men; <50 mg/dL in women
- Blood pressure >130 mm Hg systolic; >85 mm Hg diastolic
- Waist circumference >40 inches in men; >35 inches in women
- Insulin resistance or glucose intolerance

Alcohol Consumption

Moderate alcohol intake has been linked to lower occurrence of cardiovascular events. In small amounts, alcohol seems to cause vasodilation, whereas at high doses it acts as a vasoconstrictor. Current evidence does not justify encouraging nondrinkers to begin imbibing. See Table 18-6 for the decrease in cardiovascular disease risk attainable by controlling alcohol intake. See Dollars & Sense 18-1 for estimated savings from moderating alcohol intake. Heavy doses of alcohol affect the brain long term as well as short term. Alcohol use is generally associated with an approximate dose-dependent risk for hemorrhagic stroke throughout the full range of intake (Mukamal, 2007; NHLBI 2013b).

Cigarette Smoking

Among the major coronary risk factors, cigarette smoking has been shown to be particularly harmful to the heart and blood vessels, whether from active or secondhand smoke. The exact toxic components among the thousands of pharmacologically active substances present in tobacco smoke and their mechanisms affecting cardiovascular dysfunction are largely unknown, but smoking does increase LDL-C (Ambrose and Barua, 2004; NHLBI, 2013b).

CAD occurs about 10 years earlier in smokers than in nonsmokers (Brunzell, 2007). See Table 18-6 for the decrease in CVD risk attainable by smoking cessation.

$ Dollars & Sense 18-1
Drink Less, Save Money, and Health

A couple drinks a bottle of wine (two glasses for her, four for him) every night with dinner and dines in a restaurant twice a week. Assuming modest tastes in wine, $8 per bottle at the grocery and $4.50 per glass in the restaurant, their current annual outlay is $2808 for restaurant wine and $2080 for home wine.

If they implemented the cardioprotective diet plan and reduced their alcohol intake by one-half, they would save $2444 in a year while lessening the risk of cardiovascular disease.

Dietary Measures in Prevention and Treatment

Major lifestyle changes proven to be effective in reducing cardiovascular risk appear in Table 18-6. Additional actions are listed in Table 18-9. Many of the recommendations in both tables were proven effective in controlling hypertension by the DASH (Dietary Approaches to Stop Hypertension) diet, which is still recommended for hypertension control (American Dietetic Association, 2008b; National Institutes of Health, 2012). In uncomplicated Stage 1 hypertension, dietary changes serve as initial treatment before drug therapy (Appel et al, 2009).

Implementing Dietary Changes

The effect of dietary changes differs significantly among individuals, even though they may faithfully follow recommendations. Much more must be learned about gene–diet interactions before customized interventions will be available.

The DASH Diet

An 11-week clinical feeding trial of individuals with systolic blood pressure of less than 160 mm Hg and diastolic pressures from 80 to 95 mm Hg showed that dietary modification is effective in reducing blood pressure. The three diets were:

- *Control Diet* was low in fruits, vegetables, and dairy products with fat content typical of the United States (given to all participants before randomization).
- *Fruits* and *Vegetables Diet* was similar to the *Control Diet* except that it provided more fruits and vegetables and fewer snacks and sweets.
- *Combination (DASH) Diet* was rich in fruits, vegetables, and low-fat dairy foods and had reduced amounts of total fat, saturated fat, and cholesterol than either of the other two diets.

Weight reduction did not confound the results, because kilocalories were adjusted to maintain weight. Likewise, the three types of diets each contained about 3 grams of sodium, and individuals were permitted no more than three caffeinated beverages and no more than two standard alcoholic beverages per day. (See Box 18-4 for information on caffeine and heart disease.) Reported intakes of alcohol were similar across all the diets. After 8 weeks on the experimental diets, the reductions in blood pressure shown in Table 18-10 were obtained. An 8-year follow-up study showed significantly lower all-cause and stroke mortality in hypertensive adults who followed a DASH-like diet (Parikh, Lipsitz, and Natarajan, 2009).

TABLE 18-9 ■ Additional Dietary Changes That May Reduce Cardiovascular Risk

ACTION	RATIONALE	CONCERNS
Consume fatty fish (salmon, herring, trout, sardines, tuna) twice a week.	Omega-3 fatty acids are associated with a decreased risk of death from cardiac events.	Recommended for clients with and without CHD Beware of mercury hazards (see Chapter 10)
Consume 1 tbs canola or walnut oil, 0.5 tbs ground flaxseed	Plant-based sources of omega-3 fatty acids	Conversion of alpha-lipoic acid in the body produces modest amounts of docosahexaenoic acid
Take omega-3 supplements in consultation with physician	If food sources unacceptable to client for lipid management	Especially for clients with documented coronary heart disease Do not appear to lower blood pressure
Substitute 25–50 grams of soy protein (isolated soy protein, textured soy, tofu) daily for animal protein	Can reduce LDL-C by 4%–24%	If not contraindicated by risks or harms Food and Drug Administration approved a health claim for soy foods Minimal evidence of direct cardiovascular benefit Indirect benefit if reduce saturated fat and cholesterol intake Isoflavones not proven to be beneficial
Consume 5 ounces of nuts (walnuts, almonds, peanuts, macadamia, pistachios, pecans) per week.	Contain beneficial fatty acids May reduce LDL-C 6%–29%	Substitute for equal kcal from other sources to avoid weight gain.
Increase fruit and vegetable servings to 10–12 daily.	Good sources of antioxidants and potassium	Beta-carotene and vitamin C and E supplements have shown no cardioprotective benefit. Potassium intake <DRI is associated with increased B/P
Select whole oats and foods high in psyllium (e.g., Bran Buds).	Soluble fiber lowers serum LDL-C without affecting HDL-C and triglyceride concentrations.	Food and Drug Administration approved health claims for whole oats and foods containing psyllium seed husk. Consume adequate fluids.

CHD, coronary heart disease; LDL-C, low-density lipoprotein cholesterol; DRI, daily recommended intake; HDL-C, high-density lipoprotein cholesterol.
Adapted from American Dietetic Association (2008a, 2008b); American Heart Association (2013); Lichtenstein et al (2006); Theuwissen and Mensink (2008).

Box 18-4 ■ *Coffee and Heart Disease*

Coffee has more than a thousand chemicals, many formed during the roasting process that may have either beneficial or harmful effects on the cardiovascular system (Bonita, Mandarano, Shuta, and Vinson, 2007). Caffeine, found in coffee, tea, soft drinks, and chocolate, stimulates the central nervous system, releases free fatty acids from adipose tissues, and affects the kidneys, increasing urination, which could lead to dehydration. The American Heart Association states that moderate coffee drinking, 1 to 2 cups per day, does not appear to be harmful (American Heart Association 2012). The evidence is inconclusive.

Higher Risk

Three or more cups of coffee per day was significantly associated with coronary heart disease (CHD) in case–control studies (Sofi, Conti, Gori et al, 2007). Randomized controlled trials have confirmed the cholesterol-raising effect of diterpenes present in boiled coffee, which may contribute to the risk of CHD associated with drinking unfiltered coffee. Discovery of a genetic polymorphism associated with a slower rate of caffeine metabolism provides evidence that caffeine affects the risk of CHD (Cornelis, El-Sohemy, Kabagambe, and Campos, 2007). See Genomic Gem 18-3.

Lower Risk

Antioxidants in coffee might contribute to the lower risk of CHD among moderate coffee drinkers (Cornelis et al, 2007). People aged 65 years or older consuming more caffeine had a lower risk of cardiovascular disease and heart disease mortality than those who consumed less caffeine. This was not true in persons with extreme hypertension or in younger individuals (Greenberg, Dunbar, Schnoll R, et al, 2007). An inverse relationship between moderate intake of coffee, up to 4 cups, and the risk of heart failure was found in a meta-analysis of prospective studies looking at habitual coffee consumption (Mostofsky, Rice, Levitan, and Mittleman, 2012).

No Effect

A 20-year study of 128,000 men and women revealed no effect of coffee on CHD after adjusting for known risk factors (Lopez-Garcia, van Dam, Willett, et al, 2006). Neither was daily coffee consumption significantly associated with CHD in long-term prospective cohort studies involving 403,631 participants followed from 3 to 44 years (Sofi et al, 2007).

Clinical judgment on the issue of caffeine varies, so the protocol of the physician or the institution should be ascertained before providing caffeinated beverages to clients with cardiovascular diseases.

Genomic Gem 18-3
Variant Gene in Caffeine Metabolism

Evidence relating caffeine to myocardial infarction (MI) involves the cytochrome P450 gene CYP1A2 that accounts for about 95% of caffeine metabolism. See Chapter 15 for a discussion on isoenzymes.

In a Costa Rican population-based case–control study, individuals with a variant CYP1A2 gene who metabolized caffeine more slowly than normal had a 64% increased risk of nonfatal MI. Coffee intake of 4 or more cups per day

(compared with less than 1 cup per day) was associated with an increased risk of MI. This relationship existed only among individuals with the slow caffeine metabolism allele, CYP1A2*1F, and only among those younger than 59 years of age. People younger than 59 years had twice the risk of nonfatal MI and those younger than 50 years had four times the risk of healthy controls (Cornelis et al, 2006).

TABLE 18-10 ■ Reduction in Blood Pressure Compared to Control Diet

| | FRUIT AND VEGETABLE DIET | | COMBINATION (DASH) DIET | |
	Systolic	Diastolic	Systolic	Diastolic
Normotensive	2.8 mm Hg	1.1 mm Hg	5.5 mm Hg	3.0 mm Hg
Hypertensive	7.2 mm Hg	2.8 mm Hg	11.4 mm Hg	5.5 mm Hg

Source: Adapted from Appel et al (1997).

An outstanding feature of this trial was its emphasis not on limiting or restricting foods but on increasing intake of certain foods. Commonly available foods, not specialty foods containing fat substitutes, were used throughout the trial.

The DASH diet, independent of weight loss or exercise, is associated in the reduction of blood pressure among both African American and White adults (Epstein, Sherwood, Smith, et al 2012). Following a DASH diet, low in sodium and abundant in fruits and vegetables and low-fat dairy, are key recommendations in the 2010 Dietary Guidelines for Americans. Features of the DASH diet are shown in Table 18-11. The example is based on a 2000-kilocalorie diet. The daily nutrient goals of the DASH diet for this caloric level are as follows: no more than 27% fat (with no more than 6% saturated fat, and 150 mg cholesterol), 18% protein, 55% carbohydrate, no more than 2300 mg sodium (1500 mg is better for individuals with high BP, African Americans, and middle-aged and older adults), 4700 mg potassium, 1250 mg calcium, 500 mg magnesium, and 30 g fiber.

Fruits and Vegetables, Not Supplements

Atherosclerosis is thought to be related to oxidative stress characterized by lipid and protein in the vascular wall (Bonomini, Tengattini, and Fabiano, 2008). One of the earliest events promoting atherosclerosis is the oxidation of LDL that stimulates inflammatory and immunological mechanisms (Matsuura, Hughes, and Khamashta, 2008).

■ High levels of oxidized LDL have been associated with increased risk of future myocardial infarction, even after adjustment for LDL-C and other established cardiovascular risk factors (Holvoet, 2008).

TABLE 18-11 ■ The DASH Diet (based on a 2000 kilocalorie diet)

FOOD GROUP	DAILY SERVINGS	SERVING SIZES	EXAMPLES AND NOTES	SIGNIFICANCE OF FOOD GROUP TO DASH DIET
Grains and Grain Products (whole grains are recommended)	6–8	1 slice bread ½ cup dry cereal ½ cup cooked cereal, brown rice, or pasta	Whole-wheat bread, English muffin, pita bread, bagel, cereals, grits, oatmeal	Major sources of energy and fiber
Vegetables	4–5	1 cup raw leafy ½ cup cooked 6-oz juice	Tomatoes, potatoes, carrots, peas, squash, broccoli, turnip greens, collards, kale, spinach, artichokes, sweet potatoes, beans	Rich sources of potassium, magnesium, and fiber
Fruits	4–5	6 oz juice 1 medium fruit ¼ cup dried fruit ½ cup fresh, frozen, or canned fruit	Apricots, bananas, dates, oranges, grapefruit, mangoes, melons, peaches, pineapples, prunes, raisins, strawberries, tangerines	Important sources of potassium, magnesium, and fiber
Low-Fat or Nonfat Dairy Foods	2–3	8 oz milk 1 cup yogurt 1.5 oz cheese	Skim or 1% milk, skim or low-fat buttermilk, nonfat or low-fat yogurt, part-skim mozzarella cheese, nonfat cheese	Major sources of calcium and protein
Meats, Poultry, and Fish	6 or fewer	3 oz cooked meat, poultry, or fish	Select only lean; trim away visible fat, broil, roast, or boil instead of frying; remove skin from poultry	Rich sources of protein and magnesium
Nuts, Seeds, and Legumes	4–5 per week	1.5 oz or ⅓ cup nuts ½ oz or 2 tbsp seeds ½ cup cooked legumes	Almonds, filberts, mixed nuts, peanuts, walnuts, sunflower seeds, kidney beans, lentils	Rich sources of energy, magnesium, potassium, protein, and fiber
Fats and Oils	2–3	1 tsp	Canola, olive, peanut oils	Contain mainly monounsaturated fatty acids

Adapted from National Institutes of Health (2012).

- Metabolic syndrome is associated with a higher fraction of oxidized LDL and thus with higher levels of circulating oxidized LDL (Holvoet, 2008).

Hence, one might conclude that antioxidants would be effective in preventing atherosclerosis. Antioxidant-rich fruits, vegetables, and whole grains have been associated with reduced disease risk. However, beta-carotene and vitamin C and E supplements have not protected against cardiovascular events or mortality (American Dietetic Association, 2008a).

Reducing Saturated Fat Intake

About two-thirds of saturated fatty acids in the U.S. diet come from animal fats. Using nonfat or low-fat dairy products is an especially important strategy because milk fat contains more cholesterol-raising fatty acids than meat fat does (Grundy, 2006). Cooking methods also affect the fat in meat. For instance, warm water rinsing of cooked, crumbled ground beef containing 30% fat reduced its fat content by 33% to 52% (Love and Prusa, 1992). Other techniques to reduce fat in meat are shown in Figure 18-3.

Plant Sterols

Specialty foods containing plant sterols may be recommended *in prescribed amounts*. These foods are marketed as table spreads (butter substitutes), juices, yogurts, and salad dressings. **Plant sterols** (phytosterols) are compounds that structurally resemble cholesterol but are not absorbed in the human body to any extent. In the gastrointestinal tract, plant

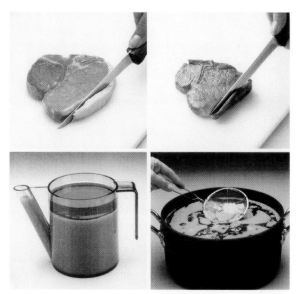

FIGURE 18-3 Selecting lean meat, trimming off visible fat, and skimming fat from meat juices reduce the amount of fat consumed. (From the National Live Stock and Meat Board, 444 North Michigan Avenue, Chicago, IL 60611, with permission.)

sterols bind with bile and cholesterol, increasing their excretion in the feces (Gropper et al, 2009). For maximum effectiveness, 2 to 3 grams daily of foods containing plant sterols should be consumed to significantly lower total cholesterol 4% to 11% and LDL cholesterol 7% to 15% while not changing HDL or triglyceride levels (Academy of Nutrition and Dietetics, 2011).

Sitosterolemia is a rare autosomal recessive disorder that is an absolute contraindication to the use of plant sterols. In this condition, both cholesterol and plant sterols are absorbed at a high rate and are not removed effectively by the liver, resulting in accelerated atherosclerosis and premature coronary artery and aortic valve disease. The possibility that plant sterols might be a risk factor for atherosclerosis in others is suggested by their presence in atheromatous plaque from individuals without absorption disorders (Academy of Nutrition and Dietetics, 2011; Patel and Thompson, 2006).

Despite their occurrence in foods, plant sterols should be monitored by the health-care provider as are drugs.

Omega-3 Fatty Acids

The regular consumption of foods rich in marine omega-3 fatty acids, **eicosapentaenoic acid (EPA)** and **docosahexaenoic acid (DHA),** may:

- Decrease occurrence of arrhythmia and sudden death
- Lower plasma triglycerides
- Slightly raise HDL levels
- Reduce homocysteine levels
- Lower blood pressure
- Reduced blood clotting tendencies

One proposed mechanism for these beneficial effects was tested with people scheduled for carotid endarterectomy who received placebo, omega-6 fatty acids as sunflower oil, or omega-3 fatty acids as fish oil. Results indicated those receiving the fish oil had more stable plaque that incorporated omega-3 fatty acids, whereas the other two groups did not (Thies, Garry, Yaqoob, et al, 2003).

Fish containing omega-3 fatty acids that are low in mercury include the following (Dietary Guidelines, 2010):

- Anchovies
- Herring
- Mackerel (Atlantic and Pacific, not king mackerel)
- Pacific oysters
- Rainbow trout
- Salmon
- Sardines

Vegetarian sources of omega-3 fatty acids include (Consumer Lab, 2013):

- Algae
- Ground flax
- Chia seeds
- Oils: canola, soy and walnut

Individuals who have hypertriglyceridemia should follow therapeutic lifestyle change (TLC), which include the dietary recommendations outlined in the 2010 Dietary Guidelines, and be given a prescription for fish oil supplements providing 2 to 4 grams of purified DHA/EPA (Academy of Nutrition and Dietetics, 2011).

The Food and Drug Administration (FDA) allows supplements containing DHA/EPA to have a label claim stating, "Supportive but not conclusive research shows that consumption of EPA and DHA omega-3 fatty acids may reduce the risk of coronary heart disease" (Consumer Lab, 2013).

Clinical studies suggest that tissue levels of long-chain omega-3 fatty acids are depressed in vegetarians, particularly in vegans. Vegetarian diets, especially the vegan, are relatively low in alpha-linolenic acid (ALA) and provide little, if any, eicosapentaenoic acid (EPA) and docosahexaenoic acid (DHA). Vegetarians are encouraged to consume flaxseeds, walnuts, canola oil, and soy in their diets as good sources of ALA (American Dietetic Association, 2009).

Conversion of ALA by the body to the more active longer-chain metabolites is less than 5% to 10% efficient for EPA and 2% to 5% for DHA. Thus, total omega-3 requirements may be higher for vegetarians than for nonvegetarians. Moreover, the balance between omega-3 and omega-6 fatty acids impacts the conversion rate. Thus, it may be wise to consult a dietitian if the client:

- Is at risk for cardiovascular disease
- Has increased need for EPA and DHA (pregnant or lactating women)
- Is likely to poorly convert ALA to EPA and DHA (persons with diabetes or neurological disorders, premature infants, elderly)

More research is needed to show a cause-and-effect relationship between alpha-linolenic acid and heart disease (American Heart Association, 2008). Figure 18-4 shows fatty acids with their common food sources.

Psyllium

Psyllium is a gelatinous substance. It is a soluble fiber, which has been demonstrated to be very effective in lowering LDL-C. If 10.2 grams per day are consumed, it has been shown to lower LDL-C on average 7% (Sports, Cardiovascular, and Wellness Nutrition, 2009). The FDA has permitted a health claim on the labels of foods containing psyllium seed husk (e.g., Kellogg's Bran Buds). The health claim states that the food, *as part of a diet low in saturated fat and cholesterol*, may reduce the risk of coronary heart disease.

To qualify, the food must provide at least 1.7 grams of soluble fiber in an amount customarily consumed.

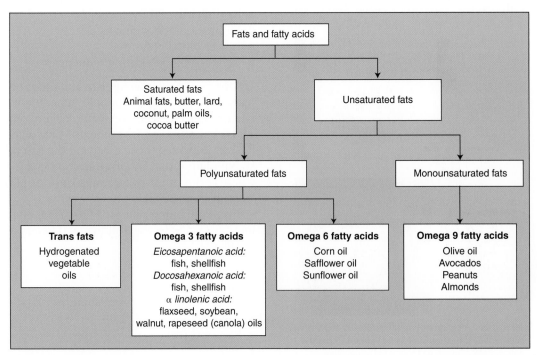

FIGURE 18-4 Fatty acids and their common food sources. Omega-3 fatty acids are particularly desirable in a heart healthy diet. (Adapted from Din JN, Newby DE, and Flapan AD: Omega 3 fatty acids and cardiovascular disease—fishing for a natural treatment. BMJ 328:30, 2004.)

To obtain the result achieved in the controlled studies on which the FDA approval was based, a person would have to consume four servings per day (U.S. FDA, 1998).

Soy Protein

Soy is a high-quality plant protein that is a source of all essential amino acids, as well as dietary fiber and iron. Clinical trials have shown that consumption of soy protein compared with other proteins such as those from milk or meat can lower total and LDL-C levels. The key is to replace some of the animal protein with soy protein. Soy protein has been found to lower cholesterol by approximately 3% to 5% (Sports, Cardiovascular, and Wellness Nutrition, 2012).

In 1999, the FDA approved a health claim for soy-containing foods stating that including soy protein in a diet low in saturated fat and cholesterol may reduce the risk of CHD by lowering blood cholesterol levels. Because 25 grams of soy protein daily in the diet is needed to show a significant cholesterol-lowering effect, to qualify for this health claim, a food must contain at least 6.25 grams of soy protein per serving (Sports, Cardiovascular, and Wellness Nutrition, 2012; U.S. FDA, 1999). Figure 18-5 shows the many choices available using soy with MyPlate.

Because soy contains phytoestrogens, clients should discuss the feasibility of adding soy products to their diets as a cardioprotective strategy with their healthcare providers.

Not all research is easily or quickly interpreted. Clinical Application 18-1 describes the search for connections between diet and disease.

Sodium-Controlled Diets

Individuals with hypertension or heart failure may need to control their sodium intake. The preference

HOW SOY FITS INTO THE USDA'S MYPLATE

The Dietary Guidelines for Americans gives science-based advice on food and physical activity choices for health. To see the full Dietary Guidelines, go to http://health.gov/dietaryguidelines/dga2010/DietaryGuidelines2010.pdf. Soyfoods can be an important part of a healthy diet as proscribed by the USDA MyPlate. Most soyfoods contain no cholesterol, little or no saturated fat, high quality protein and dietary fiber. Many soyfoods also provide essential vitamins and minerals, such as B vitamins, vitamins A and D, calcium, iron and potassium.

Grains	Vegetables	Oils	Milk	Meat & Beans
• Soy cereal • Soy grits • Soy waffles • Soy pasta • Soy bread • Soy flour Consuming at least three or more ounce-equivalents of whole grains per day can reduce the risk of several chronic diseases and may help with weight maintenance. Soy flour is part of this group. Substitute up to one-fourth of the total flour in your favorite baked product recipe.	• Green soybeans (edamame) • Canned soybeans • Soynuts One-half cup of green soybeans (edamame) contains 10 grams of soy protein. All soybeans are a good source of dietary fiber and isoflavones.	• Soybean oil (also called vegetable oil) Soybean oil is rich in polyunsaturated fat and contains only minimal saturated fat. Soybean oil is a rich source of omega-3 fatty acids. Soybean oil, labeled "vegetable oil," is a source of the antioxidant Vitamin E.	• Soy beverage • Soy cheese • Soy yogurt • Soy ice cream According to the USDA food guidelines, protein choices for those who do not consume milk products include calcium-fortified soy beverages, soybeans, soy yogurt, soy cheese and tempeh. Soy ice cream products are a part of this group, but do not contain as much calcium or protein as other options.	• Soy burgers • Soy hot dogs • Soy nuggets • Soy burger-type crumbles • Tofu • Soynuts • Canned soybeans • Green soybeans (edamame) • Soynut butter According to the USDA food guidelines, protein choices in this category include all of the above listed soyfoods. Soybeans are a source of high quality protein and include all eight of the essential amino acids.

FIGURE 18-5 How Soy Fits into the U.S. Department of Agriculture's MyPlate (United Soybean Board (USB) 2012 Soybean Guide, with permission.)

18-1

Clinical Application

The Limits of Population Studies: A Historical Perspective

Research is sometimes misinterpreted or applied prematurely. Rarely does a single study merit widespread changes in diet in the pursuit of health.

FAT INTAKE

In the 1960s, Japan and Greece had the lowest rates of heart disease among seven countries. People in those two countries were very different in their fat consumption: 10% of kilocalories in Japan and 40% on the island of Crete. On the face of these findings, fat intake might be dismissed as irrelevant to heart disease. But the Greeks derived less than 10% of kilocalories from animal protein and 33% of their kilocalories from olive oil, which is 82% monounsaturated.

MULTIPLE CAUSATION

Since 1976, Spain has experienced a decrease in cardiovascular mortality, despite increased intakes of dairy products and meat, particularly pork and poultry. If attention focused only on those foods, the rationale for the decreased mortality would be missed.

Most of the decrease in cardiovascular mortality was due to a decline in stroke mortality. Improved hypertension control, including decreased intake of salt and salt-cured foods, is thought to have influenced this trend. Other contributing factors were increased consumption of fruit and fish, reduction in cigarette smoking, and expanded access to clinical care, including a major increase in the use of aspirin as a platelet inhibitor (Serra-Majem, Ribbas, Tsesserras, et al, 1995).

RED WINE

Consumption of red wine is credited with conferring some protection against coronary heart disease (CHD). The "French Paradox" refers to the observation in the early 1990s that despite the high intake of saturated fats in their diet, there was a low incidence of CHD in the French population. This was thought to be because of the red wine intake of the French (Brannon, 2011; Catalgol, Batirel, Taga, and Ozer; Ferrieres 2004). Resveratrol is one compound found in abundance in red wine that has been identified and studied as the potential beneficial substance contributing to red wine's benefit. Resveratrol has been the subject of many studies that have shown it to potentially have cardiovascular benefits including lowering systolic blood pressure, triglyceride levels, LDL cholesterol oxidation, hgb A1C, and platelet aggregation; improved liver function and insulin sensitivity; and increasing levels of HDL-C levels (Brannon 2011; Consumer Lab, 2012; Natural Medicines Comprehensive Database, 2012). More controlled studies are necessary to make any definitive conclusions regarding the role of resveratrol in health (Catalgol et al, 2012).

IRON

Men in eastern Finland have one of the highest recorded incidences of mortality from CHD. An association was reported between high levels of stored iron (as assessed by serum ferritin levels or ratio of serum transferrin receptor to serum ferritin) and increased risk for acute myocardial infarction (Salonen, Nyyssönen, Korpela, et al, 1992; Tuomainen, Punnonen, Nyyssönen, and Salonen, 1998). Iron overload thus was hypothesized to cause the higher occurrence of CHD in men compared with women. A study in Greece also correlated high dietary iron intake with increased risk of coronary artery disease in men and women 60 years of age or older (Tzonou, Lagiou, Trichopoulou, et al, 1998).

A more detailed study found no association between total iron intake and risk of myocardial infarction after adjustment for age and gender, but the study did find high dietary intake of heme iron associated with occurrence of and mortality from myocardial infarction (Klipstein-Grosbusch, Grobbee, den Breeijen, et al, 1999). A reanalysis of Salonen's data associated increased iron intake with increased consumption of red meat (American Heart Association, 2000).

HOMOCYSTEINE

More than 30 years ago, extensive atherosclerosis was found on autopsy of individuals with elevated plasma homocysteine levels due to errors of metabolism. This autosomal recessive genetic disease, homocystinuria, occurs in about 1 of 300,000 live births with a higher prevalence in Ireland and New South Wales (Refsum, Smith, Ueland, et al, 2004).

When untreated, homocystinuria results in thromboembolic events in 50% of the clients and a 20% mortality rate before the age of 30 (Nygård, Nordrehaug, Refsum, et al, 1997). Extending investigations to general populations found plasma homocysteine levels related to heart failure (Vasan, Beiser, D'Agostino, et al, 2003), risk of stroke (Tanne et al, 2003), but also cancer mortality and all-cause mortality as well as cardiovascular mortality (Vollset, Refsum, Tverdal, et al, 2001).

Consequently, the early enthusiasm for reducing cardiovascular risk by reducing homocysteine levels has waned. Homocysteine appears to be a marker, rather than a cause, of cardiovascular disease. Therefore, routine screening for and treatment of elevated homocysteine levels to prevent cardiovascular disease is not supported by the evidence (Wierzbicki, 2007). Clinically, there is little justification for using folic acid or B vitamins in patients with established cardiovascular disease, whether or not they have elevated homocysteine levels (O'Callaghan, 2007). The American Heart Association recommends that individuals obtain their folic acid and B vitamins from foods consuming fruits and green, leafy vegetables daily (American Heart Association, 2012).

Thus, evidence accumulates slowly and must be interpreted cautiously. The many correlations found in large studies are often statistically significant but do not prove causation and may not be clinically useful. Advice to clients should be evidence based from clinical practice guidelines.

---

for salty foods is learned and culturally transmitted, even though heavy salting is no longer necessary for preservation of food. After about 3 months on a sodium-restricted diet, most individuals lose their appetite for salt. Table 18-12 lists the legal definitions for sodium and salt descriptions on labels.

Unseen contributions to sodium intake may come from beverages, over-the-counter medications, and drinking water. Table 18-13 lists sodium content of beverages. Many toothpastes and mouthwashes contain significant amounts of sodium and should not be swallowed. Over-the-counter medications that may

TABLE 18-12 ■ Labeling Regulations for Sodium Content Descriptions

TERM	LEGAL DEFINITION
Free	Less than 5 mg of sodium per serving
Salt Free	Must meet the criteria for free
Very Low* Sodium	Less than 35 mg of sodium per serving. For meals and main dishes: 35 mg or less per 100 g
Low* Sodium	Less than 140 mg of sodium per serving. Meals and main dishes: 140 mg or less per 100 g
Reduced or Less	This term means that a nutritionally altered product contains 25% less sodium than the regular, or reference, product. However, a reduced claim cannot be made on a product if its reference food already meets the requirement for a "low" claim.
Light in Sodium or Lightly Salted	May be used on food in which the sodium content has been reduced by at least 50% compared with an appropriate reference food.
Unsalted or No Added Salt	Must declare "This is not a sodium-free food" on information panel if the food is not sodium free.

*Synonyms for low include "little," "few," and "low source of."

TABLE 18-13 ■ Examples of Sodium Content of Beverages*

	REGULAR		DIET	
Beverage†	Sodium (mg)	Kilocalories	Sodium (mg)	Kilocalories
Club soda			75	0
Coffee	4	0		
Cola	15	151		
With aspartame			21	2
With saccharin			75	2
Gatorade	39	123		
Ginger Ale	25	125	130	4
Kool-Aid	0	150		
With aspartame			0	6
Lemonade	12	150		
Lemon-Lime Soda	41	149	70	4
Pepper-Type	38	151	70	0
Root Beer	49	152	170	4
Tea	2	0		

*Serving size is 12 fluid ounces.
†Sodium content may vary depending on the source of water.

contain significant amounts of sodium include analgesics, antacids, antibiotics, antitussives, laxatives, and sedatives.

Softening water can increase its sodium content.

■ Sodium in city water supplies has varied from 1.2 milligrams per liter in Seattle to 100 milligrams per liter in Phoenix.

■ "Mineral waters" contain from 8 to 172 milligrams of sodium per liter. "Read the label" is appropriate advice.

Clients who require a diet containing less than 2 grams of sodium may elect to use bottled, distilled, deionized, or demineralized water for drinking and cooking to consume preferred sodium-containing foods. Some clients prefer a daily allotment of salt in a shaker to be used as desired. If this strategy is adopted, the foods high in sodium must be limited to a greater extent than for a standardized sodium-controlled diet.

Many salt substitutes are available. Some substitute potassium for sodium and may be unsuitable for clients with kidney disease or those taking potassium-sparing diuretics or angiotensin-converting enzyme (ACE) inhibitors. Clients should consult their health-care providers about using salt substitutes. These products are for table use only and are not appropriate for cooking because they turn bitter. Salt substitutes, which are made up of different herb and spice blends and exclude salt, are excellent ways to enhance the flavor of food and make low sodium cooking more palatable.

In clinical practice, diet orders such as "no-added-salt diet" or "low-sodium diet" require clarification. Usually, a facility's diet manual defines the terms. A "no-added-salt diet" may be calculated as 4 grams of sodium and a "low-sodium diet" as 2 grams in one facility but differently in another. Diet prescriptions should be written in milligrams of sodium to achieve the desired result. Table 18-14 describes diets with sodium controlled from 2 grams to 250 milligrams per day. Figure 18-6 shows some of the seasonings permitted on a sodium-controlled diet.

Modifications for Common Conditions

Persons with heart attacks, heart failure, or stroke may require modifications in diet. Referral to the dietitian may be in order.

Myocardial Infarction

After a heart attack, the client may be in shock. One adaptive response of the body is to slow gastrointestinal function. Thus, the client may receive nothing by mouth while the shock persists. Fluid is given intravenously to maintain fluid balance and to keep an access site open for intravenous medications.

As the client recovers, the diet may progress from a 1000- to 1200-kilocalorie liquid diet to a

TABLE 18-14 ■ Sodium-Controlled Diets

DESCRIPTION	INDICATION		ADEQUACY	
These diets control sodium intake to prescribed levels.	Clients with hypertension, heart failure, fluid-retaining kidney or endocrine disease, or other edematous conditions.		The 500-mg and 250-mg diets may be deficient in some nutrients.	
Food Item or Group	**2 Grams of Sodium**	**1 Gram of Sodium**	**500 mg of Sodium**	**250 mg of Sodium**
Soups	Column A below	Column A below	Column A below	Column A below
Milk	2 cups Column B below	2 cups Column B below	Column A below	1 cup Column B below
Bread	3 slices Column B below	3 slices Column B below	Column A below	Column A below
Cereal	Column A below	1 serving Column B below	Column A below	Column A below
Fruits	Free	Free	Free	Free
Egg	1	1	1	1
Meat/Substitutes	6 oz	5 oz	4 oz	4 oz
Vegetables	Column A below	Column A below	Column A below	Column A below
Desserts	1 serving Column B below	Column A below	Column A below	Column A below
Fats and Oils	5 tsp Column B below	3 tsp Column B below	3 tsp Column B below	Column A below
Condiments	Column A below	Column A below	Column A below	Column A below
Food Group	**Column A Lower in Sodium than Column B**		**Column B Higher in Sodium than Column A**	
Soups	Unsalted broth and bouillon Low sodium canned soup Homemade soup made with allowed foods and milk allowance		Regular canned and frozen soups Dehydrated soup mixes Bouillon cubes and powder Consommé	
Milk	Commercially made low-sodium milk Low-sodium cheese		All milk from animals Yogurt Regular cheese Commercial milk products	
Breads and Cereals	Bread and crackers prepared without salt Rice, barley, and pasta without added salt Baked goods made without salt, baking soda, or baking powder Unsalted cooked cereal Puffed rice, puffed wheat, shredded wheat Cornmeal, cornstarch		Commercial mixes Frozen bread dough Instant rice and pasta mixes Regular crackers Instant and quick-cooking cereals Commercial stuffing and casserole mixes Self-rising flour and cornmeal Baked goods and quick breads made with salt, baking soda, baking powder, or egg white	
Food Group	**Column A Lower in Sodium than Column B**		**Column B Higher in Sodium than Column A**	
Fruits	Fresh, frozen, dried, or canned fruit without added sodium All fruit juices		Crystallized or glazed fruit Maraschino cherries Dried fruit with sodium preservatives	
Vegetables	Fresh, frozen without salt, low-sodium canned vegetables except those listed at right		Canned and frozen vegetables and juices Sauerkraut	
Meat, Poultry, Fish, Shellfish	Fresh, frozen, or canned low-sodium meat and poultry Low-sodium luncheon meats Eggs Low-sodium peanut butter Fresh fish Canned low-sodium tuna and salmon		Real and imitation bacon Luncheon meat Chipped or corned beef Smoked or salted meat or fish Kosher meat Frozen and powdered egg substitutes Regular peanut butter Brains, kidney, clams, lobster, crab, oysters, scallops, shrimp, and other shellfish	
Fats and Oils	Cooking oil Unsalted butter, margarine, salad dressings, and shortening		Salted butter and margarine Commercial salad dressings	
Desserts and Miscellaneous	Alcohol Coffee, coffee substitutes Lemonade Tea Low-sodium candy Unflavored gelatin Jam, jelly, maple syrup, honey Unsalted nuts and popcorn		Salted popcorn, nuts, potato chips, snacks Instant cocoa or powdered drink mixes Canned fruit drinks Commercial pastry, candy, cakes, cookies, gelatin desserts	

(continued)

TABLE 18-14 ■ Sodium-Controlled Diets (Continued)		
Food Group	**Column A Lower in Sodium than Column B**	**Column B Higher in Sodium than Column A**
Condiments and Seasonings	Sweet: allspice, almond extract, anise seed, apricot nectar, baking chocolate, cardamom, cinnamon, coriander, ginger, lemon extract, lemon juice, mace, maple extract, mint, nutmeg, orange extract, orange juice, peppermint extract, pineapple, pineapple juice, unsalted pecans, vanilla extract, unsalted walnuts, walnut extract Tangy: Basil, bay leaves, caraway seeds, cayenne pepper, chili powder, chives, cloves, curry powder, dill weed, garlic, garlic powder (not salt), green pepper, horseradish without salt, marjoram, mustard powder (not prepared), mustard seed, onion powder (not salt) onions, oregano, paprika, parsley, pepper, poppy seed, rosemary, sage, savory, sesame seeds, tarragon, thyme, turmeric	Any salt Barbecue sauce Bouillon cubes or granules Catsup Chili sauce Tartar sauce Horseradish sauce Meat extracts, sauces, and tenderizers Kitchen Bouquet Gravy and sauce mixes Monosodium glutamate Prepared mustard Olives Pickles Saccharin, other sugar substitutes containing sodium Soy sauce Teriyaki sauce Worcestershire sauce

SAMPLE MENUS FOR 2-GRAM SODIUM DIET

Breakfast	Lunch and Dinner
½ cup orange juice	3 oz chicken breast, turkey, or fish baked in lemon juice
½ cup shredded wheat	Baked potato
2 slices toast	2 tsp spread
2 tsp spread	½ cup broccoli
1 tbsp strawberry jam	Tossed salad with homemade oil and vinegar dressing
1 cup 1% milk	1 dinner roll
Sugar	½ cup sherbet
Coffee	1 cup 1% milk (day's total = 2 cups)
	Tea

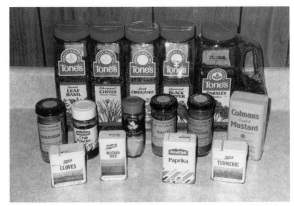

FIGURE 18-6 These are just a few of the many condiments and seasonings permissible on a sodium-restricted diet.

soft diet of small, frequent meals. Large meals can increase the workload of the heart. The diet prescription begins to implement the principles of a cardioprotective diet. As soon as possible, client education should start.

Heart Failure

For clients in heart failure, the diet order may read "as tolerated" but sodium and fluid restriction is common. Energy needs are increased due to the workload of the heart and respiratory system. Protein intakes of 1.12 to 1.37 grams per kilogram of body weight may be necessary to preserve body composition (American Dietetic Association, 2008b).

Food for the client with heart failure should be nutrient-dense, easily eaten, and easily digested. An hour's rest before meals conserves energy. Large meals, which would exert upward pressure on the chest, are undesirable. Liquid formulas, some special low-volume, nutrient-dense preparations, can be used to provide nutrients while moderating the feeling of fullness. It may be necessary to provide supplements of water-soluble vitamins and minerals that may be lost as excess fluid is excreted through treatment.

Stroke

Clients who have had a stroke may have trouble seeing their food as well as problems chewing, swallowing, and manipulating utensils. Generally, thicker, rather than thinner, liquids are easier to manage for a person with swallowing difficulty. Dry, chunky, or sticky foods are best avoided. Nurses feeding clients with hemiplegia should place the food on the unaffected side of the tongue. Turning the client's head toward the weak side while he or she is sitting upright may help with swallowing. In addition, stroke clients may be aphasic and unable to communicate their needs or desires. A speech therapist is skilled in assessing function and restorative therapy using adaptive devices for clients with dysphagia and aphasia.

Keystones

- Major modifiable risk factors for cardiovascular disease are hypertension, hypercholesterolemia, obesity, physical inactivity, diabetes mellitus, alcohol consumption, and cigarette smoking.
- Dietary modifications in cardiovascular disease most often involve cholesterol-lowering and/or blood pressure-controlling measures.
- The major target of cholesterol-lowering measures is low-density lipoprotein cholesterol (LDL-C).
- Lifestyle changes effective for hypertension control include reducing sodium intake and, if necessary, body weight.
- The most common inherited hyperlipoproteinemia is type IV, which is one cause of hypertriglyceridemia requiring restricted carbohydrate intake as well as controlled fat intake.
- Dietary treatment of chronic heart failure focuses on fluid balance and preventing malnutrition.

CASE STUDY *18-1*

Mr. Z is a 59-year-old White man who was admitted to the acute-care hospital with a diagnosis of possible myocardial infarction. Subsequent testing proved Mr. Z did not have an infarction. His medical diagnoses are Stage 1 hypertension and myocardial ischemia. He is being readied for discharge to home.

Mr. Z is vice president for sales of a large manufacturing company. His business activities involve luncheon and dinner meetings at which alcohol consumption is common. He stated he has "at least one cocktail, usually two" with lunch and with dinner.

The clinical dietitian visited Mr. Z to evaluate his food behaviors as requested by the physician. After the dietitian left, Mr. Z said to the nurse, "That diet is impossible for my situation. She just doesn't understand the business world. I don't believe there's anything wrong with my heart anyway. It was just indigestion."

Providing client care is a dynamic process. Based on the above information, the nurse added the following modifications to Mr. Z's care plan.

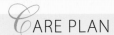 ARE PLAN

Subjective Data

Reported alcohol intake of two to four drinks per day ■ Perceived incompatibility of prescribed diet with current lifestyle ■ Stated disbelief in medical diagnosis

Objective Data

LDL-C 158 ■ B/P 150/96 ■ BMI 27

Analysis

Denial of illness and negative perception of treatment regimen as evidenced by statements to nurse.

Plan

DESIRED OUTCOMES EVALUATION CRITERIA	ACTIONS/INTERVENTIONS	RATIONALE
Client will acknowledge effect of lifestyle on health by hospital discharge.	Review pathophysiology of hyperlipoproteinemia and atherosclerosis with client.	Repeated information reinforces learning.
	Analyze with the client the possibility of partial compliance.	Perhaps the many changes required are overwhelming Mr. Z.
	Refer to clinical dietitian for repeat visit to prioritize actions and individualize diet plan.	One or two alterations might be acceptable as a starting point.
	Obtain the client's permission to discuss lifestyle changes with significant other.	Enlisting a support person might, over time, give Mr. Z reason to reconsider his options.
	Inform physician of extent of intended compliance with treatment regimen.	These statements will affect the success of treatment. It is appropriate to notify the physician and record it on the client's medical record.

The following day, the physician showed Mr. Z his laboratory results and reviewed his diagnosis and risks.

 18-1

Dietitian's Notes

The clinical dietitian revisited Mr. Z and wrote the following:

Subjective: Able to repeat the information given by physician. Does not smoke. Eats three servings of vegetables most days, some of them fried. No exercise program. Usually eats two weekday meals in a restaurant. Client consumes one to two servings of alcohol daily or twice daily. Client perceives that it is impossible to make dietary changes when he eats in restaurants.

Objective: B/P 150/96, LDL-C 158, HDL-C 36

Analysis: Harmful beliefs/attitudes about food or nutrition-related topics related to Stage 1 hypertension and myocardial ischemia as evidenced by client's reports.

Plan: Use local area restaurant menus to illustrate healthy meals—Done.

Obtain commitment to follow up with the outpatient dietitian. Appointment made.

Refer Mr. and Mrs. Z to Heart Healthy Support Group to help refocus Mr. Z's view of his health.

Critical Thinking Questions

1. How could additional assessment data regarding family history be helpful in interpreting this client's reaction? Would you expect his reaction to be different if the diagnosis of myocardial infarction had been confirmed?

2. What additional interventions have the potential to achieve the stated outcome after hospital discharge?

3. When more genomic information becomes available in the future, how might this scenario change?

Chapter Review

1. The DASH diet to reduce hypertension emphasizes:
   a. Increased amounts of fruits, vegetables, nuts, seeds, and legumes
   b. Specialty formulas as meal replacements
   c. Carbohydrate control and counting similar to that used in diabetes mellitus treatment
   d. Increased amounts of protein through low-fat dairy products and large servings of meats

2. The first action a hypertensive client should take to lower blood pressure is to:
   a. Restrict fluid to 1500 mL per day
   b. Eliminate saturated fat from the diet
   c. Lose weight if necessary
   d. Limit sodium intake to 1 gram per day

3. Lifestyle changes that are recommended to reduce cardiovascular disease risk limit saturated and *trans*-fat intake to ____ % of daily kilocalories and cholesterol to ____ milligrams per day.
   a. 45, 450
   b. 30, 300
   c. 15, 250
   d. 7, 200

4. Which of the following seasonings are permitted on a sodium-controlled diet?
   a. Catsup, horseradish, mustard, and tartar sauce
   b. Chili powder, green pepper, and caraway seeds
   c. Celery seeds, seasoned meat tenderizer, and teriyaki sauce
   d. Dry mustard, garlic, and Worcestershire sauce

5. Which of the following lifestyle changes would have the greatest effect in reducing risk of atherosclerotic cardiovascular disease?
   a. Limiting cholesterol intake to the recommended amount
   b. Consuming plant sterols in recommended amounts
   c. Limiting alcohol intake to one (women) or two (men) standard drinks per day
   d. Eating five servings of fruits and vegetables daily

Clinical Analysis

Mr. A is a 55-year-old Black man being seen in a health clinic for hypertension. His blood pressure was 152/98 3 months ago when he was first diagnosed. It has remained below that level but has not returned to normal. Today his blood pressure is 146/100.

Mr. A is 5 ft 9 in. tall and weighs 173 lb. He has a medium frame. When first diagnosed, he weighed 178 lb. A weight-loss diet with no added salt was prescribed, but progress has been slow.

Now the physician is prescribing a 2-gram sodium diet and starting Mr. A on a mild potassium-wasting diuretic. The clinic nurse is responsible for instructing the client.

1. Before he or she instructs Mr. A, which of the following actions by the nurse would best ensure his compliance with the diet?
   a. Doing a financial analysis to see if Mr. A can afford the special foods on his new diet
   b. Finding out which favorite foods Mr. A would have most difficulty giving up
   c. Listing the possible consequences of hypertension if it is not controlled
   d. Asking to see Mrs. A to instruct her on the preparation of foods for the new diet

Clinical Analysis—cont'd

2. Which of the following breakfasts would be best for Mr. A?
   a. Applesauce, raisin bran, 1% milk, and a bagel with cream cheese
   b. Canned pears, cornflakes, whole milk, and a cholesterol-free plain doughnut
   c. Cooked prunes, instant oatmeal, 2% milk, and raisin toast with margarine
   d. Orange juice, shredded wheat, skim milk, and whole-wheat toast with jelly

3. Mr. A has agreed to limit his alcohol intake to two drinks per week. He asks the nurse to recommend beverages compatible with his diet. Which of the following is the best choice?
   a. Tomato juice and bouillon
   b. Buttermilk and club soda
   c. Plain tea and fruit juice
   d. Gatorade and lemonade

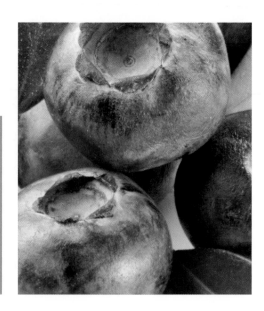

19

Diet in Renal Disease

LEARNING OBJECTIVES

After completing this chapter, the student should be able to:

- Identify the major causes of acute and chronic kidney failure.
- List the goals of nutritional care for a client with kidney disease.
- List the nutrients commonly modified in the dietary treatment of chronic kidney disease (CKD).
- Discuss the relationship among kilocaloric intake, dietary protein utilization, and uremia.
- Discuss the nutritional care of clients with kidney disease in relation to their medical treatment.

hronic kidney disease (CKD) is gradual loss of kidney function over time. The National Kidney Foundation estimates that 26 million Americans have CKD and that diabetes and hypertension are two leading causes of CKD (National Kidney Foundation 2012, 2013a).

Diet therapy for clients with kidney disease depends on an understanding of the normal function of the kidneys and basic concepts of pathophysiology of renal diseases. **Renal** means pertaining to the kidneys. The nutritional care of clients with renal disease is complex. These clients frequently must learn not just one diet in which one to seven nutrients are controlled but several different diets as their medical condition and the treatment approach change. The failure to adhere to necessary dietary changes can result in death. One aspect of working with clients with renal disease is that inattentiveness to dietary modifications can be measured objectively in weight changes or changes in blood chemistry.

Anatomy and Physiology of the Kidneys

No other organ in the human body can perform the multiple functions of the kidneys. These functions are possible because of the kidneys' internal structure.

Internal Structure

The functioning unit of the kidney is the **nephron.** Each kidney contains about a million nephrons. Figure 19-1 shows an individual nephron. Each nephron has two main parts. The first part, **Bowman's capsule,** is the cup-shaped top of the nephron. Inside Bowman's capsule is a network of blood capillaries called the **glomerulus** (plural, *glomeruli*). The second part of the nephron is the **renal tubule.** (A tubule is a small tube or canal.) The renal tubule is the ropelike portion of the nephron. This ropelike structure ends at the collecting tubule. Several nephrons usually share a single **collecting tubule.**

Functions

The kidneys assist in the internal regulation of the body by performing the following functions:

1. *Filtration:* The kidneys remove the end products of metabolism and substances that have accumulated in the blood in undesirable amounts during the **filtration** process. Substances removed from the blood include:

   - Urea
   - Creatinine

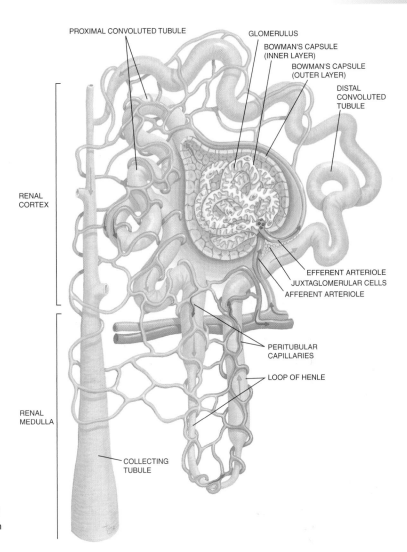

PROXIMAL CONVOLUTED TUBULE

GLOMERULUS

BOWMAN'S CAPSULE (INNER LAYER)

BOWMAN'S CAPSULE (OUTER LAYER)

DISTAL CONVOLUTED TUBULE

RENAL CORTEX

EFFERENT ARTERIOLE

JUXTAGLOMERULAR CELLS

AFFERENT ARTERIOLE

PERITUBULAR CAPILLARIES

LOOP OF HENLE

RENAL MEDULLA

COLLECTING TUBULE

FIGURE 19-1 A nephron with its associated blood vessels. The arrows indicate the direction of blood flow. (Reprinted from Scanlon, VC, and Sanders, T: *Essentials of anatomy and physiology,* 5th ed. FA Davis, Philadelphia, 2007, p. 423, with permission.)

■ Uric acid
■ Urates

Also filtered from blood are undesirable amounts of:

■ Chloride
■ Potassium
■ Sodium
■ Hydrogen ions

The **glomerular filtration rate (GFR)** is the amount of fluid filtered each minute by all the glomeruli of both kidneys and is one index of kidney function. This rate is normally about 125 milliliters per minute (Fig. 19-2).

2. *Reabsorption:* Previously filtered substances (e.g., water and sodium) needed by the body are reabsorbed into the blood in the tubules.

3. *Secretion of Ions to Maintain Acid–Base Balance:* Secretion is the process of moving ions from the blood into the urine. Secretion allows for the amount of a substance to be excreted into the urine in concentrations greater than the concentration filtered from the plasma in the glomeruli. The kidneys regulate the balance between bicarbonate and carbonic acid by the secretion and exchange of hydrogen ions for sodium ions.

4. *Excretion:* The kidneys eliminate unwanted substances from the body as urine.

5. *Renal Control of Cardiac Output and Systemic Blood Pressure:* The kidneys adapt to changing cardiac output by altering resistance to blood flow both at the beginning of the glomerulus and at the end.

6. *Calcium, Phosphorus, and Vitamin D:* The kidneys produce the active form of vitamin D, **calcitriol.** Activated vitamin D regulates the absorption of calcium and phosphorus from the intestinal tract and assists in the regulation of calcium and phosphorus levels in the blood.

7. *Erythropoietin:* The kidneys produce a hormone called **erythropoietin,** which stimulates maturation of red blood cells in bone marrow.

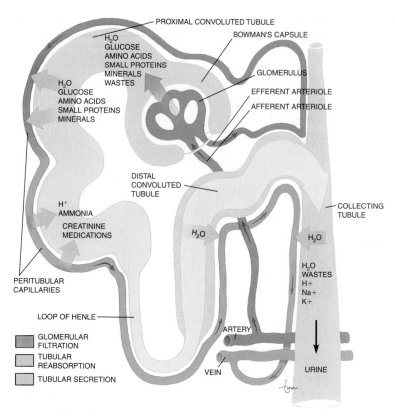

FIGURE 19-2 Schematic representation of glomerular filtration, tubular reabsorption, and tubular secretion. The renal tubule has been uncoiled, and the peritubular capillaries are shown adjacent to the tubule. (Reprinted from Scanlon, VC, and Sanders, T: *Essentials of anatomy and physiology*, 6th ed. FA Davis, Philadelphia, 2011, p. 455, with permission.)

Kidney Disease

Because the kidneys perform so many metabolic functions, kidney disease has serious consequences.

Causes

Renal disease can be caused by many factors, including:

- Trauma
- Infections
- Birth defects
- Medications
- Chronic disease (e.g., atherosclerosis, diabetes, hypertension)
- Toxic metal consumption
- See Genomic Gem 19-1.

Diabetic nephropathy is the most common cause of renal failure. A physiological stress such as a myocardial infarction (MI) or an extensive burn can precipitate renal disease by decreasing the perfusion of the kidney or markedly increasing catabolism. Clinical Application 19-1 describes the renal response after MI and the effect of reduced renal blood flow. Catabolism causes an increase in nitrogenous products and potassium, which must be excreted, overworking the kidneys. Renal disease is a feared complication of many pathologies and treatments—including radiocontrast

---

Genomic Gem 19-1
Genetic Mutations

Some kidney diseases are caused by errors in the genetic code. A genetic mutation can make it possible that a particular disease will happen. For example, high blood pressure is strongly associated with a selection of minor mutations plus lifestyle choices in diet, exercise, smoking, other environmental exposures, and kidney disease.

19-1
Clinical Application

Renal Response After a Myocardial Infarction

Immediately after a myocardial infarction (MI; commonly called a heart attack), blood flow through the systemic circulation is diminished. Systemic circulation refers to the blood flow from the left part of the heart through the aorta and all branches (arteries) to the capillaries of the tissues. Systemic circulation also includes the blood's return to the heart through the veins.

After a heart attack, blood flow to the myocardium (heart muscle) is decreased, impairing myocardial function. Less blood is delivered to the tissues. The kidneys sense the decreased cardiac output and try to compensate by reabsorption of additional water. This may lead to a fluid overload and edema. For that reason, clients who have had an MI may be on fluid restriction.

materials used in diagnostic procedures, some antibiotics, and some pain medications.

Three common conditions increase the risk of renal disease:

1. Obesity
2. Poorly controlled diabetes
3. Hypertension

Losing weight reduces the severity of diabetes and hypertension, the two leading causes of kidney failure, and helps prevent those conditions in people who have not developed them. Normalization of blood glucose and lipid levels along with blood pressure control also decrease the risk of renal disease. The Diabetes Control and Complications Trial (DCCT) and United Kingdom Prospective Diabetes Study (UKPDS) have shown that intensive diabetes therapy can significantly reduce the progression of microvascular complications in people with diabetes. It is recommended that an A1C level of 7% should be the target for individuals who are not at high risk of hypoglycemia (National Kidney Foundation, 2012).

Hypertension markedly accelerates the progression of diabetic nephropathy, and aggressive antihypertension management is able to greatly decrease the rate of fall of GFR. Some studies indicate that a higher systolic blood pressure causes kidney disease progression more than a high diastolic blood pressure (National Kidney Foundation, 2007). For those reasons, among others, all clients should be encouraged to follow their prescribed diets and always take prescribed medications.

Glomerulonephritis

A general term for an inflammation of the kidneys is **nephritis.** This is the most common type of kidney disease. Inflammation of the glomeruli is called **glomerulonephritis,** which can be either acute or chronic. This condition often follows scarlet fever or a streptococcal infection of the respiratory tract. Young children and young adults are commonly victims. Symptoms include:

■ Nausea
■ Vomiting
■ Fever
■ Hypertension
■ Blood in the urine (**hematuria**)
■ Decreased output of urine (**oliguria**)
■ Protein in the urine (**proteinuria**)
■ Edema

Recovery is usually complete. However, in some clients the disease progresses and becomes chronic. This leads to a progressive loss of kidney function. Some clients develop **anuria,** which is a total lack of urine output. Without treatment, this condition is fatal.

Specific Tubular Abnormalities

A structural problem in the renal tubules may result in abnormal reabsorption or lack of reabsorption of certain substances by the tubules. The result of a tubular abnormality is ineffective cleansing of the blood.

Nephrotic Syndrome

The result of a variety of diseases that damage the glomeruli capillary walls is called **nephrotic syndrome.** Signs of nephrotic syndrome include:

■ Proteinuria
■ Severe edema
■ Low serum protein levels
■ Anemia
■ Hyperlipidemia

Usually the higher the hyperlipidemia, the greater the proteinuria.

The disease is caused by the degenerative changes in the kidneys' capillary walls, which consequently permit the passage of albumin into the **glomerular filtrate.** Water and sodium are retained. Edema is sometimes so severe that it masks tissue wasting due to the breakdown of tissue protein stores. The degree of malnutrition is hidden until the excess fluid is removed.

Nephrosclerosis

A hardening of the renal arteries, known as **nephrosclerosis,** is caused by arteriosclerosis and results in a decreased blood supply to the kidneys. The condition is **hypertensive kidney disease** and can eventually destroy the kidney.

Progressive Nature of Kidney Failure

Kidney disease can be acute or chronic. The earliest clinical evidence of nephropathy is the appearance of low levels (30 mg/day or 20 g/min) of albumin in the urine, referred to as **microalbuminuria.**

In **acute renal failure,** the kidneys stop working entirely or almost entirely. Acute renal failure occurs suddenly and is usually temporary. It can last for a few days or weeks.

Chronic renal failure occurs when progressively more nephrons are destroyed until the kidneys simply cannot perform vital functions. Chronic renal failure occurs over time and is usually irreversible.

As individual nephrons are damaged, the remaining nephrons work harder to maintain metabolic homeostasis. As each functional nephron's workload is increased, the nephron becomes more susceptible to work overload and damage. The normal composition of the blood becomes altered when the remaining functional nephrons cannot assume any additional workload.

At such time, serum levels of **blood urea nitrogen (BUN), creatinine,** and uric acid become elevated. In some clients, even though the underlying condition (e.g., diabetes mellitus, hypertension) is treated, chronic renal disease may lead to **end-stage renal failure.** During end-stage renal failure, most or all of the kidneys' ability to produce urine and regulate blood chemistries is severely compromised.

Sodium Depletion

Often, the first sign of chronic renal failure is sodium depletion. This occurs when the kidneys lose their ability to reabsorb sodium in the tubule. Symptoms associated with sodium depletion include:

- A reduction of renal blood flow
- Dehydration
- Lethargy
- Decreased glomerular filtration rate (GFR)
- Uremia (see next section)
- Deterioration in neurological symptoms including headaches, disorientation, and, in severe cases, seizures and coma

The client's blood pressure and body weight drop. Urine volume may be increased initially in chronic renal failure. A loss of body fat and protein content is responsible for the weight loss. The client's serum albumin level may fall as protein is lost in the urine.

Sodium Retention

As kidney function further deteriorates, some of these symptoms reverse. The kidneys lose the ability to excrete sodium. When this occurs, symptoms include:

- Sodium retention
- Overhydration
- Edema
- Hypertension
- Congestive heart failure (CHF)

The body can excrete little or no urine. The GFR gradually declines in chronic renal failure. Chronic kidney disease has been formally classified into five stages based on the GFR. Table 19-1 lists the stages of CKD and describes each stage along with the corresponding GFR. Most clients with a GFR below 25 milliliters per minute will eventually require either dialysis or transplantation, regardless of the original cause of failure. Nutrition therapy for CKD is to

TABLE 19-1 ■ Stages of Chronic Kidney Disease and Glomerular Filtration Rate (GFR)

STAGE	GFR
1. Some kidney damage with normal or elevated GFR	≥90
2. Kidney damage with mildly decreased GFR	60–89
3. Moderately decreased GFR	30–59
4. Severely decreased GFR	15–29
5. Kidney failure	<15 Dialysis, transplant, hospice, or palliative care Diet may provide comfort

maintain good nutritional status (preventing malnutrition), slowing progression of the disease, and treating complications (National Institutes of Health [NIH], 2011a).

Progression to Uremia

If the client progresses to stage 5 CKD, **uremia** develops. Uremia is the name given to the toxic condition associated with renal failure. Uremia is produced by retention in the blood of nitrogenous substances normally excreted by the kidneys. The uremic client manifests many symptoms in virtually every body system as toxic waste products build up in the blood. The client may complain of:

- Fatigue
- Weakness
- Decreased mental ability
- Twitching and cramping muscles
- Anorexia
- Nausea
- Vomiting
- **Stomatitis,** an inflammation of the mouth
- Taste changes, especially for meats

To complicate matters further, gastrointestinal ulcers and bleeding are common. All of these symptoms have a direct effect on the client's willingness to eat.

Halting the Progression

Health-care professionals have known for many decades that clients with chronic renal disease who have sustained a loss of GFR may continue to lose renal function until they develop terminal renal failure. The National Kidney Disease Education Program recommends diet therapy to slow the progression of CKD by:

- Controlling blood pressure
- Reducing excessive protein intake
- Managing diabetes

Aggressive antihypertensive treatment includes reducing sodium intake to no more than 1500 mg per day and the use of angiotensin-converting enzyme (ACE) inhibitors or angiotensin receptor blockers (ARB) to slow the rate of progression of nephropathy (NIH, 2011a).

Treatment of Renal Disease

Renal functions cannot be assumed by another organ. There is no cure for chronic renal failure. However, many clients can be treated with dialysis (an artificial kidney) or a kidney transplant. Artificial kidneys have been widely used since the 1960s to treat clients with severe kidney failure.

Dialysis

Dialysis means the passage of solutes through a membrane. Two functions of the kidneys are:

1. The removal of waste products
2. The regulation of fluid and electrolyte balance

By removing waste products from the blood and assisting in the maintenance of fluid balance, dialysis reduces the symptoms of:

■ Uremia
■ Hypertension
■ Edema
■ The risk of CHF

Dialysis is usually started when GFR is less than 15 mL/minute and the client develops symptoms of severe fluid overload, high potassium levels, acidosis, or uremia. Dialysis cannot restore the lost hormonal functions of the kidney. In addition, dialysis cannot correct the anemia that occurs because of a lack of erythropoietin. Some dialysis clients still need treatment for hypertension.

Hemodialysis

During **hemodialysis,** blood is removed from the client's artery through a tube, is forced to flow over a semipermeable membrane where waste is removed, and then is rerouted back into the client's body through a vein. Before dialysis can be initiated, an access site that allows blood to be removed from the body and returned back to the body at the time of dialysis must be surgically created. Ideally, this access will be a **fistula** created several months before dialysis is anticipated.

Figure 19-3 illustrates a client undergoing a hemodialysis treatment. A solution called the **dialysate** is placed on one side of the semipermeable membrane, and the client's blood flows on the other side. The dialysate is similar in composition to normal blood plasma but may be manipulated to remove varying amounts of waste products. The client's blood has a higher concentration of urea and electrolytes than the dialysate has, so these substances diffuse from the blood into the dialysate. Sodium modeling may be used during dialysis. Modeling involves changing the concentration of sodium in the dialysate, which can improve the amount of fluid removed during the treatment. The composition of the dialysate varies according to the client's requirements.

Unit staff members usually administer in-center hemodialysis treatments for 3 to 4 hours, three times per week. Home hemodialysis is becoming more widely used in the United States. The client and a care partner learn to do the procedure in their own home. In-home treatment regimens vary from 3 to 6 days per week for 2 to 4 hours per treatment. Nocturnal hemodialysis may be done at home or in a center. These treatments are long, slow, daily, or every other day for 6 to 8 hours while the client sleeps. Dialysis is not as effective as normal kidney function because blood cleansing occurs only when clients are attached to artificial kidneys. Normal kidneys clear the blood 24 hours a day, 7 days a week.

Peritoneal Dialysis

The **peritoneum** is the lining of the abdominal cavity. During **peritoneal dialysis,** the dialysate is placed directly into the client's abdomen by means of a soft permanent catheter implanted between the abdominal wall and the peritoneum. The dialysate enters the body through a permanent catheter placed in the abdominal cavity. The peritoneum thus functions as the semipermeable membrane, allowing waste products and excess fluid to pass from blood into the dialysate. Various glucose concentrations are used in the dialysate to manipulate the amount of fluid removed.

The most common types of peritoneal dialysis are **continuous ambulatory peritoneal dialysis (CAPD)** and **continuous cycling peritoneal dialysis (CCPD).** The advantage of peritoneal dialysis is that the client's blood levels of sodium, potassium, creatinine, and nitrogen stay within a more stable range and allow for a more liberal diet than in hemodialysis. Large shifts in fluid balance are also avoided. However, part of the glucose in the dialysate is available to the client as calories. The higher the glucose concentration used, the more calories are absorbed. The decision about which treatment is best is based on the client's medical condition, lifestyle, and personal preference. For example, a client with poor personal hygiene would not be a

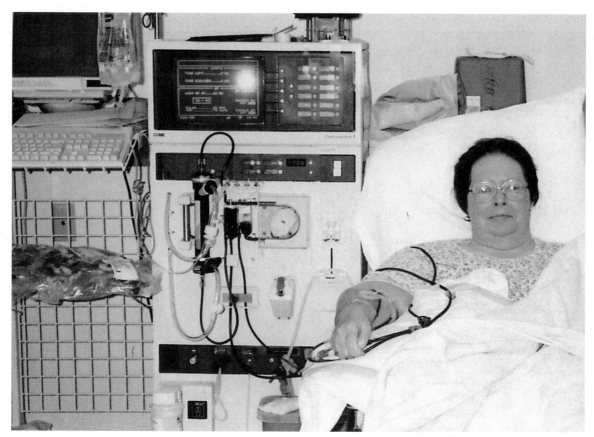

FIGURE 19-3 Client undergoing hemodialysis at dialysis center.

good candidate for peritoneal dialysis because of a high risk for infection.

CONTINUOUS AMBULATORY PERITONEAL DIALYSIS

Clients choosing CAPD are dialyzing constantly. With this method, the client instills 1.5 to 3 liters of dialysate into the abdominal cavity via a catheter. The fluid remains in the cavity for 4 to 6 hours while the client continues with activities of daily living. During this time, waste products and excess fluids diffuse through the peritoneal membrane into the dialysate. The dialysate is then drained and discarded, then replaced with fresh solution in a process called an **exchange.** Each exchange takes 30 to 40 minutes, and clients perform four to five exchanges daily to achieve good dialysis.

CONTINUOUS CYCLING PERITONEAL DIALYSIS

CCPD is a process in which the "exchanges" just described are done during the night by means of a machine. The machine automatically fills and drains the dialysate. This process takes 10 to 12 hours and so is done during sleeping hours. Clients will often do one CAPD exchange during the day in addition to the CCPD.

Kidney Transplant

Although kidney transplant can restore full renal function, it is considered a treatment, not a cure. Immunosuppressants to prevent rejection of the transplanted kidney are necessary. Some commonly used immunosuppressants are azathioprine, corticosteroids, and cyclosporine. These medications have many side effects, including diarrhea, nausea, and vomiting, which influence nutrient intake and absorption.

Nutritional Care

The nutritional needs of clients with renal diseases are changing constantly. The reason for the change is that the disease state and treatment approach are not static. Clients with kidney disease require constant assessment, monitoring, and counseling. In addition, providing quality nutritional care to these clients, who frequently must be coaxed to eat, is challenging. Anorexia, nausea, and vomiting are frequent complaints, particularly in the hospital.

Client–nurse interactions are important because nurses can influence and enhance client adherence to prescribed diets. Close communication among all members of the health-care team is vital to meeting the dynamic nutritional needs of these clients. The Academy of Nutrition and Dietetics (2013) considers coordination of care imperative in the practice guidelines for medical nutrition therapy for CKD.

Malnutrition

Malnutrition in hemodialysis clients is associated with increased mortality and morbidity. Moderate to severe malnutrition is estimated to occur in approximately 34% of clients on hemodialysis. Among the reasons for the malnutrition are:

- Increased catabolism
- Metabolic changes caused by excretion changes in different nutrients
- Decreased food intake because of restrictions and/or poor appetite
- Low economic status

Goals of Nutrition Therapy

Well-planned nutritional management is a fundamental part of any treatment plan for renal disease. Every client with renal disease requires an individualized diet based on the following goals:

- Attain and maintain optimal nutritional status.
- Prevent net protein catabolism.
- Minimize uremic toxicity.
- Maintain adequate hydration status.
- Maintain normal serum potassium levels.
- Control the progression of renal osteodystrophy (discussed later).
- Modify the diet to meet other nutrition-related concerns, such as diabetes, heart disease, gastrointestinal tract ulcers, and constipation.
- Retard the progression of renal failure and postpone the initiation of dialysis.

No single diet is appropriate for all renal clients. Every client requires individual assessment, and every client's diet will likely change over time.

Dietary Components

Several basic components need to be monitored and, if possible, controlled in renal diets:

- Kilocalories
- Protein
- Sodium
- Potassium

- Phosphorus, vitamin D, and calcium
- Fluid
- Saturated fat and cholesterol
- Iron, vitamins, and minerals

The need to restrict or encourage the consumption of any of these nutrients changes according to the client's medical status and treatment approach. For example, at one time, client control of his or her potassium intake may not be necessary, but at another time, control may be vital.

Kilocalories

Clients with renal disease need additional kilocalories. In the absence of diabetes, clients on high-kilocalorie diets are usually given all the simple carbohydrates and monounsaturated and polyunsaturated fats they will eat. *Trans*-fats are minimized. The end products of fat and carbohydrate catabolism are carbon dioxide and water. Neither of these dietary constituents imposes a burden on the client's compromised excretory ability.

Inadequate nonprotein kilocalories, however, will encourage tissue breakdown and aggravate uremia. Clients with renal insufficiency need 35 to 40 kcal/kg per day. The use of a specialized oral supplement such as Suplena®, a low-protein, high-calorie product by Abbott Laboratories, is one example of an appropriate oral supplement for clients who are unwilling or unable to eat enough food. An adequate intake of kilocalories is crucial to the success of the dietary treatment.

In addition, individuals with diabetes mellitus and renal diseases need good control of blood sugar levels. Diets for renal disease can be high in simple sugars, and clients must learn how best to distribute the sugars through the day for optimal blood glucose control. In some cases, the primary nutritional goal is to decrease uremia, and blood glucose control may become less important. Consuming enough kilocalories while adhering to the other nutrient restrictions can be difficult for clients with CKD. See the Dollars & Sense 19-1 for a recipe for a fruit smoothie that is less costly and more palatable than most commercial oral supplements.

Protein

In renal clients, a primary goal of nutritional therapy is controlling nitrogen intake. Control may mean increasing or decreasing dietary protein as the client's medical condition and treatment approach change. In addition, the kind of protein fed to the client may be important. At least 50% of the dietary protein should be of high biological value (National Kidney Foundation, 2002). Because animal products contain all the essential

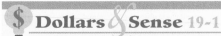

Dollars & Sense 19-1

Berry Smoothie

2 cups blueberries (fresh or frozen)
2 cups strawberries (fresh or frozen)
9 ounces silken tofu, extra firm
½ teaspoon ground ginger
2 pinches of red pepper flakes (optional)
¼ teaspoon rum extract or vanilla extract
1 tablespoon honey or agave nectar
1 teaspoon lemon juice
¼ cup ice
Use a blender to mix all ingredients thoroughly. Makes four servings.

1 cup serving contains 125 kilocalories, 1.8 grams fat, 44 mg calcium, 42 mg sodium, 100 mg phosphorus, 339 mg potassium, 22 grams carbohydrates, 6 grams fiber, and 6 grams protein. (National Kidney Foundation, 2007).

amino acids, examples of foods containing protein of high biologic value include:

- Eggs
- Meat
- Dairy products

A vegetarian diet has been proven beneficial for clients with renal failure. Human and animal models suggest that vegetarian diets that are plentiful in some plant proteins may increase survival rates and decrease proteinuria, glomerular filtration rate, renal blood flow, and histological renal damage compared with nonvegetarian diets.

Vegetarian diets by nature are high in potassium and phosphorus because of all the vegetables, whole grains, and fruits they contain. The client's goal is to eat the right combination of plant proteins while keeping potassium and phosphorus under control. A referral to a renal dietitian is indicated for these clients.

Protein restrictions are effective only if the client also consumes adequate kilocalories. Beginning renal insufficiency is usually called a predialysis and requires a restriction or modification of protein intake. Individuals with diabetes who have early stages of chronic kidney disease should eat no more than 0.8 to 1 gram protein per kilogram of body weight. For nondiabetics with CKD, 0.8 gram protein per kilogram of body weight should be consumed. (Further lowering protein to 0.6 gram in nondiabetics could be beneficial but is a difficult regimen to follow.) This reduction may actually improve measures of renal function. For this reason, dietary intervention is now instituted when microalbumin appears in the urine (NIH 2011a, 2011b).

The treatment approach influences protein requirements. Hemodialysis clients need increased protein because hemodialysis results in a loss of 1 to 2 grams of amino acids per hour of dialysis. A client on CAPD has an even higher protein need because he or she dialyzes continuously. During dialysis, protein passes out of the blood with the waste products and into the dialysate fluid. When the dialysate fluid is discarded, a significant amount of protein is lost. A high-protein diet is necessary to replenish the losses.

Sodium

The desirable sodium intake for renal clients depends on individual circumstances. Serum sodium is not a reliable indicator of sodium intake in CKD. Dietary levels of sodium are based on blood pressure and fluid balance and are also influenced by comorbidities such as congestive heart failure (National Kidney Foundation, 2002). The sodium intake of many clients with renal failure must be restricted to prevent sodium retention with consequent generalized edema. Clients need to know that high sodium intake influences thirst and therefore fluid intake. Water softeners can be a significant source of sodium, and clients may be instructed to avoid them. The National Kidney Disease Education Program recommends a sodium intake of 1500 mg per day or less (NIH 2011a).

The disease that precipitated renal failure plays a role in determining the need for sodium restriction. Because glomerulonephritis, for example, is more likely to produce hypertension and fluid retention, sodium restriction is often necessary. Low levels of sodium, absence of edema, and normal or low blood pressure commonly characterize other renal diseases, such as pyelonephritis. **Pyelonephritis** is an inflammation of the central portion of the kidney. In this situation, sodium intake may be higher than in the other groups of diseases but is individualized according to needs.

Potassium

Dietary potassium, like sodium, must be individually evaluated. **Hypokalemia** (low blood potassium level) must be avoided because it may introduce cardiac arrhythmias and eventually cardiac arrest. Boxes 19-1 and 19-2, respectively, list foods high and low in potassium. Salt substitutes are very high in potassium and should be avoided by renal clients. Water softeners may be a source of dietary potassium, and clients may be instructed to avoid water treated in such a manner. The need to restrict potassium generally increases in clients with decreased urinary output.

ACE inhibitors have been shown to reduce the level of albuminuria and the rate of progression of renal disease to a greater degree than other hypertensive agents that lower blood pressure (National Kidney Foundation, 2007). Use of ACE inhibitors may exacerbate hyperkalemia in clients with advanced renal insufficiency;

Box 19-1 ■ *High-Potassium Foods*

Clients should avoid these high-potassium foods in excess of ½ cups per day* or in the amount calculated by a dietitian.

Dairy Products
As calculated*

Meats
As calculated*

Starches
Bran cereals and bran products

Fruits
Orange, fresh
Mango, fresh
Nectarines
Papayas
Dried prunes
Avocado
Bananas

Vegetables
Bamboo shoots, fresh
Beet greens
Baked potato, with skin
Sweet potato fresh
Spinach, cooked
All others if eaten in excess of allowance*

Others
Chocolate, cocoa
Molasses
Salt substitute
Low-sodium broth
Low-sodium baking powder
Low-sodium baking soda
Nuts

*Dairy foods and meat products contain not only considerable potassium but also phosphorus and protein that need to be carefully planned in the diets of many clients.

Box 19-2 ■ *Low-Potassium Foods and Beverages**

Low-Potassium Foods

Bean sprouts, canned
Gum drops
Hard, clear candy
Nondairy topping
Honey
Jams and jellies
Jellybeans
Lollipops
Marshmallows
Suckers
Sugar
Lifesavers
Chewing gum
Poly-Rich (nondairy creamer)
Cornstarch

Low-Potassium Beverages

Carbonated beverages
Lemonade
Limeade
Cranberry juice
Popsicles (1 stick—60 mL of fluid)
Hawaiian Punch†
Kool-Aid†

Low-Potassium Unsweetened Beverages

Diet carbonated beverages
Diet lemonade
Diet Kool-Aid†

*Diabetics should not freely eat foods with sugar.
†These beverages are low in potassium but are often high in phosphorus and need to be restricted in many renal clients with a phosphorus dietary restriction.

---

therefore, when used, serum potassium levels should be monitored.

The recommended intake of potassium is 2.0 to 3.0 grams per day for most clients. If a client's potassium level is elevated (5 to 6.5 mEq/L), dietary potassium intake should be minimized to less than 2.4 grams per day. When urinary output is 100 to 500 mL and serum potassium is 5.5 to 6.5, a 40- to 60-mEq (about 1563 to 2345 mg K) intake is suggested.

In cases of anuria or when serum potassium exceeds 6.5 mEq/L, a dietary intake of 20 to 25 mEq/L (about 780 to 975 mg K) is suggested. This suggestion is for the acute, critical-care client because of its poor palatability. Fundamental to understanding medical nutritional therapy for clients with renal disease is that overrestricting a client's diet is never appropriate because of the danger of tissue catabolism and malnutrition. Before reducing diet, check the client's medications to be sure

he or she is not on potassium supplements. If the client is undergoing hemodialysis, also check the potassium level of the dialysate to see that all potassium that can be safely removed is being removed.

The potassium content of fruits and vegetables varies according to the form and the preparation method. For example, ½ cup of canned pears in heavy syrup has about 80 milligrams of potassium, and one fresh pear has about 210 milligrams. Potassium is water-soluble. For this reason, some renal clients on low-potassium diets are taught to use large amounts of water to prepare vegetables and to discard the water after cooking to decrease the vegetable's potassium content. Unfortunately, the process also decreases water-soluble vitamins. Most renal clients need renal vitamin supplements. Clients should eat fruits or vegetables in the form given on the list.

Phosphorus, Vitamin D, and Calcium

In the body, phosphorus, vitamin D, and calcium are all normally balanced. In clients with kidney disease, vitamin D cannot be activated, a situation leading to a low serum calcium level. At the same time, the kidneys cannot excrete phosphorus, a situation leading to an elevated serum phosphorus level.

When serum calcium level drops, calcium is released from the bones because of the increased secretion of **parathyroid hormone (PTH).** PTH is secreted in an effort to correct the calcium imbalance. This chain of events may lead to renal **osteodystrophy** and **vascular calcification,** which are complications of chronic renal disease. **Renal osteodystrophy** leads to faulty bone formation. **Vascular calcification** contributes to the high incidence of cardiovascular disease seen in clients with CKD.

Control of blood levels of calcium and phosphorus involves several treatment approaches. First, clients with hypocalcemia and secondary hyperparathyroidism are given activated vitamin D orally or, if they are on hemodialysis, intravenously during their treatment. Activated vitamin D cannot be given when serum calcium or phosphorus levels are very high or vascular calcification may result.

Phosphorus is a mineral found in the bones and is needed along with calcium to build strong bones. When there is extra phosphorus in the body that the kidneys cannot excrete, calcium is pulled from the bones, which can make them brittle. High phosphorus levels must be controlled with the initiation of dietary phosphorus restriction. Phosphorus is found mainly in (see Box 19-3):

- Dairy products
- High-protein foods
- Whole grain products
- Inorganic phosphate additives

The use of phosphate additives to meats, beverages, convenience foods, and many others has more than doubled in the past 10 years and will likely continue to increase. Clients must learn how to read the ingredient label to avoid as many phosphate additives as possible. Although the amount added to a given food is small, these additives are 100% absorbed, while organic phosphates found naturally in foods have a much lower absorption rate. Almost all clients with chronic renal disease, especially in stages 3 through 5, need to watch their phosphorus intake. It is recommended that they follow a diet containing 800 to 1000 mg of phosphorus per day or 10 to 12 mg per gram of protein (Academy of Nutrition and Dietetics, 2013).

Phosphate binders may be added to a client's regimen if dietary modification does not produce desired results. This is especially true for clients in stage 3 through 5 of CKD. Phosphate binders are medications that bind phosphorus in the GI tract, allowing the resulting complex to be eliminated in the stools. These medications *must* be taken while a client eats his or her meals (Academy of Nutrition and Dietetics, 2013; National Kidney Foundation, 2013b; NIH, 2011a). A **calcimimetic** may also be added to the treatment regimen. This medication acts directly on the parathyroid gland to reduce the release of PTH.

Fluid

Some predialysis (renal insufficiency) and most dialysis clients generally must restrict fluid intake because their kidneys can no longer excrete excess fluid. Table 19-2 lists guidelines for distributing fluids between meals and medications. Clients on hemodialysis are restricted to 500 to 1000 milliliters plus 24-hour urinary output. This fluid restriction allows for fluid gain of

---

Box 19-3 ■ *Foods High in Phosphorus*

Dairy Foods	Raisin bran	**Dried Beans**	Pumpkin seeds
Milk	Whole wheat	Navy beans	Sunflower seeds
Cheese	Biscuits	Kidney beans	**Other**
Cocoa	Waffles	Lima beans	Cola drinks
Condensed milk	Pancakes	Pinto beans	Chocolate
Evaporated milk	Cereals with nuts	Lentils	Toffee
Cottage cheese	Cheese crackers	Black-eyed peas	Caramel
Yogurt	Cheese curls	Soybeans	Fudge
Custard	**Meats**	**Nuts and Seeds**	Mushrooms
Ice cream	Sardines	Almonds	Molasses
Pudding	Herring	Cashews	Raisins and dates
Cream soups	Smelt	Coconut	Other dried fruits
Grains	Liver	Pecans	Casseroles with cheese or
Bran	Sweetbreads	Walnuts	cream soup
Bran flakes	Tripe/menudo	Peanuts	
Bran muffins	Egg yolk (more than	Peanut butter	
Brown rice	2 per day)		

TABLE 19-2 ■ Guidelines for Fluid-Restricted Clients

IF THE FLUID RESTRICTION IS	USE THIS AMOUNT OF FLUIDS WITH MEALS	USE THIS AMOUNT OF FLUIDS WITH MEDICATIONS
1000 mL (4 cups)*	600 mL (2½ cups)	400 mL (1½ cups)
1200 mL (5 cups)	700 mL (3 cups)	500 mL (2 cups)
1500 mL (6 cups)	1000 mL (4 cups)	500 mL (2 cups)
2000 mL (8 cups)	1000 mL (4 cups)	1000 mL (4 cups)

All foods contain some fluids, but it is especially important to count the following as part of the fluid allowance:

Milliliters of Fluid per ½ Cup

Water	120	All juices	120	Watermelon	100
Coffee	120	Soda-pop	120	Sherbet	65
Tea	120	Ice	60	Ice cream	40
Decaf Coffee	120	Gelatin	100	Ice milk	40
Milk	120	Soup	120	Popsicle	80

*All cup measures are approximations.

2 to 2½ kilograms between dialysis treatments. Pre-dialysis clients do not generally have fluid restrictions unless their clinical condition indicates a need. For clients on CAPD, fluid restriction is "as tolerated" according to their daily weight fluctuations and blood pressure.

Saturated Fat and Cholesterol

Clients with renal disease frequently have hyperlipidemia. High serum lipid levels increase the progression of renal disease, which contributes to an increased risk of cardiovascular disease. Total cholesterol levels may be increased up to tenfold. This increase is thought to be a problem, especially in clients with nephrotic syndrome, diabetes, or an **LCAT deficiency.** LCAT is an enzyme that transports cholesterol from tissues to the liver for removal from the body. Most clients with an LCAT deficiency develop progressive glomerular injury.

Significant hypertriglyceridemia is commonly present in clients with a history of renal disease. The nutritional care of clients with elevated triglycerides includes a modified fat diet, modification of carbohydrate intake and encouragement to increase exercise—as tolerated and with their physician's knowledge. Clients are counseled to avoid saturated fat and *trans* fat and to increase their intake of monounsaturated fat.

Thirty percent to 35% of the total kilocalories are provided as fat because excessive carbohydrate could worsen the hypertriglyceridemia (Moore, 2009). Simple sugars and alcohol are usually limited for the same reason. Including omega-3 fatty acids to lower the levels of high triglycerides may be helpful. The literature suggests a beneficial effect of omega-3 fatty acids, particularly from fish, and suggests that further studies are warranted (Academy of Nutrition and Dietetics Practice, 2013; National Kidney Foundation 2007).

Iron

Anemias in clients with renal disease may be due to:

■ A lack of the kidney's production of erythropoietin
■ A decreased oral iron intake, which commonly occurs as a result of dietary restriction
■ Blood loss

Epoetin alfa, a pharmaceutical form of erythropoietin, may be used to increase red blood cell production and thereby correct the anemia. The treatment for iron-deficiency anemia is oral or IV iron and an increase in dietary sources of iron.

A diagnosis of iron-deficiency anemia can be made by a laboratory measure of ferritin. **Ferritin** is the storage form of iron found primarily in the liver. A small amount of ferritin circulates in the blood and reflects the amount of iron in body stores. A laboratory value of less than 12 micrograms per liter suggests iron deficiency. KDOQI recommends that CKD clients have a serum ferritin of 100 to 800, thus ensuring adequate iron for erythropoietin-stimulated production of red blood cells. Higher levels of ferritin may indicate that inflammation or infection is present (National Kidney Foundation, 2002).

Nutritional therapy with iron supplements consists of 210 milligrams of ferrous iron salts per day divided among three to four doses. Absorption is enhanced when iron supplements are taken on an empty stomach or with vitamin C, although megadoses of vitamin C should be avoided because oxalosis may be induced, leading to kidney stones. No more than the Dietary Reference Intake for the client should be recommended (Academy of Nutrition and Dietetics Practice, 2013). In dialysis units, iron is commonly administered by intravenous (IV) line. Clients should not take oral iron if receiving IV iron.

Vitamin and Mineral Supplementation

Unless supplements are given, chronically uremic clients are prone to deficiencies of water-soluble vitamins. Losses are most notable with pyridoxine, ascorbic acid, and folic acid. Supplementation of these nutrients is recommended for clients on dialysis. Fat-soluble vitamins are not lost in the dialysate, and supplementation is not indicated except with vitamin D for another reason (see previous discussion). Because the body's ability to excrete excess fat-soluble vitamins is compromised, toxicity is a potential problem.

Teaching the Renal Diet

In 1993, the American Dietetic Association and the National Kidney Foundation introduced the National Renal Diet, a uniform renal diet that could be used across the country. The second edition, introduced in 2002, included more simple lists with more emphasis on clients' involvement in determining and managing their own diets. The edition starts with survival information and allows the dietitian to introduce new topics as client interest and blood chemistries indicate the need for further diet modification and teaching.

The importance of individualizing medical nutrition therapy for the client with chronic kidney disease cannot be overemphasized. Regular contact with a renal dietitian increases the client's ability to change established behaviors and also allows for the most liberal diet possible. Table 19-3 shows the guidelines for medical nutrition therapy of renal clients by treatment approach.

Nutrient Guidelines for Adults with Renal Disease

The nutritional care of renal clients is complex. Table 19-4 summarizes the nutrient control and the rationale for nutrient control by the stage of renal disease.

Renal Disease in Children

Growth failure is commonly seen in children with chronic renal failure treated with dialysis, but it is not an inevitable complication. Inadequate caloric consumption and metabolic acidosis are reasons for the poor growth. These children usually need to have their sodium, potassium, and protein intake rigidly controlled, and this control may contribute to poor food intake. Anorexia and emotional disturbances are also contributing factors. Continually reinforcing the rationale for medical nutrition therapy and providing meal and snack ideas and emotional support can help to improve adherence.

TABLE 19-3 ■ Selected Nutritional Parameters for Varying Levels of Kidney Failure

NUTRITIONAL PARAMETER	NORMAL KIDNEY FUNCTION	STAGES 1–4 CHRONIC KIDNEY DISEASE	STAGE 5 HEMODIALYSIS	STAGE 5 PERITONEAL DIALYSIS	TRANSPLANT
Calories (kcal/kg per day)	30–37	<60 years: 35 >60 years: 30–35	<60 years: 35 >60 years: 30–35	<60 years: 35 including calories from dialysis	Initial: 30–35 Maintenance: 25–30
Protein (grams/kg per day)	0.8	0.6–0.75 50% HBV	1.2 50% HBV	1.2–1.3 50% HBV	Initial: 1.3–1.5
Fat (percent total kcal)	30%–35% Patients considered at highest risk for cardiovascular disease: emphasis on <10% saturated fat, PUFA, MUFA, 250–300 mg cholesterol/day				
Sodium (mg/day)	<2300 mg/day*	≤1500 mg/day†	≤1500 mg/day†	≤1500 mg/day†	<2300 mg/day*; monitor medication effect
Potassium (mg/day)	Unrestricted	Correlated to laboratory values	2000–3000 (8–17 mg/kg per day)	3000–4000 (8–17 mg/ kg per day)	Unrestricted; monitor medication effect
Calcium (mg/day)	Unrestricted	1200	<2000 from diet and medications	<2000 from diet and medications	1200
Phosphorus (mg/day)	Unrestricted	Correlated to laboratory values	800–1000, adjusted for protein	800–1000, adjusted for protein	Unrestricted unless indicated
Fluid (mL/day)	Unrestricted	Unrestricted with normal urine output	1000 + urine output	Monitored; 1500–2000	Unrestricted unless indicated

Meant as guidelines only for initial assessment; individualization to patient's own metabolic status and coexisting metabolic conditions is essential for optimal care. HBV, high biological value; MUFA, monounsaturated fatty acids; PUFA, polyunsaturated fatty acids.

Source: Reprinted from Beto, JA, and Bansal, VK: Medical nutrition therapy in chronic kidney failure: Integrating clinical practice guidelines. *J Am Diet Assoc* 104:407, 2004. Copyright 2004, with permission from the American Dietetic Association. Updated sodium values based upon *2010 Dietary Guidelines for Americans and †National Institutes of Health, 2011a.

TABLE 19-4 ■ Stages of Chronic Kidney Disease, Nutrient Modification, and Rationale		
STAGE	**NUTRIENT MODIFICATION**	**RATIONALE**
1	CHO control if indicated	Control blood glucose levels.
2	Sodium Evaluate lipid levels and need to modify diet Potassium	Control blood pressure. CVD risk reduction Begin to monitor to minimize cardiac complications.
3	Phosphorus	Continue modifications of stages 1 and 2.
4	RDA for protein Potassium	Begin to monitor and treat as indicated to maximize bone health. Promote adequate and not excessive protein intake. Monitor monthly to avoid cardiac complications. All the above may slow the progression of kidney disease.
5	Highly individualized	As indicated by treatment approach, usual food intake, and laboratory values.

CHO, carbohydrate; CVD, cardiovascular disease; RDA, recommended dietary allowance.

Suggestions for improving children's intake include:

- Involving the children in selecting and preparing foods (insofar as possible)
- Serving meals in an appealing, attractive manner (e.g., serving contrasting colors and textures of foods, using decorative tableware and dishes)
- Serving small, frequent meals
- Ensuring that the child has someone with him or her at mealtime
- Planning special mealtime events such as picnics (even if they are held in the hospital playroom)

Kidney Stones

Kidney stones may be found in the bladder, kidney, ureter, or urethra. During urine formation, the urine moves from the collecting tubules into the renal pelvis. From the **renal pelvis,** the urine moves down the **ureter** and into the urinary bladder. Finally, urine passes from the bladder down the urethra and exits the body.

A stone, also called a **urinary calculus,** is a deposit of mineral salts held together by a thick, syrupy substance. A urinary calculus can block the movement of urine from the body. Symptoms of a blockage include:

- Sudden severe pain
- Chills
- Fever
- **Hematuria** (blood in the urine)
- An increased desire to urinate

A kidney stone can also pass out of the body with the urine.

Causes

The cause of most kidney stones is unknown. Some possible causes include:

- An abnormal function of the parathyroid gland
- Disordered uric acid metabolism (as in gout)
- An excessive intake of animal protein and sodium
- Immobility, being overweight
- Kidney infections (forming struvite stones)
- Genetic disorder causing cystine to leak through kidneys into the urine (cystine stones)

At higher risk for kidney stones are men, people with a sedentary lifestyle, Asians, and Whites. Typically, kidney stones occur in clients who are between ages 30 and 50. A determination of the stone's composition may lead to a restriction of dietary substrates (the substance acted on). Frequent dietary substrates of kidney stones are oxalic acid and purines. Decreased fluid intake and strongly concentrated urine or low urine volume are risk factors.

Treatment

All clients with kidney stones should drink sufficient water to keep the urine volume above 2 liters per day. About 3000 milliliters or 13 cups of water per day are necessary to produce this amount of urine. The primary reason for increasing fluid intake is to prevent formation of concentrated urine, in which crystals are more likely to combine and precipitate.

Oxalates

Calcium oxalate is the most common constituent of kidney stones. Some individuals are genetically susceptible to stone formation. A diet excluding foods high in oxalates (see Table 19-5) is frequently prescribed for clients with kidney stones if laboratory analysis shows removed or passed stone is high in oxalates. Additionally, reducing sodium to 2300 mg and limiting animal protein in the diet are recommended because excess sodium and protein cause the kidneys to excrete calcium in the urine. Having enough calcium in the diet, 800 mg per day (through food or supplements taken with food) help prevent calcium oxalate stones (NIH, 2013).

Calcium

Historically, if laboratory analysis of a surgically removed or passed stone was found to be high in calcium, a low-calcium diet was prescribed (600 milligrams per

TABLE 19-5 ■ Foods High in Oxalic Acid

	MG/100 GRAMS
Beverages	
Coffee, instant dry	143.0
Tea, brewed	12.5
Fruits	
Blackberries, raw	12.4
Gooseberries, raw	19.3
Plums, raw	11.9
Grains	
Bread, whole-wheat	20.9
Vegetables	
Beets, raw	72.2
Beets, boiled	109.0
Carrots, boiled	14.5
Green beans, raw	43.7
Green beans, boiled	29.7
Rhubarb, raw	537.0
Rhubarb, stewed	447.0
Spinach, boiled	571.0
Miscellaneous	
Cocoa, dry	623.0
Ovaltine, powder	45.9

Source: Values taken from Pennington, JA, and Douglass, JA: *Bowes and Church food values of portions commonly used*, 18th ed. Lippincott Williams & Wilkins, Philadelphia, 2004.

TABLE 19-6 ■ Purines in Food

GROUP A: HIGH CONCENTRATION (150–1000 MG/100 GRAMS)

Liver	Sardines (in oil)
Kidney	Meat extracts
Sweetbreads	Consommé
Brains	Gravies
Heart	Fish roes
Anchovies	Herring

GROUP B: MODERATE AMOUNTS (50–150 MG/100 GRAMS)

Meat, game, and fish other than those mentioned in Group A	Asparagus
	Cauliflower
Fowl	Mushrooms
Lentils	Spinach
Whole-grain cereals	
Beans	
Peas	

GROUP C: VERY SMALL AMOUNTS: NEED NOT BE RESTRICTED IN DIET OF PEOPLE WITH GOUT

Vegetables other than those mentioned above	Coffee
Fruits of all kinds	Tea
Milk	Chocolate
Cheese	Carbonated beverages
Eggs	Tapioca
Refined cereals, spaghetti, macaroni	
Butter, fats, nuts, peanut butter*	
Sugars and sweets	
Vegetable soups	

*Fats interfere with the urinary excretion of urates and should be limited if the objective is to promote excretion of uric acid.
Source: From Venes, D (ed): *Taber's cyclopedic medical dictionary*, 22nd ed. FA Davis, Philadelphia, 2013, p. 1957. Used with permission.

day). Today, it is known that kidney stones are not caused by dietary calcium. Kidney stones are of less concern with an increased calcium intake than with a decreased intake. Calcium in the digestive track binds with oxalates from foods and keeps it from entering the blood and then the urinary tract where stones can form. Consuming 800 mg of calcium per day helps prevent kidney stones and also helps maintain bone density (NIH, 2013).

Uric Acid Stones

Stones composed of uric acid form when the urine is persistently acidic. Animal protein is rich in purines, which may increase uric acid in the urine. If uric acid is concentrated in the urine, it can form a stone by itself or with calcium. Meat consumption should be limited to 6 ounces per day in individuals who form uric acid stones (NIH, 2013). Purines are sometimes a complication of **gout,** a hereditary metabolic disease that is a form of arthritis. One symptom of gout is inflammation of the joints. The metabolism of uric acid is related to dietary **purines,** a product of protein digestion. A purine-restricted diet is commonly prescribed for gout. Table 19-6 shows purines in foods. Many physicians do not prescribe a low-purine diet for gout because the condition can be more effectively controlled by medications.

Clinical Application 19-2 summarizes the recommendations for medical nutrition therapy for kidney stones.

Surgery

Surgery is sometimes necessary to remove large kidney stones. Surgical removal of the stones prevents infection, reduces pain, and prevents a loss of kidney function.

Urinary Tract Infections

One form of **urinary tract infection (UTIs)** is **cystitis,** an inflammation of the bladder. This condition is prevalent in young women. Recurrent UTI means that the individual has three or more bouts of infection per year. A general nutrition measure includes acidifying the urine by taking large doses of vitamin C. Regular intake of a cranberry juice beverage also reduces the frequency of urinary tract infections. Cranberry juice contains a substance with biologic activity that inhibits the growth of *Escherichia coli* in the urinary tract. Clients with UTIs should be encouraged to drink ample fluids.

19-2

$\mathscr{C}$linical $\mathscr{A}$pplication

Dietary Approaches to Prevent Kidney Stones

TYPE	DRINK 2–3 L OF FLUID/DAY	REDUCE SODIUM TO ≤2300 MG/DAY	LIMIT PROTEIN TO 6 OZ/DAY	CONSUME ≤800 MG OF CALCIUM/DAY	LIMIT OXALATE INTAKE FROM FOOD	DRINK CITRUS DRINKS*
Calcium oxalate	X	X	X	X	X	X
Calcium phosphate	X	X	X	X		X
Uric acid	X		X			X
Struvite	X					X
Cystine	X (or more)					X

*Studies suggest citrus drinks such as lemonade and orange juice protect against kidney stones because the citrate stops crystals from growing into stones.

Source: Adapted from National Institutes of Health, 2013 (NIH Publication No. 13-6425).

Keystones

- The basic functional unit of the kidney is the nephron.
- Millions of nephrons work together to form urine and remove unnecessary substances from the blood.
- Glomerular filtration rate (GFR) is a measure of kidney function.
- The kidneys are also the site where vitamin D_3 (calcitriol) and erythropoietin are activated.
- Kidney failure can be acute or chronic. Chronic renal disease is progressive. Treatment for kidney failure is dialysis or a kidney transplant.
- Nutritional management of clients with renal disease is a fundamental part of treatment.
- Clients with kidney disease require constant assessment, monitoring, and counseling.
- The dietary components that may need modification are kilocalories, protein, sodium, potassium, phosphorus, fluid, cholesterol, and saturated fat.
- Vitamin and mineral supplements are often prescribed for clients with renal disease.
- Frequently, the diet these clients follow must be modified as their medical condition and treatment changes.
- Some nutritional intervention is necessary for clients with kidney stones and urinary tract infections. The fluid intake of these clients should be high.

CASE STUDY *19-1*

Mr. U is a 55-year-old man who works full time and has a sedentary lifestyle. He is 5 ft 10 in. tall, has a medium frame, and weighs 68 kg. His ideal and usual weight is 76 kg. During the past 6 to 9 months, he has been anorectic and has had intermittent nausea and episodes of vomiting. He receives 4 hours of hemodialysis 3 times per week. His predialysis blood chemistry values were as follows:

- Blood urea nitrogen, 63 mg/dL
- Sodium, 135 mmol/L (135 mEq/L)
- Potassium, 4.0 mmol/L (4.0 mEq/L)
- Phosphorus, 2.0 mg/dL
- Calcium, 9.0 mg/dL

(Continued on the following page)

- Albumin, 3.3 g/dL
- Urine output ranges between 800 and 1000 mL per day.

On arrival in the hemodialysis unit today, the client complained of hopelessness and a fear of dying. He complained he cannot meet the nutritional goals set by the dietitian because he just keeps getting "sick and sicker and is afraid of dying."

The client's medical record lists religious preference as Catholic.

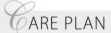 ARE PLAN

Subjective Data

Client complains of anorexia, nausea, and vomiting, a lack of hope, and a fear of dying.

Objective Data

Client tearful today. ■ Documented history of anorexia, emesis, and nausea. ■ His body weight is stable.

Analysis

Anorexia, nausea, and vomiting likely related to fear as evidenced by statement, "I have given up hope and am afraid of dying."

Plan

DESIRED OUTCOMES EVALUATION CRITERIA	ACTIONS/INTERVENTIONS	RATIONALE
The client will maintain a sense of purpose despite fear.	Assist the client/family to identify areas of hope in life.	Clients and family members who can list foods and fluids that are better tolerated will provide hope.
Involve the client actively in his own care.	Explain to the client that despite his uncomfortable symptoms, his body weight is stable.	It is more effective to begin every counseling session with a review of the client's positive behaviors.
Seeks information to reduce fear.	As client has an ongoing relationship with the dietitian, he or she may be able to expand client's repertoire of food and fluid related coping mechanisms.	Dietitians in hemodialysis centers visit clients at least monthly and frequently more often.
Help client expand spiritual self.	Ask the client if he would like you to arrange a visit from a Catholic priest or his designee.	Helping a client connect to his spiritual self helps maintain a sense of purpose despite fear.

 19-1

Dietitian's Notes

The following Dietitian's Notes are representative of the documentation found in a client's medical record.

Subjective: Visited client per nursing request today. Client asked for specific information to decrease vomiting and nausea and increase food intake. He describes his food intake as sporadic. Lately food intake has been less than he would like. He states that he has not missed any days of work due to illness. Client states that his wife has been especially helpful with meal preparation and grocery shopping, but nothing sounds good to him. Usually eats/drinks a half cup dairy, four starches, two vegetables, five meats, three fruits, and six fats. However, he is discouraged when he cannot rigidly follow this pattern every day.

Objective: Weight stable at 76 kg; Compazine (for nausea) 2 times per day as needed; albumin 3.3 g/L; blood urea nitrogen 63 mg/dL; phosphorus 2.0 mg

Analysis: Client is eating about 66 grams of protein on days he does not experience nausea and vomiting. Phosphorus of 2.0 may be related to too many phosphate binders and not eating enough. Recommend that client try eating an extra egg or two each day on the days he is not nauseated. Also, recommended he sip four cans of Nepro® (Abbott) on days he cannot eat and just to try a few sips every hour on the hour. Four cans of Nepro would provide 960 mL and 1700 kcal, and 76.2 grams of protein. Client

19-1

Dietitian's Notes—cont'd

was reminded that this would use 960 mL of his fluid allowance. Client appeared relieved to have a plan he could follow on days when he was not "up to eating."

Plan:

- Recommended client take one less phosphate binder per day until his next treatment
- Will speak again with client during his next hemodialysis treatment and provide positive reinforcement
- Client needs to consume more kcal

Daily Renal Diet Plan Goals

NUTRIENT	LEVEL	RATIONALE
Energy (kcal)	2300–2700	30–35 kcal/kg HBW
Protein (grams)	91	1.2 grams/kg HBW
Sodium (mg)	2000	Control fluid weight gain
Potassium (mg)	3000	≤40 mg/kg HBW
Phosphorus (mg)	1080 mg	10–12 mg/kg of protein
Fluid (mL)	1500–1750	750 mL plus urine output

HBW, Healthy body weight (may be called standard body weight or ideal body weight).

Critical Thinking Questions

1. Explain the relationship of each dietary modification to the signs and symptoms Mr. U is experiencing.

2. Mr. U eats only about half his needed kilocalories. What should you do?

3. Mr. U develops a stomach ulcer. What should you recommend?

4. Mr. U decides he would like to try continuous ambulatory peritoneal dialysis (CAPD). How would his diet probably change?

Chapter Review

1. Which of the following is a nutritional goal for a child with renal failure?
   a. Maintain current hydration status
   b. Promote normal growth and development
   c. Maximize uremia
   d. Stimulate client well-being

2. Kidney disease cannot be caused by:
   a. Consumption of toxic metals
   b. Consumption of 1 to 3 L a day of water
   c. Infection
   d. Trauma

3. Kilocalories usually need to be increased in protein-restricted diets because an adequate kilocalorie intake:
   a. Assists in the control of serum potassium
   b. Is necessary to prevent renal anemia
   c. Controls and prevents osteodystrophy
   d. Spares protein

4. The ____ intake from food is not monitored in renal clients.
   a. Vitamin D
   b. Fluid
   c. Protein
   d. Sodium

5. The most important nutritional consideration in treating clients with kidney stones is to:
   a. Limit calcium intake
   b. Restrict all end products of protein metabolism
   c. Restrict all food sources of calcium, oxalic acid, and purines
   d. Increase fluid intake

Clinical Analysis

1. Bill, age 10, has acute glomerulonephritis. His mother explains that Bill had a streptococcal infection 1 week before the illness. When planning Bill's care, the nurse recognizes that he needs help in understanding his diet. Bill's restrictions will include:
   a. A low-fat diet
   b. A calcium restriction
   c. A daily measurement of urine output (if any) and plan for his fluid intake
   d. A high-protein diet

2. Mr. Jones, a 49-year-old mechanic, has been admitted to the hospital with diagnosis of renal failure. Mr. Jones has been following a 40-gram protein, 2-gram sodium, 2-gram potassium, 1000-mL fluid restriction for the past 5 years. Mr. Jones is scheduled for surgery tomorrow to have a permanent fistula implanted for hemodialysis. Mr. Jones's nutritional needs will change after he is maintained on hemodialysis to:
   a. More oranges, bananas, and baked potatoes
   b. More lean meat, eggs, fish, low-fat dairy products, and peanut butter
   c. Less starches, breads, and cereals
   d. Less margarine, oil, and salad dressings

3. Mr. Jones is found to have an elevated serum phosphorus level after 6 months on hemodialysis. He should:
   a. Restrict his intake of dairy products and peanut butter
   b. Restrict his intake of red meats
   c. Increase his intake of sugar, honey, jam, jelly, and other simple sugars
   d. Discontinue his phosphate binders

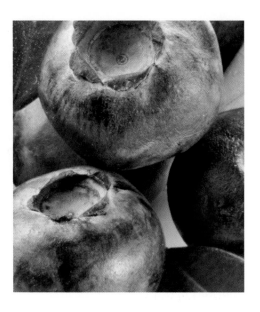

20

Diet in Digestive Diseases

LEARNING OBJECTIVES

After completing this chapter, the student should be able to:

■ Describe the preoperative limitations of specific fluids recommended by the American Society of Anesthesiologists.

■ Distinguish between the dietary preparation for gastrointestinal surgery and the dietary preparation for surgery on other body systems.

■ Compare the diet-related interventions for postprandial hypotension and dumping syndrome.

■ Identify the mealtime treatment of gastroesophageal reflux disease and hiatal hernia.

■ Explain the dietary treatment of celiac disease related to its pathophysiology.

■ Differentiate nutritional care for clients with Crohn disease from that for ulcerative colitis.

■ Relate the nutritional care for clients with hepatitis to that for cirrhosis.

■ Discriminate Wernicke encephalopathy from Korsakoff psychosis as to pathophysiology and treatment, indicating the importance of early interventions.

■ Describe the nutritional aspects of medical treatment for cholecystitis.

■ Discuss cystic fibrosis as to pathophysiology and dietary treatment.

The gastrointestinal tract functions both as a barrier to substances from the environment and as an entry point for nutrients and other substances. Many disorders that affect the gastrointestinal tract and its accessory organs (liver, gallbladder, and pancreas) influence the nutritional status of clients. Most surgical procedures have an impact on gastrointestinal tract function and require special dietary measures, both preoperatively and postoperatively. This chapter covers dietary modifications for surgical clients and for clients with common disorders and diseases of the digestive system.

Dietary Considerations with Surgical Clients

Because of its role in tissue building and healing, protein is crucial in surgical clients. Protein depletion increases the risk of:

■ Infection because the body cannot manufacture enough white blood cells

■ Shock because low serum albumin prevents the return of interstitial fluid to the blood vessels

■ Wound **dehiscence** because local edema persists and interferes with healing

Persons with diseases affecting the gastrointestinal tract are at special risk when facing surgery because such diseases interfere with nutrition. In cases involving gastrointestinal surgery, the gastrointestinal tract is incised and sutured, so postoperative feeding may be postponed to allow for healing. If the gastrointestinal tract is permanently modified, specialty nutritional care is needed to optimize use of the remaining organs. Surgical clients with liver disease also need special attention. The liver has many functions, some of which are listed in Table 20-1. Because of the liver's role in metabolizing and detoxifying drugs, clients with liver disease must be carefully managed when surgery is necessary. Moreover, some anesthetics, analgesics, and anti-infectives are toxic to the liver.

Preoperative Nutrition

Before elective surgery is undertaken, nutritional deficiencies should be identified and corrected. Poor preoperative nutritional status has been consistently linked to increased postoperative complications and poorer surgical outcome (Burden, Todd, Hill, and Lal, 2012). Many overweight or obese clients are instructed to lose weight to reduce the risks of surgery. If the client is anemic, an iron preparation may be prescribed. Other nutrients can be provided as needed. At least 2 to 3 weeks are required for objective evidence of the effectiveness of nutritional therapy.

Correction of electrolyte imbalances may be achieved more quickly if identified. A retrospective analysis of 964,263 adults undergoing major surgery in more than 200 hospitals found 75,423 patients had preoperative hyponatremia, which was associated with a

- 44% higher risk of 30-day mortality,
- 20% greater risk of major coronary events,
- 24% increased risk of wound infections,
- 17% higher risk of pneumonia than those with normal serum sodium levels (Leung, McAlister, Rogers, et al, 2012).

Although combination indices are available, preoperative albumin level is the single best indicator of

TABLE 20-1 ■ Examples of Liver Functions			
RELATED TO	**PRODUCES/PROCESSES**	**STORES**	**BREAKS DOWN**
Carbohydrate	Glucose from galactose and fructose Glucose from glycogen Glucose from glycerol and protein	Glycogen	
Fat	Fat from glucose Cholesterol Fatty acids and glycerol from cholesterol, phospholipids, and lipoproteins Lipoproteins Water-soluble bilirubin (from fat-soluble) Bile	Fat	
Protein	Albumin Some globulins Prothrombin Fibrinogen Transferrin Enzymes to convert ammonia to urea		
Vitamins	Retinol-binding protein Other transport proteins Activates thiamin Activates vitamin B_6 Processes vitamin D	A, D, E, K Thiamin Riboflavin B_6 Folic acid B_{12} Biotin	
Minerals		Iron	Worn-out red blood cells
Other			*acetaminophen* Alcohol *aldosterone* Bacteria Barbiturates Estrogen Glucocorticoids *morphine* *progesterone* Some anesthetics

postoperative complications and mortality after major surgery because impaired protein status is strongly correlated with postoperative complications. However, a low albumin level may also be caused by liver disease, inflammation, or increased blood volume rather than malnutrition. The simplest screening technique for malnutrition in preoperative clients is a thorough history and physical examination that identifies unintentional weight loss (Kudsk, 2014). Clinical Application 20-1 relates one possible cause of malnutrition in surgical clients.

Preventive nutritional support is effective for malnourished surgical clients or those whose oral intake will be compromised after surgery. In clients undergoing elective major gastrointestinal surgery, **perioperative immunonutrition** is associated with a substantial reduction in infection rates and lengths of hospital stay. These results have been found in both upper and lower gastrointestinal surgery patients, regardless of their baseline nutritional status (Braga, 2012).

Preoperative fasting protocols have been liberalized based on research showing slight risk of pulmonary aspiration with modern anesthetics. Guidelines for anesthesia administration to healthy individuals scheduled for elective procedures permit greater oral intake than in the past (Table 20-2). The guidelines do not supplant the need for individual assessment. Nor do they apply to individuals with gastrointestinal motility or metabolic disorders, individuals with potential airway problems, or women in labor.

TABLE 20-2 ■ Preoperative Fasting Recommendations to Minimize Aspiration Risk		
ORAL INTAKE	**MINIMUM FASTING TIME**	**COMMENT**
Clear liquids	2 hours	Examples: water, fruit juices without pulp, carbonated beverages, clear tea, black coffee. No alcohol
Breast milk	4 hours	For otherwise healthy neonates and infants
Infant formula and nonhuman milk	6 hours	Nonhuman milk is similar to solids in gastric emptying time.
Light meal	6 hours	Example: toast and clear liquids
Regular meal including fat or meat	8 hours	Fat and meat delay gastric emptying.
Fried or fatty foods	May require >8 hours	Amount and type of food should be considered. Fasting for >8 hours may be associated with hypoglycemia in children.

Adapted from American Society of Anesthesiologists, 2011.

Two Cochrane reviews confirmed the safety of shortened preoperative fasting in children (Brady, Kinn, Ness, et al, 2009) and adults (Brady, Kinn, and Stuart, 2003). Despite the authoritative guidelines and evidence of safety, studies suggest that providers are still using the blanket statement "NPO (nil per os, or nothing by mouth) after midnight" without regard to patient characteristics, the procedure, or the time of the procedure (Anderson and Comrie, 2009). Overall, there has been a lack of implementation of these liberalized guidelines into actual practice (Subrahmanyam and Venugopal, 2010). For the next step modifying preoperative fasting protocols, see Clinical Application 20-2. Whatever the prescribed fast, a client's compliance with it should be assessed at the time of the procedure (American Society of Anesthesiologists, 2011).

Surgery of the gastrointestinal tract demands additional bowel preparation. Anti-infectives such as *neomycin* that remain mainly in the bowel may be given to kill intestinal bacteria (Levison, 2012). Other antibiotics may be used prophylactically also. Compared to no preparation or mechanical preparation, oral antibiotic bowel preparation before elective colorectal surgery was associated with shorter postoperative length of stay and lower 30-day readmission rates, primarily due to fewer readmissions for infections (Toneva, Deierhoi, Morris, et al, 2013).

A low-fiber diet for 2 to 3 days will minimize the feces left in the bowel. All foods produce **some colonic residue** with fiber-containing foods the chief contributor. Milk is fiber-free but increases colonic residue by other mechanisms (Cunningham, 2012). Table 20-3 details a low-fiber diet.

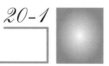

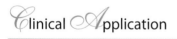

Clinical Application 20-1

Surgical clients with Rampant Dental Caries

Within a period of weeks, three clients on a gynecological surgical unit suffered postoperative wound disruptions. Each disruption was a **dehiscence,** a separation of the wound edges. Dehiscence occurs most frequently between the fifth and twelfth postoperative days. Risk factors for dehiscence include:

- Obesity
- Malnutrition
- Dehydration
- Abdominal distention
- Infection
- Increased abdominal pressure from improper deep breathing and coughing

All three clients had at least one of the risk factors. One client ran a postoperative fever, which could have been caused by infection or dehydration. The other two clients had such severely carious teeth it would have been difficult for them to chew in the months before surgery. They probably were malnourished. Marked dental caries suggest a need for a thorough nutritional assessment. Carious teeth can cause and be caused by poor eating habits.

20-2

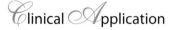
Clinical Application

Preoperative Carbohydrate Loading

Prolonged preoperative fasting in abdominal surgery results in a marked increase of insulin resistance that usually lasts for 2 to 4 weeks in uncomplicated cases. Both the metabolic response and the degree of insulin resistance following abdominal surgery are related to the magnitude of the surgery performed. Conventional preoperative fasting time may aggravate insulin resistance and promote hyperglycemia, especially because the fast is often longer than the expected 6 to 8 hours (de Aguilar-Nascimento and Dock-Nascimento, 2010).

Even after brief periods of fasting, metabolism slows to prevent starvation, one mechanism being reduced insulin sensitivity. The trauma of surgery not only provokes insulin resistance but also speeds metabolism and accelerates catabolism (Crenshaw, 2011).

The European Society for Clinical Nutrition and Metabolism recommends oral preoperative carbohydrate loading for most clients.

Providing a carbohydrate-rich beverage 2 to 3 hours before surgery did not interfere with gastric emptying and increased insulin action by 50% (Crenshaw, 2011). Gastrointestinal motility disorders such as gastroparesis, mechanical obstruction of the gastrointestinal tract, gastroesophageal reflux, and morbid obesity are examples of contraindications to this protocol (de Aguilar-Nascimento and Dock-Nascimento, 2010).

A literature review found carbohydrate drinks preoperatively in colorectal surgery to be both safe and effective. Not only was there no increased risk of aspiration, but also the carbohydrate drinks were associated with shorter hospital stays, a quicker return of bowel function, and less loss of muscle mass. A recommendation that preoperative carbohydrate drinks should be the standard in elective colorectal clients was accompanied by noting the need for further research for clients with diabetes mellitus (Jones, Badger, and Hannon, 2011).

TABLE 20-3 ■ Low-Fiber Diet

DESCRIPTION	INDICATIONS	ADEQUACY
The low-fiber diet limits milk and milk products and excludes any food made with seeds, nuts, and raw or dried fruits and vegetables. Digestibility of fiber is not appreciably altered by pureeing. The purpose of the diet is to decrease colonic contents by limiting fiber intake to 10 to 15 grams per day.	The diet can be used for severe diarrhea, partial bowel obstruction, and acute phases of inflammatory bowel diseases. Preoperatively the diet is used to minimize fecal volume and residue. Postoperatively the diet is used in the progression to a general diet. Long-term use of the diet is not recommended because it may aggravate symptoms during nonacute phases of disease.	Strict reduction in milk and milk products, vegetables, and fruits may necessitate supplementation of calcium, vitamin C, folate, and other nutrients. If used long term, a registered dietitian should be consulted regarding nutritional adequacy.

Food Group	Choose	Decrease
Milk—limit to 2 cups/day including cooking or 1.5 oz. hard cheese	Mild cheese Cottage cheese Cream cheese Yogurt with active live cultures	Strong cheese Cream Whole milk Yogurt with dried fruit, nuts
Breads and Cereals	White bread, white flour pasta, pancakes, waffles Refined cereals: cream of wheat, cream of rice, puffed rice, Rice Krispies, corn flakes Crackers without whole grains or seeds	Whole-grain breads and pasta Bread made with seeds, nuts, or bran Cracked-wheat bread Brown/wild rice
Fruits	Juice without pulp Ripe banana Cooked or canned apples, apricots, Royal Anne cherries, peaches, pears Strained fruit	Prunes and prune juice Figs Fruits not on "choose" list Dried fruit Raw fruit except banana, melon Fruit sweetened with sorbitol
Vegetables	Juice without pulp Lettuce Cooked or canned asparagus, green and wax beans, carrots, eggplant, pumpkin, spinach, acorn squash, seedless tomatoes, tomato sauce or puree, white or sweet potatoes without skin Strained vegetables	Vegetables not on "choose" list Corn Dried peas, beans, and lentils Cruciferous vegetables Greens (collard, mustard, turnip) Potato skins or chips Fried vegetables
Meat, Poultry, Fish, Shellfish, Eggs	Lean tender meat without grease: ground or well-cooked (roasted, baked, or broiled) beef, lamb, ham, veal, pork, poultry, organ meats, fish Eggs except fried Tofu	Tough, fried, fatty, or spiced meats Luncheon meats Fried eggs

TABLE 20-3 ■ Low-Fiber Diet (Continued)		
Food Group	**Choose**	**Decrease**
Fats and Oils	Smooth nut butters—2 tablespoons/day Butter, oils (canola and olive preferably) Salad dressings without seeds Margarine	All other nuts Coconut Olives
Desserts and Miscellaneous	Plain dessert made with allowed foods: fruit, ices, sherbet, ice cream, gelatin Candy: gum drops, hard candy, jelly beans, plain chocolate, marshmallows, butterscotch Sugar, molasses Jelly Salt, pepper, ground seasonings Smooth condiments Plain gravy Broth and strained soups made from recommended foods Milk sauces (deduct from milk allowance) Mayonnaise	Popcorn Seeds of any kind Whole spices Chili sauce Rich gravy Vinegar Alcohol Jam, marmalade Honey Sugar alcohols—Xylitol, sorbitol Cocoa powder
Beverages	Decaffeinated coffee Decaffeinated or herbal tea Soda	Caffeinated beverages Limit beverages with high-fructose corn syrup to 12 oz/day Alcohol

SAMPLE MENU

Breakfast	Lunch/Dinner
Strained grapefruit juice Cream of wheat Poached egg White bagel with butter and smooth jelly ½ cup milk Decaffeinated coffee	Baked halibut with clear lemon juice Twice-baked potato (no onions) Candied sweet potato (no nuts or whole spices) Canned pear and banana on lettuce French bread and spread Rice pudding (no raisins; deduct milk from allowance) Decaffeinated tea

Adapted from Academy of Nutrition and Dietetics, 2012a; Dugdale, 2011; Mayo Foundation, 2011.

Postoperative Nutrition

Intravenous fluids are continued after surgery. The usual minimum replacement is 2 liters of 5% glucose in water in 24 hours. This amount contains 100 grams of glucose and delivers 340 kilocalories. Although this will not meet a person's resting energy expenditure, it will prevent ketosis. Previously well-nourished adults generally have nutrient reserves for 3 to 4 days of semistarvation. To prevent excessive muscle protein from being used for energy, adequate nourishment should be delivered to the client within 3 days. In general, 25 kilocalories/kilogram of body weight per day is an acceptable and achievable intake.

To avoid abdominal distention, oral feedings traditionally have been delayed until **peristalsis** returns but scientific evidence supporting this practice is lacking (Charoenkwan, Phillipson, and Vutyavanich, 2007). A sure sign of peristalsis is the passage of **flatus** (gas) via the rectum. Ambulation as permitted helps clients pass the flatus and avoid uncomfortable distention. **Paralytic ileus** is a complication of abdominal surgery and other traumatic events or diseases. Peristalsis ceases and secretions and gas accumulate in the bowel, leading to distention and vomiting. Removal of secretions by suction is the usual treatment.

In many cases, early feeding of the postoperative client is the norm. Except in cases in which the bowel was handled, clients should be allowed to feed postoperatively as early as possible after ensuring return of airway reflexes (Subrahmanyam and Venugopal, 2010). In malnourished surgical clients, early oral feeding after surgery should be encouraged, but when an insufficient postoperative oral intake is anticipated, tube feeding should be initiated at once (Nespoli, Coppola, and Gianotti, 2012).

A review of studies testing the traditional practice of delaying oral intake until peristalsis returns found no significant differences in postoperative complications in major abdominal gynecological surgery clients. The women fed within 24 hours of surgery experienced more nausea but also were discharged from the hospital earlier than those treated traditionally (Charoenkwan, Phillipson, and Vutyavanich, 2007).

Clients are usually progressed from clear liquids to full liquids, a soft diet, and then a regular diet as soon as possible (see Chapter 14). The progression time varies with the client and surgical procedure. It may be hours or days. If "diet as tolerated" is ordered, the client should be asked what foods sound appealing. Sometimes a full dinner tray when the client does not feel well "turns off" the small appetite he or she has.

After gastrointestinal surgery, oral food and fluids are deferred longer than with other surgeries to allow healing. Giving the exact amount of food or fluid prescribed is important. More is not better if the client's stomach or intestine has been sutured. It is not advisable to give red liquids, such as gelatin or cranberry juice, after surgery on the mouth and throat so that vomitus is not mistaken for blood or vice versa.

For clients undergoing elective major upper gastrointestinal surgery requiring postoperative nutritional support, enteral feeding is considered as the most desirable form of postoperative feeding. Compared with parenteral nutrition, randomized controlled trials demonstrated enteral nutrition to be associated with

- Shorter hospital stays
- Lower incidence of severe or infectious complications
- Lower severity of complications
- Decreased costs (Wheble, Knight, and Khan, 2012).

Surgical removal of a part of the gastrointestinal tract, such as the stomach, duodenum, jejunum, or ileum, may result in malabsorption of specific nutrients. Similarly, realignment of parts of the tract can interfere with the digestive processes (Fig. 20-1).

Note that bile salts are absorbed in the ileum. Although the loss of bile salts in the feces may seem harmless, the body ordinarily recycles these salts over and over in the management of fats. Prolonged impaired absorption of bile salts can result in failure to absorb fat and fat-soluble vitamins.

Disorders of the Mouth and Throat

Varied conditions such as dental caries, oral surgery, surgery of the head and neck, fractured jaw, cancer chemotherapy or radiation therapy can cause difficulty with chewing and swallowing. Special feeding techniques and scrupulous oral hygiene may be required. Often the client requires a feeding tube, as covered in Chapter 14. Suggestions to manage **dysphagia** are described in Chapter 9 and interventions for anorexia appear in Chapter 21. Box 24-2 summarizes the dietary management of many symptoms.

Disorders of the Esophagus

Its sole purpose is to conduct food to the stomach, but the esophagus sometimes malfunctions. Achalasia, gastroesophageal reflux, and hiatal hernia are types of esophageal disorders.

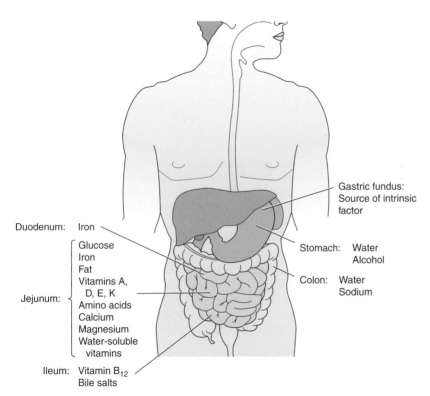

Duodenum: Iron

Jejunum:
{ Glucose
Iron
Fat
Vitamins A, D, E, K
Amino acids
Calcium
Magnesium
Water-soluble vitamins

Ileum: Vitamin B$_{12}$ Bile salts

Gastric fundus: Source of intrinsic factor

Stomach: Water
Alcohol

Colon: Water
Sodium

FIGURE 20-1 The chief sites of absorption for various nutrients. Disease or resection of an area will increase the risk of deficiency of specific nutrients. (Adapted from Scanlon, VC, and Sanders, T: *Student workbook for essentials of anatomy and physiology*, 6th ed. FA Davis, Philadelphia, 2011, p. 283, with permission.)

Achalasia

Failure of the gastrointestinal muscle fibers to relax where one part joins another is called **achalasia.** When it occurs in the **cardiac sphincter,** which separates the stomach from the esophagus, the condition is termed *cardiospasm.* Though the condition was first described more than 300 years ago, exact pathogenesis of this condition remains enigmatic. Currently, the disease is believed to be multi-factorial, with autoimmune mechanisms triggered by infection in a genetically predisposed individual leading to degeneration of inhibitory ganglia in the wall of the esophagus (Ghoshal, Daschakraborty, and Singh, 2012).

Very hot or cold foods may trigger esophageal spasm, and anxiety seems to aggravate the condition. Symptoms are described as "something sticking in my throat" and a feeling of fullness behind the sternum (breastbone). Vomiting may occur with achalasia, and aspiration of vomitus can cause pneumonia.

In mild cases, avoiding spicy foods and minimizing dietary bulk may be effective. Diets for these clients require much individual attention. Rarely does one achalasia client have intolerances for the same foods as another client. Plenty of liquids with small, frequent meals may help. Treatment of severe cases involves stretching the cardiac sphincter or surgically incising it to enlarge the passage.

Gastroesophageal Reflux Disease

Some regurgitation of stomach contents into the esophagus occurs in normal individuals. Usually the presence of stomach contents in the esophagus stimulates esophageal contractions that return the refluxed material to the stomach. If excessive reflux occurs, either in frequency or volume, or if the esophagus fails to contract in response to stomach contents, the individual has **gastroesophageal reflux disease (GERD;** also called *acid-reflux disorder*). Approximately 18% of the U.S. population reports GERD symptoms weekly (Delegge, 2014). It is the most commonly diagnosed gastrointestinal disease in physicians' office visits (Richter, Balfe, and Greene, 2011).

About 70% to 85% of infants have regurgitation within the first 2 months of life, which resolves without intervention in 95% of infants by 1 year of age. In infants, physiologic gastroesophageal reflux (GER) is treated conservatively by:

- Small, frequent feedings thickened with cereal
- Upright positioning after feeding
- Elevating the head of the bed (Schwartz, 2013)

Evidence of GERD in infants includes choking, gagging, coughing with feedings, or significant irritability (Czinn and Blanchard, 2013) along with aspiration of food into the respiratory tract or of **failure to thrive.** Regurgitation often reappears in old age due to poor muscle tone of the cardiac sphincter.

In adults, risk factors for gastroesophageal reflux are:

- Hiatal hernia with incompetent lower esophageal sphincter (Fig. 20-2)
- Medications or foods that reduce the effectiveness of the lower esophageal sphincter
- History of nasogastric intubation with a duration of more than 4 days
- Surgery on the pyloric sphincter
- Smoking
- Conditions that raise intra-abdominal pressure such as pregnancy and obesity

A clear association has been found between physically detectable reflux and higher body mass index (Hajar, Castell, Ghomrawi, et al, 2012). In addition, weight loss was dose-dependently associated with both a reduction of gastroesophageal reflux symptoms and an increased treatment success with antireflux medication in a general population in Norway (Ness-Jensen, Lindam, et al, 2013).

The stomach is normally protected from hydrochloric acid by a thick layer of mucus. Because the esophagus is not so protected, repeated bouts of gastroesophageal reflux can lead to esophagitis and ulcer formation that, when healed, may cause a stricture at the site of the scar tissue. See Peptic Ulcer later in the chapter.

The prominent symptom of gastroesophageal reflux is heartburn with pain occurring behind the breastbone. Sometimes the pain radiates to the neck and the

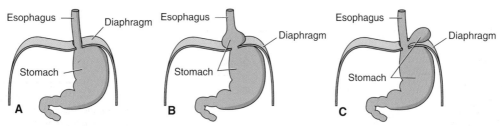

FIGURE 20-2 In hiatal hernia, the upper part of the stomach squeezes into the chest cavity through the esophageal opening in the diaphragm. *A,* Normal anatomy. *B,* Sliding hiatal hernia. *C,* Rolling hiatal hernia. (Reprinted from Williams, LS, and Hopper, PD: *Understanding medical-surgical nursing,* 4th ed. FA Davis, Philadelphia, 2011, p. 727, with permission.)

back of the throat. Lying down or bending over may increase reflux and aggravate the pain. If the passage becomes narrowed, **dysphagia** may become bothersome resulting in anorexia, malnutrition, and weight loss, and possibly leading to aspiration pneumonia.

Treatment may include medications (proton-pump inhibitors such as *osmeprazole* and histamine H_2 antagonists such as *ranitidine*) as well as diet modification.

Dietary treatment involves several principles:

- Decreasing gastric pressure on the lower esophageal sphincter (small, frequent meals)
- Normal amounts of dietary protein (associated with tightening the cardiac sphincter)
- Avoidance of foods and behaviors that relax the sphincter:
  - Fat and chocolate
  - Peppermint and spearmint
  - Caffeine, alcohol, tobacco

Timing of intake is an important self-care strategy. Avoidance of a late-night meal plays a role in prevention of nighttime reflux (Fujiwara, Arakawa, and Fass, 2012). Table 20-4 details a diet for gastroesophageal reflux. It may not be necessary to implement every element of the diet. One client with severe nighttime heartburn found that elevating the head of the bed on blocks and eliminating a predinner cocktail was enough to significantly reduce his heartburn and improve his sleep. Similarly, an expectant mother may easily identify foods that cause heartburn (increasingly uncomfortable later in pregnancy with expanding pressure on the stomach) and eliminate those for its duration.

A surgical procedure for chronic GERD is called *fundoplication*. In it the stomach fundus is wrapped around the esophagus to restore the proper gastroesophageal angle and to enhance the cardiac sphincter. The surgery can be performed through an open incision, laparoscope, or, in selected clients, transorally with an endoscope and special fasteners. In all cases, strict adherence to dietary, lifting, and activity restrictions is essential.

Following the endoscopic approach, *transoral incisionless fundoplication (TIF)*, dietary intake is limited by one group of surgeons to:

- Liquids for 2 weeks
- Soft/pureed foods for 2 weeks
- Soft low fiber diet for 2 weeks (Trad, Turgeon, and Deljkich, 2012)

Six-month follow-up of TIF in 10 community-based centers found the procedure to be safe and effective in eliminating use of proton-pump inhibitors (Bell, Mayrelis, Barnes, et al, 2012). Another multicenter 3-year follow-up reported 18% of clients had undergone revisional procedures, but no adverse effects were reported in the remainder (Muls, Eckardt, Marcjese, et al, 2012). In a tertiary care setting, however, within the 3-year follow-up period, 36% of clients had undergone revisional laparoscopic fundoplication (Witteman, Strijkers, de Vries, et al, 2012).

TABLE 20-4 ■ Diet for Gastroesophageal Reflux and Hiatal Hernia

DESCRIPTION	INDICATIONS	ADEQUACY
The diet is designed to minimize reflux through timing of intake, limiting fat, and exclusion of sphincter relaxants. Adjunctive treatment involves lifestyle changes.	Esophageal reflux, hiatal hernia, esophageal ulcers, esophagitis, esophageal strictures, heartburn	The diet may not meet the Recommended Dietary Allowance for vitamin C and iron in the premenopausal woman.

LIFESTYLE CHANGES	CHOOSE	DECREASE
Meal Pattern	Six small meals Chew thoroughly. Limit liquids with meals if causing distention or early satiety	Eating within 3 hours of bedtime
Adjunctive Therapy	Remain upright 2 hours after meals. Relax at mealtime—sit down. Use blocks to elevate head of bed 6 inches. Consider weight loss if needed. Implement appropriate regular physical activity	Lying down in the hour after eating
Food Group		
Milk	Skim or 1% fat milk, buttermilk, evaporated skim milk Skim milk cheese Low-fat or 1% cottage cheese Low-fat ice cream Sherbet Nonfat or low-fat yogurt Powdered milk Soy milk	Other milk products Hot chocolate

TABLE 20-4 ■ **Diet for Gastroesophageal Reflux and Hiatal Hernia** (Continued)

Food Group	Choose	Decrease
Breads and Cereals	Any prepared without added fat (Half of servings should be whole grains)	Pancakes, waffles, French toast Doughnuts, sweet rolls, nut breads Granola-type cereals with nuts and/or coconut
Fruits	Mild juices Any fruits prepared without fat except those on "decrease" list	Citrus fruits and juices
Vegetables	Vegetables prepared without fat except those on "decrease" list	Creamed or fried vegetables Hashed brown potatoes Garlic Onions Tomatoes, tomato juice and sauces
Meat, Poultry, Fish, Shellfish, Eggs	All prepared without added fat: 6 oz/day of: tender well-cooked lean meat, skinless poultry, fish, Eggs Soy Dried beans and peas	Higher fat meats: sausage, bacon, frankfurters, luncheon meats, canned meats and fish, duck, goose
Fats and Oils	8 tsp/day: heart healthy oils (olive, canola), mild salad dressing 2 tbsp of the following may substitute for 1 tsp of fat: light cream, sour cream, nondairy cream Vegetable pan sprays as desired Low-fat salad dressings	Fried foods Gravies and sauces Cream Regular salad dressing Shortening, lard, or oils in excess of allowance Nuts, peanut butter
Beverages	Caffeine-free herbal teas, except mint flavored	Alcohol Coffee, regular or decaffeinated Tea, regular or decaffeinated Hot chocolate Caffeinated beverages
Miscellaneous	Angel food cake Plain cakes and cookies Gelatin, popsicles Pudding made with skim milk Fat-free broth, bouillon, consommé Soup made from allowed foods Cream soup made with skim milk Sugar, honey, syrup, molasses Jam, jelly, preserves Plain candy Condiments and spices in small amounts Vanilla Vinegar	Peppermint Spearmint Spicy foods Pepper Chocolate

SAMPLE MENU

Breakfast	Lunch/Dinner
½ banana ½ cup oatmeal ½ cup skim milk 1 slice toast with jam	3 oz skinless chicken breast baked in lemon juice ½ baked potato with 1 tbsp sour cream ½ cup whole-kernel corn 3 small celery sticks Hard roll with 1 tsp spread 1 cup decaffeinated tea Baked apple made with peeled apple, cinnamon, sugar
Midmorning Snack	**Midafternoon/Evening Snack**
½ cup pineapple juice 3 graham crackers	1 cup low-fat yogurt

Sources: Academy of Nutrition and Dietetics, 2012b; Festi, Scaioli, Baldi, et al, 2009; National Digestive, April 30, 2012.

Hiatal Hernia

The *esophageal hiatus* is the opening in the diaphragm through which the esophagus is attached to the stomach. A **hiatal hernia** is a protrusion of the stomach through the esophageal hiatus into the chest cavity (see Fig. 20-2). The symptoms of hiatal hernia are similar to those of gastroesophageal reflux, and its medical treatment is the same. Persistent symptoms despite conservative treatment might lead the client to elect surgical repair of the hernia.

Disorders of the Stomach

Disorders of the stomach often require diet modification and, in some cases, surgery. The following sections concern two common disorders, gastritis and peptic ulcers, and one disorder mainly associated with diabetes mellitus, delayed gastric emptying. Also included is an exaggerated physiological response that can cause problems for older adults, postprandial hypotension.

Gastritis

Inflammation of the stomach is **gastritis** that can be acute or chronic. Worldwide, the most common cause is infection with *Helicobacter pylori* (see Peptic Ulcer Pathology later in the chapter).

Causes are characterized as:

■ Acute gastritis
   ■ Chemical injury from alcohol, aspirin, other nonsteroidal anti-inflammatory drugs **(NSAIDs),** bile reflux, or acid

   ■ Underperfusion of the gastric mucosa following trauma or sepsis
   ■ Infectious infestation, usually from *H. pylori*
■ Chronic gastritis
   ■ Atrophic autoimmune type with severe wasting of acid producing cells seen in old age and systemic autoimmune disorders such as pernicious anemia and diabetes mellitus
   ■ Atrophic multifocal type from chronic *H. pylori* infection (Delegge, 2014).

Symptoms of gastritis are:

■ Anorexia
■ Nausea
■ A feeling of fullness
■ Epigastric pain

Signs of gastritis are vomiting, perhaps of blood, and eructating (belching).

Figure 20-3 illustrates the abdominal quadrants and regions used to record signs and symptoms revealed during the assessment process. The illustration also shows the underlying soft structures contained in the quadrants and the bony structures in the regions.

More often than not, discovering which foods are responsible for the pain and discomfort of gastritis is a trial-and-error process. Tolerances vary from person to person. Suggested dietary treatments for gastritis are given in Box 20-1. Prolonged or recurrent gastritis deserves medical attention to diagnose and treat the underlying problem.

Delayed Gastric Emptying

Gastroparesis is a disorder that produces symptoms of gastric retention without physical obstruction. Peristalsis is weak, resulting in large particles of food poorly

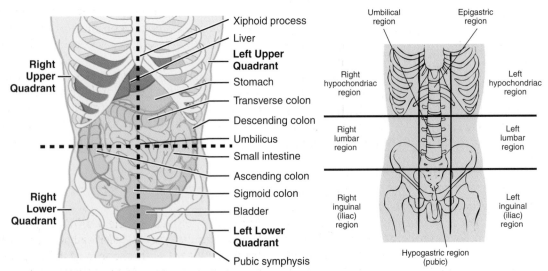

FIGURE 20-3 Abdominal quadrants and regions are used to describe locations of signs and symptoms. (Reprinted from Venes, D [ed.]: *Taber's cyclopedic medical dictionary*, 22nd ed. FA Davis, Philadelphia, 2013, pp. 4 and 2009, with permission.)

Box 20-1 ■ *Dietary Treatment for Gastritis*

Do

- Eat at regular intervals.
- Eat in a relaxed manner.
- Chew food, especially fibrous food, slowly and thoroughly.

Avoid

- Foods that cause pain
- Foods that cause gas, especially vegetables in the cabbage family (broccoli, cauliflower, and Brussels sprouts)
- Gastric irritants such as caffeine and alcohol
- NSAIDs such as *aspirin, ibuprofen,* and *naproxen*
- Strong spices, including nutmeg, pepper, garlic, and chili powder

---

prepared for digestion and in retained liquids whose exit from the stomach depends on gravity. Ingested food may remain in the stomach for a prolonged period of time and begin to putrefy. Gastroparesis is generally a disorder of the nervous innervation of the stomach or the actual muscle tissue and is seen in diabetes, Parkinson disease, and as a side effect of some medications (Delegge, 2014). Signs and symptoms include:

- **Postprandial** (after eating) upper abdominal pain
- Reduced hunger
- Fullness and bloating
- Nausea and vomiting

Fullness, upper abdominal pain, and reduced hunger correlate better with delayed gastric emptying than do nausea and vomiting (Camilleri, Bharucha, and Farrugia, 2011).

When delayed gastric emptying occurs with diabetes, it is termed *diabetic gastroparesis.* In several studies, diabetes mellitus accounted for almost one third of gastroparesis cases at tertiary centers which could reflect referral and selection bias. In contrast, a community-based study estimated that over 10 years, persons with type 1 diabetes mellitus had a 33% increased risk of developing gastroparesis compared to individuals without diabetes. For type 2 diabetes, the risk was 7.5% (Choung, Locke, Schleck, et al, 2012). Similarly, the estimated U.S. prevalence of definite diabetic gastroparesis is less than 100,000 which suggests it qualifies for "orphan drug" status to encourage development of new medications (Camilleri, Bharucha, and Farrugia, 2011).

Treatment of delayed gastric emptying focuses on the cause of the disorder: removing offending drugs, intervening appropriately in malnutrition, and controlling hyperglycemia in clients with diabetes. For most patients with mild to moderate disease, dietary intervention plays a central role in the management of gastroparesis (Keld, Kinsey, Athwal, and Lal, 2011). Unfortunately, only 32% of patients had a dietary

consultation after diagnosis of their gastroparesis, which occurred more frequently in clients who were sicker and hospitalized oftener. Also, those with type 1 diabetes were more likely to have had a nutritional consult than ones with type 2 diabetes or idiopathic gastroparesis (Parkman, Yates, Hasler, et al, 2011). Dietary interventions include:

- Eating small, frequent meals
- Replacing solids with nourishing liquids such as soups (which leave the stomach sooner than solids)
- Reducing the fat ingested (which remains in the stomach longer than carbohydrate or protein)
- Decreasing fiber intake
- Minimizing carbonated beverages
- Avoiding alcohol and tobacco smoking (Camilleri, Parkman, Shafi, et al, 2013).

A registry of clients with gastroparesis (204 **idiopathic** and 101 diabetic) found that:

- 2% followed a suggested gastroparetic diet with sufficient energy and low in fat and fiber.
- 64% consumed energy deficient diets.
- The majority consumed diets deficient in potassium; magnesium; calcium; iron; vitamins E, D, K; and folate, but just 33% were taking daily multivitamins.
- 54% were overweight or obese: 46% idiopathic, 70% diabetic ((Parkman, et al, 2011).

If adequate nutrition cannot be provided orally, jejunal feeding may be necessary. In severe cases of gastroparesis, medications may be prescribed and stimulatory techniques may be implemented.

Peptic Ulcers

Peptic ulcer disease is a common illness that affects more than 6 million people in the United States each year (Feinstein, Holman, Yorita Christensen, et al, 2010). Although most common in individuals over age 65, peptic ulcers have also occurred in infants and children.

Esophageal, gastric (stomach), and duodenal ulcers are called *peptic ulcers* and form when the mucosa is insufficiently resistant to stomach acids. If just the superficial cells are involved, the lesion is an **erosion.** If the muscular layer is involved, the person has an **ulcer.**

Pathophysiology

Approximately half of the world's population is infected with *Helicobacter pylori,* a bacterium which has been associated with chronic gastritis, peptic ulcer, and gastric cancer. Most infected people remain asymptomatic, however, and only 15% to 20% of *H.*

pylori–positive individuals develop the associated diseases (Liu, Gong, Sun, et al, 2012).

Helicobacter pylori and NSAIDs disrupt normal mucosal defense and repair, making the mucosa more susceptible to acid. NSAIDs now account for more than 50% of peptic ulcers. *H. pylori* infection is present in 50% to 70% of clients with duodenal ulcers and 30% to 50% of clients with gastric ulcers. If *H. pylori* is eradicated, peptic ulcer recurs in only 10% of clients compared with 70% recurrence in clients treated with acid suppression alone (Cohen, 2012). Contributing risk factors are caffeine consumption and use of tobacco products.

From the percentages above, it is easy to see that *H. pylori* and NSAIDs do not account for all peptic ulcer cases. A large part of NSAID use may relate to attempts to moderate the stresses of everyday life. NSAID use and resulting mucosal damage may provide an opening for opportunistic infection by *H. pylori*. The individual's psychological status, although not the major causative factor of peptic ulcer disease formerly attributed to it, may contribute to increased susceptibility of gastric mucosa to erosions and *H. pylori* infection through lifestyle choices or self-medication (Overmier and Murison, 2013).

Signs and Symptoms

Both gastric and duodenal ulcers cause epigastric pain. The pain from gastric ulcer is a burning, gnawing pain occurring 1 to 2 hours after meals and may be worsened by ingesting food. With duodenal ulcer, the pain is a burning, cramping one occurring 2 to 4 hours after eating typically relieved by antacids or food (Williams and Hopper, 2011). Pain that awakens the client at night is highly suggestive of duodenal ulcer (Cohen, 2012).

Complications

Mild to severe hemorrhage is the most common complication of peptic ulcer disease (Cohen, 2012). If the blood is vomited immediately after bleeding begins, it is bright red. If it stays in contact with digestive juices for a time, the vomitus is brown-black and granular, resembling coffee grounds. The medical term for this is *coffee-ground emesis*. Other symptoms of peptic ulcer are nausea, anorexia, and sometimes weight loss. In a meta-analysis of 16 studies involving 1633 participants, NSAID use along with *H. pylori* infection increased the risk of upper gastrointestinal bleeding 6 times (Wilkins, Khan, Nabh, and Schade, 2012).

Scar tissue from a healed ulcer can restrict the gastric outlet, causing pyloric obstruction. If the ulcer continues to erode through the entire stomach or intestinal wall, the result is a **perforated ulcer.** Leakage of gastrointestinal contents into the sterile abdominal cavity causes **peritonitis,** an inflammation of the peritoneum (the lining of the abdominal cavity).

Treatment

Medical treatment for *H. pylori* infection includes combinations of antibiotics and other drugs. Only if such treatment proves ineffective is surgery considered. No specific dietary causes or diet-based treatments have been rigorously studied in gastritis or gastric ulceration and avoidance of foods and practices that cause symptoms is recommended (Delegge, 2014).

MEDICAL

Before the advent of antiulcer medications, clients with peptic ulcers were usually advised to take antacids every 2 hours, alternating with milk and cream. Later research demonstrated that milk is a potent *inducer* of gastric acid secretion. An additional adverse effect of this treatment was **milk-alkali syndrome** (see Chapter 7).

Current guidelines suggest the use of triple antibiotic therapy as first choice treatment of *Helicobacter pylori* infection, although the eradication failure rate is more than 30%. Because of increasing resistance of pathogenic bacteria to antibiotics, probiotics have been suggested as adjunctive therapy in treatment of peptic ulcers but there is no clear evidence that probiotics increase the *H. pylori* eradication rate (Lionetti, Francavilla, Castellazzi, et al, 2012).

In *H. pylori*–infected children, yogurt promoted a normal balance of gut microflora and suppressed the *H. pylori* load (Yang and Sheu, 2012). For more information on probiotics and prebiotics, see Box 20-2.

New medications have revolutionized the treatment and are almost always effective without a drastic change in diet. In addition to antibiotics to eradicate *H. pylori*, commonly prescribed medications are:

- *cimetidine, famotidine,* and *ranitidine,* which block histamine-stimulated gastric acid secretion
- *omeprazole,* which suppresses gastric acid production

Smoking should be stopped, and alcohol consumption ceased or limited to small amounts of dilute alcohol. There is no evidence that changing the diet speeds ulcer healing or prevents recurrence (Cohen, 2012).

SURGICAL

When surgery is necessary, the ulcer is removed, and the remaining gastrointestinal tract is sutured together. Surgical procedures designed to eliminate the diseased area include gastroduodenostomy (stomach and duodenum anastomosed) and gastrojejunostomy (stomach and jejunum anastomosed). **Anastomosis** is the surgical

Box 20-2 ■ *Probiotics and Prebiotics*

Fermented foods have been considered health-promoting for centuries. More than 2000 years ago, Plinius the Old recommended fermented milk to treat acute gastritis (Vandenplas, Salvatore, Vieira, et al, 2007).

Probiotics are food products or oral supplements containing a sufficient number of viable microorganisms to improve the intestinal microbial balance of the host to potentially confer health benefits. To be effective, the selected microorganisms must exhibit resistance to low pH, bile salts, and pancreatic enzymes and thus survive passage through the upper gastrointestinal tract (Tejero, Rowland, Rastall, and Gibson, 2014).

There is no consensus about the minimum number of microorganisms that must be ingested to obtain a beneficial effect; however, a probiotic should typically contain several billion microorganisms to increase the chance that adequate gut colonization will occur (Williams, 2010).

The traditional delivery method for probiotics is in dairy products, but new technologies using spray or freeze-drying extend shelf life and permit the use of tablets and capsules. Those dietary supplements are not routinely tested by government agencies (see Chapter 15) but ConsumerLab's (2013) voluntary certification program tests for viability of the organisms, lack of potentially harmful organisms, and appropriate disintegration. An added advantage of supplements is the possibility of providing nondairy probiotic products for people who are lactose intolerant or vegetarian (Tejero, Rowland, Rastall, and Gibson, 2014); however, trace amounts of milk proteins may be present in *Lactobacilli* or *Bifidobactrium* strains because the culture media contain milk proteins (ConsumerLab, 2013).

Despite the health benefits attributed to probiotics, only specific strains of organisms have been tested. Results cannot be generalized to other strains. Suggested modes of action are by:

- Lowering intestinal pH
- Decreasing colonization and invasion by pathogenic organisms
- Modifying the host immune response (Williams, 2010).

Sufficient consistent data exist to conclude that certain probiotics, under certain conditions, and in certain target populations, are beneficial in the management of infectious diarrhea in infants, travelers' diarrhea, antibiotic-associated diarrhea, and necrotizing enterocolitis (Johnston, Goldenberg, Vandvik, et al, 2011; Kale-Pradhan, Jassal, and Wilhelm, 2010; Videlock and Cremonini, 2012; Wolvers, Antoine, Myllyluoma, et al, 2010). For information on necrotizing enterocolitis, see Chapter 11. In addition, probiotics have been effective in reducing antibiotic-associated diarrhea and reducing the incidence of the most serious form, *Clostridium difficile* infection, by 66% (Friedman, 2010; Johnston, Ma, Goldenberg, et al, 2012).

The use of probiotics in constipation, irritable bowel syndrome, inflammatory bowel disease, and extra-intestinal infections requires more studies (Vandenplas, Veereman-Wauters, De Greef, et al, 2011). In addition, caution regarding safety is warranted in clients with compromised immunity, premature infants, those with short bowel syndrome, those with indwelling medical devices, elderly patients, the chronically debilitated, and those with cardiac valve disease (Snydman, 2008; Thomas, Greer, et al, 2010). Long-term effects of probiotic interventions are largely unknown and the current literature is not able to answer specific questions about their safety with confidence (Hempel, Newberry, Ruelaz, et al, 2011).

Probiotics are found in fermented or aged milk and milk products, other fermented products, breast milk, and supplements. Food sources of probiotics not only enhance the probiotic's stability by buffering stomach acid but also provide other nutrients. The most reliable food source is yogurt labeled "live and active culture." To earn this seal, the product must contain at least 100 million bacteria per gram of yogurt at the time it is made and must not have been heat treated because heat kills the bacteria. Many yogurts contain both starter cultures and additional bacteria presumed to be probiotic (Douglas and Sanders, 2008). Most labels do not differentiate the amounts of the bacterial strains contained in the product, making it difficult to choose a proven product for a given condition.

Analysis of commercial probiotic products in the U.S. marketplace in 2009 discovered only 4 of 13 products were correctly labeled in terms of quantity of viable bacteria, identification of species, and cross contamination by species not on the label. These findings suggest the need for adequate control of probiotic production as well as periodical screenings by competent organizations to monitor the effect of storage on product quality (Drago, Rodighiero, Celeste, et al, 2010).

When choosing to use probiotics in the treatment or prevention of gastrointestinal disease, the type of disease and probiotic species (strain) are the most important factors to take into consideration (Ritchie, and Romanuk, 2012). In addition, to retain their viability, bacteria-derived probiotics should not be consumed within 2 hours of antibiotics (Williams, 2010).

Prebiotics are nondigestible food ingredients that selectively stimulate the favorable growth and/or activity of one or more indigenous probiotic bacteria to benefit the host (Thomas, Greer, et al, 2010). Prebiotics are specialized ingredients that target specific bacteria, not food fiber in general. Some foods that could be prebiotic sources are artichokes, asparagus, bananas, chicory, garlic, leeks, onions, tomatoes, and wheat (Douglas and Sanders, 2008; Dryden and Seidner, 2014; Tejero, Rowland, Rastall, and Gibson, 2014).

connection between tubular structures. Figure 20-4 illustrates these two procedures.

After gastric surgery, parenteral and enteral feedings are used singly or in combination. If enteral feeding is used, the tube must be inserted beyond the area that was resected (removed). Nutritional care includes delivering nutrients to ensure maximal utilization of the remaining functions of the gastrointestinal tract. After a client is advanced to an oral diet, he or she may experience **dumping syndrome,** a complication of a surgical procedure that removes, disrupts, or bypasses the pyloric sphincter. Clinically significant dumping

syndrome occurs in 10% of clients following gastric surgery that alters the stomach's reservoir function (Delegge, 2014). Clinical Application 20-3 describes the dumping syndrome in more detail.

Postprandial Hypotension

Postprandial hypotension is a drop in systolic blood pressure of 20 mm Hg or more within 2 hours after beginning a meal. Postprandial hypotension occurs in up to one-third of older people but virtually never occurs

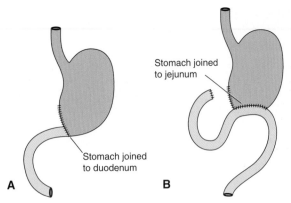

FIGURE 20-4 Common gastric resection procedures. *A*, Gastroduodenostomy or Billroth I procedure. *B*, Gastrojejunostomy or Billroth II procedure. (Reprinted from Williams, LS, and Hopper, PD: *Understanding medical-surgical nursing*, 4th ed. FA Davis, Philadelphia, 2011, p. 738, with permission.)

Clinical Application 20-3

Dumping Syndrome

The pyloric sphincter normally allows only small amounts of gastric contents into the duodenum at a time. After the pyloric sphincter is surgically removed, concentrated liquid is suddenly "dumped" into the intestine. Depending on the time elapsed after a meal dumping syndrome is characterized as

- Early (30–60 minutes **postprandial**)
  - Abdominal pain and cramping, bloating, diarrhea due to large osmolar load in small intestine
  - Hypotension, tachycardia, dizziness due to compensatory fluid shifts
- Late (longer than 60 minutes postprandial)
  - Carbohydrate load increases blood glucose
  - Hypersecretion of insulin produces rapid decrease in blood glucose
  - Sweating, shakiness, difficulty concentrating, decreased consciousness, hunger (Delegge, 2014)

Dumping syndrome is most often associated with a total or partial gastrectomy involving resection of two-thirds of the stomach. The same signs and symptoms can occur in a client after **vagotomy** or one receiving enteral feeding if the nasogastric tube is accidentally carried down into the duodenum.

Treatment includes medications, dietary modification, and surgical reconstruction.

Medications that may be helpful are:

- *acarbose*, which delays and reduces glucose absorption;
- *loperamide*, which decreases gut motility; and
- *octreotide*, which can delay gastric emptying and small bowel transit and inhibit insulin production and postprandial vasodilation (Delegge, 2014).

Dietary treatment of the dumping syndrome attempts to delay gastric emptying and to distribute the increased osmolality to the bowel over time. Table 20-5 depicts a diet to prevent or treat dumping syndrome.

in younger people. It is more likely to occur in people who have high blood pressure or disorders that impair the brain centers controlling the autonomic nervous system (Bakris, 2007).

Symptoms and complications include:

- Dizziness
- Light-headedness
- Falls
- Disturbed speech
- Vision changes
- Angina pectoris
- Stroke

The mechanism is not clearly understood but appears to be secondary to a blunted sympathetic response to a meal (Luciano, Brennan, and Rothberg, 2010). Normally the body compensates for the increased blood flow to the digestive tract following meals, but in the elderly, the mechanisms maintaining adequate circulation to the rest of the body become less effective. Greater effects are seen when the stomach empties more rapidly.

To prevent postprandial hypotension, a person should:

- Drink 12 to 18 ounces of water 15 minutes before eating for fluid enhancement
- Limit carbohydrate intake
- Take frequent small meals
- Lie in a semirecumbent position for 90 minutes after eating
- Schedule antihypertensive medications between rather than just before meals (Harvard Medical School, 2010; Luciano, Brennan, and Rothberg, 2010).

Special dietary additives or medications to delay gastric emptying are sometimes prescribed.

Disorders of the Intestines

To obtain satisfactory diagnostic radiographic or endoscopic studies of the bowel, it must be emptied. This is usually accomplished by a low fiber/clear liquid diet followed by laxatives. Explaining the procedures and the necessity for them helps to gain the client's cooperation. For inpatients, the nurse should ensure that the client receives maximum nourishment when tests are completed for the day. Frequently, another series of tests is scheduled for the next day.

Problems with Elimination

Several problems with frequency and consistency of bowel movements are common. These include irritable bowel syndrome, diarrhea, and constipation.

TABLE 20-5 ■ Diet for Dumping Syndrome

DESCRIPTION	INDICATIONS	ADEQUACY
This diet consists of six small feedings, high in protein and fat and low in simple sugars.	This diet and adjunct therapy, used after surgical removal of the pyloric sphincter or other treatments that speed gastric emptying, is designed to prevent rapid emptying of hypertonic gastric contents into the small intestine. Examples of such operative procedures include vagotomy, pyloroplasty, hemigastrectomy, total gastrectomy, esophagogastrectomy, Whipple procedure, gastroenterostomy, and gastrojejunostomy. As the body adapts to its new condition, specific foods may be tolerated later in convalescence.	Deficiencies secondary to surgery or malabsorption may require supplementation. Among the nutrients likely to be needed are the vitamins B_{12}, D, and folic acid and the minerals calcium and iron.

LIFESTYLE CHANGES	CHOOSE	DECREASE
Meal Pattern	Six small servings. Eat slowly and chew thoroughly.	Fluids with meals. Very hot or cold foods that stimulate peristalsis
Adjunctive Therapy	Lie down for ½ to 1 hour after meals. Fiber supplements (pectin, guar gum) that form gels with carbohydrates are effective for hypoglycemia by decreasing glucose absorption and increasing intestinal transit time (Delegge, 2014).	
Food Group		
Milk	LactAid Aged cheese (>90 days)	Milk if lactose intolerant*
Breads and Cereals	White, whole-wheat, rye, Jewish, Italian, and Vienna breads* Rolls, crackers, biscuits, and muffins (milk-free)* Any cooked or dry cereal, milk-free* Rice, noodles, spaghetti, macaroni	Frosted breads Sweet rolls, doughnuts, coffeecake Bread made with milk (unless tolerated)* Sugar-sweetened cereal Cereal containing milk*
Fruits	Fresh, frozen, or unsweetened canned fruits, banana Juices, fresh, frozen, canned, unsweetened, between meals only	Sweetened canned or frozen juices and fruits, dried fruit Raw fruits unless tolerated Juices with meals
Vegetables	Any as tolerated Juices between meals only	Those causing discomfort Juices with meals
Meat Group	Any as tolerated	None
Fats and Oils	Milk-free margarine if lactose intolerant* Oils Vegetable shortening	Any containing milk unless tolerated*
Desserts and Miscellaneous	Artificially sweetened gelatin Angel food and sponge cakes Salt, pepper, spices as tolerated Mustard, catsup, pickles, relishes as tolerated Artificially sweetened beverages Decaffeinated tea and coffee, herbal tea Dietetic jam and jelly	Sugar-containing cakes, pies, cookies, ice cream*, sherbet* Seasonings that cause discomfort Caffeine-containing beverages Sugar, honey, syrup, molasses Jam, jelly Candy

SAMPLE MENU

30 Minutes Before Breakfast	30 Minutes Before Lunch
Decaffeinated beverage Artificial sweetener	1 cup LactAid*
Breakfast	**Lunch/Dinner**
½ banana 1 egg, poached 1 tsp milk-free margarine Dietetic jelly	3 oz roast pork Barley with butter ½ cup squash ½ cup fruit cocktail, drained
1½ Hours After Breakfast	**½ Hour After Meal**
Orange juice	Decaffeinated beverage Artificial sweetener
Midmorning Snack	
1 slice whole-wheat toast	

*If lactose restriction is necessary.

Irritable Bowel Syndrome

This is a chronic **functional** gastrointestinal disorder characterized by a combination of abdominal pain or discomfort and altered bowel habits at least three times a month over at least 3 months for which other gastrointestinal causes have been excluded. **Irritable bowel syndrome (IBS)** is estimated to affect 10% to 15% of the population, about twice as many women as men, usually in people younger than 45 years (National Digestive Diseases Information Clearinghouse (NDDIC), July 2, 2012).

The physiological basis for many of the symptoms is distention of the bowel (Gibson and Shepherd, 2010). Clients are symptomatic during the day but not while sleeping. The most common signs and symptoms of irritable bowel syndrome are:

- Cramping
- Bloating, abdominal distention
- Abdominal pain, often relieved by passage of flatus or stool
- Constipation or diarrhea or alternating episodes of both
- Mucus in stools

The causes of IBS are not well understood. Researchers believe a combination of physical and mental health problems can lead to IBS (NDDIC, July 2, 2012). Up to two-thirds of individuals with IBS believe their symptoms to be diet-related and modify their consumption to avoid food triggers. In most cases, reported food intolerances are not substantiated by formal testing for food allergies, malabsorption, or **celiac disease** (Schwartz and Semrad, 2014), but screening for celiac disease is recommended in specific circumstances (Harris, 2012).

Treatment for IBS is symptomatic. In general, a balanced diet with few restrictions is advised. Avoidance of specific carbohydrates (fructose, lactose) and sugar alcohols (sorbitol, Xylitol) may prove helpful (Schwartz and Semrad, 2014). A novel and exceptionally thorough implementation of those strategies involves the Low FODMAP Diet (see Clinical Application 20-4). Clients should be reassured that IBS is a **benign** condition that does not permanently harm the intestines (NDDIC, July 2, 2012).

Diarrhea

Passage of liquid or unformed feces, diarrhea, is an important cause of morbidity and mortality in the elderly and in children (see Chapter 11). Most instances of diarrhea in adults are self-limiting and resolve without treatment or the need for extensive medical workup. In many cases, the cause of diarrhea cannot be found. If an adult is in little jeopardy from an electrolyte imbalance, self-treatment for diarrhea following the conservative regimen listed in Table 20-6 is appropriate. Oral Rehydration Solutions can be used (see Chapter 8 for Pedialyte). Also, Dollars & Sense 20-1 shows a homemade oral rehydration fluid recipe.

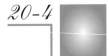

20-4

Clinical Application

Low FODMAP Diet

The Low FODMAP (**f**ermentable **o**ligosaccharides, **d**isaccharides, **m**onosaccharides, **a**nd **p**olyols) diet, accepted as an effective strategy for managing symptoms of irritable bowel syndrome (IBS) in Australia, has sparked interest worldwide. The targets of restriction are short-chain carbohydrates that have been shown to induce IBS symptoms of abdominal pain, bloating, flatus, and diarrhea due to their poor absorption, osmotic activity, and rapid fermentation. Up to 86% of clients with IBS have achieved relief of overall gastrointestinal symptoms from the Low FODMAP Diet (Barrett, 2013).

The richest sources of the FODMAPs are:

- Fructooligosaccharides (fructans)—wheat, rye, onions, garlic, artichokes
- Galactoligosaccharides (GOS)—legumes (soy, beans, chickpeas, lentils), cabbage, Brussels sprouts
- Lactose—milk, dairy products, beer, prepared soups and sauces
- Fructose—honey, apples, dates, mangoes, papaya, pears, prunes, watermelon, high fructose corn syrup
- Sorbitol—apples, pears, stone fruits, sugar-free mints/gums
- Mannitol—mushrooms, cauliflower, sugar-free mints/gums (Barrett and Gibson, 2012; Thomas, Nanda, and Shu, 2012).

Not all FODMAPs will trigger symptoms for all clients. Only those that are malabsorbed are likely to be clinically significant:

- Fructans and GOS are always malabsorbed and fermented by intestinal **microflora.** This process results in gas production and associated flatulence in healthy people. With the altered gut flora, motility disorders, and hypersensitivity in IBS, the symptoms may be that much more evident.
- The remaining FODMAP carbohydrates will only induce symptoms in the proportion of clients with IBS that malabsorb them. A significant rise in breath hydrogen following ingestion of the test sugar (e.g., fructose) demonstrates poor absorption with subsequent fermentation by intestinal microflora.
  - When breath tests are undertaken, a Low FODMAP Diet can be implemented without restricting sugars the person absorbs well. This individualizes the diet and avoids unnecessary restrictions.
  - If breath testing is unavailable, a trial of a full Low FODMAP diet can be conducted. This is usually recommended for 4 to 6 weeks, after which structured rechallenges with the potentially well absorbed carbohydrates (lactose, fructose, sorbitol, and mannitol) can begin.

20-4

*C*linical *A*pplication—cont'd

Low FODMAP Diet

In a crossover trial using researcher-provided low- or high-FODMAP diets, subjects with IBS had higher levels of breath hydrogen on both diets (four times greater with the high FODMAP intake) than did healthy volunteers. In daily questionnaires, the IBS clients also reported significantly more gastrointestinal symptoms with the high-FODMAP diet compared with the one with restricted content (Ong, Mitchell, Barrett, et al, 2010).

The Low FODMAP Diet is not simple to implement correctly. Lactose is only a FODMAP in individuals with lactase insufficiency (see Chapter 9). Fructose requires an alternate method of absorption when its amount exceeds that of glucose (Marcason, 2012). Individualizing the diet is particularly important for vegetarians, who may depend on legumes for protein intake, but may also highlight to clients that they can cope with garlic as a minor ingredient or wheat products occasionally, which would

expand the nutritional composition of the diet long term. The key issue is the total FODMAPS ingested at a meal, not the individual items. Additionally, FODMAPs have prebiotic effects due to the production of short-chain fatty acids after fermentation. Therefore, all clients should be encouraged to try to reintroduce FODMAPs to a level that they can comfortably tolerate.

The low-FODMAP diet requires a registered dietitian's expertise both to maximize compliance with instigating the complete list of FODMAP sources and to avoid an overly restricted approach. The latter is of great import in the event the diet is successful and likely to be followed long term. Considerable evidence supports the efficacy of the low-FODMAP diet for IBS, suggesting that this should be the first dietary strategy tried (Barrett and Gibson, 2012).

TABLE 20-6 ■ Self-Treatment for Diarrhea*		
TIME	ORAL INTAKE	COMMENTS
First 12 hours	Water or oral hydration solutions at room temperature	Easily absorbed fluids to maintain hydration
Second 12 hours	Clear liquids, no caffeine or extremes of temperature	If up to 5% body weight lost; if more than 5% lost, seek medical attention
		Very hot, very cold, or caffeinated beverages stimulate peristalsis
Third 12 hours	Full liquids	Experiment with milk in case lactose intolerance has developed
Fourth 12 hours	Soft diet	Include applesauce or banana for pectin; rice, pasta, and bread without fat (digested by enzymes usually unaffected by gastroenteritis)
By 48th hour	Regular diet	Seek medical treatment if diarrhea has not resolved and regular diet is not tolerated. Other reasons for medical attention: dehydration, abdominal distension, fever, bloody stools.

*Appropriate for healthy adults.

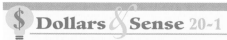
$ **Dollars** & **Sense** 20-1

Homemade Oral Rehydration Fluid Recipe

½ to 1 level teaspoon salt (should taste no saltier than tears)
6 to 8 level teaspoons sugar
5 cups (1000 mL) clean drinking water, boiled and cooled if necessary

Stir the mixture until the salt and sugar dissolve. Store in a cool place. Discard after 24 hours and replace with a new batch.

The cost is infinitesimal compared with purchased, bottled solutions, but the ingredients must be measured carefully. A weak solution is unlikely to be harmful, but one that is too strong can be hazardous.

Alternatively, a standard rehydrating sports drink, such as Gatorade, can be turned into a rehydration solution by mixing 8 ounces of the sports drink with 8 ounces of clean water and adding a ¼ teaspoon of salt. This results in a solution with roughly the same electrolyte concentration as Pedialyte.

Adapted from Lawrence, 2011; Nurse Courtney, 2012; World Gastroenterology Organization, 2012.

Medical consultation becomes important if diarrhea:

■ lasts for more than 3 days,
■ causes severe pain in the abdomen or rectum,
■ provokes a fever of 102°F or higher,
■ produces blood in the stool or black, tarry stools, or
■ is accompanied by signs of dehydration.

In addition to these concerns, if a client has medical conditions for which fasting, dehydration, or infectious disease is a hazard, a physician should be consulted.

TRAVELER'S DIARRHEA

The classic definition of traveler's diarrhea is passage of at least three unformed stools per day plus one or more signs or symptoms of an enteric infection (nausea, vomiting, fever, abdominal pain, cramps, fecal urgency). Traveler's diarrhea is a self-limited infection that affects approximately 40% of travelers to developing countries (Connor, 2013) with women more susceptible than men (Hill and Beeching, 2010).

Individuals with traveler's diarrhea experience approximately 24 hours of disability barring complications. More than 60% of traveler's diarrhea cases are caused by a variety of bacterial enteropathogens but noroviruses are also an important cause of morbidity among travelers. Rainy seasons are associated with a higher risk than dry seasons for traveler's diarrhea caused by most enteric bacterial pathogens, with the opposite true for viruses (de la Cabada Bauche and DuPont, 2011). Destination is the most significant risk factor for developing traveler's diarrhea in

- High-risk areas of South Asia, Sub-Saharan Africa, and Latin America
- Moderate-risk areas of Southeast Asia, the Middle East, Oceania, and the Caribbean (Paredes-Paredes, Flores-Figueroa, Dupont, 2011)

Other risk factors are:

- Immunocompromised states
- Lowered gastric acidity
- Genetic susceptibility (see Genomic Gem 20-1)

Traveler's diarrhea is transmitted by food and drinks contaminated with bacteria, viruses, or parasites. Overall levels of sanitation at the travel destination, including individual eating establishments, are strong predictors for contracting traveler's diarrhea (Hill and Beeching, 2010).

To minimize risk, people should avoid:

- Drinking tap water and ice made from it
- Foods washed in water and served raw
- Unpasteurized milk
- Sauces and salsas
- Uncooked seafood
- Raw or poorly cooked meats
- Foods from street vendors (especially risky)

Usually safe foods and beverages include:

- Carbonated bottled beverages (if the seal is intact)
- Food cooked and served piping hot
- Dry foods such as bread and cereal

Genomic Gem 20-1
Traveler's Diarrhea

Traditional risk factors do not explain the individual differences in susceptibility to traveler's diarrhea among visitors to developing countries. Host genetic studies have demonstrated that single nucleotide polymorphisms in the genes encoding for lactoferrin, osteoprotegerin, and interleukin-10 are associated with small but increased risks for diarrhea and enteric pathogens (Hill and Beeching, 2010).

In contrast, persons with mutations of the *FUT2* gene are immune to norovirus infection. The recognition of individual variations in susceptibility to traveler's diarrhea will aid in customizing prophylactic medication regimens and standby treatments (Cabada and White, 2008).

Between 5% and 10% of travelers with traveler's diarrhea will later develop irritable bowel syndrome. The risk of developing postinfectious IBS is five times higher in returning travelers who had traveler's diarrhea than travelers who did not, with more than 50% of the cases persisting for longer than 5 years (de la Cabada Bauche and DuPont, 2011). Many experts advise all people who travel to high-risk areas to take curative antimicrobial agents selected according to the usual contaminants in destination countries with them for self-treatment of illness. Although hygiene measures are credited with limited impact (Kollaritsch, Paulke-Korinek, and Wiedermann, 2012), thorough hand washing can't hurt if the wash water is not contaminated.

OTHER CAUSES

Diarrhea may be iatrogenic (produced by treatment) accompanying antibiotic therapy or tube feeding. In the acute hospital setting, especially critical care units, diarrhea is a common complication of enteral feeding, but in long-term care settings, constipation frequently accompanies tube feeding. Fiber can play a role in reducing stool frequency when it is high, and increasing it when it is low, thereby potentially ameliorating both diarrhea and constipation through a combination of soluble and insoluble fiber in the enteral feeding. Because of reported side effects associated with certain single fiber sources with very high or very low degrees of solubility and fermentability, experts caution against their use (Engfer, Green, and Silk, 2008).

Probiotics have accelerated recovery from acute infectious diarrhea and have prevented antibiotic-associated diarrhea (see Box 20-2). An often overlooked cause of diarrhea, celiac disease, is addressed in Chapter 9, Clinical Application 20-5, and Genomic Gem 20-2.

Constipation

Each person develops a usual bowel pattern, so that a bowel movement every day or every second or third day may be perfectly normal for a given individual. **Constipation** refers to a decrease in a person's normal frequency of defecation, especially if the stool is hard, dry, or difficult to expel. Female sex, older age, low fiber diet, a sedentary lifestyle, malnutrition, **polypharmacy**, and a lower socioeconomic status have all been identified as risk factors for constipation (Alame and Bahna, 2012). Review of National Health and Nutrition Examination Survey (**NHANES**) data on 10,914 adults revealed constipation rates of 10.2% for women and 4.0% for men. After adjusting for many variables, low liquid consumption remained a predictor of constipation for both genders in this group; however, dietary fiber intake was not a predictor (Markland, Palsson, Goode, et al, 2013).

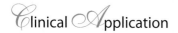

20–5

Clinical Application

Case–Finding and Diagnosis: Celiac Disease (Gluten-Sensitive Enteropathy, Nontropical Sprue)

This illness is classically diagnosed in a child who presents with **steatorrhea** after gluten-containing cereals (wheat, rye, barley) are added to the diet. Oats may be problematic because they can pick up gluten from other grains during milling.

Up to 3 million Americans have celiac disease. An analysis of the 2009–10 NHANES data of 7798 persons aged six years or older found celiac disease, diagnosed serologically or clinically, in 35 individuals, 29 of whom were unaware of the condition (Rubio-Tapia, Ludvigsson, Brantner, et al, 2012). Many adults have the disease for a decade or more before they are diagnosed (National Digestive, January 27, 2012) as personally detailed by six registered nurses who suffered or witnessed such delayed and erroneous diagnoses (McCabe, Toughill, Parkhill, et al, 2012).

The proliferation of serologic testing is likely to promote earlier diagnosis. In a Canadian study, median age at diagnosis increased from 2 years before serologic testing became available to 9 years of age after its use. The marked increase in the incidence of celiac disease between time periods was attributed to the improved detection of nonclassic presentations, particularly in older children. Although the incidence of classic celiac disease did not decrease, many children with atypical gastrointestinal presentations and those in high-risk groups with mild symptoms were identified because of serological testing. Some of the children only recognized their presenting symptoms in retrospect after a gluten-free diet alleviated them (McGowan, Castiglione, and Butzner, 2009).

At presentation:

■ Younger children are seen with diarrhea and failure to thrive. Older children are seen with short stature, anemia, neurological problems, dental enamel defects, and even constipation.
■ Adults present with anemia or are discovered through endoscopies to evaluate symptoms not suggestive of celiac disease.
■ A previous diagnosis of irritable bowel syndrome is common (Green and Jabri, 2006; Harris, 2012).
■ Prevalence of biopsy-proven celiac disease in cases meeting diagnostic criteria for IBS was more than four times of that in controls without IBS (Ford, Chey, Talley, et al, 2009).
■ Gluten sensitivity also has a skin manifestation, *dermatitis herpetiformis*. Virtually all of the individuals with this burning, itching rash have celiac disease (Semrad, 2014).

The gold standard for definitive diagnosis of celiac disease is a biopsy of the small intestine. In all cases, the client should consume a gluten-containing diet until the diagnostic testing has been completed.

Genomic Gem 20–2

Celiac Disease

The prevalence of celiac disease in the general population with no known risk factors is 1 in 133 people. In **first-degree relatives** (parent, sibling, child) of those with the disease the prevalence is 1 in 22. Genetic predisposition to celiac disease is strongly linked to genes that encode inherited human leukocyte antigen (HLA), specifically alleles HLA-DQ2 and HLA-DQ8. These alleles are found in one-third of the general population. Having either is necessary but not sufficient for disease development. Non-HLA genes are thought to play a role as well (McCabe, Toughill, Parkhill, et al, 2012).

Although about 30% to 40% of Caucasians carry the essential genetic factors, fewer than 3% develop the disease (Green and Jabri, 2006). Genetic testing is useful to exclude the diagnosis of celiac disease in individuals already following a gluten-restricted diet or when duodenal biopsy findings are equivocal and to evaluate risk in first-degree relatives of someone with celiac disease (Semrad, 2014).

Because only a few genetically susceptible individuals develop celiac disease, its etiology is considered to be multifactorial involving a combination of:

■ Genetic predisposition
■ Ingestion of gluten (see Chapter 9)

■ An autoimmune response that produces chronic inflammation of the small intestine

At present, a strict gluten-restricted diet is the only treatment. Selecting such a diet should become easier because in 2013, the FDA published the first regulation defining "gluten-free" for voluntary food labeling that covers other terms such as "no gluten," "without gluten," and "free of gluten." Such foods must contain less than 20 parts per million of gluten. Manufacturers have 1 year to bring their labels into compliance (U.S. Food and Drug Administration, August 2, 2013).

In the future, new forms of treatment may include:

■ Use of gluten-degrading enzymes to be ingested with meals,
■ Development of alternative, gluten-free grains by genetic modification,
■ Inhibitors of intestinal permeability to prevent gluten entry across the epithelium,
■ Different forms of immunotherapy,
■ Vaccination (Semrad, 2014; Setty, Hormaza, and Guandalini, 2008).

Changes in bowel habits should be investigated thoroughly to discover or rule out disease. It is important to rule out a colonic malignancy as the cause of constipation, especially in an elderly client with a dramatic change in bowel habits. Caregivers must be particularly vigilant with clients unable to communicate. A fatal bowel perforation and **peritonitis** in a client with dementia resulted from impacted feces (Craft and Prahlow, 2011).

Constipation may precede the development of somatic motor symptoms of Parkinson disease by several years (Cersosimo and Benarroch, 2012). Other early gastrointestinal symptoms of Parkinson disease are dysphagia and delayed gastric emptying (Rayner and Horowitz, 2013).

Medications that commonly cause constipation include:

■ Opiates
■ Aluminum- or calcium-containing antacids
■ Anticholinergic agents
■ Antidepressants
■ Antiemetics
■ Calcium channel blockers
■ Diuretics
■ Iron and calcium supplements
■ NSAIDs
■ Sympathomimetics
■ Tricyclic antidepressants (Alame and Bahna, 2012).

After disease conditions causing constipation have been ruled out, a search for deficits in the following areas may suggest some of these changes:

■ Gradually increase dietary fiber (see Clinical Calculation 20-1).

■ Drink adequate water.
■ Exercise regularly.
■ Have a warm drink with breakfast.
■ Evacuate at a regular time (usually after a meal to take advantage of the body's programming).

When dietary interventions and lifestyle modifications fail, further testing may be warranted. The many possible causes contributing to constipation include mechanical, metabolic, neurologic, and muscular pathologies (Alame and Bahna, 2012). In some cases of fecal impaction, the client may experience diarrhea. Clinical Application 20-6 explains this paradox.

Inflammatory Bowel Diseases (IBDs)

Normally, the immune cells protect the body from infection. In people with IBD, however, because the immune system mistakes food, bacteria, and other materials in the intestine for foreign substances, it attacks the cells of the intestines. In the process, the body sends white blood cells into the lining of the intestines where they produce chronic inflammation and a cascade of nutritional effects.

IBDs are complex, multifactorial disorders in which the body loses its tolerance to its own gut microorganisms. The gut has many tiers of defense against incursion by luminal microbes, including the epithelial barrier, and the innate and adaptive immune responses. These components are all tightly interrelated, and to develop disease requires breakdown at several checkpoints (Cho and Brant, 2011).

An estimated 1.4 million persons in the United States have IBD. The peak age at onset is 15 to 30 years,

20-1

Clinical Calculation

Constipation and Fiber Intake

Achieving the recommended fiber intake of 21 to 38 grams per day is a matter of prudent choices at every meal. Listed below are examples of high fiber foods on the left and foods in the same category on the right with less fiber.

HIGHER FIBER FOODS	GRAMS OF FIBER	LOWER FIBER FOODS	GRAMS OF FIBER
Breakfast			
All-bran buds, ⅓ cup	13	Corn flakes, 1 cup	1
Orange sections, 1 cup	4	Orange juice from frozen concentrate, 1 cup	0
Lunch			
Wendy's chili, small	5	Campbell's microwavable chicken noodle soup, 1 cup	2
Raw apple with skin, 2 ¾" diameter	4	Raw apple peeled, 2 ¾" diameter	2
Dinner			
Whole wheat spaghetti, 1 cup cooked	6	White spaghetti, 1 cup cooked	3
Banana, 1 cup sliced	4	Watermelon 1 cup diced	1
Totals	**36**		**9**

Many other foods also contribute to fiber intake and can be evaluated via labels or at http://ndb.nal.usda.gov or http://nutritiondata.self.com. Individuals who wish to correct constipation without medications should determine their present fiber intake and increase it gradually to the Recommended Dietary Allowance while also drinking *sufficient water.*

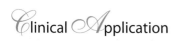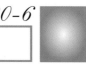

Clinical Application 20-6

Distinguishing Diarrhea From Fecal Impaction

If a client usually is constipated and then has diarrhea, the nurse should check the rectum for impacted stool. The stool will be dry and hard and the client will not be able to pass it unassisted. The diarrheal stool is passed around the impaction.

As in many cases, prevention is preferable to diagnosis and treatment. Institutionalized clients should be monitored for elimination problems. Frequency and consistency of bowel movements should be charted and appropriate interventions implemented before impaction results.

although IBD may occur at any age (Centers for Disease Control and Prevention [CDC], July 15, 2011). The incidence of IBD continues to rise, both in low- and in high-incidence areas. Also, increased incidence among migrants from low-incidence to high-incidence areas within the same generation suggests a strong environmental influence (Latella, Fiocchi, and Caprili, 2010).

The two most common IBDs are **Crohn disease (CD),** also known as *ileitis* or *regional enteritis*, and **ulcerative colitis.** The two diseases share some similar characteristics but also have major differences (see Tables 20-7 and 20-8).

TABLE 20-7 ■ Similarities Between Crohn Disease and Ulcerative Colitis

Etiology	Loss of tolerance to intestinal bacteria
Theories	Autoimmune interaction of genetic susceptibility and environment
Familial links	Between 5% and 16% of IBD clients have a **first-degree relative** with IBD (Halme, Paavola-Sakki, Turunen, et al, 2006). See Genomic Gem 20-3.
Contributing dietary factors	Increased animal protein intake strongest influence Refined sugars, fatty foods, fast foods Diet likely influences susceptibility but dietary interventions inadequate to reverse disease
Geographic factors	Higher frequency in urban communities compared with rural areas Decreased disease in southern latitudes presumably related to vitamin D (Jussila, Virta, Salomaa, et al, 2012; Khalili, Huang, Ananthakrishnan, et al, 2012; see Chapter 6 for other connections)
Signs and symptoms	Diarrhea, abdominal pain Weight loss Decreased bone mineral density
Associated conditions	Arthritis, joint pain Eye irritation Kidney stones Liver disease

TABLE 20-8 ■ Differences Between Crohn Disease (CD) and Ulcerative Colitis (UC)

	CD	UC
Location	Anywhere in gastrointestinal tract, most often terminal ileum	Large intestine
Distribution	Diseased areas alternate with healthy tissue	Usually starts in rectum and spreads upward in continuous pattern
Lesions	Involves all layers of intestinal wall	Confined to mucosal and submucosal layers
Associated Conditions*	Problems with skin Gallstones	Osteoporosis Colon cancer if entire colon affected over 8 to 10 years
Environmental Factors	Associated with smoking No strong association between childhood passive smoke exposure and the development of CD	Associated with nonsmoking (see Box 20-3 for possible pathophysiology) Sibling pairs discordant for both smoking and IBD subtype almost always show CD in the smoking and UC in the nonsmoking mate (Halme et al, 2006) No evidence for childhood passive smoke exposure protecting against ulcerative colitis
Nutrient Deficiencies in >50% of Clients	Folate Vitamin D	Iron
Complications	Blockage of the intestine due to swelling and scar tissue (most common) Fistulas, abscesses	Toxic megacolon
Prognosis After Surgery	Disease recurs†	Cured

*Uncertain pathophysiology; may be result of inflammation.
†Postoperative maintenance is disappointing. Smoking cessation is the only effective measure.
Sources: Centers for Disease Control and Prevention, July 15, 2011; Dryden and Seidner, 2014; Jones, Osterman, Bewtra, and Lewis, 2008; NDDIC, January 18, 2011 and November 15, 2011.

The concept of "bowel rest" has been abandoned, and IBD patients are now advised to eat a diet as unrestricted as possible. Likewise, avoiding every food that causes an upset is unwise (Cabré and Domènech, 2012). General goals for nutritional care of IBD clients include the following:

- The prevention and correction of malnutrition through screening and monitoring
- The prevention of osteoporosis
- In children, the promotion of optimal growth and development

Specific actions to achieve those goals include the following:

- Avoiding foods that clearly worsen symptoms
- Taking small, frequent meals

Genomic Gem 20-3
Inflammatory Bowel Disease

Genome-wide association studies account for 23% of the heritability in Crohn disease (CD) and 16% in ulcerative colitis. More than 50% of inflammatory bowel disease (IBD) susceptibility **loci** have also been associated with other inflammatory and autoimmune diseases (Khor, Gardet, and Xavier, 2011), with as many as 14 susceptibility loci shared between IBD and celiac disease (Cho and Brant, 2011). Approximately 30% of IBD-related genetic loci are shared between CD and ulcerative colitis, indicating that these diseases engage common pathways and may be part of a mechanistic continuum (Khor, Gardet, and Xavier, 2011).

If a disease is entirely due to genes, its concordance in identical (*monozygotic*) twins would approach 100% and that in nonidentical (*dizygotic*) twins 50%. If, on the other hand, the disease is fully dependent on extrinsic and acquired factors, then its concordance would be similar in both types of twins (Halme et al, 2006). Identical twins more often have IBD, especially CD, than do fraternal twins. The concordance rate in monozygotic twins of 30% to 35% in CD compared with 10% to 15% in ulcerative colitis suggests that nongenetic factors may have a more important role in ulcerative colitis than in CD (Khor et al, 2011).

For both CD and ulcerative colitis:

1. Genetic mutation encodes susceptibility. More than 70 loci have been identified for Crohn disease.
2. A trigger initiates inflammation (see below and Box 20-3).
3. Intolerance to normal gut microorganisms develops.

One gene involved in CD encodes for a bacterial defense peptide expressed in ileal mucosa, the site most affected in CD (Dryden and Seidner, 2014). Another identified inherited defect found in clients with CD is a mutation of a gene on chromosome 16, which results in abnormal chronic inflammation in response to bacteria such as *Escherichia coli* in the digestive tract (Thomas and Greer, 2010).

One suggested trigger is dietary change, specifically adoption of the Western diet. IBD cases in Japan have increased significantly over the past 3 decades with total kilocalories from fat and animal protein displacing those from rice. Refined sugars, fatty foods, and fast foods all enhance development of CD and ulcerative colitis (Dryden and Seidner, 2014). Among sources of animal protein, high consumption of meat or fish but not of eggs or dairy products was associated with IBD risk in French middle-aged women (Jantchou, Morois, Clavel-Chapelon, et al, 2010).

Box 20-3 ■ *Possible Explanation for Smoking's Relation to Ulcerative Colitis*

Smoking cigarettes protects against ulcerative colitis, improves its course after disease onset, and reduces its extent, even in the presence of mutant alleles (Manolakis, Kapsoritakis, Kapsoritaki, et al, 2013). Smokers who quit the habit experienced an increase in disease activity, hospital admissions, and the need for major medical therapy (oral steroids, immunosuppressants) within the first years following smoking cessation. Most large and recent studies show smoking decreases risk of colectomy in ulcerative colitis clients (Bastida and Beltrán, 2011).

Introducing nicotine to clients with ulcerative colitis, however, has not brought the positive results anticipated (Bernstein, 2010), which may relate to the mode of delivery. Nicotine is rapidly and extensively metabolized, primarily in the liver via the cytochrome P450 enzyme pathway. When nicotine is ingested orally, bioavailability is low (20% to 44%). Topical administration of nicotine directly into the colon by enema or delayed release oral capsule formulations decrease the systemic absorption and side effects of the drug and may be clinically beneficial (Bastida and Beltrán, 2011).

One mechanism suggested in explaining the influence of smoking on ulcerative colitis relates to the disposal of hydrogen sulfide that is produced by colonic bacteria. Hydrogen sulfide is increased in the feces of ulcerative colitis clients. Cysteine and methionine,

sulfur-containing amino acids, function as substrates for hydrogen sulfide production by colonic bacteria (Rowan, Docherty, Coffey, and O'Connell, 2009). If not rapidly detoxified, hydrogen sulfide would be expected to damage the intestinal mucosa.

The main product of hydrogen sulfide metabolism by the colonic mucosa is thiosulfate (Blachier, Davila, Mimoun, et al, 2010). Investigation using rat cecum mucosa, demonstrated the influence of cyanide (found in higher concentrations in the serum of cigarette smokers than in nonsmokers) on the metabolism of hydrogen sulfide. In the presence of cyanide, the major metabolite of sulfide metabolism was thiocyanate rather than thiosulfate (Wilson, Mudra, Furne, and Levitt, 2008). Therefore, the protection afforded in ulcerative colitis clients by smoking may be achieved by cyanide diverting hydrogen sulfide toward an inert compound (Rowan et al, 2009).

Some authors reported a worsening in clinical outcomes among ulcerative colitis clients who quit smoking, whereas improvement of disease activity occurred in ex-smokers who resumed the habit (Cabré and Domènech, 2012). Of 15 clients with refractory disease who resumed "low-dose" smoking, 14 were able to maintain prolonged clinical remission off steroids (Calabrese, Yanai, Shuster, et al, 2012).

- Drinking adequate fluids
- Avoiding caffeine and alcohol
- Taking vitamin/mineral supplements
- Eliminating dairy foods if lactose intolerant
- Limiting excess fat
- Reducing carbohydrates and high-fiber foods during flares (Brown, Rampertab, and Mullin, 2011)

Box 20-4 provides some facts about IBD in children. Table 20-9 lists general uses of nutritional modalities for IBD.

Nutritional Therapy

Beyond general goals, the nutritional care of clients with IBD must be individualized according to the nutritional

Box 20-4 ■ *Inflammatory Bowel Diseases in Children*

About 10% of IBD cases occur in individuals younger than 18 years (Centers for Disease Control, July 15, 2011). Investigation of growth retardation should consider an IBD etiology because the Crohn disease is typically heralded by an unexplained slowing of linear growth before the diagnosis is established (Cooper, Mones, and Heird, 2014). Growth failure is common at presentation in Crohn disease but less common in ulcerative colitis. Consequences of poor nutrition and prolonged corticosteroid use result in a significant reduction in final adult height of almost 1 in 5 children (Heuschkel, Salvestrini, Beattie, et al, 2008).

Treatment with enteral formulas is effective in restoring growth. Children treated with exclusive enteral nutrition have better growth velocity than those treated with glucocorticoids (Ezri, Marques-Vidal, and Nydegger, 2012). Restoration and maintenance of pre-illness growth pattern indicate successful therapy (Griffiths, 2009).

TABLE 20-9 ■ Nutritional Care in Inflammatory Bowel Disease

	CROHN DISEASE	ULCERATIVE COLITIS
Oral Intake	Following exacerbation: low-fat, low-fiber, high-protein, high-kilocalorie in small frequent feedings Progress to normal diet as tolerated Avoid foods high in **oxalate** (see Chapter 6)	As unrestricted and balanced as possible
Enteral Feeding By mouth or feeding tube	Primary therapy in active disease and in children with impaired growth As effective as steroids in inducing remission in children	Not proven as primary therapy or for maintenance
Parenteral Nutrition Evidence-based guidelines do not recommend as primary treatment	Induces remission effectively but rarely maintains it In chronic disease, for clients with a very short gut, prolonged ileus or obstruction, or anastomotic fistulas	Lower remission rates than in Crohn disease Maintenance rates of <15%
Probiotics	Little evidence of benefit	Certain strains may be beneficial

Sources: Academy of Nutrition and Dietetics, 2012c; Alastair, Emma, and Emma, 2011; Cabré and Domènech, 2012; Dryden and Seidner, 2014.

status of the individual, the location and extent of the disease, and the surgical and medical treatments. Although certain food choices enhance risk of IBD, elimination of individual food items will not likely alter the course of the disease (Dryden and Seidner, 2014). To maintain nutritional status, foods should not be eliminated from the diet without a fair trial. Restrictions should be limited to foods that produce gas or loose stools. Suspected foods should be tried in small amounts to determine tolerance levels.

CROHN DISEASE

Tolerances and intolerances to food vary among clients. Researchers could not ascertain specific foods that should be avoided by all CD patients. In fact, for a number of the items, the same food that was beneficial for one group of subjects was detrimental to others (Triggs, Munday, Hu, et al, 2010).

Two interventions might prove helpful:

- A food-symptom diary followed by a customized elimination diet for 2 to 4 weeks (Brown and Roy, 2010)
- A semivegetarian diet (Chiba, Abe, Tsuda, et al, 2010) (see Box 20-5)

ULCERATIVE COLITIS

Dietary modification is usually based on client tolerance and avoidance of irritating foods. Because ulcerative colitis is a complex, multifactorial disease, no single cause or single intervention holds the key to management. Box 20-6 describes one aspect of metabolism in the gut relating to ulcerative colitis pathophysiology, which might eventually have an impact on management of the disease.

Surgical Treatment

Surgery may be recommended when IBD becomes medically unmanageable. The portion of the bowel that is inflamed can be surgically resected but may cause major nutritional complications.

ILEOSTOMY

In an **ileostomy,** the end of the remaining portion of the small intestine (the **ileum**) is attached to a surgically

Box 20-5 ■ *Semivegetarian Diet for Crohn Disease*

This diet was designed to increase the number of beneficial bacteria in the bowel. Foods known to increase beneficial bacteria include green tea and unrefined brown rice. Because most prebiotics are plant-based, a vegetarian diet served as the basis for the intervention.

Elements of the diet include:

- A basic lacto-ovo-vegetarian diet
- Fish once a week, half-size serving
- Meat once every 2 weeks, half-size serving
- Eating between meals discouraged
- Green tea encouraged
- No food item prohibited

The diet was complementary to and did not supplant medical treatment. A small 2-year study demonstrated the semivegetarian diet to be significantly better than an omnivorous diet in preventing relapse in Crohn disease. Under the semivegetarian diet, remission was maintained at 100% at 1 year and 92% at 2 years (Chiba, Abe, Tsuda, et al, 2010).

Box 20-6 ■ *Colonic Sulfur Metabolism in Ulcerative Colitis*

Aside from the broad causality of the Western diet, an interesting approach distinguishing ulcerative colitis from Crohn disease concerns sulfur metabolism in the large intestine. Hydrogen sulfide is the sulfur derivative that has attracted the most attention in the context of colonic health but whether it is detrimental or beneficial remains in debate. It is the most generally suspected sulfated compound in the etiology of colonic disorders and inflammation. Hydrogen sulfide is among the most hazardous gases in industrial applications, exhibiting toxicity to different organs at low concentrations, with increasing concentrations being fatal. There is ample evidence that hydrogen sulfide at physiological concentrations is genotoxic and induces DNA damage as well as inflammatory responses (Carbonero, Benefiel, Alizadeh-Ghamsari, and Gaskins, 2012).

Several lines of evidence point to sulfur-reducing bacteria or exogenous hydrogen sulfide as potential players in the etiology of intestinal disorders, especially inflammatory bowel diseases and colorectal cancer. Sulfated compounds in the colon are either inorganic (e.g., sulfates, sulfites) or organic (e.g., host mucins and the dietary amino acids methionine and cysteine). Studies using human feces indicate that organic sulfur-containing compounds provide a more efficient source for sulfide production than inorganic sulfate, with meat being a particularly important source. Elevated concentrations of cysteine are found in red meat, eggs, and milk (Carbonero et al, 2012).

Given that most of the colonic disorders for which a potential pathogenic role for sulfide exists are gene–environment disorders,

it is logical to envision how common polymorphisms in host genes encoding components of the sulfide oxidation pathway might underlie ineffective epithelial sulfide detoxification and thereby predispose certain individuals to chronic sulfide-generated inflammation or genotoxicity (Carbonero et al, 2012).

Food sources of inorganic sulfate include commercial breads, dried fruits, vegetables, nuts, fermented beverages, and brassica vegetables (Carbonero et al, 2012). Between 2.8 and 2.6 times the risk of relapse from remission in ulcerative colitis has been linked to intakes of high sulfur or sulfate intakes (Jowett, Seal, Pierce, et al, 2004). A suggested mechanism relates to colonic bacteria producing hydrogen sulfide from sulfur-containing amino acids (Tilg and Kaser, 2004) as well as intake of foods containing sulfite as a preservative (Magee, Edmond, Tasker, et al, 2005). Clients with ulcerative colitis showed a fundamental difference in gut sulfide metabolism compared with those without that diagnosis (Ohge, Furne, Springfield, et al, 2005) and evidence implicates sulfate-reducing bacteria as an environmental factor in ulcerative colitis (Rowan, Docherty, Coffey, and O'Connell, 2009).

The extent to which these mechanisms unfold in clients with ulcerative colitis remains to be clarified. Understanding the exact nature of hydrogen sulfide's interactions with the colon makes pharmacological modulation of its production and metabolism potential targets for treatment of a multitude of colonic conditions in the future (Medani, Collins, Docherty, et al, 2011). Box 20-3 details another slant on hydrogen sulfide metabolism related to ulcerative colitis.

---

established opening in the abdominal wall called a **stoma,** from which the intestinal contents are discharged. This results in a shorter gut that may create additional nutritional hazards for the client (Clinical Application 20-7).

An ileostomy produces liquid drainage containing active enzymes that irritate the skin. In addition, nutrient losses are great. A loss of as much as 2 liters of fluid per day immediately after surgery is possible. Over time, the bowel adapts to some extent, and drainage decreases to 300 to 500 milliliters. This amount, however, is more than the 100 to 200 milliliters of water lost in the normal stool. In addition to fluid and electrolyte losses, ileostomy clients have decreased fat, bile acid, and vitamin B_{12} absorption. Clinical Application 20-8 describes innovations for controlling ileostomy drainage.

20-7

Clinical Application

Short Bowel Syndrome

The small intestine is approximately 20 feet long and may be resected for Crohn disease as well as for obstructions, tumors, and traumatic injuries. Short bowel syndrome is malabsorption resulting from extensive resection of the small bowel, usually the loss of more than two-thirds of its length. The location of the missing bowel is significant:

- Following jejunal resection, the ileum adapts by increasing the length and absorptive function of its villi permitting gradual improvement of nutrient absorption, a process that may take 2 years.
- If the ileum is resected, its function of bile acid and vitamin B_{12} absorption cannot be replaced by the remaining bowel.

Immediately after surgery, diarrhea is typically severe, with significant electrolyte losses requiring parenteral nutrition and intensive

monitoring of fluid and electrolytes. As clients recover, enteral nutrition should be reintroduced as soon as possible to enhance intestinal adaptation. Nutritional treatment of short bowel syndrome is intensive and requires ongoing consultation with an expert dietitian. Typically, clients with

- more than 1 meter of remaining jejunum may survive on small low carbohydrate feedings that are high in fat and protein
- less than 100 centimeters of remaining jejunum and those with excessive fluid and electrolyte losses require lifelong parenteral nutrition (Ruiz, 2012).

Vitamin and mineral status is watched carefully. Among the interventions are special preparations of fat-soluble vitamins and of magnesium without diarrheal side effects (Jeejeebhoy, 2014).

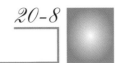

Clinical Application 20-8

Continent Ileostomies

Ordinarily if an ileostomy is performed, the client must wear an appliance to contain the drainage. Other procedures afford a measure of control of the drainage.

Continent ileostomies sometimes can be constructed from the remaining intestine, creating an intestinal reservoir or pouch just inside the abdominal wall. The pouch is emptied by inserting a catheter into the stoma several times a day.

Sometimes an ileoanal anastomosis is done so that the anal sphincter can be used to control elimination. Even after the bowel adapts to its shorter length, the client has 7 to 10 bowel movements per day.

It is important for all health-care providers to know which procedure has been performed so that the surgeon's and client's expectations can be reinforced when teaching the client.

COLOSTOMY

A **colectomy** is the surgical removal of part or all of the colon. Depending on the pathology, the surgeon may connect the remaining bowel to allow evacuation through the anus or make an artificial opening in the abdominal wall to allow the passage of waste. In a **colostomy,** a part of the large intestine is resected, and a stoma is created in the abdominal wall. Clients who have surgery to divert intestinal contents through the abdominal wall often suffer psychological trauma in addition to the physical change.

In contrast to an ileostomy, a colostomy after the convalescent period may be so continent that a dry dressing is all that is necessary to cover the stoma. The client may do daily irrigations or not, as the surgeon suggests. Sometimes, after the initial learning process, the client knows best.

DIETARY GUIDELINES FOR OSTOMY CLIENTS

A soft or general diet is usually served to ostomy clients after recovery from surgery with restrictions based on individual tolerance. Stringy, high-fiber foods are initially avoided until a definite tolerance has been demonstrated and then are best tried in small amounts one at a time. Stringy, high-fiber foods include:

■ Celery, corn, cabbage, coleslaw, peas, sauerkraut, spinach
■ Coconut, dried fruit, membranes on citrus fruits, pineapple
■ Popcorn, nuts, seeds, and skins of fruits and vegetables.

In addition, some clients avoid **cruciferous** vegetables, beans, fish, eggs, beer, and carbonated beverages because they produce excessive odor or gas. Certain

foods may be therapeutic because they thicken the stool: applesauce, banana, cheese, creamy peanut butter, pasta, white bread, and white rice.

Clients with ostomies should be encouraged to:

■ Eat at regular intervals.
■ Chew food well to avoid blockage at the stoma site.
■ Drink adequate amounts of fluid.
■ Avoid foods that produce excessive gas, loose stools, offensive odors, or undesirable bulk.
■ Avoid excessive weight gain that will affect the stoma.

Diverticular Disease

A **diverticulum** (plural: diverticula) is an outpouching of intestinal membrane through a weakness in the intestine's muscular layer, chiefly in the colon (Fig. 20-5). Once thought to be a condition nearly confined to the elderly, rates of hospitalization in the United States between 1998 and 2005 for acute diverticulitis increased most rapidly for 18- to 44-year-old clients (Etzioni, Mack, Beart, and Kaiser, 2009).

Of environmental factors contributing to diverticular disease, dietary fiber deficiency has received the most attention, although data are limited and conflicting. Whether a deficiency is causative or not, fiber may improve symptoms and decrease complications. Other dietary factors that may increase risk of diverticular disease are:

■ Red meat intake
■ Obesity
■ Alcohol consumption (Strate, 2012)

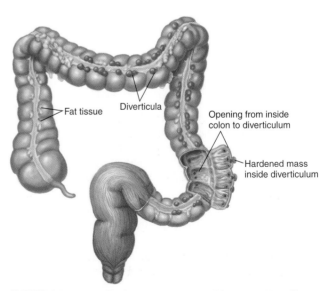

FIGURE 20-5 Diverticula of the colon. (Reprinted from Venes, D [ed.]: *Taber's cyclopedic medical dictionary*, 22nd ed. FA Davis, Philadelphia, 2013, p. 715, with permission.)

Contrary to a long-standing belief, avoidance of seeds and nuts to reduce risk is not supported by the literature. A large cohort study of 47,000 male health professionals followed over an 18-year period found no association between a diet high in corn, seeds, or nuts and subsequent risk of developing diverticulitis (Weizman and Nguyen, 2011). Individual clients however, may dispute the reports in the literature, steadfastly maintaining those foods increase symptoms and choosing to avoid them.

Diverticulosis

The presence of diverticula is called **diverticulosis.** A common location is the point at which a blood vessel enters the intestinal muscle. A proposed causative factor in diverticulosis is the increased force needed to propel insufficient intestinal contents through the lumen.

Frequently a person with diverticulosis has no signs or symptoms. After a diagnosis of diverticulosis, a high-fiber diet of 30 grams per day is advised. This should be accompanied by an adequate fluid intake.

Diverticulitis

When diverticula become inflamed, the condition is termed diverticulitis. An endoscopic view is shown in Figure 20-6. These clients typically present with left lower quadrant pain, fever, and elevated white blood count. The diagnosis is confirmed on computed tomography scan (Weizman and Nguyen, 2011).

Initial therapy for uncomplicated diverticulitis is supportive, including monitoring, bowel rest, and antibiotics. Diet is advanced through clear liquids, soft, and general menus as the client's condition improves. After that, a high-fiber diet as for diverticulosis is prescribed. Clients should receive detailed instructions on the incorporation of fiber into the diet after they have followed a low-fiber diet. Fiber should be reintroduced gradually

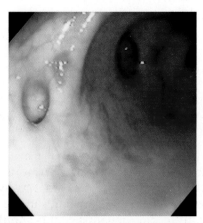

FIGURE 20-6 Diverticulitis, seen endoscopically. (Reprinted from Venes, D [ed.]: *Taber's cyclopedic medical dictionary*, 22nd ed. FA Davis, Philadelphia, 2013, p. 715, with permission.)

to avoid the abdominal cramping, bloating, and gas pains that can occur with drastic changes in fiber intake.

Diseases of the Liver

Some of the many functions of the liver are listed in Table 20-1. Major liver diseases, hepatitis and cirrhosis, often require careful nutritional management as part of a complex treatment regimen.

Hepatitis

Inflammation of the liver, or **hepatitis,** can result from viral infections, alcohol, drugs, or toxins. Acetaminophen poisoning accounts for approximately 50% of acute liver failure cases in the United States and Great Britain (Hinson, Roberts, and James, 2010). The overdose may be a deliberate suicide attempt or accidental, sometimes involving multiple drugs containing acetaminophen. Other hepatotoxic substances including alcohol contribute additively to the risk of acetaminophen toxicity (Vallerand, Sanoski, and Deglin, 2013).

Viral hepatitis is caused by infection with any of at least five distinct viruses: hepatitis A virus (HAV), hepatitis B virus (HBV), hepatitis C virus (HCV), hepatitis D virus (HDV), and hepatitis E virus (HEV). Most viral hepatitis infections in the United States are attributable to HAV, HBV, and HCV (CDC, June 5, 2012). Table 20-10 compares those three types by mode of transmission, high-risk populations, and vaccine availability.

Notable epidemics involved:

■ Hepatitis A, transmitted by green onions, infected 601 persons, of whom three died. One gravely ill client survived after a liver transplant (Wheeler, Vogt, Armstrong, et al, 2005). A smaller outbreak was attributed to sushi bars in Japan (Tekeuchi, Kobayashi, Matui, 2006). Hepatitis A is also discussed in Chapter 13.

■ Acute hepatitis B, diagnosed in 31 residents of four assisted living facilities in Virginia, was traced to infection control lapses while performing assisted monitoring of blood glucose (CDC, May 18, 2012). Similar breaks in procedure were identified in North Carolina, where all eight residents of an assisted living facility who contracted acute hepatitis B (and six of them died of hepatitis complications) were assisted in blood glucose monitoring by staff, whereas none of the residents performing their own glucose monitoring were infected (CDC, February 18, 2011).

■ Hepatitis C infections occurred in two clients about 6 months after they received transplanted kidneys from the same deceased donor (CDC, December 23, 2011).

TABLE 20-10 ■ Common Types of Viral Hepatitis		
	HEPATITIS A	**HEPATITIS B**	**HEPATITIS C***
Cases of Chronic Disease	Usually complete recovery	About 1.2 million Americans have chronic hepatitis b, 50% of asian descent About ⅔ unaware of status	About 3.2 million Americans have chronic hepatitis c
Usual Mode of Transmission	Fecal–oral: contaminated water, shellfish, raw produce Rarely, blood products, parenteral equipment	Body fluids Rare—transplanted organs Inanimate objects contaminated with body fluids including medical equipment, razors, toothbrushes, acupuncture and tattoo needles Virus is stable on environmental surfaces at least 7 days	Parenteral equipment: medical, religious, recreational Rarely: sexual contact, perinatal transmission, transplanted organs
High-Risk Populations	Household and sexual contacts of acute cases Contacts with diapered children in day care Travelers to areas with endemic disease Men who have sex with men Injecting drug users	Household and sexual contacts of infected persons, including perinatal Injecting drug users Heterosexuals with multiple partners Men who have sex with men Long-term international travelers in close contact with local people Health-care and public-safety workers exposed to blood in their work Hemodialysis clients Assisted living residents receiving assistance with blood glucose monitoring if aseptic technique not followed	Individuals who share injecting equipment Health-care workers using parenteral equipment (needle-stick accidents) HIV-infected men who have sex with men
Vaccine	Yes, if at least 12 months of age Routine vaccination recommended in all 50 states	Yes, universal vaccination of infants beginning at birth Screening of pregnant women; immunoprophylaxis to infants born to infected women; those of unknown infection status Vaccination of previously unvaccinated children, adolescents, organ transplant recipients Vaccination of high-risk adults Effective at least 15 years; booster not recommended	No; the 6 genotypes and approximately 100 subtypes of the virus impede development of effective vaccines

*Most common bloodborne infection in United States.
Adapted from Centers for Disease Control and Prevention, February 18, 2011, July 19, 2011, July 22, 2011, August 19, 2011, December 23, 2011, May 18, 2012, June 5, 2012; Heymann, 2008; Kim, 2011; London, 2011; Sanyal, Mullen, and Bass, 2010; Vallerand, et al, 2013.

Signs and Symptoms

Regardless of type or cause, symptoms are:

- Anorexia
- Nausea
- Epigastric discomfort
- Fatigue
- Weakness

Signs of hepatitis are vomiting, diarrhea, and jaundice caused by the inability of the liver to convert fat-soluble bilirubin to a water-soluble (conjugated) form. The degree of jaundice gives a rough estimate of the severity of the disease. Physical examination shows an enlarged and tender liver and an enlarged spleen.

Treatment

No current medications can cure hepatitis, but combinations of interferon and antiviral drugs are used to modify its course. The medications have significant side effects that require careful monitoring (Heyman, 2008). Therefore, the cornerstones of treatment are:

- Bed rest
- Abstinence from alcohol and other substances toxic to the liver
- Optimum nutrition to permit the liver to heal

Convalescence may take from 3 weeks to 3 months. Clients on bed rest, especially debilitated clients with hepatitis, are more susceptible to **pressure ulcers** than the average client because of decreased synthesis of albumin and the globulins. If the client abstains from alcohol, the hepatitis is often reversible. Full recovery is measured by the return of liver function tests to normal and may take more than a year.

Nutritional Care

A high-kilocalorie, high-protein, moderate-fat diet is frequently prescribed for hepatitis clients:

- Up to 400 grams of carbohydrate provides energy intake
- Up to 100 grams of protein promotes healing
- Up to 35% of kilocalories in fat utilizes a dense energy source; emulsified fats in dairy products and eggs may be better tolerated than other fats
- Up to 3 to 3.5 liters of fluid intake per day

Coaxing a person with hepatitis to accept such a substantial meal pattern is an enormous task because of the anorexia and nausea that typify the disease. Because the nausea is often less in the morning than later in the day, hepatitis clients should be encouraged to eat a big breakfast. **Standard (polymeric)** oral feedings that are high in kilocalories and protein may be prescribed for between-meal feedings (see Chapter 14).

Cirrhosis of the Liver

Cirrhosis of the liver is the twelfth leading cause of death in the United States, responsible for more than 27,000 deaths each year. The most common causes of cirrhosis are alcoholism and chronic viral hepatitis. The only treatment for end-stage liver disease that affects survival is liver transplantation (Sanyal, Mullen, and Bass, 2010).

In **cirrhosis,** the liver becomes scarred and ineffective at regeneration. The major nutritional effects of alcoholism are summarized in Clinical Application 20-9, and its connection to mortality is described in Clinical Application 20-11.

Several barriers interfere with alcoholism case–finding:

- Alcoholism's multiple and varied manifestations
- The health-care provider's personal definition of alcoholism
- Denial by the client and family

Clinical Application 20-12 shows two brief, effective screening tools to identify possible alcohol misusers. In more than 250,000 veterans surveyed by mail, brief alcohol screening questionnaires predicted hospitalizations for alcohol-related gastrointestinal conditions within the follow-up times of 2 to 3.75 years (Au, Kivlahan, Bryson, et al, 2007; Lembke, Bradley, Henderson, et al, 2011). Such specific information might be useful in counseling clients. Regardless of the tool or free-form used, health-care providers should assess lifestyle factors that contribute to illness and note should be made of the client's definition of a drink which may not match that of a **standard drink.**

Although not the only factor involved, genetics seems to contribute to the way in which alcoholic liver disease progresses (see Genomic Gem 20-4).

Pathophysiology

Alcohol needs no digestion. It is absorbed rapidly, 20% from the stomach and 80% from the small intestine. Immediately after absorption, alcohol is carried throughout the body. In the liver, which is subjected to higher concentrations than other organs, it is metabolized at the rate of ½ ounce of alcohol per hour. This refers to the alcohol content, not the whole beverage. This rate cannot be rushed, and giving coffee or other stimulants to an inebriated person induces not sobriety but merely alert intoxication.

If the liver is not able to repair the damage caused by alcohol, dying liver cells are replaced by scar tissue. Figure 20-7 traces the path from cell death to several

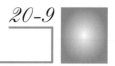

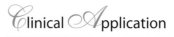

20-9

Clinical Application

Nutritional Effects of Alcoholism

Alcoholism is a disease of alcohol consumption that produces tolerance, physical dependence, and characteristic organ pathology in the body. Associating the numerous functions of the liver (Table 20-1) with the facts that (1) the liver is the main organ for ethanol metabolism and (2) alcohol is toxic to all body cells, including those of the gastrointestinal tract, the nutritional havoc accompanying alcoholism becomes obvious. In addition, persons with alcoholism take up to 50% of their daily kilocalories as ethanol resulting in a high rate of nutritional deficiencies (Beier, Landes, Mohammad, and McClain, 2014).

Thiamin deficiency almost always accompanies alcoholism. It can be caused by

- Inadequate intake
- Decreased hepatic storage
- Impairment of intestinal absorption (Beier, Landes, Mohammad, and McClain, 2014).

See Chapter 6 for information on beriberi. Wernicke–Korsakoff syndrome (Clinical Application 20-10) is a neurological complication of thiamin deficiency.

These are examples of other vitamin deficiencies associated with alcoholism:

- Vitamin A at all stages of the disease; caution is urged with supplements that can cause hepatotoxicity (Beier et al, 2014; Xerophthalmia secondary to alcoholic malnutrition was diagnosed in a 47-year-old man who complained of diminished night vision; Roncone, 2006)
- Vitamin D from several causes including impaired metabolism by the liver
- Riboflavin, which may be related to skin and mucous membrane abnormalities (Beier et al, 2014)

Also associated with alcoholism are deficiencies of these minerals:

- Magnesium, which is increasingly excreted even after moderate alcohol intake
- Zinc that may contribute to poor wound healing or liver regeneration, skin lesions, and altered mental status
- Selenium that correlates with the severity of liver disease (Beier et al, 2014; see refeeding syndrome in Chapter 22.)

Awareness of the wide range of nutritional effects of alcoholism should stimulate case–finding. Interruption of the downward spiral in health caused by alcohol can literally be lifesaving.

cardinal signs of cirrhosis. Because the liver has multiple functions, one pathological change reinforces another. The most common complications include portal hypertension, esophageal varices, and hepatic encephalopathy (Sanyal, Mullen, and Bass, 2010).

The signs and symptoms of cirrhosis appear in Box 20-7. Esophageal varices occur in approximately one-half the clients with cirrhosis. One of the most serious complications of portal hypertension is variceal hemorrhage that occurs in about one-third

20-10

Clinical Application

Wernicke–Korsakoff Syndrome

These disorders of the central nervous system, caused by thiamin deficiency, are diagnosed mainly in alcoholics but also occasionally in malnourished clients with no history of alcohol abuse, including women with **hyperemesis gravidarum** (see Chapters 6 and 10). In one study, half the clients with Wernicke–Korsakoff syndrome were not alcoholics and two of the nonalcoholics were diagnosed with Wernicke–Korsakoff syndrome only at autopsy (Ogershok, Rahman, Nestor, Brick, et al, 2002).

Wernicke encephalopathy is an acute neuropsychiatric condition caused by inadequate thiamin supplied to the brain. When caused by dietary deficiency, it can usually be successfully treated with small doses of oral or subcutaneous thiamin and rarely progresses to Korsakoff psychosis.

In contrast, Wernicke encephalopathy caused by the combination of thiamine deficiency and alcohol abuse probably interferes with adequate thiamine transport at a number of sites in the body, including the blood–brain barrier. In these cases thiamine deficiency treatment may require up to 1 gram of thiamine intravenously in the first 24 hours to be treated successfully. If it is undiagnosed or inadequately treated, it is likely to proceed to the chronic state, Korsakoff psychosis (Thomson, Guerrini, and Marshall, 2012).

Korsakoff psychosis is the result of damage to the brain tissue, and thiamin given at this stage will not reverse the effects (Beier et al, 2014). These clients display an abnormal mental state in which memory and learning are affected out of proportion to other cognitive functions in an otherwise alert and responsive client. There have been no trials of other nutrients and indeed, no studies have been done to test whether Wernicke encephalopathy, treated with the full recommended dose of thiamine, prevents the development of Korsakoff psychosis or reduces its incidence (Thomson et al, 2012).

The continuum of symptoms in clients is referred to as Wernicke–Korsakoff syndrome. They include:

- **Ataxia**
- Weakness of the muscles that control the eyes, producing
  - Double vision (*diplopia*)
  - Abnormal movements of the eyeball (*nystagmus*)
- Disorientation
- Short-term memory loss

Residual impairments such as *nystagmus* (involuntary eye movements) or *ataxia* affect about 60% of the clients. Of 49 individuals with Wernicke encephalopathy complicating hyperemesis gravidarum, just 29% achieved complete remission (Chiossi, Neri, Cavazzuti, et al, 2006).

An understanding that thiamin is essential to energy production from glucose is critical for health-care providers. Administering a simple solution of glucose intravenously can precipitate symptoms of Wernicke–Korsakoff syndrome if the client is thiamin-deficient.

20-11

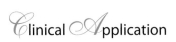 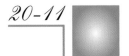

Clinical Application

Alcohol Contributes to Mortality

Alcohol is the eighth leading cause of mortality globally. In 2004, alcohol was responsible for 2.3 million deaths, representing 3.8% of all deaths. Alcohol use is a major risk factor for mortality, with more than 30 International Classification of Diseases codes with alcohol in their names and more than 200 codes listing alcohol as a component cause (Shield, Gmel, Kehoe-Chan, et al, 2013).

In 2005, for persons aged 15 to 64 years in the United States, alcohol was responsible for 55,974 deaths representing 9.0% of all deaths. These deaths were 12.0% of all deaths of men, and 4.1% of all deaths of women. For this analysis, death before age 65 years was defined as premature (Shield et al, 2013).

Many consequences of alcohol abuse, such as cirrhosis, can take years to develop, but not acute alcohol toxicity. Ingesting a large quantity of ethanol (or a smaller quantity of alcohols not intended for beverages) in a short time can kill within a few hours. Alcohol poisoning is especially heartbreaking when it kills a young person whose companions let the victim "sleep it off" through ignorance or fear of retribution. Teaching young people about the hazards of alcohol and counseling adult clients about the responsible use of alcohol are appropriate health-teaching functions in all settings.

of clients with esophageal varices (Smith, 2010). In 30% to 50% of clients, esophageal hemorrhage is fatal during the first occurrence (Sanyal, Mullen, and Bass, 2010).

The end result of cirrhosis is liver failure, which can lead to hepatic coma. See hepatic encephalopathy in Clinical Application 20-13.

Dietary Treatment for Cirrhosis

The prevalence of malnutrition in cirrhosis has been estimated to range from 65% to 100%. Restriction of dietary protein was long considered a mainstay in the management of liver disease and hepatic encephalopathy until studies showed the strategy was not only ineffective but possibly harmful (Bémeur, Desjardins, and Butterworth, 2010). Contrary to previous recommendations, protein intake in patients with cirrhosis of the liver should not be diminished but rather increased to prevent protein malnutrition (Ambühl, 2011).

In general, nutrition in clients with stable cirrhosis features these key components:

- Avoidance of alcohol
- Ingestion of four to six meals per day
- Late evening snack to avoid fasting-associated catabolism

20-12

Clinical Application

Questionnaires for Identifying Alcohol Misuse

The **CAGE Questionnaire** is a screening instrument to identify a need for a diagnostic work-up. Its advantages are its simplicity and its proven accuracy in clinical studies. It also focuses on the behavioral effects of drinking rather than on the number of drinks consumed (O'Brien, 2008). The four questions are:

C—Have you ever had a need to CUT BACK on your drinking?
A—Have people ANNOYED YOU with criticism about your drinking?
G—Have you ever felt GUILTY about your drinking?
E—Have you ever needed to start the day with a drink? (an EYE-OPENER)

A score of 2 to 3 "yes" answers indicates a high index of suspicion and a score of 4 is virtually diagnostic for alcoholism (O'Brien, 2008).

The **AUDIT-C Questionnaire** focuses on the amount and frequency of alcohol consumption. It asks, all within the past year:

1. How often did you have a drink* containing alcohol?
   a. Never = 0
   b. 2 to 4 times per month = 2
   c. 2 to 3 times a week = 3
   d. 4 or more times a week = 4

2. How many drinks did you have on a typical day when you were drinking?
   a. None, I do not drink = 0
   b. 1 or 2 = 0
   c. 3 or 4 = 1
   d. 5 or 6 = 2
   e. 7 to 9 = 3
   f. 10 or more = 4

3. How often did you have six or more drinks on one occasion?
   a. Never = 0
   b. Less than monthly = 1
   c. Monthly = 2
   d. Weekly = 3
   e. Daily or almost daily = 4

Men with AUDIT-C scores of 9 or greater were shown to be at increased risk for all adverse gastrointestinal outcomes, including new-onset pancreatitis in the subsequent 2 years. Women with scores of 9 or greater were at increased risk for hospitalization with a gastrointestinal diagnosis (Lembke et al, 2011). The AUDIT-C assesses drinking in the past year but does not differentiate lifetime abstainers from previous high-risk or problem drinkers who may have quit drinking because of other illnesses.

*A standard drink is 0.5 oz. of alcohol found in 12 oz. of beer, 5 oz. of wine, or 1.5 oz. distilled spirits.

Genomic Gem 20-4

Alcoholic Liver Disease

The metabolism of alcohol varies widely among human ethnic populations. Both genetic and environmental factors may have an impact on the outcome. Evidence does support some genetic components. For instance, individuals with high-activity alcohol dehydrogenase or low-activity aldehyde dehydrogenase 2 are at lower risk of alcoholism than other individuals (Stover and Gu, 2014).

Studies have revealed a substantial contribution of genetic factors to the evolution of alcoholic liver disease. Identical twins have a threefold higher disease concordance than do fraternal twins (Stickel and Hampe, 2012).

A particular genotype was strongly overrepresented in German clients with alcoholic liver cirrhosis relative to alcoholic clients without liver damage. The population attributable risk of cirrhosis in alcoholic carriers of the involved variation on the allele was estimated at 26.6%. (Stickel, Buch, Lau, et al, 2011).

- Protein intake of 1.0 to 1.2 grams per kilogram of body weight
- Sufficient kilocalories to avoid muscle catabolism
- Monitored vitamin status and appropriate supplementation
- Sodium restriction based on **ascites** level

The dietary management of these clients, particularly those with end-stage liver disease, is complex and constantly changing, requiring the continuing services of an expert dietitian.

Gallbladder Disease

On the underside of the liver is a small pouchlike organ called the **gallbladder.** Its function is to concentrate and store bile until needed for digestion. The liver secretes 600 to 800 milliliters of bile per day that the gallbladder, by eliminating the water content, reduces to 60 to 160 milliliters. Bile functions to emulsify large fat droplets into smaller droplets, exposing greater surface area to the action of lipase.

Causative Factors

The presence of gallstones is called **cholelithiasis** (Fig. 20-8). About 15% of men and 30% of women in the United States have gallstones. Often the diagnosis is made during an abdominal ultrasound examination for other reasons. Progression from asymptomatic to symptomatic disease is relatively low in Western countries, ranging from 10% to 25% over a period of

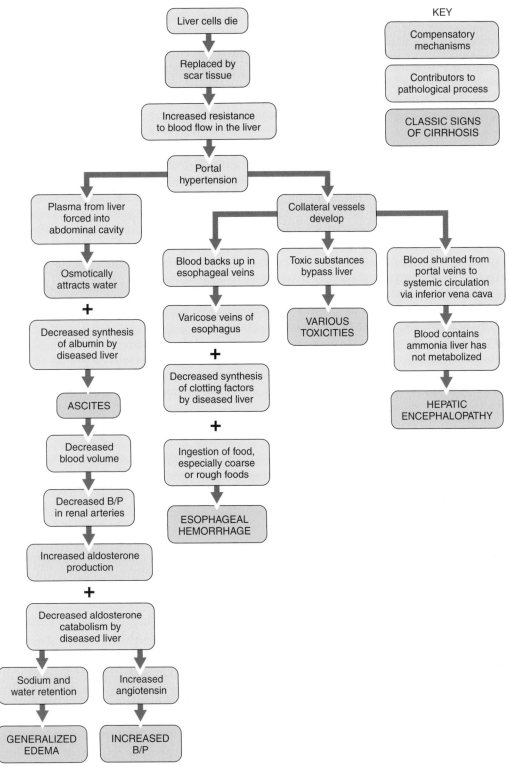

FIGURE 20-7 Progression of pathology leading to the classic signs and symptoms of cirrhosis of the liver. Many other manifestations appear given the multiple functions of the liver.

5 to 15 years (Behari and Kapoor, 2012). When the gallbladder becomes inflamed from irritation by stones (90% of the cases), parasitic infection, or prolonged fasting associated with parenteral nutrition, the condition is labeled **cholecystitis.**

More than 85% of gallstones in developed countries are composed of crystalized cholesterol, and the other 15% are comprised of calcium crystals with bilirubin (pigment stones). Cholesterol gallstone disease is a metabolic problem, which correlates with

Box 20-7 ■ *Signs and Symptoms of Cirrhosis*

Symptoms	Signs
■ Anorexia	■ Abdominal distention
■ Epigastric pain	■ Vomiting
■ Nausea that worsens as the day goes on	■ **Steatorrhea**
	■ Jaundice
	■ Ascites
	■ Edema
	■ Gastrointestinal bleeding

lipid abnormalities, diabetes mellitus, and adiposity but without a definite association with hypercholesterolemia (Stinton and Shaffer, 2012).

Gallstone disease **phenotypes** likely result from the complex interaction of genetic factors, chronic overnutrition with carbohydrates, depletion of dietary fiber, and other not fully defined environmental factors including physical inactivity and infections. This hypothesis is supported by the profound increases of cholesterol gallstone prevalence rates in Native Americans, postwar European countries, and current urban centers in East Asia, all of which are associated with the Western diet

(Stokes, Krawczyk, and Lammert, 2011). Risk factors for gallstone formation are as follows:

- Unmodifiable
  - Female gender and hormonal links to oral contraceptives, estrogen therapy
  - Ethnicity (Box 20-8)
  - Family history
  - Genetics (see Genomic Gem 20-5)
  - Increasing age
- Modifiable
  - Obesity, especially abdominal, even in children
  - Dyslipidemia
  - Rapid weight loss
  - Sedentary lifestyle
  - Parenteral nutrition and extensive fasting, possibly due to gallbladder stasis (Stinton and Shaffer, 2012)

A long fast between the evening meal and the first meal of the next day is a modifiable risk factor. Two health-promoting strategies include:

1. Taking a light bedtime snack
2. Drinking two glasses of water on arising if breakfast will be delayed

20-13

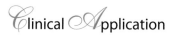

Clinical Application

Hepatic Encephalopathy

The pathophysiologic basis of this liver-caused brain disease is unclear but general agreement exists that ammonia plays a key role (Bémeur, Desjardins, and Butterworth, 2010).

Ammonia is produced by intestinal bacteria and by digestive enzymes breaking down protein. Even if the person consumes no protein foods, the bacteria work on the castoff cells of the gastrointestinal tract and on the blood from gastrointestinal bleeding, which is common in alcoholic cirrhosis. Ordinarily, the liver degrades ammonia to urea, which is excreted in urine by the kidneys, but in liver failure, blood ammonia levels rise. Ammonia is toxic to all cells, including those of the liver and the brain.

Some signs and symptoms of hepatic encephalopathy can be observed before the onset of coma, including:

- Personality changes
- Irritability
- Weakness
- Apathy
- Confusion
- Sleepiness

   More specific signs are:

- *Asterixis*, involuntary jerking movements of the hand when the arm is outstretched,
- *Fetor hepaticus*, a fecal odor to the breath
- Coma

   Primary treatment of hepatic encephalopathy is administration of *lactulose*. This drug, given orally or by enema, acidifies the large

intestine. The change in pH causes ammonia to be converted to ammonium ions, which are not absorbed but eliminated in the feces. If *lactulose* is not sufficient, the antibiotic *neomycin* (that remains in the lumen of the intestine) may be added to decrease the bacteria present (Levison, 2012).

   The goal of nutritional management of clients with hepatic encephalopathy should be to promote protein synthesis by supplying ample amounts of amino acids. Only in cases of severe protein intolerance should protein be restricted and then for as short a time as possible with supplemental branched-chain amino acids (isoleucine, leucine, and valine) administered until normal protein intake is resumed (Beier et al, 2014).

   Early research suggested a benefit to altering the ratio of **aromatic** to **branched-chain amino acids (BCAA)** in hepatic encephalopathy. Branched-chain amino acids do not require oxidation by the liver and are available for direct use by other tissues. Some evidence shows supplementation with BCAAs may delay the progression of cirrhosis. High cost as well as poor palatability due to the bitter taste are barriers to compliance (Beier et al, 2014).

   If branched-chain amino acids are selected as therapy, special preparations low in aromatic amino acids are available for enteral or oral feeding. Hepatic-Aid II® is one of the latter. Aspartame (NutraSweet®) also contains phenylalanine, an aromatic amino acid that may have to be avoided as well.

   Mild hepatic encephalopathy has responded to probiotics, prebiotics, and combination of both (synbiotics). The treatment may simply consist of a yogurt supplement (Beier et al, 2014).

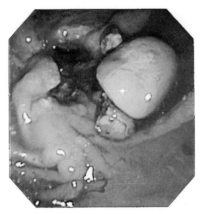

FIGURE 20-8 Gallstones seen endoscopically (original magnification × 3). (Reprinted from Venes, D [ed.]: *Taber's cyclopedic medical dictionary*, 22nd ed. FA Davis, Philadelphia, 2013, p. 987, with permission.)

Box 20-8 ■ *Ethnic Variations in the Prevalence of Gallstones*

Group	Percent
■ American Indian women	■ 64–73
■ Canadian Indian women	■ 62
■ North American Indian men	■ 29.5
■ Mexican American women	■ 27
■ White American women	■ 17
■ Black American women	■ 14
■ White American men	■ 8.6
■ Black American men	■ 5.3

Source: Stinton and Shaffer, 2012

Genomic Gem 20-5

Gallbladder Disease

Gallstones are caused by a combination of genetic and environmental risk factors. The analysis of more than 40,000 Swedish twin pairs with gallstones demonstrated that genetic factors account for 25% of the phenotypic variance (Stokes, Krawczyk, and Lammert, 2011).

Building on earlier studies, recent genome-wide research has identified multiple lithogenic genes, two in particular, as major genetic determinants of gallstones in humans (Krawczyk, Wang, Portincasa, and Lammert 2011).

Either practice stimulates the gallbladder to empty, thus decreasing the likelihood of very concentrated bile. Evidence for a liberal water intake preventing gallstone formation is rated as speculative (Popkin, D'Anci, and Rosenberg, 2010) but, with few exceptions, is likely to be harmless.

An association was found between consumption of 5 ounces of nuts weekly and decreased gallbladder disease, perhaps because of the influence of nuts on lipid levels which has been extensively investigated (Ros, 2010).

Symptoms and Treatment

The cardinal symptom of gallbladder disease is pain after ingestion of fat caused by spasms of the gallbladder. The pain is located in the right upper quadrant and often radiates to the right shoulder.

Dietary Modifications

During an acute attack, a full-liquid diet with minimal fat is recommended. For chronic gallbladder disease, the client should limit fat and obese clients should lose weight. Some clients obtain relief with the restriction of dietary fat; others do not. A reasonable approach to fat restriction is to:

- select skim milk dairy products,
- limit fats or oils to 3 teaspoons per day, and
- consume no more than 6 ounces of very lean meat per day.

Another approach is to eliminate foods that cause symptoms. Clients usually can identify foods that cause them pain. Fried foods are the worst offenders. Gas-forming foods also are often poorly tolerated. Table 20-11 identifies some foods that are low in fat and some that are high in fat.

Medical and Surgical Treatments

Asymptomatic gallstones are usually just monitored. Surgery is the preferred option to treat symptomatic gallbladder disease, but medical management may be recommended to allow inflammation to subside, for individuals who are poor surgical risks, or for individuals who wish to delay surgery to accommodate their priorities.

The usual surgical procedure in the United States is laparoscopic **cholecystectomy.** Clients and physicians still may opt for removal of the gallbladder through the traditional open incision if the stones are large or the gallbladder is infected. The removal of the stones without the gallbladder is a *cholecystotomy*.

After traditional cholecystectomy, the client may initially receive nothing by mouth or clear liquids. Then the diet is progressed as tolerated. Following laparoscopic cholecystectomy, clients may receive a general diet immediately.

Later in convalescence, balanced meals should be well tolerated because bile enters the duodenum continuously. Clients who become nauseated and suffered pain after eating certain foods preoperatively, however, may continue to avoid them postoperatively because of the association.

Two alternate, less invasive treatments have been devised to treat gallstones. One technique involves an oral agent to dissolve the stones, *ursodiol*. This is

TABLE 20-11 ■ Comparison of Fat Content of Selected Foods

LOW-FAT FOODS	FAT (GRAMS)	HIGH-FAT FOODS	FAT (GRAMS)
Starch/Breads			
Angel food cake, 1/12	<1	Pecan pie, 1/6 of pie	24
Italian bread, 1 slice	<1	Bread stuffing, 1/2 cup	13
English muffin, 1	1	Danish pastry	12
Raisin toast, 1 slice	1	Croissant, 1	12
Pancake, 4-inch, 1	2	Glazed raised doughnut, 1	13
Meats, Fish, and Poultry			
Beef round, 3 oz lean roasted	9	Beef prime rib, 3 oz lean only	24
Chicken breast, 3 oz roasted, without skin	9	Chicken, deep-fried thigh, 1	14
Boiled ham, 3 oz	9	Spare ribs, 3 oz	24
Tuna, 1/2 cup water-packed	6	Tuna, 1/2 cup oil-packed, drained	24
Fruits and Vegetables			
Banana, 8¾ inch long, 1	1	Avocado, 1	30
Raisins, 1 cup	1	Coconut, dried, 1 cup	50
Potato, baked, 1	<1	French fried potato, 2 × 3½ inches, 15 pieces	12
Onion, raw, sliced, 1 cup	<1	French fried onion rings, 4	10
Milk Products			
Cottage cheese, 1%, 1/2 cup	1	Cottage cheese, 4%, 1/2 cup	5
Mozzarella, part skim, 1 oz	5	Cheddar, 1 oz	9
Skim milk, with added milk solids, 1 cup	1	Whole milk, 1 cup	8
Frozen yogurt, low-fat, 1 cup	4	Ice cream, regular, hard, vanilla, 1 cup	14
Fast Foods*			
Arby's			
Junior Roast Beef sandwich	8	Beef'n Cheddar sandwich	20
McDonald's			
Hamburger	9	Quarter Pounder with cheese	26
Subway			
6-inch roast beef	5	6-inch tuna	25
Wendy's			
Ultimate Chicken Grill sandwich	10	Spicy Chicken sandwich	22

*Check with the restaurant. Recipes may be revised.

indicated for cholesterol stones only, not pigment stones, only those less than 1.5 centimeters in diameter, and in cases where reformation of stones is not expected—for instance, when caused by rapid weight loss (RxList, 2013).

Another method is to break up the stones using shock waves through a procedure called *lithotripsy*. It is used infrequently because it is labor-intensive, requires expensive equipment, and, compared with laparoscopic procedures, less universally effective.

Diseases of the Pancreas

In addition to the endocrine secretions, insulin, glucagon, and somatostatin, the **pancreas** secretes at least 10 digestive enzymes including amylase, lipase, trypsin, and chymotrypsin. It also secretes bicarbonate to aid electrolyte balance. Because of those many secretions, diseases of the pancreas create major nutritional consequences. Two important disorders of the pancreas affecting nutrition are pancreatitis and cystic fibrosis.

Pancreatitis

Normally, the pancreatic enzymes necessary for digestion are inactive in the pancreas and become activated only on entering the duodenum. Otherwise, the active enzymes would digest the pancreas itself. In **pancreatitis,** the retained pancreatic enzymes become activated and do digest the pancreatic tissue. In severe cases, the enzymes escape into the general circulation causing inflammation in distant organs.

Acute Pancreatitis

In the United States, about 75% to 85% of acute pancreatitis cases are attributed to alcohol abuse or gallstones. In women, a gallstone affecting the distal common bile-pancreatic duct is predominant; in men, alcohol abuse (Raina and O'Keefe, 2014). Pancreatitis can also be hereditary (see Genomic Gem 20-6).

The characteristic symptom of acute pancreatitis is excruciating pain in the left upper quadrant. Nausea and vomiting accompany an attack. Laboratory tests reveal elevated levels of serum amylase and lipase.

Genomic Gem 20-6

Hereditary Pancreatitis

This condition affects clients with genetic mutations that predispose them to pancreatitis. It is diagnosed either by detecting a causative gene mutation or by the presence of chronic pancreatitis in two **first-degree** or in three **second-degree relatives,** in two or more generations, without precipitating factors and with a negative work-up for known causes of chronic pancreatitis (Patel, Eppolito, and Willingham, 2013).

Approximately 68% to 81% of clients with hereditary pancreatitis have an **autosomal dominant** disorder caused by mutations in a trypsinogen gene. These individuals may display symptoms in childhood or adolescence. They suffer with the symptoms typical of pancreatitis and may have long delays in time to diagnosis. Frequently, the disease becomes chronic (Patel, Eppolito, and Willingham, 2013).

Other genetic causes involve

■ A complex inheritance pattern affecting a pancreatic secretory trypsin inhibitor
■ Mutations in the cystic fibrosis gene. See Genomic Gem 20-7.

Not all mutations causing hereditary pancreatitis have been detected, however (Patel, Eppolito, and Willingham, 2013) and a client may have multiple affected genes (Sultan, Werlin, and Venkatasubramani, 2012).

Complicating the pathophysiology even more, both disease-causing or protective traits have been identified for mutations in different trypsinogen genes (Nitsche, Simon, Weiss, et al, 2011).

About 75% of clients with acute pancreatitis have mild cases and relatively benign, self-limited courses. Nutritionally, mild pancreatitis may be treated with:

■ Nothing by mouth for 48 hours to avoid stimulating the pancreas
■ Aggressive hydration with intravenous fluids
■ Clear liquids after pain has been controlled and nausea and vomiting cease
■ Low-fat, soft diet
■ Soft to general diet over 3 or 4 days if satisfactory progress (Raina and O'Keefe, 2014)

In the remaining 25% of clients, the disease develops into severe pancreatitis. These clients display an intense systemic inflammatory response and often develop multiple organ failure resulting in a 5% to 50% mortality rate depending on access to modern intensive care unit management. Protein deficiency can occur within the first week unless nutrition support is begun. Enteral nutrition within 5 days of the onset of symptoms has prevented progression of complications and improved outcomes (Raina and O'Keefe, 2014).

The goal of nutritional support is to meet the elevated metabolic demands as much as possible without stimulating pancreatic secretion and self-digestion. The more distally the feeding enters the gut, the less it stimulates pancreatic secretions, resulting in mortality rates of 5% to 6% in two studies. A jejunal feeding tube with a gastric decompression lumen is recommended to be placed with radiologic or endoscopic confirmation (Raina and O'Keefe, 2014).

In general feedings should:

■ Begin as early as possible following admission to the hospital
■ Consist of a high-protein, low-fat, **semielemental formula**
■ Start slowly, 20 to 25 mL/hour for 24 hours
■ Increase in 25-mL increments to goal of 25 kcal/kg/**ideal body weight**/day (Raina and O'Keefe, 2014)

Clients should be monitored for complications of enteral feedings: residual gastric secretions and diarrhea. For additional information on maintaining enteral nutrition, see Chapter 14.

Studies have shown that enteral nutrition is less expensive than parenteral nutrition when treating acute pancreatitis. More important, analysis of eight randomized controlled trials demonstrated that total enteral nutrition was significantly superior to parenteral nutrition in treating severe acute pancreatitis regarding

■ Mortality
■ Infectious complications
■ Organ failure
■ Surgical intervention (Yi, Ge, Zhao, et al, 2012).

Chronic Pancreatitis

In chronic pancreatitis, persistent inflammation results in permanent structural damage with fibrosis and ductal strictures. Chronic pancreatitis has long been thought to be mainly associated with immoderate alcohol consumption. The fact that only about 10% of heavy drinkers develop chronic pancreatitis not only suggests that other environmental factors, such as tobacco smoke, are potent additional risk factors, but also that the genetic component of pancreatitis is more common than previously presumed (Nitsche, Simon, Weiss, et al, 2011).

In the United States, fewer than half the cases of chronic pancreatitis result from alcoholism, and 15% to 25% are **idiopathic.** Other known causes include hereditary pancreatitis, autoimmune pancreatitis, hyperparathyroidism, and obstruction of the main pancreatic duct (Freedman, 2012).

Most often, these clients present with severe abdominal pain that may last many hours or several days. Episodes typically subside spontaneously after 6 to 10 years as the cells that secrete digestive enzymes are destroyed. Because fat malabsorption does not occur until pancreatic enzyme secretions are reduced by 90%, **steatorrhea** is a late-appearing sign. Likewise glucose intolerance emerges late in the disease but leads to diabetes in 20% to 30% of clients (Freedman, 2012).

General dietary management principles depend on the stage of disease but progressively are likely to include:

■ Total abstinence from alcohol (and, although not dietary, from smoking)
■ Small, frequent nutritionally balanced meals, avoiding fatty foods
■ Vitamin-mineral supplements as appropriate
■ If underweight
  ■ 35 kilocalories per kilogram of body weight daily
  ■ 1.0 to 1.5 grams of protein per kilogram of body weight per day
■ Pancreatic enzyme supplements, which help but do not substitute for normal function
■ Jejunal tube feeding
■ Rarely, short-term parenteral nutrition to replace nutrient stores
■ Monitoring for and treating brittle diabetes resulting from loss of **endogenous** insulin and glucagon secretions (Raina and O'Keefe, 2014).

Cystic Fibrosis

Originally considered a disease of childhood because of limited life expectancy, **cystic fibrosis (CF)** is increasingly seen in adults, currently affecting 30,000 children and adults in the United States (70,000 worldwide). More than 45% of the CF patient population is aged 18 or older, but more than 70% of clients are diagnosed by age 2 (Cystic Fibrosis Foundation, undated) indicating long-term health-care management issues are the norm. Prevalence estimates have increased with the spread of newborn screening and recognition of clients with milder forms of disease (Patel, Eppolito, and Willingham, 2013).

CF is the most common life-threatening genetic disease in the White population. In the United States, it occurs in about 1:3300 White births, 1:15,300 Black births, and 1:32,000 Asian American births (Rosenstein, 2012). As indicated in Genomic Gem 20-7, multiple possibilities for developing the disease lead to variations in disease severity.

Case–Finding

By January 2010, all states and the District of Columbia had implemented newborn screening for CF (Boyle and McColley, 2011). Early diagnosis from screening produces long-term improvements in height-for-age and reductions in chronic malnutrition. Screening tests are not perfect, however, and the variable expression of the disease merits investigation if the clinical signs and symptoms warrant, even if the screening test was negative.

Examples of arrival at a CF diagnosis through other signs and symptoms are seen in the following cases:

■ Cerebral hemorrhage in a male infant (Hamid and Khan, 2007)
■ Facial nerve paralysis in a 10-week-old infant (Cameron, Lodes, and Gershan, 2007)
■ Hematoma in the leg of 2½ month old girl after intramuscular vaccination (Ngo, Van Pelt, Labarque, et al, 2011).

Genomic Gem 20-7
Cystic Fibrosis

Cystic fibrosis is inherited in an **autosomal recessive** pattern because of mutations in the *cystic fibrosis transmembrane conductance regulator* (*CFTR*) gene located on chromosome 7. The most common gene mutation, F508del, occurs in about 70% of cystic fibrosis alleles, but more than 1900 less common mutations have been reported (Rosenstein, 2012). Hence, clinical expression and severity of the disease are understandably highly variable. The CFTR protein is a chloride channel in the epithelial tissue of most of the lumens of the body where it significantly affects secretions and sodium and water balance.

The severe phenotypes of cystic fibrosis are usually associated with high concentrations of sweat chloride, early onset of pancreatic insufficiency, meconium ileus at birth, and severe lung disease, whereas mild phenotypes present with less involved pathology. Some clients have single-organ manifestations such as pancreatitis, chronic sinusitis, or congenital bilateral absence of the vas deferens that may be due to partial CFTR protein dysfunction (Rosenstein, 2012).

A new drug that for the first time can improve CFTR function at a cellular level, *ivacaftor,* has been approved for use in cystic fibrosis clients with a G551D mutation in their CTFR gene (Vallerand, et al, 2013). That particular mutation occurs in about 4% of those with cystic fibrosis. The drug is a CFTR potentiater that increases the time that activated CFTR channels at the cell surface remain open (Ramsey, Davies, McElvaney, et al, 2011). In clinical trials, the drug improved lung function as indicated by sweat chloride levels within weeks of beginning therapy (Boyle and Elborn, 2011). *Ivacaftor* may also affect the gastrointestinal tract because the substantial weight gains in all age groups was more than might be expected from controlling lung infections (Boyle and McKone, 2012). Efforts are ongoing with other mutations contributing to cystic fibrosis.

Pathophysiology

The chief cause of morbidity and mortality in cystic fibrosis is obstruction of exocrine glands with thick mucus. Affecting multiple organ systems, cystic fibrosis is characterized by:

■ Pulmonary dysfunction and infection
■ Pancreatic impairment contributing to malnutrition
■ Elevated sweat chloride
■ Male infertility.

In the lungs, the stagnant secretions become a hospitable environment for bacteria. As a result, lung infection is the most common cause of death. The prevalence of methicillin-resistant *Staphylococcus aureus* (MRSA) in the respiratory tract of individuals with CF has increased dramatically. A study of more than 19,000 clients with CF found that, after adjustment for covariates associated with severity of illness, MRSA was associated with a 25% higher risk of death than in CF clients without MRSA in their respiratory tracts (Dasenbrook, Checkley, Merlo, et al, 2010).

Obstruction by viscid material in the lumen of the glands interferes with the digestive secretions of the pancreas. Fat malabsorption results in the passage of bulky, fatty, foul-smelling feces and protein malabsorption, which leads to stunted growth (deficit in height for age).

The sweat of a CF client has more sodium chloride than normal. A sweat chloride level greater than 60 milliequivalents per liter is diagnostic of CF, but other criteria in combination also can be used in doubtful cases. During fever or hot weather, the high sodium chloride content of the sweat increases the risk of electrolyte imbalance.

Treatment

■ Supportive care is the foundation of CF treatment with the overall goal that every client should achieve normal growth (Kalnins and Wilschanski, 2012). Greater weight at age 4 years was associated with greater height, better lung function, and better survival through age 18 years verifying that a focus on nutrition early in life is crucial (Boyle and Singh, 2011).
■ With appropriate pancreatic enzyme replacement, most clients can maintain a reasonable nutritional status with a normal diet. Advanced pulmonary manifestations may require enteral feeding not only to maintain weight and growth but because better nutritional status improves muscle strength and lung function (Cooper, Mones, and Heard, 2014). Pulmonary congestion and infections are treated as required.

CF clients have specific physiological changes related to nutrition:

■ Resting energy expenditure is 25% to 80% greater than normal due to the work of breathing.

■ Fat-soluble vitamins are poorly absorbed.
  ■ Up to 50% of clients have vitamin A deficiency; 18% have visual defects.
  ■ Osteoporosis is widespread due to vitamin D malabsorption, lack of sunlight, and liver impairment (Patel and Johnson, 2014). Aside from bone health, higher serum levels of vitamin D in children with CF were associated with better lung function (Boyle and Singh, 2011).
■ Riboflavin needs are increased because of the client's high-energy expenditure. Riboflavin deficiency manifested as stomatitis in three children, 2- to 10-years-old, with cystic fibrosis. In addition, the children had deficiencies of thiamin, pyridoxine, and iron (McCabe, 2001).
■ Iron and zinc deficiencies are common (Patel and Johnson, 2014).

Nutritional care is ongoing for CF clients. Some considerations pertinent to planning include providing:

■ A high protein diet composed of 35% to 40% of kilocalories from fat to meet energy needs that may be 120% to 150% of those normally recommended for their age (Patel and Johnson, 2014)
■ Enteral tube feeding, usually delivered as overnight feeds to provide approximately 30% to 50% of estimated daily energy requirements
■ Supplemental pancreatic enzyme therapy to control symptoms and permit adequate food intake for normal growth and weight gain despite not completely correcting nutrient malabsorption
■ Yearly monitoring of serum vitamin A, E, and D levels and supplementation as needed; hypervitaminosis A has been reported following lung transplantation from unclear mechanisms (Kalnins, and Wilschanski, 2012)
■ Possible inclusion of high-fat, low-carbohydrate formulas (*Pulmocare*®, Abbott) that produce less carbon dioxide than with normal CHO intake to decrease the work of the lungs (Cooper, et al, 2014)
■ Appetite stimulants may enhance weight gain but may not improve lung function (Cooper, et al, 2014)
■ Adequate salt intake and monitoring of electrolytes. Infants with CF who feed on breast milk or formula and live in a high-temperature environment are at increased risk for hyponatremia, even when receiving a higher salt intake in accordance with recommendations (Guimarães, Schettino, Camargos, and Penna, 2012)

Those are just the nutritional considerations. Clients with CF may also have extensive pulmonary medications to take and multiple treatments to perform. Motivated clients may spend 2 to 3 hours a day performing therapies (Boyle and McColley, 2011). Health-care providers should offer options to improve a client's care and let the individual and family decide whether it is too troublesome to implement an additional strategy (VandenBranden, 2011).

Keystones

- Recommended preoperative intake allows clear fluids up to 2 hours before anesthesia, breast milk 4 hours, infant formula and nonhuman milk 6 hours.

- In addition to the preparation for general surgery, the client about to undergo gastrointestinal surgery may be asked to consume a low-fiber diet for several days to decrease amount of feces and to ingest poorly absorbed anti-infective agents to decrease the number of microorganisms in the bowel.

- Dumping syndrome and postprandial hypotension require similar dietary interventions. Meals should be dry, frequent, and low in simple sugars. Lying down after eating helps retain stomach contents for a longer time.

- For gastroesophageal reflux (GERD) and hiatal hernia, meals should be small and frequent with normal protein and limited fat. Remaining upright after eating encourages movement of stomach contents into the duodenum.

- Celiac disease develops in a genetically predisposed individual in whom exposure to dietary gluten leads to damage to the small intestine. The treatment is a gluten-free diet for life.

- In Crohn disease, enteral feeding is the primary mode of therapy in active disease with modifications of oral intake and parenteral nutrition useful in other situations. For ulcerative colitis, parenteral nutrition and probiotics are sometimes effective. If a surgical stoma is constructed, the client may need to avoid stringy, high-fiber foods and those producing excessive odor.

- Keys to nutritional treatment of hepatitis and cirrhosis of the liver are abstinence from alcohol and optimum nutrition. Clients often have the best appetite at breakfast.

- Thiamin deficiency causes Wernicke encephalopathy, which can be precipitated by administration of glucose to the thiamin-deficient client. It is possible to halt the progression of Wernicke encephalopathy with appropriate thiamin therapy, whereas Korsakoff psychosis involves pathological changes in the brain tissue that cannot be reversed by thiamin treatment.

- Cholecystitis is treated medically with a low-fat diet. To prevent cholelithiasis, eating breakfast or drinking two glasses of water on arising empties the gallbladder of concentrated bile that results from a long overnight fast.

- In cystic fibrosis, mutations on a gene controlling chloride transport cause thick secretions that clog the lungs and pancreas. Adequate intake and pancreatic enzyme supplements are used to prevent malnutrition.

CASE STUDY 20-1

An outpatient, Ms. C, a 40-year-old White woman, has just been evaluated for right upper quadrant pain. The pain occurs after meals and radiates to the right shoulder. Ms. C has noticed her stools have become pale gray in the past 2 months.

Ultrasound examination of the gallbladder showed the presence of numerous stones. None is obstructing the duct system yet.

Ms. C is a single parent of four children, aged 4 to 17 years, and is employed as a secretary. If surgery does become necessary, she would like to delay it until the youngest child is in school. For that reason, she is electing medical management.

Usual food intake: no breakfast; coffee and doughnut mid-morning; "this week's special" lunch-meat sandwich and chips at noon; casseroles for dinner.

Stated she does not know much about nutrition, that she shops as her mother did and that she cooks food her children will eat. Rarely buys fresh fruits or vegetables because of the cost.

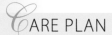ARE PLAN

Subjective Data

Pain in right upper quadrant immediately after eating ■ Pale stools for 2 months by history ■ Usual intake: high fat, low fiber ■ Admitted lack of knowledge about nutrition

Objective Data

Gallstones per ultrasound ■ Measured height 5 ft 4 in. ■ Measured weight 165 lb ■ BMI 28.3. ■ B/P 139/89

Analysis

Need for diet instruction related to prescribed low-fat diet for cholecystitis as evidenced by self-report ■ Potential increased risk for surgical complications related to overweight and prehypertension

Plan

DESIRED OUTCOMES EVALUATION CRITERIA	ACTIONS/INTERVENTIONS	RATIONALE
Client will verbalize foods to avoid on low-fat diet by end of teaching session.	Explain low-fat diet, adapting to client's lifestyle. Provide written instructions for client to take home.	Having written instructions available as a teaching tool structures the session and may stimulate questions the client would not think of otherwise. Taking the material home will reinforce the instruction.
Client will state means to modify meals to accommodate prescribed diet by end of teaching session.	Explore Ms. C's preferences for adding fiber to her diet.	Soluble fiber will combine with cholesterol, which comprises most gallstones, and carry it out of the body. Building on the client's choices increases the chances of compliance.
Client will think through her ability to implement the diet and voice hesitations by the end of this visit.	Obtain client's reaction to diet and offer alternatives to her present meal pattern.	Considering the client's wishes affirms her status as an individual. Personalizing the diet for her circumstances will increase the chances of success.
	Suggest Ms. C either eat breakfast or drink two glasses of water first thing in the morning.	Either of these actions will stimulate the gallbladder to empty the concentrated bile that has accumulated overnight.
Client will accept referral to social worker to maximize nutrition for self and family.	Make appointment with social worker for Ms. C before she leaves today.	Completing arrangements before the client leaves avoids the possibility of procrastination.

 20-1

Social Worker's Notes

The following Social Worker's Notes are representative of the documentation found in a client's medical record.

Referred by nurse instructing client on low-fat diet for cholecystitis

Subjective: Head of household of five; divorced 6 months; ex-husband unemployed and behind on child support

Objective: Earning slightly more than minimum wage per paycheck stub

Analysis: Eligible for Head Start and Supplemental Nutrition Assistance Program (SNAP)

Plan: Identify barriers to participation; assist with applications; encourage attendance at nutrition education sessions provided by Head Start

Critical Thinking Questions

1. How important is dietary modification for the children? How might the interventions be modified for them?

2. If Ms. C were not in such a dire financial situation and ineligible for assistance, what other approaches to improving the family's nutritional intake could be tried?

3. How would you follow up on Ms. C's implementation of the low-fat diet as well as her overweight and prehypertension (assuming other measurements confirm the readings)?

Chapter Review

1. Which of the following foods is allowed for a preoperative client on a low-fiber diet?
   a. Bologna sandwich
   b. Corn on the cob
   c. Canned peaches
   d. Banana-nut waffles

2. The American Society of Anesthesiologists' guidelines suggest which of the following intakes is permissible for healthy individuals undergoing elective procedures?
   a. Water and apple juice until 1 hour before the procedure
   b. Plain tea and unbuttered toast with clear jelly 6 hours before scheduled surgery
   c. Infant formula or breast milk 4 hours before an elective procedure begins
   d. Light meal containing meat at 5 a.m. before a procedure scheduled for noon

3. Clients who have had resection of the ileum should be monitored for:
   a. Iron-deficiency anemia
   b. Fat-soluble vitamin deficiency
   c. Calcium and phosphorus deficiency
   d. Vitamin B_{12} deficiency

4. A client with cirrhosis of the liver should be asked if he or she experienced ____ before ordering a diet.
   a. A headache
   b. Vomiting of blood
   c. A recent course of antibiotic therapy
   d. Hives

5. Which of the following meal components is likely to lessen symptoms of the dumping syndrome?
   a. Mashed fresh strawberries
   b. Orange sherbet
   c. Salt-free tomato juice
   d. Whole-wheat toast with dietetic jelly

Clinical Analysis

Mr. W is a 55-year-old White man admitted to the acute care unit for jaundice and ascites secondary to cirrhosis of the liver. He has gained 15 pounds in the past 3 weeks, and his serum sodium is 125 mEq/L. He is a diagnosed alcoholic who has been through a detoxification program several times in the past 5 years. The dietitian has instructed Mr. W on a 1500-mg sodium diet with a fluid restriction of 1000 mL per day.

1. When the nurse does the beginning of shift assessment, Mr. W says he tried "cutting down on salt" when he started gaining weight, but it didn't work. Which of the following statements best reflects a good understanding of Mr. W's pathology and treatment?
   a. Just cutting out added salt is not enough, because many foods are naturally high in sodium.
   b. Fluids are always restricted with a low-sodium diet.
   c. The ascites is caused by the inability of the liver to produce water-soluble bilirubin.
   d. Besides retaining sodium, Mr. W has ascites due to decreased blood pressure in the liver.

2. Mr. W vomits immediately after his next meal. The physician then orders a hydrating solution of 5% dextrose in water intravenously. If thiamin is not included in that order, the nurse should inquire about it because:
   a. Thiamin is necessary to predigest the dextrose for immediate absorption.
   b. Deficiency of thiamin causes delirium tremens.
   c. Intravenous glucose without thiamin in the cirrhosis client can precipitate the Wernicke–Korsakoff syndrome.
   d. Thiamin prevents folic acid stores from being diluted by the hydrating solution.

3. Ms. M has been diagnosed with gastroesophageal reflux disease. Dietary instructions should include taking:
   a. Normal amounts of protein to help tighten the cardiac sphincter.
   b. Mint teas to counteract the bitter taste caused by reflux of gastric contents into the esophagus.
   c. Small amounts of wine with dinner to aid in relaxation and enjoyment of the meal.
   d. Whole milk products to increase the kilocalorie density of the diet.

21

Diet and Cancer

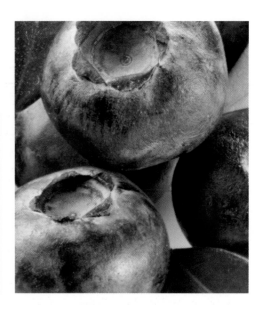

LEARNING OBJECTIVES

After completing this chapter, the student should be able to:

- Explain how normal cells become cancerous.
- Relate nutritional factors to the incidence of cancers at the most common sites.
- Summarize dietary guidelines for the prevention of cancer.
- Compare the New American Plate to MyPlate (Chapter 1) as to its potential value as a teaching tool.
- Interpret the lack of validation of population correlations of fruit and vegetable intake with cancer occurrence in more focused research.
- Identify measures to increase oral intake for anorexic clients with cancer.
- Discuss strategies to prevent infections in the immunosuppressed client.
- List four classes of drugs that may be used to affect food intake and weight in clients with cancer.
- Describe three approaches to increase oral intake for a cancer client with mouth ulcerations.
- Define *cachexia* and correlate its characteristics with the challenges of managing the condition.

ancer has been known and described for thousands of years. Amazingly, one substance now linked to prevention was used as a treatment in ancient Rome, where crushed cabbage leaves were applied to cancerous ulcers (Albert-Puleo, 1983). Now cabbage is one of the cruciferous vegetables in the diet associated with reduced risk of cancer.

Definitions and Statistics

Cancer means "crab," for the creeping way in which it spreads. Cancer is a general term for more than 200 types of malignant neoplasms.

Terminology

A **neoplasm** is a new and abnormal formation of tissue (tumor) that grows at the expense of the healthy organism.

- **Benign** tumors are localized but potentially dangerous if situated in vital organs.
- **Malignant** (cancerous) tumors infiltrate surrounding tissue and spread to distant parts of the body.
- **Sarcomas** arise from connective tissue, such as muscle or bone and are more common in young people.
- **Carcinomas** occur in epithelial tissue, including cancers of the lung, breast, prostate, and colon, and are more common in older people.

Characteristics common to all types of cancer are uncontrolled growth and the ability to spread to distant sites (**metastasize**). Clinical Application 21-1 summarizes the transformation of normal cells into cancer cells.

To determine the severity of a client's disease, both microscopic and macroscopic measures are used. Although particular cancers have specific systems, in general, the scales for both run from one (least severe) to four (most severe).

■ **Grade** of malignancy refers to the extent to which the cells under the microscope resemble normal cells, with Grade 1 most like normal cells and Grade 4 least like them.
■ **Stage** of disease refers to the physical location of the tumor, with Stage I localized and Stage IV involving distant metastases.

Incidence and Mortality

In the United States, more than 30% of cancer deaths are attributed to smoking, and an estimated 35% are due to poor nutrition, physical inactivity, and obesity

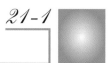

Clinical Application   *21-1*

Transformation of Normal Cells Into Cancer Cells

Cancer is basically uncontrolled replication of cells. Normal cells divide in the processes of growth and maintenance but stop dividing at appropriate points.

Apoptosis, a process of programmed cell death, is necessary to the maintenance of healthy tissue. Apoptosis eliminates cells that are aged, dysfunctional, or damaged by external stimuli, and thus potential cancer cells. When this housekeeping process fails, cancer may result.

Transformation of normal cells into cancer cells is a two-step process:

1. The first step is **initiation.** In this step, physical forces, chemicals, biological agents, or errors in replication alter a cell's DNA.
2. The second step is **promotion,** which activates the altered genes, allowing uncontrolled cell growth.

The time between initiation and promotion in some cases is 10 to 30 years but may be shorter if a mutated gene is inherited from a parent. Those are rare cases, amounting to about 5% to 10% of all cancers (Eggert, 2011). See Genomic Gem 21-1.

Substances that enhance the expression of the altered gene are called promoters. They must be present at high levels for a prolonged period. Promoters are tissue-specific, such as saccharin for cancer of the urinary bladder (in rats) and bile acids for colon cancer. In contrast to initiation, which results in permanent change, the process of promotion is reversible. Reducing exposure to high levels of promoters allows the body to repair the damaged cells.

Genomic Gem 21-1

Growth and Suppression of Malignant Cells

Proto-oncogenes support the growth and division of normal cells. When a proto-oncogene's DNA is altered and the gene is activated, it is called an oncogene. Only one of the two **alleles** of a gene needs to be converted to an oncogene to cause malignant transformation. Thus, the oncogene is dominant over its corresponding proto-oncogene.

Other genes called **tumor suppressor genes** act to inhibit the growth of malignant cells. A tumor suppressor gene can function even if one of its alleles is mutated. The cause of the mutation may be spontaneous or inherited. If the mutation is inherited, the person is vulnerable to the loss of protection should the paired allele also mutate.

Many inherited cancers involve tumor suppressor gene mutations. Mutations in *BRCA1* and *BRCA2* lead to high risk for breast and ovarian cancer as well as significantly increased susceptibility to pancreatic, prostate, and male breast cancer. *BRCA2* belongs to the tumor suppressor gene family, and the protein encoded by this gene is involved in the repair of chromosomal damage (Pisanò, Mezzolla, Galante, et al, 2011).

Cancer results from accumulated inherited and/or acquired genetic mutations causing oncogene activation, tumor suppressor gene inactivation, and production of **telomerase.** Cancers of the breast, lung, kidney, colon, and cervix are believed to have multifactorial origins. It is also thought that mutations in at least four genes are required for cancer to develop (Eggert, 2011).

Genetic differences also have an impact on treatment selections. Variations in CYP2D6 (see Chapter 15) can be used as biomarkers to predict response to tamoxifen therapy in breast cancer clients because CYP2D6 converts tamoxifen to an anticancer agent (Pierce, McCabe, White, and Clancy, 2012).

(American Cancer Society [ACS], 2013). Cancer is the second most common cause of death in the United States after heart disease.

The incidence of the three most common cancers for men (prostate, lung/bronchus, colorectal) and women (breast, lung/bronchus, colorectal) of different ethnicities is illustrated in Figure 21-1. The factors that drive these disparities as well as the causes of cancer are complex and often incompletely understood. Certain cancers appear in great numbers in particular countries. Clinical Application 21-2 summarizes some of these findings. For all groups, cancer of lung and bronchus is the chief cause of cancer deaths (ACS, 2013).

This chapter:

■ Describes some examples of the associations that have been found between diet and cancer
■ Explains some of the variability of effects of diet due to differences in the human phenotypes
■ Shows the difficulty of generalizing dietary behaviors to adopt or to avoid with the goal of preventing cancer

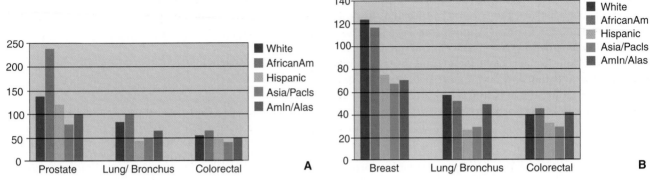

FIGURE 21-1 The three most common cancers for men (*A*) and women (*B*) in the United States, 2005–2009. These are age-adjusted rates per 100,000 persons. The race/ethnicity groupings are White, African American, Hispanic/Latino, Asian American/Pacific Islander, and American Indian/ Alaskan native. (Data derived from American Cancer Society, 2013.)

21-2

Clinical Application

Diet–Cancer Links in Various Populations

Residents of a given country experience similar environmental factors, including diet. They also may have **genes** that are similar compared with those found in people elsewhere.

■ Stomach cancer is common where nitrates and nitrites are prevalent in food and water and where cured and pickled foods are popular. These areas include Korea, Japan, and China.

■ High consumption of processed meat, but not of other meats (i.e., red meat, fish and poultry), was associated with about a 50% increased risk of stomach cancer in 61,433 Swedish women followed for 18 years (Larsson, Bergkvist, and Wolk, 2006).

■ Changing the staple diet of Black South Africans from sorghum to maize (corn) caused an epidemic of squamous carcinoma of the esophagus attributed to fungi growing freely on maize that contribute to the production of nitrosamines (Isaacson, 2005).

Studies of immigrants are especially enlightening. People that move from countries with low rates of specific cancers to areas with high rates, or the reverse, almost invariably achieve the rates of the new homeland within a few generations (Wallace, Martin, and Ambs, 2011; Willett and Giovannucci, 2014). In Japan, the incidence of stomach cancer is higher and the incidence of prostate and colon cancer is lower than those in the United States. In second-generation Japanese immigrants to the United States, however, the distribution of cancers becomes similar to that of other Americans.

Groups with similar lifestyles also provide information linking diet to cancer incidence. Among Seventh Day Adventists, those consuming vegan diets had a 16% lower risk of all cancers and a 34% lower risk of female-specific cancers whereas lacto-ovo-vegetarians had a 25% lower risk of gastrointestinal cancers (Tantamango-Bartley, Jaceldo-Siegl, Fan, and Fraser, 2013).

Diet and Cancer Development

New insights into the benefits obtained from foods show that:

■ Food can provide benefits beyond its intrinsic nutrient content (see Functional Foods in Chapter 1)
■ Individual differences affect ability to realize these benefits (Isaak and Siow, 2013)

Genetic variants that influence nutrient metabolism have been identified, but individual variants have not been conclusively linked to the risk of multifactorial diseases such as cancer and cardiovascular disease (Hesketh, 2012). Foods contain thousands of bioactive molecules that have the potential to alter gene and protein expression. Developing personalized

nutrition for cancer prevention and therapy will require:

■ Understanding **genotypes** and **phenotypes**
■ Identifying bioactive food components that can favorably intervene in cellular processes

Bioactive food components with anticancer potential can affect the expression of genes involved in cell proliferation, differentiation, and death that are frequently altered in cancer. Few studies have addressed the influence of dietary components on these mechanisms, particularly on the phenotype of humans, and thus the exact mechanisms through which diet mediates an effect on cancer prevention remains unclear (Ong, Moreno, and Ross, 2012).

Until the era of personalized nutrition arrives, the American Cancer Society has issued general recommendations to decrease cancer risk (Box 21-1). The ACS Guidelines are consistent with guidelines from the American Heart Association and the American Diabetes Association for the prevention of coronary heart disease and diabetes, as well as for general health promotion (Kushi, Doyle, McCullough, et al, 2012). The New American Plate (Fig. 21-2) exemplifies the guidelines.

Not to be considered as recommendations but only to note the complexity of prescribing preventive diets for cancer, the following information is included. The

ability of one well-defined group to ignore much of this nutritional advice and still post low incidence rates for cancer appears in Box 21-2.

Dietary Habits Linked to Cancer

Table 21-1 shows four dietary conditions that are convincingly related to cancers arising in specific organs. Many other items have been studied that may be related to particular cancers but the evidence is not as

---

Box 21-1 ■ *Recommendations to Decrease Cancer Risk*

For Community Action

- Increase access to healthful foods in schools, worksites, and communities.
- Decrease access to and marketing of foods and drinks of low nutritional value, particularly to youth.
- Provide safe, enjoyable, and accessible environments for physical activity in schools and workplaces, and for transportation and recreation in communities.

For Individual Choices

- Maintain a healthy weight throughout life. Be as lean as possible without being underweight.
  - Avoid excess weight gain at all ages. For the overweight person, even a small amount of weight loss has health benefits.
  - Limit intake of high-calorie foods and drinks.

- Adopt a physically active lifestyle. Some activity above one's usual level can produce health benefits.
  - Adults: 150 minutes of moderate-intensity or 75 minutes of vigorous-intensity activity per week, preferably distributed throughout the week.
  - Children and teens: 1 hour of moderate or vigorous physical activity daily with vigorous activity 3 days per week.
  - Limit sedentary behavior: sitting, lying down, screen-based entertainment.
- Consume a healthy diet, emphasizing plant food sources.
  - Choose amounts to maintain a healthy weight.
  - Limit intake of processed meat and red meat.
  - Consume at least 2½ cups of vegetables and fruits daily.
  - Select whole grains in preference to refined grain products.
- If alcohol is chosen, limit consumption to one **standard drink** per day for women and two for men.

Adapted from American Cancer Society, August 20, 2012.

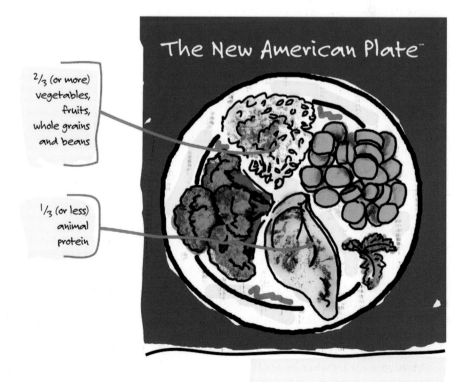

FIGURE 21-2 Vegetables, fruits, whole grains, and beans cover two-thirds (or more) of the New American Plate with the remaining one-third (or less) of the plate reserved for fish, poultry, meat, and low-fat dairy foods. (The New American Plate® is a registered trademark of the American Institute for Cancer Research, 2000. Reprinted with permission.)

Box 21-2 ■ *Comparing Amish Diets to American Cancer Society Recommendations*

The Amish are seen as living a simple life characterized by wholesome, often family-produced foods. The Amish eschew modern conveniences, electricity, automobiles, and telephones and are less likely to use tobacco than other Americans. One might assume the agrarian lifestyle would stimulate healthy diets, but not necessarily. In reality, compared with the U.S. Department of Agriculture Dietary Guidelines, the Amish tend to eat high-carbohydrate and high-fat foods with a relatively high intake of refined sugar.

A group of Amish adults in Ohio had a significantly lower age-adjusted cancer incidence rate of 389.5 compared with non-Amish with a rate of 649.9 per 100,000. A capsule comparison of their behavior to that recommended by the American Cancer Society is as follows.

	Amish Men	**Amish Women**	**Non-Amish Men**	**Non-Amish Women**
Maintaining a healthy weight	Mean BMI 27.6	Mean BMI 30.1	Mean BMI 29.4	Mean BMI 29.2
Consuming a healthy diet that emphasizes plant sources	Fruit/vegetable servings/day 3.8	Fruit/vegetable servings/day 2.6	Fruit/vegetable servings/day 3.3	Fruit/vegetable servings/day 3.2
Limiting alcohol consumption	1 drink/week or less 55%	1 drink/week or less 85%	1 drink/week or less 16%	1 drink/week or less 60%

Physical activity was not assessed, but the Amish likely surpassed the non-Amish because of the dearth of motorized devices. Avoiding alcohol misuse may account for some of the difference in cancer incidence. Other lifestyle factors such as reduced tobacco use, alone or combined with diet and genetics, may help to explain the lower cancer incidence rates among these Ohio residents.

Adapted from American Cancer Society, August 20, 2012; Cuyun Carter, Katz, Ferketich, et al, 2011; Purnell, 2013.

TABLE 21-1 ■ **Dietary Habits Convincingly Linked to Particular Cancers**

CANCER SITE	OVERWEIGHT-OBESITY	RED OR PROCESSED MEAT	ALCOHOL	SALT-PRESERVED FOODS
Breast	X (postmenopausal)		X	
Colon	X	X	X	
Endometrium	X			
Esophagus	X (adenocarcinoma)		X*	
Gallbladder	X			
Kidney	X			
Larynx			X*	
Liver			X*	
Mouth			X*	
Pharynx			X	X
Prostate		X		
Stomach		X		X

*Especially in cigarette smokers.
Data from Chang and Adami, 2006; D'Elia, Rossi, Ippolito, et al, 2012; De Stefani, Boffetta, Ronco, et al, 2012; Ge, Feng, Shen, et al, 2012; Larsson, et al, 2006; Raina and O'Keefe, 2014; Willett and Giovannucci 2014.

strong as for the ones listed. Numerous factors can impede certainty in nutrition research:

- Inconsistent results from small studies or varying designs
- Isolated nutrients or foods studied, thus oversimplifying the nutritive process
- Interventions too small, durations too short to produce an effect
- Individuals assumed to be equal in specific characteristics who are not (Genomic Gem 21-2)

Obesity

Rapid growth rates before puberty contribute to future risk of cancers. In the Japanese, traditionally short of stature, rapid gains in height during the past several decades correspond to increases in breast and colon cancer rates (Willett and Giovannucci, 2014).

Accumulation of body fat in adulthood contributes to cancers of the colon, kidney, pancreas, endometrium, gallbladder, and adenocarcinoma of the esophagus. Regarding breast cancer, premenopausal women with

Genomic Gem 21-2
Individual Differences in Metabolism

Many studies have related diet to risk of cancer, but frequently the follow-up intervention studies did not show the expected protection against cancer, possibly because the biological diversity of the participants was not controlled. Genetics also impacts the mobilization of the body's defenses. Individuals vary in their metabolizing enzymes to activate potential **carcinogens** and, in defense of the body, to counter **oxidative stress** and to repair damaged DNA. The ability to manage and prevent oxidative stress depends upon functioning endogenous and exogenous antioxidant defense systems, both of which may be influenced by individual genetic variation (Da Costa, Badawi, and El-Sohemy, 2012).

Individuals identified as *slow acetylators* of the NAT2 enzyme have decreased risk of various cancers because of reduced activation of carcinogens. For instance, a decreased risk for bladder cancer was associated with high cruciferous vegetable intake in persons with *GSTM1*-null or *NAT2*-slow genotypes (Lin, Kamat, Gu, et al, 2009).

The opposite effect has also been documented. People who were classified as *fast acetylators* of the NAT2 enzyme, and who consumed meat more than 3 times a week had increased risk of colorectal cancer (da Silva, Felipe, de Lima, et al, 2011).

The carcinogen does not have to be consumed. Even exposure to cooking oil fumes containing relatively high amounts of heterocyclic amines has been related to a greater than twofold increase in lung cancer in never-smoking females with *NAT2 fast acetylator* genotype (Chiou, Wu, Chien, et al, 2005).

greater body fat have reduced risk whereas in postmenopausal women, there is a positive but weak association between adiposity and breast cancer. For colon cancer, increasing waist-to-hip ratio is associated with increased risk regardless of body mass index (Willett and Giovannucci, 2014).

Therefore, some of the association between dietary fat intake and cancer may be explained by excess energy intake, leading to overweight and obesity. Strong evidence refutes a link between total fat intake during midlife and breast cancer. Additional evidence is needed to confirm an association between animal fat or red meat intake during adolescence or premenopausal years and risk of premenopausal breast cancer (Willett and Giovannucci, 2014).

Strong evidence remains to support the link between animal fat consumption and risk of aggressive or advanced prostate cancer. Recent studies of colon cancer, however, suggest the association with animal fat may relate to factors in red meat other than its fat content (Willett and Giovannucci, 2014).

Similarly, an important consideration in carcinogenesis is abnormal glucose and insulin metabolism especially in obese sedentary persons. High **glycemic index** diets have been associated with pancreatic cancer

and endometrial cancer and require further research (Willett and Giovannucci, 2014).

Red or Processed Meat

Red meat intake has been linked with risk of cancers of the colon, rectum, and prostate. Heterocyclic aromatic amines (HCAs), formed by high-temperature cooking of muscle meats, are well-known risk factors for colorectal cancer. HCA intake is positively associated with risk of colorectal adenoma (a precursor of colorectal cancer) regardless of phenotype affecting the metabolizing enzymes (Barbir, Linseisen, Hermann, et al, 2012). The amount of HCAs in a meal can be reduced by:

- Marinating meat for at least 30 minutes before cooking with a mixture of vinegar, lemon juice, or wine with herbs and spices
- Using low-temperatures on the grill or employing high-moisture cooking, such as stewing and pot-roasting
- Cutting off charred portions before serving (American Institute for Cancer Research, 2013).

For someone interested in reducing meat intake, Dollars & Sense 21-1 offers an alternative burger.

Dollars & Sense 21-1
Easy and Inexpensive Veggie Burger

This recipe uses spices liberally. Other choices might be just as tasty or more so if fresh herbs are used. Salt is absent. Frying until crispy is necessary to hold the shape.

- 1 cup cooked unsalted beans well drained (black are good, others worth trying)
- ½ cup chopped raw onion (compensates for lack of salt)
- ⅛ tsp. powdered garlic
- ½ tsp. dried thyme
- ½ tsp. dried rosemary
- ½ tsp. dried parsley
- ½ tsp. Mrs. Dash Caribbean Citrus Salt-free Seasoning (or other flavor)
- ¼ tsp. black pepper
- ½ slice sour dough bread torn into ¼ inch crumbs
- 1 egg, beaten
- 2 tbsp. canola or olive oil for frying

Mash beans with potato masher or fork. Stir in rest of ingredients except egg and oil. If desired, taste at this point (before raw egg is added) and adjust seasoning. Add egg and mix well. Heat oil in skillet. Shape mixture into two patties. Fry in skillet over medium heat with adequate space between. Try to turn just once to keep intact. Cooking aromas suggest when first side is browned.

Slide out of skillet onto whole-wheat buns. Serve with usual burger condiments.

Assuming other ingredients or substitutes are on hand, the cost for beans, onion, egg, breadcrumbs, and buns was $2.14 for two bean burgers.

Alcohol

Risk for the cancers associated with alcohol (Table 21-1) increases significantly with the consumption of more than two drinks per day. The risks are equal whether the drink is 12 ounces of beer, 5 ounces of wine, or 1.5 ounces of liquor. Substantial evidence indicates one or two drinks per day increases the risk of breast cancer. Women at high risk of breast cancer might reasonably consider abstaining from alcohol. Most evidence indicates high intake of alcohol increases the risk of colorectal cancer (Willett and Giovannucci, 2014).

In cases of upper gastrointestinal cancer, the carcinogenic effects of alcohol may be caused by direct contact; in cancer of the liver, by toxicity. The mechanisms through which alcohol is related to breast and colon cancer are unclear, but one possibility involves the well-established antifolate effects of alcohol (Willett and Giovannucci, 2014).

Salt-Preserved Foods

Dietary salt intake was directly associated with risk of gastric cancer in prospective population studies involving 268,718 participants followed for 6 to 15 years, with progressively increasing risk as intake increased. The association was stronger in the Japanese population, and higher consumption of selected salt-rich foods was also associated with greater risk (D'Elia, Rossi, Ippolito, et al, 2012).

Another systemic review concluded that dietary salt intake is positively associated with the risk of gastric cancer but noted that some salty foods are also high in nitrites, also related to gastric cancer. In addition, most studies assessed salt intake by questionnaire rather than 24-hour urinary sodium excretion, which is recommended by the World Cancer Research Fund as the best measurement of salt intake. Several mechanisms through which salt intake may increase gastric cancer risk have been suggested without attaining consensus (Ge, Feng, Shen, et al, 2012).

A Diet to Prevent Cancer

The campaign to improve fruit and vegetable intake for general health continues (Fig. 21-3), but behavior change comes slowly. A 2007 survey found that 29% of participants were aware of the "5 a Day" campaign and 39% reported consuming at least 5 servings of fruits and vegetables daily (Erinosho, Moser, Oh, et al, 2012). Isolating the effects of vegetables and fruits from lifestyle is also problematic. People who eat large amounts of vegetables and fruits also tend to eat less meat and to be physically active.

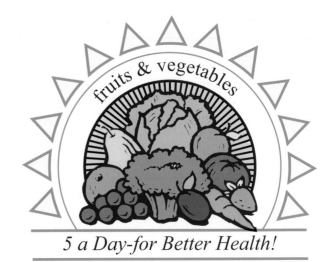

FIGURE 21-3 National 5 a Day program logo. The program logo and slogan are registered service marks. To use them, food industry and state health authority partners sign a license agreement to follow guidelines that maintain the scientific integrity of all messages and other communications to the public. (Reprinted from Foerster, SB, et al: California's "5 a Day—for Better Health" campaign: An innovative population-based effort to effect large-scale dietary change. *Am J Prev Med* 11:124, 1995, with permission.)

Changing Emphasis on Fruits and Vegetables

Still included in the ACS recommendations (see Box 21-1) is consumption of 2½ cups of fruits and vegetables daily. Scientific emphasis on overall fruit and vegetable intake to prevent cancer has been moderated because large prospective studies showed weak or absent effects on cancer risk, perhaps because all fruits and vegetables were lumped together for analysis. In addition, potatoes and some fruit juices have high glycemic indexes and increase insulin secretion (see obesity section earlier in this chapter). Furthermore, in the United States, 29% of fruit is consumed as juices and 27% of vegetable consumption comprises potatoes and potato products (Willett and Giovannucci, 2014).

Although blanket protection against cancer by fruits and vegetables is unlikely, as sources of beneficial phytochemicals, certain fruits and vegetables may bolster defenses against specific cancers. Among promising areas of study are:

- Tomato or lycopene-containing foods and prostate cancer
- Cruciferous vegetables (broccoli, cabbage, cauliflower, Brussels sprouts) for prostate, bladder, and lung cancer
- Allium vegetables (garlic, onion, leeks, chives, scallions) and gastric cancer
- Folate-rich fruits and vegetables and colon cancer
- Citrus fruits and lung cancer (Willett and Giovannucci, 2014).

In a population at high risk for gastric cancer, vitamin C supplementation, with or without anti–*Helicobacter pylori* treatment, was associated with regression of precancerous lesions (Levine and Padayatty, 2014). Nonetheless, much remains to be learned about the effects of food components on body cells. For instance, garlic and its associated allyl sulfur constituent may function as antioxidants in normal cells but cause a pro-oxidant event in cancer cells (Milner, Toner, and David, 2014).

Complicating the interpretation of the evidence is the concept that dietary patterns can result in synergistic and antagonistic interactions among bioactive components that likely contribute to the inconsistencies in observed biologic responses to functional foods. For that reason, researchers are cautioned to consider the total diet when investigating a functional food or **nutraceutical** (Milner, Toner, and Davis, 2014).

Additionally, the focus on identifying bioactive components in fruits and vegetables with the goal of developing single agents using a pharmacologic approach has been criticized on the basis that no chemopreventive strategies that are standard of care in medical practice have resulted from that approach. Rather, development of a highly consistent tomato-based food product rich in anticancer phytochemicals for clinical trials targeting specific cancers, particularly the prostate, is suggested (Tan, Thomas-Ahner, Grainger, et al, 2010).

Balance, Moderation, and Variety—Again

Unfortunately, there is no nutritional bulletproof vest against cancer. Population studies that found links between vegetable and fruit intakes and decreased cancer cases investigated whole foods. Whether the specific components can be proven to prevent cancer remains to be seen. For most people, including generous amounts of plant products in the diet is a healthful strategy.

Consumption of vegetables and fruits is especially important if they replace other more kilocaloric dense foods. On the other hand, if the produce is fried or served with rich sauces, or the fruit is converted to high-kilocaloric beverages, the goal of reaching and maintaining a healthy weight will be thwarted.

As noted in Clinical Application 21-3, the best-intended use of supplements can result in surprising adverse effects. Taking a single nutrient in large amounts clearly is harmful for some groups.

Nutrition for Cancer Clients

A cancer survivor is anyone who has been diagnosed with cancer, from the time of diagnosis through the rest of his or her life. The 5-year survival rate is the

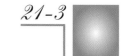

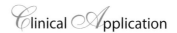

Clinical Application *21-3*

More Is Not Better: Beta-Carotene and Lung Cancer

Carotene, the precursor of vitamin A, is present in many green and deep-yellow vegetables. Vitamin A helps maintain epithelial tissue, protects against oxidation, may influence host **immune** defenses, and assists in the control of cellular differentiation, a process that is faulty in the rapidly growing cancer cell.

Observational studies found people with lower rates of lung cancer:

■ Consumed more fruits and vegetables
■ Had higher serum beta-carotene concentrations

Connecting knowledge about the functions of vitamin A and those observational findings, researchers designed clinical trials using supplements. In Finland, when testing beta-carotene and vitamin E as cancer-preventive agents for lung cancer, the intervention produced surprising findings:

■ A 16% *increase* in lung cancer, and
■ An 8% *increase* in total mortality in the beta-carotene group (Alpha-tocopherol, Beta-carotene Cancer Prevention Study Group, 1994).

In another trial, beta-carotene and retinol were given to men and women who had been heavy smokers and to men with extensive occupational asbestos exposure. The results were similar:

■ A 28% higher than expected incidence of lung cancer, and
■ A 17% higher mortality (Omenn, Goodman, Thornquist, et al, 1994, 1996).

This research showed that beta-carotene can have pro-oxidant effects under certain conditions, such as high oxygen pressures and oxidative stress found in the lungs of smokers (Kamat and Lamm, 2002). The fact that beta-carotene supplements were associated with increased morbidity and mortality from lung cancer, however, should not deter someone from consuming vegetables rich in this nutrient.

Box 21-3 outlines some of the factors to consider when confronted with research findings concerning nutrition. There are no guarantees, however, even with an optimal diet and favorable lifestyle, that an individual will not develop cancer.

percentage of persons still living 5 years after diagnosis. The 5-year relative survival rate for all cancers combined is now approximately 68%. Among Whites, it is about 69%, among Blacks, about 59%. For the five cancers most commonly diagnosed in adults, the 5-year survival rates were as follows:

■ Breast, 75%
■ Bladder, 74%
■ Prostate, 69%
■ Colorectal, 51%
■ Lung, 13% (National Institutes of Health, March 29, 2013)

Box 21-3 ■ *Research Findings: Probabilities, Not Certainties*

There is a natural progression in research (from descriptive to experimental studies) that reflects increasing certainty that the findings display reality. Unfortunately, the significance and practical applications of research results are often overstated and publicized in the general press before being reviewed and replicated by other scientists. A single study may be interesting but should not be the basis for radical behavior changes. Peer scientists should examine all research for its strengths and weaknesses. Possible shortcomings affecting all research include the following:

- Inaccurate measurements. Recall data from questionnaires, although showing statistical differences in large studies, may not accurately reflect dietary intake or other behaviors. Even blood levels may be insensitive to small differences and may not correlate with cellular levels in certain organs.
- Imperfect statistical controls. Although extraneous variables are often held constant by statistical manipulation, the process is not perfect, and all extraneous variables may not have been considered.
- Incorrect assumptions. An underlying physiological basis for a given effect increases the credibility of research. New methods to test physiological effects often challenge earlier assumptions and conclusions. For instance, the mechanism supporting the value of cranberry juice in decreasing bladder infections was determined to be inhibition of *Escherichia coli*. The earlier anecdotal evidence regarding cranberry juice was dismissed by scientists who assumed that the mechanism of action would be acidification of urine, and cranberry juice did not make that much difference in pH.

The following table lists some types of studies (descriptive, correlational, and experimental), their distinguishing qualities, and examples of individual studies focusing on nutrition.

Type of Study	Characteristics	Application to Nutrition	Limitations	Example
Descriptive	Reports naturally occurring events	Examines a population in relation to presence of risk factors, average intake of nutrients, cancer rates and mortality, utilization of health care, etc.	Cannot establish causation Diet is just one of many influences on health outcomes Even less certainty results if the population is diverse	Body mass index increased steadily in all race, sex, and education groups from 1997 to 2008, and Blacks (particularly women) had a consistently higher BMI than their White counterparts (Jackson, Szklo, Yeh, et al, 2013)
Correlational	Compares phenomena in groups with particular outcomes	Determines the existence of systematic relationships between consumption of specific foods or supplements and cancer occurrence	Correlation does not establish causation. An untested variable may be causing the relationship	
Cross-Sectional	Compares behavior of different groups using the same measures at one point in time		The point in time may not be typical	Young adults who placed high importance on alternative production practices (organic, local, sustainable, and nonprocessed foods) consumed significantly more fruits and vegetables, dietary fiber and significantly fewer added sugars and sugar-sweetened beverages than those who placed low importance on these practices (Pelletier, Laska, Neumark-Sztainer, and Story, 2013)
Case-Control	Compares reported behavior by case clients with reported behavior by a control group of similar people without the illness		Controls may differ from cases in significant ways that were not considered and inability to recall behavior accurately	After adjustment for waist circumference, waist-to-hip ratio, total energy intake, sex, age, and education, there was a positive dose–response relationship between reflux esophagitis and intake of calcium, meat, oils, and salt (Wu, Zhao, Ai, et al, 2013)
Prospective (Cohort)	Measures phenomena of interest in a large population; much later compares those with a particular outcome to those without it in relation to the earlier determined practice	Determines usual diet and other pertinent traits of large group of people at point A; waits until illness of interest develops in an adequate number of the people, then	Requires large groups to obtain sufficient cases May take years for illness of interest to develop, and diet may have changed in the interim	After a mean follow-up of 69,310 women for 11 years, drinking 2 to 3 cups of tea per day was associated with a 21% reduced risk of digestive system cancers in nonsmoking, non-alcohol-drinking Chinese women (Nechuta, Shu, Li, et al, 2012)

Box 21-3 ■ Research Findings: Probabilities, Not Certainties—cont'd

Type of Study	Characteristics	Application to Nutrition	Limitations	Example
		compares the groups with and without disease in relation to the early diet		
Experimental	Compares results of an intervention administered to one group but not to another	Administers vitamin or specific food to one group, placebo or none to another; measures changes in illness, symptoms, blood levels	Component selected for intervention may not be the one that gave the effect when whole foods are investigated	
Cell and Tissue Cultures			Laboratory results may not be duplicated in animals or humans	Lutein or zeaxanthin modulates inflammatory responses in cultured retinal pigment epithelial cells in response to photooxidation (Bian, Gao, Zhou, et al, 2012)
Animals			Large doses may be used that are unrealistic to extrapolate to humans	Both calorie restriction and treadmill exercise reduced adiposity by 35% to 40% and serum leptin levels by 80% in obese mice, but only calorie restriction increased adiponectin and insulin sensitivity (Wheatley, Nogueira, Perkins, Hursting, 2011)
Humans			Difficult to shield participants from knowing their intervention or control status. In a crossover design, each person serves as his or her own control. May take a long time to see an effect. Ethical considerations limit the withholding of treatment from the control group	In a crossover trial using researcher-provided low- or high-FODMAP diets, subjects with irritable bowel syndrome had higher levels of breath hydrogen on both diets (four times greater with the high FODMAP intake) than did healthy volunteers (Ong, Mitchell, Barrett, et al, 2010)

In summary, careful reading of research reports is required to make wise judgments about the applicability to health practices. Occasionally, an intervention trial is terminated early to permit an obviously effective treatment to be extended to the control group, as in the folic acid–neural tube defect study (MRC Vitamin Study Research Group, 1991) or to prevent harm, as in the beta-carotene/vitamin A–lung cancer trial (Redlich, Blaner, Van Bennekum, et al, 1998). Even in these rare situations, the complete reasons for the effect shown by the overwhelming evidence are not always clear. A broad perspective is necessary to guide a person's behavior toward healthy choices for a lifetime.

Given advances in early detection and treatment, the number of cancer survivors in the United States is estimated to exceed 12 million. Approximately 1 in every 25 Americans is a cancer survivor, and about 68% of Americans diagnosed with cancer now live more than 5 years. Their nutritional needs change over the course of survivorship (Rock, Doyle, Demark-Wahnefried, et al, 2012). The number of survivors also increases the risk of developing another primary cancer over time (August and Huhmann, 2014). The trajectory of cancer survivorship is marked by three general phases:

1. Active treatment and recovery
2. Living after recovery (those who are disease-free or have stable disease)
3. Advanced cancer and end of life (Rock et al, 2012)

Malnutrition in cancer clients affects prognosis and choices of treatment. For any given type of tumor, survival is shorter in clients with significant pretreatment weight loss (more than 10% of usual body weight). Conversely, excess weight is estimated to contribute to 14% of cancer deaths in men and 20% in women (August and Huhmann, 2014).

Nutrition and Physical Activity During Active Treatment and Recovery

All of the major modalities of cancer treatment, including surgery, radiation, and chemotherapy, can significantly affect nutritional needs by:

■ Altering usual eating habits
■ Adversely affecting digestion, absorption, and metabolism of food

Nutritional assessment should begin as soon after diagnosis as possible and should consider treatment goals (cure, control, or palliation) while focusing on both the current nutritional status and anticipated nutrition-related symptoms (Rock et al, 2012). The physical changes evoked by treatments are only part of the difficulty encountered in adequately nourishing cancer clients. Likely to also affect food intake are psychological factors such as pain, anxiety, depression, and social isolation (August and Huhmann, 2014).

During active cancer treatment, the overall goals of nutritional care should be to:

■ Prevent or resolve nutrient deficiencies
■ Achieve or maintain a healthy weight
■ Preserve lean body mass
■ Minimize nutrition-related side effects
■ Maximize quality of life including an individualized exercise prescription (Rock et al, 2012)

Randomized controlled trials have demonstrated that aerobic exercise significantly reduced cancer-related fatigue during and postcancer therapy. In relation to diagnosis, exercise decreased fatigue in clients with breast or prostate cancer but not in those with hematological malignancies. Aerobic exercise significantly reduced fatigue but resistance training and alternative forms of exercise did not (Cramp and Byron-Daniel, 2012)

Concerns that the estrogenic activity of isoflavones may have adverse effects on breast cancer recurrence have been assuaged. Soy foods consumed at levels comparable to those in Asian populations have no detrimental effects on risk of breast cancer recurrence and in some cases significantly reduce the risk (Magee and Rowland, 2012). A moderate amount of soy is 1 to 2 standard servings of whole soy foods, such as tofu, soy milk, and edamame (American Institute for Cancer Research, 2012).

Living After Recovery

Determining exactly when a cancer's aberrant cell division began is difficult because of:

■ Cancer's long development time
■ The complex interaction between cancer cells and the body's defenses

Equating the beginning of the cancer with the date of diagnosis is measureable but misleading. Consequently, it may be too much to expect that lifestyle changes after diagnosis would make a major difference in the client's outcome.

Nevertheless, during this posttreatment phase, setting and achieving lifelong goals for weight management, a physically active lifestyle, and a healthy diet are important to promote overall health, quality of life, and longevity. Although cancer survivorship is a relatively new area of study, current evidence supports recommendations in three basic areas: weight management, physical activity, and dietary pattern (Rock et al, 2012).

Weight Management

The ACS advises cancer survivors to achieve and maintain a healthy weight. Individuals who are overweight or obese should limit consumption of high-caloric foods and beverages and increase physical activity to promote weight loss (Rock et al, 2012).

Observational studies of female breast cancer consistently find that adiposity is associated with a 30% increased risk of mortality (Patterson, Cadmus, Emond, and Pierce, 2010). While it is true that obese women with breast cancer have poorer survival rates than women of normal weight with breast cancer, no study has elucidated the causal mechanism (Protani, Coory, and Martin, 2010).

Physical Activity

The ACS advises cancer survivors to engage in regular physical activity, to avoid inactivity, and return to normal daily activities as soon as possible after diagnosis. Specifically, the ACS recommends 150 minutes of exercise per week, including strength training at least 2 days per week (Rock et al, 2012).

The American College of Sports Medicine concurs with the ACS with the caveat to consult with the medical staff to assess tumor site–specific issues. Receiving particular mention are clients with breast cancer, prostate cancer, intestinal stomas, and morbidly obesity. The National Comprehensive Cancer Network, which produces evidence-based standards of care guidelines, recommends that certain survivor groups (e.g., clients with comorbidities, recent major surgery, functional or anatomical deficits, or substantial deconditioning) obtain referral to physical therapy to facilitate exercise during fatigue (Wolin, Schwartz, Matthews, et al, 2012).

In short, individual assessment underlies safe implementation of an exercise program in cancer survivors. Many survivors can safely begin a low- to moderate-intensity exercise program, such as walking, without supervision or exercise specialist evaluation. Oncology professionals should feel comfortable prescribing exercise to cancer survivors, with advice to start with light-intensity exercises, progress slowly, and allow the survivor's symptoms to guide the process (Wolin et al, 2012). Results of studies linking physical activity after diagnosis to outcomes are shown in Table 21-2.

Dietary Patterns

The ACS advises cancer survivors to consume a diet that is high in vegetables, fruits, and whole grains and to follow the Guidelines on Nutrition and Physical Activity for Cancer Prevention summarized in Box 21-1 (Rock et al, 2012). Despite efforts to find a "magic bullet" among micronutrients, none has been demonstrated to be effective in humans with an established cancer. Similarly, no proven role exists for nutritional pharmacologic supplements (August and Huhmann, 2014).

Prospective observational studies have shown that increased exercise after diagnosis and avoidance of a Western pattern diet are associated with reduced risk of cancer recurrence and improved overall survival in early-stage colorectal cancer after standard therapy (Meyerhardt, 2011).

Advanced Cancer and End of Life

A diagnosis of cancer does not necessarily mean that the person will die of cancer. For instance, women with low-grade localized endometrial cancer were most likely to die of cardiovascular disease, whereas women with high-grade advanced cancer were most likely to die of endometrial cancer. For the entire population, risk of death from cardiovascular causes surpasses the risk of death from endometrial cancer 5 years after diagnosis (Ward, Shah, Saenz, et al, 2012).

That is not to minimize the fact that in 2013, 580,350 deaths from cancer were expected to occur in the United States (ACS, 2013). Those clients should receive the best care available with emphasis on maximizing the quality of their remaining life.

Diet and Exercise

Recommendations for nutrition and physical activity in those who are living with advanced cancer are best based on individual nutrition needs and physical abilities. To the extent possible, physical activity should be encouraged. Anorexia and fatigue may begin a cycle of inactivity that ultimately results in greater loss of muscle mass and consequent inability to be active (Gullett, Mazurak, Hebbar, and Ziegler, 2011).

Although advanced cancer is sometimes accompanied by substantial weight loss, it is not inevitable that individuals with cancer lose weight or experience malnutrition. In general, the goal should be to optimize nutritional state and encourage repair of tissues not only during cancer surgery or procedures but throughout the course of cancer therapy to decrease morbidity and increase quality of life.

Many clients with advanced cancer choose to adapt their food choices and meal patterns to meet nutritional needs and to manage cancer symptoms or treatment side effects. Additional nutritional supplementation such as nutrient-dense beverages and foods can be consumed by those who cannot eat or drink enough to maintain sufficient energy intake. The use of enteral nutrition and parenteral nutrition support should be individualized with recognition of overall treatment goals (control or palliation) and the associated risks of medical complications and/or ethical dilemmas. The evidence of a benefit from exercise for survivors of advanced cancer is insufficient to make general recommendations (Rock et al, 2012).

Modalities of nutritional support for cancer clients are shown in Table 21-3. The goal of nutrition intervention is to support anabolism, body composition,

TABLE 21-2 ■ Effect of Postdiagnosis Physical Activity on Cancer Survival					
SITE	NUMBER OF STUDIES	NUMBER OF SUBJECTS	EFFECT ON RECURRENCE	EFFECT ON MORTALITY	SOURCE
Breast	6	12,108	Reduced by 41%	Reduced breast cancer deaths by 34% Reduced all-cause mortality by 41%	Ibrahim EM, and Al-Homaidh A, 2011
Colorectal	1	2293		The equivalent of 150 minutes per week of walking lowered all-cause mortality 42%	Campbell, Patel, Newton, et al, 2013
Prostate	1	2705		≥3 hours per week of vigorous activity lowered all-cause mortality 46% Normal to very brisk walking ≥90 minutes/week lowered all-cause mortality 49%	Kenfield, Stampfer, Giovannucci, and Chan, 2011

TABLE 21-3 ■ Nutritional Therapies for Cancer Clients

	INDICATIONS	CLINICAL RESULTS	PRECAUTIONS
Oral	Impaired GI tract Special metabolic needs	Enhanced long-term oral intake Weight maintenance Preservation of lean body mass Improved quality of life	Dietitian's conversion of prescribed diet to acceptable meal plan is critical to success
Enteral	Obstruction/defect in GI tract Limited absorptive capacity Chemoradiotherapy for head and neck cancer	Weight gain Benefits perioperative clients with functional GI tract and inability to meet nutritional needs orally for 7–10 days Decreased infectious complications than with PN No effect on survival Prevents dehydration and interference with treatment due to inflammation of the mouth	Monitor swallowing ability to discontinue artificial feeding when appropriate
Parenteral	Intensive anticancer therapy Intolerance of oral/enteral feedings >14 days Malnourished clients before chemotherapy or surgery Bone marrow transplant clients Severe gastrointestinal injury in clients with cured/controlled cancer	Improved nutrient laboratory values Reduced incidence of wound healing complications Increased risk of perioperative infections, chiefly pneumonia and bacteremia	Routine use in chemotherapy or radiation clients gives no advantage in response to therapy, complications, or mortality In most cases, inappropriate if life expectancy is less than 40–60 days
Pharmacotherapy			
Anabolic Steroids	*oxandrolone*	FDA*-approved therapeutic option for increasing lean body mass in cachectic clients	Schedule III controlled substance
Appetite Stimulants	*megestrol* *cyproheptadine* *dronabinol*	Weight gain, much of it fat Improved quality of life	
Antidepressant Drugs		Relief of anorexia Possible weight gain	Major depression occurs in about 25% of cancer clients
Antiemetic Drugs		Optimal dosing can control vomiting in 70%–90% of chemotherapy clients	Clients often do not mention nausea unless specifically asked
NSAIDs		Reduces resting energy expenditure Preserves body fat	Well-tolerated with minimal side effects
Stimulant	*methylphenidate*	Relief of anorexia Relief of depression	Causes anorexia in clients without cancer

*U.S. Food and Drug Administration
Adapted from August and Huhmann, 2014; Gullett, Mazurak, Hebbar, and Ziegler, 2011; Pronsky and Crowe, 2012.

functional status, and quality of life. When designed in a structured, formal nutrition care process, nutrition support can be effective in clients with cancer who are:

■ Receiving active anticancer treatment
■ Moderately to severely malnourished
■ Expected to be unable to ingest or absorb adequate nutrients
   ■ For 7 to 14 days in perioperative clients
   ■ For 14 days or longer in nonsurgical clients (August and Huhmann, 2014)

Enteral and parenteral nutrition are covered in detail in Chapter 14. Suggestions to mitigate costs of enteral nutrition appear as Dollars & Sense 21-2. Care of the client with terminal illness is the subject of Chapter 24.

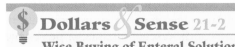
$ Dollars & Sense 21-2

Wise Buying of Enteral Solutions

For individuals receiving enteral nutrition at home, a bit of shopping among store brands at drug store chains may produce significant savings. Look for products containing the same kilocalories per milliliter as prescribed.

Food assistance programs may cover costs.

Although it is possible to make a homemade solution from pureed foods, it is not recommended. Cancer clients may be immunocompromised. The commercially prepared solutions are less subject to contamination than a homemade feeding.

Common Nutritional Problems

Some nutritional problems in cancer clients are due to the disease, and others are due to treatment modalities. Common problems affecting the consumption of meals and nourishment of cancer clients are early satiety and anorexia, taste alterations, local effects in the mouth, nausea, vomiting, diarrhea, and altered immune response. Cachexia is a wasting condition seen in cancer and other diseases.

EARLY SATIETY AND ANOREXIA

Although they may look starved, cancer clients may take a few bites of food and declare that they are full. They may say that they have no appetite at all. The main source of this symptom is the cancer itself, by mechanisms that are beginning to be understood. Control of the disease improves the appetite.

Sometimes, however, the physical pressure from the tumor or **third-space** fluid accumulation may give a feeling of fullness. Relieving that problem may improve food intake.

Some additional factors may interfere with appetite. The psychological stress of dealing with cancer may produce anxiety or depression. The person may be grappling with a body image change or may be going through the grieving process for the loss of a body function or the potential loss of life itself.

Interventions
- Encourage eating whether hungry or not.
- Exercise appropriately before meals.
- Serve small, frequent, attractive meals.
- For inpatients, serve favorite foods from home or a family-shared meal.
- For children, serve food in shapes or decorated with the child's name.
- Vary supplement flavors to prevent taste fatigue.
- Offer 1 ounce of a complete supplement every hour.
- Add nutrients to regular foods.
    - 1⅓ cups (or whatever amount satisfies) of instant dry skim milk powder in 1 quart of liquid milk increases the nutrient density, with little or no change in palatability.
    - 1 tablespoon of dry skim milk powder in mashed potatoes or puddings.

TASTE ALTERATIONS

Cancer clients may have changes in taste perceptions, particularly a decreased threshold for bitterness. Accordingly, they will often say that beef and pork taste bitter or metallic. Some clients report a decreased sensation of sweet, salty, and sour tastes, and they desire increased seasonings. These taste changes are caused by the cancer and the various modes of therapy. In some cases, taste acuity returns 2 to 3 months after cessation of treatment. Changes induced by radiation treatments however, may be permanent (August and Huhmann, 2014).

Interventions
- Provide oral hygiene before meals to freshen the mouth.
- Offer lemon-flavored beverages to improve taste sensations.
- Cook in a microwave oven or in glass utensils to minimize the metallic taste.
- Offer plastic table service if metal utensils are a problem.
- Serve eggs, fish, poultry, and dairy products that may be better received than beef or pork.
- Serve meat cold or at room temperature to lessen the bitter taste.
- Add sweet sauces and marinades to the meat to improve its palatability.

LOCAL EFFECTS IN THE MOUTH

Because of the rapid cellular turnover in the oral mucosa, chemotherapy induces **stomatitis** in more than 50% of outpatients (August and Huhmann, 2014). Also, clients being treated with radiation for head and neck cancers often experience inflammation or ulcers in the mouth, decreased and thick saliva, and swallowing difficulty. Any of these conditions may interfere with nutritional intake.

Interventions
- For all: provide oral hygiene, before and after meals.
- For mouth ulcerations, try the following strategies:
    - Serve soft, mild foods.
    - Top foods with sauces, gravies, and dressings, which may make foods easier to eat.
    - Serve cream soups and milk, which provide much nutrition for the volume ingested.
    - Serve cold foods, which have a somewhat numbing effect and may be better tolerated than hot food.
    - Include liquids with meals to help wash down the food.
    - Introduce drinking straws, which may detour liquids around mouth ulcerations.
    - Avoid these irritants (a highly recommended strategy): hot items, salty or spicy foods, acidic juices, and alcohol (even in mouthwash).
    - If necessary, seek an anesthetic mouthwash, which can be prescribed. If the mouth is anesthetized, clients should be instructed to chew slowly and carefully to avoid biting their lips, tongue, or cheeks.

- For dry mouth, try the following strategies:
  - Include adequate hydration to help keep the mouth moist.
  - Present food with lubricants, such as gravy, butter, margarine, milk, beer, or bouillon to aid intake.
  - Consider synthetic salivas, but they have caused allergic reactions (Kandala and Playfor, 2003). In addition, many clients prefer sips of water to the synthetic products.
  - Offer sugarless hard candy, chewing gum, or popsicles to stimulate saliva production.
- For swallowing difficulty, try the following strategies (see also the section on dysphagia in Chapter 9):
  - Advise the client to make swallowing a conscious act (inhaling, swallowing, and exhaling) to lessen the risk of choking.
  - Suggest experimenting with head position, which may ease the dysphagia. Tilting the head backward or forward may help.
  - Serve foods that are nonsticky and of even consistency to minimize swallowing difficulty. Lumpy gravy and mixed vegetables, for example, are hard to manage.
  - Suggest dunking bread products in beverages to help lubricate the passage.
  - Refer to a speech therapist as necessary.

NAUSEA, VOMITING, AND DIARRHEA

This triad of symptoms often accompanies radiation treatment or chemotherapy, as well as certain types of tumors. Because the gastrointestinal tract cells are normally replaced every few days, these rapidly dividing cells are more vulnerable to cancer treatments than other body cells. Not all clients suffer these side effects to the same extent, and the effects generally cease when the treatment is completed. See also Table 21-3 for antiemetic therapy.

Cancer treatment regimens that include radiation therapy to the abdomen have the potential to disturb the indigenous gut flora, causing diarrhea, enteritis, and colitis in more than 80% of recipients of that therapy (Visich and Yeo, 2010). Some clients are disabled by diarrhea but reluctant to seek help, perhaps believing their situation is normal. Both during and after treatment ends, questions about specific symptoms could bring to light a condition amenable to correction.

Radiation enteritis involves injury to the intestine. Clients at greater risk of radiation enteritis are those:

- Who are thin
- Who have had previous abdominal surgery
- Who have hypertension, diabetes mellitus, or pelvic inflammatory disease
- Who receive chemotherapy along with the radiation

Interventions

For nausea and vomiting, try the following strategies:

- Offer the client dry crackers before rising.
- Schedule meals at times of the day when nausea is least.
- Serve liquids 30 to 60 minutes after solid food.
- Limit fats in the diet to promote gastric emptying.
- Teach the client to eat slowly and chew thoroughly.
- Suggest the client rest after eating.
- Recommend the client save favorite foods for times of feeling well to avoid food aversion.
- Instruct the client to take antiemetics and analgesics as prescribed. Pain also causes nausea.
- Advise the client or caregiver to minimize strong cooking odors by
  - Selecting milder foods.
  - Ventilating the kitchen.
  - Preparing food in a microwave oven or by boil-in-bag methods.

For diarrhea, try the following strategies:

- Add pectin-containing (apple, banana) foods to the client's intake.
- Implement a low-fiber diet (see Chapter 20).
- Test for and treat lactose intolerance.
- Consult with a dietitian about special feedings.
- Investigate the feasibility of probiotic therapy. Randomized clinical trials have demonstrated efficacy of probiotic preparations VSL #3 and Lactobacillus case DN-114 001 in decreasing the incidence and grade of radiation therapy-induced diarrhea (Visich and Yeo, 2010).

ALTERED IMMUNE RESPONSE

Sometimes antineoplastic agents suppress the client's immune system. Clients receiving them are at risk for overwhelming infections from organisms that would not affect other persons. Clients receiving radiation therapy or radiation as part of bone marrow transplantation also are at high risk for infections and need to be protected from all organisms, even those that are harmless to most healthy people. Clinical Application 21-4 relates the role of the aging immune system to cancer.

Interventions

Depending on the client's condition, the following strategies may be used.

- Institute protective isolation to minimize exposure to microorganisms.
- Observe strict procedures for food safety and sanitation (see Chapter 13).

Some providers attempt to limit exposure to microorganisms by restricting unpasteurized, uncooked,

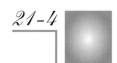

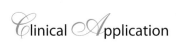

Role of the Immune System in Cancer

Age is the most important risk factor for tumorigenesis. More than 60% of new cancers and more than 70% of cancer deaths occur in persons older than 65 years. Many lines of evidence point to the most important factor simply being the passage of time, allowing the accumulation of damage from **free radicals,** viruses, carcinogens, or other agents causing mutations that favor the development of cancer (Fulop, Larbi, Kotb, et al, 2011). Immune competence tends to decrease with age, a phenomenon termed *immunosenescence,* implying that decreased immunosurveillance against cancer could also contribute to increased disease in the elderly (Pawelec, Derhovanessian, and Larbi, 2010).

The immune system can recognize and eliminate tumor cells, but the tumors also can interfere with and evade immune responses through multiple mechanisms. The increased incidence of cancer in AIDS clients and organ transplant clients on immunosuppressive drugs demonstrates the consequence of a weakened immune system.

Part of the body's immune defense is provided by certain white blood cells called **T-lymphocytes.** These cells have the task of recognizing foreign materials, including cancer cells, as "nonself" and acting to destroy the invaders. Some of the T-lymphocytes develop into killer cells, which bind to the foreign cell membrane and release lysosomal enzymes into the foreign cell to destroy it.

The T-lymphocytes mature in the **thymus** gland in the chest, hence the name, thymic lymphocytes. Possibly contributing to the development of cancer in the elderly is the deterioration of the immune system, since the thymus gland begins to shrink at sexual maturity and by age 50 only 10% of the original gland remains.

Present knowledge only suggests that the age-related immune alterations are likely to favor the development of tumors. There is little direct evidence that age-associated immune response changes are really important for controlling the development and progression of cancer (Fulop, et al, 2011).

and unwashed foods, but the effectiveness of this dietary approach has not been substantiated with direct proof (Fox and Freifeld, 2012). Analysis of three randomized controlled trials involving 197 chemotherapy subjects found no evidence of effect of a low-bacterial diet in the neutropenic client at the same time noting that "no evidence of effect" is not the same as "evidence of no effect." No recommendation for clinical practice could be made on the basis of the available evidence. More high-quality research is needed (van Dalen, Mank, Leclercq, et al, 2012).

CACHEXIA

A state of malnutrition and wasting is called **cachexia,** but muscle wasting due to cancer differs from that which occurs in starvation and aging. Also seen in other advanced diseases, a degree of cancer-induced cachexia is experienced by up to 80% of advanced-stage cancer clients. Incidence of cachexia is partly dependent on the site of the primary cancer, often occurring with gastrointestinal, pancreatic, thoracic, and head and neck malignancies (Gullett et al, 2011). Gastrointestinal malignancy is associated with the largest losses: 50% of muscle mass and protein content and 30% to 40% of body fat. Clients with solid tumors can lose as much as 1.34 kilogram of fat free mass in 4 weeks (August and Huhmann, 2014).

Cachexic clients are shown to have:

- Increased muscle protein synthesis and that is outpaced by the rate of protein degradation
- Increased basal metabolic rate and total energy expenditure
- Increased inflammation and insulin resistance
- Decreased fat mass, muscle mass, strength, and function (Evans, 2010)

Current research implicates an inflammatory reaction to the tumor that is predominantly local but may also be systemic as the basis for cancer-induced cachexia. Diagnostic components are weight loss, low kilocaloric intake, and serum C-reactive protein, a nonspecific measure of systemic inflammation (Gullett et al, 2011).

Cachexia results from a complex cascade of physiologic and metabolic derangements involving synthesis, storage, and degradation of all three macronutrients:

- Despite protein depletion, protein turnover remains normal or is even increased.
- Depletion of fat stores results from increased turnover of glycerol and fatty acids.
- Alterations in carbohydrate metabolism are often associated with glucose intolerance and diminished insulin sensitivity (August and Huhmann, 2014).

The result is inefficient utilization of whatever nutrients are supplied to the client. Weight loss seen in cachexic clients cannot be reversed by increased nutrient intake alone and usually continues despite supplementation (August and Huhmann, 2014). Figure 21-4 shows a woman with cachexia.

Interventions

Depending on the cachectic client's condition and wishes and the provider's judgment, the following strategies to improve nutrition may be implemented.

- Best choice—aggressive treatment of the cancer
- Appropriately treat symptoms interfering with nutritional intake (see Chapter 24)
- Reassure client that poor appetite is caused by the cancer not by his or her lack of effort
- Encourage available medications (see Table 21-3) to improve the quality of life

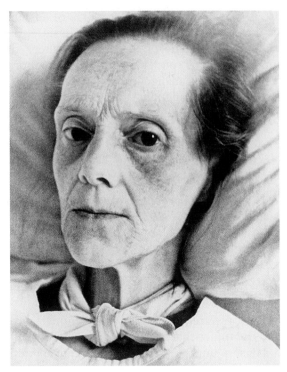

FIGURE 21-4 This woman is cachectic, showing signs of malnutrition and wasting. (Reproduced from *Nutrition Today*, 16(3), cover, © Williams & Wilkins, 1981, with permission.)

■ In selected clients, supplementation with omega-3 fatty acids (fish oil) or protein may be advised (Gullett et al, 2011)

The Charting Tip in Box 21-4 advocates forethought when documenting cancer clients' at-home treatments and diet plans.

One should not expect identical disease outcomes in different people. Just as human beings vary in characteristics, so do cancers differ from one another. Much of the difference in treatment outcomes for clients with cancer stems from variations in tumor biology. Those differences dictate spread of the tumor and its sensitivity to treatments (Burstein and Schwartz, 2008).

Box 21-4 ■ *Charting Tip*

When admitting a client who provides much of his or her own care at home, try to learn all about treatments and dietary preferences and document them. If the client becomes less self-sufficient after surgery or after beginning cancer therapy, the staff will not have to ask multiple questions before providing care. Recording this information ensures that others besides the nurse who obtained it will be able to meet the client's needs.

Keystones

■ Cancer develops in two steps: initiation that alters a cell's genes and promotion that then activates the altered genes to begin their unruly growth locally and at distant sites.

■ Alcohol intake plus overweight and obesity, caused by poor diet and inactivity, are related to breast and colon cancer occurrence. Red or processed meat intake is related to prostate cancer occurrence. Smoking, not diet, is the major factor in lung cancer occurrence, the deadliest of the most common cancers.

■ The best dietary advice to prevent cancer: avoid obesity, stay physically active, consume a healthy plant-based diet with limited red and processed meats, and drink minimal amounts of alcohol if at all.

■ The New American Plate® includes amounts and sample foods in the graphic but omits specific reference to dairy foods. MyPlate includes online resources to assist in implementation. Depending on the learner's motivation and abilities, either could serve as a starting point for instruction.

■ Studying fruits and vegetables in general may not contain sufficient items that really might be of benefit. In more focused studies, the selected study components are likely an infinitesimal part of the whole food from which it comes. A study may be too short to account for the long lead-time in cancer development. The people studied likely differ in genetic makeup, that may affect nutrient utilization.

■ The anorexic client with cancer could benefit from appropriate exercise before meals, small amounts of complete nutritional supplements hourly, added dry milk powder to appropriate foods, and efforts to make mealtime special and pleasurable.

Keystones—cont'd

- Protective isolation is common for clients with altered immune responses. Dietary strategies to protect the immunosuppressed client are directed at strict adherence to food safety and sanitation procedures. Some providers may wish to limit the client's access to unpasteurized, uncooked, and unwashed foods.

- Appetite stimulants may succeed in increasing a cancer client's weight (mostly fat) and are credited with increasing the quality of life. An anabolic steroid has been approved to increase lean body mass in cancer clients. Antidepressants and a stimulant may also relieve anorexia.

- Nutrient intake in clients with mouth ulcerations may be enhanced by using straws to bypass the sores; by serving cool, smooth, bland nutrient-dense foods; and by avoiding acidic, salty, and spicy foods.

- Cachexia is a wasting condition thought to be caused by an inflammatory response to the tumor. The result is a complex cascade of physiologic and metabolic derangements involving synthesis, storage, and degradation of all three macronutrients. Weight loss in cachexic clients cannot be reversed by increased nutrient intake alone. Controlling the cancer is the best method of reversing cachexia.

CASE STUDY *21–1*

Ms. Z is a 67-year-old White widow who had a lumpectomy for breast cancer yesterday. If no complications arise, she is scheduled for discharge tomorrow. The nurse providing her morning care asked how she felt.

"Terrible."

"Do you need something for pain?"

"No, I had something a little while ago. I'm just overwhelmed. This happened so fast. I don't know how I'm going to manage all I have to do. The doctor said I was a good candidate for lumpectomy but I don't know how I will get to radiation therapy. He also said I should lose weight. What good will that do—I've already got cancer!"

"Had cancer. It's gone, remember?"

The nurse continued to explore Ms. Z's risk factors conversationally. She eats the typical Western diet, red meat about every other day, a glass of wine, maybe two, daily with dinner. It was a habit she and her husband had until his death from colon cancer 9 months ago shortly after they retired and moved south. Ms. Z is 5 ft 4 in. tall and weighs 175 lb. She has no children, no relatives in the area, and no church affiliation.

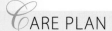 ARE PLAN

Subjective Data

Uncertain of ability to obtain radiation treatment ■ Lacks information about risk factors for breast cancer ■ Feeling overwhelmed; widowed <1 year

Objective Data

Admission weight 175 pounds, height 5 ft, 4 in. ■ BMI 30.1

Analysis

Lack of resources related to procuring cancer treatment; lack of information related to breast cancer prevention

(Continued on the following page)

Plan

DESIRED OUTCOMES EVALUATION CRITERIA	ACTIONS/INTERVENTIONS	RATIONALE
Client will formulate plan to attend radiation therapy by discharge.	Refer to social worker to be seen today.	Ensuring that client has a bridge to continuing therapy will increase likelihood of completing the regimen.
Client will acknowledge three risk factors for breast cancer pertinent to her situation.	Teach that obesity and alcohol are recognized risk factors for breast cancer.	Acknowledging personal risk factors for breast cancer is the first step to changing behavior.
	Point out that • diet is only one of many possible factors leading to cancer. • physical activity has been linked to decreases in recurrence of breast cancer. • lifestyle changes may prevent a second primary cancer in her unaffected breast that has been subjected to the same risk factors as the operated breast.	Recognizing the many factors that play a role in developing cancer should alleviate regrets and guilt about the cause of her cancer.
	Present or review information on a healthy diet according to the American Cancer Society.	Focusing on what can be done now and in the future to change her risk factors offers a measure of control to the client and encourages a positive outlook.

21-1

Social Worker's Notes

The following Social Worker's Notes are representative of the documentation found in a client's medical record. The social worker, after interviewing Ms. Z, wrote the following:

Subjective: Lacks transportation to radiation therapy. Widowed, without social support system in place. States that the doctor recommended weight reduction.

Objective: Coherent. Ready to accept advice.

Analysis: Immediate need is transportation to and from radiation therapy.

Secondary need is social support system to cope with diagnosis and lifestyle changes.

Plan: Set up transportation with American Cancer Society (ACS).

Recommend follow-up with support group at ACS.

𝒞ritical 𝒯hinking 𝒬uestions

1. What additional assessment data might impact the design of Ms. Z's nutritional care plan?

2. Was the nurse's statement, "Had cancer. It's gone..." a wise reply? Why or why not?

3. Do you think there is a relationship between Ms. Z's cancer and that of Mr. Z's illness and death? Why or why not?

Chapter Review

1. Research has identified which of the following factors as possibly explaining the conflicting results reported concerning dietary intakes and cancer development?
   a. Erroneous classification of the tumor types
   b. A time frame that extends over too many years
   c. Too large a sample of people recruited to the study
   d. Genetic differences in the metabolism of the people studied

2. Cruciferous vegetables that are thought to protect against cancer are:
   a. Corn, lima beans, and peas
   b. Carrots, green beans, and tomatoes
   c. Brussels sprouts, bean sprouts, and water chestnuts
   d. Broccoli, cauliflower, and cabbage

3. Which of the following foods is likely to be well received by a cancer client with mouth ulcerations?
   a. Hot chicken noodle soup
   b. Orange juice with orange sherbet
   c. Vanilla milkshake
   d. Soda crackers with cream cheese

4. All of the following interventions except one are likely to assist a client with cancer who suffers from anorexia. Which is the *exception*?
   a. Confining the diet to full liquids
   b. Sipping complete nutritional supplements hourly between meals
   c. Serving meals attractively
   d. Exercising as possible before meals

5. Heterocyclic aromatic amines (HCAs), formed by high-temperature cooking of muscle meats, are well-known risk factors for
   a. Breast cancer
   b. Colorectal cancer
   c. Lung cancer
   d. Prostate cancer

Clinical Analysis

Ms. R is a 70-year-old widow under treatment for breast cancer. She is being cared for by her daughter, Ms. S, with assistance from a home health-care service. Despite fairly good oral intake at the daughter's urging, Ms. R continues to lose weight and now carries 95 lb on her 5-ft, 4-in. frame. Her main complaint regarding food is its bitter taste.

1. Ms. S asks why her mother continues to lose weight when she is taking half the meals and more than half the supplements offered. Which of the following replies by the nurse would be most appropriate?
   a. "Your mother must be too active and using more calories than she is taking in."
   b. "Probably the medications are dehydrating her. We should increase her fluid intake."
   c. "Frequently the tumor short-circuits the body's metabolism so that nutrients cannot be used normally."
   d. "She doesn't take in enough protein to prevent loss of muscle. We should try supplements of amino acid powders."

2. Ms. S expressed interest in learning what she could do to lessen her own chances of developing a malignancy of the breast. Which of the following suggestions have the best evidence for preventing breast cancer?
   a. Limit intake of red, processed, or charbroiled meats.
   b. Maintain a normal weight and minimize or avoid alcohol intake.
   c. Gradually increase fiber intake to 25 grams per day, accompanied by adequate fluid intake.
   d. Eat a variety of colorful fruits and vegetables every day.

3. Which of the following interventions could alleviate the bitter tastes Ms. R is experiencing?
   a. Cooking meats in the microwave oven in glass dishes
   b. Limiting the intake of dairy products
   c. Selecting only very tender cuts or ground beef
   d. Cooking fish outside on the grill to eliminate odors

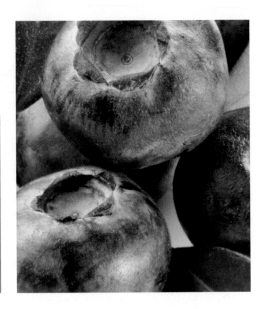

22

Nutrition in Critical Care

LEARNING OBJECTIVES

After completing this chapter, the student should be able to:

- List four hypermetabolic conditions that increase resting energy expenditure and hence kilocaloric requirements.
- Describe how metabolism differs in starvation and hypermetabolism.
- Discuss the effects of impaired respiratory function on nutritional status and appropriate nutritional therapy.
- List six recommendations for the safe refeeding of malnourished clients.

*P*atients admitted to critical care units have life-threatening injuries and illnesses. Acute conditions may include severe burns, trauma, and infections. The most likely chronic conditions related to admission to critical care units are respiratory and cardiac problems. This chapter focuses on clients admitted with respiratory problems. Chapter 18 focused on cardiac care. The body responds to life-threatening injuries and illnesses with a hypermetabolic response. The provision of nutritional care for these clients is a challenge. Under- or overfeeding these clients may result in a loss of lean body mass and death, respectively.

Stress and Critical Care

Metabolically the body responds to starvation by decreasing energy expenditure and to hypermetabolism by increasing energy expenditure. Some of the major complications seen in critical care include:

- Inflammation
- Sepsis (blood infection)
- Gastrointestinal (GI) effects
- Wounds
- Fluid imbalances
- Multisystem organ failure

The Stress of Starvation

The physical stress of starvation alters nutrient needs. Biologically, our bodies evolved to cope with periods of feast or famine. Our response to the stress of starvation evolved slowly over the course of millions of years. The human body's response to food deprivation allowed a person to survive despite inadequate food for longer periods than after other physical assaults.

Uncomplicated starvation means that the client is experiencing food deprivation without an underlying disease state. During uncomplicated starvation, clients expend about 70% of the kilocalories they normally need to maintain body weight. Because of the biochemical adaptation to starvation, these clients require fewer kilocalories than is normal for their height and weight.

The breakdown or catabolism of nutrient stores to meet energy needs characterizes our initial response to starvation. Every cell within the human body needs a constant supply of energy to function. During starvation, a series of four chemical reactions occurs to meet each cell's energy needs:

1. **Glycogenolysis** is the breakdown of glycogen (the liver's carbohydrate stores). This breakdown releases glucose into the bloodstream. However, the body's limited glycogen stores last only a few hours.
2. **Gluconeogenesis** is the production of glucose from noncarbohydrate stores (only the glycerol portion of

triglycerides and amino acids derived from proteins in muscle and organ mass). The primary source of glucose in early starvation is the increased rate of gluconeogenesis, which causes a reduction of lean body mass.

3. **Lipolysis** is the breakdown of adipose tissue for energy. This breakdown releases free fatty acids into the bloodstream. In prolonged starvation, adaptive mechanisms conserve body protein stores by enabling a greater proportion of energy needs to be met by increased fatty acids, with a decreased requirement for glucose.

4. **Ketosis** is the accumulation of ketone bodies: acetone, beta-hydroxybutyric acid, and acetoacetic acid. Ketosis results from the incomplete metabolism of fatty acids, generally from carbohydrate deficiency, and occurs commonly in starvation. The body utilizes some ketone bodies for energy during prolonged starvation to meet the central nervous system's need for glucose. This use of ketones reduces, but does not eliminate, the need for glucose.

These chemical reactions are summarized in Figure 22-1.

Each body cell needs glucose, fatty acids, or the end products of fatty acids and amino acids for energy. Body cells need fuel constantly. Amino acids can be utilized for energy, but only after the liver converts them into glucose or fat. Specific organs have a preference for glucose as a fuel source. The brain, for example, prefers glucose for energy. Some cells can also utilize ketone bodies for energy. The brain will use ketone bodies but prefers glucose. For the most part, the human body can use only a small part of the fat molecule, the glycerol portion, to manufacture glucose. Therefore, after the liver's glycogen stores are depleted, body protein stores must be continually broken down to supply the brain with glucose during starvation.

The heart, kidney, and skeletal muscle tissues prefer fatty acids and ketone bodies for their fuel sources. As a result, even if a starving person is fed glucose (as in intravenous feeding); some fat is still needed to prevent the breakdown of adipose tissue. A balance of the end products of fat and carbohydrate metabolism is necessary for survival.

In prolonged starvation, most body organs switch to a less preferred fuel source. Even the brain increasingly uses more ketone bodies for energy after adaptation to starvation than before. The breakdown of muscle tissue continues in prolonged starvation but at a much lower rate. The human body also becomes more efficient in reusing amino acids for protein synthesis. Thus, urea nitrogen excretion decreases during prolonged starvation.

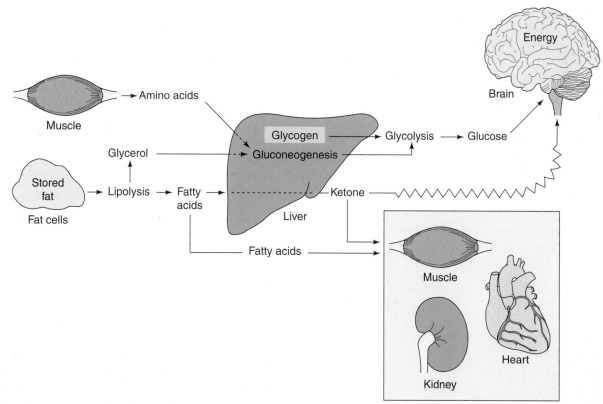

FIGURE 22-1 Origin of fuel and fuel consumption during starvation. The primary source of glucose in early starvation (after the depletion of glycogen stores) is the increased rate of gluconeogenesis. In prolonged starvation, adaptive mechanisms conserve protein by enabling a greater proportion of energy needs to be met by ketone bodies, with a decreased requirement for glucose.

The rate of tissue breakdown in prolonged starvation also decreases because the metabolic rate and total energy expenditure decrease to conserve energy and prolong life. The catabolic or starved individual spontaneously decreases physical activity, increases sleep, and has a lower body temperature. All of these adaptations during prolonged starvation serve one purpose—to prolong life. The human body gets "more miles per gallon" as a result of individual body organs switching to a less preferred fuel source.

Hypermetabolism

An abnormal increase in the rate at which fuel or kilocalories are burned is called **hypermetabolism.** Characteristics of this condition are:

- Increased metabolic rate
- Negative nitrogen balance
- Hyperglycemia
- Increased oxygen consumption

Box 22-1 discusses the benefits of intensive insulin therapy in critical care clients. The body increasingly uses protein obtained from internal body stores (lean body mass) to meet energy needs and depletes lean body mass.

Hormonal Response

The stress response in hypermetabolism is also mediated by hormones. The catecholamines, glucagon, and cortisol oppose insulin and are typically referred to as counter-regulatory hormones. Collectively these hormones influence glucose and fat metabolism by causing the breakdown of glycogen and amino acids to produce glucose and triglycerides from body fat stores. The body produces glucose so it has the fuel to respond to stress. Two other hormones, aldosterone and

antidiuretic hormone, also respond to stress, and result is the retention of both water and sodium.

Metabolic Response

The metabolic response of the immune system to infection or injury is called the **inflammatory response.** The signs and symptoms of inflammation include:

- Swelling
- Redness
- Heat
- Pain

C-reactive protein (CRP) is released by the liver during acute phase of the inflammatory response and alters:

- Metabolism
- Heart rate
- Blood pressure
- Body temperature
- Immune cell function

CRP is frequently measured in critical care clients. One practical application of this metabolic response is that an individual's kilocalorie and protein intake may be sufficient, but their pre-albumin level remains depressed. The negative nitrogen balance seen cannot be prevented because metabolic processes during stress promote protein breakdown. The inflammatory response needs to run its course before anabolism begins again.

Early Feeding

When to start nutritional rehabilitation of the critical client is under debate. For example, when treating clients with burn injuries some physicians keep clients NPO (non per os) for the first 24 to 72 hours after admission, and others initiate tube feedings within 4 hours. Here, an important consideration is that **peristalsis,** the wavelike motion that propels food through the GI tract, ceases in some burn clients. Until peristalsis returns, the client's stomach should not be the site of choice for a tube feeding.

In addition, other critically ill clients may have an ileus caused by muscle paralysis or an obstruction. Physicians who do feed clients early insert the feeding tube into the client's intestines past the ileus and deliver a very slow, continuous-drip feeding. The slow, continuous drip minimizes the likelihood of the feeding collecting in the intestines.

Some institutions have a policy of measuring **gastric residual volume (GRV)** in clients with gastric tube feedings. To measure stomach contents that have not been absorbed, the nurse will periodically suction the stomach's gastric contents utilizing a large bore syringe. Institutions will have varying policies regarding nursing

---

Box 22-1 ■ *Intensive Insulin Therapy in Critically Ill Clients*

Hyperglycemia and insulin resistance are common in critically ill clients because of hormonal response to a severe stress. Even if a client has not had diabetes before the stressor, hyperglycemia frequently becomes problematic. Intensive insulin therapy to maintain blood glucose at or below 110 mg per deciliter was implemented because it was thought to reduces morbidity and mortality among critically ill clients. This level of glucose control is possible only with close monitoring and an insulin drip. Follow-up studies are demonstrating that strict blood sugar control, with ranges between 80 and 180 mg/dL, does not reduce mortality rates. The current recommendation by the American College of Physicians is to maintain blood sugar levels between 140 and 180 mg/dL for clients in both the medical and surgical intensive care units (Qaseem, Humphrey, Chou, et al, 2011).

intervention if GRV is 250 mL or greater. Studies have demonstrated that tube feedings should not be stopped or reduced in clients with an isolate GRV of 250 mL when the client demonstrates no other signs of feeding intolerance (Makic, VonRueden, Rauen, and Chadwick, 2011). Overestimating feeding intolerances by nurses can result in undernourishment in clients.

If the critically ill client is adequately fluid resuscitated, then enteral nutrition should be started within 24 to 48 hours after surgery or admission to the critical care unit. Enteral nutrition is associated with a reduction in infectious complications and may reduce length of stay as opposed to parenteral nutrition.

Although early enteral feeding offers many advantages, in many cases it is not medically feasible. A functioning GI tract is a prerequisite to enteral feeding. These conditions preclude the use of enteral feedings:

■ Low mesenteric blood (ischemic bowel)
■ Severe hypotension
■ Perforate bowel
■ Peritonitis
■ Chemotherapy- or radiation-induced mucositis
■ Multisystem organ failure

For these clients, intravenous nutrition is obligatory. Clinical Calculation 22-1 demonstrates the calculation of a sample central parenteral solution. See Dollars & Sense 22-1 for information regarding the cost of intensive care treatment.

Examples of Hypermetabolism

Cancer, major surgery, burns, infections, and trauma are the physical stressors that have the greatest impact

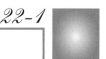

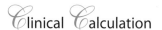

Calculating a Sample Central Parenteral Nutrition (CPN) Solution

These are the steps for calculating the total kilocalories and grams of protein in the following CPN solution: 500 cc D_{50}, 500 cc amino acids 10%, 250 cc lipid 10%.

DEXTROSE
$$D_{50} = 0.50 \times 500 \text{ mL} = 250 \text{ grams of dextrose}$$
$$250 \text{ grams} \times 3.4 \text{ kcal/gram} = 850 \text{ kcal}$$

AMINO ACIDS
$$500 \text{ mL} \times 0.10 = 50 \text{ grams of protein}$$
$$50 \text{ grams of protein} \times 4 \text{ kcal/gram} = 200 \text{ kcal}$$

LIPIDS
$$250 \text{ mL} \times 1.1 \text{ kcal/mL} = 275 \text{ kcal}$$

TOTAL KCALORIES
$$850 \text{ from dextrose} + 200 \text{ from protein} + 275 \text{ from lipid} = 1325 \text{ kcal}$$

$ Dollars & Sense 22-1

Cost of Intensive Care Stay

Admissions to intensive care units results in burdening expense for hospitals as well as for the client. Average daily direct costs range from $1436 to $1759 with higher acuity of illness costing more per day (Dahl, Wajtal, Breslow, et al, 2012). Providing nutrition to the critically ill contributes to the cost of admission. Clients who require central parenteral nutrition will require placement of a central venous access device, specialized IV formula, and specialized equipment to deliver the solution which all have associated costs. The Academy of Nutrition and Dietetics (2013) has confirmed that the use of enteral tube feeding reduces the cost of medical care in the critically ill client when compared to the use of CPN.

on metabolism. The needs of clients with cancer are described in Chapter 21. This section of this chapter focuses on the nutritional needs of clients experiencing surgery, burns, infections and fevers, and trauma. Nutritional support during extreme stress is needed to decrease the length of the stress, prevent complications, and minimize suffering.

SURGERY

Uncomplicated minor surgery increases the surgical client's kilocaloric requirement by only 5%. Surgery needed to repair soft tissue trauma requires a 14% to 37% increase in kilocalories. A surgical client with complications may require a large increase in kilocalories.

BURNS

Major burns are the most extreme state of stress a client can sustain and produce a hypermetabolic state that raises kilocaloric needs higher than those of most other stresses. Kilocaloric requirements may be as high as 8000 calories per day. Even a client who was well nourished before becoming burned may rapidly develop protein–calorie malnutrition. The degree to which the metabolic rate increases is directly related to the body surface area burned. The percentage of body surface area burned is determined by totaling the percentages in Figure 22-2A. Figure 22-2B illustrates first (superficial)-, second (partial thickness)-, and third-degree (full-thickness) burns. Burn clients may remain in a hypermetabolic state for many weeks to months. One study showed that resting energy expenditure (REE) remains elevated at 130% to 140% of the predicted value for 3 years following a burn (Rojas, Finnerty, Radhakrishnan, and Herndon, 2012).

An increase in waste products in some clients with burns requires an increase in fluids. Extra fluids help the kidneys eliminate waste products. Capillary

Rule of Nines

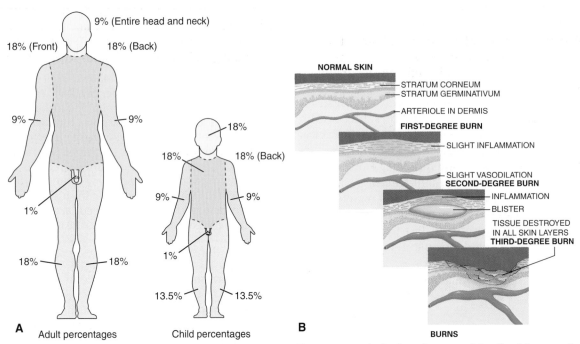

FIGURE 22-2 *A,* The percentage of body surface area burned is determined by comparing the body surface area of the client's burns to the percentages given in the chart. For example, if a client has extensive burns over both legs, the total body surface area burned would be 36% (18% for the first leg plus 18% for the second leg). (Reprinted from Venes, D [ed]: *Taber's Cyclopedic Medical Dictionary,* 21st ed. FA Davis, Philadelphia, 2010, by Beth Anne Willert, MS, Illustrator, with permission.) *B,* Burns are classified as first degree, second degree, and third degree. (Reprinted from Thomas, CL [ed]: *Taber's Cyclopedic Medical dictionary,* 18th ed. FA Davis, Philadelphia, 1997, p. 278, by Beth Anne Willert, MS, Illustrator, with permission.)

permeability is increased in burn clients; thus, plasma proteins, fluids, and electrolytes escape into the burn area and interstitial space. This shift reduces the volume of plasma, so fluid volume needs to be replaced. Adults with burns greater than 15% of total body surface area and children with greater than 10% total body surface area will require intravenous fluids resuscitation (Rowley-Conway, 2013). The formula that is used to calculate fluid resuscitation needs in adults within the first 24 hours is called the Parkland Formula. It is important for the nurse to realize that the formula is only a guide to fluid resuscitation. The nurse is still responsible for assessing the client for adequate perfusion and circulation by monitoring vital signs, capillary refill, urine output, and laboratory values. The volume may need to be adjusted to a higher or lower rate based on the client's response to the fluid (see Clinical Calculation 22-2).

Burn clients are particularly susceptible to **sepsis,** the state in which disease-producing organisms are present in the blood. Sepsis is a medical emergency that causes an overwhelming, uncontrolled, systemic inflammatory response (Robson and Daniels, 2013). Major sepsis further increases a client's metabolic rate. Clients with indwelling catheters and central venous access devices are at risk for sepsis. Sepsis, of course, is not limited to burn clients; clients with surgical trauma

22-2

Clinical Calculation

Parkland Formula

4 × client's weight in kilograms × percentage of burn = total fluid volume to be infused over the first 24 hours. Half of the volume is infused over the first 8 hours and the rest of the volume is infused over the next 16 hours.

A 186-pound man sustained second- and third-degree burns over 20% of his body after pouring gasoline on burning leaves and tree limbs.

STEP ONE: CALCULATE WEIGHT IN KILOGRAMS

186 pounds ÷ 2.2 = 85 kilograms in body weight

STEP TWO: CALCULATE FLUID NEEDS FOR THE FIRST 24 HOURS

4 × 85 kilograms × 20 BSA = 6800 mL/24 hours

STEP THREE: CALCULATE FLUID VOLUME TO BE INFUSED OVER FIRST 8 HOURS

Half the volume is infused over the first 8 hours
[6800 mL ÷ 2 = 3400 mL]

3400 mL ÷ 8 hours = 425 mL/hour × 8 hours then the remaining volume
3400 mL ÷ 16 hours = 213 mL/hour × 16 hours

or infections such as pneumonia or urinary tract infections may also suffer from sepsis.

For all burn clients, a nutritional assessment is essential to minimize complications and allow nutritional therapy to be evaluated effectively. The food intake of these clients should be monitored and documented. The kilocalories and grams of protein consumed or taken intravenously should be monitored per the facility's policy.

A high-protein, high-kilocalorie diet is ordered for most burn clients as soon as oral intake is medically feasible. Often the diet is initially offered in six small meals. Complete nutritional oral supplements are commonly used to increase the client's kilocaloric and protein intake. The protein content of the diet can be increased by providing a between-meal feeding high in protein, a serving of 2 eggs at breakfast, and a 4-ounce serving of meat at both lunch and supper. If the client drinks a full 8 ounces of milk with each meal, this further increases the protein content of the diet.

TRAUMA

Trauma is a physical injury or wound caused by an external violence. Stab and gunshot wounds, multiple fractures, and injuries acquired in motor vehicle accidents are examples of trauma. Victims of traumas may become hypermetabolic, depending on the severity of the injury, and vitamin and mineral supplements may be necessary.

Vitamin C plays a role in wound healing, and its administration restores healing. Vitamin C functions as a cofactor in the hydroxylation of proline into collagen and enhances cellular and humoral response to stress. Studies have demonstrated that administering 500 milligrams of vitamin C in conjunction with zinc and arginine improved the rate of pressure ulcer healing (Sinno, Lee, and Khachemoune, 2011).

Vitamin A, calcium, and zinc are also important in wound healing. Vitamin A enhances fibroplasia and collagen accumulation in wounds. Calcium is needed for calcium-dependent collagenases, iron for the formation of collagen, and zinc as a cofactor for enzymes responsible for cellular proliferation.

INFECTIONS AND FEVER

Malnutrition decreases resistance to infection, and infection aggravates malnutrition by depleting body nutrient stores. Fever characteristically accompanies infection but can also result from a variety of causes. The body needs extra kilocalories and fluids during fever because it takes more energy to support the higher metabolic rate. Infection may result in:

■ Decreased food intake and absorption of nutrients
■ Altered metabolism
■ Increased excretion of nutrients

Extra protein is also needed to produce antibodies and white blood cells to fight the infection. Perspiration entails a loss of fluids from the body, and many clients with fever have increased perspiration. Fluid may also be lost in vomiting and diarrhea and needs to be replaced.

Protein and Kilocalorie Needs

The client with hypermetabolism has an increased need for protein. Kilocalorie intake should maintain energy balance without overfeeding. Many critical care clients have GI problems and poor food intake.

Protein

Injury or illness requires active protein formation. These states all require a constant supply of protein:

■ Surgical wound healing
■ Tissue repair
■ Replacement of red blood cells and plasma protein lost in hemorrhage
■ Immune response to infection

The extent of hypermetabolism and catabolism depends on the degree of injury and client response to the injury.

PROTEIN NEEDS

The protocol for calculating a client's protein requirement varies from institution to institution. For noncritical care clients, 0.8 to 1.2 grams of protein per kg of ideal body weight (IBW) or actual body weight (ABW) formula is often used. For critical care clients 1.2 to 2 grams of protein per kilogram per day or higher in burns or multitrauma clients is used (McClave, Martindale, Vanek, et al, 2009).

URINE ASSESSMENT OF PROTEIN STATUS

Total urinary excretion of nitrogen increases with the client's stress level. Urinary creatinine measurements may be used to estimate muscle protein reserves. One problem common to the use of all urinary measurements is the completion of an accurate 24-hour urine collection. Nurses are typically responsible for collecting a 24-hour urine specimen from the client. If even one voiding is discarded, the measurement will be inaccurate.

Kilocalories

Clients who are hypermetabolic have an increased need for kilocalories. Clients lose weight because an increased need for energy coupled with a possibly inadequate energy intake and/or protein intake promotes weight loss.

KILOCALORIE NEEDS

Energy expenditure is the number of kilocalories that an individual uses to meet the body's demand for fuel. The gold standard for measuring energy expenditure is indirect calorimetry (see Chapter 6). However, many facilities lack the equipment and trained personnel to complete this procedure. Each organization usually has a protocol to follow to calculate the number of kilocalories to be initially delivered via nutritional support. The client is then monitored closely to determine metabolic response to the initial kilocalorie estimate.

The number of required kilocalories is typically calculated by either kcal/kg or one of several different predictive formulas. Three of these formulas are discussed here. The first method is outlined in Clinical Calculation 22-3. Clinical Calculation 22-4 presents guidelines to follow for parenteral feedings.

Propofol is a commonly used medication to sedate mechanically ventilated clients. This medication is administered parenterally in a 10% fat emulsion. It is important to consider the number of calories derived from fat in this medication and include them when assessing the total overall kilocalories the client received.

EQUATIONS

Three different equations to predict kilocaloric need are discussed.

Harris–Benedict Equation

Although the Harris–Benedict equation is still widely used to estimate REE for critically ill clients, the American Dietetic Associations' Evidence-Based Library discourages its use. Because of the continued use

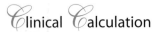

22-3

Clinical Calculation

Calculating Kilocalories

Kilocalories are typically estimated using the following:
   If overweight, use maximum ideal body weight (IBW):
   If underweight, use actual body weight (ABW):
   If within the IBW range, use ABW:
   Ideal body weight is calculated based on the following:

Female = 100 pounds for 5 feet and 5 pounds for each inch over 5 feet ± 10%

Male = 106 pounds for 5 feet and 6 pounds for each inch over 5 feet ± 10%

Energy needs are calculated as follows:

   Critical care: 20 to 30 kcal/kg* (25–35 for ventilated clients)

---

*Noncritical care: 25 to 35 kcal/kg.

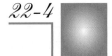

22-4

Clinical Calculation

Parenteral Guidelines for Macronutrients

Parenteral guidelines for macronutrient distribution include:

DEXTROSE
1. Initiate at 3 grams/kg or 300 mL of D_{70} (210 grams)
2. Maximum of 5 grams/kg in stressed clients
3. Maximum of 7 to 8 grams/kg in nonstressed clients
4. Assess tolerance with repeated blood glucose monitoring

LIPIDS
1. Initiate with 30% of total kilocalories as fat.
2. Maximum of 0.5 to 1.0 gram/kg in stressed clients
3. Maximum of 2.5 grams/kg in nonstressed clients
4. Maximum of 40% to 50% of total kcal in any client
5. Assess tolerance with triglyceride levels and if greater than 300 mg/dL, hold lipid

PROTEIN
1. Give full protein requirement the first day in clients without hepatic or renal impairment.

---

in many institutions, a brief explanation of the equation is presented in Clinical Calculation 22-5. The Harris–Benedict equation has been found to be within 15% of measured energy expenditure by indirect calorimetry for mechanically ventilated clients if the formula is adjusted by multiplying the factor of 1.2 (DeWaele et al, 2012).

Stress Factors

When using the Harris–Benedict equation, the use of stress factors is common. Research has shown that different types of stress increase kilocaloric needs differently. A stress factor is a number assigned to a given pathological state to predict how much a client's kilocaloric need has increased as a result of the type of stress the client is experiencing.

Table 22-1 lists various types of physical stress and the stress factor used for each disease state. Stress factors are used most often with the Harris–Benedict equation. The Ireton–Jones (1992 version) equation considers stress factors in the equation.

As the table shows, a client with burns more than 50% of the body has a stress factor of 2.0. This means kilocaloric need is twice (200%) his or her resting energy expenditure. In contrast, the stress factor after minor surgery is 1.05. This means a client who has had minor surgery needs only 5% more kilocalories than his or her REE. Depending on the physical activity of the client, a factor for this is sometimes used. Stress factors are convenient to use in estimating kilocaloric needs when using predictive equations for clients with multiple stressors.

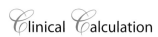

22-5

Clinical Calculation

Calculating Kilocaloric Needs Using the Harris–Benedict Predictive Equation

MALE CLIENT

Energy Need = Resting Energy Expenditure (REE) × Activity Factor × Stress Factor

Step 1: Use the following **Harris–Benedict equation** to calculate the male client's resting energy expenditure:

REE = 66 + (13.7 × weight in kg) + (5 × height in cm) – (6.8 × age)

Step 2: Multiply an activity factor by the client's REE (see Table 22-2).

REE × Activity Factor

Step 3: Multiply the answer obtained in step 2 by the appropriate stress factor (Table 22-1).

REE × Activity Factor × Stress Factor

FEMALE CLIENT

Energy Need = REE × Activity Factor × Stress Factor

Step 1: Use the following Harris–Benedict equation to calculate the female client's resting energy expenditure:

REE = 655 + (9.6 × weight in kg) + (1.7 × height in cm) – (4.7 × age)

Step 2: Multiply an activity factor by the client's REE (see Table 22-2).

REE × Activity Factor

Step 3: Multiply the answer obtained in step 2 by the appropriate stress factor (see Table 22-1).

REE × Activity Factor × Stress Factor

EXAMPLE CALCULATION

Assume you need to estimate the kilocaloric need of a 154-lb (70-kg) man who is 5 ft 5 in. (165 cm) tall and 25 years old. Assume he is confined to bed and has a fractured long bone.

Sample calculation for step 1:
70-kg man who is 165 cm tall and 25 years old

REE = 66 + (13.7 × 70) + (5 × 165) – (6.8 × 25)
REE = 66 + 959 + 825 – 170
REE = 1680

Sample calculation for step 2:

REE × Activity Factor
1680 × 1.2
2016

Sample calculation for step 3:

Answer from step 2 × Stress Factor
2016 × 1.35
2721.6 = client's estimated energy need

TABLE 22-1 ■ Stress Factors Used to Determine Kilocalories with Harris–Benedict Equation

STRESSOR	FACTOR
Surgery	1.1–1.3
Anabolism	1.5–1.75
For each degree F above 98.6°	1.07
Cancer	1.6
Soft tissue trauma	1.14–1.37
Long bone fracture	1.6
Burns (0%–20% of body surface area)	1.25
Burns (20%–40% of body surface area)	1.5
Burns (>40% of body surface area)	1.85
Peritonitis	1.2–1.5
Major sepsis	1.4–1.8

TABLE 22-2 ■ Activity Factors Commonly Used to Calculate a Client's Activity Kilocalories

Little or no activity	1.2
Light activity	1.375
Moderate activity	1.55
Very active	1.725
Exceedingly active	1.9

Ireton–Jones, 1992

Another equation is the Ireton–Jones, 1992 version. Clinical Calculation 22-6 provides the formula used to estimate energy expenditure with this equation. This equation includes stressors for the ventilator dependant, burned, and trauma client.

Mifflin–St. Jeor

Yet another equation is the Mifflin–St. Jeor. Clinical Calculation 22-7 provides the formula used to estimate energy expenditure with this equation. The Mifflin–St. Jeor formula takes into account activity factors.

Predictive equations are used to initially determine a client's kilocaloric goal rate. Without indirect calorimetry, the best method to determine if too much or too little energy is being given to a client is to closely monitor body weight, laboratory values (especially pre-albumin), nutritional intake, and sometimes blood gases at predetermined intervals.

It is important to recognize that calculating nutritional needs for intensive care clients requires specialized training and the calculations will be performed by registered dietitians in collaboration with the physician and pharmacists. The nurse is responsible for accurate, timely, and safe administration and as stress factors change the nurse can report these findings to the medical team.

The B vitamins help release the chemical energy stored in foods. Whenever a client requires increased

Clinical Calculation 22-6

Ireton–Jones (IJ), 1992 Equation

An explanation of the equation components is followed by example equations.

    (A) = Age in years
    (W) = Weight in kilograms
    (S) = Sex; male = 1; female = 0

DIAGNOSIS OF TRAUMA
        (T) = present = 1; absent = 0

DIAGNOSIS OF BURN
        (B) = present = 1; absent = 0

BODY MASS INDEX (BMI) >27
        (0) = present = 1; absent = 0

CLIENT WHO IS BREATHING SPONTANEOUSLY
$$IJ_{(s)} = 629 - 11(A) + 25(W) - 609(0)$$

CLIENT WHO IS VENTILATOR DEPENDENT
$$IJ_{(V)} = 1925 - 10(A) + 5(W) + 281(S) + 292(T) + 851(B)$$

Clinical Calculation 22-7

Mifflin–St. Jeor

An explanation of the equation components is followed by example equations.

    (A) = Age in years
    (W) = Weight in kilograms
    (H) = Height in centimeters

MEN
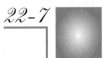
$$REE = (9.99 \times W) + (6.25 \times H) - (4.92 \times A) + 5$$

WOMEN
$$REE = (9.99 \times W) + (6.25 \times H) - (4.92 \times A) - 161$$

Once REE is calculated the result can be multiplied by the stress factors in Table 22-1 and the activity factors in Table 22-2.

kilocalories, the need for the B-vitamin complex automatically increases. When anabolism or the building of body tissue is indicated, vitamin C requirements are increased.

Hypermetabolic clients usually need to build up depleted tissue stores. It is estimated that critically ill clients can lose 2% of their muscle mass per every 24 hours and some clients can lose up to 50% of their muscle mass during one intensive care unit stay (Aversa, Alamdari, and Hasselgren, 2011). Critically ill clients may have increased micronutrient needs, but research is lacking to make specific recommendations.

Gastrointestinal Complication

Ulcers and some intestinal diseases are aggravated by stress. A client may report that he or she has specific food intolerances when under stress but that the same food is easily tolerated at other times. This change is partially due to impairment of GI function during episodes of stress and the use of some medications. Decreased motility can cause the development of anorexia, abdominal distention, gas pains, and constipation. These symptoms may contribute to food intolerances or reduced food intake.

Food Intake

The volume of food a client consumes and the desire to prepare food are influenced by stress. The time at which food is eaten also may be important. The best approach is to offer small frequent meals or oral nutritional supplements between meals.

Nutrition and Respiration

The scientific literature addresses the relationship between good nutrition and respiration:

Respiration refers to the exchange of gases (oxygen and carbon dioxide) between a living organism and its environment. The air or oxygen inhaled and the carbon dioxide exhaled is the act of ventilation.

Ventilation means breathing.

Pulmonary means concerning or involving the lungs.

Chronic obstructive pulmonary disease (COPD) refers to a group of lung diseases with a common characteristic of chronic airflow obstruction. COPD has become the fourth leading cause of death in the United States.

Respiratory failure is an acute or chronic disease caused by an imbalance between the amount of gases entering the lungs and the demand of body cells for gases, resulting in tissue hypoxia.

Acute respiratory failure is an imbalance caused by a disease that affects ventilation in a client who has a healthy lung and normal alveoli.

Chronic respiratory failure results from a disease in the bronchial structures or functioning (alveoli) structures of the lung. Malnutrition is commonly seen in clients with respiratory diseases.

Acute respiratory distress syndrome (ARDS) is often caused by conditions such as pneumonia and is characterized by a rapid onset of dyspnea and severe deficits in gas exchange. O_2 saturation reflects the percentage of hemoglobin saturated with oxygen and is an indicator of inadequate oxygen delivery to tissues. Normal oxygen (O_2) saturation in adults is usually 95% to 100% in adults and 95% in the elderly. Critical O_2 saturation is equal or less than 75%.

Effects of Impaired Nutritional Status on Respiratory Function

Poor nutrition is related to inadequate pulmonary function in five important ways:

1. Clients with respiratory diseases or inadequate respiratory function frequently have an inadequate food intake, which is related to anorexia, shortness of breath (SOB), or GI distress. Shortness of breath during food preparation and consumption of meals may limit kilocaloric intake. Inadequate oxygen delivery to the cells causes fatigue. Impaired GI tract motility is common in clients with respiratory diseases (see the following section).
2. Kilocaloric requirements are often increased in clients with pulmonary disease. It has been estimated that clients with COPD utilized 10 times the amount of calories to breath than those without pulmonary disease. As a result of the combined effects of decreased food intake and increased energy requirements, weight loss is commonly seen in these clients.
3. A client's catabolism can affect pulmonary function. When kilocaloric intake is decreased, the body begins to break down muscle stores, including those of the respiratory muscles. A loss in the lean mass of any muscle affects the muscle's function. The lung's structure itself is thus affected as a result of catabolism often referred to as pulmonary cachexia. Malnutrition may also result in decreased lung tissue cell replacement or growth.
   GI distress is common in clients with pulmonary disease and is related to malnutrition. A loss of GI structure including muscle mass may lead to hemorrhage and paralytic ileus. **Paralytic ileus** is the temporary cessation of peristalsis and contributes to decreased food intake and the feeling of anorexia. In addition, paralytic ileus may lead to a translocation of bacteria. Decreased peristalsis in the GI tract fosters the movement (translocation) of bacteria from the GI tract into the bloodstream. This translocation, in turn, leads to sepsis, or bloodborne infection, a sometimes fatal complication.
4. Malnutrition increases the risk of respiratory tract infections. Lung infection is frequently the cause of death in pulmonary clients. In severe malnutrition, the body decreases the production of antibodies, which are necessary to fight infection. Also, as a result of starvation, the lungs decrease production of pulmonary phospholipid (a fatlike substance). Phospholipids assist in keeping the lung tissue lubricated and help to protect the lungs from any inhaled disease-producing organisms.
5. Improved nutritional status has been shown to be associated with a better ability to wean clients from ventilators. A ventilator is a machine that provides gases under pressure to clients who are unable to breathe on their own because of an insufficient number of ventilations or inspired volume amounts for cellular respiration.
   Clients on ventilators do not have to use their respiratory muscles to breathe. Active muscle movement stimulates muscle growth through protein stimulus. This is the same principle that applied to physical exercise increasing muscle size. To some extent, all the respiratory muscles **atrophy,** or waste away, due to inactivity while a client is artificially breathing.

Clients on ventilators are usually weaned slowly from these machines as their conditions improve. Some experts have attributed clients' ability to be successfully weaned from ventilators to an increase in protein synthesis. Good nutrition stimulates respiratory muscle growth.

In mechanically ventilated clients, there is good data to indicate that once a client is extubated, swallowing dysfunction and a real risk of aspiration is present in most clients and may last up to several days.

Nutritional Therapy

Respiratory disease can affect food intake and nutrient utilization. Many clients with respiratory diseases also have problems with water balance.

Energy Nutrient Utilization

Care must be taken not to overfeed clients with reduced respiratory function. Excess intake can raise the demand for oxygen and the production of carbon dioxide beyond the client's capacity. The total number of kilocalories fed to the pulmonary client should be closely monitored. A nutritional assessment helps estimate the client's kilocaloric need and assists in therapy. Clients should be advised to consume high-carbohydrate, high-protein diets (Shepherd, 2010).

Research has shown that in individuals with COPD, the presence of lower body mass index (BMI; $<20 \text{ kg/m}^2$) may be as high as 30%, and the risk of COPD-related death doubles with weight loss (www.adaevidencelibrary.

com). This means these clients require close monitoring with appropriate follow-up. Too many kilocalories may increase carbon dioxide production and too few kilocalories may result in a weight loss and contribute to a decreased body mass with a subsequent poor outcome. Kilocalories are typically given on the low side of the 25 to 35 kcal/kg initially and increased slowly.

Vitamins and Minerals

Clients who have had a poor nutrient intake are at risk for nutrient deficits. Even if intake is adequate, nutritional depletion may occur in severe COPD clients, resulting in a need for supplementation of vitamins and minerals. Specific nutrients depleted in pulmonary disease include:

- Iron
- Vitamin A
- Vitamin C
- Vitamin D
- Vitamin E
- Selenium

Usually electrolyte levels are closely monitored in ICU clients because of fluid imbalances and the occurrence of **respiratory acidosis** and **respiratory alkalosis.** Some clients' intravenous solutions require daily manipulation to correct imbalances of electrolytes.

An adequate intake of vitamins A and C is essential for helping to prevent pulmonary infections and decrease the extent of lung tissue damage. The diet should include foods high in vitamin A, such as:

- Fortified milk
- Dark green or yellow fruits and vegetables
- Some breakfast cereals (check the label)
- Cheese
- Eggs

The diet should include foods high in vitamin C, such as:

- Citrus fruits and juices
- Strawberries
- Fortified breakfast cereals (check the label) should also be included.

Sources of vitamins A and C should be carefully chosen to ensure that they do not contribute to gas production.

Low bone density is problematic in many clients with COPD. Among the reasons for this are glucocorticosteroid therapy, reduced physical activity, a history of tobacco use, an inadequate calcium and vitamin D intake, and the pulmonary disease process itself.

Fat

The COPD client needs to be conscientious regarding fat intake. Fat metabolism generates less CO_2 than metabolism of carbohydrates, which is a benefit to the client. Clients with COPD tend to retain higher levels of CO_2, which can worsen respiratory distress. When choosing fats, the client needs to be advised to consume monounsaturated and polyunsaturated fats while avoiding *trans* fatty acids and saturated fats. Some studies have suggested that omega-3 fatty acids may have protective antioxidant effects on the lungs, but further studies need to be conducted. Excess fat intake can lead to weight gain and increased adipose tissue around the midsection, which can increase respiratory effort in the COPD client.

Water, Phosphorus, and Magnesium

Water balance and serum phosphorus levels need to be closely monitored. Clients with COPD and acute respiratory failure often need fluid restriction. Fluid restriction assists in the control of **pulmonary edema** or a movement of fluid into interstitial lung tissue.

Low serum phosphorus levels or hypophosphatemia are often seen in clients who are respirator-dependent. Phosphorus leaves the intracellular space and moves into the extracellular space during starvation. Serum phosphorus levels are in the normal or near-normal range at this point.

With refeeding, phosphate moves back into the intracellular space. At this point, the serum phosphorus level may drop below normal. If this occurs, it is crucial that the client receive phosphate replacement. Because acute hypophosphatemia has been reported to cause respiratory failure, serum phosphorus levels should be monitored in all clients receiving aggressive nutritional support. A magnesium deficiency appears to cause a loss of muscle strength and should, therefore, be monitored closely.

Feeding Techniques

Many of these clients lack the energy to eat. Complaints of fatigue are common. The GI distress experienced by these clients contributes to the anorexia. Box 22-2 lists interventions that can be used to improve nutrition in COPD clients.

Box 22-2 ■ *Interventions for Clients with COPD*

- Avoid gas causing foods such as carbonated beverages, cruciferous foods, and fried foods.
- Ensure adequate daily calcium intake.
- Encourage clients to eat little amounts frequently. Encourage six small energy dense meals a day.
- Maintain adequate hydration to assist in thinning secretions.
- Choose foods that are easily prepared and chewed.
- Advise clients to clear their airways prior to eating.
- Limit sodium intake to prevent water retention.
- Chew slowly to avoid swallowing air.
- Drink fluid between meals.
- Sit upright at a table for all meals.
- Wear oxygen via nasal cannula during meals to increase oxygen level.

Refeeding Syndrome

Refeeding is the reintroduction of kilocalories and nutrients by oral or other routes. **Refeeding syndrome** is a detrimental state that results when a previously severely malnourished person is reintroduced to food and nutrients improperly. Complications with refeeding can occur regardless of the route by which nutrients are delivered, whether oral, enteral, or parenteral.

The term *refeeding syndrome* has been used to describe a series of metabolic and physiological reactions that occur in some malnourished clients when nutritional rehabilitation is begun. Improper refeeding of a chronically malnourished client can result in congestive heart failure (CHF) and respiratory failure. Clients at risk include those with:

- Alcoholism
- Chronic weight loss
- Hyperglycemia, or insulin-dependent diabetes mellitus

Included also are clients on:

- Chronic antacid or
- Diuretic therapy

Elderly persons living alone who choose not to eat or are unable to eat because of progressive infirmity are likely candidates. Any incompetent mentally or physically challenged adult or abused child who has not been eating, either by choice or because of neglect, is also at risk of experiencing refeeding syndrome.

Starvation leads to both a loss of the lean body mass in the heart and respiratory muscles and decreased insulin secretion. When carbohydrate intake is low, the pancreas adapts by decreasing insulin secretion. With the reintroduction of carbohydrates into the diet, insulin secretion will increase. The increased insulin secretion is associated with increased sodium and water retention.

Other hormones are also activated with carbohydrate feeding. As a result of hormone action, increases in metabolic rate, oxygen consumption, and carbon dioxide production occur. The net effect of these metabolic changes is an increased workload for the cardiopulmonary system. Refeeding may increase the work of the cardiopulmonary system beyond its diminished capacity (due to the loss of lean body mass) and cause CHF and respiratory failure.

Starvation also leads to an increase in extracellular fluid and an increased loss of intracellular phosphorus, potassium, and magnesium. The degree of intracellular loss of these minerals reflects the degree of loss of lean body mass. Before refeeding, serum phosphorus and magnesium levels may remain in the lower range of normal, whereas the intracellular and total body stores of these minerals are depleted.

After refeeding, these minerals are redistributed from the extracellular to the intracellular compartments. Repeated laboratory measurements taken after refeeding is started may show low serum levels of phosphorus, magnesium, and potassium. Failure to correct for these mineral deficiencies may be fatal for the client.

Principles of Safe Refeeding

Health-care workers need to be aware of the dangers of refeeding a severely malnourished or starved client. Starved or severely malnourished clients may be seen in outpatient settings as well as in hospital intensive care units and long-term care facilities. The recommendations in Clinical Application 22-1 may help health-care workers avoid the refeeding syndrome.

Refeeding the malnourished client requires a team effort. A careful diet history taken by the dietitian can assist in the identification of clients likely to become victims of refeeding syndrome. Indications of a significantly altered status include changes in:

- Taste
- Appetite
- Intake
- Weight
- Consumption of a special diet

Correction of electrolyte abnormalities by the physician before implementing nutritional support can prevent death. Careful observation and monitoring by the nutritional support service can identify early signs of this syndrome. Open and prompt communication among all health-care team members may be crucial to the client's survival.

22-1

$\mathscr{C}$linical $\mathscr{A}$pplication

Recommendations for Refeeding the Malnourished Client

These seven points are broad guidelines for working with malnourished clients.

1. Health-care professionals need first to recognize clients at risk. Refeeding syndrome occurs in:
   - Clients with frank starvation, including war victims undergoing repletion
   - Chronically ill clients who are malnourished
   - Clients on prolonged intravenous dextrose solutions without other modes of nutritional support
   - Hypermetabolic clients who have not received nutritional support for 1 to 2 weeks
   - Clients who report prolonged fasting
   - Obese clients who report a recent loss of a considerable amount of weight
   - Chronic alcoholics
   - Clients with anorexia nervosa
2. Health-care workers practicing in outpatient settings not directly under the supervision of a physician need to develop a referral plan in the event they suspect a client is a likely candidate for refeeding syndrome. These clients require the expertise of a physician.
3. A physician needs to test for and correct all electrolyte abnormalities before initiating nutritional support, whether by the oral, enteral, or parenteral route. Many physicians depend on other health-care workers to assist in the monitoring of:
   - Serum phosphorus
   - Magnesium
   - Potassium values

For nurses practicing within hospitals, this means notifying the physician on receipt of laboratory test results showing low serum levels of these minerals. It is especially important to notify the physician before implementing changes in:
- Tube feeding
- Oral diets
- The rate of intravenous nutrition

4. The physician needs to restore circulatory volume and to monitor pulse rate and intake and output before initiating nutritional support. Again, many physicians depend on nurses and other health-care workers to assist in monitoring these signs.
5. The kilocaloric delivery to a previously starved client should be slow. Tube-fed and parenterally fed clients who have been previously malnourished need to be closely monitored for the following items:
   - Rate
   - Total volume
   - Concentration of kilocalories delivered
     These items should be increased one at a time:
   - Concentration
   - Volume
   - Rate of kilocaloric intake
6. Stepwise advancement to a higher kilocaloric intake should not occur unless the client is metabolically and physiologically stable.
7. Electrolytes should be monitored before nutritional support is started and at designed intervals thereafter.

Keystones

- Hypermetabolism differs from starvation in that resting energy expenditure (REE) increases during hypermetabolism and decreases during a prolonged state of starvation.
- Major surgery, severe infections, fever, major burns, and severe trauma are all examples of hypermetabolic states.
- Respiratory status profoundly affects nutrient need and utilization as well as food intake.
- Nutritional support can decrease catabolism of the respiratory muscles, improve immune function, minimize carbon dioxide production, and improve the likelihood of successfully weaning clients who are on mechanical respirators.
- Refeeding a previously starved client involves some risks. Refeeding may increase the work of the cardiorespiratory system beyond its diminished capacity and cause congestive heart failure and respiratory failure.

CASE STUDY *22-1*

Mr. X is a 48-year-old man who was admitted to the intensive care unit (ICU) with a diagnosis of bilateral pneumonia that was resistant to a 10-day prior course of antibiotic therapy. On admission, the client presented in acute distress: clammy to touch; weak; and unable to sit on examination table without assistance and support. Recumbent vital signs revealed the following: blood pressure 110/65; pulse 120 and weak; respiratory rate 28 breaths per minute and shallow; and sublingual temperature of 102.5°F. Medical history obtained from client was unremarkable and, in particular, no history of prior respiratory distress, smoking, or exposure to inhalation of toxic substances such as asbestoses.

His O_2 saturation was 50 on admission and his PCO_2 53. Imaging studies showed diffuse bilateral pulmonary infiltrates and small to moderate bilateral plural effusions. His albumin level was 2.5. Based on these findings and the blood gases, mechanical ventilation was instituted.

Mr. X is 5 ft 11 in. tall and weighs 140 lb (63.6 kg). His body mass index is 19.5. He reported a 9-lb weight loss over the past 3 weeks. He admits to living a sedentary lifestyle and reports a poor food intake. He states that his wife died about 6 months ago, and since then he has quit eating much. Mr. X admits his personal hygiene has also been poor. The neighbor brought him to the hospital and stated Mr. X appeared to have lost "a lot of weight."

An orally placed feeding tube with the tip placed in the stomach was inserted and placement was confirmed by diagnostic imaging. His kilocaloric need was estimated to be 1590 to 2226 based on 25 to 35 kcal/kg and his actual body weight. His protein needs were estimated to be 1.2 to 1.5 grams/kg or 75.8 to 95.4 grams/day, also based on his actual body weight.

The dietitian recommended a formula with a 1.5 kcal/mL concentration. A 24-hour continuous feeding of 1435 total milliliters at 59 mL per hour was recommended as a goal. An initial rate of 20 mL per hour with a gradual increase of 10 mL every 8 hours as tolerated was set until the goal rate was reached. In addition, 750 mL water would be needed to meet fluid needs and should be used to flush the tube, as tolerated by the client.

On the third day of his hospital stay, the client's phosphorus, potassium, and magnesium, which had been in the normal range on admission, dropped below normal. These electrolytes were replaced intravenously by physician's order. The client remained and tolerated the tube feeding without problems for the next 6 days.

The physician started to wean the client from the mechanical ventilator 24-hours ago as his pneumonia related-symptoms responded well to the intravenous antibiotic treatment. The client states he does not know why he got so ill.

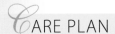ARE PLAN

Subjective Data
Denies knowledge of the relationship among lifestyle behaviors and infection ■ Reported significant weight loss and very poor food intake and sedentary behaviors

Objective Data
BMI = 19.5 on admission ■ Mechanical ventilation for the past 8 days second to pneumonia ■ Tube feeding well tolerated since admission ■ On admission visually presented with dirty hands, soiled clothing, and body odor

Analysis
Client's condition related to poor personal hygiene as a result of grieving and knowledge deficit

Plan

DESIRED OUTCOMES EVALUATION CRITERIA	ACTIONS/INTERVENTIONS	RATIONALE
Client expresses feelings about loss.	Actively listen to the client, particularly when he mentions his wife.	Client needs much assistance learning to ask for help.
Client seeks social support	Offer social services referral.	The social worker will be able to determine client's eligibility for treatment and match Mr. X's financial resources to specific doctors or programs.
Client states that good nutrition and moderate exercise, and proper hygiene are important for disease resistance,	Explain the relationship between lifestyle behaviors and resistance to infectious disease.	Knowledge is the first step to behavioral change.
	Offer client a referral to the dietitian to discuss healthful eating and easily prepared meals.	The dietitian has reliable educational materials suitable for most populations.

22-1

Social Worker's Notes

The following Social Worker's Notes are representative of the documentation found in a client's medical record.

Met with client per physician and nursing request. Although we did discuss his wife's death, client did not express grief or sadness. Also, phoned client's next closest relative, a sister living out-of-state. She indicated concern with her brother's inability to move forward with his life. She claims that before her sister-in-law's death, her brother was a well-groomed, cheerful person. At first, she denied any family history of mental illness. After some discussion, she admitted that her mother had committed suicide when she and her brother were very young. Long-term counseling and possibly medication are indicated. Mr. X has mental health coverage. Recommend referral to psychiatrist and possibly discharge to outpatient mental health program per the psychiatrist's evaluation.

22-2

Dietitian's Follow-up Notes

The following Dietitian's Notes are representative of the documentation found in a client's medical record.

Spoke with client initially 1 day after his present hospital admission to assess his nutritional needs and write recommendations. At that time, client was tearful about his poor health habits. He did not mention much about his deceased spouse except to say she died 6 months ago.

Concur with social worker's note. Client does not currently appear able to meet his own nutritional needs on discharge. Will defer education until after psychiatrist's evaluation. In the meantime, client is consuming sips of clear liquids only as he is still in the process of being weaned from the ventilator. The client agreed to try a complete liquid supplement, a few sips every hour. The client needs much encouragement.

Critical Thinking Questions

1. After 2 days of monitoring, the client's kilocalorie and protein intake and despite encouragement to eat from the nurses and the dietitian, the client refuses to eat much food. His kilocalorie intake is less than 500, with only 12 grams of protein. What would you recommend?

2. The client has concerns regarding access and preparation of foods at home. What suggestions would you give the client? What referrals can be made?

3. You question the client's mental competence. What should you do?

Chapter Review

1. The following is true about clients who have a life-threatening injury or illness:
   a. Their resting energy expenditure is about 70% of the kilocalories normally needed to maintain body weight.
   b. They have a decreased need for fluids.
   c. Biologically, their organs do not adapt to their increased need for kilocalories by switching to a less preferred fuel source.
   d. They need 0.8 to 1.2 grams of protein per kilogram of actual body weight.

2. Which of these conditions does not increase a client's resting energy expenditure?
   a. Infection
   b. Chronic obstructive pulmonary disease
   c. Starvation
   d. Burn

3. A burn client's need for kilocalories is related to:
   a. The amount of protein eaten
   b. The total body surface area burned
   c. The volume of food tolerated
   d. The amount of existing nutrient stores

4. Malnutrition is commonly seen in clients with pulmonary disease for all but one of the following reasons. Identify the exception.
   a. Many of these clients have a decreased food intake.
   b. Many of these clients expend more kilocalories to breathe.
   c. Many of these clients have impaired gastrointestinal tract function.
   d. Many of these clients have an extraordinary ability to fight infection.

5. Experts advocate the following when refeeding a malnourished client:
   a. Immediately pushing kilocalories and protein to replenish lost stores
   b. Progressing the rate, volume, and concentration of a tube feeding as rapidly as possible
   c. Full participation of all members of the health-care team to manage commonly seen metabolic abnormalities
   d. Correction of the hyperphosphatemia seen during the refeeding of a malnourished client

Clinical Analysis

1. Mr. L is suffering from second- and third-degree burns over 40% of his body. His physician has decided to use topical agents and leave the wound open to air. In the first 30 to 40 days postburn, the health-care team is planning nutritional support. The best supplemental feedings for the client would be:
   a. A high-fat feeding such as a milkshake made with ½ cup skim milk and 1 cup of ice cream
   b. A high-carbohydrate feeding such as soda with added honey
   c. A polymeric (complete nutritional) supplement that is acceptable to the client
   d. A high-kilocalorie dessert such as apple pie, cake, or ice cream

2. Mrs. J is an alcoholic who has previously reported that she has not eaten "food" for at least the past 3 months. She stated that her primary source of kilocalories has been alcohol. After her treatment for alcohol withdrawal on another unit, she was transferred to the unit where you work. The physician has ordered a high-kilocalorie, high-protein diet. So far, she has eaten 100% of the three high-kilocalorie, high-protein trays she has received while on your unit. While reviewing the client's laboratory values, you notice her serum phosphorus, magnesium, and potassium levels have just recently decreased. Mrs. J's depressed phosphorus values may be related to:
   a. A movement of phosphorus into the extracellular space
   b. A total compartmental depletion of phosphorus
   c. A lack of phosphorus in Mrs. J's present dietary intake
   d. A movement of phosphorus into the intracellular space

3. Mr. C is a heavy smoker. He was recently admitted to your unit with carbon dioxide retention and a diagnosis of chronic obstructive pulmonary disease. He complains of gas pains. The client will not derive benefit from:
   a. Caffeinated beverages
   b. Broccoli, onions, peas, melons, and cabbage
   c. Six small meals
   d. Custard, hot cooked cereals, bananas, ground meats, and mashed potatoes

23

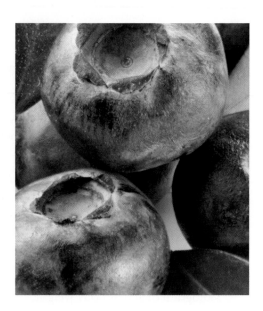

Diet in HIV and AIDS

LEARNING OBJECTIVES

After completing this chapter, the student should be able to:

■ Define AIDS and HIV and list transmission routes for the virus.

■ List nutrition-related complications seen in clients infected with HIV and, for each complication, describe interventions to improve nutritional status.

■ Discuss why malnutrition is commonly seen in clients with HIV or AIDS.

■ Describe why each client with AIDS needs an individualized nutritional assessment.

$\mathcal{A}$cquired **immune deficiency syndrome (AIDS)** is a life-threatening disease and a major public health issue. The **human immunodeficiency virus (HIV)** causes AIDS. The impact of this virus on our society is and will continue to be a challenge. In 2011, 34 million people were living with HIV globally, with 2.5 million newly affected (World Health Organization, 2012). This chapter discusses the prevention, diagnosis, and treatment of HIV **infection.** HIV is complicated by the side effects of medications, coinfections with other infectious disease, wasting, and lipodystrophy. The course of AIDS is often complicated by malnutrition. For these reasons, a major portion of this chapter is devoted to the nutritional care of clients infected with HIV.

Human Immunodeficiency Virus

The human immunodeficiency virus attacks both the immune system and the nervous system. **Immunity** refers to resistance to or protection against a specified disease.

When the HIV virus enters the bloodstream, it begins to attack cells with a specific protein called CD_4 on their surfaces. CD_4 is present on lymphocytes. Health-care providers may also refer to T cells when discussing HIV/AIDS. The terms *T cells* and *CD_4* are often used interchangeably. Lymphocytes are the main source of the body's immune capability, which involves humoral immunity produced by B cells and cell-mediated immunity produced by T cells. CD_4 levels decrease as the HIV disease progresses.

A healthy, uninfected person usually has 500 to 1000 CD_4 cells/mm^3. The HIV virus enters the cell, conscripts its DNA, and reprograms it to reproduce the virus. Loss of CD_4 function leaves an individual susceptible to infections and certain cancers. Evidence shows that the AIDS virus may also attack the nervous system, causing damage to the brain. See Box 23-1 for route of HIV transmission and prevention strategies.

Acquired Immune Deficiency Syndrome

AIDS is defined by the presence of HIV infection and a low level of white blood cells or T cells of less than 200 cells in every microliter of blood. It is a disease complex characterized by a collapse of the body's natural immunity against disease. Every part of the human body may be affected.

On average, HIV takes about 10 to 15 years, without treatment, to progress to AIDS. The survival rate for newly diagnosed clients initiating therapy in 2005 is now estimated to be decades (see Box 23-2). Many

Box 23-1 ■ *HIV Transmission and Prevention*

Primary Transmission

- Primarily transmitted through unprotected sexual contact with infected partner; anal sex increases risk
- Sharing needles or syringes
- Infants born to HIV-infected mothers

Less Common Route of Transmission

- Being accidently stuck with HIV-contaminated needle
- Receiving blood products or organ transplants
- Being bitten by an HIV-positive person
- Contact between broken skin, wounds, or mucous membranes with HIV-positive blood or body fluids

Ways HIV Is Not Transmitted

- Air or water
- Insect bites
- Saliva, tears, or sweat
- Casual contact such has hugs or handshakes

Prevention

- Be aware of HIV status
- Limit sexual partners
- Correct and consistent use of condoms if sexually activity
- Don't share needles
- Health-care workers should utilize Universal Precaution when exposed to blood or bodily fluids (see Fig. 23-1)

Box 23-2 ■ *HIV in Aging Population*

The Centers for Disease Control and Prevention (2011) reports that the percentage of people living with stage 3 HIV or AIDS aged 65 years or older increased from 45.4% in 2008 to 57.7% in 2010. Special considerations need to be made with the aging population who are living with HIV/AIDS. **Frailty** is a syndrome that is characterized by a progressive decline in system functions including physical, social, and cognitive attributes (Mohandas, Reifsnyder, Jacobs, and Fox, 2011). Frailty often results in loss of independence with increased nursing home admissions and an increase in illness and death. Clinical manifestations include low endurance, poor strength, impaired balance, and low physical activity (Shah, Hilton, Myers, et al, 2012). Older people will undergo natural age-related changes such as loss of muscle mass, and it is unknown how the virus will affect this progression. The older population with HIV may see an increase in complications related to both age and comorbidities such as preexisting heart disease or dementia (Kirk and Bidwell-Goetz, 2009).

No Known Cure

Dramatic but expensive treatment advances have changed the health-care community's view of AIDS. The use of highly active antiretroviral therapy (HAART) has decreased mortality rates. However, findings indicate that in the vast majority of clients receiving HAART who had undetectable levels of HIV-1 RNA in plasma, the virus has not been eradicated. Clients will require treatments continuously for the rest of their lives. Also, HAART is not a treatment option for much of the world's population. Sadly, the medications are too costly.

Signs and Symptoms

The natural history of HIV infection is divided into three phases:

1. Acute infection
2. Clinical latency
3. AIDS

Acute Infection Phase

An HIV-infected individual may experience no symptoms or develop an acute flulike illness, with symptoms appearing from 2 to 4 weeks to up to 3 months after exposure to the virus. This is often referred to as acute retroviral syndrome (ARS) or primary HIV infection. Typically, the symptoms are not severe enough for the infected individual to seek medical attention. During this early phase, there are higher levels of the virus circulating in the blood, which can make the virus more easily transmittable. It is important to note that not every person infected with HIV will develop these symptoms.

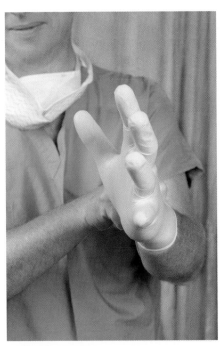

FIGURE 23-1 A health-care worker donning a pair of beige latex gloves to protect himself from body fluids.

clients still progress to end-stage AIDS because of the development of multidrug-resistant HIV virus (Eyawo, Fernandes, Brandson, et al, 2011). Progression of the disease may also be contributed to the inability to adhere to or access to antiretroviral (medication) therapy.

Clinical Latency Stage

This stage may also be referred to as *asymptomatic HIV* or the *chronic HIV* stage. The individual may be **asymptomatic** for years after becoming infected with the virus. This stage can last an average of 10 years. About 25% of HIV-infected people do not know they are infected, and the danger lies in their ability to infect others unknowingly. Even though the person may be symptom-free, viral replication continues. Clients may seek health care with minor infections and wasting syndrome, unaware of their HIV infection.

If the infection is untreated, CD_4 cells decline steadily during the latency stage.

AIDS

A diagnosis of AIDS is made whenever a person is HIV infected and has a CD_4 count of less than 200 cells/mm³ or the emergence of opportunistic infections a healthy immune system would normally prevent (Moss, 2012). Nutrition-related AIDS defining illnesses include wasting, nutrient malabsorption, and oropharyngeal and esophageal *candidiasis* (thrush).

The Epidemic

The AIDS epidemic started in Africa, and the first cases of the syndrome were described in the United States in the early 1980s. Untreated case fatality rates initially approached 100%. With the introduction of HAART, the HIV-related death rate has declined 70% since 1995.

The epidemic increasingly affects persons infected through heterosexual contact, women, minorities, and the poor. These affected groups are usually diagnosed at a later stage of infection when related disease is present and often delay care for themselves because they must care for others or have competing subsistence needs for their time and resources. Gay and bisexual men are still the most severely affected by HIV. Genomic Gem 23-1 provides insight into why certain racial, sexually oriented, and ethnic groups are more severely affected by this virus.

Complications of HIV Infection

The HIV-infection complications explained in this text include opportunistic infections such as thrush, tuberculosis (TB), and *Pneumocystis* pneumonia; gastrointestinal dysfunction; AIDS dementia complex; organ dysfunction; wasting; and lipodystrophy. Boxes 23-3 and 23-4 discuss characteristics of AIDS and the common problems these clients experience.

Genomic Gem 23-1

HIV Infections by Race, Sexual Orientation, and Ethnicity

The Centers for Disease Control and Prevention monitors statistics in relation to HIV in the United States. The number of new infections among young, Black, gay, and bisexual men was roughly twice that of Whites and Hispanic/Latinos. Although Black men represent only 12% to 14% of the population, they accounted for 44% of all new HIV infections among adults and adolescents in 2010.

For some time, the continent of Africa has the highest prevalence of HIV infection in the world. Why would this be so? Sexual behavior, lack of education, family structure, and poverty cannot explain why more than 66% of the world's 33 million people infected with HIV live in sub-Saharan Africa.

Researchers have recently found a mutation in the Duffy antigen receptor expression (DARC). This mutation gives profound protection against some malaria species and became almost universal in the African population (Ramsuran, Kulkarni, He, et al, 2011). Unfortunately, this mutation leads to significantly increased susceptibility to HIV-1 infection in those of African heritage and paradoxically to prolonged survival in HIV-1-infected individuals. This mutation may explain both the high incidence and prevalence of HIV in those of African heritage. Researchers think the gene variant arose tens of thousands of years ago, in response to a deadly strain of malaria.

Box 23-3 ■ *Signs and Symptoms of AIDS*

AIDS is characterized by:

- Fatigue
- Anorexia
- Diarrhea
- Weight loss
- Fever
- Decreased white blood cell count, or **leukopenia**
- Muscle wasting

Box 23-4 ■ *Conditions Seen in Clients with HIV/AIDS*

Common problems associated with AIDS include:

- Opportunistic infections
- Gastrointestinal dysfunction
- Tumors
- AIDS dementia complex (ADC)
- Organ dysfunction

Opportunistic Infections

Parasitic, bacterial, viral, and fungal organisms are everywhere in our environment. A healthy person's immune system keeps these organisms in check and under control. AIDS places the client at high risk for certain infections, called **opportunistic infections.** Following the guidelines for safe food handling is especially important for this population. Opportunistic infections commonly seen in clients with AIDS include thrush, TB, and *Pneumocystis* pneumonia.

Thrush

A physical assessment may show signs of **thrush,** a thick whitish coating on the tongue or in the throat that may be accompanied by sore throat (see Fig. 23-2). Thrush is a fungal infection that can cause oral ulcers, frequent fevers, and gastrointestinal inflammation. Basic teaching for mouth care by the health educator should include the following information:

- Use a prescribed antifungal medication as directed. The client should not eat for 30 minutes after treatment (Wyndham, 2012).
- Use a cotton swab instead of a toothbrush if brushing is painful or causes bleeding. Commercial mouthwash may cause discomfort or pain.
- Avoid hot foods.
- Try soft foods, such as scrambled eggs, cottage cheese, mashed potatoes, mashed winter squash, puddings, custards, milk, juices (not citrus), and canned fruits such as peaches, pears, apricots, and bananas.
- Cut meat into small pieces or grind or blend it.
- Supplement the diet with a complete oral nutritional supplement.
- Use a straw.
- Tilt the head forward or backward to ease swallowing.
- Avoid any food that causes discomfort. Fried, spicy, sour, salty, and sticky foods may not be tolerated, such as chips, nuts, seeds, raw vegetables, peanut butter, pickles, citrus fruits and juices, and tomatoes.

Tuberculosis

TB is spread from person to person through tiny airborne particles. By sharing surroundings with a person who has active pulmonary TB, a susceptible person may inhale the disease-producing bacteria. Fortunately, most people who have inhaled these particles never become contagious or develop active TB. Even a healthy immune system cannot kill all the particles. HIV infection weakens the body's immune system and makes it more likely that the individual who has inhaled TB-related particles will develop active TB. It is estimated that 8.7 million people contracted TB in 2011 with 13% of those coinfected with HIV (Kondro, 2012).

Pneumocystis Pneumonia

Pneumonia, characterized by shortness of breath, fatigue, and anorexia, is also common in AIDS clients. About 60% of AIDS clients are infected with one type of pneumonia-causing organism, called *Pneumocystis jiroveci,* formerly called *Pneumocystis carinii,* hence the name **Pneumocystis pneumonia (PCP).** PCP is the most common pulmonary opportunistic infection in clients with HIV. The organisms settle in the person's lungs, causing progressively worsening breathing problems and eventually leading to death. Many times clients with this infection are too tired to cook meals.

Gastrointestinal Dysfunction

The gastrointestinal tract is a common site for expression of HIV-related symptoms. The client may feel pain in the mouth or esophagus due to the growth of opportunistic infections. The client may have difficulty swallowing because of open lesions or sores.

AIDS commonly affects both the small and large intestine. The enzymes necessary for digestion and absorption in the wall of the small intestine may be lacking or present in insufficient amounts. Malabsorption may occur with diarrhea. Gut failure may follow. Medications to control these infections also contribute to the gastrointestinal dysfunction.

AIDS Dementia Complex

AIDS dementia complex (ADC) is the most common HIV-caused central nervous system illness associated with AIDS. Research is demonstrating that 50% of clients with AIDS have some degree of neurological impairment (Neurologic Disorders, 2011). Early symptoms of ADC are difficulty concentrating, slowness in thinking and response, and memory impairment. Behavioral symptoms include social withdrawal, apathy, and personality changes. Older adults affected with HIV are more susceptible to depression, dementia, and Alzheimer disease (Cahill and Valadez, 2013). Motor symptoms include clumsiness of gait, difficulty with fine motor movements, and poor balance and coordination. Clients frequently become so mentally impaired that they cannot procure and prepare their own meals.

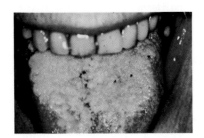

CANDIDIASIS

FIGURE 23-2 Thrush may cause mouth pain and interfere with nutritional intake. A soft diet may be helpful.

Organ Dysfunction

AIDS affects many organs in the body, leading to organ dysfunction. Diseases of the gallbladder, liver, and kidneys are seen in some AIDS clients:

Cholecystitis, inflammation of the gallbladder, can occur in conjunction with certain opportunistic infections seen in AIDS clients.

Hepatomegaly, an enlarged liver, is frequently seen, and symptoms include pain, fever, and abnormal liver function test results, especially of the alkaline phosphatase level. Liver disease is one of the leading causes of mortality in HIV-positive clients and is often attributed to the use of HAART (Cahill and Valadez, 2013).

Pancreatitis, inflammation of the pancreas, has also been noted in some infected clients.

AIDS can lead to **end-stage renal failure** within weeks.

Wasting

AIDS wasting syndrome is characterized primarily by involuntary weight loss, consisting of both lean and fat body mass. Despite treatment with medication, wasting remains a leading AIDS-defining event and is associated with high morbidity and mortality. Analysis of body composition, measurement of soft tissue volumes (muscle, fat, and organ), and diagnostic imaging of adipose tissue distribution make it possible to define wasting syndrome in terms of total weight loss and tissue compartment loss.

Wasting may be caused by undernutrition or nutrient malabsorption. The body does not compensate by decreasing resting energy expenditure as it does during starvation in wasting. Thus, kcalorie need remains elevated, and when accompanied by anorexia, the result is a high fatality rate. AIDS-related wasting syndrome is described as a 10% weight loss from baseline in a 6-month period with diarrhea or chronic weakness and fever for more than 30 days without a known cause.

Lipodystrophy

Lipodystrophy, an adverse effect of HAART, is a syndrome causing peripheral fat wasting and fat accumulation centrally. Metabolic abnormalities in total cholesterol, increased low-density lipoprotein, and increased triglycerides may necessitate that clients modify their diets accordingly. Box 23-5 describes the signs and symptoms of lipodystrophy.

Treatment

A variety of new medications show some promise of killing or inhibiting the activity of the HIV virus. Clinical Application 23-1 discusses medication treatment for

---

Box 23-5 ■ *Signs and Symptoms of Lipodystrophy*

Characteristics of lipodystrophy:

- Increasing abdominal girth
- Decreasing fat in the extremities and face
- Advent of a buffalo hump
- Breast enlargement
- Increased serum triglyceride levels
- Increased glucose levels
- Increased insulin levels
- Increased blood pressure

AIDS. Clients with HIV and AIDS take multiple prescribed medications, and almost all these clients need extensive counseling on food and medication interactions. Resistance training may be beneficial for these clients, especially those who are losing lean body mass. Realistically, health-care intervention can only suppress most infections for these clients, not cure them.

In 2013, the World Health Organization recognized news that a child born with traces of the HIV virus appeared to be "functionally cured," without detectable virus, at age 18 months through treatment with triple antiretroviral therapy within the first 30 hours of birth. Further research is required.

Other medications may be useful in reversing the nutritional decline and sequelae associated with AIDS: Marinol (dronabinol), and Megace (megestrol acetate) have both been shown to have significant efficacy in:

- Appetite stimulation
- Increased kilocalorie intake
- Reversing weight loss
- Improving a client's sense of well-being

Meal plans to support medication regimens include not only meal timing but also carbohydrate, fat, and protein distribution and symptoms management strategies.

Prevention and Counseling

All states and the District of Columbia have specific laws regarding HIV testing. Screening for HIV should be part of routine medical screening with an option to decline. In 2013, the U.S. Preventative Service Task Force released guidelines advising that adolescents and adults aged 15 to 65 years be tested for HIV. It is also recommended that clients who may be younger or older who are high risk be tested. It is important that no client be tested without informed consent. Every client must be notified either verbally or in writing before the screening. Notification of a positive HIV test finding may create a crisis for the individual. A person who has had pretest counseling is more prepared and likely to cope better.

Counseling the individual on how best to fight the virus is important; for example, the HIV-positive

23-1

Clinical Application

Medications Used for HIV and AIDS

Drug therapy for clients with HIV has increased in complexity. There are currently six classes of antiretroviral medications used during the initial treatment of an HIV-positive patient including nucleoside reverse transcriptase inhibitors (NRTIs), which can also come as a dual NRTIs, nonnucleoside reverse transcriptase inhibitors (NNRTIs), protease inhibitors (PIs), CCR5 antagonists, integrase strand transfer inhibitors (INSTIs), and fusion inhibitors (FIs). Lifelong medication therapy with combinations of these medications may be required for management and presents challenges to nutritional status by introducing potential interactions with food, body metabolism, and side effects. The following table lists common medications used in HIV/AIDS, typical dosing, and food tips.

Common Medications Used in HIV/AIDS

MEDICATION	DOSING	FOOD TIPS
GENERIC NAME		
PIs		
ritonavir	Twice a day	Take with a full meal
		Complications may include diarrhea, lipodystrophy, elevated lipids, and hyperbilirubinemia
		Avoid alcohol
		Avoid antacids
zidovuldine	Twice a day	Take with food, preferably nonfat
		Take 400 IU vitamin E every day to decrease bone marrow suppression
NNRTIs		
efavirenz	Daily at bedtime	Take on an empty stomach; 1 hour before or 2 hours after a meal
		Take with a full glass of water
		Teratogenic to fetus
rilpivirine	Daily	Avoid taking antacids
		For optimal absorption, it is recommended that the medication be taken with a regular meal
INSTIs		
raltegravir	Twice daily	May cause an increase in cholesterol and triglyceride levels
		Nausea and diarrhea
NRTIs		
tenofovir	Daily	May decrease bone density
		May cause lactic acidosis
		May worsen renal failure
emtricitabine	Daily	No interaction with meals
		May increase low-density lipoprotein cholesterol and triglycerides
FI		
enfuvirtide	Twice daily subcutaneous	Nausea and vomiting
Fusion Inhibitors		
maraviroc	Twice daily	Hepatotoxicity
		Nausea and vomiting
		No interaction with meals

How are the drugs mentioned in the table combined? Typically the patient will take a combination of antiretrovirals based on efficacy, toxicity, pill burden, dosing frequency, drug–drug interactions, and comorbidities. Preferred regimens include:

- NNRTI-based regimen:
  - *Efavirenz, tenofovir, and emtricitabine*
- PI-based regimen:
  - *Atazanavir/ritonavir plus tenofovir/emtricitabine*
- INSTI-based regimen
  - *Raltegravir plus tenofovir/emtricitabine*

It is important to note that many of the medications now come as a combination tablet.

Adapted from Guideline for the Use of Antiviral Agents in HIV-1-Infected Adults and Adolescents. Available at http://aidsinfo.nih.gov/contentfiles/lvguidelines/adultandadolescentgl.pdf.

individual needs to receive all current immunizations to boost his or her immunity. Behaviors that interfere with wellness and reduce immunity include:

- Drinking alcohol
- Smoking
- Illegal drug use
- Poor nutrition

They should be discouraged. Adequate rest and exercise can improve general good health and should be encouraged.

Nutrition and HIV Infection

Nutritional management is both a preventive and a therapeutic treatment in HIV infection. A malnourished client has a limited ability to fight infection. A well-nourished individual infected with the HIV virus is better able to resist opportunistic infections and tolerate the side effects of treatment. Good nutritional status may influence response to medications by:

■ Decreasing the incidence of adverse drug reactions
■ Providing nutrients for reactions evoked by medications
■ Supporting organ functions

Worldwide, few people who have advanced disease are receiving antiretroviral treatment. Micronutrient supplements have been proposed as a low-cost intervention that may slow the progression of HIV disease. The impact of micronutrient supplementation may be less in the developed nations of the world because the general population is less likely to be malnourished.

Malnutrition in AIDS Clients

Malnutrition in clients with HIV/AIDS causes a number of physiological alterations that may lead to decreased resistance to infection and is an important predictor of morbidity and mortality. People who are malnourished are six times more likely to die than those who are adequately nourished. A well-balanced diet is essential to optimal immune function (see Box 23-6).

Malabsorption

Diarrhea and malabsorption are probably the major nutrition-related problems for AIDS clients. Diarrhea is also a side effect of antiretroviral medications.

Mucosal atrophy and decreased digestive enzyme activity contribute to the malabsorption and diarrhea seen in persons with AIDS. Carbohydrate and fat malabsorption are frequently seen in AIDS clients

with diarrhea. Gastrointestinal problems such as diarrhea may occur in children with HIV infection due to disaccharide intolerance rather than to enteric infection with known pathogens.

Malabsorption of fat, simple sugars, and vitamin B_{12} occurs in clients with intestinal infections. AIDS clients who have diarrhea or malabsorption clearly have additional vitamin and mineral needs. Clinicians should measure 25-hydroxy vitamin D levels as an indicator of fat-soluble vitamin absorption. Studies have demonstrated that vitamin D supplementation may help slow HIV disease progression and improve quality of life (Mehta, Mugusi, MMed, Spiegleman, Villamor et al, 2011).

Initially, dietary treatment involves identification of the cause of the diarrhea and a determination of which nutrients the client cannot absorb. The concentration of hydrogen in the breath can be measured after oral lactose or sucrose administration to determine whether the client is intolerant to either of these sugars. An elevated breath hydrogen level implies intolerance because hydrogen is primarily a product of metabolism of these sugars by colon bacteria.

Fecal microbiological evaluations and intestinal biopsies are used to determine absorptive capability. In some clients infected with HIV, malabsorption of sucrose, maltose, lactose, and fat has been documented, even in the absence of diarrhea.

Clients with a form of carbohydrate intolerance may benefit from either a lactose-restricted or a disaccharide-free diet. A disaccharide-free diet is indicated for severe intolerance to sugar. Sucrose needs to be broken down into glucose and fructose (lactose into glucose and galactose; maltose into glucose and glucose) before absorption is possible.

A disaccharide-free diet excludes most fruits and vegetables and many starches and is nutritionally inadequate. Vitamin C is deficient, and daily supplementation is recommended. Some of these clients may tolerate a small amount of sugar, but they usually need assistance in understanding their tolerance level. A lactose-free diet may be sufficient for clients who are deficient only in lactase.

A low-fat diet may be necessary to control **steatorrhea.** Several additional meal-planning tips are suggested to promote the client's well-being and to control malabsorption:

■ Fluids should be encouraged to maintain hydration when large fluid volume is lost in stools.
■ Yogurt and other foods that contain the *Lactobacillus acidophilus* culture may be helpful if bacteria overgrowth is a problem secondary to long-term anti-infective use.
■ Small, frequent meals make the best use of a limited absorptive capacity of the gut.
■ A multivitamin supplement is indicated to increase the amount of vitamin available for absorption.

Box 23-6 ■ *Effects of Malnutrition*

Malnutrition causes numerous physiological alterations within the body. Some of the changes include:

■ Increased gut permeability, which allows more alien material to be absorbed into the body
■ Decreased intestinal secretions; some of these secretions are necessary for the proper digestion and absorption of food
■ Changes in intestinal flora, which may affect the utilization of nutrients
■ Hormonal imbalances
■ Decreased ability to repair tissue; the body ceases to replace and repair tissue because it lacks the raw materials to do so

- Oral liquid nutritional supplements may be helpful.
- Aggressive nutritional support such as enteral and parenteral nutrition, if appropriate, should be considered.
- Pancreatic enzymes (Pancrecarb) may be prescribed as indicated.
- Sorbitol, which is used as a sweetening agent in both sugar-free candies and some medications, has been shown to cause diarrhea and should be avoided.
- Caffeine should be avoided because it stimulates peristalsis.
- Fiber-containing supplements may be useful.

In some situations, the malabsorption is highly resistant to treatment. Nutritional therapy goals should maximize client comfort. The benefits of overly restricting the client's diet may not suffice to offset the resulting loss in client comfort in an incurable situation.

Increased Nutritional Requirements

There is an increase in Resting Energy Expenditure of 5% to 17% in clients with HIV/AIDS, but their total energy expenditure is thought to be similar to a healthy person (Academy of Nutrition and Dietetics, 2013). HIV wasting and secondary infections increase resting energy expenditure and increase kilocalorie, protein, and certain mineral and vitamin requirements.

Historically, dietitians have used the Harris–Benedict equation and multiplied the appropriate stress and activity factors to estimate kilocaloric requirements. Many software programs in use are still based on this equation. The Academy of Nutrition and Dietetics in its Evidenced Based Library recommends that kilocaloric needs be measured by indirect calorimetry. If this technology is not available, using formulas such as Harris–Benedict equation or Mifflin–St. Jeor equation are appropriate methods for estimating the client's energy needs.

Hypometabolism

Not all clients with AIDS become hypermetabolic. Hypometabolic clients need a gradual increase in kilocalories and a lower kilocalorie:nitrogen ratio. These clients should also be monitored for refeeding syndrome.

Decreased Food Intake

Anorexia can be a major problem for many clients with AIDS. A poor food intake may be the result of fever, respiratory infections, drug side effects, gastrointestinal complications, oral and esophageal pain, and emotional stress. Clients with ADC may experience mechanical problems with eating.

Nutritional Care in AIDS

Manifestations of the HIV virus vary greatly from one client to another. Therefore, nutritional care must be tailored to each client's unique set of symptoms. Quality nutritional care starts with screening.

Screening

Screening HIV-infected clients for nutritional problems is a crucial component of quality client care. Early indicators of decreased nutritional status include decreases in usual body weight, low weight for height, a low albumin level, and a body mass index (BMI) less than 20.

The following should be included in the assessment process:

- A baseline measure of percent body fat and lean body mass to monitor disease progression
- Recent food intake
- Comorbidities and opportunistic infection
- Oral or gastrointestinal symptoms
- Barriers the client may have to safe nutritious food
- Lack of food and poor food choices, which are linked to transmission of HIV infection and a poor response to treatment

Referral to a social worker is always indicated to address these challenging issues.

Planning Nutrient Delivery

In keeping with the general principle "if the gut works, use it," every effort should be made to feed the client orally. The following dietary modifications to oral intake may be helpful:

- Changing the meal plan, which may resolve the anorexia commonly seen in AIDS clients
- Offering small, frequent feedings
- Serving food cold or at room temperature, which may help some clients consume more kilocalories
- Modifying seasonings and kilocaloric density, which may improve intake
- Modifying texture, which may assist the client with poor chewing ability or oral lesions

If the client is unable to consume sufficient nutrients from table foods, supplemental feedings or other enteral feedings should be considered. The type of malnutrition should influence the food and supplements offered, which the dietitian usually determines.

If the client is unable to consume sufficient nutrients orally and the gut is working, a tube feeding may be considered. Percutaneous endoscopic gastrostomy (PEG) tubes are often used. If the gut is not functioning properly, peripheral parenteral nutrition (PPN) or central parenteral nutrition (CPN) may be considered. The goal should always be to prolong living, not to prolong dying. A client has the right to refuse any alternative-feeding route offered.

Monitoring

To ensure that adequate nutrients are being consumed, body weight, waist circumference, and nutritional intake should be monitored every few weeks along with BMI and percent body fat. The loss of lean tissue central to body metabolism may be present throughout the disease process, regardless of weight maintenance, suggesting that weight is not a good early indicator of declining nutritional status. Throughout this process, health-care workers should maintain a supportive, nonjudgmental approach, which is the key to establishing a trusting relationship.

Client Teaching

An assessment of the client's knowledge level and understanding of an individualized meal plan is appropriate. All AIDS clients need instruction on food safety because low immune system functioning makes them much more susceptible to food-borne illnesses. Education will minimize the likelihood of opportunistic infection. Instructions on dietary modifications including nutrient-dense meals and the use of supplemental feedings are also indicated (see Box 23-7).

Food Faddism and Quackery

Some clients with AIDS are vulnerable to both food faddism and quackery because they become desperate to try anything that arouses hope.

Food faddism is an unusual pattern of food behavior enthusiastically adapted by its adherents.

Food quackery is the promotion for profit of a medical scheme or remedy that is unproved or known to be false.

Health-care educators need to carefully balance and consider the danger of unusual food behaviors versus taking away any hope the client may have. Clients may tune out educators if they perceive that their beliefs and feelings are discounted without sensitivity. Some unusual food behaviors are not harmful, and some food behaviors can result in negative health consequences (see Dollars & Sense 23-1).

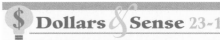

$ Dollars & Sense 23-1

No Money for Food

The client with limited resources who spends money on dietary supplements and herbal products of limited health benefits and spends little or no money on food will develop malnutrition.

A reliable desktop reference and carefully chosen Internet sites can help the health educator recommend what is appropriate. Care must be taken by health educators not to use Internet sites that sell questionable products.

Follow-Up Care

The nutritional status of a client may depend on appropriate follow-up care. A referral should be made to a community agency, a home health-care program, an outpatient clinic, or a dietitian to provide continuity of care.

Box 23-7 ■ *Counseling the Client with HIV and AIDS*

These nutritional principles are important to discuss with AIDS clients soon after the initial diagnosis:

■ Review the principles of safe food handling and storage with the client.
■ Review MyPlate guidelines as a basis for dietary intake.
■ Discuss considering multivitamin and mineral supplement.
■ Discourage inappropriate weight loss; many HIV clients lose lean body mass first and fat second. Address prevention, restoration, and maintenance of optimal body composition with emphasis on lean tissue. Encourage physical activity.
■ If indicated, encourage more and frequent meals to increase energy intake. Teach regarding consuming foods with high nutrient density. Snacks, complete nutritional supplements, and intravenous feedings may be necessary.

■ Suggest increasing whole-grain and fiber intake, which may include soluble-fiber supplementation.
■ Discuss potential medication–nutrition interactions.
■ Review use of nutrient supplements and potential interactions with nonprescription and herbal supplements.
■ Address food and nutrition security issues. Refer to the social worker if the client lacks enough food.
■ During counseling, evaluate signs and symptoms and tailor counseling to the client's unique needs. In addition, closely monitor the client's blood lipids, triglyceride, glucose, and cholesterol levels and recommend modification of the diet as indicated.

Keystones

- The AIDS epidemic is worldwide.
- Although HAART treatment has reduced mortality rates, no cure has been found for AIDS.
- Transmittal routes include blood-to-blood, perinatal, and sexual contact.
- Health-care professionals can protect themselves from AIDS by using extreme care when handling blood and equipment that has been in contact with blood; practicing safe sexual behaviors can help to protect everyone from AIDS.
- HIV attacks the immune system and leaves its victims defenseless against opportunistic infections.
- AIDS is a disease with many clinical complications.
- Nutritional management is both a preventive and a therapeutic treatment in clients infected with HIV.
- Increased nutrient needs, decreased food intake, and impaired nutrient absorption contribute to the malnutrition seen in AIDS clients.

CASE STUDY *23–1*

Ms. S is a 30-year-old woman who acquired HIV from her drug-abusing husband and subsequently infected their son in utero. She could not believe the test results when she was first told. Now she is seeking nutritional information to allow her to increase her chance for a quality life and her son's chance to survive infancy. Her knowledge of basic nutrition is good. She expressed some concern about transportation and has already missed one of her prenatal visits because her husband sold their car for money to buy drugs. She is also unable to go to the grocery store easily. She is 5 ft 6 in. tall and weighs 120 lb. All her laboratory work was within normal limits. Percent body fat is 25%.

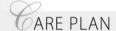

CARE PLAN

Subjective Data

Lack of information on relationship of nutrition to AIDS ■ Concrete goals established

Objective Data

HIV-positive tests, both mother and infant ■ Percent body fat, 25%

Analysis

Lack of information related to modifying AIDS progression and changing unhealthy home environment

Plan

DESIRED OUTCOMES EVALUATION CRITERIA	ACTIONS/INTERVENTIONS	RATIONALE
Client will verbalize areas in which nutrition could affect AIDS development.	Reinforce need for regular, balanced meals. Emphasize adequate kcalories.	The stress of receiving this diagnosis may impede use of previously learned information.
	Instruct Ms. S to keep home environment clean, especially kitchen, bathroom, and basements, where molds and fungi could thrive.	Organisms that are harmless to persons with normal immune systems can cause opportunistic infections in HIV-infected persons.
	Teach client to monitor herself and her son for changes in health related to food intake or digestion.	Discovering beginning malabsorption problems would permit treatment before malnutrition becomes apparent.
Client will monitor her percent body fat.	Explain the relationships among percent body fat, percent lean body mass, and exercise.	Exercise can prevent a loss of lean body mass.
		Weight can be stable, but body fat content can increase.
Client will keep her medical appointments and obtain groceries as needed.	Refer to social worker for help with transportation and food assistance programs.	The social worker has knowledge of available local resources.

23-1

Social Worker's Note

If the client is an inpatient, the social worker typically writes in the discharge planning section of the medical record. If the client is an outpatient, the social worker typically phones the physician's office directly with a solution to the problem and writes a short note to be placed in the medical record.

I met with the client, who described a sad home situation. We discussed the need for her to remove herself and unborn child from her present environment. I arranged for client to move into a shelter for abused women. She agreed to do this immediately.

23-2

Dietitian's Notes

The following Dietitian's Notes are representative of the documentation found in a client's medical record.

Subjective: Met with the client, who expressed an interest in making improvements to her diet. She currently eats three times each day and does not avoid any of the major food groups. She does not take a multivitamin/mineral supplement.

Objective: 5 ft 6 in. Percent body fat 25%; 120 lb

Analysis: Ideal body weight range 117 to 143 lb. Weight in kg is 54.5 kg. Estimated kcal need at 25 to 35 kcal/kg and

54.5 kg equals 1363 to 1907. Estimated protein need at 1.0 to 1.5 grams/kg equals 54.4 to 82 grams. Client's reported food intake, based on a 24-hour dietary recall and cross-checked with a food frequency, showed a kcalorie intake between 1400 and 1600. Her usual protein intake is between 40 and 50 grams per day. We discussed options for the client to increase her protein intake.

Plan: Recommend the addition of one cup of low-fat yogurt or milk per day. Client agreed to do this.

𝒞ritical 𝒯hinking 𝒬uestions

1. The client has developed mouth sores from thrush and would like you to arrange for her to have TPN. She claims it is just too painful to eat. What would you recommend?

2. The client's child has been diagnosed HIV positive. During a home visit, you notice the kitchen is filthy. You instruct the client on food safety and sanitation. On a return visit, despite prior instruction on food safety, you notice that the client's kitchen is still not clean. The client claims she is too tired to clean. What do you do?

3. The client went to a health food store and purchased several bottles of vitamin pills and herbal supplements. She believes she can take these in lieu of eating. What should you do?

Chapter Review

1. The health-care worker's best insurance against HIV transmission on the job is:
   a. Frequent hand washing
   b. Universal precautions
   c. Body substance isolation
   d. Adherence to all food safety policies and procedures

2. A client on HAART can partially compensate for fat redistribution syndrome by:
   a. Taking medications as prescribed
   b. Taking supplemental vitamins and minerals
   c. Consuming a low-fat diet
   d. Exercising

3. Compared with wasting, cachexia is:
   a. A slower process
   b. The result of both a protein and kilocalorie deficit
   c. Always the result of a poor food intake
   d. Best treated by the inclusion of 400 additional kilocalories per day

4. Clinicians measure _____ as an indicator of fat-soluble vitamin absorption.
   a. Folate
   b. Zinc
   c. 25-hydroxy vitamin D
   d. Glucose

5. Educating a client with AIDS about food safety is important:
   a. To minimize the risk of rare tumors
   b. To prevent body fat redistribution
   c. To enhance renal function
   d. To prevent opportunistic infections

Clinical Analysis

1. Mr. Y, a 45-year-old Black man, was diagnosed as HIV-positive 1 month ago. His height is 6 ft 0 in., and his weight is 178 lb and stable. He reports no signs or symptoms and has not seen a physician yet. He wants to know what he should eat. As the nurse during this first visit, you might discuss:
   a. The many benefits of HAART
   b. Food safety, exercise, good nutrition, and the importance of follow-up with a physician
   c. The expected outcome and potential complications
   d. Vitamin and mineral supplementation, increased kilocaloric needs, and the treatment for malabsorption

2. Carlos, a 25-year-old Hispanic man, presents with severe diarrhea. He was diagnosed with HIV about 8 years ago. He has five to six watery stools each day that do not appear to be related to his medications. His height is 5 ft 10 in., and his weight is 140 lb (usual weight is 175 lb). He is an inpatient, and the physician has ordered a stool culture, but the results are not back. You recommend:
   a. Extra fluids with meals to prevent dehydration
   b. A clear-liquid, complete nutritional supplement
   c. A high-fat and high-fiber diet to provide both kilocalories and bulk to his diet
   d. Six small meals with a milkshake between meals to push kilocalories and protein

3. Dave, a 36-year-old White man, complains of fatigue. He is often too tired to cook and has little interest in food. He lives alone and is on disability. His CD$_4$ cell count is 400, and his viral load is 100,000. You recommend:
   a. Tube feeding
   b. Referral to a social service agency
   c. Meals-on-Wheels
   d. Six small meals daily

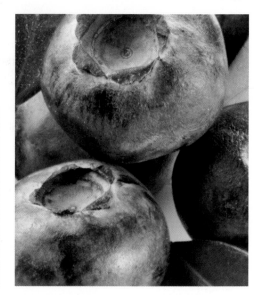

24

Nutritional Care of the Terminally Ill

LEARNING OBJECTIVES

After completing this chapter, the student should be able to:

- Differentiate between palliative and curative nutritional care.
- State appropriate nutritional screening questions for the terminally ill client.
- List at least two appropriate dietary management techniques for symptom control for each of the following: anemia, anorexia, bowel obstruction, cachexia, constipation, cough, dehydration, diarrhea, dysgeusia, esophageal reflux, fever, fluid accumulation, hiccups, incontinence, jaundice and hepatic encephalopathy, migraine headache, nausea and vomiting, pruritus, stomatitis, weakness, wounds and pressure sores, and **xerostomia.**
- State appropriate assessment questions for a terminally ill client.
- Discuss the ethical and legal considerations for feeding a terminally ill client.

This chapter discusses clients who have been certified by physicians to be terminally ill. An individual is considered terminally ill if he or she has a medical prognosis of 6 months or less based on the usual disease progression. Although a physician can estimate life expectancy based on disease progression, this is not an exact science. A client diagnosed with a terminal disease may live longer than or not as long as predicted because the disease may not follow its usual progression. Individuals who have been certified by a physician as terminally ill can elect to use the hospice benefit under federal guidelines. Hospice is the major health-care program for the terminally ill in the United States.

Although health-care workers have received much training on how to reverse the effects of disease, we have received much less training on how to assist our clients with dying. With changes in the health-care system bringing decreased lengths of hospital stays, an increasing number of clients will again be cared for in their homes. Training health-care workers to provide home care for terminally ill clients is becoming essential.

Nutritional and dietary issues are at the center of some ethical questions concerning the care of these clients. Health-care professionals need to address clients' values, goals of care, and preferences with regard to treatment to truly become client advocates.

Dealing with Death

Our culture emphasizes the enjoyment of life. At the beginning of the 20th century, most people died at home, and many died young. Death was a part of everyday life. Over the past 50 years, most people have died in hospitals or long-term care facilities. Often an ambulance is called if a person is dying.

The Dying Process

Death is an unavoidable part of the life cycle. Both physiological and psychological changes occur as part of the dying process. The client's age, diagnosis, and physical condition influence physiological changes. Regardless of the underlying disease, cardiopulmonary failure is the final cause of death. Pulmonary and circulatory failure may be gradual or sudden. The major signs and symptoms in the final days and hours of life include:

■ Cessation of eating and drinking
■ Oliguria and incontinence
■ Muscle weakness
■ Difficulty in breathing
■ Cyanosis
■ Decreased mental alertness
■ Changes in vital signs

Hospice team members may describe clients with a terminal diagnosis as actively dying. An actively dying client has a life expectancy of a few hours or a few days. The reason for the actively dying designation is to determine staff needs.

Cessation of Eating and Drinking

Life will soon cease when a client's eating and drinking diminishes critically. Oral intake dwindles because a client has no desire to eat or because disease prevents digestion. This greatly decreased oral intake is often worrisome to family members.

Health-care workers need to counsel family members that dehydration at this time is believed to have a euphoric effect and is not painful. Clinical Application 24-1 discusses the physiological responses to fluid restriction. Fluids and comfort care such as the following actions can reduce the thirst sensations from dehydration:

■ Ice chips
■ Lubricating the lips with moistened gauze or a water-soluble product. Avoid products such as Vaseline that can dry mucosa (Couch, Mead, & Walsh, 2013).
■ Small amounts of food and water

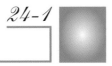

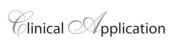

Physiological Response to Fluid Restriction

Young, healthy, active individuals who are deprived of water develop thirst, dry mouth, and headache, followed by fatigue; cognitive impairment occurs as dehydration progresses and becomes severe with abnormal electrolytes, rising blood urea nitrogen, and hemoconcentration. If water is not taken, renal failure is likely.

In terminally ill clients, dehydration results in the same signs and symptoms. However, studies have shown metabolic changes may produce a sedative effect on the brain just before death. In cases where the evidence strongly suggests that hydration or feeding does not provide benefit, the health-care team has a responsibility to explain this to the client and/or family.

Hospice nurses working with terminal clients were asked to rate the quality of death in clients, using a scale of 0 equaling a very bad death and 9 being a very good death, rated the death of those that voluntarily refused both food and fluid at an 8 (Fuhrman, 2008).

Withholding and minimizing hydration can have the desirable effect of reducing:

■ Disturbing oral secretions
■ Bronchial secretions
■ Need for frequent urination
■ Cough from diminished pulmonary congestion

It is uncompassionate to force food or fluids on a client who is actively dying.

Oliguria and Incontinence

Because oral intake is usually decreased for several days before death, urine output is often diminished and may cease. The color of the urine may become very dark. A period of incontinence often precedes the oliguria, and anuria occurs. General fatigue, muscle weakness, and decreased mental acuity are among the reasons for the incontinence. Bedding should be changed as quickly as possible to avoid skin irritation. Death usually occurs within 48 to 72 hours after urine output stops.

Difficulty in Breathing

Most clients have some difficulty breathing before death. Caregivers may become alarmed when they hear a loud, hoarse, and bubbling sound. These sounds are caused by the passage of breath through pharyngeal and pulmonary secretions that lodge at the back of the client's throat. These sounds have been referred to as the "death rattle" because studies have demonstrated that approximately 75% of clients will die within 48 hours of this symptom developing (Kompanje, van der Hoven, and Bakker, 2008). It is believed that the client does not experience increased suffering, but the symptom can be distressing for loved ones. Interventions that can be used to reduce symptoms and maintain a clear airway include elevating the head of the bed, positioning the client on his or her side and frequent turning, discontinuing artificial hydration, and use of anticholinergic medication such as scopolamine in order to decrease the amount of secretions (Hipp and Letizia, 2009). Suctioning is not recommended because it can cause discomfort in the client. All terminally ill clients do not have these sounds with respiration. Some clients experience apnea (a temporary cessation of breathing). A change such as these in breathing is an indicator that life will soon cease.

Cyanosis

Slightly bluish, grayish, or dark purple discoloration of the skin caused by poor oxygenation is called **cyanosis.** The client's feet, legs, hands, and groin feel cold. Many health-care workers believe this is one of the most useful indicators that the end of life is approaching. Slowed circulation and decreased tissue perfusion cause these signs.

Decreased Mental Alertness

The amount of blood reaching the brain, lungs, liver, and kidneys decreases as general circulation slows. Sleepiness, apathy, disorientation, confusion, restlessness, and finally a decreased level of consciousness that frequently progresses to a sleeplike state are among the signs that death is imminent.

Changes in Vital Signs

Signs of impeding death include:

- A decrease in body temperature
- A rise and then a decrease in pulse rate
- A rise and then a decrease in respirations
- A fall in blood pressure

Death occurs when there is no pulse and respiration ceases.

Family members and caregivers of terminally ill clients often express fear at the thought of being alone with an actively dying client. For this reason, health-care workers often remain with the client and their loved ones during this time. Some health-care workers resist working with the terminally ill because they think that they cannot cope with this experience. However, death is not always a painful experience. Health-care workers who share the death experience with a client and the client's family often describe the experience as rewarding and profound.

Palliative Versus Curative Care

Palliative care has been defined as the active total care of an individual when curative measures are no longer considered an option by either the medical team or the client. The goal of curative care is arresting the disease. The goal of palliative care is the relief of symptoms to alleviate or ease pain and discomfort. Emphasis in palliative care is placed on addressing:

- Pain and symptom control
- Spiritual and psychological support
- Improving quality of life

These concerns are common in dying clients. Palliative care is defined by the World Health Organization (2013) as "An approach that improves the quality of life of patients and their families facing the problems associated with life-threatening illness, through the prevention and relief of suffering by means of early identification and impeccable assessment and the treatment of pain and other problems physical, psychosocial and spiritual." Palliative care programs address and include the client and family members in the plan of care and care can be provided at any time during the course of the disease, not just at the end of life.

Hospice dates back to medieval times. During the crusades, travelers needed a place to stop for comfort. The Knights of Hospitallers of the Order of St. John of Jerusalem in the twelfth century sheltered the sick and religious pilgrims. They established hospices in England, Germany, Italy, Cyprus, and Rhodes. The soul, mind, and spirit were considered as much in need of help as the body.

Around the fifteenth century, anatomical and surgical practices developed. Physicians moved into hospitals that emphasized curative treatments. Monks and nuns remained in cloisters and cared for the people the physicians could not heal, including the disabled, the chronically ill, and the terminally ill.

During the eighteenth and nineteenth centuries, great advances in curative treatments occurred, and hospitals became highly specialized in acute life-threatening situations. Hospitals were less able to offer shelter to people nearing life's end. At the same time, caring for the terminally ill became less a private or religious function and more a public and governmental one.

The modern hospice has its roots in the late nineteenth century, when a place of shelter for the incurably ill was founded in Dublin. The British physician Dr. Cicely Saunders inspired the hospice movement in the United States. Dr. Saunders is noted for her work in pain control and for the founding of St. Christopher's Hospice in London in 1967. The first operational hospice program in the United States was established in New Haven, Connecticut, in the early 1970s.

Hospice philosophy includes the belief that death is a natural aspect of life. Hospice is committed to the philosophy that persons have the right to die in the setting of their choice and to be as comfortable as possible. Central to the hospice philosophy is the idea that palliative care is appropriate when treatment of the client's disease becomes ineffective and irrelevant.

In 2011, it was estimated that 1.65 million people received hospice services and 66% of those patients died at home with their family or loved ones providing their primary care (National Hospice and Palliative Care Organization, 2012).

Nutrition Screening

All palliative care begins with the establishment of the goals of care. Studies suggest that what terminally ill clients want is to:

- Have their pain and other symptoms relieved
- Improve their quality of life
- Avoid being a burden to their family
- Have a close relationship with loved ones
- Maintain a sense of control

The goal of palliative nutritional care is to assist the client and caregiver with any food-related concerns. These difficulties may be related to uncomfortable symptoms and attitudes and beliefs held about food. Screening the client with a terminal illness for food-related concerns is the first step. There are major differences between screening a client who is undergoing curative or preventive treatment and screening a terminally ill client who is receiving palliative care.

First, the health-care worker needs to ascertain if the client has any symptoms that may be diminished by nutritional intervention. Second, the attitudes and beliefs of the client or caregiver about food need to be examined. Some clients and their caregivers have difficulty accepting that the terminally ill client frequently eats much less than is needed to sustain life. Box 24-1 is an example of a nutrition screening form for the client with a terminal condition.

Health-care professionals, clients, and family members frequently want to discuss the use of an intravenous or tube feedings in a terminally ill client during the screening process. The use of any artificial feeding should always be considered but is often inconsistent with treatment goals. For example, in the case of a client with dementia who has dysphagia or stops eating, placement of a percutaneous endoscopic gastrostomy (PEG) tube may be considered but should not be routinely used if dysphagia is caused by end-stage disease or for the sole purpose of prolonging life (Parker and Power, 2013). If the treatment goal of the client is to reduce suffering and enhance the quality of life, a PEG tube may not assist in meeting this goal. The position of the Academy of Nutrition and Dietetics is that individuals have the right to request or refuse nutrition and hydration as medical treatment. This refusal includes PEG tube placement. If death is imminent and feeding will not alter the condition, the health-care provider should consider whether nutrient support will be burdensome (American Dietetic Association, 2008).

Box 24-1 ■ *Sample Nutrition Screening Form

Name _____ Caregiver's Name _____
Date _____ Diagnosis _____

1. Have you had any concerns about weight changes or food intake?

   No _____ Yes _____ Describe _____

2. For clients on tube feedings or parenteral feedings only: Have your feedings created or increased discomfort, diarrhea, distension, other?

   Type: _____ Amount _____ Infusion rate _____

3. Do you feel your symptoms could be decreased or controlled through dietary change?

   No _____ Yes _____ Describe _____

4. Do you feel diet or nutritional supplement would benefit you or your disease process?

   No _____ Yes _____ Type _____

5. Do you believe that your diet caused your disease or will slow the progression of your disease?

   No _____ Yes _____ Describe _____

6. Do you find eating enhances comfort?

   No _____ Yes _____

7. What concerns do you have regarding your diet intake?

   _____

8. Would you (client or caregiver) like to discuss food-related concerns with the dietitian?

   No _____ Yes _____

*For printing, available on DavisPlus.

Assessment

During the nutritional assessment, every question posed to the client or caregiver should have a purpose. Health-care workers generally need to know the results of laboratory tests, diagnostic procedures, physical examinations, and anthropometric measures as well as the level of immune function and food intake information to determine a client's nutritional status; however, this may have no value in the provision of nutritional care for a terminally ill client.

For example, why ask if a client drinks milk? Is it to estimate if the client is meeting the calcium, riboflavin, and vitamin D allowances? If it is determined that the client's milk intake is suboptimal, would anything be done about the inadequacy? If the client has diarrhea with severe abdominal cramping after the ingestion of milk, however, a recommendation to drink lactose-free milk would be appropriate. Unless the client will experience relief from bothersome symptoms, it is best not to recommend behavioral changes that may be difficult for the client to make. On the other hand, if the client expresses concern about the nutritional adequacy of his or her diet, nutrition education is not contraindicated (see Box 24-1).

Intervention and Symptom Control

Box 24-2 describes appropriate dietary management for symptom control for a client with a terminal illness. If a health-care worker feels uncomfortable discussing these issues with the client or lacks the time to counsel the client, a referral to the dietitian is indicated.

Ethical and Legal Considerations

Many of the legal and ethical issues concerning health-care delivery and health-care provider–client relations involve the provision of nutrition and hydration. In the past, before the development of tube feedings and intravenous feedings, the inability to eat and drink by mouth meant death from progressive body wasting. Although humans can survive several weeks without food, lack of water can result in death within 3 to 5 days (Ruxton, 2012).

Now a decision needs to be made whether to feed a client. A client may experience a more comfortable death if he or she is slightly dehydrated. On the other

---

Box 24-2 ■ *Dietary Management for Symptom Control*

Anemia

- Recommend a vitamin C source with red meats and iron-fortified foods.
- Discourage use of coffee, tea, and chocolate if the client has gastrointestinal bleeding.
- Recommend a multivitamin supplement if the client desires and the primary care provider approves but avoid megadose vitamins.

Anorexia

- Discuss practical issues with the client or caregiver, such as food attitudes, social aspects of eating, food preferences, and beliefs about food.
- Encourage concentration on the sensual pleasures of eating, such as table setting, garnishes, smells, and socialization.
- Evaluate the client's desire for a sense of well-being.
- Suggest use of small, frequent feedings.
- Educate the caregiver to recognize early signs of malnutrition and provide protein supplements, make food accessible, and encourage eating as desired by the client and caregiver if the client's prognosis is more than a few weeks.
- Evaluate the client's acceptance of a liquid diet and recommend complete oral nutritional supplements.
- Teach the caregiver that the client has the right to self-determination and may refuse to eat or drink when actively dying. The caregiver should continue to offer nourishment as a sign of love and caring but not harass the client to eat or drink.

Bowel Obstruction

- NPO (nothing by mouth) may be indicated; limited clear liquids may be possible.
- Encourage small meals low in fiber and residue if oral intake is not contraindicated.
- Encourage the client to eat slowly, chew food well, and rest after each meal if oral intake is not contraindicated.
- Recommend dry feedings if oral intake is not contraindicated.
- Recommend avoidance of sugary fatty foods, alcohol, and foods with a strong odor.

Cachexia

- Teach relaxation techniques and encourage use before mealtime.
- Encourage the client and the caregiver to concentrate on the sensual pleasures of eating such as setting an attractive table

and plate and using food garnishes and providing an appetizing eating environment by removing bedpans and emesis basin before serving the food.
- Evaluate client for dysgeusia and dysphagia and xerostomia.

Constipation

- Encourage high-fiber foods (bran, whole grains, fruits, vegetables, nuts, and legumes) if an adequate fluid intake can be maintained.
- Instruct the client to avoid high-fiber foods if dehydration or an obstruction is suspected or anticipated.
- Assess the client's fluid intake and recommend an increased intake if needed.
- Recommend taking 1 to 2 ounces of a special recipe with the evening meal: 2 cups applesauce, 2 cups unprocessed bran (All-Bran®), and 1 cup of 100% prune juice. Refrigerate this mixture between uses and discard after 5 days if not used.
- Suggest limiting cheese and high-fat, sugary foods (doughnuts, cakes, pies, cookies) that may be constipating.
- Discontinue calcium and iron supplements if they contribute to constipation.
- Review the client's medications. If the client is taking bulking agents (milk of magnesia, magnesium citrate, Metamucil®, or Golytely®), a large fluid intake is essential. Suggest the client or caregiver mask the taste of these medications in applesauce, mashed potatoes, gravy, orange juice, and nectars.

Cough

- Encourage fluids and ice chips.
- Recommend hard candy, including sour balls.
- Have the client try tea and coffee to dilate pulmonary vessels.

Dehydration

- Encourage intake of fluids such as juices, ice cream, gelatin, custards, puddings, and soups if the client's life expectancy is more than a few days.
- Encourage the client to try creative beverages such as orange sherbet and milkshake.
- Consider a nasogastric tube feeding for fluid delivery only after a discussion with other team members, client, and caregivers. Plain water and foods high in electrolytes can be delivered via a tube feeding.

Box 24-2 ■ *Dietary Management for Symptom Control—cont'd*

- Consider a parenteral line only after a tube feeding is considered and rejected and after an in-depth discussion with the team members, client, and family. Client goals, expectations, and quality-of-life issues should all be very carefully considered. Parenteral lines for the delivery of nutrients and water are rarely indicated in terminally ill clients.

Diarrhea

- Consider modification of the diet to omit lactose, gluten, or fat if related to diarrhea.
- Suggest a decrease in dietary fiber content.
- Consider the omission of gas-forming vegetables if an association between the consumption of these foods and diarrhea can be ascertained.
- Consider the use of a low-residue diet.
- Encourage consumption of high-potassium foods (bananas, tomato juice, orange juice, potatoes) if the client is dehydrated.
- Recommend dry feedings (drink fluids 1 hour before or 30–60 minutes after meals).
- Encourage intake of medium-chain triglycerides and a diet high in protein and carbohydrates for steatorrhea due to pancreatic insufficiency.
- Consider the use of a complete oral nutritional supplement to provide adequate nutrient composition while helping the client overcome mild-to-moderate malabsorption.
- For copious diarrhea or diarrhea combined with a coccyx decubitus, consider use of a clear-liquid complete nutritional supplement or a predigested oral nutritional supplement.

Dysgeusia (abnormal taste)

- Encourage oral care before mealtime.
- Evaluate whether the client experiences a bitter, sweet, or no taste after food consumption.
- If foods taste bitter, encourage consumption of poultry, fish, milk and milk products, and legumes. Recommend the use of marinated meats and poultry in juices or wine. Sour and salty foods are generally not liked when a client experiences a bitter taste. Cook food in a glass or porcelain container to improve taste. Recommend a decreased use of red meats, sour juices, coffee, tea, tomatoes, and chocolate. The use of a modular protein supplement may be helpful if the client's protein intake is suboptimal.
- If foods taste sweet, recommend sour juices, tart foods, lemon juice, vinegar, pickles, spices, herbs, and the use of a modular carbohydrate supplement.
- If food has no taste, recommend foods served at room temperature, highly seasoned foods, and sugary foods.

Dyspnea (difficulty breathing)

- Encourage intake of coffee, tea, and chocolate. These foods are bronchodilators that increase blood pressure, dilate pulmonary vessels, increase glomerular filtration rate, and thus break up and expel pulmonary secretions and fluids.
- Encourage use of a soft diet. Liquids are usually better tolerated than solids. Cold foods are often better accepted than hot foods.
- Recommend small, frequent feedings.
- Encourage ice chips, frozen fruit juices, and popsicles; these are often well accepted.
- Consider the use of a complete high-fat, low-carbohydrate nutritional supplement. This decreases carbon dioxide retention and assists in breathing.

Esophageal Reflux

- Recommend small feedings.
- Discourage consumption of foods that lower esophageal sphincter pressure, such as high-fat foods, chocolate, peppermint, spearmint, and alcohol.
- Encourage the client to sit up while eating and for 1 hour afterward.
- Recommend avoidance of food within 3 hours before bedtime.
- Teach relaxation techniques.

Fever

- Recommend a high fluid intake.
- Consider a tube feeding for severe dehydration to maintain hydration after a discussion with team members. This is not recommended if death is imminent (hours/days).
- Recommend high-protein, high-caloric foods.

Fluid Accumulation

- Recommend a mild sodium restriction (<2 grams/day). Recommend a lower sodium restriction only if this is the wish of the client.
- Discourage a fluid restriction unless the client has significant hyponatremia.
- Provide a list of foods high in protein and potassium.

Hiccups

- Recommend smaller meals and slow eating.
- Discourage the use of a straw.
- Recommend the client swallow a large teaspoon of granulated sugar.

Hypoglycemia

- Assess the client's and caregiver's knowledge about diabetes and hypoglycemia.
- Determine if the client is truly insulin dependent as part of the admission assessment process.
  The following suggest true insulin dependence:
  - Introduction of insulin soon after the diagnosis
  - A history of previous ketoacidosis
  - Use of more than one daily dose of insulin for years
- Evaluate the client's expressed desire for extent of medical care. The primary guide for determining the level of nutritional intervention is the wish of the client.
- Determine the last time the client experienced the signs of a hypoglycemic episode. Many of these clients have deficiencies in the counter-regulatory hormones, especially epinephrine, and may lapse into a coma without any warning signs. Caregivers need to be informed of this potential complication. Educate the client and/or caregiver on the treatment of hypoglycemia.
- Monitor the client's blood glucose level. A suitable range for blood sugars would be 127 to 309 mg/dL in the hospice population.
- Encourage consumption of 30 to 50 grams of carbohydrate every 3 hours to prevent starvation ketosis. Each of the following is equal to 30 to 50 grams of carbohydrate: ¾ cup of Carnation Instant Breakfast®, 1 cup of regular gelatin, 1 cup of vanilla ice cream, 1½ cups of ginger ale, 1 cup of orange juice, 1 cup of apple juice.

Incontinence

- Discourage intake of coffee, tea, and carbonated beverages containing caffeine, especially before bedtime.
- Continue to encourage adequate fluid intake during the day.

(continued)

Box 24-2 ■ *Dietary Management for Symptom Control—cont'd*

Jaundice and Hepatic Encephalopathy

- Encourage a high-carbohydrate diet.
- Encourage a protein-restricted diet only if the client desires.
- Specialized oral nutritional supplements for clients with liver disease are often ineffective for the terminally ill but may be beneficial when the client desires to "live long enough to _____."
- Evaluate for the presence of esophageal varices. If present, provide soft foods.

Nausea and Vomiting

- Discuss practical issues with the client and caregiver such as food attitudes, social aspects of eating, and unpredictable food preferences.
- Recommend the client restrict fluids to 1 hour before or after meals to prevent early satiety.
- Assess if sweet, fried, or fatty foods are poorly tolerated; recommend avoidance if necessary.
- Evaluate if starchy foods such as crackers, breads, potatoes, rice, and pasta are better tolerated. Encourage increased consumption if helpful.
- Encourage the client to eat slowly, chew food well, and rest after each meal because these behaviors may increase food intake.
- Recommend the client is not subjected to offensive odors during food preparation.
- Recommend that the person who has recently experienced severe nausea and vomiting try one to two bites of food per hour.
- Emphasize the sensual aspects of food, including appearance (serve garnished food on attractive tableware), odor of environment (remove bedpans and emesis basins from room), taste (cater to the client's likes and dislikes), and the importance of companionship during mealtime.
- Recommend the avoidance of food if nausea and vomiting become severe and food makes the client feel worse. Feeding may not be desirable if death is expected within hours or a few days and the effects of partial dehydration or the withdrawal of nutrition support will not adversely alter client comfort.
- Use of ginger to reduce effects of nausea.

Migraine Headaches

- Recommend that the client eat at regular intervals. Hunger or missed meals can trigger a migraine headache.
- Recommend that the highly motivated client keep a food diary and record the onset of any headaches. Migraine headaches can be triggered by one or many foods. Common food offenders include many common food additives, processed meats, peanuts and peanut products, soybeans, yeast, chocolate, aged cheeses, seasonings, caffeine, some types of alcohol, and flavorings.

Pruritus (severe itching)

- Recommend avoidance of known allergy foods.
- Encourage adequate fluid intake.
- Encourage adequate consumption of vitamin A and vitamin C (Cowdell, 2009).
- Encourage adequate consumption of protein and fatty acids.

Stomatitis (inflammation of the mouth)

- Consider a multivitamin supplement with folic acid and vitamin B_{12}.
- Recommend avoidance of spicy, acidic, rough, hot, and salty foods.
- Recommend a consistency modification, such as pureed, soft, or liquid.
- Consider the use of a complete nutritional supplement.
- Recommend creamy foods, white sauces, and gravies.
- Consider between-meal supplements, such as milkshakes, eggnogs, and puddings.
- Recommend meals be served when the client's pain is under control.
- Recommend good oral care before and after meals.

Weakness

- Recommend a multivitamin-mineral supplement with folic acid, vitamin B_{12}, and iron.
- Encourage high-potassium foods (bananas, cantaloupe, milk, baked winter squash, etc.) if the client vomits easily.
- Recommend a modification in the food's consistency (mechanical soft or full liquid) to decrease the energy cost of eating.

Wounds and Pressure Sores

- Recommend the caregiver cater to the client's food preferences.
- Use of aggressive nutritional support is rarely effective but may be appropriate if the client and family desire quantity. For example, "I want to live and see my _____."
- Correct elevated glucose levels to increased risk of infection.
- Evaluate the use of a multivitamin and mineral supplement that contains zinc and vitamin C. Because excess dietary zinc impedes healing, do not routinely recommend a zinc supplement without assessment information.
- Encourage protein and caloric intake equal to estimated needs only if the client desires and is able.
- Encourage the client to dip foods in gravy, margarine, butter, and olive oil to increase calorie intake.

Xerostomia (dry mouth)

- Encourage frequent sips of water or ice chips.
- Recommend the use of sugar-free chewing gum.
- Use of organic acids such as ascorbic acid (vitamin C), citric acid (acid in citrus fruits), and malic acid (acid in apples and pears) if the client does not have stomatitis (Davies and Hall, 2011).
- Consider a modification of food consistency such as soft, mechanical soft, or full liquids.
- Recommend avoidance of extremely hot or cold foods. Foods served at room temperature are generally better tolerated.
- Recommend creamy foods, white sauces, and gravies.
- Encourage the client to dip foods in gravy, margarine, butter, olive oil, coffee, and broth.
- Consider the need for a complete liquid nutritional supplement between meals.

hand, efforts to hydrate some clients (not those actively dying) may offer a benefit. This is controversial. Sometimes a client, significant other, or physician thinks that artificial hydration may promote client comfort and prolong life in a given situation.

Perhaps a client's vital signs had been fluctuating and are now stable. Ethicists use rational processes for determining the most morally desirable course of action in the face of conflicting value choices. The process of choosing an ethical course of action involves:

■ Medical goals and proportionality
■ Client preferences
■ Quality of life
■ Contextual features

Contextual features are the characteristics of a given situation.

Medical Care Goals and Proportionality

The medical care goals that apply to the client with a terminal illness include:

■ Relieving symptoms, pain, and suffering
■ Preventing untimely death ("I want to live long enough to....")
■ Improving functional status or maintaining compromised status
■ Educating and counseling the client and his or her significant others regarding the client's condition and prognosis
■ Avoiding harming the client in the course of care
■ Promoting health and preventing disease not related to the terminal disease

The physician is responsible for the initial education and counseling of clients regarding their condition and prognosis.

The principle of proportionality is an important ethical consideration in the treatment of terminally ill clients. **Proportionality** means a medical treatment is ethically mandatory to the extent that it is likely to confer greater benefits than burdens to the client. For example, many experts believe that a client who is actively dying and is slightly dehydrated has a more comfortable death. Dehydration has been reported to reduce:

■ A client's secretions and excretions
■ Breathing problems
■ Emesis
■ Incontinence

Dehydration can sedate the brain just before death. Greatly diminished oral intake or its cessation is one of the signs that death is imminent. In another context, a client who is terminally ill but whose condition is

stable and enjoys many activities of daily living may appreciate or request education on how to maintain hydration. A nutritional intervention is appropriate if the client would receive greater benefits than burdens.

Client Preference

The most important ethical principle to consider is the client's right to self-determination. Some individuals may perceive suffering as an important means of personal growth or a religious experience. Other individuals may hope a miracle cure will be discovered for his or her disease. Others may be ready for and accepting of death. Health-care workers have a responsibility to provide a combination of emotional support and technical nutritional advice on how best to achieve each client's goals.

Quality of Life

The most fundamental goal of medical care is an improvement in the quality of life for those who seek care. If improvement is not possible, a goal of medical care is maintenance of the same quality of life or slowing a decline in quality of life. Oral feeding is part of being human and associated with human dignity. Some clients derive some pleasure from the sensual aspect of food and the socialization that accompanies meals. Food conveys emotional, spiritual, sociological, and biological meanings.

If food remains enjoyable for a client with a terminal illness, the health-care worker should encourage mealtimes to be shared with loved ones. If eating is not a pleasant experience, however, it should not be overemphasized. Families and loved ones need to be educated that the loss in desire to eat and drink is a natural part of the dying process (Barrocas, Geppert, Durfee, et al, 2010).

Contextual

Every terminally ill client has his or her own story, with both a history and a future. A client's decision to eat or not to eat is part of his or her narrative. Two examples can illustrate why eating issues should always be given consideration when formulating a care plan.

Client 1 lives in a rooming house without air-conditioning; his family does not want to get involved; he does not have cooking facilities; he refuses to eat the meals delivered to him from the Senior Nutrition Center; and he insists that he wants to die at home. Client 1 refuses to eat.

Client 2 lives with his male companion in a beach house; his friend carries him every day to the beach to watch the sunset; meals are prepared for him by his companion and many other neighbors and friends.

Client 2 tries to eat a small amount at least six times a day.

The willingness to eat is part of each man's story. The contextual features in a client's situation often relate to food acceptance. In Client 1's situation, the health-care worker may offer a valuable service by reassuring the client that he will not be abandoned because he refuses to eat. The fear of abandonment is among the most frequently cited apprehensions of dying. Even if a client refuses to eat, health-care workers should remain supportive. The client may change his or her mind. The health-care worker should not consider the rejection of food as a sign of personal or professional failure.

A consideration of a client's medical goals, preferences, quality of life, and contextual features may provide a framework for resolution of ethical dietary issues. Hospice programs have interdisciplinary care teams, and the interdisciplinary team conference is the best arena in which to discuss ethical feeding conflicts.

Legal Issues

The issue of whether to discontinue food and fluid to a client with a terminal illness first emerged in the 1960s. Clients have the legal right to refuse treatment, including artificial feedings. This right is based on the Fourteenth Amendment to the Constitution, which refers to the right to liberty, including the right to be left alone and not invaded or treated against one's will. Courts have recognized that competent adults have the right to refuse treatment, including artificial feeding.

Each state may exert its authority to expand the individual's right to liberty, however, based on other concepts. The preservation of life, the prevention of suicide, the protection of innocent third parties (such as minor children), and the protection of the ethical integrity and professional discretion of the medical profession are among these concepts. Health-care workers need to be familiar with the laws in their individual states and the policies and procedures of the organization for which they work.

They should also know their professional organization's standards of practice. In some states, a charge of battery can be made if a client is fed artificially against his or her wishes. In some states, a charge of negligence can be made if clients are allowed to intentionally starve themselves to death. Situations such as these should be discussed at the interdisciplinary team meeting or brought to the risk manager's attention. (The risk manager is hired by a health-care organization to identify, evaluate, and correct potential risks of injuring clients, staff, visitors, or property.)

With incompetent adult clients, caretakers and family should try to ascertain the client's wishes from past written and oral statements and actions. State laws differ as to whether nutrition and hydration are medically obligatory or medically optional. Some clients may wish for the withdrawal of antibiotics and ventilators but wish to continue nutritional support. This situation may occur when an individual has a PEG tube in place because of an inability to swallow, such as may occur with cancer of the esophagus.

What can health-care workers legally do if the client is incompetent and the family wants the feeding tube removed? What can the health-care worker legally do if family members disagree about whether to have the feeding tube removed? When in doubt, the best advice is to continue to feed the client until the health-care team, the institution's ethics committee, or the facility's risk manager reviews the case. The artificial feeding can be stopped at a future time if the decision is changed, but a deceased person cannot be brought back to life.

Individuals may make their wishes known in writing through advance directives, such as a living will or durable power of attorney. An **advance directive** is a signed document in which the client has specified what type of medical care is desired should he or she lose the ability to make decisions. A **durable power of attorney** for health care is a document in which the client gives another person power to make medical treatment and related personal care decisions for him or her. It can be used as an addition to the advance directive. Health-care workers are responsible for becoming familiar with a client's advance directive, durable power of attorney, and living will. In the event that a client does not have a written directive, the next of kin or guardian should be consulted about a probable preference for the level of nutritional intervention.

General Considerations

Palliative care does not automatically preclude aggressive nutritional support. The client's informed preference for the level of nutrition intervention is important. If the client wants maximal nutrition support and the policy of the organization is not to provide parenteral nutrition or tube feedings for terminally ill clients, the client has the right to be informed of the name of a facility that will provide this service. Artificial feeding generally is not desirable if death is expected within hours or a few days.

The effects of partial dehydration and the withdrawal of nutritional support will not adversely alter the client's comfort. Enteral or parenteral feeding would probably worsen the client's condition, symptoms, or discomfort when shock, pulmonary edema, diarrhea, or aspiration is a potential or actual complication. The client or surrogate needs to be informed of these facts when he or she requests maximal support.

Keystones

- Death is an aspect of life.
- If we want to help the dying, we must examine our own attitudes toward death.
- Treatment for terminally ill clients is palliative.
- The goal of care is symptomatic relief to reduce or alleviate pain.
- Nutritional intervention can frequently alleviate or reduce the pain and suffering of a terminally ill client.
- The use of oral feedings should always be given consideration over tube and parenteral feedings.
- Oral feeding is ordinary care, whereas tube feedings and parenteral nutrition are considered by some to be extraordinary care.
- In the United States, the client's expressed desire is the primary guide for determining the extent of nutritional and hydration therapy.
- The U.S. Constitution guarantees clients the right to self-determination.
- Ethical and legal dilemmas should be brought to the attention of the interdisciplinary team, the risk manager, or the facility's ethics committee promptly.
- Artificial feeding should never be stopped unless one of these parties has investigated the situation and made a legal and ethical determination that the feeding should cease.
- Each health-care worker has an obligation to know his or her client's advance directive, durable power of attorney, and living will documentation.

CASE STUDY *24–1*

Ms. Z is a 60-year-old woman who has a diagnosis of amyotrophic lateral sclerosis (ALS), also called Lou Gehrig disease, with a prognosis of less than 6 months. The client has at least two swallowing impediments. She is unable to dislodge food that collects under her tongue, in cheeks, and on her hard palate. She does not have adequate swallow control (the bolus goes down before she wants it to). Because of these impediments, Ms. Z is unable to tolerate thin liquids, and the maintenance of hydration and aspiration are of concern to the caregiver. Ms. Z is alert, oriented, and highly educated. She saw a television program that led her to believe that a high-protein diet would delay the progression of ALS. She would like instruction on a high-protein diet.

CARE PLAN

Subjective Data

Client believes a high-protein diet will delay the progression of her ALS. ■ Caregiver is concerned about the danger of aspiration and the maintenance of hydration.

Objective Data

Diagnosis: ALS with a prognosis of less than 6 months ■ Lack of swallowing control

Analysis

Related to lack of desired information about foods high in protein as evidenced by verbal statements. ■ Deficient knowledge related to a lack of understanding of how to increase and/or maintain hydration with the client's swallowing impediments as evidenced by the caregiver's verbal statements.

(Continued on the following page)

Plan

DESIRED OUTCOMES EVALUATION CRITERIA	ACTIONS/INTERVENTIONS	RATIONALE
The client will indicate how she can incorporate foods high in protein and of semisolid or pureed consistency into her diet.	Refer to dietitian.	Because a 70- to 80-g protein diet would most likely not harm the client and would make her feel in control, instruction on the diet is appropriate.
The caregiver will verbalize how to reduce the likelihood of aspiration by following safety precautions for clients with dysphagia.	Discuss feeding issues with the caregiver such as the correct body positioning and eating conditions.	The risk of aspiration is high in clients with dysphagia.
	Eliminate distractions.	
	Position individual in an upright position (90 degrees at the hip) with feet flat on floor.	
	Give semiliquids in very small amounts (syringe) and only after food has been cleared from the mouth.	
	Feed the client very small bites.	
	Encourage several dry swallows between bites of food.	
	If the Adam's apple rises, it is likely the food is being swallowed and not deposited in the cheeks.	
	A wet-sounding voice with a gurgle may mean food is resting on the vocal cords.	

24-1

Dietitian's Notes

The following Dietitian's Notes are representative of the documentation found in a client's medical record.

Subjective: The client requested a high-protein diet because she believes it may delay the progression of her ALS. Client reports an intake of one poached egg, thickened whole milk, one slice of bread softened with gelatin, and one cup of thickened orange juice at breakfast. For lunch client has a half banana, half a tuna or chicken salad sandwich (bread softened with gelatin the night before). For dinner the client has ½ cup of pureed casserole (beef stew or macaroni and cheese with ½ cup of added pureed vegetables), and a glass of thickened whole milk. She drinks at least three glasses of thickened water each day. She believes she is 5 ft tall and weighs 90 lb. She denies a declining body weight.

Objective: Hospice client

Analysis: Ideal body weight 90 to 100 lb. Estimated kcalorie needs at actual body weight of 41 kg and 20 to 30 kcal/kg equals 820 to 1230 kcal. Estimated protein needs at 1.2 grams/kg equals 49 grams. Client's reported protein intake is about 55 grams per day and her kcalorie intake is about 1251 kcal per day. Client is currently eating about 1.1 grams of protein/kg of body weight. Reassured client and her daughter that her current intake is already high in protein and both her stable body weight and reported food intake are within current guidelines. Both were reassured with the assessment.

Plan: No further action is necessary; however, my phone number was provided, and both parties were encouraged to call with any further food-related issues.

Critical Thinking Questions

1. The client's swallowing disorders are becoming more severe. Ms. Z is capable of eating only very small bites of food very slowly. The client's daughter is her caregiver, and she states, "It has been taking me 2 hours to feed my mother each meal. If I go any faster, she chokes. My husband is becoming very resentful and has asked me to make a decision. He says I can't continue to spend all day with my mother and ignore him." What would you say to this caregiver?

2. The caregiver believes the client is still mentally alert and oriented, although the client cannot communicate. The client has progressed to the point where she has lost all motor function. She cannot talk or walk and has lost the use of her hands. The client's physician now believes Ms. Z has an ileus (paralysis of the bowel). Why does this mean the client cannot be fed orally? What are the treatment options? Who needs to be informed of the treatment options?

Chapter Review

1. A diet prescription consistent with palliative care goals is:
   a. Forty grams of protein for liver failure
   b. Low-cholesterol, low-saturated-fat diet for hyperlipidemia
   c. Gluten-free diet for diarrhea and celiac disease
   d. High-calorie, high-protein diet for anorexia in an actively dying client

2. An appropriate nutritional screening question for a client with a terminal illness is:
   a. "How many times a day do you eat?"
   b. "How much weight have you lost in the past month?"
   c. "Do you look forward to meals?"
   d. "Do you include a green or yellow vegetable in your diet each day?"

3. The most important ethical principle to consider when a decision must be made about whether or not to feed a client is:
   a. The client's right to self-determination
   b. The principle of proportionality
   c. The client's medical goals
   d. The client's quality of life

4. Which recommendation would be appropriate for a client with end-stage congestive heart failure who requests dietary advice?
   a. Recommend a low-potassium diet
   b. Recommend a 1000 mL fluid restriction
   c. Monitor the client's fluid intake and output
   d. Recommend a 1- or 1.5-gram sodium diet

5. The intervention appropriate for a terminally ill client with dyspnea who requests dietary treatment is:
   a. Encourage a high-fiber diet
   b. Consider a high-fat, low-carbohydrate complete nutritional supplement
   c. Recommend fresh fruits, whole grains, and vegetables
   d. Encourage avoidance of caffeine

Clinical Analysis

1. Mr. O is actively dying. Mr. O's wife is concerned because her husband adamantly refuses all food and fluids. The nurse should:
   a. Call the doctor and request an order for a tube feeding
   b. Call the doctor and request an order for an intravenous feeding
   c. Instruct the caregiver to be more creative in the type of food and fluids she gives the client
   d. Counsel the caregiver that oral intake often ceases near the end of life

2. Mrs. P has terminal brain cancer and insulin-dependent diabetes mellitus; her life expectancy is a few days. She and her caregiver have been self-monitoring her blood glucose levels. The caregiver is quite concerned because Mrs. P's blood glucose levels are running between 400 and 500 mg/dL. Historically, the client claims to have followed her 1200-kcalorie diet faithfully. Recently, her appetite is markedly reduced, and her blood glucose levels are elevated. The physician has been contacted and refuses to increase the client's insulin further but recommends to Mrs. P's caregiver to stop monitoring the client's blood glucose levels. The nurse should:
   a. Encourage the caregiver to offer Mrs. P frequent sips of clear liquid fruit juices (about 30 grams of carbohydrate every 3 hours)
   b. Encourage the caregiver to continue to offer the client the 1200-kcalorie diet to avoid a hypoglycemic episode
   c. Recommend the caregiver look for a new doctor because obviously the doctor does not know how to treat clients with insulin-dependent diabetes
   d. Contact the hospice medical director and ask for an order to increase the client's insulin

3. Mr. J has a partial bowel obstruction and shows signs of dehydration. He has an order for Metamucil® as needed (prn). The nurse should immediately recommend:
   a. Eating high-fiber foods such as bran, whole grains, fruits, and vegetables
   b. Discontinuing the use of Metamucil®
   c. Increasing the dose of Metamucil®
   d. Eating cheese, cakes, pies, cookies, and doughnuts

APPENDIX A   Dietary Reference Intakes for Individuals: Recommended Dietary Allowances, Adequate Intakes, Acceptable Macronutrient Distribution Ranges, and Tolerable Upper Intake Levels.

Dietary Reference Intakes (DRIs): Recommended Dietary Allowances (RDAs) and Adequate Intakes (AIs), Vitamins (Food and Nutrition Board, Institute of Medicine, National Academies)

LIFE STAGE GROUP	VITAMIN A (mcg/d)a	VITAMIN C (mg/d)	VITAMIN D (mcg/d)b,c	VITAMIN E (mg/d)d	VITAMIN K (mcg/d)	THIAMIN (mg/d)	RIBOFLAVIN (mg/d)	NIACIN (mg/d)e	VITAMIN B6 (mg/d)	FOLATE (mcg/d)f	VITAMIN B12 (mcg/d)	PANTOTHENIC ACID (mg/d)	BIOTIN (mcg/d)	CHOLINE (mg/d)g
Infants														
0–6 mo	400*	40*	10*	4*	2.0*	0.2*	0.3*	2*	0.1*	65*	0.4*	1.7*	5*	125*
7–12 mo	500*	50*	10*	5*	2.5*	0.3*	0.4*	4*	0.3*	80*	0.5*	1.8*	6*	150*
Children														
1–3 y	300	15	15	6	30*	0.5	0.5	6	0.5	150	0.9	2*	8*	200*
4–8 y	400	25	15	7	55*	0.6	0.6	8	0.6	200	1.2	3*	12*	250*
Males														
9–13 y	600	45	15	11	60*	0.9	0.9	12	1.0	300	1.8	4*	20*	375*
14–18 y	900	75	15	15	75*	1.2	1.3	16	1.3	400	2.4	5*	25*	550*
19–30 y	900	90	15	15	120*	1.2	1.3	16	1.3	400	2.4	5*	30*	550*
31–50 y	900	90	15	15	120*	1.2	1.3	16	1.3	400	2.4	5*	30*	550*
51–70 y	900	90	15	15	120*	1.2	1.3	16	1.7	400	2.4h	5*	30*	550*
>70 y	900	90	20	15	120*	1.2	1.3	16	1.7	400	2.4h	5*	30*	550*
Females														
9–13 y	600	45	15	11	60*	0.9	0.9	12	1.0	300	1.8	4*	20*	375*
14–18 y	700	65	15	15	75*	1.0	1.0	14	1.2	400i	2.4	5*	25*	400*
19–30 y	700	75	15	15	90*	1.1	1.1	14	1.3	400i	2.4	5*	30*	425*
31–50 y	700	75	15	15	90*	1.1	1.1	14	1.3	400i	2.4	5*	30*	425*
51–70 y	700	75	15	15	90*	1.1	1.1	14	1.5	400	2.4h	5*	30*	425*
>70 y	700	75	20	15	90*	1.1	1.1	14	1.5	400	2.4h	5*	30*	425*
Pregnancy														
14–18 y	750	80	15	15	75*	1.4	1.4	18	1.9	600i	2.6	6*	30*	450*
19–30 y	770	85	15	15	90*	1.4	1.4	18	1.9	600i	2.6	6*	30*	450*
31–50 y	770	85	15	15	90*	1.4	1.4	18	1.9	600i	2.6	6*	30*	450*
Lactation														
14–18 y	1200	115	15	19	75*	1.4	1.6	17	2.0	500	2.8	7*	35*	550*
19–30 y	1300	120	15	19	90*	1.4	1.6	17	2.0	500	2.8	7*	35*	550*
31–50 y	1300	120	15	19	90*	1.4	1.6	17	2.0	500	2.8	7*	35*	550*

Note: This table (adapted from the DRI reports, see www.nap.edu) presents Recommended Dietary Allowances (RDAs) in **bold type** and Adequate Intakes (AIs) in ordinary type followed by an asterisk (*). An RDA is the average daily dietary intake level—sufficient to meet the nutrient requirements of nearly all (97%–98%) healthy individuals in a group. It is calculated from an Estimated Average Requirement (EAR). If sufficient scientific evidence is not available to establish an EAR, and thus calculate an RDA, an AI is usually developed. For healthy breastfed infants, an AI is the mean intake. The AI for other life stage and gender groups is believed to cover the needs of all healthy individuals in the groups, but lack of data or uncertainty in the data prevent being able to specify with confidence the percentage of individuals covered by this intake.

aAs retinol activity equivalents (RAEs). 1 RAE = 1 mcg retinol, 12 mcg-β-carotene, 24 mcg-α-carotene, or 24 mcg-β-cryptoxanthin. The RAE for dietary provitamin A carotenoids is twofold greater than retinol equivalents (RE), whereas the RAE for preformed vitamin A is the same as RE.

bAs cholecalciferol. 1 mcg cholecalciferol = 40 IU vitamin D.

cUnder the assumption of minimal sunlight.

dAs α–tocopherol. α–Tocopherol includes *RRR*-α–tocopherol, the only form of α–tocopherol that occurs naturally in foods, and the 2*R*-stereoisomeric forms of α–tocopherol (*RRR*-, *RSR*-, *RRS*-, and *RSS*-α–tocopherol) that occur in fortified foods and supplements. It does not include the 2*S*-stereoisomeric forms of α–tocopherol (*SRR*-, *SSR*-, *SRS*-, and *SSS*-α–tocopherol), also found in fortified foods and supplements.

eAs niacin equivalents (NE). 1 mg of niacin = 60 mg of tryptophan; 0–6 months = preformed niacin (not NE).

fAs dietary folate equivalents (DFE). 1 DFE = 1 mcg food folate = 0.6 mcg of folic acid from fortified food or as a supplement consumed with food = 0.5 mcg of a supplement taken on an empty stomach.

gAlthough AIs have been set for choline, there are few data to assess whether a dietary supply of choline is needed at all stages of the life cycle, and it may be that the choline requirement can be met by endogenous synthesis at some of these stages.

hBecause 10% to 30% of older people may malabsorb food-bound B$_{12}$, it is advisable for those older than 50 years to meet their RDA mainly by consuming foods fortified with B$_{12}$ or a supplement containing B$_{12}$.

iIn view of evidence linking folate intake with neural tube defects in the fetus, it is recommended that all women capable of becoming pregnant consume 400 mcg from supplements or fortified foods in addition to intake of food folate from a varied diet.

It is assumed that women will continue consuming 400 mcg from supplements or fortified food until their pregnancy is confirmed and they enter prenatal care, which ordinarily occurs after the end of the periconceptional period—the critical time for formation of the neural tube.

Sources: Dietary Reference Intakes for Calcium, Phosphorous, Magnesium, Vitamin D, and Fluoride (1997); *Dietary Reference Intakes for Thiamin, Riboflavin, Niacin, Vitamin B$_6$, Folate, Vitamin B$_{12}$, Pantothenic Acid, Biotin, and Choline* (1998); *Dietary Reference Intakes for Vitamin C, Vitamin E, Selenium, and Carotenoids* (2000); *Dietary Reference Intakes for Vitamin A, Vitamin K, Arsenic, Boron, Chromium, Copper, Iodine, Iron, Manganese, Molybdenum, Nickel, Silicon, Vanadium, and Zinc* (2001); *Dietary Reference Intakes for Water, Potassium, Sodium, Chloride, and Sulfate* (2005); and *Dietary Reference Intakes for Calcium and Vitamin D* (2011). These reports may be accessed at www.nap.edu.

Copyrighted by the National Academy of Sciences, used with permission.

Dietary Reference Intakes (DRIs): Recommended Dietary Allowances (RDAs) and Adequate Intakes (AIs), Elements (Food and Nutrition Board, Institute of Medicine, National Academies)

LIFE STAGE GROUP	CALCIUM (mg/d)	CHROMIUM (mcg/d)	COPPER (mcg/d)	FLUORIDE (mg/d)	IODINE (mcg/d)	IRON (mg/d)	MAGNESIUM (mg/d)	MANGANESE (mg/d)	MOLYBDENUM (mcg/d)	PHOSPHORUS (mg/d)	SELENIUM (mcg/d)	ZINC (mg/d)	POTASSIUM (g/d)	SODIUM (Lcg/d)	CHLORIDE (g/d)
Infants															
0–6 mo	200*	0.2*	200*	0.01*	110*	0.27*	30*	0.003*	2*	100*	15*	2*	0.4*	0.12*	0.18*
7–12 mo	260*	5.5*	220*	0.5*	130*	11	75*	0.6*	3*	275*	20*	3	0.7*	0.37*	0.57*
Children															
1–3 y	700	11*	340	0.7*	90	7	80	1.2*	17	460	20	3	3.0*	1.0*	1.5*
4–8 y	1000	15*	440	1*	90	10	130	1.5*	22	500	30	5	3.8*	1.2*	1.9*
Males															
9–13 y	1300	25*	700	2*	120	8	240	1.9*	34	1250	40	8	4.5*	1.5*	2.3*
14–18 y	1300	35*	890	3*	150	11	410	2.2*	43	1250	55	11	4.7*	1.5*	2.3*
19–30 y	1000	35*	900	4*	150	8	400	2.3*	45	700	55	11	4.7*	1.5*	2.3*
31–50 y	1000	35*	900	4*	150	8	420	2.3*	45	700	55	11	4.7*	1.5*	2.3*
51–70 y	1000	30*	900	4*	150	8	420	2.3*	45	700	55	11	4.7*	1.3*	2.0*
>70 y	1200	30*	900	4*	150	8	420	2.3*	45	700	55	11	4.7*	1.2*	1.8*
Females															
9–13 y	1300	21*	700	2*	120	8	240	1.6*	34	1250	40	8	4.5*	1.5*	2.3*
14–18 y	1300	24*	890	3*	150	15	360	1.6*	43	1250	55	9	4.7*	1.5*	2.3*
19–30 y	1000	25*	900	3*	150	18	310	1.8*	45	700	55	8	4.7*	1.5*	2.3*
31–50 y	1000	25*	900	3*	150	18	320	1.8*	45	700	55	8	4.7*	1.5*	2.3*
51–70 y	1200	20*	900	3*	150	8	320	1.8*	45	700	55	8	4.7*	1.3*	2.0*
>70 y	1200	20*	900	3*	150	8	320	1.8*	45	700	55	8	4.7*	1.2*	1.8*
Pregnancy															
14–18 y	1300	29*	1000	3*	220	27	400	2.0*	50	1250	60	12	4.7*	1.5*	2.3*
19–30 y	1000	30*	1000	3*	220	27	350	2.0*	50	700	60	11	4.7*	1.5*	2.3*
31–50 y	1000	30*	1000	3*	220	27	360	2.0*	50	700	60	11	4.7*	1.5*	2.3*
Lactation															
14–18 y	1300	44*	1300	3*	290	10	360	2.6*	50	1250	70	13	5.1*	1.5*	2.3*
19–30 y	1000	45*	1300	3*	290	9	310	2.6*	50	700	70	12	5.1*	1.5*	2.3*
31–50 y	1000	45*	1300	3*	290	9	320	2.6*	50	700	70	12	5.1*	1.5*	2.3*

Note: This table (table adapted from the DRI reports; see www.nap.edu) presents Recommended Dietary Allowances (RDAs) in **bold type** and Adequate Intakes (AIs) in ordinary type followed by an asterisk (*). An RDA is the average daily dietary intake level—sufficient to meet the nutrient requirements of nearly all (97%–98%) healthy individuals in a group. It is calculated from an Estimated Average Requirement (EAR). If sufficient scientific evidence is not available to establish an EAR, and thus calculate an RDA, an AI is usually developed. For healthy breastfed infants, an AI is the mean intake. The AI for other life stage and gender groups is believed to cover the needs of all healthy individuals in the groups, but lack of data or uncertainty in the data prevent being able to specify with confidence the percentage of individuals covered by this intake.

Sources: Dietary Reference Intakes for Calcium, Phosphorous, Magnesium, Vitamin D, and Fluoride (1997); Dietary Reference Intakes for Thiamin, Riboflavin, Niacin, Vitamin B_6, Folate, Vitamin B_{12}, Pantothenic Acid, Biotin, and Choline (1998); Dietary Reference Intakes for Vitamin C, Vitamin E, Selenium, and Carotenoids (2000); and Dietary Reference Intakes for Vitamin A, Vitamin K, Arsenic, Boron, Chromium, Copper, Iodine, Iron, Manganese, Molybdenum, Nickel, Silicon, Vanadium, and Zinc (2001); Dietary Reference Intakes for Water, Potassium, Sodium, Chloride, and Sulfate (2005); and Dietary Reference Intakes for Calcium and Vitamin D (2011). These reports may be accessed at www.nap.edu.

Copyrighted by the National Academy of Sciences, used with permission.

Dietary Reference Intakes (DRIs): Recommended Dietary Allowances (RDAs) and Adequate Intakes (AIs), Total Water and Macronutrients (Food and Nutrition Board, Institute of Medicine, National Academies)

LIFE STAGE GROUP	TOTAL WATER[a] (L/d)	CARBOHYDRATE (g/d)	TOTAL FIBER (g/d)	FAT (g/d)	LINOLEIC ACID (g/d)	α-LINOLENIC ACID (g/d)	PROTEIN[b] (g/d)
Infants							
0–6 mo	0.7*	60*	ND	31*	4.4*	0.5*	9.1*
7–12 mo	0.8*	95*	ND	30*	4.6*	0.5*	11.0
Children							
1–3 y	1.3*	130	19*	ND[c]	7*	0.7*	13
4–8 y	1.7*	130	25*	ND	10*	0.9*	19
Males							
9–13 y	2.4*	130	31*	ND	12*	1.2*	34
14–18 y	3.3*	130	38*	ND	16*	1.6*	52
19–30 y	3.7*	130	38*	ND	17*	1.6*	56
31–50 y	3.7*	130	38*	ND	17*	1.6*	56
51–70 y	3.7*	130	30*	ND	14*	1.6*	56
>70 y	3.7*	130	30*	ND	14*	1.6*	56
Females							
9–13 y	2.1*	130	26*	ND	10*	1.0*	34
14–18 y	2.3*	130	26*	ND	11*	1.1*	46
19–30 y	2.7*	130	25*	ND	12*	1.1*	46
31–50 y	2.7*	130	25*	ND	12*	1.1*	46
51–70 y	2.7*	130	21*	ND	11*	1.1*	46
>70 y	2.7*	130	21*	ND	11*	1.1*	46
Pregnancy							
14–18 y	3.0*	175	28*	ND	13*	1.4*	71
19–30 y	3.0*	175	28*	ND	13*	1.4*	71
31–50 y	3.0*	175	28*	ND	13*	1.4*	71
Lactation							
14–18 y	3.8*	210	29*	ND	13*	1.3*	71
19–30 y	3.8*	210	29*	ND	13*	1.3*	71
31–50 y	3.8*	210	29*	ND	13*	1.3*	71

Note: This table (taken from the DRI reports, see www.nap.edu) presents Recommended Dietary Allowances in **bold type** and Adequate Intakes (AI) in ordinary type followed by an asterisk (*). An RDA is the average daily dietary intake level; sufficient to meet the nutrient requirements of nearly all (97%–98%) healthy individuals in a group. It is calculated from an Estimated Average Requirement (EAR). If sufficient scientific evidence is not available to establish an EAR, and thus calculate an RDA, an AI is usually developed. For healthy breastfed infants, an AI is the mean intake. The AI for other life stage and gender groups is believed to cover the needs of all healthy individuals in the groups, but lack of data or uncertainty in the data prevent being able to specify with confidence the percentage of individuals covered by this intake.

[a]Total water includes all water contained in food, beverages, and drinking water.

[b]Based on grams of protein per kilogram of body weight for the reference body weight, e.g., for adults 0.8 g/kg body weight for the reference body weight.

[c]Not determined.

Source: Dietary Reference Intakes for Energy, Carbohydrate, Fiber, Fat, Fatty Acids, Cholesterol, Protein, and Amino Acids (2002/2005) and Dietary Reference Intakes for Water, Potassium, Sodium, Chloride, and Sulfate (2005). The report may be accessed at www.nap.edu.

Copyrighted by the National Academy of Sciences, used with permission.

Dietary Reference Intakes (DRIs): Acceptable Macronutrient Distribution Ranges (Food and Nutrition Board, Institute of Medicine, National Academies)

MACRONUTRIENT	RANGE (% OF ENERGY)		
	CHILDREN, 1–3 Y	CHILDREN, 4–18 Y	ADULTS
Fat	30–40	25–35	20–35
n-6 polyunsaturated fatty acids[a] (linoleic acid)	5–10	5–10	5–10
n-3 polyunsaturated fatty acids[a] (α-linolenic acid)	0.6–1.2	0.6–1.2	0.6–1.2
Carbohydrate	45–65	45–65	45–65
Protein	5–20	10–30	10–35

[a]Approximately 10% of the total can come from longer-chain n-3 or n-6 fatty acids.

Source: Dietary Reference Intakes for Energy, Carbohydrate, Fiber, Fat, Fatty Acids, Cholesterol, Protein, and Amino Acids (2002/2005). The report may be accessed at www.nap.edu.

Copyrighted by the National Academy of Sciences, used with permission.

Dietary Reference Intakes (DRIs): Acceptable Macronutrient Distribution Ranges (Food and Nutrition Board, Institute of Medicine, National Academies)

MACRONUTRIENT	RECOMMENDATION
Dietary Cholesterol	As low as possible while consuming a nutritionally adequate diet
Trans fatty acids	As low as possible while consuming a nutritionally adequate diet
Saturated fatty acids	As low as possible while consuming a nutritionally adequate diet
Added sugars[a]	Limit to no more than 25% of total energy

[a]Not a recommended intake. A daily intake of added sugars that individuals should aim for to achieve a healthful diet was not set.

Source: Dietary Reference Intakes for Energy, Carbohydrate, Fiber, Fat, Fatty Acids, Cholesterol, Protein, and Amino Acids (2002/2005). The report may be accessed at www.nap.edu.

Copyrighted by the National Academy of Sciences, used with permission.

Dietary Reference Intakes (DRIs): Tolerable Upper Intake Levels (ULs), Vitamins (Food and Nutrition Board, Institute of Medicine, National Academies)

LIFE STAGE GROUP	VITAMIN A (mcg/d)[a]	VITAMIN C (mg/d)	VITAMIN D (mcg/d)	VITAMIN E (mg/d)[b,c]	VITAMIN K	THIAMIN	RIBOFLAVIN	NIACIN (mg/d)[c]	VITAMIN B6 (mg/d)	FOLATE (mcg/d)[c]	VITAMIN B12	PANTOTHENIC ACID	BIOTIN	CHOLINE (g/d)	CAROTENOIDS[d]
Infants															
0-6 mo	600	ND[e]	25	ND	ND	ND	ND	ND	ND	ND	ND	ND	ND	ND	ND
7-12 mo	600	ND	38	ND	ND	ND	ND	ND	ND	ND	ND	ND	ND		ND
Infants															
1-3 y	600	400	63	200	ND	ND	ND	10	30	300	ND	ND	ND	1.0	ND
4-8 y	900	650	75	300	ND	ND	ND	15	40	400	ND	ND	ND	1.0	ND
Males															
9-13 y	1700	1200	100	600	ND	ND	ND	20	60	600	ND	ND	ND	2.0	ND
14-18 y	2800	1800	100	800	ND	ND	ND	30	80	800	ND	ND	ND	3.0	ND
19-30 y	3000	2000	100	1000	ND	ND	ND	35	100	1000	ND	ND	ND	3.5	ND
31-50 y	3000	2000	100	1000	ND	ND	ND	35	100	1000	ND	ND	ND	3.5	ND
51-70 y	3000	2000	100	1000	ND	ND	ND	35	100	1000	ND	ND	ND	3.5	ND
>70 y	3000	2000	100	1000	ND	ND	ND	35	100	1000	ND	ND	ND	3.5	ND
Females															
9-13 y	1700	1200	100	600	ND	ND	ND	20	60	600	ND	ND	ND	2.0	ND
14-18 y	2800	1800	100	800	ND	ND	ND	30	80	800	ND	ND	ND	3.0	ND
19-30 y	3000	2000	100	1000	ND	ND	ND	35	100	1000	ND	ND	ND	3.5	ND
31-50 y	3000	2000	100	1000	ND	ND	ND	35	100	1000	ND	ND	ND	3.5	ND
51-70 y	3000	2000	100	1000	ND	ND	ND	35	100	1000	ND	ND	ND	3.5	ND
>70 y	3000	2000	100	1000	ND	ND	ND	35	100	1000	ND	ND	ND	3.5	ND
Pregnancy															
14-18 y	2800	1800	100	800	ND	ND	ND	30	80	800	ND	ND	ND	3.0	ND
19-30 y	3000	2000	100	1000	ND	ND	ND	35	100	1000	ND	ND	ND	3.5	ND
31-50 y	3000	2000	100	1000	ND	ND	ND	35	100	1000	ND	ND	ND	3.5	ND
Lactation															
14-18 y	2800	1800	100	800	ND	ND	ND	30	80	800	ND	ND	ND	3.0	ND
19-30 y	3000	2000	100	1000	ND	ND	ND	35	100	1000	ND	ND	ND	3.5	ND
31-50 y	3000	2000	100	1000	ND	ND	ND	35	100	1000	ND	ND	ND	3.5	ND

Note: A Tolerable Upper Intake Level (UL) is the highest level of daily nutrient intake that is likely to pose no risk of adverse health effects to almost all individuals in the general population. Unless otherwise specified, the UL represents total intake from food, water, and supplements. Due to a lack of suitable data, ULs could not be established for vitamin K, thiamin, riboflavin, vitamin B$_{12}$, pantothenic acid, biotin, and carotenoids. In the absence of a UL, extra caution may be warranted in consuming levels above recommended intakes. Members of the general population should be advised not to routinely exceed the UL. The UL is not meant to apply to individuals who are treated with the nutrient under medical supervision or to individuals with predisposing conditions that modify their sensitivity to the nutrient.

[a] As preformed vitamin A only.

[b] As α-tocopherol; applies to any form of supplemental-α-tocopherol.

[c] The ULs for vitamin E, niacin, and folate apply to synthetic forms obtained from supplements, fortified foods, or a combination of the two.

[d] β-Carotene supplements are advised only to serve as a provitamin A source for individuals at risk of vitamin A deficiency.

[e] ND = Not determinable due to lack of data of adverse effects in this age group and concern with regard to lack of ability to handle excess amounts. Source of intake should be from food only to prevent high levels of intake.

Sources: Dietary Reference Intakes for Calcium, Phosphorous, Magnesium, Vitamin D, and Fluoride (1997); Dietary Reference Intakes for Thiamin, Riboflavin, Niacin, Vitamin B$_6$, Folate, Vitamin B$_{12}$, Pantothenic Acid, Biotin, and Choline (1998); Dietary Reference Intakes for Vitamin C, Vitamin E, Selenium, and Carotenoids (2000); Dietary Reference Intakes for Vitamin A, Vitamin K, Arsenic, Boron, Chromium, Copper, Iodine, Iron, Manganese, Molybdenum, Nickel, Silicon, Vanadium, and Zinc (2001); and Dietary Reference Intakes for Calcium and Vitamin D (2011). These reports may be accessed at www.nap.edu.

Dietary Reference Intakes (DRIs): Tolerable Upper Intake Levels (ULs), Elements (Food and Nutrition Board, Institute of Medicine, National Academies)

LIFE STAGE GROUP	ARSENIC[a]	BORON (mg/d)	CALCIUM (mg/d)	CHROMIUM	COPPER (mcg/d)	FLUORIDE (mg/d)	IODINE (mcg/d)	IRON (mg/d)	MAGNESIUM (mg/d)[b]	MANGANESE (mg/d)	MOLYBDENUM (mcg/d)	NICKEL (mg/d)	PHOSPHORUS (g/d)	SELENIUM (mcg/d)	SILICON[c]	VANADIUM (mg/d)[d]	ZINC (mg/d)	SODIUM (g/d)	CHLORIDE (g/d)
Infants																			
0–6 mo	NDe	ND	1000	ND	ND	0.7	ND	40	ND	ND	ND	ND	ND	45	ND	ND	4	ND	ND
7–12 mo	ND	ND	1500	ND	ND	0.9	ND	40	ND	ND	ND	ND	ND	60	ND	ND	5	ND	ND
Children																			
1–3 y	ND	3	2500	ND	1000	1.3	200	40	65	2	300	0.2	3	90	ND	ND	7	1.5	2.3
4–8 y	ND	6	2500	ND	3000	2.2	300	40	110	3	600	0.3	3	150	ND	ND	12	1.9	2.9
Males																			
9–13 y	ND	11	3000	ND	5000	10	600	40	350	6	1100	0.6	4	280	ND	ND	23	2.2	3.4
14–18 y	ND	17	3000	ND	8000	10	900	45	350	9	1700	1.0	4	400	ND	ND	34	2.3	3.6
19–30 y	ND	20	2500	ND	10,000	10	1100	45	350	11	2000	1.0	4	400	ND	1.8	40	2.3	3.6
31–50 y	ND	20	2500	ND	10,000	10	1100	45	350	11	2000	1.0	4	400	ND	1.8	40	2.3	3.6
51–70 y	ND	20	2000	ND	10,000	10	1100	45	350	11	2000	1.0	4	400	ND	1.8	40	2.3	3.6
>70 y	ND	20	2000	ND	10,000	10	1100	45	350	11	2000	1.0	3	400	ND	1.8	40	2.3	3.6
Females																			
9–13 y	ND	11	3000	ND	5000	10	600	40	350	6	1100	0.6	4	280	ND	ND	23	2.2	3.4
14–18 y	ND	17	3000	ND	8000	10	900	45	350	9	1700	1.0	4	400	ND	ND	34	2.3	3.6
19–30 y	ND	20	2500	ND	10,000	10	1100	45	350	11	2000	1.0	4	400	ND	1.8	40	2.3	3.6
31–50 y	ND	20	2500	ND	10,000	10	1100	45	350	11	2000	1.0	4	400	ND	1.8	40	2.3	3.6
51–70 y	ND	20	2000	ND	10,000	10	1100	45	350	11	2000	1.0	4	400	ND	1.8	40	2.3	3.6
>70 y	ND	20	2000	ND	10,000	10	1100	45	350	11	2000	1.0	3	400	ND	1.8	40	2.3	3.6
Pregnancy																			
14–18 y	ND	17	3000	ND	8000	10	900	45	350	9	1700	1.0	3.5	400	ND	ND	34	2.3	3.6
19–30 y	ND	20	2500	ND	10,000	10	1100	45	350	11	2000	1.0	3.5	400	ND	ND	40	2.3	3.6
31–50 y	ND	20	2500	ND	10,000	10	1100	45	350	11	2000	1.0	3.5	400	ND	ND	40	2.3	3.6
Lactation																			
14–18 y	ND	17	3000	ND	8000	10	900	45	350	9	1700	1.0	4	400	ND	ND	34	2.3	3.6
19–30 y	ND	20	2500	ND	10,000	10	1100	45	350	11	2000	1.0	4	400	ND	ND	40	2.3	3.6
31–50 y	ND	20	2500	ND	10,000	10	1100	45	350	11	2000	1.0	4	400	ND	ND	40	2.3	3.6

Note: A Tolerable Upper Intake Level (UL) is the highest level of daily nutrient intake that is likely to pose no risk of adverse health effects to almost all individuals in the general population. Unless otherwise specified, the UL represents total intake from food, water, and supplements. Due to a lack of suitable data, ULs could not be established for chromium and silicon. In the absence of a UL, extra caution may be warranted in consuming levels above recommended intakes. Members of the general population should be advised not to routinely exceed the UL. The UL is not meant to apply to individuals who are treated with the nutrient under medical supervision or to individuals with predisposing conditions that modify their sensitivity to the nutrient.

aAlthough the UL was not determined for arsenic, there is no justification for adding arsenic to food or supplements.

bThe ULs for magnesium represent intake from a pharmacological agent only and do not include intake from food and water.

cAlthough silicon has not been shown to cause adverse effects in humans, there is no justification for adding silicon to supplements.

dAlthough vanadium in food has not been shown to cause adverse effects in humans, there is no justification for adding vanadium to food, and vanadium supplements should be used with caution. The UL is based on adverse effects in laboratory animals; these data could be used to set a UL for adults, but not children and adolescents.

eND = Not determinable due to lack of data of adverse effects in this age group and concern with regard to lack of ability to handle excess amounts. Source of intake should be from food only to prevent high levels of intake.

Sources: Dietary Reference Intakes for Calcium, Phosphorous, Magnesium, Vitamin D, and Fluoride (1997); *Dietary Reference Intakes for Thiamin, Riboflavin, Niacin, Vitamin B6, Folate, Vitamin B12, Pantothenic Acid, Biotin, and Choline* (1998); *Dietary Reference Intakes for Vitamin C, Vitamin E, Selenium, and Carotenoids* (2000); *Dietary Reference Intakes for Vitamin A, Vitamin K, Arsenic, Boron, Chromium, Copper, Iodine, Iron, Manganese, Molybdenum, Nickel, Silicon, Vanadium, and Zinc* (2001); *Dietary Reference Intakes for Water, Potassium, Sodium, Chloride, and Sulfate* (2005); and *Dietary Reference Intakes for Calcium and Vitamin D* (2011). These reports may be accessed at www.nap.edu.

Copyrighted by the National Academy of Sciences, used with permission.

APPENDIX B Academy of Nutrition and Dietetics Exchange Lists for Diabetes

Legend:

* = More than 3 grams of dietary fiber per serving.

† = Extra fat, or prepared with added fat (count as 1 starch + 1 fat).

\# = 480 milligrams or more of sodium per serving; 600 milligrams or more of sodium per serving for combination food main dishes/meals and fast food main dishes/meals.

Starch List

Bread

FOOD	SERVING SIZE	FOOD	SERVING SIZE
Bagel, large (about 4 oz)	¼ (1 oz)	Pancake, 4 in. across, ¼ in. thick	1
†Biscuit, 2 ½ in. across	1	Pita, 6 in. across	½
Bread		Roll, plain, small	1 (1 oz)
*reduced calorie	2 slices (1 ½ oz)	†Stuffing, bread	⅓ cup
white, whole-grain, pumpernickel, rye, unfrosted raisin	1 slice (1 oz)	†Taco shell, 5 in. across	2
Chapatti, small, 6 in. across	1	Tortilla, corn, 6 in. across	1
†Cornbread, 1 ¾-in. cube	1 (1 ½ oz)	Tortilla, flour, 6 in. across	1
English muffin	½	Tortilla, flour, 10 in. across	⅓ tortilla
Hot dog bun or hamburger bun	½ (1 oz)	†Waffle, 4-in. square or 4 in. across	1
Naan, 8 × 2 in.	¼		

Cereals and Grains

FOOD	SERVING SIZE	FOOD	SERVING SIZE
Barley, cooked	⅓ cup	Grits, cooked	½ cup
Bran, dry		Kasha	½ cup
*oat	¼ cup	Millet, cooked	⅓ cup
*wheat	½ cup	Muesli	¼ cup
*Bulgar (cooked)	½ cup	Pasta, cooked	⅓ cup
Cereals		Polenta, cooked	⅓ cup
*bran	½ cup	Quinoa, cooked	⅓ cup
cooked (oats, oatmeal)	½ cup	Rice, white or brown, cooked	⅓ cup
puffed	1 ½ cups	Tabbouleh (tabouli), prepared	½ cup
shredded wheat, plain	½ cup	Wheat germ, dry	3 tbsp
sugar-coated	½ cup	Wild rice, cooked	½ cup
unsweetened, ready-to-eat	¾ cup		
Couscous	⅓ cup		
Granola			
low-fat	¼ cup		
†regular	¼ cup		

Starchy Vegetables

FOOD	SERVING SIZE	FOOD	SERVING SIZE
Cassava	⅓ cup	*Pumpkin, canned, no sugar added	1 cup
Corn	½ cup	Spaghetti/pasta sauce	½ cup
on cob, large	½ cob (5 oz)	*Squash, winter (acorn, butternut)	1 cup
*Hominy, canned	¾ cup	*Succotash	½ cup
*Mixed vegetables with corn, peas, or pasta	1 cup	Yam, sweet potato, plain	½ cup
*Parsnips	½ cup		
*Peas, green	½ cup		
Plantain, ripe	⅓ cup		
Potato			
baked with skin	¼ large (3 oz)		
boiled, all kinds	½ cup or ½ medium (3 oz)		
†mashed, with milk and fat	½ cup		
French fried (oven-baked)	1 cup (2 oz)		

Crackers and Snacks

FOOD	SERVING SIZE	FOOD	SERVING SIZE
Animal crackers	8	Popcorn	
Crackers		*†with butter	3 cups
†round, butter type	6	*no fat added	3 cups
saltine type	6	*lower fat	3 cups
†sandwich style, cheese or peanut butter filling	3	Pretzels	¾ oz
†whole-wheat regular	2–5 (¾ oz)	Rice cakes, 4 in. across	2
*whole-wheat lower fat or crisp breads	2–5 (¾ oz)	Snack chips	
Graham cracker, 2 ½ in. square	3	fat-free or baked (tortilla, potato), baked pita chips	15–20 (¾ oz)
Matzo	¾ oz	†regular (tortilla, potato)	9–13 (¾ oz)
Melba toast, about 2 × 4-in. piece	4 pieces		
Oyster crackers	20		

Beans, Peas, and Lentils

The choices on this list count as 1 starch + 1 lean meat.

FOOD	SERVING SIZE	FOOD	SERVING SIZE
*Baked beans	⅓ cup	*Peas, cooked (black-eyed, split)	½ cup
*Beans, cooked (black, garbanzo, kidney, lima, navy, pinto, white)	½ cup	*#Refried beans, canned	½ cup
*Lentils, cooked (brown, green, yellow)	½ cup		

Fruit List

Fruit

The weight listed includes skin, core, seeds, and rind.

FOOD	SERVING SIZE	FOOD	SERVING SIZE
Apple, unpeeled, small	1 (4 oz)	Apricots	
Apples, dried	4 rings	canned	½ cup
Applesauce, unsweetened	½ cup	dried	8 halves
		*fresh	whole (5 ½ oz)

Fruit—cont'd

FOOD	SERVING SIZE	FOOD	SERVING SIZE
Banana, extra small	1 (4 oz)	Mango, small	½ fruit (5 ½ oz) or ½ cup
*Blackberries	¾ cup	Nectarine, small	1 (5 oz)
Blueberries	¾ cup	*Orange, small	1 (6 ½ oz)
Cantaloupe, small	⅓ melon or 1 cup cubed (11 oz)	Papaya	½ fruit or 1 cup cubed (8 oz)
Cherries		Peaches,	
sweet, canned	½ cup	canned	½ cup
sweet, fresh	12 (3 oz)	fresh, medium	1 (6 oz)
Dates	3	Pears	
Dried fruits (blueberries, cherries,	2 tbsp	canned	½ cup
cranberries, mixed fruit, raisins)		fresh, large	½ (4 oz)
Figs		Pineapple	
dried	1 ½	canned	½ cup
*fresh	1 ½ large or 2 medium (3 ½ oz)	fresh	¾ cup
Fruit cocktail	½ cup	Plums	
Grapefruit		canned	½ cup
large	½ (11 oz)	dried (prunes)	3
sections, canned	¾ cup	small	2 (5 oz)
Grapes, small	17 (3 oz)	*Raspberries	1 cup
Honeydew melon	1 slice or 1 cup cubed (10 oz)	*Strawberries	1 ¼ cup whole berries
*Kiwi	1 (3 ½ oz)	*Tangerines, small	2 (8 oz)
Mandarin oranges, canned	¾ cup	Watermelon	1 slice or 1 ¼ cups cubes (13 ½ oz)

Fruit Juice

FOOD	SERVING SIZE	FOOD	SERVING SIZE
Apple juice/cider	½ cup	Orange juice	½ cup
Fruit juice blends, 100% juice	⅓ cup	Pineapple juice	½ cup
Grape juice	⅓ cup	Prune juice	⅓ cup
Grapefruit juice	½ cup		

Milk List

Milk and Yogurts

FOOD	SERVING SIZE	COUNT AS
Fat-free (skim) or low-fat (1%)		
Milk, buttermilk, acidophilus milk, Lactaid®	1 cup	1 fat-free milk
Evaporated milk	½ cup	1 fat-free milk
Yogurt, plain or flavored with artificial sweetener	⅔ cup (6 oz)	1 fat-free milk
Reduced-fat (2%)		
Milk, acidophilus milk, kefir, Lactaid®	1 cup	1 reduced-fat milk
Yogurt, plain	⅔ cup (6 oz)	1 reduced-fat milk
Whole		
Milk, buttermilk, goat's milk	1 cup	1 whole milk
Evaporated milk	½ cup	1 whole milk
Yogurt, plain	1 cup (8 oz)	1 whole milk

Dairy-Like Foods

FOOD	SERVING SIZE	COUNT AS
Chocolate milk		
fat-free	1 cup	1 fat-free milk + 1 carbohydrate
whole	1 cup	1 whole milk + 1 carbohydrate
Eggnog, whole milk	½ cup	1 carbohydrate + 2 fats
Rice drink		
flavored, low-fat	1 cup	2 carbohydrates
plain, fat-free	1 cup	1 carbohydrate
Smoothies, flavored, regular	10 oz	1 fat-free milk + 2 ½ carbohydrates
Soy milk		
light	1 cup	1 carbohydrate + ½ fat
regular, plain	1 cup	1 carbohydrate + 1 fat
Yogurt		
and juice blends	1 cup	1 fat-free milk + 1 carbohydrate
low-carbohydrate (less than 6 grams carbohydrate per serving)	⅔ cup (6 oz)	½ fat-free milk
with fruit, low-fat	⅔ cup (6 oz)	1 fat-free milk + 1 carbohydrate

Nonstarchy Vegetable List

In general, 1 nonstarchy vegetable choice is:
- ½ cup of cooked vegetables or vegetable juice
- 1 cup of raw vegetables

Amaranth or Chinese spinach	*Carrots	Kohlrabi	Soybean sprouts
Artichoke	Cauliflower	Leeks	Spinach
Artichoke hearts	Celery	Mixed vegetables (without corn, peas, or pasta)	Squash (summer, crookneck, zucchini)
Asparagus	*Chayote	Mung bean sprouts	Sugar snap peas
Baby corn	Coleslaw, packaged, no dressing	Mushrooms, all kinds, fresh	*Swiss chard
Bamboo shoots	Cucumber	Okra	Tomato
Bean sprouts	Daikon	Onions	Tomatoes, canned
Beans (green, wax, Italian)	Eggplant	Pea pods	#Tomato sauce
Beets	Gourds (bitter, bottle, luffa, bitter melon)	*Peppers (all varieties)	#Tomato/vegetable juice
#Borscht	Green onions or scallions	Radishes	Turnips
Broccoli	Greens (collard, kale, mustard, turnip)	Rutabaga	Water chestnuts
*Brussels sprouts	Hearts of palm	#Sauerkraut	Yard-long beans
Cabbage (green, bok choy, Chinese)	Jicama		

Meat and Meat Substitutes List

Lean Meats and Meat Substitutes

FOOD	SERVING SIZE	FOOD	SERVING SIZE
Beef: Select or Choice grades trimmed of fat: ground round, roast (chuck, rib, rump), round, sirloin, steak (cubed, flank, porterhouse, T-bone), tenderloin	1 oz	Fish, fresh or frozen, plain: catfish, cod, flounder, haddock, halibut, orange roughy, salmon, tilapia, trout, tuna	1 oz
#Beef jerky	½ oz	#Fish, smoked: herring or salmon (lox)	1 oz
Cheeses with 3 grams of fat or less per oz	1 oz	Game: buffalo, ostrich, rabbit, venison	1 oz
Cottage cheese	¼ cup	#Hot dog with 3 grams of fat or less per oz (8 dogs per 14 oz package) *Note: May be high in carbohydrate.*	1
Egg substitutes, plain	¼ cup		
Egg whites	2		

Lean Meats and Meat Substitutes—cont'd

FOOD	SERVING SIZE	FOOD	SERVING SIZE
Lamb: chop, leg, or roast	1 oz	Salmon, canned	1 oz
Organ meats: heart, kidney, liver *Note: May be high in cholesterol.*	1 oz	Sardines, canned	2 small
		#Sausage with 3 grams of fat or less per oz	1 oz
Oysters, fresh or frozen	6 medium	Shellfish: clams, crab, imitation shellfish, lobster, scallops, shrimp	1 oz
Pork, lean #Canadian bacon rib or loin chop/roast, ham, tenderloin	 1 oz 1 oz		
		Tuna, canned in water or oil, drained	1 oz
Poultry, without skin: chicken, Cornish hen, domestic duck or goose (well-drained of fat), turkey	1 oz	Veal: loin chop, roast	1 oz
Processed sandwich meats with 3 grams of fat or less per oz: chipped beef, deli thin-sliced meats, turkey ham, turkey kielbasa, turkey pastrami	1 oz		

Medium-Fat Meat and Meat Substitutes

FOOD	SERVING SIZE	FOOD	SERVING SIZE
Beef: corned beef, ground beef, meatloaf, Prime grades trimmed of fat (prime rib), short ribs, tongue	1 oz	Lamb: ground, rib roast	1 oz
		Pork: cutlet, shoulder roast	1 oz
Cheeses with 4–7 grams of fat per oz: feta, mozzarella, pasteurized processed cheese spread, reduced-fat cheeses, string	1 oz	Poultry: chicken with skin; dove, pheasant, wild duck, or goose; fried chicken; ground turkey	1 oz
		Ricotta cheese	2 oz (¼ cup)
Egg *Note: High in cholesterol, limit to 3 per week.*	1	#Sausage with 4–7 grams of fat per oz	1 oz
Fish, any fried type	1 oz	Veal, cutlet (no breading)	1 oz

High-Fat Meat and Meat Substitutes

FOOD	SERVING SIZE	FOOD	SERVING SIZE
Bacon #pork #turkey	 2 slices (16 slices per lb or 1 oz each, before cooking) 3 slices (½ oz each before cooking)	#Hot dog: turkey or chicken (10 per 1 lb package)	1
		Pork: ground, sausage, spareribs	1 oz
		Processed sandwich meats with 8 grams of fat or more per oz: bologna, hard salami, pastrami	1 oz
Cheese, regular: American, bleu, brie, cheddar, hard goat, Monterey jack, queso, and Swiss	1 oz each before cooking	#Sausage with 8 grams fat or more per oz: bratwurst, chorizo, Italian, knockwurst, Polish, smoked, summer	1 oz
#†Hot dog: beef, pork, or combination (10 per 1 lb-sized package)	1		

Plant-Based Proteins

FOOD	SERVING SIZE	COUNT AS
"Bacon" strips, soy-based	3 strips	1 medium-fat meat
*Baked beans	⅓ cup	1 starch + 1 lean meat
*Beans, cooked: black, garbanzo, kidney, lima, navy, pinto, white	½ cup	1 starch + 1 lean meat
*"Beef" or "sausage" crumbles, soy-based	2 oz	½ carbohydrate + 1 lean meat
"Chicken" nuggets, soy-based	2 nuggets (1½ oz)	½ carbohydrate + 1 medium-fat meat
*Edamame	½ cup	½ carbohydrate + 1 lean meat
Falafel (spiced chickpea and wheat patties)	3 patties (about 2 in. across)	1 carbohydrate + 1 high-fat meat

(continued)

Plant-Based Proteins—cont'd

FOOD	SERVING SIZE	COUNT AS
Hot dog, soy-based	1 (1 ½ oz)	½ carbohydrate + 1 lean meat
*Hummus	⅓ cup	1 carbohydrate + 1 high-fat meat
*Lentils, brown, green, or yellow	½ cup	1 carbohydrate + 1 lean meat
*Meatless burger, soy-based	3 oz	½ carbohydrate + 2 lean meats
*Meatless burger, vegetable- and starch-based	1 patty (about 2 ½ oz)	1 carbohydrate + 2 lean meats
Nut spreads: almond butter, cashew butter, peanut butter, soy nut butter	1 tbsp	1 high-fat meat
*Peas, cooked: black-eyed and split peas	½ cup	1 starch + 1 lean meat
*#Refried beans, canned	½ cup	1 starch + 1 lean meat
"Sausage" patties, soy-based	1 (1 ½ oz)	1 medium-fat meat
Soy nuts, unsalted	¾ oz	½ carbohydrate + 1 medium-fat meat
Tempeh	¾ cup	1 medium-fat meat
Tofu	4 oz (½ cup)	1 medium-fat meat
Tofu, light	4 oz (½ cup)	1 lean meat

Fat List

Unsaturated Fats—Monounsaturated Fats

FOOD	SERVING SIZE	FOOD	SERVING SIZE
Avocado, medium	2 tbsp (1 oz)	mixed (50% peanuts)	6 nuts
Nut butters (*trans*-fat–free): almond butter, cashew butter, peanut butter (smooth or crunchy)	1 ½ tsp	peanuts	10 nuts
		pecans	4 halves
		pistachios	16 nuts
Nuts		Oil: canola, olive, peanut	1 tsp
almonds	6 nuts	Olives	
Brazil	2 nuts	black (ripe)	8 large
cashews	6 nuts	green, stuffed	10 large
filberts (hazelnuts)	5 nuts		
macadamia	3 nuts		

Unsaturated Fats—Polyunsaturated Fats

FOOD	SERVING SIZE	FOOD	SERVING SIZE
Margarine: lower-fat spread (30%–50% vegetable oil, *trans*-fat–free)	1 tbsp	Oil: made from soybean and canola oil—Enova	1 tsp
Margarine: stick, tub (*trans*-fat–free), or squeeze (*trans*-fat–free)	1 tsp	Plant stanol esters	
		light	1 tbsp
		regular	2 tsp
Mayonnaise		Salad dressing	
reduced fat	1 tbsp	#reduced fat	2 tbsp
regular	1 tsp	*Note: May be high in carbohydrate.*	
Mayonnaise-style salad dressing		#regular	1 tbsp
reduced fat	1 tbsp	Seeds	
regular	2 tsp	flaxseed, whole	1 tbsp
Nuts		pumpkin, sunflower	1 tbsp
pignola (pine nuts)	1 tbsp	sesame seeds	1 tbsp
walnuts, English	4 halves	Tahini or sesame paste	2 tsp
Oil: corn, cottonseed, flaxseed, grape seed, safflower, soybean, sunflower	1 tsp		

Saturated Fats

FOOD	SERVING SIZE	FOOD	SERVING SIZE
Bacon, cooked, regular or turkey	1 slice	light	1 ½ tbsp
Butter		whipped	2 tbsp
reduced fat	1 tbsp	whipped, pressurized	¼ cup
stick	1 tsp	Cream cheese	
whipped	2 tsp	reduced fat	1 ½ tbsp (¾ oz)
Butter blends made with oil		regular	1 tbsp (½ oz)
reduced fat or light	1 tbsp	Lard	1 tsp
regular	1 ½ tsp	Oil: coconut, palm, palm kernel	1 tsp
Chitterlings, boiled	2 tbsp (½ oz)	Salt pork	¼ oz
Coconut, sweetened, shredded	2 tbsp	Shortening, solid	1 tsp
Coconut milk		Sour cream	
light	⅓ cup	reduced fat or light	3 tbsp
regular	1 ½ tbsp	regular	2 tbsp
Cream			
half and half	2 tbsp		
heavy	1 tbsp		

Free Foods List

Most foods on this list should be limited to three servings (as listed here) per day. Spread out the servings throughout the day. Food and drink choices listed here without a serving size can be eaten whenever you like.

Low-Carbohydrate Foods

FOOD	SERVING SIZE	FOOD	SERVING SIZE
Cabbage, raw	½ cup	Gum	
Candy, hard (regular or sugar-free)	1 piece	Jam or jelly, light or no sugar added	2 tsp
Carrots, cauliflower, or green beans, cooked	¼ cup	Rhubarb, sweetened with sugar substitute	½ cup
Cranberries, sweetened with sugar substitute	½ cup	Salad greens	
Cucumber, sliced	½ cup	Sugar substitutes (artificial sweeteners)	
Gelatin		Syrup, sugar-free	2 tbsp
dessert, sugar-free unflavored			

Modified-Fat Foods With Carbohydrate

FOOD	SERVING SIZE	FOOD	SERVING SIZE
Cream cheese, fat-free	1 tbsp (½ oz)	Mayonnaise-style salad dressing	
Creamers		fat-free	1 tbsp
nondairy, liquid	1 tbsp	reduced-fat	1 tsp
nondairy, powdered	2 tsp	Salad dressing	
Margarine spread		fat-free or low fat	1 tbsp
fat-free	1 tbsp	fat-free, Italian	2 tbsp
reduced fat	1 tsp	Sour cream, fat-free or reduced-fat	1 tbsp
Mayonnaise		Whipped topping	
fat-free	1 tbsp	light or fat-free	2 tbsp
reduced fat	1 tsp	regular	1 tbsp

Condiments

FOOD	SERVING SIZE	FOOD	SERVING SIZE
Barbecue sauce	2 tsp	Salsa	¼ cup
Catsup (ketchup)	1 tbsp	#Soy sauce, light or regular	1 tbsp
Honey mustard	1 Tbsp	Sweet and sour sauce	2 tsp
Horseradish		Sweet chili sauce	2 tsp
Lemon juice		Taco sauce	1 tbsp
Miso	1 ½ tsp	Vinegar	
Mustard		Yogurt, any type	2 tbsp
Parmesan cheese, freshly grated	1 tbsp		
Pickle relish	1 tbsp		
Pickles			
#dill	1 ½ medium		
sweet, bread and butter	2 slices		
sweet, gherkin	¾ oz		

Drinks/Mixes

The foods on this list without a serving size can be consumed in any moderate amount.

- #Bouillon, broth, consommé
- Bouillon or broth, low-sodium
- Carbonated or mineral water
- Club soda
- Cocoa powder, unsweetened (1 tbsp)
- Coffee, unsweetened or with sugar substitute

- Diet soft drinks, sugar-free
- Drink mixes, sugar-free
- Tea, unsweetened or with sugar substitute
- Tonic water, diet
- Water
- Water, flavored, carbohydrate-free

Seasonings

Any food on this list can be consumed in any moderate amount.

- Flavoring extracts (for example, vanilla, almond, peppermint)
- Garlic
- Herbs, fresh or dried
- Nonstick cooking spray

- Pimento
- Spices
- Hot pepper sauce
- Wine, used in cooking
- Worcestershire sauce

Combination Foods List

Entrees

FOOD	SERVING SIZE	COUNT AS
#Casserole type (tuna noodle, lasagna, spaghetti with meatballs, chili with beans, macaroni and cheese)	1 cup (8 oz)	2 carbohydrates + 2 medium-fat meats
#Stews (beef/other meats and vegetables)	1 cup (8 oz)	1 carbohydrate + 1 medium-fat meat + 0–3 fats
Tuna salad or chicken salad	½ cup (3½ oz)	½ carbohydrate + 2 lean meats + 1 fat

Frozen Meals/Entrees

FOOD	SERVING SIZE	COUNT AS
#**Burrito (beef and bean)	1 (5 oz)	3 carbohydrates + 1 lean meat + 2 fats
#Dinner-type meal	Generally 14–17 oz	3 carbohydrates + 3 medium-fat meats + 3 fats
#Entree or meal with less than 340 calories	About 8–11 oz	2–3 carbohydrates + 1–2 lean meats
Pizza		
#cheese/vegetarian, thin crust	¼ of a 12-in. (4 ½–5 oz)	2 carbohydrates + 2 medium-fat meats
#meat topping, thin crust	¼ of a 12-in. (5 oz)	2 carbohydrates + 2 medium-fat meats + 1 ½ fats
#Pocket sandwich	1 (4 ½ oz)	3 carbohydrates + 1 lean meat + 1–2 fats
#Pot pie	1 (7 oz)	2 ½ carbohydrates + 1 medium-fat meat + 3 fats

Salads (Deli-Style)

FOOD	SERVING SIZE	COUNT AS	FOOD	SERVING SIZE	COUNT AS
Coleslaw	½ cup	1 carbohydrate + 1½ fats	#Potato salad	½ cup	1 ½–2 carbohydrates + 1–2 fats
Macaroni/pasta salad	½ cup	2 carbohydrates + 3 fats			

Soups

FOOD	SERVING SIZE	COUNT AS
#Bean, lentil, or split pea	1 cup	1 carbohydrate + 1 lean meat
#Chowder (made with milk)	1 cup (8 oz)	1 carbohydrate + 1 lean meat + 1 ½ fats
#Cream (made with water)	1 cup (8 oz)	1 carbohydrate + 1 fat
#Instant	6 oz prepared	1 carbohydrate
#with beans or lentils	8 oz prepared	2 ½ carbohydrates + 1 lean meat
#Miso soup	1 cup	½ carbohydrate + 1 fat
#Ramen noodle	1 cup	2 carbohydrates + 2 fats
Rice (congee)	1 cup	1 carbohydrate
#Tomato (made with water)	1 cup (8 oz)	1 carbohydrate
#Vegetable beef, chicken noodle, or other broth type	1 cup (8 oz)	1 carbohydrate

Fast Foods List

Breakfast Sandwiches

FOOD	SERVING SIZE	COUNT AS
#Egg, cheese, meat, English muffin	1 sandwich	2 carbohydrates + 2 medium-fat meats
#Sausage biscuit sandwich	1 sandwich	2 carbohydrates + 2 high-fat meats + 3 ½ fats

Main Dishes/Entrees

FOOD	SERVING SIZE	COUNT AS
*#Burrito (beef and beans)	1 (about 8 oz)	3 carbohydrates + 3 medium-fat meats + 3 fats
#Chicken breast, breaded and fried	1 (about 5 oz)	1 carbohydrate + 4 medium-fat meats
Chicken drumstick, breaded and fried	1 (about 2 oz)	2 medium-fat meats
#Chicken nuggets	6 (about 3½ oz)	1 carbohydrate + 2 medium-fat meats + 1 fat
#Chicken thigh, breaded and fried	1 (about 4 oz)	½ carbohydrate + 3 medium-fat meats + 1 ½ fats
#Chicken wings, hot	6 (5 oz)	5 medium-fat meats + 1 ½ fats

Asian

FOOD	SERVING SIZE	COUNT AS
#Beef/chicken/shrimp with vegetables in sauce	1 cup (about 5 oz)	1 carbohydrate + 1 lean meat + 1 fat
#Egg roll, meat	1 (about 3 oz)	1 carbohydrate + 1 lean meat + 1 fat
Fried rice, meatless	½ cup	1 ½ carbohydrates + 1 ½ fats
#Meat and sweet sauce (orange chicken)	1 cup	3 carbohydrates + 3 medium-fat meats + 2 fats
*#Noodles and vegetables in sauce (chow mein, lo mein)	1 cup	2 carbohydrates + 1 fat

Pizza

FOOD	SERVING SIZE	COUNT AS
Pizza		
#cheese, pepperoni, regular crust	⅛ of a 14-in. (about 4 oz)	2½ carbohydrates + 1 medium-fat meat + 1 ½ fats
#cheese/vegetarian, thin crust	¼ of a 12-in. (about 6 oz)	2½ carbohydrates + 2 medium-fat meats + 1 ½ fats

Sandwiches

FOOD	SERVING SIZE	COUNT AS
#Chicken sandwich, grilled	1	3 carbohydrates + 4 lean meats
#Chicken sandwich, crispy	1	3 ½ carbohydrates + 3 medium-fat meats + 1 fat
Fish sandwich with tartar sauce	1	2 ½ carbohydrates + 2 medium-fat meats + 2 fats
Hamburger		
#large with cheese	1	2 ½ carbohydrates + 4 medium-fat meats + 1 fat
regular	1	2 carbohydrates + 1 medium-fat meat + 1 fat
#Hot dog with bun	1	1 carbohydrate + 1 high-fat meat + 1 fat
Submarine sandwich		
#less than 6 grams fat	6-in. sub	3 carbohydrates + 2 lean meats
#regular	6-in. sub	3 ½ carbohydrates + 2 medium-fat meats + 1 fat
Taco, hard or soft shell (meat and cheese)	1 small	1 carbohydrate + 1 medium-fat meat + 1 ½ fats

Salads		
FOOD	**SERVING SIZE**	**COUNT AS**
**##Salad, main dish (grilled chicken type, no dressing or croutons)	Salad	1 carbohydrate + 4 lean meats
Salad, side (no dressing or cheese)	Small (about 5 oz)	1 vegetable

Sides/Appetizers		
FOOD	**SERVING SIZE**	**COUNT AS**
†French fries, restaurant style	small	3 carbohydrates + 3 fats
	medium	4 carbohydrates + 4 fats
	large	5 carbohydrates + 6 fats
#Nachos with cheese	small (about 4 ½ oz)	2 ½ carbohydrates + 4 fats
#Onion rings	1 serving (about 3 oz)	2 ½ carbohydrates + 3 fats

Desserts		
FOOD	**SERVING SIZE**	**COUNT AS**
Milkshake, any flavor	12 oz	6 carbohydrates + 2 fats
Soft-serve ice cream cone	1 small	2 ½ carbohydrates + 1 fat

Alcohol List

ALCOHOLIC BEVERAGE	SERVING SIZE	COUNT AS
Beer		
light (4.2%)	12 fl oz	1 alcohol equivalent + ½ carbohydrate
regular (4.9%)	12 fl oz	1 alcohol equivalent + 1 carbohydrate
Distilled spirits: vodka, rum, gin, whiskey 80 or 86 proof	1 ½ fl oz	1 alcohol equivalent
Liqueur, coffee (53 proof)	1 fl oz	½ alcohol equivalent + 1 carbohydrate
Sake	1 fl oz	½ alcohol equivalent
Wine		
dessert (sherry)	3 ½ fl oz	1 alcohol equivalent + 1 carbohydrate
dry, red or white (10%)	5 fl oz	1 alcohol equivalent

Sweets, Desserts, and Other Carbohydrates List

Beverages, Soda, and Energy/Sports Drinks		
FOOD	**SERVING SIZE**	**COUNT AS**
Cranberry juice cocktail	½ cup	1 carbohydrate
Energy drink	1 can (8.3 oz)	2 carbohydrates
Fruit drink or lemonade	1 cup (8 oz)	2 carbohydrates
Hot chocolate		
regular	1 envelope added to 8 oz water	1 carbohydrate + 1 fat
sugar-free or light	1 envelope added to 8 oz water	1 carbohydrate
Soft drink (soda), regular	1 can (12 oz)	2 ½ carbohydrates
Sports drink	1 cup (8 oz)	1 carbohydrate

Brownies, Cake, Cookies, Gelatin, Pie, and Pudding

FOOD	SERVING SIZE	COUNT AS
Brownie, small, unfrosted	1 ¼ in. square, ⅞ in. high (about 1 oz)	1 carbohydrate + 1 fat
Cake		
angel food, unfrosted	¹⁄₁₂ of cake (about 2 oz)	2 carbohydrates
frosted	2-in. square (about 2 oz)	2 carbohydrates + 1 fat
unfrosted	2-in. square (about 1 oz)	1 carbohydrate + 1 fat
Cookies		
(chocolate chip)	2 cookies (2¼ in. across)	1 carbohydrate + 2 fats
gingersnap	3 cookies	1 carbohydrate
sandwich, with crème filling	2 small (about ⅔ oz)	1 carbohydrate + 1 fat
sugar-free	3 small or 1 large (¾–1 oz)	1 carbohydrate + 1–2 fats
vanilla wafer	5 cookies	1 carbohydrate + 1 fat
Cupcake, frosted	1 small (about 1 ¾ oz)	2 carbohydrates + 1–1 ½ fats
Fruit cobbler	½ cup (3½ oz)	3 carbohydrates + 1 fat
Gelatin, regular	½ cup	1 carbohydrate
Pie		
commercially prepared fruit, 2 crusts	⅙ of 8-in. pie	3 carbohydrates + 2 fats
pumpkin or custard	⅛ of 8-in. pie	1 ½ carbohydrates +1 ½ fats
Pudding		
regular (made with reduced-fat milk)	½ cup	2 carbohydrates
sugar-free or sugar- and fat-free (made with fat-free milk)	½ cup	1 carbohydrate

Candy, Spreads, Sweets, Sweeteners, Syrups, and Toppings

FOOD	SERVING SIZE	COUNT AS
Candy bar, chocolate/peanut	2 "fun size" bars (1 oz)	1½ carbohydrates + 1 ½ fats
Candy, hard	3 pieces	1 carbohydrate
Chocolate "kisses"	5 pieces	1 carbohydrate + 1 fat
Coffee creamer		
dry, flavored	4 tsp	½ carbohydrate + ½ fat
liquid, flavored	2 Tbsp	1 carbohydrate
Fruit snacks, chewy (pureed fruit concentrate)	1 roll (¾ oz)	1 carbohydrate
Fruit spreads, 100% fruit	1 ½ tbsp	1 carbohydrate
Honey	1 tbsp	1 carbohydrate
Jam or jelly, regular	1 tbsp	1 carbohydrate
Sugar	1 tbsp	1 carbohydrate
Syrup		
chocolate	2 tbsp	2 carbohydrates
light (pancake type)	2 tbsp	1 carbohydrate
regular (pancake type)	1 tbsp	1 carbohydrate

Condiments and Sauces

FOOD	SERVING SIZE	COUNT AS
Barbeque sauce	3 tbsp	1 carbohydrate
Cranberry sauce, jellied	¼ cup	1 ½ carbohydrates
#Gravy, canned or bottled	½ cup	½ carbohydrate + ½ fat
Salad dressing, fat-free, low-fat, cream-based	3 tbsp	1 carbohydrate
Sweet and sour sauce	3 tbsp	1 carbohydrate

Doughnuts, Muffins, Pastries, and Sweet Breads

FOOD	SERVING SIZE	COUNT AS
Banana nut bread	1-in. slice (2 oz)	2 carbohydrates + 1 fat
Doughnut		
cake, plain	1 medium (1½ oz)	1½ carbohydrates + 2 fats
yeast type, glazed	3¾ in. across (2 oz)	2 carbohydrates + 2 fats
Muffin (4 oz)	¼ muffin (1 oz)	1 carbohydrate + ½ fat
Sweet roll or Danish	1 (2½ oz)	2½ carbohydrates + 2 fats

Frozen Bars, Frozen Desserts, Frozen Yogurt, and Ice Cream

FOOD	SERVING SIZE	COUNT AS
Frozen pops	1	½ carbohydrate
Fruit juice bars, frozen, 100% juice	1 bar (3 oz)	1 carbohydrate
Ice cream		
fat-free	½ cup	1½ carbohydrates
light	½ cup	1 carbohydrate + 1 fat
no sugar added	½ cup	1 carbohydrate + 1 fat
regular	½ cup	1 carbohydrate + 2 fats
Sherbet, sorbet	½ cup	2 carbohydrates
Yogurt, frozen		
fat-free	⅓ cup	1 carbohydrate
regular	½ cup	1 carbohydrate + 0–1 fat

Granola Bars, Meal Replacement Bars/Shakes, and Trail Mix

FOOD	SERVING SIZE	COUNT AS
Granola or snack bar, regular or low-fat	1 bar (1 oz)	1½ carbohydrates
Meal replacement bar	1 bar (1⅓ oz)	1½ carbohydrates + 0–1 fat
Meal replacement bar	1 bar (2 oz)	2 carbohydrates + 1 fat
Meal replacement shake, reduced calorie	1 can (10–11 oz)	1½ carbohydrates + 0–1 fat
Trail mix		
candy/nut-based	1 oz	1 carbohydrate + 2 fats
dried fruit-based	1 oz	1 carbohydrate + 1 fat

APPENDIX C   Answers to Questions

Chapter 1. Nutrition in Human Health

Chapter Review
1. d **2.** b **3.** a **4.** c **5.** d

Clinical Analysis
1. d **2.** b **3.** a

Chapter 2. Carbohydrates

Chapter Review
1. b **2.** c **3.** c **4.** d **5.** a

Clinical Analysis
1. c **2.** d **3.** a

Chapter 3. Fats

Chapter Review
1. c **2.** b **3.** c **4.** b **5.** c

Clinical Analysis
1. d **2.** a **3.** c

Chapter 4. Proteins

Chapter Review
1. a **2.** c **3.** b **4.** b **5.** d

Clinical Analysis
1. d **2.** c **3.** a

Chapter 5. Energy Balance

Chapter Review
1. c **2.** a **3.** c **4.** b **5.** d

Clinical Analysis
1. d **2.** d **3.** b

Chapter 6. Vitamins

Chapter Review
1. c **2.** d **3.** a **4.** a **5.** b

Clinical Analysis
1. d **2.** c **3.** b

Chapter 7. Minerals

Chapter Review
1. b **2.** c **3.** a **4.** c **5.** d

Clinical Analysis
1. a **2.** b **3.** d

Chapter 8. Water

Chapter Review
1. d **2.** a **3.** c **4.** b **5.** b

Clinical Analysis
1. c **2.** d **3.** c

Chapter 9. Digestion, Absorption, Metabolism, and Excretion

Chapter Review
1. d **2.** a **3.** c **4.** b **5.** b

Clinical Analysis
1. c **2.** d **3.** a

Chapter 10. Life Cycle Nutrition: Pregnancy and Lactation

Chapter Review
1. b **2.** a **3.** c **4.** a **5.** d

Clinical Analysis
1. c **2.** b. **3.** d

Chapter 11. Life Cycle Nutrition: Infancy, Childhood, and Adolescence

Chapter Review
1. c **2.** b **3.** c **4.** b **5.** d

Clinical Analysis
1. c **2.** c **3.** a

Chapter 12. Life Cycle Nutrition: The Mature Adult

Chapter Review
1. b **2.** d **3.** b **4.** a **5.** d

Clinical Analysis
1. b **2.** b **3.** c

Chapter 13. Food Management

Chapter Review
1. c **2.** a **3.** d **4.** b **5.** a

Clinical Analysis
1. b **2.** a **3.** c

Chapter 14. Nutrient Delivery

Chapter Review
1. c **2.** a **3.** c **4.** b **5.** a

Clinical Analysis
1. c **2.** c **3.** a

Chapter 15. Interactions: Food and Nutrients Versus Medications and Supplements

Chapter Review
1. b **2.** d **3.** c **4.** d **5.** a

Clinical Analysis
1. c **2.** a **3.** c

Chapter 16. Weight Management

Chapter Review
1. a **2.** b **3.** d **4.** b **5.** b

Clinical Analysis
1. a **2.** b **3.** c

Chapter 17. Diet in Diabetes Mellitus and Hypoglycemia

Chapter Review
1. a **2.** b **3.** d **4.** b **5.** a

Clinical Analysis
1. c **2.** a **3.** b

Chapter 18. Diet in Cardiovascular Disease

Chapter Review
1. a **2.** c **3.** d **4.** b **5.** d

Clinical Analysis
1. b **2.** d **3.** c

Chapter 19. Diet in Renal Disease

Chapter Review
1. b **2.** b **3.** d **4.** a **5.** d

Clinical Analysis
1. c **2.** b **3.** a

Chapter 20. Diet in Digestive Diseases

Chapter Review
1. c **2.** b **3.** d **4.** b **5.** d

Clinical Analysis
1. a **2.** c **3.** a

Chapter 21. Diet and Cancer

Chapter Review
1. d **2.** d **3.** c **4.** a **5.** b

Clinical Analysis
1. c **2.** b **3.** a

Chapter 22. Diet in Critical Care

Chapter Review
1. c **2.** c **3.** b **4.** d **5.** c

Clinical Analysis
1. c **2.** d **3.** b

Chapter 23. Diet in HIV And AIDS

Chapter Review
1. b **2.** d **3.** a **4.** c **5.** d

Clinical Analysis
1. b **2.** b **3.** b

Chapter 24. Nutritional Care of The Terminally Ill

Chapter Review
1. c **2.** c **3.** a **4.** d **5.** b

Clinical Analysis
1. d **2.** a **3.** b

APPENDIX D   Glossary

This glossary contains commonly used terms as well as terms that appear in **boldface** in the book.

Abdominal circumference (girth)—Distance around the trunk at the umbilicus.

Abdominal obesity—Excess body fat located between the chest and pelvis.

Abortifacient—Anything used to cause or induce an abortion.

Absorption—The movement of the end products of digestion from the gastrointestinal tract into the blood and/or lymphatic system.

Accreditation—Process by which a nongovernmental agency recognizes an institution for meeting established criteria of quality.

Acculturation—Process of adopting the values, attitudes, and behaviors of another culture.

Acetone—A ketone body found in urine, which can be due to the excessive breakdown of stored body fat.

Acetyl CoA—Important intermediate byproduct in metabolism formed from the breakdown of glucose, fatty acids, and certain amino acids.

Acetylcholine—A chemical necessary for the transmission of nervous impulses.

Achalasia—Failure of the gastrointestinal muscle fibers to relax where one part joins another.

Achlorhydria—Absence of free hydrochloric acid in the stomach.

Acidosis—Condition that results when the pH of the blood falls below 7.35; may be caused by diarrhea, uremia, diabetes mellitus, respiratory depression, and certain drug therapies.

Acquired immune deficiency syndrome (AIDS)—A disease complex caused by a virus that attacks the immune system and causes neurological disease and permits opportunistic infections and malignancies.

Acrodermatitis enteropathica—Rare autosomal recessive disease that causes zinc deficiency through an unknown mechanism of absorptive failure; fatal if untreated.

Acute illness—A sickness characterized by rapid onset, severe symptoms, and a short course.

Acute renal failure—Condition that occurs suddenly, in which the kidneys are unable to perform essential functions; usually temporary.

Adaptive thermogenesis—The adjustment in energy expenditure the body makes to a large increase or decrease in kilocalorie intake of several days' duration.

Additive—A substance added to food to increase its flavor, shelf life, and/or characteristics such as texture, color, and aroma.

Adequate Intake (AI)—The average observed or experimentally defined intake by a defined population or subgroup that appears to sustain a defined nutritional state; incorporates information on the reduction of disease risk; may be used as a goal for an individual's nutrient intake if an EAR or RDA cannot be set.

Adipose cells—Cells in the human body that store fat.

Adipose tissue—Tissue containing masses of fat cells.

Adolescence—Time from the onset of puberty until full growth is reached.

ADP (adenosine diphosphate)—A substance present in all cells involved in energy metabolism. Energy is released when molecules of ATP, another compound in cells, release a phosphoric acid chain and become ADP. The opposite chemical reaction of adding the third phosphoric acid group to ADP requires much energy.

Adrenal glands—Small organs on the superior surface of the kidneys that secrete many hormones, including epinephrine (adrenalin) and aldosterone.

Advanced directive—A signed document in which the client has specified what type of medical care is desired should he or she lose the ability to make decisions.

Aerobic exercise—Training methods such as running or swimming that require continuous inspired oxygen.

Afferent—Proceeding toward a center, as arteries, veins, lymphatic vessels, and nerves.

Afferent arteriole—Small blood vessel through which blood enters the glomerulus (functional unit of the kidney).

Aflatoxin—A naturally occurring food contaminant produced by some strains of *Aspergillus* molds; found especially on peanuts and peanut products.

AIDS dementia complex (ADC)—A central nervous system disorder caused by the human immunodeficiency virus.

ALA—*See* Alpha-linolenic acid.

Albumin—A plasma protein responsible for much of the colloidal osmotic pressure of the blood.

Aldosterone—An adrenocorticoid hormone that increases sodium and water retention by the kidneys.

Alimentary canal—The digestive tube extending from the mouth to the anus.

Alkaline phosphatase—An enzyme found in highest concentration in the liver, biliary tract epithelium, and bones; enzyme levels are elevated in liver, bone, and biliary disease.

Alkalosis—Condition that results when the pH of the blood rises above 7.45; may be caused by vomiting, nasogastric suctioning, or hyperventilation.

Allele—One of two or more different genes containing specific inheritable characteristics that occupy corresponding positions (loci) on paired chromosomes; an individual possessing a pair of identical alleles, either dominant or recessive, is homozygous for this gene.

Allergen—Substance that provokes an abnormal, individual hypersensitivity.

Allergy—State of abnormal, individual hypersensitivity to a substance.

Alopecia—Hair loss, especially of the head; baldness.

Alpha-linolenic acid (ALA)—A polyunsaturated omega-3 fatty acid found in some plants.

Alpha-tocopherol equivalent (α-TE)—The measure of vitamin E; 1 milligram of alpha-tocopherol equivalent equals 1.5 International Units of natural alpha-tocopherol or 2.2 IU of synthetic vitamin.

Amenorrhea—Absence of menstruation; normally occurs before puberty, after menopause, and during pregnancy and lactation.

Amino acids—Organic compounds that are the building blocks of protein; also the end products of protein digestion.

Amniotic fluid—Albuminous liquid that surrounds and protects the fetus throughout pregnancy.

Amylase—A class of enzymes that splits starches—for example, salivary amylase, pancreatic amylase.

Anabolic phase—The third and last phase of stress; characterized by the building up of body tissue and nutrient stores; also called recovery phase.

Anabolism—The building up of body compounds or tissues by the synthesis of more complex substances from simpler ones; the constructive phase of metabolism.

Anaerobic exercise—A form of physical activity such as weight lifting or sprinting that does not rely on continuous inspired oxygen.

Anaphylaxis—Exaggerated, life-threatening hypersensitivity response to a previously encountered antigen; in severe cases, produces bronchospasm, vascular collapse, and shock.

Anastomosis—The surgical connection between tubular structures.

Anemia—Condition of less-than-normal values for red blood cells or hemoglobin, or both; result is decreased effectiveness in oxygen transport; causes may include inadequate iron intake, malabsorption, and chronic or acute blood loss.

Anencephaly—Congenital absence of the brain; cerebral hemispheres missing or reduced to small masses; fatal within a few weeks.

Angina pectoris—Severe pain and a sense of constriction about the heart caused by lack of oxygen to the heart muscle.

Angiotensin II—End product of complex reaction in response to low blood pressure; effect is vasoconstriction and aldosterone secretion.

Anion—An ion with a negative charge.

Anorexia—Loss of appetite.

Anorexia nervosa—A mental disorder characterized by a 25% loss of usual body weight, an intense fear of becoming obese, and self-starvation.

Anorexia of aging—Loss of appetite in an elderly individual related to physiologic, social, psychological, or medical causes.

Anorexigenic—Causing loss of appetite.

Antagonist—A substance that counteracts the action of another substance.

Anthropometric measurements—Physical measurements of the human body such as height, weight, and skinfold thickness; used to determine body composition and growth.

Anthropometry—The science of measuring the human body.

Antibody—A specific protein developed in the body in response to a substance that the body senses to be foreign.

Anticholinergic—An agent that blocks parasympathetic nerve impulses, thereby causing dry mouth, blurred vision due to dilated pupils, and decreased gastrointestinal and bronchial secretions.

Antidiuretic hormone (ADH)—Hormone formed in the hypothalamus and released from the posterior pituitary in response to blood that is too concentrated; effect is return of water to the bloodstream by the kidney.

Antigen—Protein or oligosaccharide marker on surface of cells; body can detect foreign antigens on organisms, foods, and transplanted tissues.

Anti-insulin antibodies (AIAs)—A protein found to be elevated in persons with insulin-dependent diabetes mellitus.

Antineoplastic drug—A drug that combats tumors.

Antioxidant—A substance that prevents or inhibits the uptake of oxygen; in the body, antioxidants prevent tissue damage; in foods, antioxidants prevent deterioration.

Antiretroviral—Substance or drug that stops or suppresses the activity of retroviruses such as human immunodeficiency virus (HIV).

Anuria—A total lack of urine output.

Apoferritin—A protein found in intestinal mucosal cells which combines with iron to form ferritin; it is always found attached to iron in the body.

Apolipoproteins—Protein components of lipoproteins that assist in regulating lipid metabolism; apo A, the primary high-density lipoprotein apoprotein, is inversely related to the risk for developing coronary artery disease.

Appetite—A strong desire for food or for a pleasant sensation, based on previous experience, that causes one to seek food for the purpose of tasting and enjoying.

Aquaporin—Water transport proteins, found in many cell membranes, that serve as water-selective channels and explain the speed at which water moves across cell membranes.

Arachidonic acid—An omega-6 polyunsaturated fatty acid present in peanuts; precursor of prostaglandins.

Ariboflavinosis—Condition arising from a deficiency of riboflavin in the diet.

Aromatic amino acids—Phenylalanine, tryptophan, tyrosine; ratio to branched-chain amino acids altered in liver failure.

Arrhythmia—Irregular heartbeat.

Arteriosclerosis—Common arterial disorder characterized by thickening, hardening, and loss of elasticity of the arterial walls; also called "hardening of the arteries."

Arthritis—Inflammatory condition of the joints, usually accompanied by pain and swelling.

Ascites—Accumulation of serous fluid in the peritoneal (abdominal) cavity.

Ascorbic acid—Vitamin C; *ascorbic* literally means "without scurvy."

Ash—The residue that remains after an item is burned; usually refers to the mineral content of the human body.

Aspartame—Artificial sweetener composed of aspartic acid and phenylalanine; 180 times sweeter than sucrose; brand names: Equal®, Nutrasweet®.

Aspergillus—Genus of molds that produce aflatoxins.

Aspiration—The state in which a substance has been drawn into the nose, throat, or lungs.

Assessment—An organized procedure to gather pertinent facts.

Astrocyte—A supporting cell of the central nervous system that contributes to the blood–brain barrier.

Asymptomatic—Without symptoms.

Ataxia—Defective muscular coordination, especially seen in voluntary movement attempts.

Atherosclerosis—A form of arteriosclerosis characterized by the deposit of fatty material inside the arteries; major factor contributing to heart disease.

Atom—Smallest particle of an element that has all the properties of the element. An atom consists of the nucleus, which contains protons (positively charged particles), neutrons (particles with no electrical charge), and surrounding electrons (negatively charged particles).

Atopy—Genetic predisposition to develop allergy primarily involving immunoglobulin E (IgE) antibodies; a child with two atopic parents has a 75% chance of similar symptoms; a child with one atopic parent has a 50% chance.

ATP (adenosine triphosphate)—Compound in cells, especially muscle cells, that stores energy; when needed, enzymes break off one phosphoric acid group, which releases energy for muscle contraction.

Atrophy—Decrease in size of a normally developed organ or tissue.

Autoimmune disease—A disorder in which the body produces an immunologic response against itself.

Autonomy—Achieving independence; the psychosocial developmental task of the toddler.

Autosomal dominant gene—Dominant gene on any chromosome except X or Y; autosomal dominant inheritance: trait or disease transmitted from one parent even if the matching gene from the other parent is normal; example: familial hypercholesterolemia.

Autosomal recessive inheritance—Non–sex-linked pattern of inheritance in which an affected gene must be received from both parents for the individual to be affected; examples: **cystic fibrosis, phenylketonuria (PKU), galactosemia,** sickle cell disease. Note that the chance of normal, carrier, or affected children is the same with every pregnancy. Having had an affected child does not mean the offspring of next three pregnancies will be normal or carriers (see Fig. 4-2).

Avidin—Protein in raw egg white that inhibits the B vitamin biotin.

Bacteria—Single-celled microorganisms that lack a true nucleus; may be either harmless to humans or disease producing.

Bacteriostat—Agent that prevents bacteria from growing and multiplying but does not necessarily kill them.

Balanced diet—A diet including sufficient foods from each of the major food groups daily; one containing all the essential nutrients in required amounts.

Bariatric surgery—Surgery performed to treat and control obesity.

Barium enema—Series of x-ray studies of the colon used to demonstrate the presence and location of polyps, tumors, diverticula, or positional abnormalities. The client is first administered an enema containing a radio-opaque substance (barium) that enhances visualization when the film is exposed.

Barium swallow—The primary diagnostic tool for direct visualization of the swallowing mechanism is called the *cookie swallow* or *modified barium swallow*. During this procedure, the client consumes three items of different viscosities. Each item contains a contrast medium that allows all phases of the swallowing mechanism to be visualized in x-rays. A physician is always present during this procedure.

Basal ganglia—Four masses of gray matter located in the cerebrum; contribute to the subconscious aspects of voluntary movement; inhibit tremors.

Benign—Not recurrent or progressive; nonmalignant; benign tumor may be life threatening in crucial tissue such as the brain.

Beriberi—Disease caused by deficiency of vitamin B_1 (thiamin).

Beta-carotene—Carotenoid with the greatest provitamin A activity.

Beta-endorphin—Chemical released in the brain during exercise that produces a state of relaxation.

Bicarbonate—Any salt containing the HCO_3^- anion; blood bicarbonate is a measure of alkali (base) reserve of the body; bicarbonate of soda is sodium bicarbonate ($NaHCO_3$).

Bile—Yellow secretion of the liver that alkalinizes the intestine and breaks large fat globules into smaller ones to facilitate enzyme digestive action.

Binge-eating disorder—Eating disorder in which the patient eats excess amounts of food and calories and does not purge.

Binging—Eating to excess; eating from 5000 to 20,000 kilocalories per day.

Bioavailability—The rate and extent to which an active drug or nutrient or metabolite enters the general circulation, permitting access to the site of action; measured by concentration of the drug in body fluids or by the magnitude of the pharmacologic response.

Bioelectric impedance—Indirect measure of body fatness based on differences in electrical conductivity of fat, muscle, and bone.

Biological value—Scoring system of how well food proteins can be converted into body protein; eggs are norm of 100% of nitrogen being retained.

Biotin—B-complex vitamin widely available in foods.

Bladder—A body organ, also called the urinary bladder, which receives urine from the kidneys and discharges it through the urethra.

Blood–brain barrier—Specialized cells lining the brain capillaries that separate the brain from the circulatory system, thus protecting it from harmful substances.

Blood pressure—Force exerted against the walls of blood vessels by the pumping action of the heart.

Blood urea nitrogen (BUN)—The amount of nitrogen present in the blood as urea, often elevated in renal disorders; may be referred to as serum urea nitrogen (SUN).

B-lymphocytes (B-cells)—White blood cells that protect against infection by inducing antibody production; *see* Humoral immunity.

Body frame size—Designation of a person's skeletal structure as small, medium, or large; used to determine healthy body weight (HBW).

Body image—The mental image a person has of himself or herself.

Body mass index (BMI)—Weight in kilograms divided by the square of height in meters; BMIs of 19 to 24 are considered normal.

Body substance isolation—A situation in which all body fluids should be considered contaminated and treated as such by all health-care workers.

Bolus—A mass of food that is ready to be swallowed or a single dose of feeding or medication.

Bolus feeding—Giving a 4- to 6-hour volume of a tube feeding within a few minutes.

Bomb calorimeter—A device used to measure the energy content of food.

Botulism—An often fatal form of food intoxication caused by the ingestion of food containing poisonous toxins produced by the microorganism *Clostridium botulinum*.

Bowman capsule—The cuplike top of an individual nephron; functions as a filter in the formation of urine.

Branched-chain amino acids—Leucine, isoleucine, lysine, valine; sometimes used as therapy for hepatic coma.

Buffer—A substance that can react to offset excess acid or excess alkali (base) in a solution; blood buffers include carbonic acid, bicarbonate, phosphates, and proteins, including hemoglobin.

Bulimia—Excessive food intake followed by extreme methods, such as self-induced vomiting and the use of laxatives, to rid the body of the foods eaten.

C-reactive protein (CRP)—An abnormal protein produced by the liver in response to acute inflammation that is strongly associated with future vascular events.

Cachexia—State of malnutrition and wasting seen in chronic conditions such as cancer, AIDS, malaria, tuberculosis, and pituitary disease.

Calcidiol—25-hydroxyvitamin D [25(OH)D]; inactive form of vitamin D produced in the liver; circulating half-life of 15 days; serum level is best indicator of vitamin D status, reflecting vitamin D (from sun, food, and dietary supplements but not vitamin D stored in body tissues).

Calcification—Process in which tissue becomes hardened with calcium deposits; necessary for bone anabolism; pathological in vitamin D toxicity.

Calcitonin—Hormone produced by the thyroid gland that slows the release of calcium from the bone when serum calcium levels are high.

Calcitriol—1,25-dihydroxyvitamin D [1,25(OH)$_2$D]; physiologically active form of vitamin D produced primarily in the kidney; circulating half-life of 15 hours; serum levels typically not decreased until severe deficiency because of regulation by parathyroid hormone.

Calorie—A measurement unit of energy; unit equaling the amount of heat required to raise or lower the temperature of 1 gram of water 1° Celsius.

Campylobacter—Flagellated, gram-negative bacteria; important cause of diarrheal illnesses.

Candida albicans—Microscopic fungal organism normally present on skin and mucous membranes of healthy people; cause of thrush, vaginitis, opportunistic infections.

Capillary—Minute vessel connecting arteriole and venule; vessel wall acts as semipermeable membrane to exchange substances between blood and lymph and interstitial fluid.

Carbohydrate—Any of a group of organic compounds, including sugar, starch, and cellulose, which contains only carbon, oxygen, and hydrogen.

Carbonic acid—Aqueous solution of carbon dioxide; carbon dioxide in solution or in blood is carbonic acid.

Carcinogen—Any substance or agent that causes the development of or increases the risk of cancer.

Carcinoma—A malignant neoplasm that occurs in epithelial tissue.

Cardia—Upper orifice of the stomach connecting with the esophagus.

Cardiac arrhythmia—Irregular heartbeat.

Cardiac sphincter—Smooth muscle band at the lower end of the esophagus; prevents reflux of stomach contents.

Cardiomyopathy—Disease of heart muscle; may be primary due to unknown cause or secondary to another cardiac disorder or systemic disease.

Carotene—One of several yellow to red antioxidant pigments that are precursors to vitamin A.

Carotenemia—Excess carotene in the blood, producing yellow skin but not discoloring the whites of the eyes.

Carotenoid—Group of more than 500 red, orange, or yellow pigments found in fruits and vegetables, about 50 of which are precursors of vitamin A; includes carotene, which is such a precursor, and lycopene, which is not.

Casein—Principal protein in cow's milk.

Catabolism—The breaking down of body compounds or tissues into simpler substances; the destructive phase of metabolism.

Catalyst—A substance that speeds up a chemical reaction without entering into or being changed by the reaction.

Cataract—Clouding of the lens of the eye.

Cation—An ion with a positive charge.

Cecum—The first portion of the large intestine between the ileum and the ascending colon.

Celiac disease (gluten-sensitive enteropathy)—An intolerance to dietary gluten, which damages the intestine and produces diarrhea and malabsorption.

Cell—The smallest functional unit of structure in all plants and animals.

Cellular immunity—Delayed immune response produced by T-lymphocytes, which mature in the thymus gland; examples of this type of response are rejection of transplanted organs and some autoimmune diseases.

Central parenteral nutrition (CPN)—Parenteral nutrition delivered into a large-diameter vein, usually the superior vena cava adjacent to the right atrium.

Cerebrovascular accident (CVA)—An abnormal condition in which the brain's blood vessels are occluded by a thrombus, an embolus, or hemorrhage, resulting in damaged brain tissue; stroke.

Cesarean delivery—Delivery of a baby through a surgical incision made into the mother's abdomen and uterus.

Chelating agent—A chemical compound that binds metallic ions into a ring structure, inactivating them; used to remove poisonous metals from the body.

Chemical digestion—Digestive process that involves the splitting of complex molecules into simpler forms.

Chemical reaction—The process of combining or breaking down substances to obtain different substances.

Chlorophyll—The green plant pigment necessary for the manufacture of carbohydrates.

Cholecalciferol—Vitamin D$_3$, formed when the skin is exposed to sunlight; further processed by the liver and kidneys; may be reported as serum 25-hydroxy-cholecalciferol.

Cholecystitis—Inflammation of the gallbladder.

Cholecystokinin—A hormone secreted by the duodenum; stimulates contraction of the gallbladder (releases bile) and the secretion of pancreatic juice.

Cholelithiasis—The presence of gallstones.

Cholestasis—Blockage of the flow of bile due to liver disease or obstructions in the duct system.

Cholesterol—A fatlike substance made in the human body and found in foods of animal origin; associated with an increased risk of heart disease.

Choline—Vitamin-like organic compound recognized as an essential nutrient; required for normal carbohydrate and fat metabolism and involved in protein metabolism.

Chronic illness—A sickness persisting for a long period that shows little change or a slow progression over time.

Chronic obstructive pulmonary disease (COPD)—A group of chronic diseases with a common characteristic of chronic airflow obstruction.

Chronic renal failure—An irreversible condition in which the kidneys cannot perform vital functions.

Chvostek's sign—Spasm of facial muscles following a tap over the facial nerve in front of the ear; indication of tetany.

Chylomicron—A lipoprotein that carries triglycerides in the bloodstream after meals.

Chyme—The mixture of partly digested food and digestive secretions found in the stomach and small intestine during digestion of a meal.

Chymotrypsin—A protein-splitting enzyme produced by the pancreas; active in the intestine.

Cirrhosis—Chronic disease of the liver in which functioning cells degenerate and are replaced by fibrosed connective tissue.

Client-care conference—A meeting that includes all health-care team members and may include the client or a significant other to review and update the client's nursing care plan.

Clostridium botulinum—An anaerobic (grows without air) organism that produces a poisonous toxin; the cause of botulism.

Clostridium perfringens—A bacterium that produces a poisonous toxin that causes a food intoxication; the symptoms are generally mild and of short duration and include intestinal disorders.

Cobalamin—Vitamin B_{12}; essential for proper blood formation.

Coenzyme—A substance that combines with an enzyme to activate it.

Cognitive—Of, relating to, or involving conscious mental activities such as thinking, understanding, learning, and remembering.

Colectomy—Surgical removal of part or all of the colon.

Collagen—Fibrous insoluble protein found in connective tissue.

Collecting tubule—The last segment of the renal tubule; follows the distal convoluted tubule. Several nephrons usually share a single collecting tubule.

Colloidal osmotic pressure (COP)—Pressure produced by plasma and cellular proteins.

Colon—The large intestine from the end of the small intestine to the rectum.

Colonic residue—Total solid material in the large intestine after digestion, including insoluble fiber, secretions, shed cells, and microorganisms. Fiber is the chief contributor to colonic residue and residual substance manageable by diet.

Colostomy—Surgical procedure in which an opening to the large intestine is constructed on the abdomen.

Comorbidity—A disease coexisting with the primary disease.

Complementation—Principle of meal planning advocating combining plant foods within a meal so that it contains all the essential amino acids; now applied to daily intake rather than to single meals.

Complement system—Series of about 25 proteins that work to "complement" the activity of antibodies in destroying bacteria; also helps to rid the body of antigen–antibody complexes; in carrying out these tasks, it induces an inflammatory response.

Complete protein—A protein containing all essential amino acids that humans need; usually found in animal sources such as milk, meat, eggs, and fish.

Complex carbohydrate—A carbohydrate composed of many molecules of $C_6H_{12}O_6$ joined together; polysaccharide; includes starch, glycogen, and fiber.

Compound—Two or more elements united chemically in specific proportions.

Compound fat—Substance obtained when one of the fatty acids joined to the glycerol molecule is replaced by another molecule, such as a protein.

Conditionally essential nutrient—Substance normally manufactured by the body; in certain situations, the body cannot manufacture an optimal amount.

Consanguinous union—Marriage of blood relatives; usually meaning second cousins or closer; genetic influence in unions between more distant relatives likely to differ only slightly from that in the general population.

Constipation—Decrease in a person's normal frequency of defecation; stool is often hard, dry, or difficult to expel.

Contamination iron—Iron that leaches from cookware into the food; in special circumstances, can become hazardous.

Continuous ambulatory peritoneal dialysis (CAPD)—A form of self-dialysis in which the dialysate is allowed to remain in the abdominal cavity for 4 to 6 hours before replacement.

Continuous feeding—Enteral feeding in which the formula drips slowly throughout the prescribed time span.

Contraindication—Any circumstance under which treatment should not be given.

Coronary heart disease (CHD)—Disease resulting from the decreased flow of blood through the coronary arteries to the heart muscle.

Coronary occlusion—Blockage of one or more branches of the coronary arteries, which supply the heart muscle with oxygen and nutrients.

Creatine—Nonprotein substance synthesized in the body from arginine, glycine, and methionine; combines with phosphate to form creatine phosphate, which is stored in muscle tissue as an energy source.

Creatinine—Nonprotein nitrogenous end product of creatine metabolism; because creatinine is excreted by the kidneys, serum creatinine levels are used to detect and monitor renal disease and to estimate muscle protein reserves.

Cretinism—A congenital condition resulting from a lack of thyroid secretions; characterized by a stunted and malformed body and arrested mental development.

Crohn disease—Inflammatory disease appearing in any area of the bowel in which diseased areas can be found alternating with healthy tissue.

Cross-contamination—The spreading of a disease-producing organism from one food, person, or object to another food, person, or object.

Cruciferous—Belonging to a botanical mustard family; includes broccoli, Brussels sprouts, cabbage, cauliflower, kale, kohlrabi, and Swiss chard.

Crystalluria—The presence of crystals in the urine; may be caused by the administration of sulfonamides.

Culture—The learned, shared, and transmitted values, beliefs, and norms of a particular group that guides its thinking, decisions, and actions in patterned ways.

Cyclical variation—A recurring series of events during a specified period.

Cystic fibrosis—Hereditary disease often affecting the lungs and pancreas in which glandular secretions are abnormally thick.

Cysteine—Sulfur-containing amino acid often lacking in legumes.

Cystitis—Inflammation of the bladder.

Cytochrome P450 enzymes—Group of genetically determined enzymes that help to metabolize fat-soluble vitamins, steroids, fatty acids, and other substances and to detoxify drugs and environmental pollutants. Example: CYP3A4 depicts family (3), subfamily (A), and number (4).

Cytokine—One of more than 100 proteins mainly produced by white blood cells that function in inflammatory and specific immune responses.

Deamination—Metabolic process whereby nitrogen is removed from an amino acid.

Deciliter (dL)—100 milliliters or $1/_{10}$ liter.

Decubitus ulcer—A pressure sore on the lower back, such as a bedsore.

Dehiscence—Separation of the edges of a surgical incision.

Delusion—False belief that is firmly maintained despite obvious proof to the contrary.

Dementia—The impairment of intellectual function that usually is progressive and interferes with normal social and occupational activities.

Dental caries—The gradual decay and disintegration of the teeth; a dental cavity is a hole in a tooth caused by dental caries.

Dental plaque—Colorless and transparent gummy mass of microorganisms that grows on the teeth, predisposing them to decay.

Deoxyribonucleic acid (DNA)—the hereditary material in humans and almost all other organisms; protein substance in the cell nucleus that directs all the cell's activities, including reproduction.

Desired outcome—The behavioral or physical change in a client that indicates the achievement of a nursing goal.

Development—Gradual process of changing from a simple to a more complex organism; involves psychosocial and physical changes, not only an increase in size.

Dextrose—Another name for the simple sugar glucose.

DHA—*See* Docosahexaenoic acid.

Diabetes insipidus—Increased water intake and increased urine output resulting from inadequate secretion of antidiuretic hormone (ADH) by the posterior pituitary or by failure of the kidney tubules to respond to ADH; underlying causes can be tumor, surgery, trauma, infection, radiation injury, or congenital anomaly.

Diabetes mellitus—Disease caused by insufficient insulin secretion by the pancreas or insulin resistance by body tissues causing excess glucose in the blood and deranged carbohydrate, fat, and protein metabolism.

Diabetic neuropathy—Degeneration of peripheral nerves occurring in diabetes; possible causes are microscopic changes in blood vessels or metabolic defects in nerve tissue.

Diacetic acid—A ketone body found in the urine; can be due to the excessive breakdown of stored body fat.

Diagnostic—Relating to scientific and skillful methods to establish the cause and nature of a sick person's illness.

Dialysate—In renal failure, the fluid used to remove or deliver compounds or electrolytes that the failing kidney cannot excrete or retain in proper concentrations.

Dialysis—The process of diffusing blood across a semipermeable membrane to remove toxic materials and to maintain fluid, electrolyte, and acid–base balances in cases of impaired kidney function or absence of the kidneys.

Dialysis dementia—A neurological disturbance seen in clients who have been on dialysis for a number of years.

Diastolic pressure—Pressure exerted against the arteries between heartbeats; the lower number of a blood pressure reading.

Dietary fiber—Material in foods, mostly from plants, that the human body cannot break down or digest.

Dietary recall, 24-hour—Description of what a person has eaten for the previous 24 hours.

Dietary Reference Intake (DRI)—Four nutrient-based reference values that can be used for assessing and planning diets for the healthy general population; refer to average daily intakes for 1 or more weeks; include Estimated Average Requirements (EARs), Recommended Dietary Allowances (RDAs), Adequate Intakes (AIS), and Tolerable Upper Intake Levels (ULs).

Dietary status—Description of what a person has been eating; his or her usual intake.

Digestion—The process by which food is broken down mechanically and chemically in the gastrointestinal tract into forms simple enough for intestinal absorption.

Diglyceride—Two fatty acids joined to a glycerol molecule.

Dilutional hyponatremia—Low serum sodium due not to an absolute lack of sodium but to an excess of water.

Diplopia—Double vision.

Disaccharide—A simple sugar composed of two units of $C_6H_{12}O_6$ joined together; examples include sucrose, lactose, and maltose.

Disulfide linkage—Specific chemical bond joining amino acids; in hair, skin, and nails, holds amino acids in their distinct shapes.

Diverticulitis—Inflammation of a diverticulum.

Diverticulosis—Presence of one or more diverticula.

Diverticulum—A sac or pouch in the walls of a tubular organ; pl., diverticula.

DNA—*See* Deoxyribonucleic acid.

Docosahexaenoic acid (DHA)—A polyunsaturated omega-3 fatty acid found in fish oils.

Dopamine—Catecholamine synthesized by the adrenals; immediate precursor in the synthesis of norepinephrine.

Double-blind—Technique of scientific investigation in which neither the investigator nor the subject knows what treatment, if any, the subject is receiving.

Double bond—A type of chemical connection in which, for example, a fatty acid has two neighboring carbon atoms, each lacking one hydrogen atom.

Drink—An alcoholic beverage; *see* Standard drink.

Dual-energy x-ray absorptiometry (DEXA)—Diagnostic test using two x-ray beams to determine body composition; used to measure bone mineral density as an indicator of osteopenia and osteoporosis.

Duct—A structural tube designed to allow secretions to move from one body part to another body part.

Dumping syndrome—A condition in which the contents of the stomach empty too rapidly into the duodenum; mostly occurs in patients who have had gastric resections.

Duodenum—The first part of the small intestine between the stomach and the jejunum.

Durable power of attorney—A document in which the client gives another person power to make medical treatment and related personal care decisions for him or her.

Dysgeusia—Abnormal taste.

Dysphagia—Difficulty swallowing; component of many diseases from Alzheimer disease and other neurological disorders to tumors of the head and neck.

Dysphoria—A speech disorder characterized by hoarseness.

Dyspnea—Difficulty breathing.

Eclampsia—An obstetrical emergency involving hypertension, proteinuria, and convulsions appearing after the twentieth week of pregnancy.

Eczema—Skin inflammation, acute or chronic; caused by external (chemical irritation or microbial invasion) or internal (genetic or psychological) factors.

Edema—The accumulation of excessive amounts of fluid in interstitial spaces.

Edentulous—The state of having no teeth.

Efferent—Directed away from a center; used to describe arteries, veins, lymphatic vessels, and nerves.

Efferent arteriole—Small blood vessel by which blood leaves the nephron.

Efficacy—Ability of a drug or treatment to achieve the desired effect.

Eicosapentaenoic acid (EPA)—Omega-3 fatty acid found in fish oils.

Electrocardiogram (ECG)—A graphic record produced by an electrocardiograph that shows the electrical activity of the heart.

Electroencephalogram (EEG)—The record obtained from an electroencephalograph that shows the electrical activity of the brain.

Electrolyte—An element or compound that when dissolved in water separates (dissociates) into ions that are capable of conducting an electrical current; acids, bases, and salts are common electrolytes.

Element—A substance that cannot be separated into simpler parts by ordinary means.

Elemental and semielemental formula—Formula that contains either totally or partially hydrolyzed nutrients.

Embolus—A circulating mass of undissolved matter in a blood or lymphatic vessel; may be composed of tissues, fat globules, air bubbles, clumps of bacteria, or foreign bodies, including pieces of medical devices.

Embryo—A developing infant in the prenatal period between the second and eighth weeks inclusive.

Empty kilocalories—Refers to a food that contains kilocalories and almost no other nutrients.

Emulsification—The physical breaking up of fat into tiny droplets.

Emulsifier—A molecule that attracts both water- and fat-soluble molecules.

Emulsion—One liquid evenly distributed in a second liquid with which it usually does not mix.

Encephalopathy—Generalized brain dysfunction with varying degrees of impairment of speech, cognition, orientation, and arousal.

Endemic—The constant presence of a disease or infectious agent within a given geographic area; the usual prevalence of a given disease within such an area.

Endogenous—Produced within or caused by factors within the organism.

Endoscope—A device consisting of a tube and an optical system for observing the inside of a hollow organ or cavity.

Endothelium—Flat cells lining blood and lymphatic vessels, the heart, and various body cavities; produce compounds affecting vascular lumen and platelets.

End-stage renal failure—A state in which the kidneys have lost most or all of their ability to maintain internal homeostasis and produce urine.

Energy—The capacity to do work.

Energy balance—A situation in which kilocaloric intake equals kilocaloric output.

Energy expenditure—The amount of fuel the body uses for a specified period.

Energy imbalance—Situation in which kilocalories eaten do not equal the number of kilocalories used for energy.

Energy nutrients—The chemical substances in food that are able to supply fuel; refers collectively to carbohydrate, fat, and protein.

Enrichment—The addition of nutrients previously present in a food but removed during food processing or lost during storage.

Enteral nutrition—Nutrition provided through the gastrointestinal tract via a tube, catheter, or stoma that delivers nutrients distal to the oral cavity.

Enteric-coated—A type of drug preparation designed to dissolve in the intestine rather than in the stomach.

Enteritis—Inflammation of the intestines, particularly the small intestine.

Enzyme—Complex protein produced by living cells that acts as a catalyst.

EPA—*See* Eicosapentaenoic acid.

Epidemic—Affecting or tending to affect a disproportionately large number of individuals within a population, community, or region at the same time; excessively prevalent or widespread.

Epilepsy—Disease marked by repetitive abnormal electrical discharges within the brain; signs and symptoms vary with type: partial, generalized, or unclassified.

Epinephrine—Hormone of the adrenal gland; produces the fight-or-flight response.

Epithelial tissue—A type of tissue that forms the outer layer of skin and lines body surfaces opening to the outside; functions include protection, absorption, and secretion.

Ergocalciferol—Vitamin D_2 formed by the action of sunlight on plants.

Ergot poisoning—Poisoning resulting from excessive use of the drug ergot or from the ingestion of grain or grain products infected with the *Claviceps purpurea* fungus.

Erikson, Erik—Psychologist who devised a theory of human development consisting of eight stages of life, each with a psychosocial developmental task to be mastered.

Erosion—Destruction of the surface of a tissue, either on the external surface of the body or internally.

Erythropoietin—Hormone released by the kidney to stimulate red blood cell production.

Esophagostomy—A surgical opening in the esophagus.

Esophagus—A muscular canal extending from the mouth to the stomach.

Essential amino acid—One of the amino acids that cannot be manufactured by the human body; must be obtained from food or artificial feeding.

Essential (primary) hypertension—Elevated blood pressure that develops without apparent cause.

Essential nutrient—A substance found in food that must be present in the diet because the human body lacks the ability to manufacture it in sufficient amounts for optimal health.

Estimated Average Requirement (EAR)—Intake that meets the estimated nutrient need of 50% of the individuals in a life-stage and gender group; used to set the RDA and to assess or plan the intake of groups.

Ethanol—Grain alcohol; ounces of ethanol in beverages can be estimated with the conversion factors of 0.045 for beer, 0.121 for wine, and 0.409 for liquor.

Ethnocentrism—Belief that one's own culture and worldview is superior to anyone else's.

Etiology—The cause of a disease.

Evaporative water loss—Insensible water loss through the skin.

Exchange—A defined quantity of food on the Academy of Nutrition and Dietetics Exchange List for Diabetes (see Appendix B) or on another exchange list.

Exchange List—A food guide used in clinical practice to aid in meal planning.

Excretion—The elimination of waste products from the body in feces, urine, exhaled air, and perspiration.

Exogenous—Outside the body.

External muscle layer—Muscle layer of the alimentary canal.

External water loss—Water lost to the outside of the body.

Extracellular fluid—Fluid found between the cells and within the blood and lymph vessels.

Extrinsic factor—Vitamin B_{12}, necessary for proper red blood cell development.

Failure to thrive (FTT)—Medical diagnosis for infants who fail to gain weight appropriately or who lose weight; also applied to elderly who lose ability to care for themselves.

Fasting—The state of having had no food or fluid enterally or no parenteral nutrition.

Fasting blood sugar (FBS)—Blood glucose measured in the fasting state; normal values are 70 to 100 mg per deciliter.

Fat-free mass—Lean body mass plus nonfat components of adipose tissue.

Fatty acid—Part of the structure of a fat.

Fatty liver—Accumulation of lipids in the liver cells; may be reversible if the cause, of which there are many, is removed.

Feedback cycle—Control system of many bodily functions involving the interaction between a stimulus and an effect; in positive feedback, the effect increases the stimulus as uterine contractions increasing oxytocin secretion; in negative feedback, the effect decreases the stimulus as blood levels of thyroid hormone decrease secretion of thyroid-stimulating hormone.

Ferric iron—Oxidized iron, which is less absorbable from the gastrointestinal tract than ferrous iron; abbreviated Fe^{3+}.

Ferritin—An iron–phosphorus–protein complex formed in the intestinal mucosa by the union of ferric iron with apoferritin; the form in which iron is stored in the tissues, mainly in liver, spleen, and bone marrow cells.

Ferrous iron—The more absorbable form of iron for humans; abbreviated Fe^{2+}.

Fetal alcohol syndrome (FAS)—A condition characterized by mental and physical abnormalities in an infant caused by the mother's consumption of alcohol during pregnancy.

Fetus—The human child in utero from the third month until birth; also applicable to the later stages of gestation of other animals.

Fiber, dietary—Material in foods, mostly from plants, that the human body cannot break down or digest.

Fibrin—Insoluble protein formed from fibrinogen by the action of thrombin; forms the meshwork of a blood clot.

Fibrinogen—Protein in blood essential to the clotting process; also called Factor I; *see* Fibrin.

Filtration—The process of removing particles from a solution by allowing the liquid to pass through a membrane or other partial barrier.

First-degree relatives—An individual's parents, siblings, or children.

First pass effect—Process whereby drugs are extensively metabolized by the small intestine or liver enzymes; result is that less drug reaches the systemic circulation.

Flatus—Gas in the digestive tract, averaging 400 to 1200 milliliters per day.

Flavonoids—Nonnutritive antioxidant compounds that occur naturally in certain foods such as onions, apples, tea, and red wine; inhibit oxidation of low-density lipoprotein in laboratory experiments.

Flow phase—The second phase in the stress response; marked by pronounced hormonal changes.

Fluorosis—Condition due to excessive prolonged intake of fluoride; tissues affected are teeth and bones.

FODMAPs—Fermentable **O**ligosaccharides, **D**isaccharides, **M**onosaccharides, **A**nd **P**olyols; carbohydrates that are known to cause symptoms in patients with IBS because of their poor absorption, osmotic activity, and rapid fermentation.

Folate—B vitamin necessary for DNA formation and proper red blood cell formation; form occurring in foods and body tissues.

Folic acid—B vitamin necessary for DNA formation and proper red blood cell formation; oxidized form used to fortify foods and in supplements.

Food acceptance record—A checklist that indicates food items accepted or rejected by the client.

Food allergy—Sensitivity to a food that does not cause a negative reaction in most people.

Food faddism—An unusual pattern of food behavior enthusiastically adapted by its adherents.

Food frequency—A usual food intake or a description of what an individual usually eats during a typical day.

Food infection—Infection acquired through contact with food or water contaminated with disease-producing microorganisms.

Food insecurity—Limited or uncertain availability of nutritionally adequate and safe foods; uncertain ability to acquire food either sometimes or always.

Food intoxication—An illness caused by the consumption of a food in which bacteria have produced a poisonous toxin.

Food quackery—The promotion for profit of a medical scheme or remedy that is unproven or known to be false.

Food record—A diary of a person's self-reported food intake.

Fortification—Process of adding nutritive substances not naturally occurring in the given food to increase its nutritional value; for example, milk fortified with vitamins A and D.

Free radicals—Atoms or molecules that have lost an electron and vigorously pursue its replacement; in doing so, free radicals can damage normal cell constituents.

Fructose—A monosaccharide found in fruits and honey; a simple sugar.

Functional disease—One for which anatomic abnormality is not apparent; opposite of organic disease.

Functional foods—Foods or food components that have additional health or physiological benefits over and above the normal nutritional value they provide.

Fundus—Larger part of a hollow organ; the part of the stomach above its attachment to the esophagus.

Galactose—A monosaccharide derived mainly from the breakdown of the sugar in milk, lactose; a simple sugar.

Galactosemia—Lack of an enzyme needed to metabolize galactose; absolute contraindication to breastfeeding.

Gallbladder—A pear-shaped organ on the underside of the liver that concentrates and stores bile.

Gastric bypass—A surgical procedure that routes food around the stomach.

Gastric lipase—An enzyme in the stomach that aids in the digestion of fats.

Gastric residual volume (GRV)—The volume of unabsorbed enteral feeding in the stomach.

Gastric stapling—A surgical procedure on the stomach to induce weight loss by reducing the size of the stomach; also known as gastroplasty.

Gastrin—A hormone secreted by the gastric mucosa; stimulates the secretion of gastric juice.

Gastritis—Inflammation of the stomach.

Gastroesophageal reflux (acid-reflux disorder) (GERD)—Regurgitation of stomach contents into the esophagus.

Gastroparesis—Partial paralysis of the stomach.

Gastrostomy—A surgical opening in the stomach.

Gene—Basic unit of heredity; linear segment of deoxyribonucleic acid (DNA) that occupies a specific location on a specific chromosome; provides the instructions for protein synthesis.

Generativity—The seventh of Erikson's developmental stages, in which the middle-aged adult guides the next generation.

Generic name—The name given to a drug by its original developer; usually the same as the official name given to it by the Food and Drug Administration.

Genetic code—Hereditary instructions for building proteins; analogous to software that dictates the processing of information by the computer.

Genetic susceptibility—Likelihood of an individual developing a given trait as determined by heredity.

Genomics—The study of an organism's complete set of DNA; regarding nutrition, the study of how different foods may interact with specific genes to increase the risk of common chronic diseases.

Genotype—Total of the hereditary information present in an organism whether or not expressed in the individual's phenotype (*see* Phenotype).

Geriatrics—Branch of medicine involved in the study and treatment of diseases of the elderly.

Gestation—Time from fertilization of the ovum until birth; in humans, the length of gestation is usually 38 to 42 weeks.

Gestational diabetes (GDM)—Hyperglycemia and altered carbohydrate, protein, and fat metabolism related to the increased physiological demands of pregnancy.

Globin—The simple protein portion of hemoglobin.

Glomerular filtrate—The fluid that has been passed through the glomerulus.

Glomerular filtration rate (GFR)—An index of kidney function; the amount of filtrate formed each minute in all the nephrons of both kidneys.

Glomerulonephritis—Inflammation of the glomeruli.

Glomerulus—The network of capillaries inside the Bowman capsule.

Glossitis—Inflammation of the tongue.

Glucagon—A hormone secreted by the alpha cells of the pancreas; increases the concentration of glucose in the blood.

Gluconeogenesis—The production of glucose from noncarbohydrate sources such as amino acids and glycerol.

Glucose—A monosaccharide (simple sugar) commonly called the blood sugar; the same as dextrose.

Glucose tolerance test—A test of blood and urine after the patient receives a concentrated dose of glucose; used to diagnose abnormalities of glucose metabolism.

Gluteal-femoral obesity—Excess body fat centered around an individual's buttocks, hips, and thighs.

Gluten—A type of protein found in wheat, rye, and barley; may contaminate oats through processing.

Gluten-sensitive enteropathy (celiac disease)—An intestinal disorder caused by an abnormal response following the consumption of gluten.

Glycemic index—A measure of how much the blood glucose level increases following consumption of a particular food that contains a given amount of carbohydrate.

Glycerol—The backbone of a fat molecule; pharmaceutical preparation is glycerin.

Glycogen—The form in which carbohydrate is stored in liver and muscle.

Glycogenolysis—The breakdown of glycogen.

Glycosuria—Glucose in the urine.

Glycosylated hemoglobin—Hemoglobin to which a glucose group is attached; in diabetes mellitus, if the blood glucose level has not been controlled over the previous 120 days, the glycosylated hemoglobin level is elevated.

Goiter—Enlargement of the thyroid gland characterized by pronounced swelling in the neck.

Goitrogens—Substances that block the absorption of iodine, thereby causing goiter; found in cabbage, rutabaga, and turnips, but only related to goiter in cassava.

Gout—A hereditary metabolic disease that is a form of acute arthritis and is marked by inflammation of the joints.

GRAS List—Food additives categorized by the U.S. Food and Drug Administration to be **G**enerally **R**ecognized **A**s **S**afe.

Growth—Progressive increase in size of a living thing that entails the synthesis of new protoplasm and multiplication of cells.

Gut failure—Impaired absorption due to structural damage to the small intestine; symptoms include diarrhea, malabsorption, and unsuccessful absorption of oral food.

Halal—Pertaining to food prepared and served according to Islamic dietary laws.

Half-life—In drug therapy, time required by the body to metabolize or inactivate half the amount of a substance.

Harris–Benedict equation—A formula commonly used to estimate resting energy expenditure in a stressed client.

Health—The state of complete physical, mental, and social well-being, not just the absence of disease or infirmity.

Healthy body weight (HBW)—Estimate of a weight suitable for an individual based on frame size and height and weight tables.

Heart failure—Inability of heart to circulate blood sufficiently to meet body's needs; peripheral edema is an early sign of right sided failure usually due to lung disease; difficulty breathing is an early sign of left sided failure usually a consequence of myocardial infarction.

Hematocrit—Percentage of total blood volume that is red blood cells; normal levels are 40% to 54% for men, 37% to 47% for women.

Hematuria—Blood in the urine.

Heme—The iron-containing portion of the hemoglobin molecule.

Heme iron—Iron bound to hemoglobin and myoglobin in meat, fish, and poultry; 10% to 30% of the iron in these foods is absorbed.

Hemochromatosis—A genetic disease of iron metabolism in which iron accumulates in the tissues.

Hemodialysis—A method for cleansing the blood of wastes by circulating blood through a machine that contains tubes made of synthetic semipermeable membranes.

Hemoglobin—The iron-carrying pigment of the red blood cells; carries oxygen from the lungs to the tissues.

Hemolysis—Rupture of red blood cells releasing hemoglobin into the plasma; causes include bacterial toxins, chemicals, inappropriate medications, vitamin E deficiency.

Hemolytic anemia—An abnormal reduction in the number of red blood cells due to hemolysis.

Hemosiderin—An iron oxide–protein compound derived from hemoglobin; a storage form of iron.

Hemosiderosis—Condition resulting from excess deposits of hemosiderin, especially in the liver and spleen; caused by destruction of red blood cells, which occurs in diseases such as hemolytic anemia, pernicious anemia, and chronic infection.

Heparin—A chemical, found naturally in many tissues, that inhibits blood clotting by preventing the conversion of prothrombin to thrombin; also given as an anticoagulant medication.

Hepatic portal circulation—A subdivision of the vascular system in which blood from the digestive organs and spleen circulates through the liver before returning to the heart.

Hepatitis—Inflammation of the liver, caused by viruses, drugs, alcohol, or toxic substances.

Hepcidin—Hormone synthesized by the liver that regulates iron metabolism; released in response to high body iron levels to inhibit iron transport in the duodenum and to prevent release of stored iron.

Heterozygous—Having dissimilar pairs of genes, one from each parent, for any hereditary characteristic; genes, one from each parent, governing a particular trait; the dominant gene will produce the given trait in the individual.

Hiatal hernia—A protrusion of part of the stomach into the chest cavity.

High-density lipoprotein (HDL)—A plasma protein that carries fat in the bloodstream to the tissues or to the liver to be excreted; elevated blood levels are associated with a decreased risk of heart disease.

High-fructose corn syrup (HFCS)—Corn syrup that has been enzymatically processed to convert some of its glucose into fructose to produce a desired sweetness; principal sweetener used in processed foods and beverages because it costs less than sucrose.

Hives (urticaria)—Sudden swelling and itching of skin or mucous membranes, often caused by allergies; if the respiratory tract is involved, may be life threatening.

Homeostasis—Tendency toward balance in the internal environment of the body, achieved by automatic monitoring and regulating mechanisms.

Homozygous—Having two identical genes, one from each parent, governing a particular trait; necessary condition to produce a disease caused by a recessive gene, such as sickle cell anemia.

Hormone—A substance produced by cells of the body that is released into the bloodstream and carried to target sites to regulate the activity of other cells and organs.

Human immunodeficiency virus (HIV)—The virus that causes AIDS.

Humoral immunity—Development of antibodies to specific antigens by the B-lymphocytes, some of which retain the ability to recognize the antigen if it is encountered again; basis of immunizations.

Humulin—Exact duplicate of human insulin manufactured by altering bacterial DNA.

Hunger—The sensation resulting from a lack of food, characterized by dull or acute pain around the lower part of the chest; in global context, insufficient quantity of food where minimum kilocalorie intake is not met.

Hydrochloric acid (HCl)—Strong acid secreted by the stomach that aids in protein digestion.

Hydrogenation—The process of adding hydrogen to a fat to make it more highly saturated.

Hydrolysis—A chemical reaction that splits a substance into simpler compounds by the addition of water; in hydrolyzed infant formulas, whole proteins are split into smaller pieces.

Hydrostatic pressure—The pressure created by the pumping action of the heart on the fluid in the blood vessels.

Hyperbilirubinemia—Excessive bilirubin in the blood; bilirubin is produced by the breakdown of red blood cells.

Hypercalcemia—A serum calcium level that is too high; in adults, more than 5.5 milliequivalents per liter.

Hypercholesterolemia—Excessive cholesterol in the blood.

Hyperemesis gravidarum—Severe nausea and vomiting persisting after the fourteenth week of pregnancy of unknown etiology.

Hyperglycemia—An elevated level of glucose in the blood; fasting value above 110 milligrams per deciliter, depending on measuring technique used.

Hyperglycemic hyperosmolar nonketotic syndrome (HHNS)—Life-threatening complication of NIDDM characterized by blood glucose levels greater than 600 milligrams per deciliter, absence of or slight ketosis, profound cellular dehydration, and electrolyte imbalances.

Hyperkalemia—Excessive potassium in the blood; greater than 5.0 milliequivalents per liter of serum in adults.

Hyperlipoproteinemia—A group of acquired and inherited disorders causing increased lipoproteins and lipids in the blood; also referred to as hyperlipidemia.

Hypermetabolism—An abnormal increase in the rate at which fuel or kilocalories are burned.

Hypernatremia—An excess of sodium in the blood; greater than 145 milliequivalents per liter of serum in adults.

Hyperparathyroidism—Excessive secretion of parathyroid hormone, causing changes in the bones, kidney, and gastrointestinal tract.

Hyperphosphatemia—Excessive amount of phosphates in the blood; in adults, greater than 4.7 milligrams per 100 milliliters of serum.

Hypertension—Condition of elevated blood pressure; diagnosed if blood pressure is greater than 140/90 on three successive occasions or if person is receiving antihypertensive medication.

Hypertensive disorders of pregnancy—Blood pressure greater than 140 mm Hg systolic or greater than 90 mm Hg diastolic occurring in pregnancy;

subcategories are chronic hypertension, gestational hypertension, preeclampsia, and eclampsia.

Hypertensive kidney disease—A condition in which vascular or glomerular lesions cause hypertension but not total renal failure.

Hyperthyroidism—Oversecretion of thyroid hormones, which increases the metabolic rate above normal.

Hypertonic—A solution that contains more particles and exerts more osmotic pressure than the plasma.

Hypervitaminosis—Condition caused by excessive intake of vitamins.

Hypocalcemia—A depressed level of calcium in the blood; less than 4.5 milliequivalents per liter of serum in adults.

Hypoglycemia—A depressed level of glucose in the blood; less than 70 milligrams per deciliter.

Hypokalemia—Potassium depletion in the circulating blood; less than 3.5 milliequivalents per liter of serum in adults.

Hyponatremia—Too little sodium per volume of blood; less than 135 milliequivalents per liter of serum in adults.

Hypophosphatemia—Too little phosphate per volume of blood; in adults, less than 2.4 milligrams per 100 milliliters of serum.

Hypothalamus—A portion of the brain that helps to regulate water balance, thirst, body temperature, carbohydrate and fat metabolism, and sleep.

Hypothyroidism—Undersecretion of thyroid hormones; reduces the metabolic rate.

Hypotonic—A solution that contains fewer particles and exerts less osmotic pressure than the plasma does.

Iatrogenic malnutrition—Excessive or deficit intake of one or more nutrients induced by the oversight or omissions of health-care workers.

Ideal body weight—Person's projected healthy weight based on height, frame, and gender; for information about MetLife's development of the tables, see http://www.halls.md/ideal-weight/met.htm.

Identity—The fifth developmental task in Erikson's theory, in which the adolescent decides on an appropriate role.

Idiopathic—Without a recognizable cause.

Ileocecal valve—The valve between the ileum and cecum.

Ileostomy—Surgical procedure in which an opening to the small intestine (ileum) is constructed on the abdomen.

Ileum—The lower portion of the small intestine.

Immune—Produced by, involved in, or concerned with resistance or protection against a specified disease.

Immune system—The organs in the body responsible for fighting off substances interpreted as foreign.

Immunity—The state of being protected from a particular disease, especially an infectious disease.

Immunoglobulin—Blood proteins with known antibody activity; five types of immunoglobulins have been identified: IgA, IgD, IgE, IgG, and IgM.

Immunosuppressive agent—Medication that interferes with the body's ability to fight infection.

Impaired glucose tolerance (IGT)—A type of classification for hyperglycemia; for persons who have a glucose intolerance but do not meet the criteria for classification as having diabetes.

Implantation—Embedding of the fertilized egg in the lining of the uterus 6 or 7 days after fertilization.

Incidence—The frequency of occurrence of any event or condition over a given time and in relation to the population in which it occurs.

Incomplete protein—Protein lacking one or more of the essential amino acids that humans need; found primarily in plant sources such as grains and vegetables; gelatin is an animal product but is an incomplete protein.

Incubation period—The time it takes to show disease symptoms after exposure to the causative organism.

Indication—A circumstance that indicates when a treatment should or can be used.

Indoles—Compounds found in vegetables of the cruciferous family that activate enzymes to destroy carcinogens.

Industry—The fourth stage of development in Erikson's theory in which the school-age child learns to work effectively.

Infant botulism—Neurological toxicity caused by ingestion of *Clostridium botulinum* spores from honey or soil-contaminated foods; infant's intestinal tract flora cannot suppress the spores; also called intestinal botulism.

Infection—Entry and development of parasites or entry and multiplication of microorganisms in the bodies of persons or animals; may or may not cause signs and symptoms.

Inflammatory response—The metabolic response of the immune system to infection or injury.

Initiation—The first step in the cell's becoming cancerous, when physical forces, chemicals, or biologic agents permanently alter the cell's DNA.

Initiative—The third stage of development in Erikson's theory in which the preschooler learns to set and achieve goals.

Insensible water loss—Water that is lost invisibly through the lungs and skin.

Insoluble—Incapable of being dissolved in a given substance.

Insulin—Hormone secreted by the beta cells of the pancreas in response to an elevated blood glucose level.

Insulin resistance—A disorder characterized by elevated levels of both glucose and insulin; thought to be related to a lack of insulin receptors.

Intact feeding—A feeding consisting of nutrients that have not been predigested.

Intact nutrients—Nutrients that have not been predigested.

Integrity—The final stage of Erikson's theory of psychosocial development, in which the older adult learns to look back on his or her life as worthwhile.

Intermittent feeding—Giving a 4- to 6-hour volume of a tube feeding over 20 to 30 minutes.

Intermittent peritoneal dialysis—Method of dialysis treatment in which the dialysate remains in a patient's abdominal cavity for about 30 minutes and then drains from the body by gravity.

International normalized ratio (INR)—measure of standardized prothrombin time; used to monitor anticoagulation effects of warfarin; normal individual = 1; therapeutic range for anticoagulation = 2 to 3, meaning client's blood takes 2 to 3 times as long as normal to clot.

International unit (IU)—Individually scaled measure of vitamins A, D, and E agreed to by a committee of scientists; also used for some hormones, enzymes, and biologicals such as vaccines.

Interstitial fluid—Extracellular fluid located between the cells.

Intimacy—The sixth stage of development in Erikson's theory, in which the young adult builds reciprocal, caring relationships.

Intracellular fluid—Fluid located within the cells.

Intravascular fluid—Fluid found in the blood and lymph vessels.

Intravenous—Through a vein.

Intrinsic factor—Specific protein-binding factor secreted by the stomach, necessary for the absorption of vitamin B_{12}.

Invisible fat—Dietary fats that cannot be seen easily; hidden fats in foods such as baked goods, peanut butter, emulsified milk, and so forth.

Ion—An atom or group of atoms carrying an electrical charge; an ion with a positive charge is called a cation; an ion with a negative charge is called an anion.

Ionic bond—A chemical bond formed between atoms by the loss and gain of electrons.

Iron deficiency—State of inadequate iron stores measured by laboratory tests such as serum ferritin and transferrin saturation; may progress to anemia when the person's hemoglobin value drops.

Irrigation—Flushing a prescribed solution through a tube or cavity.

Irritable bowel syndrome—Diarrhea or alternating constipation-diarrhea with no discernible organic cause.

Islet cell antibody—A protein found to be elevated in a person with insulin-dependent diabetes mellitus.

Islets of Langerhans—Clusters of cells in the pancreas including alpha, beta, and delta cells; alpha cells produce glucagon, beta cells produce insulin, and delta cells produce somatostatin.

Isotonic—A solution that has the same osmotic pressure as blood plasma.

Isotretinoin—Vitamin A metabolite used to treat severe acne, requiring strict contraceptive protocols in fertile women because the metabolite can cause birth defects.

Jaundice—Yellowing of skin, whites of eyes, and mucous membranes due to excessive bilirubin in the blood; causes may be obstructed bile duct, liver disease, or hemolysis of red blood cells.

Jejunoileal bypass—A surgical procedure that removes a portion of the small intestine, bypassing about 90% of it.

Jejunostomy—A surgical opening into the jejunum.

Jejunum—The second portion of the small intestine.

Joule—A measurement of energy; amount of energy needed to raise the temperature of 1 gram of cool, dry air by 1.8°F (1.0°C).

Kaposi sarcoma—A type of cancer often related to the immunocompromised state that accompanies AIDS; characterized by multiple areas of cell proliferation, initially in the skin and eventually in other body sites.

Keshan disease—Deterioration of the heart due to selenium deficiency, but heart failure not reversible by supplementation; named for the province of Keshan, China; fatality rate as high as 80%; in mice, linked to a mutation of an avirulent virus to a virulent one producing myocardial disease; virulent strain then caused heart disease in mice not selenium-deficient.

Keto acid—Amino acid residue left after deamination.

Ketoacidosis—Acidosis due to an excess of ketone bodies.

Ketone—Any of a class of organic compounds characterized by a carbonyl group attached to two carbon atoms; example: acetone, used in nail polish remover and paint remover.

Ketone body—Any of the three compounds (acetoacetic acid, acetone, and *B*-hydroxybutyric acid) that are normal intermediates in lipid metabolism; accumulate in blood and urine in abnormal amounts in conditions of impaired metabolism.

Ketonuria—The presence of ketone bodies in the urine.

Ketosis—Accumulation of ketone bodies in the blood; result of incomplete metabolism of fatty acids, generally from carbohydrate deficiency or malfunctioning carbohydrate metabolism.

Kilocaloric density—The kilocalories contained in a given volume of a food.

Kilocalorie (Kcal)—A measurement unit of energy; the amount of heat required to raise 1 kilogram of water 1° Celsius; on food labels: Calorie.

Kilocalorie:nitrogen ratio—A mathematical relationship expressed as the number of kilocalories per gram of nitrogen provided in a feeding.

Kilojoule—A measurement unit of energy required to move a mass of one kilogram with an acceleration of one meter per second; one kilocalorie equals 4.184 kilojoules.

Konzo—An irreversible paralytic disease of the lower extremities caused by consumption of inadequately processed cassava roots that contain cyanide along with a diet deficient in sulphur-based amino acids.

Korsakoff psychosis—Amnesia, often seen in chronic alcoholism, caused by degeneration of the thalamus due to thiamin deficiency; characterized by loss of short-term memory and inability to learn new skills.

Kosher—pertaining to food prepared and served according to Jewish dietary laws.

Krebs cycle—A complicated series of reactions that results in the release of energy from carbohydrates, fats, and proteins, also known as the TCA (tricarboxylic acid) cycle.

Kussmaul respirations—Pattern of rapid and deep breathing due to the body's attempt to correct metabolic acidosis by eliminating carbon dioxide through the lungs.

Kwashiorkor—Severe protein deficiency in child after weaning; symptoms include edema, pigmentation changes, impaired growth and development, and liver pathology.

Lactalbumin—Simple soluble protein found in greater concentration in human breast milk than in cow's milk; easily absorbed by the infant.

Lactase—An intestinal enzyme that converts lactose into glucose and galactose.

Lactational amenorrhea—Absence of menstrual cycle in a mother who is fully breastfeeding.

Lacteal—The central lymph vessel in each villus.

Lactose—A disaccharide found mainly in milk and milk products.

Large intestine—The part of the alimentary canal that extends from the small intestine to the anus.

LCAT deficiency—A lack of LCAT (lecithin-cholesterol acyltransferase), an enzyme that transports cholesterol from the tissues to the liver for removal from the body.

Lean body mass—Also called fat-free mass; the weight of the body minus the fat content but including essential fats that are associated with the central nervous system, the viscera, the bone marrow, and cell membranes.

Legumes—Plants that have nitrogen-fixing bacteria in their roots; a good alternative to meat as a protein source; examples are dried beans, lentils.

Lesion—Area of diseased or injured tissue.

Leukopenia—Abnormal decrease in the number of white blood corpuscles; usually below 5000 per cubic millimeter.

Life expectancy—The probable number of years that persons of a given age may be expected to live.

Limiting amino acid—Particular essential amino acid lacking or undersupplied in a food that classifies the food as an incomplete protein.

Linoleic acid—An essential fatty acid.

Lipectomy—Surgical removal of adipose tissue.

Lipid—Any one of a group of fats or fat-like substances that are insoluble in water; includes true fats (fatty acids and glycerol), lipoids, and sterols.

Lipoid—Substances resembling fats but containing groups other than glycerol and fatty acids that make up true fats; example: phospholipids.

Lipolysis—The breakdown of adipose tissue for energy.

Lipoprotein—Combination of a protein with lipid components such as cholesterol, phospholipids, and triglycerides.

Lipoprotein lipase—An enzyme that breaks down chylomicrons.

Liposuction—Surgical removal of adipose tissue through a vacuum hose.

Listeriosis—Bacterial infection caused by *Listeria monocytogenes* that is particularly virulent for fetuses; transmitted from the mother to the fetus in utero or through the birth canal; outbreaks associated with raw or contaminated milk, soft cheeses, contaminated vegetables, and ready-to-eat meats; others at risk include the elderly, those with impaired immune systems, and farm workers.

Liver—A digestive organ that aids in the metabolism of all the energy nutrients, screens toxic substances from the blood, manufactures blood proteins, and performs many other important functions.

Locus, loci (pl.)—In genetics, the site of a gene on a chromosome.

Loop of Henle—The segment of the renal tubule that follows the proximal convoluted tubule.

Low birth weight (LBW)—Characterizing an infant that weighs less than 2500 g (5.5 lb) at birth.

Low-density lipoprotein (LDL)—A plasma protein containing more cholesterol and triglycerides than protein; elevated blood levels are associated with increased risk of heart disease.

Luminal effect—Drug-induced changes within the intestine that affect the absorption of nutrients and drugs without altering the intestine.

Lycopene—A red pigmented carotenoid with powerful antioxidant functions but no provitamin A activity; found in tomatoes and various berries and fruits.

Lymph—A body fluid collected from the interstitial fluid all over the body and returned to the bloodstream via the lymphatic vessels.

Lymphatic system—All the structures involved in the transportation of lymph from the tissues to the bloodstream.

Lysine—Amino acid often lacking in grains.

Macrocytic anemia—Anemia in which the red blood cells are larger than normal; one characteristic of pernicious anemia also found in folic acid deficiency.

Macrophage—Monocyte (see Fig. 8-13) that has left the circulation and settled in a tissue such as the spleen, lymph nodes, and tonsils; with neutrophils, major phagocytic cells of immune system.

Major minerals—Those present in the body in quantities greater than 5 grams (approximately 1 teaspoonful); humans need at least 100 milligrams daily (approximately ⅙₀ teaspoonful); also called macrominerals.

Malabsorption—Inadequate movement of digested food from the small intestine into the blood or lymphatic system.

Malignant—Tumor that infiltrates surrounding tissue and spreads to distant sites of the body.

Malnutrition—Poor nutrition; results when the body's cells receive either an excess or a deficiency of one or more nutrients.

Maltase—An intestinal enzyme that converts maltose into glucose.

Maltose—A disaccharide produced when starches are broken down by the body into simpler units; two units of glucose joined together.

Marasmus—Malnutrition due to a protein and kilocalorie deficit.

Mastication—The process of chewing.

Mechanical digestion—The digestive process that involves the physical breaking down of food into smaller pieces.

Median—Statistical measure of central tendency; in a ranked set, value above which and below which are an equal number of values.

Medical foods—Foods formulated to be consumed or administered enterally under the supervision of a physician intended for the specific dietary management of a disease or condition, which have distinctive nutritional requirements.

Medical Nutrition Therapy (MNT)—Provision of nutrient, dietary, and nutrition education based on a comprehensive nutritional assessment by a registered dietitian (RD); can offer cost-effective health benefits in disease management and medication optimization.

Megadose—Dose providing 10 times or more of the recommended dietary allowance.

Megaloblastic anemia—Anemia characterized by large immature red blood cells in the bloodstream that cannot carry oxygen properly; occurs in folic acid deficiency and pernicious anemia.

Melatonin—Hormone produced from the amino acid tryptophan by the pineal gland in the brain; stimulates the onset and duration of sleep; used to treat sleep disorders and jet lag.

Menaquinone—Vitamin K that is synthesized by intestinal bacteria; also called vitamin K_2.

Meninges—Three membranes covering the brain and spinal cord; from the outside named the dura, arachnoid, and pia maters.

Meningocele—Congenital protrusion of the meninges through a defect in the skull or the spinal column.

Meningoencephalocele—Protrusion of the brain and its coverings through a defect in the skull.

Menkes disease—Metabolic defect blocking the absorption of copper in the gastrointestinal tract.

Meta-analysis—Statistical procedure for combining data from a number of studies to analyze therapeutic effectiveness.

Metabolic syndrome—Combination of atherosclerotic risk factors, including dyslipidemia, insulin resistance, obesity, and hypertension, that produces an increased risk for coronary artery disease.

Metabolism—The sum of all physical and chemical changes that take place in the body; the two fundamental processes involved are anabolism and catabolism.

Metabolite—Any product of metabolism; 4229 human serum metabolites commonly detected and quantified (with today's technology) in the human serum metabolome have recently been cataloged for use by researchers.

Metastasis—The "seeding" of cancer cells to distant sites of the body; spread via blood or lymph vessels or by spilling into a body cavity.

Methionine—Sulfur-containing amino acid often lacking in legumes.

Microalbuminuria—Small amounts of protein in the urine. Detected by a laboratory using methods more sensitive than traditional urinalysis.

Microflora—Resident bacteria in the intestinal tract; functions include assisting in the development of the immune system and protecting the host from foreign microbes.

Microgram—One-millionth of a gram or one-thousandth of a milligram; abbreviated mcg.

Micronize—To pulverize a substance into very tiny particles.

Microvilli—Microscopic, hairlike rodlets (resembling bristles on a brush) covering the edge of each villus.

Midarm circumference—Measure of the distance around the middle of the upper arm; used to assess body protein stores.

Milk-alkali syndrome—Condition characterized by high blood calcium and a more alkaline urine that predisposes to the precipitation of calcium in the kidney; caused by ingestion of excessive absorbable alkali and milk; associated with the milk and cream and antacid treatment of peptic ulcers used years ago.

Milliequivalent (mEq)—Unit of measure used for determining the concentration of electrolytes in solution; expressed as milliequivalents per liter.

Milling—The process of grinding grain into flour.

Milliosmole—Unit of measure for osmotic activity.

Mineral—An inorganic element or compound occurring in nature; in the body, some minerals help regulate bodily functions and are essential to good health.

Mixed malnutrition—The result of a deficiency or excess of more than one nutrient.

Modified diet—A term used in health-care institutions to mean the food served to a client has been altered or changed from that served to clients on regular diets, usually by physician order.

Modular supplement—A nutritional supplement that contains a limited number of nutrients, usually only one.

Mold—Any of a group of parasitic or other organisms living on decaying matter; fungi.

Molecule—The smallest quantity into which a substance may be divided without loss of its characteristics.

Monoamine oxidase inhibitor (MAOI)—A class of drugs that may have critical interactions with foods.

Monocyte—White blood cell (see Fig. 8-3) that circulates in the bloodstream for about 24 hours before settling into tissues to become a macrophage; with macrophages, provide a defense against foreign antigens.

Monoglyceride—One fatty acid joined to a glycerol molecule.

Monosaccharide—A simple sugar composed of one unit of $C_6H_{12}O_6$; examples include glucose, fructose, and galactose.

Monounsaturated fat—A lipid in which the majority of fatty acids contain one carbon-to-carbon double bond.

Morbid obesity—BMI greater than 39.

Morbidity—The state of being diseased; number of cases of disease in relation to population.

Mortality—State of being subject to death; the death rate; number of deaths per unit of population.

Motility—Power to move spontaneously.

Mucosa—A mucous membrane that lines body cavities.

Mucosal effect—Drug-induced changes within the intestine that affect the absorption of drugs or nutrients by damaging the tissues.

Mucus—A thick fluid secreted by the mucous membranes and glands.

Multiparous—Having borne more than one child.

Mutation—Permanent transmissible change in a gene; natural mutation produces evolutionary change in organisms; induced mutation results from exposure to environmental influences such as physical forces, chemicals, or biologic agents.

Mycotoxin—A substance produced by mold growing in food that can cause illness or death when ingested by humans or animals.

Myelin sheath—Fatty covering surrounding the long appendages of some nerves; serves to increase the transmission speed of impulses.

MyPlate—U.S. Department of Agriculture food guide using the visual cues of a divided plate and a glass to represent the proportions of healthy foods for consumers.

Myocardial infarction (MI)—Area of dead heart muscle; usually the result of coronary occlusion.

Myocardium—The heart muscle.

Myoglobin—A protein located in muscle tissue that contains and stores oxygen.

Myxedema—A condition that occurs in older children and adults, resulting from hypofunction of the thyroid gland characterized by a drying and thickening of the skin and slowing of physical and mental activity.

Narcolepsy—A chronic condition consisting of recurrent attacks of drowsiness and sleep.

Nasoduodenal tube (ND tube)—A tube inserted via the nose into the duodenum.

Nasogastric tube (NG tube)—A tube inserted via the nose into the stomach.

Nasojejunal tube (NJ tube)—A tube inserted via the nose into the jejunum.

Necrotizing enterocolitis—A condition in premature infants in which intestinal cells die and fall off.

Neonate—Infant from birth to age 28 days.

Neoplasm—A new and abnormal formation of tissue (tumor) that grows at the expense of the healthy organism.

Nephritis—General term for inflammation of the kidneys.

Nephron—The structural and functional unit of the kidney.

Nephropathy—A kidney disease characterized by inflammation and degenerative lesions.

Nephrosclerosis—A hardening of the renal arteries; may be caused by arteriosclerosis of the kidney arteries.

Nephrotic syndrome—The end result of a variety of diseases that cause the abnormal passage of plasma proteins into the urine.

Neuropathy—Any disease of the nerves.

Neural tube defects—A birth defect of the brain, spine, or spinal cord; includes spina bifida and anencephaly.

NHANES—National Health and Nutrition Examination Survey, a nationally representative cross-sectional survey of civilian noninstitutionalized population of the United States; conducted by the Centers for Disease Control and Prevention's National Center for Health Statistics; the interview includes demographic, socioeconomic, dietary, and health-related questions; the examination component consists of medical, dental, and physiological measurements, as well as laboratory tests.

Niacin—A B vitamin that functions as a coenzyme in the production of energy from glucose; obtained from meat or produced from the amino acid tryptophan, present in milk, eggs, and meat; also called nicotinic acid.

Niacin equivalent (NE)—Measure of niacin activity; equal to 1 milligram of preformed niacin or 60 milligrams of tryptophan.

Night blindness—Vision that is slow to adapt to dim light; caused by vitamin A deficiency or hereditary factors or, in the elderly, by poor circulation.

Nitrogen—Colorless, odorless, tasteless gas forming about 80% of Earth's air.

Nitrogen balance—The difference between the amount of nitrogen ingested and that excreted each day; when intake is greater, a positive balance exists; when intake is less, a negative balance exists.

Nitrogen-fixing bacteria—Organisms that absorb nitrogen from the air, which, upon the death of the bacteria, is released for legume plants to use in the anabolism of protein.

Nomogram—A chart that shows a relationship between numerical values.

Nonessential—In nutrition, refers to a chemical substance or nutrient the body normally can manufacture in sufficient amounts for health.

Nonessential amino acid—Any amino acid that can normally be synthesized by the body in sufficient quantities.

Nonheme iron—Iron that is not bound to hemoglobin or myoglobin; all the iron in plant sources.

Norwalk virus norovirus—A causative organism that is responsible for more than 50% of the reported cases of epidemic viral gastroenteropathy. The incubation period ranges from 18 to 72 hours, and the outbreaks are usually self-limiting; influenzalike intestinal symptoms last for 24 to 48 hours.

NSAID—Nonsteroidal anti-inflammatory drug; examples: aspirin, ibuprofen, naproxen, as well as agents available by prescription.

Nulliparous—Never having borne a child.

Nursing action (intervention)—Specific care to be administered, including physical and psychological care, teaching, counseling, and referring.

Nursing-bottle syndrome—A condition in which an infant has many dental caries caused by drinking milk or other sweet liquids during sleep.

Nutraceutical—Food component used for medicinal purposes; Ex: vitamins, minerals, amino acids; regulated under Dietary Supplement Health Education Act of 1994 (see Chapter 15).

Nutrient—Chemical substance supplied by food that the body needs for growth, maintenance, and/or repair.

Nutrient density—The concentration of nutrients in a given volume of food compared with the food's kilocalorie content.

Nutrigenetics—Detection of gene variants within an individual to identify environmental factors that trigger dysfunction or disease; part of the initiation of food allergies and **celiac disease**.

Nutrigenomics—Study of the interaction between one's diet and his or her genes in order to alter susceptibilities to disease and responses to foods.

Nutrition—Science of food and its relationship to health; processes of taking in and utilizing nourishment.

Nutrition support service—A team service for clients on enteral and parenteral feedings that assesses, monitors, and counsels these clients.

Nutritional assessment—The evaluation of a client's nutritional status based on a physical examination, anthropometric measurements, laboratory data, and food intake information.

Nutritional status—Condition of the body as it relates to the intake and use of nutrients.

Obese—Body mass index (BMI) of 30 kg/m² or more; muscular person may exceed BMI of 30 kg/m² but not be obese.

Obesity—Excessive amount of fat on the body; for women, a fat content greater than 30%; for men, a fat content greater than 25%.

Obesogens—Chemical in the environment that may have an effect on obesity.

Objective data—Findings verifiable by another through physical assessment or diagnostic tests, also termed signs.

Obligatory excretion—Minimum amount of urine production necessary to keep waste products in solution, amounting to 400 to 600 milliliters per day.

Oliguria—A decreased output of urine.

Oncogene—Carcinogenic gene that stimulates excessive reproduction of the cell.

Opportunistic infection—Infection caused by normally nonpathogenic organisms in a host with decreased resistance.

Opsin—A protein that combines with vitamin A to form rhodopsin, a chemical in the retina necessary for vision.

Optic nerve—The second cranial nerve, which transmits impulses for the sense of sight.

Oral cavity—The cavity in the skull bounded by the mouth, palate, cheeks, and tongue.

Oral rehydration solution—Oral fluid that prevents or treats dehydration.

Organ—Somewhat independent body part having specific functions; examples: stomach, liver.

Orthostatic hypotension—A drop in blood pressure producing dizziness, fainting, or blurred vision when arising from a lying or sitting position or when standing motionless in a fixed position.

Osmolality—Measure of osmotic pressure exerted by the number of dissolved particles per weight of liquid; usually reported clinically as mOsm/kg.

Osmolarity—Measure of osmotic pressure exerted by the number of dissolved particles per volume of liquid; usually reported clinically as mOsm/L.

Osmosis—The movement of water across a semipermeable cell membrane from an area with fewer particles to one with more particles.

Osmotic demyelinating disease—Brain pathology caused by too rapid correction of hyponatremia resulting in motor nerve dysfunction including quadriplegia; more common in malnourished and debilitated clients.

Osmotic pressure—The pressure that develops when a concentrated solution is separated from a less-concentrated solution by a semipermeable membrane.

Osteoarthritis—Progressive deterioration of the cartilage in the joints; risk factors are aging, obesity, occupational or athletic abuse of joints, and trauma.

Osteoblasts—Bone cells that build bone.

Osteocalcin—Vitamin K–dependent protein; second most abundant protein in bone but its function is not yet clearly defined.

Osteoclasts—Bone cells that break down bone.

Osteodystrophy—Defective bone formation.

Osteomalacia—Adult form of rickets.

Osteopenia—Bone mineral density 1 to 2.5 standard deviations below the mean of healthy young adults.

Osteoporosis—Bone mineral density more than 2.5 standard deviations below the mean of young adults.

Ostomy—A surgically formed opening to permit passage of urine or bowel contents to the outside.

Overnutrition—The result of an excess of one or more nutrients in the diet.

Overweight—Body mass index from 25 kg/m² to 29.99 kg/m².

Ovum—The egg cell that, after fertilization by a sperm cell, develops into a new individual.

Oxalates—Salts of oxalic acid found in some plant foods; bind with the calcium in the plant, making it unavailable to the body.

Oxidation—The process in which a substance is combined with oxygen.

Oxidative stress—Cellular damage caused by oxygen-derived free radical formation; potential damage can be decreased by antioxidants.

Oxytocin—A hormone produced by the posterior pituitary gland in the brain; effects are uterine contractions and release of milk.

Pancreas—An abdominal gland that secretes enzymes important in the digestion of carbohydrates, fats, and proteins; also secretes the hormones insulin and glucagon.

Pancreatic lipase—An enzyme produced by the pancreas; used in fat digestion.

Pancreatitis—Inflammation of the pancreas.

Pantothenic acid—A B-complex vitamin found in almost all foods; deficiencies from lack of food have not been documented.

Paralytic ileus—A temporary cessation of peristalsis that causes an intestinal obstruction.

Paralytic shellfish poisoning—Disease caused by the consumption of poisonous clams, oysters, mussels, or scallops.

Parasite—An organism that lives within, upon, or at the expense of a living host.

Parathyroid hormone (PTH)—Hormone secreted by the parathyroid glands; regulates calcium and phosphorus metabolism in the body.

Parenteral feeding—Administration of nutrients by a route other than the gastrointestinal tract, such as subcutaneously, intravenously, intramuscularly, or intradermally.

Parenteral nutrition (PN)—Provision of nutrients through a vein (intravenously) into a large diameter vein. (see Chapter 14)

Paresthesia—Abnormal or unpleasant sensation resulting from nerve injury; described as a feeling of numbness, prickliness, stinging, or burning.

Parietal—Two bones that form the sides and roof of the skull; also two lobes of the cerebrum lying roughly under those bones.

Parity—Condition of having carried a pregnancy to viability (20 weeks or 500-gram birth weight) regardless of whether resulted in a live birth; nulliparous—never carried a child to viability; multiparous—more than once.

Parotid glands—One of the salivary glands of the mouth, located just below and in front of the ears; the mumps virus causes infectious parotitis.

Pathogen—Any disease-producing agent, especially a virus, bacterium, fungus, or other microorganism.

Pectin—Purified carbohydrate obtained from peel of citrus fruits or apple pulp; gels when cooked with sugar at correct pH to thicken jelly and jam; contained in mashed raw apple, applesauce, firm banana; recommended for diarrhea to contribute firmness to stools.

Pellagra—Deficiency disease due to lack of niacin and tryptophan; characterized by the three Ds: dermatitis, diarrhea, and dementia.

Pepsin—An enzyme secreted in the stomach that begins protein digestion.

Pepsinogen—The antecedent of pepsin; activated by hydrochloric acid, a component of gastric juice.

Peptidases—Enzymes that assist in the digestion of protein by reducing the smaller molecules to single amino acids.

Peptide bond—Chemical bond that links two amino acids in a protein molecule.

Percutaneously—Affected through the skin.

Perforated ulcer—Condition in which an ulcer penetrates completely through the stomach or intestinal wall, spilling the organ's contents into the peritoneal cavity.

Perinatal—Period beginning after the 28th week of pregnancy and ending 28 days after birth.

Periodontal disease—Disorder of the gingiva (gums) and the supporting structures of the teeth.

Perioperative immunonutrition—Provision of nutritional support before, during, and after surgery using enteral preparations modified by the addition of specific nutrients, such as arginine, omega-3 fatty acids, and others, which have been shown to upregulate the immune response, to control inflammatory response, and to improve gut function after surgery.

Peripheral parenteral nutrition (PPN)—An intravenous feeding via a vein away from the center of the body, usually in the hand or forearm.

Peristalsis—A wavelike muscular movement that propels food along the alimentary canal.

Peritoneal dialysis—Method of removing waste products from the blood by injecting the flushing solution into a client's abdomen and using the client's peritoneum as the semipermeable membrane.

Peritoneum—The membrane that covers the internal abdominal organs and lines the abdominal cavity.

Peritonitis—Inflammation of the peritoneal cavity.

Pernicious anemia—Inadequate red blood cell formation due to lack of intrinsic factor from the stomach, which is required for the absorption of vitamin B_{12}; leads to neural deterioration.

Pesticides—A chemical used to kill insects or rodents.

Petechiae—Pinpoint, flat, round, red lesions caused by intradermal or submucosal hemorrhage.

P-glycoprotein—Cell membrane pump influencing cellular uptake and release of chemicals; affects relative susceptibility or resistance of cells to drug therapy.

pH—*Potential of Hydrogen*; a scale representing the relative acidity or alkalinity of a solution; a value of 7 is neutral, less than 7 is acidic, and greater than 7 is alkaline.

Pharmacodynamics—Study of drugs and their actions on living organisms; the clinical effects of the drugs.

Pharmacokinetics—The study of the action of drugs, emphasizing absorption time, duration of effect, distribution in the body, and method of excretion.

Pharynx—Muscular passage between the oral cavity and the esophagus.

Phenotype—Observable properties of an organism; blood type is completely inherited; other phenotypes can be altered by environmental agents.

Phenylalanine—Essential amino acid, which is indigestible if a person lacks a particular enzyme. Accumulation of phenylalanine in the blood can lead to mental retardation.

Phenylketonuria (PKU)—Hereditary disease caused by the body's failure to convert phenylalanine to tyrosine because of a defective enzyme.

Phlebotomy—Puncturing or surgical opening of a vein to withdraw blood.

Phospholipid—Diglyceride containing phosphorus; primary lipid constituent of cell membranes; examples include lecithin and myelin.

Photosynthesis—Process through which plants containing chlorophyll are able to manufacture carbohydrates from carbon dioxide and water using the sun's energy.

Phylloquinone—Vitamin K_1, found in foods.

Phytic acid—A substance found in grains that forms an insoluble complex with calcium; phytates.

Phytochemicals—Nonnutritive food components that provide medical or health benefits including the prevention or treatment of a disease.

Phytonadione—Synthetic, water-soluble pharmaceutical form of vitamin K_1; can be administered orally or by injection.

Pica—The craving to eat nonfood substances such as dirt and laundry starch.

Pitting edema—Usually of the skin of the extremities; firm pressure by a finger produces an indentation that remains for 5 seconds.

Placebo—Drug or treatment used as inactive control in a test of therapy; "placebo effect" attributed to positive response caused by subject's expectations.

Placenta—The organ in the uterus through which the unborn child exchanges carbon dioxide for oxygen and wastes for nourishment; lay term is afterbirth.

Plant sterols—Compounds, structurally similar to cholesterol, that in prescribed amounts interfere with the absorption of cholesterol and thus lower low-density lipoprotein cholesterol levels; marketed as table spreads (butter substitutes) and salad dressings.

Plaque—Accumulation of material; in lining of arteries, obstructs blood flow; on crowns of teeth, forerunner of dental caries and periodontal disease.

Plasma—The liquid portion of the blood including the clotting elements.

Plasma transferrin receptor—Measure of iron status; increases even in mild deficiency; unaffected by inflammation.

Plumbism—Lead poisoning.

Pneumocystis pneumonia—A type of lung infection frequently seen in AIDS patients; caused by the organism *Pneumocystis jiroveci,* formerly called *Pneumocystis carinii.*

Polycythemia—Increase in red blood cells; may be physiologic due to demand for oxygen-carrying capacity or pathologic as in *polycythemia vera,* a chronic, life-shortening disorder of unknown etiology involving hematologic stem cells.

Polydipsia—Excessive thirst.

Polymer—A natural or synthetic substance formed by combining two or more molecules of the same substance.

Polymorphism—Occurrence of more than one form in a life cycle; variation in alleles within a species.

Polypeptide—A chain of amino acids linked by peptide bonds that form proteins.

Polyphagia—Excessive appetite.

Polypharmacy—Concurrent use of a large number of drugs, increasing risk of interactions; especially likely in client with many diseases treated by multiple health-care providers.

Polysaccharide—Complex carbohydrates composed of many units of $C_6H_{12}O_6$ joined together; examples important in nutrition include starch, glycogen, and fiber.

Polyunsaturated fat—A fat in which the majority of fatty acids contain more than one carbon-to-carbon double bond; intake is associated with a decreased risk of heart disease.

Polyuria—Excessive urination.

Positive feedback cycle—Situation in which a condition provokes a response that worsens the condition; example: low blood pressure due to a failing heart stimulates the kidney to save sodium and water, increasing fluid retention that further overloads the failing heart.

Postprandial—Following a meal.

Potable water—Water that is safe for drinking, free of harmful substances.

Potassium pump—Proteins located in cell membranes that provide an active transport mechanism to move potassium ions across a membrane to their area of greater concentration; moves potassium ions into the cells.

Prebiotic—Nondigestible food ingredients that encourage the growth of favorable intestinal microorganisms.

Precursor—A substance from which another substance is derived.

Preeclampsia—Hypertension and proteinuria, appearing after the twentieth week of pregnancy.

Preformed vitamin—A vitamin already in a complete state in ingested foods, as opposed to a provitamin, which requires conversion in the body to be in a complete state.

Pressure ulcer—Tissue breakdown from external force impairing circulation.

Prevalence—The number of cases of a disease or condition present in a specified population at a given time.

Primary amenorrhea—Delay of menarche (initial menstrual period) until after age of 16 or absence of secondary sex characteristics after age 14.

Primary malnutrition—A nutrient deficiency due to poor food choices or a lack of nutritious food to eat.

Primary prevention—The implementation of practices that are likely to avert the occurrence of disease; nutrition example: maintaining a healthy body weight.

Principle of complementarity—Combining incomplete-protein foods so that each supplies the amino acids lacking in the other.

Prion—A proteinaceous infectious agent, extremely difficult to destroy; resistant to heat, pressure cooking, ultraviolet light, irradiation, bleach, formaldehyde, and weak acids; even autoclaving at 135° for 18 minutes does not eliminate infectivity.

Probiotic—Live microbial food supplements that improve the microbial balance of the intestine, mainly by reinforcing the intestinal mucosal barrier against harmful agents.

Prognosis—Probable outcome of an illness based on client's condition and natural course of the disease.

Promotion—The second step in a cell turning cancerous, through the action of environmental substances on the altered, initiated gene.

Proportionality—A medical treatment is ethically mandatory to the extent that it is likely to confer greater benefits than burdens to the client.

Prostaglandins—Long-chain, unsaturated fatty acids mostly synthesized in the body from arachidonic acid; have hormone-like effects.

Protein—Nutrient necessary for building body tissue; composed of carbon, hydrogen, oxygen, and nitrogen (and sometimes with sulfur, phosphorus, or iron); amino acids represent the basic structure of proteins.

Protein binding sites—Various sites in the body tissues to which drugs may become attached, rendering the drug temporarily inactive.

Protein-calorie malnutrition (PCM)—Condition in which the person's diet lacks both protein and kilocalories.

Protein-energy malnutrition (PEM)—Condition in which the person's diet lacks both protein and kilocalories. Also termed protein-calorie malnutrition (PCM).

Proteinuria—Protein in the urine.

Prothrombin—A protein essential to the blood-clotting process; manufactured by the liver using vitamin K.

Protocol—A description of steps to be followed when performing a procedure or providing care for a particular condition.

Proto-oncogene—Gene that in the normal cell stimulates growth and maintenance; when mutated, becomes an oncogene.

Provitamin—Inactive substance that the body converts to an active vitamin.

Provitamin A—Carotenoids that are precursors of vitamin A, the most powerful of which is beta-carotene.

Proximal convoluted tubule—The first segment of the renal tubule.

Psychology—The science of mental processes and their effects on behavior.

Psychosis—Severe mental disturbance with personality derangement and loss of contact with reality.

Psychosocial development—The maturing of an individual in relationships with others and within himself or herself.

Ptyalin—A salivary enzyme that breaks down starch and glycogen to maltose and a small amount of glucose; also known as salivary amylase.

Puberty—The period of life at which the physical ability to reproduce is attained.

Pulmonary—Concerning or involving the lungs.

Pulmonary edema—The accumulation of fluid in the lungs.

Pulse pressure—The difference between systolic and diastolic blood pressure; normally 30 to 40 mm Hg; narrows in insufficient fluid volume and widens in excessive fluid volume.

Purging—The intentional clearing of food out of the human body by vomiting and/or using enemas, laxatives, and/or diuretics.

Purines—One of the end products of the digestion of some nitrogen-containing compounds.

Pyelonephritis—An inflammation of the central portion of the kidney.

Pyloric sphincter—The sphincter muscle guarding the opening between the stomach and small intestine.

Pyridoxine—Pharmaceutical name for vitamin B_6.

Pyruvate—An intermediate in the metabolism of energy nutrients.

Quality assurance—A planned and systematic program for evaluating the quality and appropriateness of services rendered.

Quetelet index—Body mass index.

Radiologist—Physician with special training in diagnostic imaging and radiation treatments.

Rancid—Having the rank smell and sour taste of stale fat or oil from decomposition.

Rate—The speed or frequency of an event per unit of time.

Rationale—Reason certain actions are likely to achieve a desired outcome; in nursing, ideally based on research indicating a nursing action was effective in similar circumstances.

Rebound scurvy—Vitamin C deficiency produced in a person following cessation of megadosing due to a habitually lessened rate of absorption.

Recessive trait—One that requires two recessive genes for the trait, one from each parent, for the trait to be expressed (to be manifested) in the individual.

Recommended Dietary Allowance (RDA)—Intake that meets the needs of 97% to 98% of the individuals in a life stage and gender group; intended as a goal for daily intake by individuals, not for assessing adequacy of an individual's nutrient intake.

Rectum—The lower part of the large intestine.

Refeeding—The reintroduction of kilocalories and nutrients into a patient either orally or parenterally.

Refeeding syndrome—A detrimental state that results when a previously severely malnourished person is reintroduced to food and/or nutrients and kilocalories improperly.

Regurgitate—To cause to flow backward, as with an infant "spitting up."

Relative risk—In epidemiological studies, the ratio of the frequency of a certain disorder in groups exposed and groups not exposed to a particular hereditary or environmental factor.

Renal—Pertaining to the kidney.

Renal corpuscle—Refers collectively to both Bowman's capsule and the glomerulus.

Renal exchange lists—A specialized type of exchange list for clients with kidney disease who require restriction of one or more of the following: protein, sodium, phosphorus, and potassium.

Renal osteodystrophy—Defective bone development caused by phosphorus retention, a low or normal serum calcium level, and increased parathyroid activity.

Renal pelvis—A structure inside the kidney that receives urine from the collecting tubules.

Renal threshold—The blood glucose level at which glucose begins to spill into the urine.

Renal tubule—The second major portion of the nephron; appears ropelike.

Renin—An enzyme produced by the kidney that catalyzes the conversion of angiotensinogen to angiotensin I.

Rennin—An enzyme that coagulates milk.

Reservoir—Place that an infectious agent normally lives and multiplies so that it can be transmitted to a susceptible host.

Residue—Trace amount of any substance in a product at the time of sale; substance remaining in the bowel after absorption.

Respiration—The exchange of oxygen and carbon dioxide between a living organism and the environment.

Respirator—A machine used to assist respiration.

Respiratory acidosis—Blood pH less than 7.35 caused by pulmonary disease, characterized by a retention of carbon dioxide.

Respiratory alkalosis—Blood pH greater than 7.45 caused by pulmonary disease, characterized by a loss of carbon dioxide.

Resting energy expenditure (REE)—The amount of fuel the human body uses at rest for a specified period of time; often used interchangeably with basal metabolic rate (BMR).

Retina—Inner lining of eyeball that contains light-sensitive nerve cells; corresponds to film in camera.

Retinal—Form of vitamin A specifically required for vision.

Retinoic acid syndrome—Characteristic fetal deformities, including small ears or no ears, abnormal or missing ear canals, brain malformation, and heart defects caused by excessive preformed vitamin A or isotretinoin.

Retinoids—Group of structurally similar compounds possessing the biological activity of all-*trans* retinol including retinol, retinal, retinoic acid, retinyl ester, and synthetic analogues.

Retinol—One of the active forms of preformed vitamin A.

Retinol Activity Equivalent (RAE)—Measure of vitamin A activity that considers both preformed vitamin A (retinol) and its precursor (carotene); 1 RAE equals 3.3 international units from animal foods or 20 international units from the beta-carotene in plant foods.

Retinopathy—Any disorder of the retina.

Retrolental fibroplasia (RLF)—A disease of the vessels of the retina present in premature infants; often caused by exposure to high postnatal oxygen concentration.

Rhabdomyolysis—Breakdown of muscle fibers resulting in myoglobin in the bloodstream; some components are toxic to kidney and can cause kidney damage.

Rhodopsin—Light-sensitive protein in the retina that contains vitamin A; also called visual purple.

Riboflavin—Coenzyme in the metabolism of protein; also called vitamin B_2.

Ribonucleic acid (RNA)—Nucleic acid that controls protein synthesis in all living cells; HIV/RNA is the genetic material of human immunodeficiency virus.

Rickets—Disease caused by a deficiency of vitamin D that affects the young during the period of skeletal growth, resulting in bones that are abnormally shaped and weak.

Ritter syndrome—An inflammatory skin disease seen in newborns, characterized by pustules that fill with a straw-colored fluid and become encrusted.

Rooting reflex—The infant's natural response to a stroke on its cheek, which turns the head toward that side to nurse.

Rotavirus—Most common cause of infectious enteritis in human infants; survives for long periods on hard surfaces, in contaminated water, and on hands.

Roux-en-Y—A surgical connection between the distal end of the small bowel and another organ such as the stomach.

Rugae—Folds of mucosa of organs such as the stomach.

Salivary amylase—An enzyme that initiates the breakdown of starch in the mouth.

Salivary glands—The glands that secrete saliva into the mouth.

Salmonella—A genus of bacteria responsible for many cases of foodborne illness.

Salmonellosis—A bacterial infection manifested by the sudden onset of headache, abdominal pain, diarrhea, nausea, and vomiting. Fever is almost always present. Contaminated food is the predominant method of transmission.

Sarcoma—A malignant neoplasm that occurs in connective tissue such as muscle or bone.

Satiety—The feeling after consuming food that enough has been eaten; the sensation of satisfaction.

Saturated fat—A fat in which the majority of fatty acids contain no carbon-to-carbon double bonds.

Scurvy—Disease due to deficiency of vitamin C marked by bleeding problems and, later, by bony skeleton changes.

Seasonal variation—Refers to differences during spring, summer, fall, and winter.

Sebaceous gland—Oil-secreting gland of the skin; most sebaceous glands have a hair follicle associated with them.

Second-degree relative—A relative sharing one-quarter of an individual's genes; examples: grandparent, grandchild, uncle, aunt, nephew, niece, half-sibling.

Secondary diabetes—A World Health Organization classification for diabetes when the hyperglycemia occurs as a result of another disorder.

Secondary hypertension—High blood pressure that develops as the result of another condition.

Secondary malnutrition—A nutrient deficiency due to improper absorption and distribution of nutrients.

Secondary prevention—Institution of monitoring techniques to discover incipient diseases early to enhance the opportunity to control their effects; nutrition example: testing blood glucose levels to diagnose prediabetes.

Secretin—A hormone that stimulates the production of bile by the liver and the secretion of sodium bicarbonate juice by the pancreas.

Self-efficacy—The extent to which a person believes he or she has the ability to perform a particular task or behavior.

Self-monitoring of blood glucose (SMBG)—A procedure that persons with diabetes follow to test their own blood glucose levels.

Sensible water loss—Visible water loss through perspiration, urine, and feces.

Sensitivity—Characteristic of diagnostic test; the proportion of people correctly identified as having the condition in question; a score of 100% would indicate that all the affected persons were identified by the test.

Sepsis—A condition in which disease-producing organisms are present in the blood.

Sequelae—Conditions following and resulting from a disease; sequel.

Serosa—A serous membrane that covers internal organs and lines body cavities.

Serotonin—A body chemical that assists the transmission of nerve impulses; it produces constriction of blood vessels and is thought to be related to sleep.

Serum—The liquid portion of the blood minus the clotting elements.

Serum transferrin—Globulin in the blood that binds and transports iron; level increases in early iron deficiency, before hemoglobin and hematocrit readings drop.

Shelf life—The duration of time a product can remain in storage without deterioration.

Shigella—Organisms causing intestinal disease; spread by fecal-oral transmission from a client or carrier via direct contact or indirectly by contaminated food.

SIAD (syndrome of inappropriate antidiuresis)—Dilutional hyponatremia resulting from diverse pathologies (central nervous system disorders, certain lung diseases, some tumors, particular drugs). Formerly called syndrome of inappropriate secretion of antidiuretic hormone (SIADH).

Signs—*See* Objective data.

Simple carbohydrate—Composed of one or two units of $C_6H_{12}O_6$; includes the monosaccharides (glucose, fructose, and galactose) and the disaccharides (sucrose, lactose, and maltose).

Simple fat—Lipids that consist of fatty acids or a simple filler such as a hydroxyl (OH) molecule joined to glycerol.

Small for gestational age (SGA)—Infant weighing less at birth than considered normal for the calculated length of the pregnancy.

Small intestine—The part of the alimentary canal between the stomach and the large intestine, where most absorption of nutrients occurs.

Sodium pump—Proteins located in cell membranes that provide an active transport mechanism to move sodium ions across a membrane to their area of greater concentration; moves sodium ions out of the cells and water follows.

Solubility—The ability of one substance to dissolve into another in solution.

Soluble—Able to be dissolved.

Solute—The substance that is dissolved in a solvent.

Solvent—A liquid holding another substance in solution.

Somatostatin—A hormone produced by the delta cells of the islets of Langerhans that inhibits both the release of insulin and the production of glucagon.

Specific gravity—The weight of a substance compared to an equal volume of a standard substance; usual standard for liquids is water; its specific gravity set at 1.000.

Specificity—Characteristic of diagnostic test; the proportion of people correctly identified as not having the condition in question; a score of 100% would indicate that all of the unaffected persons were identified by the test.

Sphincter—A circular band of muscles that constricts a passage.

Spina bifida—Congenital defect in spinal column whereby the vertebrae fail to close; clinical manifestations may or may not include protrusion of the meninges outside the spinal canal.

Spore—A form assumed by some bacteria that is highly resistant to heat, drying, and chemicals.

Sprue—Chronic form of malabsorption syndrome affecting the small intestine; subcategories: tropical and nontropical.

Standard (polymeric) formula—An oral or enteral feeding that contains all the essential nutrients in a specified volume.

Standard drink—0.5 oz. of alcohol found in 12 oz. of beer, 5 oz. of wine, or 1.5 oz. distilled spirits.

Staphylococcus aureus—One of the most common species of bacteria, which produces a poisonous toxin. The main reservoir is nose and throat discharge. Food can act as a vehicle for transmission, so proper hand washing is an essential means of control.

Starches—Polysaccharides; many units of $C_6H_{12}O_6$ joined together; complex carbohydrates.

Steatorrhea—The presence of greater than normal amounts of fat in the stool, producing foul-smelling, bulky excrement.

Sterol—Substance related to fats and belonging to the lipoids; for example, cholesterol.

Stimulus control—The identification of cues that precede a behavior and rearranging daily activities to avoid such cues.

Stoma—A surgically created opening in the abdominal wall.

Stomach—The portion of the alimentary canal between the esophagus and small intestine.

Stomatitis—An inflammation of the mouth.

Stress—Any threat to a person's mental or physical well being.

Stress factor—A number used to predict how much a client's kilocalorie need has increased as a result of a disease state.

Subcutaneously—Beneath the skin.

Subdural hematoma—Collection of blood under the outermost membrane covering the brain and spinal cord; usually resulting from head injury.

Subjective data—Experiences the client reports, also termed symptoms.

Submucosa—Structural layer of the alimentary canal below the mucosa; contains tissues and blood vessels.

Sucrase—An enzyme in the intestinal mucosa that splits sucrose into glucose and fructose.

Sucrose—A disaccharide; one unit of glucose and one unit of fructose joined together; ordinary white table sugar.

Superior vena cava—One of the largest diameter veins in the human body; used to deliver parenteral nutrition.

Supplemental Feeding Program for Women, Infants, and Children (WIC)—Federal program providing nutrition education and supplemental food to low-income pregnant or breastfeeding women and children up to 5 years of age.

Symptoms—*See* Subjective data.

System—An organized grouping of related structures or parts.

Systolic pressure—Pressure exerted against the arteries when the heart contracts; the upper number of the blood pressure reading.

Tapeworm—A parasitic intestinal worm that is acquired by humans through the ingestion of raw seafood or undercooked beef or pork.

Tardive dyskinesia—Neurological syndrome involving involuntary, slow, rhythmic, movements often seen in the mouth and tongue; side effect of psychotropic drugs, especially phenothiazines.

Target heart rate—Seventy percent of maximum heart rate (number of heartbeats per minute); a person's target heart rate can be objectively determined by a stress test. Individuals can estimate their target heart rate by subtracting their age from 220 and multiplying the difference by 70%. A person's target heart rate is the rate at which the pulse should be maintained for at least 20 minutes during aerobic exercise.

Telomerase—enzyme that helps repair cell damage that occurs to the end of the DNA molecule during each cycle of cell division; cancer cells have telomerases that allow infinite repair to the DNA strands, contributing to their immortality.

Teratogenic—Capable of causing abnormal development of the embryo; results in a malformed fetus.

Term infant—One born between the beginning of the 38th week through the 42nd week of gestation.

Tertiary prevention—Use of treatment techniques after a disease has occurred to prevent complications or to promote maximum adaptation; nutrition example: interventions to treat swallowing disorders to maintain nourishment and avoid choking incidents.

Tetany—Muscle contractions, especially of the wrists and ankles, resulting from low levels of ionized calcium in the blood; causes include parathyroid deficiency, vitamin D deficiency, and alkalosis.

Therapeutic index—Maximum tolerated dose of a drug divided by the minimum curative dose; a narrow index indicates greater potential for adverse side effects.

Thermic effect of exercise (TEE)—The number of kilocalories used above resting energy expenditure as a result of physical activity.

Thermic effect of foods (diet-induced thermogenesis, specific-dynamic action)—The energy cost to extract and utilize the kilocalories and nutrients in foods; the heat produced after eating a meal.

Thiamin—Coenzyme in the metabolism of carbohydrates and fats; vitamin B_1.

Thiaminase—An enzyme in raw fish that destroys thiamin.

Third-space losses—Sequestering of fluid in body cavities such as the chest and abdomen; in the abdominal cavity, it produces ascites.

Thoracic—Pertaining to the chest, or thorax.

Threonine—Essential amino acid often lacking in grains.

Thrombus—A blood clot that obstructs a blood vessel; obstruction of a vessel of the brain or heart is among the most serious effects.

Thrush—An infection caused by the organism *Candida albicans;* characterized by the formation of white patches and ulcers in the mouth and throat.

Thymus—Gland in the chest, above and in front of the heart, that contributes to the immune response, including the maturation of T-lymphocytes.

Thyroid-stimulating hormone (TSH)—A hormone secreted by the pituitary gland that stimulates the thyroid gland to secrete thyroxine and triiodothyronine; thyrotropin.

Thyrotropin-releasing factor (TRF)—Stimulates the secretion of thyroid-stimulating hormone; produced in the hypothalamus.

Thyroxine (T_4)—A hormone secreted by the thyroid gland; increases the rate of metabolism and energy production.

Tissue—A group or collection of similar cells and their similar intercellular substance that acts together in the performance of a particular function.

T-lymphocytes (T-cells)—White blood cells that recognize and fight foreign cells such as cancer; thymic lymphocytes.

Tolerable Upper Intake Level (UL)—Highest average daily intake by an individual that is unlikely to pose risks of adverse health effects in 97% to 98% of individuals in specified life-stage and gender group; ordinarily refers to intake from food, fortified food, water, and supplements.

Tolerance level—The highest dose at which a residue causes no ill effects in laboratory animals.

Toxoplasmosis—Infection with the protozoan *Toxoplasma gondii;* when infected in utero, infant may suffer mental retardation, blindness, and epilepsy.

Trace minerals—Those present in the body in amounts less than 5 grams; daily intake of less than 100 milligrams needed; also called microminerals or trace elements.

Traction—The process of using weights to draw a part of the body into alignment.

Transcellular fluid—Located in body cavities and spaces; constantly being secreted and absorbed; examples: cerebrospinal fluid, pericardial fluid, pleural fluid.

Transferrin—Protein in the blood that binds and transports iron.

Trauma—A physical injury or wound caused by an external force; an emotional or psychological shock that usually results in disordered behavior.

Triceps skinfold—Measure of skin and subcutaneous tissue over the triceps muscle in the upper arm; used in body fat assessment.

Trichinella spiralis—A wormlike parasite that becomes embedded in the muscle tissue of pork.

Trichinosis—The infestation of *Trichinella spiralis,* a parasitic roundworm, transmitted by eating raw or insufficiently cooked pork.

Triglyceride—Three fatty acids joined to a glycerol molecule.

Triiodothyronine (T_3)—A hormone secreted by the thyroid gland that increases the rate of metabolism and energy production.

Trousseau sign—Spasms of the forearm and hand upon inflation of the blood pressure cuff; sign of tetany or lack of ionized calcium in the blood.

Trust—First stage of Erikson's theory of psychosocial development, in which the infant learns to rely on those caring for it.

Trypsin—An enzyme formed in the intestine that assists in protein digestion.

Tryptophan—An essential amino acid, often lacking in legumes; serves as provitamin for the production of niacin by the liver.

Tubular reabsorption—The movement of fluid back into the blood from the renal tubule.

Tubule—A small tube or canal.

Tumor suppressor gene—Gene that inhibits growth and division of the cell.

Turgor—Resilience of skin; when pinched, quickly returns to original shape in well-hydrated young person; test for deficient fluid volume that is not reliable for elderly clients.

Type 1 diabetes—Persons with this disorder must take insulin to survive and are prone to ketoacidosis; formerly called insulin-dependent diabetes mellitus (IDDM) and juvenile diabetes.

Type 2 diabetes—Although some persons with this disorder take insulin, it is not necessary for their survival; formerly called non–insulin-dependent diabetes (NIDDM) and adult-onset diabetes mellitus.

Tyramine—A monoamine present in various foods that will provoke a hypertensive crisis in persons taking monoamine oxidase inhibitors (MAOIs).

Ulcer—An open sore or lesion of the skin or mucous membrane.

Ulcerative colitis—Inflammatory disease of the large intestine that usually begins in the rectum and spreads upward in a continuous pattern.

Ultrasound bone densitometer—Machine that uses sound waves to estimate bone density as a screening test.

Uncomplicated starvation—A food deprivation without an underlying stress state.

Undernutrition—The state that results from a deficiency of one or more nutrients.

Underwater weighing—Most accurate measure of body fatness.

Universal precautions—A list of procedures developed by the Centers for Disease Control and Prevention for when blood and certain other body fluids should be considered contaminated and treated as such.

Unsaturated fat—A fat in which the majority of fatty acids contain one or more carbon-to-carbon double bonds.

Urea—The chief nitrogenous constituent of urine; the final product, along with CO_2, of protein metabolism.

Uremia—A toxic condition produced by the retention of nitrogen-containing substances normally excreted by the kidneys.

Ureter—The tube that carries urine from the kidney to the bladder.

Urinary calculus—A kidney stone, or deposit of mineral salts.

Urinary tract infection (UTI)—The condition in which disease-producing microorganisms invade a client's bladder, ureter, or urethra.

USDA Dietary Guidelines—Guidelines for health promotion issued by the U.S. Department of Agriculture and U.S. Department Health and Human Services; revised in 2010.

U.S. Pharmacopeia (USP)—Compendium of standards of strength and purity for drugs; issued and revised periodically by a national committee.

Usual food intake—A description of what a person habitually eats.

Vaginitis—Inflammation of the vagina, most often caused by an infectious agent.

Vagotomy—surgical cutting of vagus nerve to reduce gastric acid secretion; achieving similar results by the use of medications is termed medical vagotomy.

Vasopressin—Antidiuretic hormone; abbreviated ADH.

Ventilation—Process by which gases are moved into and out of the lungs; two aspects of ventilation are inhalation and exhalation.

Very low-calorie diet (VLCD)—Diet that contains less than 800 kilocalories per day.

Very low-density lipoprotein (VLDL)—A plasma protein containing mostly triglycerides with small amounts of cholesterol, phospholipid, and protein; transports triglycerides from the liver to tissues.

Villi—Multiple minute projections on the surface of the folds of the small intestine that absorb fluid and nutrients; plural of villus.

Virus—Very small noncellular parasite that is entirely dependent on the nutrients inside host cells for its metabolic and reproductive needs.

Viscera—Internal organs enclosed in a cavity.

Visible fat—Dietary fat that can be easily seen, such as the fat on meat or in oil.

Vitamin—Organic substance needed by the body in very small amounts; yields no energy and does not become part of the body's structure.

Waist-to-hip ratio (WHR)—Waist measurement divided by hip measurement; if greater than 0.8 in women or greater than 0.95 in men, indicates increased risk of health problems related to obesity.

Warfarin—Anticoagulant that interferes with the liver's synthesis of vitamin K–dependent clotting factors II, VII, IX, and X.

Water intoxication—Excess intake or abnormal retention of water.

Weight cycling—The repeated gain and loss of body weight.

Wernicke–Korsakoff syndrome—A disorder of the central nervous system resulting from thiamine deficiency; often seen in chronic alcoholism; signs and symptoms include motor, sensory, and memory deficits.

Wernicke encephalopathy—Inflammatory, hemorrhagic, degenerative lesions in several areas of the brain resulting in double vision, involuntary eye movements, lack of muscle coordination, and mental deficits; caused by thiamin deficiency, often seen in chronic alcoholism but also in gastrointestinal tract disease and hyperemesis gravidarum.

Whey—Component of milk; in human milk, contains soluble proteins that are easily digested; major whey protein in breast milk is alpha-lactalbumin, with an amino acid pattern much like that of the body tissues.

Whipple procedure—Pancreatoduodenectomy; surgical procedure for cancer of the head of the pancreas; removal of the head of the pancreas, lower portion of common bile duct, most of duodenum, and possibly part of stomach.

WIC—*See* Supplemental Feeding Program for Women, Infants, and Children.

Wilson disease—Rare genetic defect of copper metabolism that permits copper to accumulate in various organs; inherited as an autosomal recessive trait.

Xerophthalmia—Drying and thickening of the epithelial tissues of the eye; can be caused by vitamin A deficiency.

Xerostomia—Dry mouth caused by decreased salivary secretions.

X-linked inheritance—Hereditary pattern involving a gene on the X chromosome; in females, a dominant gene or two recessive genes will cause the trait to be manifested; in males, with only one X chromosome, the trait will be manifested whether the gene is dominant or recessive.

APPENDIX E Bibliography

Chapter 1

Academy of Nutrition and Dietetics: Position of the Academy of Nutrition and Dietetics: Functional Foods. J Am Diet Assoc 113: 1096, 2013.

Ahluwalia, IB, D'Angelo, D, Morrow, B, and McDonald, JA: Association between acculturation and breastfeeding among Hispanic women: data from the pregnancy risk assessment and monitoring system. J Hum Lact 28:167, 2012.

American Dietetic Association: Choose Your Foods: Exchange Lists for Diabetes. Chicago, American Dietetic Association, 2008.

American Dietetic Association: Food nutrient data for choose your foods: exchange lists for diabetes, 2007. Accessed August 20, 2013. Available at www.eatright. org/search.aspx?search=Exchange%20lists

American Dietetic Association: Position of the American Dietetic Association: Functional Foods. J Am Diet Assoc 109:735, 2009.

Bliss, RM: Fully cooked emergency aid food. Agricultural Res 59:4, 2011.

Bliss, RM: Monitoring food-supply nutrients. Agricultural Res 60:8, 2012.

Boone-Heinonen, J, Gordon-Larsen, P, Kiefe, CI, et al: Fast food restaurants and food stores: longitudinal associations with diet in young to middle-aged adults: the CARDIA study. Arch Intern Med 171:1162, 2011.

Brambila-Macias, J, Shankar, B, Capacci, S, et al: Policy interventions to promote healthy eating: A review of what works, what does not, and what is promising. Food Nutr Bull 32:365, 2011.

Brown, L, Edwards, J, and Hartwell, H, A taste of the unfamiliar. Understanding the meanings attached to food by international postgraduate students in England. Appetite 54:202, 2010.

Brunner, HG: The variability of genetic disease. N Eng J Med 367:1350, 2012.

Buzzell, PR, and Pintauro, SJ: Bioelectrical impedance analysis interactive tutorial. University of Vermont Department of Nutrition and Food Sciences. Accessed July 17, 2012. Available at nutrition.uvm.edu/bodycomp/bia/lesson4.html

Caccialanza, R, Klersy, C, Cereda, E, et al: Nutritional parameters associated with prolonged hospital stay among ambulatory adult patients. CMAJ 182:1843, 2010. Accessed July 9, 2012. Available at www.ncbi. nlm.nih.gov/pubmed/20940233

Center for School, Health and Education: Understanding hunger and obesity and the role for school-based health care. American Public Health Association, Washington, DC, September 2011. Accessed July 11, 2012. Available at www.schoolbasedhealthcare.org/WP-content/uploads/2011/09/APHA4_article_HungerObesity_9_14_FINAL2.pdf

Centers for Disease Control and Prevention: Fact Sheet: Trends in diabetes prevalence among American Indian and Alaska native children, adolescents, and young adults—1990–1998. Diabetes Public Health Resource, Updated May 20, 2011. Accessed July 24, 2012. Available at www.cdc.gov/diabetes/pubs/factsheets/aian.htm

Centers for Disease Control and Prevention: Quick stats: life expectancy at birth, by race and sex—United States, 1970–2007. Morb Mortal Wkly Rep 59:1185, September 17, 2010. Accessed December 12, 2012. Available at www.cdc.gov/mmwr/preview/mmwrhtml/mm5936a9. htm?s_cid=mm5936a9_e

Centers for Disease Control and Prevention: State-specific trends in fruit and vegetable consumption among adults—United States, 2000—2009. Morb Mortal Wkly Rep 59:1125, September 10, 2010. Accessed December 12, 2012. Available at www.cdc.gov/mmwr/preview/mmwrhtml/mm5935a1.htm?s_cid=mm5935a1_e

Coleman-Jensen, A, Nord, M, Andrews, M, and Carlson, S: Household Food Security in the United States in 2010 (ERR-125). U.S. Department of Agriculture Economic Research Service, Washington, DC, September 2011. Accessed July 10, 2012. Available at www.ers.usda. gov/media/121076/err125_2_.pdf

Crowe, KN, and Francis, C: Position of the Academy of Nutrition and Dietetics: functional foods. J Acad Nutr Diet. 113, 1096, 2013.

Dubock, A: Genetically modified foods: scientific perspective and controversies. Albert Einstein College of Medicine Continuing Medical Education. Accessed December 4, 2012. Available at www.cyberounds.com/cmecontent/art508.html

Durham, S, and Avant, S: ARS and CGIAR: Working to provide international food security. Agricultural Research 59:4, 2011.

Ely, JJ, Zavaskis, T, and Wilson, SL: Diabetes and stress: an anthropological review for study of modernizing populations in the US-Mexico border region. Rural and Remote Health 11:1758, 2011. Accessed July 23, 2012. Available at www.ncbi.nlm.nih.gov/pubmed/21905760

Fanzo, JC, and Pronyk, PM: A review of global progress toward the Millennium Development Goal 1 hunger target. Food Nutr Bull 32:144, 2011.

Fong, M, Braun, KL, and Tsark, JU: Improving Native Hawaiian health through community-based participatory research. Californian J Health Promotion 1(Special Issue: Hawaii), 132, 2003.

Gavrilova, NS, and Gavrilov, LA: Search for mechanisms of exceptional human longevity. Rejuvenation Res 13:262, 2010.

Going, S, Hingle, M, and Farr, J: Body composition. In Ross, AC, Caballero, B, Cousins, RJ, et al (eds): Modern Nutrition in Health and Disease, ed 11. Lippincott Williams & Wilkins, Philadelphia, 2014.

Gropper, SS, and Smith, JL: Advanced Nutrition and Human Metabolism, ed 6. Wadsworth, Belmont, CA, 2013.

Gunderson, C: Food assistance programs. In Ross, AC, Caballero, B, Cousins, RJ, et al (eds): Modern Nutrition in Health and Disease, ed 11. Lippincott Williams & Wilkins, Philadelphia, 2014.

Hagey, R: The phenomenon, the explanations and the responses: Metaphors surrounding diabetes in urban Canadian Indians. Soc Sci Med 18:265, 1984.

Hausman, DB, Fischer, JG, and Johnson, MA: Nutrition in centenarians. Maturitas 68:203, 2011.

Jackson, LE: Understanding, eliciting and negotiating clients' multicultural health beliefs. Nurse Pract 18:30, 1993.

Jacquier, C, Bonthoux, F, Baciu, M, and Ruffieux, B: Improving the effectiveness of nutritional information policies: assessment of unconscious pleasure mechanisms involved in food-choice decisions. Nutr Rev 70:118, 2012.

Kanwar, J, Taskeen, M, Mohammad, I, Huo, C, et al: Recent advances on tea polyphenols. Front Biosci (Elite Ed) 4: 111, 2012.

Kovacevich, DS, Boney, AR, Braunschweig, CL, et al: Nutrition risk classification: A reproducible and valid tool for nurses. Nutr Clin Pract 12:20, 1997.

Lee, H: The role of local food availability in explaining obesity risk among young school-aged children. Soc Sci Med 74:1193, 2012.

Li, Y, Kong, D, Bao, B, Ahmad, A, et al: Induction of cancer cell death by isoflavone: the role of multiple signaling pathways. Nutrients 3:877, 2011.

Liu, B, Mao, Q, Cao, M, and Xie, L: Cruciferous vegetables intake and risk of prostate cancer: a meta-analysis. Int J Urol 19:134, 2012.

Majewska-Wierzbicka, M, and Czeczot, H: [Flavonoids in the prevention and treatment of cardiovascular diseases]. Pol Merku Lekarski 32:50, 2012.

Mechanick, JI, Marchetti, AE, Apovian, C, and Benchimol, AK: Diabetes-specific nutrition algorithm: a transcultural program to optimize diabetes and prediabetes care. Curr Diab Rep 12:180, 2012.

Milner, J, Toner, C, and Davis, CD: Functional foods and nutraceuticals in health promotion. In Ross, AC, Caballero, B, Cousins, RJ, et al (eds): Modern Nutrition in Health and Disease, ed 11. Lippincott Williams & Wilkins, Philadelphia, 2014.

Moran, JM, Lavado-Garcia, JM, and Pedrera-Zamorano, JD: Methods for nurses to measure body composition. Rev Lat Am Enfermagem 19:1033, 2011.

Nicoletti, M: Nutraceuticals and botanicals: overview and perspectives. Int J Food Sci Nutr 63 Suppl 2, 2012.

O'Brien, D: ARS in Africa: building trust and fighting poverty. Agricultural Res 59: 16, 2011.

O'Brien, D: Corn: boosting vitamin A levels in corn to fight hunger. Agricultural Res 58: 12, 2010.

Ordovas, JM, Kaput, J, and Corella, D: Nutrition in the genomics era: cardiovascular disease risk and the Mediterranean diet. Mol Nutr Food Res 51:1293, 2007.

Othman, RA, Moghadasian, MH, and Jones, PJ: Cholesterol-lowering effects of oat β-glucan. Nutr Rev 69:299, 2011.

Padela, AI, Gunter, K, Killawi, A, and Heisler, M: Religious values and healthcare accommodations: voices from the American Muslim community. J Gen Intern Med 27: 708, 2012.

Pignolo, RJ: Exceptional human longevity. Cyberounds CME, July 12, 2010. Accessed April 14, 2012. Available at www.cyberounds.com/cmecontent/art475.html?pf=yes

Purnell, LD: Transcultural Health Care: A Culturally Competent Appoach, ed 4. FA Davis, Philadelphia, 2013.

Rasmussen, LG, Winning, H, Savorani, F, et al: Assessment of the effect of high or low protein diet on the human urine metabolome as measured by NMR. Nutrients 4:112, 2012.

Riscuta, G, and Dumitrescu, RG: Nutrigenomics: implications for breast and colon cancer prevention. Methods Mol Biol 863:343, 2012.

Ronald, P: Plant genetics, sustainable agriculture and global food security. Genetics 188:11, 2011.

Rosenmoller, DL, Gasevic, D, Seidell, J, and Lear, SA: Determinants of changes in dietary patterns among Chinese immigrants: a cross-sectional analysis. Int J Behav Nutr Phys Act 8:42, 2011. Accessed July 29, 2012. Available at www.ncbi.nlm.nih.gov/pmc/articles/PMC3118129/?tool=pubmed

Sayre, R, Beeching, JR, Cahoon, EB, Egesi, C, et al: The BioCassava plus program: biofortification of cassava for sub-Saharan Africa. Annu Rev Plant Biol 62:251, 2011.

Seeram, NP: Berry fruits for cancer prevention: current status and future prospects. J Agric Food Chem 56:630, 2008.

Shintani, T, Beckham, S, Tang, BS, et al: Waianae Diet Program: long-term follow-up. Hawaii Med J 58:117, 1999.

Shintani, TT, Hughes, CK, Beckham, S, and O'Connor, HK: Obesity and cardiovascular risk intervention through the ad libitum feeding of traditional Hawaiian diet. Am J Clin Nutr 53:1647S, 1991.

Sowattanangoon, N, Kochabhakdi, N, and Petrie, KJ: Buddhist values are associated with better diabetes control in Thai patients. Int J Psychiatry Med 38:481, 2008.

Stoltzfus, RJ: Iron interventions for women and children in low-income countries. J Nutr 141:756S, 2011.

Uauy, R, Hawkesworth, S, and Dangour, AD: Food-based dietary guidelines for healthier populations: international considerations. In Ross, AC, Caballero, B, Cousins, RJ, et al (eds): Modern Nutrition in Health and Disease, ed 11. Lippincott Williams & Wilkins, Philadelphia, 2014.

U.S. Department of Agriculture: MyPlate style guide and conditions of use for the icon. Washington, DC, June 2011.

U.S. Department of Agriculture and U.S. Department of Health and Human Services: Dietary Guidelines for Americans, ed 7. U.S. Government Printing Office, Washington, DC, 2010.

U.S. Department of Health and Human Services: National standards on culturally and linguistically appropriate services (CLAS). April 12, 2007. Accessed July 23, 2012. Available at minorityhealth.hhs.gov/templates/browse.aspx?lvl=2&lvlID=15

U.S. Food and Drug Administration: Food Standards Under the 1938 Food, Drug, and Cosmetic Act: Bread and Jam. Updated April 14, 2009. Accessed December 12, 2012. Available at www.fda.gov/AboutFDA/WhatWeDo/History/ProductRegulation/ucm132892.htm

Velasco C, García E, Rodríguez V, Frias L, et al: Comparison of four nutritional screening tools to detect nutritional risk in hospitalized patients: a multicentre study. Eur J Clin Nutr 65:269, 2011.

Wang, Y, Lim, H, and Caballero, B: Use and interpretation of anthropometry. In Ross, AC, Caballero, B, Cousins, RJ, et al (eds): Modern Nutrition in Health and Disease, ed 11. Lippincott Williams & Wilkins, Philadelphia, 2014.

Widener, MJ, Metcalf, SS, and Bar-Yam, Y: Developing a mobile produce distribution system for low-income urban residents in food deserts. J Urban Health 89:733, 2012.

Wood, M: What's in your blood? The ongoing hunt for metabolites. Agricultural Res 60: 10, 2012.

World Food Program: Facts blast. May 2011. Accessed July 12, 2012. Available at http://documents.wfp.org/stellent/groups/public/documents/communications/wfp187701.pdf

Yao, S, and Flores, A: Improving rice, a staple crop worldwide. Agricultural Res 58:4, 2010.

Yates, AA: Dietary Reference Intakes: rationale and applications. In Shils, ME, Shike, M, Ross, AC, et al (eds): Modern Nutrition in Health and Disease, ed 10. Lippincott Williams & Wilkins, Philadelphia, 2006.

Zhang, Y: The molecular basis that unifies the metabolism, cellular uptake and chemopreventive activities of dietary isothiocyanates. Carcinogenesis 33:2, 2012.

Chapter 2

Academy of Nutrition and Dietetics Position Paper: Use of Nutritive and Nonnutritive Sweeteners. J Acad Nutr Diet 112:5, 2012.

American Dietetic Association: ADA's nutrition trends survey result. J Am Diet Assoc 102:7(Suppl), 2002.

American Dietetic Association Position Paper: Health Implications of Dietary Fiber, J Am Diet Assoc 108:10, 2008.

American Diabetes Association and American Dietetic Association: Exchange lists for meal planning. American Dietetic Association, Alexandria, VA, 2003.

American Diabetes Association and American Dietetic Association: Choose Your Foods: Exchange Lists for Diabetes. American Dietetic Association, Alexandria, VA, 2009.

Aspartame Information Center. Accessed June 2008. Available at www.aspartame.org

Bachman, JL, et al: Sources of food group intakes among the U.S. population, 2001–2002. J Am Diet Assoc 108: 804, 2008.

Duyff, LD: American Dietetic Association Complete Food and Nutrition Guide, ed 2. John Wiley and Sons, Hoboken, NJ, 2002.

Ervin, RB, and Ogden, CL: Consumption of added sugars among US adults, 2005–2010, NCHS Data Brief Number 122, May 2013.

Food and Nutrition Board, National Academy of Science, Institute of Medicine: Dietary Reference Intakes for Energy, Carbohydrate, Fiber, Fat, Fatty Acids, Cholesterol, Protein, and Amino Acids. National Academy Press, Washington, DC, 2005.

Fowler, MJ: Classification of diabetes: not all hypoglycemia is the same. Clin Diabetes 25:74, 2007.

Goran, M: High fructose corn syrup and diabetes prevalence: a global perspective. Global Public Health, November 27, 2012.

Gottschlich, MM (ed): The A.S.P.E.N. Nutrition Support Core Curriculum: A Case-based Approach—The Adult Patient. American Society for Parenteral and Enteral Nutrition, Silver Spring, MD, 2007.

Holt, R, Roberts, G, and Scully, C: Dental damage, sequelae, and prevention. BMJ 320:1719, 2000.

Korol, DL: Enhancing cognitive function across the life span. Ann N Y Acad Sci 959:167, 2002.

Nielson, SJ, and Popkin, BM: Patterns and trends in food portion sizes, 1977–1998. JAMA 289:450, 2003.

Roberts, RO, Roberts, LA, Geda, YE, et al: Relative intake of macronutrients impacts risk of mild cognitive impairment or dementia. J Alzheimers Dis 32:329, 2012.

Uhlman, M, and Ridder, K: Nutrition information, questionable serving sizes confuse Americans. Salt Lake City Tribune, October 20, 2002.

U.S. Department of Agriculture: Continuing survey of food intake by individuals, 1994–1996. Accessed April 2005. Available at www.usda.gov.

U.S. Department of Agriculture: Dietary Guidelines for Americans 2010. Accessed October 2012. Available at www.dietaryguidelines.gov.

U.S. Department of Agriculture: MyPlate. Accessed October 2012. Available at www.ChooseMyPlate.gov.

U.S. Department of Agriculture: FDA food labeling Guide 2009. Accessed October 2012. Available at www.fda.gov/Food/GuidanceRegulation/GuidanceDocumentsRegulatoryInformation/LabelingNutrition/ucm2006828.htm

Valeo, T: Controlling blood glucose may fend off cognitive decline. The Dana Foundation, 2009 podcast transcript. Accessed October 2012. Available at www.dana.org/Publications/Brainwork/Details.aspx?id=43776

Weight Control Information Network, National Institute of Diabetes and Digestive and Kidney Diseases: Weight-loss and nutrition myths, how much do you really know? (Publication No. 04-4561). March 2009. Accessed March 2013. Available at www.win.niddk.nih.gov/publications/PDFs/Myths.pdf

Yaffe, K, Blackwell, T, Kanaya, AM, et al: Diabetes, impaired fasting glucose and development of cognitive impairment in older women. Neurology 63, 658, 2004.

Chapter 3

Agricultural Research Service Dietary Guidelines Committee: Dietary Guidelines for Americans 2000. Accessed December 2012. Available at www.ars.usda.gov/dgac

American Dietetic Association: International Dietetics and Nutrition Terminology (IDNT) Reference Manual. American Dietetic Association, Chicago, 2008.

American Dietetic and Diabetic Associations: Exchange Lists for Meal Planning. American Dietetic Association, Chicago, 2003.

Blundell, JE, and Stubbs, J: Diet composition and the control of food intake in humans. In Bray, GA,

Bouchard, C (eds): Handbook of Obesity: Etiology and Pathophysiology. Marcel Dekker, New York, 2004.

Caballero, B: A nutrition paradox—underweight and obesity in developing countries. N Engl J Med 352:1514, 2005.

Carlson, A, and Frazao, E: Are healthy foods really more expensive? It depends on how you measure the price. USDA Economic Information Bulletin Number 96, May 2012.

Centers for Disease Control and Prevention, Polyunsaturated Fats and Monounsaturated Fats. Accessed December 2012. Available at www.cdc.govnutrition/everyone/basics/fat/unsaturatedfat.html..

Chanmugan, P, Guthrie, JF, Cecilio, S, et al: Did fat intake in the United States really decline between 1989–1991 and 1994–1996? J Am Diet Assoc 103:867, 2003.

Cunningham, E, and Marason, W: Should my client's diet contain plant sterol/sterol esters to lower cholesterol? J Am Diet Assoc 102:81, 2002.

Dausch, J: Trans-fatty acids: A regulatory update. J Am Diet Assoc 102:18, 2002.

Food and Nutrition Board, Institute of Medicine: Dietary Reference Intakes for Energy, Carbohydrate, Fiber, Fat, Fatty Acids, Cholesterol, Protein, and Amino Acids. National Academy Press, Washington, DC, 2002/2005.

Frisardi, V, Panza, F, Seripa, D, Imbimbo, BP, et al: Nutraceutical properties of Mediterranean diet and cognitive decline: possible underlying mechanisms. J Alzheimers Dis. 22(3):715, 2010.

Gottschlich, MM (ed): The A.S.P.E.N. nutrition support core curriculum: A case-based approach—the adult patient. American Society for Parenteral and Enteral Nutrition, Silver Spring, MD, 2007.

Hise, ME, and Brown, JC: Lipids. In The A.S.P.E.N. nutrition support core curriculum: A case-based approach—the adult patient. American Society for Parenteral and Enteral Nutrition, Silver Spring, MD, 2007.

International Food Information Council (IFIC) and The Food and Drug Administration (FDA): The benefits of balance: Managing fat in your diet. International Food Information Council and Food and Drug Administration, Washington, DC, 1998.

Kendler, BS: Recent nutritional approaches to the prevention and therapy of cardiovascular disease. Prog Cardiovasc Nurs 12:3, 1997.

Koletzko, B, Baker, S, Cleghorn, G, Neto, UF, et al: Global Standard for the Composition of Infant Formula: Recommendations of an ES,PGHAN Coordinated International Expert Group. J Pediatric Gastroent and Nutr, 41:584, 2005.

Lichtenstein, AH: Trans fatty acids and hydrogenated fat: What do we know? Nutr Today 30:102, 1995.

Lichtenstein, AH, Kennedy, E, Barrier, P, et al: Dietary fat consumption and health. Nutr Rev 56:53, 1998.

Morris, MC: Consumption of fish and n-3 fatty acids and risk of incident Alzheimer disease. Arch Neurol 60:940, 2003.

National Institutes of Health, National Heart, Lung, and Blood Institute: Clinical Guidelines on the Identification and Treatment of Overweight and Obesity in Adults. U.S. Department of Health and Human Services, Bethesda, MD, 1998.

Pearson, TA, Blair, SN, Daniels, SR, et al: AHA Guidelines for Primary Prevention of Cardiovascular Disease and Stroke: 2002 Update. Consensus panel guide to comprehensive risk reduction for adult patients without coronary or other vascular diseases. Circulation 106: 388, 2002.

Roberts, RO, Cerhan, JR, Geda, YE, Knopman, DS, et al: Polyunsaturated fatty acids and reduced odds of MC,I: the Mayo Clinic Study of Aging. J Alzheimers Dis, 21(3):853, 2010.

Solfrizzi, V, Panza, F, Frisardi, V, Seripa, D, et al: Diet and Alzheimer's disease risk factors or prevention: the current evidence. Expert Rev. Neurother. 11(5):677, 2011.

Tucker, KL, Hallfrisch, J, Qiao, N, et al: The combination of high fruit and vegetable and low saturated fat intakes is more protective against mortality in aging men than is either alone: Baltimore longitudinal study of aging. J Nutr 135:556, 2005.

U.S. Department of Agriculture: Dietary Guidelines for Americans, 2010. Accessed August 6, 2012. Available at www.usda.gov/dietaryguidelines/dga

U.S. Department of Agriculture: Dietary saturated fat and cardiovascular health: A review of the evidence. Nutrition Insights 44, 2011.

U.S. Department of Agriculture, Center for Nutrition Policy and Health Promotion: Nutrition insights: The role of nuts in a healthy diet. Accessed December 2008. Available at www.usda.gov/cnpp

World Health Organization: Years of healthy life can be increased 5–10 years. Accessed December 2012. Available at www.who.int/mediacentre/releases/pr84/en/print.html

Wiese, HF, Hansen, AE, and Adam, DJD: Essential fatty acids in infant nutrition. J Nutr 58:345, 1958.

Willett, WC: Diet, nutrition, and the prevention of cancer. In Shils, ME (ed): Modern Nutrition in Health and Disease, ed 9. Williams & Wilkins, Baltimore, 1999.

Chapter 4

American Dietetic Association: Exchange lists for Diabetes American Dietetic Association, Chicago, 2008.

American Dietetic Association: Food nutrient data for choose your foods: exchange lists for diabetes, 2007. Accessed December 6, 2012. Available at www.eatright.org/search.aspx?search=Exchange%20lists

Amit, M: Vegetarian diets in children and adolescents. Paediatr Child Health 15:303, 2010.

Atherton, PJ, Etheridge, T, Watt, PW, et al: Muscle full effect after oral protein: time-dependent concordance and discordance between human muscle protein synthesis and mTORC1 signaling. Am J Clin Nutr 92:1080, 2010.

Benson, JM, and Therrell, BL, Jr: History and current status of newborn screening for hemoglobinopathies. Semin Perinatol 34:134, 2010.

Benton, MJ, Whyte, MD, and Dyal, BW: Sarcopenic obesity: strategies for management. Am J Nurs 111: 38, 2011.

Blau, N, van Spronsen, FJ, and Levy, HL: Phenylketonuria. Lancet. 376:1417, 2010.

Bouchlariotou, S, Tsikouras, P, and Maroulis, G: Undiagnosed maternal phenylketonuria: Own clinical experience and literature review. J Matern Fetal Neonatal Med 22:943, 2009.

Bradbury, JH, Cliff, J, and Denton, IC: Uptake of wetting method in Africa to reduce cyanide poisoning and konzo from cassava. Food Chem Toxicol 49:539, 2011.

Breen, L, and Phillips, SM: Nutrient interaction for optimal protein anabolism in resistance exercise. Curr Opin Clin Nutr Metab Care 15:226, 2012.

Brooks, N, Cloutier, GJ, Cadena, SM, et al: Resistance training and timed essential amino acids protect against the loss of muscle mass and strength during 28 days of bed rest and energy deficit. J Appl Physiol 105:241, 2008.

Camp, KM, Lloyd-Puryear, MA, and Huntington, KL: Nutritional treatment for inborn errors of metabolism: indications, regulations, and availability of medical foods and dietary supplements using phenylketonuria as an example. Mol Genet Metab. 107:3, 2012.

Carvalho, NF, Kenney, RD, Carrington, PH, and Hall, DE: Severe nutritional deficiencies in toddlers resulting from health food milk alternatives. Pediatrics 107:E46, 2001.

Centers for Disease Control and Prevention: Announcement: Sickle Cell Awareness Month—September, 2010. Morb Mortal Wkly Rep 59:1147, September 10, 2010. Accessed November 17, 2012. Available at www.cdc.gov/mmwr/preview/mmwrhtml/mm5935a5.htm?s_cid=mm5935a5_e

Centers for Disease Control and Prevention: Data and Statistics. Updated September 16, 2011. Accessed November 17, 2012. Available at www.cdc.gov/NCBDDD/sicklecell/data.html

Cliff, J, Muquingue, H, Nhassico, D, et al: Konzo and continuing cyanide intoxication from cassava in Mozambique. Food Chem Toxicol 49:631, 2011.

Debaun, MR, and Telfair, J: Transition and sickle cell disease. Pediatrics 130:926, 2012.

Elsas, LJ, and Acosta, PB: Inherited metabolic disease: amino acids, organic acids, and galactose. In Ross, AC, Caballero, B, Cousins, RJ, et al (eds): Modern Nutrition in Health and Disease, ed 11. Lippincott Williams & Wilkins, Philadelphia, 2014.

Evans, WJ: Skeletal muscle loss: cachexia, sarcopenia, and inactivity. Am J Clin Nutr 91:1123S, 2010.

Fong, C-T: Amino acid and organic acid metabolism disorders. Merck Manual, February 2010. Accessed November 22, 2012. Available at www.merckmanuals.com/professional/pediatrics/inherited_disorders_of_metabolism/amino_acid_and_organic_acid_metabolism_disorders.html#v1100917

Fourreau, D, Peretti, N, Hengy, B, et al: Pediatric nutrition: Severe deficiency complications by using vegetable beverages, four cases report [article in French]. Presse Med 42:e37, 2013.

Gropper, SS, and Smith, JL: Advanced Nutrition and Human Metabolism, ed 6. Wadsworth, Belmont, CA, 2013.

Guo, JJ, Yang H, Qian, H, et al: The effects of different nutritional measurements on delayed wound healing after hip fracture in the elderly. J Surg Res 159:503, 2010.

Hanley, WB: Finding the fertile woman with phenylketonuria. Eur J Obstet Gynecol Reprod Biol 137:131, 2008.

Harmon, KG, Drezner, JA, Klossner, D, and Asif, IM: Sickle cell trait associated with a RR, of death of 37 times in National Collegiate Athletic Association football athletes: a database with 2 million athlete-years as the denominator. Br J Sports Med 46:325, 2012.

Hughes, GJ, Ryan, DJ, Mukherjea, R, and Schasteen, CS: Protein digestibility-corrected amino acid scores (PDCAAS) for soy protein isolates and concentrate: criteria for evaluation. J Agric Food Chem 59:12707, 2011.

Katayama, M, and Wilson, LA: Utilization of soybeans and their components through the development of textured soy protein foods. J Food Sci 73:S158, 2008.

Katz, KA, Mahlberg, MJ, Honig, PJ, and Yan, AC: Rice nightmare: kwashiorkor in two Philadelphia-area infants fed Rice Dream beverage. J Am Acad Dermatol 52:S69, 2005.

Koch, R: Maternal phenylketonuria and tetrahydrobiopterin. Pediatrics 122:1367, 2008.

Koch, R, Moseley, K, and Guttler, F: Tetrahydrobiopterin and maternal PK,U. Mol Genet Metab 86:S139, 2005.

Matthews, DE: Proteins and amino acids. In Ross, AC, Caballero, B, Cousins, RJ, et al (eds): Modern Nutrition in Health and Disease, ed 11. Lippincott Williams & Wilkins, Philadelphia, 2014.

Mazariegos, GV, Morton, DH, Sindhi, R, et al: Liver transplantation for classical maple syrup urine disease: long-term follow-up in 37 patients and comparative United Network for Organ Sharing experience. J Pediatr 160:116, 2012.

Mitchell, JJ, Trakadis, YJ, and Scriver, CR: Phenylalanine hydroxylase deficiency. Genet Med 13:697, 2011.

Morley, JE: Protein-energy undernutrition. Merck Manual, October 2012. Accessed November 27, 2012. Available at www.merckmanuals.com/professional/nutritional_disorders/undernutrition/protein-energy_undernutrition.html?qt=ketones for energy&alt=sh

National Collegiate Athletic Association: Background on sickle cell trait and the NCAA. September 9, 2010. Accessed November 18, 2012. Available at www.ncaa.org/wps/wcm/connect/public/NCAA/Resources/Latest+News/2010+news+stories/September+latest+news/Background+on+sickle+cell+trait+and+the+NCAA

National Heart, Lung, and Blood Institute: Food exchange lists. June 28, 2013. Accessed June 28, 2013. Available at www.nhlbi.nih.gov/health/public/heart/obesity/lose_wt/fd_exch.htm

Ngudi, DD, Kuo, YH, Van Montagu, M, and Lambein, F: Research on motor neuron diseases konzo and neurolathyrism: trends from 1990 to 2010. PLoS Negl Trop Dis 2012;6:e1759, 2012.

Nzwalo, H, and Cliff, J: Konzo: from poverty, cassava, and cyanogen intake to toxico-nutritional neurological disease. PLoS Negl Trop Dis 5:e 1051, 2011. Accessed November 13, 2012. Available at www.ncbi.nlm.nih.gov/pmc/articles/PMC3125150

Olowoyeye, A, and Okwundu, CI: Gene therapy for sickle cell disease. Cochrane Database Syst Rev. 2010 Aug 4:CD007652.

Pasiakos, SM, and McClung, JP: Supplemental dietary leucine and the skeletal muscle anabolic response to essential amino acids. Nutr Rev 69:550, 2011.

Piercecchi-Marti, MD, Louis-Borrione, C, Bartoli, C, et al: Malnutrition, a rare form of child abuse: Diagnostic criteria. J Forensic Sci 51:670, 2006.

Prick, BW, Hop, WC, and Duvekot, JJ: Maternal phenylketonuria and hyperphenylalaninemia in pregnancy: pregnancy complications and neonatal sequelae in untreated and treated pregnancies. Am J Clin Nutr 95:374, 2012.

Ramirez-Zea, M, and Caballero, B: Protein-energy malnutrition. In Ross, AC, Caballero, B, Cousins, RJ, et al (eds): Modern Nutrition in Health and Disease, ed 11. Lippincott Williams & Wilkins, Philadelphia, 2014.

Rice, A: The peanut solution. New York Times, September 2, 2010. Accessed November 30, 2012 at www.nytimes.com/2010/09/05/magazine/05Plumpy-t.html?pagewanted=all

Seyler, J, and Layman, DK: The role of protein in overall health: quality, quantity, and timing considerations. Scan's Pulse (Continuing Education approved by Academy of Nutrition and Dietetics) 31:3, 2012.

Tierney, EP, Sage, RJ, and Shwayder, T: Kwashiorkor from a severe dietary restriction in an 8-month infant in suburban Detroit, Michigan: case report and review of the literature. Int J Dermatol 49:500, 2010.

Tipton, KD: Efficacy and consequences of very-high-protein diets for athletes and exercisers. Proc Nutr Soc 70:205, 2011.

Trefz, FK, and Belanger-Quintana, A: Sapropterin dihydrochloride: a new drug and a new concept in the management of phenylketonuria. Drugs Today (Barc) 46:589, 2010.

U.S. Department of Agriculture: Peas and beans are unique foods, June 22, 2011. Accessed February 18, 2013. Available at www.choosemyplate.gov/food-groups/dry_beans_peas_table.html

U.S. Department of Agriculture: What counts as an ounce equivalent in the protein foods group? June 4, 2011. Accessed February 18, 2013. Available at www.choosemyplate.gov/food-groups/proteinfoods_counts_table.html

van Loon, LJ: Leucine as a pharmaconutrient in health and disease. Curr Opin Clin Nutr Metab Care 15:71, 2012.

Van Winckel M, Vande Velde, S, De Bruyne, R, and Van Biervliet, S: Clinical practice: vegetarian infant and child nutrition. Eur J Pediatr 170:1489, 2011.

Venes, D (ed): Tabor's Cyclopedic Medical Dictionary, ed 21. FA Davis, Philadelphia, 2009.

Vernon, HJ, Koerner, CB, Johnson, MR, et al: Introduction of sapropterin dihydrochloride as standard of care in patients with phenylketonuria. Mol Genet Metab 100:229, 2010.

Wells, J: Can Plumpy'nut solve global hunger? Accessed December 1, 2012. Available at www.cnbc.com/id/48894202/Can_Plumpy_Nut_Solve_Global_Hunger

Widaman, KF: Phenylketonuria in children and mothers: genes, environments, behavior. Curr Dir Psychol Sci 18:48, 2009.

Wild, T, Rahbarnia, A, Kellner, M, et al: Basics in nutrition and wound healing. Nutrition 26:862, 2010.

Chapter 5

Centers for Disease Control and Prevention: How much physical activity do adults need? 2011. Accessed December 29, 2012 at www.cdc.gov/physicalactivity/everyone/guidelines/adults.html

Centers for Disease Control and Prevention: Low-energy-dense foods and weight management: cutting calories while controlling hunger. Reasearch to Practice Series, No. 5. Accessed December 20, 2012 at www.cdc.gov/nccdphp/dnpa/nutrition/pdf/r2p_energy_density.pdf

Dalee-Grave, R, Calugi, S, Centis, E, El Ghoch, M, & Marchesini, G: Cognitive-behavioral strategies to increase the adherence to exercise in the management of obesity. J Obes 2011. Accessed February 20, 2014. Available at http://www.hindawi.com/journals/jobe/2011/348293

Jamurtas, AZ, Tofas, T, Fatouros, I, et al: The effects of low and high glycemic index foods on exercise performance and beta-endorphin responses. J Int Soc Sports Nutr 8:15, 2011.

Kreymann, G, Adolph, M, and Mueller, MJ: Energy expenditure and energy intake—Guidelines on Parenteral Nutrition, Chapter 3. German Med Sci (e-journal) 7:Doc25, 2013. Accessed February 20, 2014. Available at www.egms.de/static/en/journals/gms/2009-7/000084.shtml

O'Riordan, CF, Metcalf, BS, Perkins, JM, and Wilkin, TJ: Reliability of energy expenditure prediction equations in the weight management clinic. J Hum Nutr Dietetics 23:169, 2010.

Scott, CB: Glucose and fat oxidation: bomb calorimeter be damned. Scientific World Journal 2012:375041, 2012.

Shrapnel, B: Is energy density a useful concept for understanding and preventing obesity? Nutr Dietetics 67:281, 2010.

Sum, S, Mayer, L, and Warren, MP: Bone mineral density accrual determines energy expenditure with refeeding in anorexia nervosa and supersedes return of menses. J Osteoporosis 7, 2011.

U.S. Department of Agriculture and U.S. Department of Health and Human Services: Dietary Guidelines for Americans 2010, ed 7. Washington, DC: U.S. Government Printing Office, December 2010.

U.S. Department of Agriculture, Agricultural Research Service: Energy intakes: percentage of energy from protein, carbohydrate, fat, and alcohol, by gender and age. What we eat in America, NHANES 2009–2010, 2012. Retrieved on December 21, 2012 at www.ars.usda.gov/ba/bhnrc/fsrg

Walpole, SC, Prieto-Merino, D, Edwards, P, Cleland, G, Stevens, G, and Roberts, I: The weight of nations: an estimation of adult human biomass. BMC Public Health 12:439, 2012.

World Health Organization: Obesity and overweight, 2013. Accessed June 9, 2013. Available at www.who.int/mediacentre/factsheets/fs311/en/

World Health Organization: Physical activity and adults, 2014. Accessed January 19, 2014. Available at www.who.int/dietphysicalactivity/factsheet_adults/en/index.html

Chapter 6

American Academy of Pediatrics: Controversies concerning vitamin K and the newborn. Pediatrics 112:191, 2003. Reaffirmed May 2009. Accessed January 24, 2013. Available at http://pediatrics.aappublications.org/content/124/2/845.full

Andres, E, and Serraj, K: Optimal management of pernicious anemia. J Blood Med 3: 97, 2012. Accessed February 9, 2013. Available at www.ncbi.nlm.nih.gov/pmc/articles/PMC3441227

Ashourian, N, and Mousdicas, N: Pellagra-like dermatitis. N Engl J Med 354:1614, 2006.

Banka, S, Ryan, K, Thomson W, and Newman, WG: Pernicious anemia—genetic insights. Autoimmun Rev 10:455, 2011.

Bartlett, PC, Morris, JG, Jr, and Spengler, J: Foodborne illness associated with niacin: report of an outbreak linked to excessive niacin in enriched cornmeal. Public Health Rep 97:258, 1982.

Becker, DA, Ingala, EE, Martinez-Lage, M, et al: Dry beriberi and Wernicke's encephalopathy following gastric lap band surgery. J Clin Neurosci 19:1050, 2012.

Bello, S, Neri, M, Riezzo, I, et al: Cardiac beriberi: morphological findings in two fatal cases. Diagn Pathol 6:8, 2011. Accessed January 31, 2013. Available at www.ncbi.nlm.nih.gov/pmc/articles/PMC3034660

Bemeur, C, and Butterworth, RF: Thiamin. In Ross, AC, Caballero, B, Cousins, RJ, et al (eds): Modern Nutrition in Health and Disease, ed 11. Lippincott Williams & Wilkins, Philadelphia, 2014.

Ben-Zvi, GT, and Tidman, MJ: Be vigilant for scurvy in high-risk groups. Practitioner 256:23, 2012.

Berry, RJ, Bailey, L, Mulinare, J, et al: Fortification of flour with folic acid. Food Nutr Bull 31(Suppl 1):S22, 2010.

Blank, S, Scanlon, KS, Sinks, TH, et al: An outbreak of hypervitaminosis D associated with the overfortification of milk from a home-delivery dairy. Am J Public Health 85:656, 1995.

Bliss, RM: Monitoring food-supply nutrients. Agricultural Research 60:8, 2012.

Brazy, PC: Hartnup disease. Merck Manual. Modified August 2010. Accessed February 4, 2013. Available at www.merckmanuals.com/professional/pediatrics/congenital_renal_transport_abnormalities/hartnup_disease.html?qt=Hartnup diseaseandalt=sh#v1098310

Brouwer, I, and Verhoef, P: Folic acid fortification: Is masking of vitamin B_{12} deficiency what we should really worry about? Am J Clin Nutr 86:897, 2007. Accessed February 10, 2013. Available at http://ajcn.nutrition.org/content/86/4/897.long

Cahill, LE, and El-Sohemy, A: Haptoglobin genotype modifies the association between dietary vitamin C and serum ascorbic acid deficiency. Am J Clin Nutr 92:1494, 2010.

Camadoo, L, Tibbot, R, and Isaza, F: Maternal vitamin D deficiency associated with neonatal hypocalcaemic convulsions. Nutr J 6:23, 2007.

Cannell, JJ, Zasloff, M, Garland, CF, et al: On the epidemiology of influenza. Virol J 5:29, 2008.

Carmel, R: Cobalamin (vitamin B_{12}). In Ross, AC, Caballero, B, Cousins, RJ, et al (eds): Modern Nutrition in Health and Disease, ed 11. Lippincott Williams & Wilkins, Philadelphia, 2014.

Carmel, R, Bellevue, R, and Kelman, Z: Low cobalamin levels associated with sickle cell disease: contrasting origins and clinical meanings in two instructive patients. Am J Hematol 85: 436, 2010. Accessed February 10, 2013. Available at www.ncbi.nlm.nih.gov/pmc/articles/PMC2992813

Carvalho, NF, Kenney, RD, Carrington, PH, and Hall, DE: Severe nutritional deficiencies in toddlers resulting from health food milk alternatives. Pediatrics 107:E46, 2001.

Cashman, KD, and Kiely, M: Towards prevention of vitamin D deficiency and beyond: knowledge gaps and research needs in vitamin D nutrition and public health. Br J Nutr 106:1337, 2011.

Caudill, M, da Costa, K-A, Zeisel, S, and Hornick, B: Elevating awareness and intake of choline. Nutr Today 46:235, 2011.

Centers for Disease Control and Prevention: Neurologic impairment in children associated with maternal dietary deficiency of cobalamin—Georgia, 2001. Morb Mortal Wkly Rep 52:61, 2003. Accessed February 9, 2013 at www.cdc.gov/mmwr/PDF/wk/mm5204.pdf

Centers for Disease Control and Prevention: Trends in tuberculosis—United States, 2011. 61:181, March 23, 2012. Accessed January 17, 2013. Available at www.cdc.gov/mmwr/preview/mmwrhtml/mm6111a2.htm

Chatterjee, M, and Speiser, PW: Pamidronate treatment of hypercalcemia caused by vitamin D toxicity. J Pediatr Endrocrinol Metab 20:1241, 2007.

Chitambar, CR, and Antony, AC: Hematologic aspects of iron deficiency and less common nutritional anemias. In Ross, AC, Caballero, B, Cousins, RJ, et al (eds): Modern Nutrition in Health and Disease, ed 11. Lippincott Williams & Wilkins, Philadelphia, 2014.

Chung, M, Lee, J, Terasawa, T, et al: Vitamin D with or without calcium supplementation for prevention of cancer and fractures: an updated meta-analysis for the U.S. Preventive Services Task Force. Ann Intern Med 155:827, 2011.

Cole, JA, Warthan, MM, Hirano, SA, et al: Scurvy in a 10-year-old boy. Pediatr Dermatol 28:444, 2011.

Consumer Lab: Product Review: Multivitamin and multimineral supplements review. Updated Novermber 10, 2012. Accessed February 16, 2013. Available at www.consumerlab.com/news/multivitamin_review_report/06_16_2011

Cylwik, B, and Chrostek, L: Disturbances of folic acid and homocysteine metabolism in alcohol abuse [article in Polish]. Pol Merkur Lekarski 30:295, 2011.

da Silva, VR, Mackey, AD, Davis, SR, and Gregory, JF, III: Vitamin B_6. In Ross, AC, Caballero, B, Cousins, RJ, et al (eds): Modern Nutrition in Health and Disease, ed 11. Lippincott Williams & Wilkins, Philadelphia, 2014.

Delanghe, JR, Langlois, MR, De Buyzere, ML, and Torck, MA: Vitamin C deficiency and scurvy are not only a dietary problem but are codetermined by the haptoglobin polymorphism. Clin Chem 53:1397, 2007.

Dhar, M, Bellevue, R, and Carmel, R: Pernicious anemia with neuropsychiatric dysfunction in a patient with sickle cell anemia treated with folate supplementation. N Engl J Med 348:2204, 2003.

Dubock, A: Genetically modified foods: scientific perspective and controversies. Albert Einstein College of Medicine Continuing Medical Education. Accessed December 4, 2012. Available at www.cyberounds.com/cmecontent/art508.html

Essa, E, Velez, MR, Smith, S, et al: Cardiovascular magnetic resonance in wet beriberi. J Cardiovasc Magn Reson 13: 41, 2011.

Evans, JR, and Lawrenson, JG: Antioxidant vitamin and mineral supplements for preventing age-related macular degeneration. Cochrane Database Syst Rev 13;6: CD000253, June 2012.

Evans, JR, and Lawrenson, JG: Antioxidant vitamin and mineral supplements for slowing the progression of age-related macular degeneration. Cochrane Database Syst Rev 14;11:CD000254, November 2012.

Fattal-Valevski A, Kesler A, Sela BA, et al: Outbreak of life-threatening thiamine deficiency in infants in Israel caused by a defective soy-based formula. Pediatrics 115:e233, 2005. Accessed January 31, 2013. Available at http://pediatrics.aappublications.org/content/115/2/e233.long

Food and Agriculture Organization of the United Nations: Vitamin A. Human Vitamin and Mineral Requirements. FAO/WHO, Bangkok, Thailand, 2002. Accessed January 14, 2013. Available at www.fao.org/docrep/004/Y2809E/y2809e0d.htm#bm13

Fukushima, R, and Yamazaki, E: Vitamin C requirement in surgical patients. Curr Opin Clin Nutr Metab Care 13:669, 2010.

Gerlach, AT, Thomas, S, Stawicki, SP, et al: Vitamin B_6 deficiency: a potential cause of refractory seizures in adults. JPEN J Parenter Enteral Nutr 35:272, 2011.

Goselink, RJ, Harlaar, JJ, Vermeij, FH, et al: Beriberi after bariatric surgery [article in Dutch]. Ned Tijdschr Geneeskd 155:A4500, 2012.

Gropper, SS, and Smith, JL: Advanced Nutrition and Human Metabolism, ed 6. Wadsworth, Belmont, CA, 2013.

Guez, S, Chiarelli, G, Menni, F, et al: Severe vitamin B_{12} deficiency in an exclusively breastfed 5-month-old Italian infant born to a mother receiving multivitamin supplementation during pregnancy. BMC Pediatr 12:85, 2012.

Guyton, JR, and Bays, HE: Safety considerations with niacin therapy. Am J Cardiol 99:22C, 2007.

Heimburger, DC: Clinical manifestations of nutrient deficiencies and toxicities. In Ross, AC, Caballero, B, Cousins, RJ, et al (eds): Modern Nutrition in Health and Disease, ed 11. Lippincott Williams & Wilkins, Philadelphia, 2014.

Hemilä, H, and Chalker, E: Vitamin C for preventing and treating the common cold. Cochrane Database Syst Rev 1: CD000980. Published online January 31, 2013. Acccessed January 30, 2013. Available at http://summaries.cochrane.org/CD000980/vitamin-c-for-preventing-and-treating-the-common-cold

Holick, MF, Binkley, NC, Bischoff-Ferrari, HA, et al: Evaluation, treatment and prevention of vitamin D deficiency: an Endocrine Society clinical practice guideline. J Clin Endocrinol Metab 96:1911, 2011.

Holland, S, Silberstein, SD, Freitag, F, et al: Evidence-based guideline update: NSAIDs and other complementary treatments for episodic migraine prevention in adults: report of the Quality Standards Subcommittee of the American Academy of Neurology and the American Headache Society. Neurology 78:1346, 2012.

Imai, N, Kubota, M, Saitou, M, et al: Increase of serum vascular endothelial growth factors in wet beriberi: two case reports. Intern Med 51:929, 2012.

Jagielska, G, Tomaszewicz-Libudzic, EC, and Brzozowska, A: Pellagra: A rare complication of anorexia nervosa. Eur Child Adolesc Psychiatry 16:417, 2007.

Johnston, CS, and Bowling, DL: Stability of ascorbic acid in commercially available orange juices. J Am Diet Assoc 102:525, 2002.

Johnston, CS, and Hale, JC: Oxidation of ascorbic acid in stored orange juice is associated with reduced plasma vitamin C concentrations and elevated lipid peroxides. J Am Diet Assoc 105:106, 2005.

Jones, G: Vitamin D. In Ross, AC, Caballero, B, Cousins, RJ, et al (eds): Modern Nutrition in Health and Disease, ed 11. Lippincott Williams & Wilkins, Philadelphia, 2014.

Khasru, MR, Yasmin, R, Salek, AK, et al: Acute hypervitaminosis A in a young lady. Mymensingh Med J 19:294, 2010.

Kirkland, J: Niacin. In Ross, AC, Caballero, B, Cousins, RJ, et al (eds): Modern Nutrition in Health and Disease, ed 11. Lippincott Williams & Wilkins, Philadelphia, 2014.

Klein, EA, Thompson, IM, Jr, Tangen, CM, et al: Vitamin E and the risk of prostate cancer: the Selenium and Vitamin E Cancer Prevention Trial (SELECT). JAMA 306:1549, 2011.

Kowalski, TE, Falestiny, M, Furth, E, and Malet, PF: Vitamin A hepatotoxicity: A cautionary note regarding 25,000 IU supplements. Am J Med 97:523, 1994.

Lachner, C, Steinle, NI, and Regenold, WT: The neuropsychiatry of vitamin B_{12} deficiency in elderly patients. J Neuropsychiatry Clin Neurosci 24:5, 2012.

Lerner, V, and Kanevsky, M: Acute dementia with delirium due to vitamin B_{12} deficiency: A case report. Int J Psychiatry Med 32:215, 2002.

Levine, M, and Padayatty, SJ: Vitamin C. In Ross, AC, Caballero, B, Cousins, RJ, et al (eds): Modern Nutrition in Health and Disease, ed 11. Lippincott Williams & Wilkins, Philadelphia, 2014.

Li, R, Byers, K, and Walvekar, RR: Gingival hypertrophy: A solitary manifestation of scurvy. Am J Otolaryngol 29:426, 2008.

Linus Pauling Institute: Choline. Updated August 18, 2009. Accessed February 12, 2013 at http://lpi.oregonstate.edu/infocenter/othernuts/choline/index.html#deficiency

MacDonald, A, and Forsyth, A: Nutritional deficiencies and the skin. Clin Exp Dermatol 30:388, 2005.

Malloy, PJ, Zhou, Y, Wang, J, et al: Hereditary vitamin D-resistant rickets (HVDRR) owing to a heterozygous mutation in the vitamin D receptor. J Bone Miner Res 26:2710, 2011.

Martí, N, Mena, P, Cánovas, JA, et al: Vitamin C and the role of citrus juices as functional food. Nat Prod Commun 4:677, 2009.

Maruani A, Labarthe F, Dupré T, et al: Hypercarotenaemia in an infant [article in French]. Ann Dermatol Venereol 137:32, 2010.

Mayo-Wilson, E, Imdad, A, Herzer, K, et al: Vitamin A supplements for preventing mortality, illness, and blindness in children aged under 5: systematic review and meta-analysis. BMJ 343:d5094, 2011.

McLaren, DS, and Frigg, M: Sight and Life Manual on Vitamin A Deficiency Disorders (VADD), ed 2. Sight and Life, Basel, Switzerland, 2001.

Mertens, MT, and Gertner, E: Rheumatic manifestations of scurvy: a report of three recent cases in a major urban center and a review. Semin Arthritis Rheum 41:286, 2011.

Messamore, E: Niacin subsensitivity is associated with functional impairment in schizophrenia. Schizophr Res 137:180, 2012.

Miksad, R, de Lédinghen, V, McDougall, C, et al: Hepatic hydrothorax associated with vitamin A toxicity. J Clin Gastroenterol 34:275, 2002.

Milea, D, Cassoux, N, and LeHoang, P: Blindness in a strict vegan [letter]. N Engl J Med 342:897, 2000.

Mock, DM: Biotin. In Ross, AC, Caballero, B, Cousins, RJ, et al (eds): Modern Nutrition in Health and Disease, ed 11. Lippincott Williams & Wilkins, Philadelphia, 2014.

Mohr, SB, Garland, CF, Gorham, ED, et al: Ultraviolet B and incidence rates of leukemia worldwide. Am J Prev Med 41:68, 2011.

Morris, MS, Picciano, MF, Jacques, PF, and Selhub, J: Plasma pyridoxal 5'-phosphate in the US, population: the National Health and Nutrition Examination Survey, 2003–2004. Am J Clin Nutr 87:1446, 2008.

Morse, JW, Morse, SJ, and Patterson, J: Niacin reaction: Common vitamin, uncommon ED, diagnosis. Am J Emerg Med 17:320, 1999.

Moyer, VA, and U.S. Preventive Services Task Force: Prevention of falls in community-dwelling older adults: U.S. Preventive Services Task Force recommendation statement. Ann Intern Med 157:197, 2012.

Muoki, PN, Makokha, AO, Onyango, CA, and Ojijo, NK: Potential contribution of mangoes to reduction of vitamin A deficiency in Kenya. Ecol Food Nutr 48:482, 2009.

Murphy, C, Bangash, IH, and Varma, A: Dry beriberi mimicking the Guillain-Barre syndrome. Pract Neurol 9:221, 2009.

Nadalin, S, Bureti-Tomljanovi, A, and Rubesa, G: Niacin skin flush test: A research tool for studying schizophrenia. Psychiatr Danub 22:14, 2010.

National Institutes of Health, Office of Dietary Supplements: Dietary supplement fact sheet: Multivitamin/mineral supplements. Reviewed January 7, 2013. Accessed February 14, 2013. Available at http://ods.od.nih.gov/factsheets/MVMS-HealthProfessional

National Institutes of Health, Office of Dietary Supplements: Dietary supplement fact sheet: Vitamin C. Reviewed June 24, 2011a. Accessed January 30, 2013. Available at http://ods.od.nih.gov/factsheets/VitaminC-HealthProfessional

National Institutes of Health, Office of Dietary Supplements: Dietary supplement fact sheet: Vitamin D. Reviewed June 24, 2011b. Accessed January 18, 2013. Available at http://ods.od.nih.gov/factsheets/VitaminD-HealthProfessional

Oldham, MA, and Ivkovic, A: Pellagrous encephalopathy presenting as alcohol withdrawal delirium: A case series and literature review. Addict Sci Clin Pract. 2012; 7: 12. Accessed February 4, 2013. Available at www.ncbi.nlm.nih.gov/pmc/articles/PMC3542555

Pandev, S, Lin, Y, Collier-Tenison, S, and Bodden, J: Social factors determining the experience of blindness among pregnant women in developing countries: The case of India. Health Soc Work 37:157, 2012.

Patel, AB, and Prabhu, AS: Hartnup disease. Indian J Dermatol 53:31, 2008. Accessed February 4, 2013. Available at www.ncbi.nlm.nih.gov/pmc/articles/PMC2784584

Pawlak, R, Parrott, SJ, Raj, S, et al: How prevalent is vitamin B_{12} deficiency among vegetarians? Nutr Rev 71:110, 2013.

Perrine, CG, Sharma, AJ, Jefferds, ME, et al: Adherence to vitamin D recommendations among US infants. Pediatrics 125:627, 2010.

Perry, CA, and Caudill, MA: Biotin: critical for fetal growth and development yet often overlooked. Nutr Today 47:79, 2012.

Popovich, D, McAlhany, A, Adewumi, AO, and Barnes, MM: Scurvy: Forgotten but definitely not gone. J Pediatr Health Care 23:405, 2009.

Preston, AM, Rodríguez, C, Rivera, CE: Plasma ascorbate in a population of children: influence of age, gender, vitamin C intake, BMI and smoke exposure. P R Health Sci J 25:137, 2006.

Reddy, HL, Doane, SK, Keil, SD, et al: Development of a riboflavin and ultraviolet light-based device to treat whole blood. Transfusion 53(Suppl 1):131S, 2013.

Reinhardt, D, Giambarba, C, and Raimondi, S: Alcohol, acid, vitamins and heart [article in German]. Praxis (Bern 1994) 100(12):733, 2011.

Riaz, MN, Asif, M, and Ali, R: Stability of vitamins during extrusion. Crit Rev Food Sci Nutr 49:361, 2009.

Roman, GC: Nutritional disorders of the nervous system. In Ross, AC, Caballero, B, Cousins, RJ, et al (eds): Modern Nutrition in Health and Disease, ed 11. Lippincott Williams & Wilkins, Philadelphia, 2014.

Ronald, P: Plant genetics, sustainable agriculture and global food security. Genetics 188:11, 2011.

Ross, AC: Vitamin A. In Ross, AC, Caballero, B, Cousins, RJ, et al (eds): Modern Nutrition in Health and Disease, ed 11. Lippincott Williams & Wilkins, Philadelphia, 2014.

Said, HM, and Ross, AC: Riboflavin. In Ross, AC, Caballero, B, Cousins, RJ, et al (eds): Modern Nutrition in Health and Disease, ed 11. Lippincott Williams & Wilkins, Philadelphia, 2014.

Saiga, H, Shimada, Y, and Takeda, K: Innate immune effectors in mycobacterial infection. Clin Dev Immunol 2011: 347594. Accessed January 16, 2013. Available at www.ncbi.nlm.nih.gov/pmc/articles/PMC3025378

Schwalfenberg, GK: Solar Radiation and Vitamin D: Mitigating environmental factors in autoimmune disease. J Environ Public Health 2012: 619381. Accessed January 15, 2013. Available at www.ncbi.nlm.nih.gov/pmc/articles/PMC3317188

Sherwin, JC, Reacher, MH, Dean, WH, and Ngondi, J: Epidemiology of vitamin A deficiency and xerophthalmia in at-risk populations. Trans R Soc Trop Med Hyg 106:205, 2012.

Shin, JS, Choi, MY, Longtine, MS, and Nelson, DM: Vitamin D effects on pregnancy and the placenta. Placenta 31:1027, 2010.

Staggs, CG, Sealey, WM, McCabe, BJ, et al: Determination of the biotin content of select foods using accurate and sensitive HPLC/avidin binding. J Food Compost Anal 17:767, 2004. Accessed February 12, 2013. Available at www.ncbi.nlm.nih.gov/pmc/articles/PMC1450323

Stover, PJ: Folic acid. In Ross, AC, Caballero, B, Cousins, RJ, et al (eds): Modern Nutrition in Health and Disease, ed 11. Lippincott Williams & Wilkins, Philadelphia, 2014.

Stroh, C, Weiher, C, Hohmann, U, Meyer, F, et al: Vitamin A deficiency (VAD) after a duodenal switch procedure: a case report. Obes Surg 20:397, 2010.

Suba, Z: Light deficiency confers breast cancer risk by endocrine disorders. Recent Pat Anticancer Drug Discov 7:337, 2012.

Suttie, JW: Vitamin K. In Ross, AC, Caballero, B, Cousins, RJ, et al (eds): Modern Nutrition in Health and Disease, ed 11. Lippincott Williams & Wilkins, Philadelphia, 2014.

Swanson, AM, and Hughey, LC: Acute inpatient presentation of scurvy. Cutis 86:205, 2010.

Tang, AM, Smit, E, and Semba, RD: Nutrition and infectious diseases. In Ross, AC, Caballero, B, Cousins, RJ, et al (eds): Modern Nutrition in Health and Disease, ed 11. Lippincott Williams & Wilkins, Philadelphia, 2014.

Touger-Decker, R, Radler, DR, and DePaola, DP: Nutrition and dental medicine. In Ross, AC, Caballero, B, Cousins, RJ, et al (eds): Modern Nutrition in Health and Disease, ed 11. Lippincott Williams & Wilkins, Philadelphia, 2014.

Traber, MG. Vitamin E. In Ross, AC, Caballero, B, Cousins, RJ, et al (eds): Modern Nutrition in Health and Disease, ed 11. Lippincott Williams & Wilkins, Philadelphia, 2014.

Trumbo, PR: Pantothenic acid. In Ross, AC, Caballero, B, Cousins, RJ, et al (eds): Modern Nutrition in Health and Disease, ed 11. Lippincott Williams & Wilkins, Philadelphia, 2014. University of Washington: What factors influence skin synthesis of vitamin D? Osteo Ed June 4, 2009. Accessed January 18, 2013. Available at http://depts.washington.edu/osteoed/faqs.php?faqID=109

Vallerand, AH, Sanoski, CA, and Deglin, JH: Davis's Drug Guide for Nurses, ed 13. FA Davis, Philadelphia, 2013.

Van Mieghem, T, Van Schoubroeck, D, Depiere, M, et al: Fetal cerebral hemorrhage caused by vitamin K deficiency after complicated bariatric surgery. Obstet Gynecol 112:434, 2008.

Velandia, B, Centor, RM, McConnell, V, and Shah, M: Scurvy is still present in developed countries. J Gen Intern Med. 23:1281, 2008.

Viuda-Martos, M, Fernández-López, J, Sayas-Barbera, E, et al: Citrus co-products as technological strategy to reduce residual nitrite content in meat products. J Food Sci 74:R93, 2009.

Wagner, CL, and Greer, FR: Prevention of rickets and vitamin D deficiency in infants, children, and adolescents. Pediatrics 122:1142, 2008. Accessed February 14, 2013. Available at http://pediatrics.aappublications.org/content/122/5/1142.long

Wagner, DA, Schatz, R, Coston, R, et al: A new ^{13}C breath test to detect vitamin B_{12} deficiency: A prevalent and poorly diagnosed health problem. J Breath Res 5:046001, 2011. Accessed February 8, 2013. Available at www.ncbi.nlm.nih.gov/pmc/articles/PMC3204151

Ward, LM, Gaboury, I, Ladhani, M, and Zlotkin, S, Vitamin D–deficiency rickets among children in Canada. CMAJ 177:161, 2007.

Watkins, D, and Rosenblatt, DS: Update and new concepts in vitamin responsive disorders of folate transport and metabolism. J Inherit Metab Dis 35:665, 2012.

Weisberg, P, Scanlon, KS, Li, R, and Cogswell, ME: Nutritional rickets among children in the United States: Review of cases reported between 1986 and 2003. Am J Clin Nutr 80(Suppl 6):1697S, 2004. Accessed January 17, 2013. Available at http://ajcn.nutrition.org/content/80/6/1697S.long

Willett, WC, and Stampfer, MJ: Foundations of a healthy diet. In Ross, AC, Caballero, B, Cousins, RJ, et al (eds): Modern Nutrition in Health and Disease, ed 11. Lippincott Williams & Wilkins, Philadelphia, 2014.

Wolpowitz, D, and Gilchrest, BA: The vitamin D questions: How much do you need and how should you get it? J Am Acad Dermatol 54:301, 2006.

Yamazaki, E, Horikawa, M, and Fukushima, R: Vitamin C supplementation in patients receiving peripheral parenteral nutrition after gastrointestinal surgery. Nutrition 27:435, 2011.

Zalesin, KC, Miller, WM, Franklin, B, et al: Vitamin A deficiency after gastric bypass surgery: An underreported postoperative complication. J Obes 2011:760695. Accessed January 11, 2013. Available at www.ncbi.nlm.nih.gov/pmc/articles/PMC2943134

Zeisel, SH: Choline. In Ross, AC, Caballero, B, Cousins, RJ, et al (eds): Modern Nutrition in Health and Disease, ed 11. Lippincott Williams & Wilkins, Philadelphia, 2014.

Chapter 7

Afrin, LB: Fatal copper deficiency from excessive use of zinc-based denture adhesive. Am J Med Sci 340:164, 2010.

Airola, G, Allais, G, Castagnoli Gabellari, I, et al: Non-pharmacological management of migraine during pregnancy. Neurol Sci 3(Suppl 1):S63, 2010.

Aldenhoven, M, Klomp, LW, van Hasselt, PM, et al: From gene to disease; Menkes disease: Copper deficiency due to an ATP7A-gene defect [article in Dutch]. Ned Tijdschr Geneeskd 151:2266, 2007.

Amit, M: Vegetarian diets in children and adolescents. Paediatr Child Health 15:303, 2010.

Arsenic in your food. Consumer Rep November: 22, 2012.

Auwaerter, PG: Is zinc a cure for the common cold? Not yet. Medscape Infectious Diseases. March 3, 2011. Accessed September 17, 2012. Available at www.medscape.com/viewarticle/738285

Ayus, JC, Achinger, SG, and Arieff, A: Brain cell volume regulation in hyponatremia: Role of sex, age, vasopressin, and hypoxia. Am J Physiol Renal Physiol 295:F619.

Bailey, JL, Sands, JM, and Franch, HA: Water, electrolytes, and acid-base metabolism. In Ross, AC, Caballero, B, Cousins, RJ, et al (eds): Modern Nutrition in Health and Disease, ed 11. Lippincott Williams & Wilkins, Philadelphia, 2014.

Bank, IM, Shemie, SD, Rosenblatt B, et al: Sudden cardiac death in association with the ketogenic diet. Pediatr Neurol 39:429, 2008.

Banner, B, Schaeffer, S, Badillo, RB, et al: Multiple lead appendoliths following ingestion of lead shot: Time course and removal by laporoscopic appendectomy. Clin Toxicol (Phila) 50:266, 2012.

Beier, JI, Landes, S, Mohammad, M, and McClain, CJ: Nutrition in liver disorders and the role of alcohol. In Ross, AC, Caballero, B, Cousins, RJ, et al (eds): Modern Nutrition in Health and Disease, ed 11. Lippincott Williams & Wilkins, Philadelphia, 2014.

Bradford, PG, Gerace, KV, Roland, RL, and Chrzan, BG: Estrogen regulation of apoptosis in osteoblasts. Physiol Behav 99:181, 2010.

Brna, P, Gordon, K, Dooley, JM, and Price, V: Manganese toxicity in a child with iron deficiency and polycythemia. J Child Neurol 26:891, 2011.

Brown, MJ, and Margolis, S: Lead in drinking water and human blood lead levels in the United States. Morb Mortal Wkly Rep 61:1, 2012. Accessed September 29, 2012. Available at www.ncbi.nlm.nih.gov/pubmed/22874873

Btaiche, IF, Yeh, AY, Wu, IJ, and Khalidi, N: Neurologic dysfunction and pancytopenia secondary to acquired copper deficiency following duodenal switch: case report and review of the literature. Nutr Clin Pract 26:583, 2011.

Bunta, AD: It is time for everyone to own the bone. Osteoporos Int 22(Suppl 3):477, 2011.

Calvez J, Poupin N, Chesneau C, et al: Protein intake, calcium balance and health consequences. Eur J Clin Nutr 66:281, 2012.

Centers for Disease Control and Prevention: Announcement: Response to the advisory committee on childhood lead poisoning prevention report, low level lead exposure harms children: A renewed call for primary prevention. Morb Mortal Wkly Rep 61:383, May 25, 2012a. Accessed September 28, 2012. Available at www.cdc.gov/mmwr/preview/mmwrhtml/mm6120a6.htm?s_cid=mm6120a6_e

Centers for Disease Control and Prevention: Bottled water and fluoride, Reviewed and Updated January 7, 2011. Accessed September 15, 2012. Available at www.cdc.gov/fluoridation/fact_sheets/bottled_water.htm

Centers for Disease Control and Prevention: CDC Grand rounds: Dietary sodium reduction—time for choice. Morb Mortal Wkly Rep 61:89, May 25, 2012b. Accessed December 13, 2012. Available at www.cdc.gov/mmwr/preview/mmwrhtml/mm6105a2.htm?s_cid=mm6105a2_w

Centers for Disease Control and Prevention: Childhood lead poisoning associated with tamarind candy and folk remedies—California, 1999–2000. Morb Mortal Wkly Rep 51:684, 2002. Accessed September 27. 2012 at www.cdc.gov/mmwr/preview/mmwrhtml/mm5131a3.htm

Centers for Disease Control and Prevention: Chlorine gas exposure at a metal recycling facility—California, 2010. Morb Mortal Wkly Rep 60:951, July 22, 2011. Accessed September 15, 2012. Available at www.cdc.gov/mmwr/preview/mmwrhtml/mm6028a3.htm?s_cid=mm6028a3_w

Centers for Disease Control and Prevention: Community water fluoridation: Questions and answers, Reviewed and Updated December 16, 2011. Accessed September 14, 2012. Available at www.cdc.gov/fluoridation/fact_sheets/cwf_qa.htm#top

Centers for Disease Control and Prevention: Death of a child after ingestion of a metallic charm—Minnesota, 2006. Morb Mortal Wkly Rep 55:340, March 31, 2006. Accessed September 27, 2012. Available at www.cdc.gov/mmwr/preview/mmwrhtml/mm5512a4.htm

Centers for Disease Control and Prevention: Deaths associated with hypocalcemia from chelation therapy—Texas, Pennsylvania, and Oregon, 2003–2005. Morb Mortal Wkly Rep 55:204, March 3, 2006. Accessed September 28, 2012. Available at www.cdc.gov/mmwr/preview/mmwrhtml/mm5508a3.htm

Centers for Disease Control and Prevention: Elevated serum aluminum levels in hemodialysis patients associated with the use of electric pumps—Wyoming, 2007. Morb Mortal Wkly Rep 57:689, 2008. Accessed December 15, 2012 at www.cdc.gov/mmwr/preview/mmwrhtml/mm5725a4.htm?s_cid=mm5725s4_e

Centers for Disease Control and Prevention: Fatal pediatric lead poisoning—New Hampshire, 2000. Morb Mortal Wkly Rep 50:457, 2001. Accessed September 27, 2012 at www.cdc.gov/mmwr/preview/mmwrhtml/mm5022a1.htm

Centers for Disease Control and Prevention: Infant lead poisoning associated with use of tiro, an eye cosmetic from Nigeria—Boston, Massachusetts, August 3, 2012. Accessed September 27, 2012. Available at www.cdc.gov/mmwr/preview/mmwrhtml/mm6130a3.htm?s_cid=mm6130a3_w

Centers for Disease Control and Prevention: Lead poisoning in pregnant women who used Ayurvedic medications from India—New York City, 2011–2012. Morb Mortal Wkly Rep 61:641, August 24, 2012. Accessed September 27, 2012. Available at www.cdc.gov/mmwr/preview/mmwrhtml/mm6133a1.htm?s_cid=mm6133a1_w

Centers for Disease Control and Prevention: Lead poisoning of a child associated with use of a Cambodian amulet—New York City, 2009. Morb Mortal Wkly Rep 60:69, January 28, 2011. Accessed September 27, 2012. Available at www.cdc.gov/mmwr/preview/mmwrhtml/mm6003a2.htm

Centers for Disease Control and Prevention: Overview: Infant formula and fluorosis, Reviewed and Modified April 27, 2012. Accessed September 15, 2012. Available at www.cdc.gov/fluoridation/safety/infant_formula.htm

Centers for Disease Control and Prevention: Refugee health guidelines: lead screening, Reviewed March 29, 2012. Accessed September 27, 2012. Available at www.cdc.gov/immigrantrefugeehealth/guidelines/lead-guidelines.html

Cerulli, J, Grabe, DW, Gauthier, I, et al: Chromium picolinate toxicity. Ann Pharmacother 32:428, 1998.

Chitambar, CR, and Antony, AC: Hematologic aspects of iron deficiency and less common nutritional anemias. In Ross, AC, Caballero, B, Cousins, RJ, et al (eds): Modern Nutrition in Health and Disease, ed 11. Lippincott Williams & Wilkins, Philadelphia, 2014.

Christensen, NK, et al: Juniper ash as a source of calcium in the Navajo diet. J Am Diet Assoc 98:333, 1998.

Chung, RT, Misdraji, MD, and Sahani, DV: Case 33—2006: A 43-year-old man with diabetes, hypogonadism, cirrhosis, arthralgias, and fatigue. N Engl J Med 355:1812, 2006.

Clarke, B: Normal bone anatomy and physiology. Clin J Am Soc Nephrol 3(Suppl 3):S131, 2008.

Cleveland, LM, Minter, ML, Cobb, KA, et al: Lead hazards for pregnant women and children: Part 1. Am J Nurs 108:40, 2008.

Collins, JF: Copper. In Ross, AC, Caballero, B, Cousins, RJ, et al (eds): Modern Nutrition in Health and Disease, ed 11. Lippincott Williams & Wilkins, Philadelphia, 2014.

De Nijs, RN: Glucocorticoid-induced osteoporosis: A review on pathophysiology and treatment options. Minerva Med 99:23, 2008.

Doherty, K, Connor M, and Cruickshank, R: Zinc-containing denture adhesive: A potential source of excess zinc resulting in copper deficiency myelopathy. Br Dent J 210:523, 2011.

Doumouchtsis, SK, Martin, NS, and Robins, JB: "Veterinary" diagnosis of lead poisoning in pregnancy. BMJ 333:1302, 2006.

Emder, PJ, and Jack, MM: Iodine-induced neonatal hypothyroidism secondary to maternal seaweed consumption: A common practice in some Asian cultures to promote breast milk supply. J Paediatr Child Health 47:750, 2011.

Eward, WC, Darcey, D, Dodd, LG, and Zura, RD: Case report: lead toxicity associated with an extra-articular retained missile 14 years after injury. J Surg Orthop Adv 20:241, 2011.

Fairweather-Tait, SJ, Fox, TE, and Mallilin, A: Balti curries and iron. BMJ 310:1368, 1995.

Fenton, TR, Tough, SC, Lyon, AW, et al: Causal assessment of dietary acid load and bone disease: A systematic review and meta-analysis applying Hill's epidemiologic criteria for causality. Nutr J 10:41, 2011.

Fewtrell, MS, Bishop, NJ, Edmonds, CJ, et al: Aluminum exposure from parenteral nutrition in preterm infants: Bone health at 15-year follow-up. Pediatrics 124:1372, 2009.

Fini M, Giavaresi G, Salamanna F, et al: Harmful lifestyles on orthopedic implantation surgery: A descriptive review

on alcohol and tobacco use. J Bone Miner Metab 29:633, 2011.

Frankel, EP: Primary hemochromatosis. Merck Manual. Revised November 2009. Accessed September 10, 2012. Available at www.merckmanuals.com/professional/hematology_and_oncology/iron_overload/primary_hemochromatosis.html

Fritzsche, J, Borisch, C, and Schaefer, C: Case report: High chromium and cobalt levels in a pregnant patient with bilateral metal-on-metal hip arthroplasties. Clin Orthop Relat Res 470:2325, 2012.

Garrison, SR, Allan, GM, Sekhon, RK, et al: Magnesium for skeletal muscle cramps. Cochrane Database Syst Rev. 2012 Sep 12;9:CD009402.

Geller, JL, Hu, B, Reed, S, et al: Increase in bone mass after correction of vitamin D insufficiency in bisphosphonate-treated patients. Endocr Pract 14:293, 2008.

Gibson, RS, Donovan, UM, and Heath, aL: Dietary strategies to improve the iron and zinc nutriture of young women following a vegetarian diet. Plant Foods Hum Nutr 51:1, 1997.

Goddard, AF, James, MW, McIntyre, AS, and Scott, BB: Guidelines for the management of iron deficiency anaemia. Gut 60:1309, 2011.

Gropper, SS, and Smith, JL: Advanced Nutrition and Human Metabolism, ed 6. Wadsworth, Belmont, CA, 2013.

Grossman, JM: Osteoporosis prevention. Curr Opin Rheumatol 23:203. 2011.

Grubb, M, Gaurav, K, and Panda, M: Milk-alkali syndrome in a middle-aged woman after ingesting large doses of calcium carbonate: a case report. Cases J 16:8198, 2009.

Hackley, G, and Katz-Jacobson, A: Lead poisoning in pregnancy: A case study with implications for midwives. J Midwifery Women's Health 48:30, 2003.

Hamidi, M, Boucher, BA, Cheung, AM, et al: Fruit and vegetable intake and bone health in women aged 45 years and over: A systematic review. Osteoporos Int 22:1681, 2011.

Harrison-Findik, DD: Gender-related variations in iron metabolism and liver diseases. World J Hepatol 2:302, 2010.

Harrison-Findik, DD: Is the iron regulatory hormone hepcidin a risk factor for alcoholic liver disease? World J Gastroenterol 15:1186, 2009.

Hassan, HA, Netchvolodoff, C, and Raufman, JP: Zinc-induced copper deficiency in a coin swallower. Am J Gastroenterol 95:2975, 2000.

Healthy People 2020. Oral health. Updated September 6, 2012. Accessed September 17, 2012. Available at www.healthypeople.gov/2020/topicsobjectives2020/overview.aspx?topicid=32

Heaney, RP: Bone biology in health and disease. In Ross, AC, Caballero, B, Cousins, RJ, et al (eds): Modern Nutrition in Health and Disease, ed 11. Lippincott Williams & Wilkins, Philadelphia, 2014.

Heimburger, DC: Clinical manifestations of nutrient deficiencies and toxicities. In Ross, AC, Caballero, B, Cousins, RJ, et al (eds): Modern Nutrition in Health and Disease, ed 11. Lippincott Williams & Wilkins, Philadelphia, 2014.

Hiroz, P, Antonino, A, Doerig, C, Pache, I, and Moradpour, D: A primer on Wilson disease for the general practitioner [article in French]. Rev Med Suisse 7:1690, 2011.

Holick, MF, Siris, ES, Binkley, N, et al: Prevalence of vitamin D inadequacy among postmenopausal North American women receiving osteoporosis therapy. J Clin Endocrinol Metab 90:3215, 2005.

Hsieh, CT, Liang, JS, Peng, SS, and Lee, WT: Seizure associated with total parenteral nutrition-related hypermanganesemia. Pediatr Neurol 36:181, 2007.

Institute of Medicine: Dietary reference intakes for vitamin a, vitamin k, arsenic, boron, chromium, copper, iodine, iron, manganese, molybdenum, nickel, silicon, vanadium, and zinc. National Academy of Sciences, Washington, DC, 2001. Accessed September 8, 2012. Available at www.nap.edu/catalog.php?record_id=10026

Institute of Medicine: Dietary reference intakes tables and application, Last Updated: 9/12/2011. Accessed September 1, 2012. Available at www.iom.edu/Activities/Nutrition/SummaryDRIs/DRI-Tables.aspx

International Osteoporosis Foundation: One minute osteoporosis risk awareness test. Undated. Accessed August 29, 2012. Available at www.iofbonehealth.org/one-minute-osteoporosis-risk-awareness-test

Jackson, BP, Taylor, VF, Pumshon, T, and Cottingham, KL: Arsenic concentration and speciation in infant formulas and first foods. Pure Appl Chem 84:215, 2012.

Jeejeebhoy, KN: Short bowel syndrome. In Ross, AC, Caballero, B, Cousins, RJ, et al (eds): Modern Nutrition in Health and Disease, ed 11. Lippincott Williams & Wilkins, Philadelphia, 2014.

Johnson, LE: Iodine deficiency and toxicity. Merck Manual. Revised August 2008a. Accessed September 12, 2012. Available at www.merckmanuals.com/professional/nutritional_disorders/mineral_deficiency_and_toxicity/iodine.html?qt=endemic goiter&alt=sh

Johnson, LE: Iron deficiency and toxicity. Merck Manual. Revised August 2008b. Accessed September 10, 2012. Available at www.merckmanuals.com/professional/nutritional_disorders/mineral_deficiency_and_toxicity/iron.html#v886400

Kaleita, TA, Kinsbourne, M, and Menkes, JH: A neurobehavioral syndrome after failure to thrive on chloride-deficient formula. Dev Med Child Neurol 33:626, 1991.

Kemi, VE, Kärkkäinen, MU, Karp, HJ, et al: Increased calcium intake does not completely counteract the effects of increased phosphorus intake on bone: an acute dose-response study in healthy females. Br J Nutr 99:832, 2008.

Kemi, VE, Rita, HJ, Kärkkäinen, MU, et al: Habitual high phosphorus intakes and foods with phosphate additives negatively affect serum parathyroid hormone concentration: a cross-sectional study on healthy premenopausal women. Public Health Nutr 12:1885, 2009.

Kew, MC: Prevention of hepatocellular carcinoma. Ann Hepatol 9:120, 2010.

King, JC, and Cousins, RJ: Zinc. In Ross, AC, Caballero, B, Cousins, RJ, et al (eds): Modern Nutrition in Health and Disease, ed 11. Lippincott Williams & Wilkins, Philadelphia, 2014.

Kodama, H, Fujisawa, C, and Bhadhprasit, W: Inherited copper transport disorders: Biochemical mechanisms, diagnosis, and treatment. Curr Drug Metab 13:237, 2012.

Kolnick, L, Harris, BD, Choma, DP, and Choma, NN: Hypercalcemia in pregnancy: A case of milk-alkali syndrome. J Gen Intern Med 26:939, 2011.

Kumar, A, and Jazieh, AR: Case report of sideroblastic anemia caused by ingestion of coins. Am J Hematol 66:126, 2001.

Kurland, ES, Schulman, RC, Zerwekh, JE, et al: Recovery from skeletal fluorosis (an enigmatic, American case). J Bone Miner Res 22:163, 2007.

Laurberg, P: Iodine. In Ross, AC, Caballero, B, Cousins, RJ, et al (eds): Modern Nutrition in Health and Disease, ed 11. Lippincott Williams & Wilkins, Philadelphia, 2014.

Lichtin, AE: Iron deficiency anemia. Merck Manual. Revised May 2013. Accessed July 10, 2013. Available at www.merckmanuals.com/professional/hematology_and_oncology/anemias_caused_by_deficient_erythropoiesis/iron_deficiency_anemia.html?qt=serum transferrin&alt=sh

Mast, AE, Schlumpf, KS, Wright, DJ, et al: The impact of HFE mutations on haemoglobin and iron status in individuals experiencing repeated iron loss through blood donation. Br J Haematol 156: 388, 2012.

Maurel, DB, Boisseau, N, Benhamou, CL, and Jaffre, C: Alcohol and bone: Review of dose effects and mechanisms. Osteoporos Int 23:1, 2012.

Meyer, PA, Pivetz, T, Digman, TA, et al: Surveillance for elevated blood lead levels among children—United States, 1997–2001. Morb Mortal Wkly Rep 52:SS10, 2003. Accessed September 27, 2012 at www.cdc.gov/mmwr/PDF/ss/ss5210.pdf.

Moreno-Jiménez, E, Esteban, E, and Peñalosa, JM: The fate of arsenic in soil-plant systems. Rev Environ Contam Toxicol 215:1, 2012.

Nada, A, Ahmed, AM, Vilallonga, R, et al: A giant euthyroid endemic multinodular goiter with no obstructive or compressive symptoms. Case Report Med 620480, 2011. Accessed September 12, 2012. Available at www.hindawi.com/journals/crim/2011/620480

National Kidney Foundation: Diet and kidney stones. Updated September 2011. Accessed July 15, 2013. Available at www.kidney.org/atoz/content/diet.cfm

National Osteoporosis Foundation: Fast facts. Undated. Accessed August 28, 2012. Available at www.nof.org/node/40

National Institutes of Health, Office of Dietary Supplements: Dietary supplement fact sheet: Calcium. Reviewed August 1, 2012. Accessed August 27, 2012. Available at http://ods.od.nih.gov/factsheets/Calcium-HealthProfessional

National Institutes of Health, Office of Dietary Supplements: Dietary supplement fact sheet: Iron. Reviewed August 24, 2007. Accessed October 4, 2012. Available at http://ods.od.nih.gov/factsheets/Iron-HealthProfessional

National Institutes of Health, Office of Dietary Supplements: Multivitamin/mineral supplements. Reviewed January 12, 2012. Accessed November 11, 2012. Available at http://ods.od.nih.gov/factsheets/MVMS-HealthProfessional

National Institutes of Health, Office of Dietary Supplements: Selenium. Reviewed October 11, 2011. Accessed September 21, 2012. Available at ods.od.nih.gov/factsheets/Selenium-HealthProfessional

Nishiwaki, S, Iwashita, M, Goto, N, et al: Predominant copper deficiency during prolonged enteral nutrition through a jejunostomy tube compared to that through a gastrostomy tube. Clin Nutr 30:585, 2011.

Nyenwe, EA, and Dagogo-Jack, S: Iodine deficiency disorders in the iodine-replete environment. Am J Med Sci 337:37, 2009.

Olympio, KP, Goncalves, C, Günther, WM, and Bechara, EJ: Neurotoxicity and aggressiveness triggered by low-level lead in children: A review. Pan Am J Public Health 26:266, 2009.

O'Malley, GF: Iron poisoning. Merck Manual. Revised April 2009. Accessed September 11, 2012. Available at www.merckmanuals.com/professional/injuries_poisoning/poisoning/iron_poisoning.html?qt=iron poisoning&alt=sh

Patel, AB, Mamtani, M, Badhoniya, N, and Kulkarni, H: What zinc supplementation does and does not achieve in diarrhea prevention: a systematic review and meta-analysis. BMC Infect Dis 11:122, 2011.

Pawa, S, Khalifa, AJ, Ehrinpreis, MN, et al: Zinc toxicity from massive and prolonged coin ingestion in an adult. Am J Med Sci 336:430, 2008.

Pelclova, D, Sklensky, M, Janicek, P, and Lach, K: Severe cobalt intoxication following hip replacement revision: Clinical features and outcome. Clin Toxicol (Phila) 50:262, 2012.

Perrine, CG, Herrick, K, Serdula, MK, and Sullivan, KM: Some subgroups of reproductive age women in the United States may be at risk for iodine deficiency. J Nuti 140:1489, 2010.

Perumal, V, Alkire, M, and Swank, ML: Unusual presentation of cobalt hypersensitivity in a patient with a metal-on-metal bearing in total hip arthroplasty. Am J Orthop 39:E39, 2010.

Polyzois, I, Nikolopoulos, D, Michos, I, et al: Local and systemic toxicity of nanoscale debris particles in total hip arthroplasty. J Appl Toxicol 32:255, 2012.

Poole, RL, Hintz, SR, Mackenzie, NI, and Kerner, JA, Jr: Aluminum exposure from pediatric parenteral nutrition: Meeting the new FDA regulation. JPEN J Parenter Enteral Nutr 32:242, 2008.

Poole, RL, Pieroni, KP, Gaskari, S: Aluminum in pediatric parenteral nutrition products: Measured versus labeled content. J Pediatr Pharmacol Ther 16:92, 2011.

Pringsheim, T, Davenport, W, Mackie, G, et al: Canadian Headache Society guideline for migraine prophylaxis. Can J Neurol Sci 39(2 Suppl 2):S1, 2012.

Raiten, DJ, Namasté, S, and Brabin, B: Considerations for the safe and effective use of iron interventions in areas of malaria burden—executive summary. Int J Vitam Nutr Res 81:57, 2011.

Ronald, P: Plant genetic, sustainable agriculture, and global food security. Genetics 188:11, 2011.

Ronis, MJ, Mercer, K, Chen, JR: Effects of nutrition and alcohol consumption on bone loss. Curr Osteoporos Rep 9:53, 2011.

Rosado, JL, Díaz, M, González, K, et al: The addition of milk or yogurt to a plant-based diet increases zinc bioavailability but does not affect iron bioavailability in women. J Nutr 135:465, 2005.

Rosin, A: The long-term consequences of exposure to lead. Isr Med Assoc J 11:689, 2009.

Roush, K: Prevention and treatment of osteoporosis in postmenopausal women: A review. Am J Nurs 111:26, 2011.

Rude, RK: Magnesium. In Ross, AC, Caballero, B, Cousins, RJ, et al (eds): Modern Nutrition in Health and Disease, ed 11. Lippincott Williams & Wilkins, Philadelphia, 2014.

Sahni, V, Léger, Y, Panaro, L, et al: Case report: A metabolic disorder presenting as pediatric manganism. Environ Health Perspect 115:1776, 2007.

Saliba, W, El Fakih, R, and Shaheen, W: Heart failure secondary to selenium deficiency, reversible after supplementation. Int J Cardiol 141:e26, 2010.

Sardesai, VM: Molybdenum: An essential trace element. Nutr Clin Pract 8:277, 1993.

Science, M, Johnstone, J, Roth, DE, et al: Zinc for the treatment of the common cold: A systematic review and meta-analysis of randomized controlled trials. CMAJ 184:E5, 2012.

Shaikh, MG, Anderson, JM, Hall, SK, Jackson, MA: Transient neonatal hypothyroidism due to a maternal vegan diet. J Pediatr Endocrinol Metab 16:111, 2003.

Shannon, M: Severe lead poisoning in pregnancy. Ambul Pediatr 3:37, 2003.

Shannon, M, and Graef, J: Hazard of lead in infant formula [letter]. N Engl J Med 326:137, 1992.

Simonsen, LO, Harbak, H, and Bennekou, P: Cobalt metabolism and toxicology—A brief update. Sci Total Environ 432:210, 2012.

Singh, M, and Das, RR: Zinc for the common cold. Cochrane Database Syst Rev 16:CD001364, 2011.

Smith, HM, Farrow, SJ, Ackerman, JD, et al: Cardiac arrests associated with hyperkalemia during red blood cell transfusion: A case series. Anesth Analg 106:1062, 2008.

Sterns, RH, Hix, JK, and Silver, S: Treatment of hyponatremia. Curr Opin Nephrol Hypertens. 19:493, 2010.

Sunde, RA: Selenium. In Ross, AC, Caballero, B, Cousins, RJ, et al (eds): Modern Nutrition in Health and Disease, ed 11. Lippincott Williams & Wilkins, Philadelphia, 2014.

Swaminathan, K: A hidden history of heartburn: The milk-alkali syndrome. Indian J Pharmacol 43:78, 2011.

Talebi, M, Savadi-Oskouei, D, Farhoudi, M, et al: Relation between serum magnesium level and migraine attacks. Neurosciences (Riyadh) 16:320, 2011.

Tredici P, Grosso E, Gibelli B, et al: Identification of patients at high risk for hypocalcemia after total thyroidectomy. Acta Otorhinolaryngol Ital 31:144, 2011.

Trocello, JM, Hinfray, S, Sanda, N, et al: An unrecognized cause of myelopathy associated with copper deficiency: The use of denture cream [article in French]. Rev Neurol (Paris) 167:537, 2011.

Tsukamoto, S, Maruyama, K, Nakagawa, H, et al: Fatal hyperkalemia due to rapid red cell transfusion in a critically ill patient. J Nippon Med Sch 76:258, 2009.

Tucker, KL, Morita, K, Qiao, N, et al: Colas, but not other carbonated beverages, are associated with low bone mineral density in older women: The Framingham Osteoporosis Study. Am J Clin Nutr 84:936, 2006.

Tucker, KL, and Rosen, CJ: Prevention and management of osteoporosis. In Ross, AC, Caballero, B, Cousins, RJ, et al (eds): Modern Nutrition in Health and Disease, ed 11. Lippincott Williams & Wilkins, Philadelphia, 2014.

Tymitz, K, Magnuson, T, and Schweitzer, M: Bariatric surgery. In Ross, AC, Caballero, B, Cousins, RJ, et al (eds): Modern Nutrition in Health and Disease, ed 11. Lippincott Williams & Wilkins, Philadelphia, 2014.

Urbano, AM, Ferreira, LM, and Alpoim, MC: Molecular and cellular mechanisms of hexavalent chromium-induced lung cancer: An updated perspective. Curr Drug Metab 13:284, 2012.

U.S. Environmental Protection Agency: Arsenic in drinking water. Updated March 6, 2012. Accessed September 25, 2012. Available at water.epa.gov/lawsregs/rulesregs/sdwa/arsenic/index.cfm

U.S. Federal Trade Commission: Docket #D-3758 Decision and Order, July 11, 1997. Accessed September 23, 2012. Available at www.ftc.gov/os/1997/07/nutritid.pdf

U.S. Food and Drug Administration: Arsenic. Updated September 21, 2012. Accessed September 24, 2012. Available at www.fda.gov/Food/FoodSafety/FoodContaminantsAdulteration/Metals/ucm280202.htm

U.S. Food and Drug Administration: FDA proposes "action level" for arsenic in apple juice. July 12, 2013. Accessed July 12, 2013. Available at www.fda.gov/NewsEvents/Newsroom/PressAnnouncements/ucm360466.htm

U.S. Food and Drug Administration: FDA requires new safety measures for oral sodium phosphate products to reduce risk of acute kidney injury. December 11, 2008. Accessed September 3, 2012 at www.fda.gov/NewsEvents/Newsroom/PressAnnouncements/2008/ucm116988.htm

U.S. Food and Drug Administration: Guidance for Industry: Bottled Water: Arsenic; Small Entity Compliance Guide. Updated August 24, 2011. Accessed September 24, 2012. Available at www.fda.gov/Food/GuidanceComplianceRegulatoryInformation/GuidanceDocuments/ChemicalContaminantsandPesticides/ucm151384.htm

U.S. Food and Drug Administration: Guidance for Industry: Iron-Containing Supplements and Drugs: Label Warning Statements Small Entity Compliance Guide. Updated July 18, 2011. Accessed September 11, 2012. Available at www.fda.gov/Food/GuidanceComplianceRegulatoryInformation/GuidanceDocuments/DietarySupplements/ucm073014.htm

U.S. Food and Drug Administration: Public Health Advisory: Loss of Sense of Smell With Intranasal Cold Remedies Containing Zinc. June 16, 2009. Accessed September 18, 2012. Available at www.fda.gov/Drugs/DrugSafety/PostmarketDrugSafetyInformationforPatientsandProviders/DrugSafetyInformationforHeathcareProfessionals/PublicHealthAdvisories/ucm166059.htm

U.S. National Library of Medicine: Genetics Home Reference, HFE. Published September 3, 2012. Accessed September 10, 2012. Available at ghr.nlm.nih.gov/condition/hemochromatosis

Valadez-Vega, C, Zúñiga-Pérez, C, Quintanar-Gómez, S: Lead, cadmium and cobalt (Pb, Cd, and Co) leaching of glass-clay containers by pH effect of food. Int J Mol Sci 12:2336, 2011.

Vallerand, AH, Sanoski, CA, and Deglin, JH: Davis's Drug Guide for Nurses, ed 13. FA Davis, Philadelphia, 2013.

Van Sickle, D, Wenck, MA, Belflower, A, et al: Acute health effects after exposure to chlorine gas released after a train derailment. Am J Emerg Med 27:1, 2009.

Vassilev, ZP, Marcus, SM, Ayyanathan, K, et al: Case of elevated blood lead in a South Asian family that has used Sindoor for food coloring. Clin Toxicol (Phila) 43:301, 2005.

Vraets, A, Lin, Y, and Callum, JL: Transfusion-associated hyperkalemia. Transfus Med Rev 25:184, 2011.

Waked, A, Geara, A, and El-Imad, B: Hypercalcemia, metabolic alkalosis and renal failure secondary to calcium bicarbonate intake for osteoporosis prevention—"modern" milk alkali syndrome: a case report. Cases J 6:6188, 2009.

Weaver, CM, and Heaney, RP: Calcium. In Ross, AC, Caballero, B, Cousins, RJ, et al (eds): Modern Nutrition in Health and Disease, ed 11. Lippincott Williams & Wilkins, Philadelphia, 2014.

Weiss, G: Genetic mechanisms and modifying factors in hereditary hemochromatosis. Nat Rev Gastroenterol Hepatol 7:50, 2010.

Wessling-Resnick, M: Iron. In Ross, AC, Caballero, B, Cousins, RJ, et al (eds): Modern Nutrition in Health and Disease, ed 11. Lippincott Williams & Wilkins, Philadelphia, 2014.

Whyte, MP, Totty, WG, Lim, VT, and Whitford, GM: Skeletal fluorosis from instant tea. J Bone Miner Res 23:759, 2008.

Wier, HA, and Kuhn, RJ: Aluminum toxity in neonatal parenteral nutrition: What can we do? Ann Pharmacother 46:137, 2012.

World Health Organization: Micronutrient deficiencies. 2012. Accessed October 11, 2012. Available at www.who.int/nutrition/topics/idd/en/index.html

World Health Organization: Zinc supplementation in the management of diarrhea. Updated December 13, 2011. Accessed September 18, 2012. Available at www.who.int/elena/titles/zinc_diarrhoea/en

Yakoob, MY, Theodoratou, E, Jabeen, A, et al: Preventive zinc supplementation in developing countries: impact on mortality and morbidity due to diarrhea, pneumonia and malaria. BMC Public Health 13(Suppl):S23, 2011.

Yang, XE, Chen, WR, Feng, Y: Improving human micronutrient nutrition through biofortification in the soil-plant system: China as a case study. Environ Geochem Health 29:413, 2007.

Zhou, Y, and Brittin, HC: Increased iron content of some Chinese foods due to cooking in steel woks. J Am Diet Assoc 94:1153, 1994.

Zhu, K, Meng, X, and Kerr, DA: The effects of a two-year randomized, controlled trial of whey protein supplementation on bone structure, IGF-1, and urinary calcium excretion in older postmenopausal women. J Bone Miner Res 26:2298, 2011.

Zimmermann, MB: Iodine deficiency. Endocr Rev 30:376, 2009.

Zimmermann, MB, and Andersson, M: Prevalence of iodine deficiency in Europe in 2010. Ann Endocrinol (Paris) 72:164, 2011.

Chapter 8

Almond, CS, Shin, AY, Fortescue, EB, et al: Hyponatremia among runners in the Boston Marathon. N Engl J Med 352:1550, 2005.

Anderko, L, Chalupka, S, Gray, WA, and Kesten, K: Greening the "proclamation for change": healing through sustainable health care environments. Am J Nurs 113:52, 2013.

Bailey, JL, Sands, JM, and Franch, HA: Water, electrolytes, and acid-base metabolism. In Ross, AC, Caballero, B, Cousins, RJ, et al (eds): Modern Nutrition in Health and Disease, ed 11. Lippincott Williams & Wilkins, Philadelphia, 2014.

Becker, JA, and Stewart, LK: Heat-related illness. Am Fam Physician 83:1325, 2011. Accessed July 21, 2013. Available at www.aafp.org/afp/2011/0601/p1325.html

Centers for Disease Control and Prevention: Heat illness among high school athletes—United States, 2005–2009. Morb Mortal Wkly Rep 59:1009, August 20, 2010. Accessed October 31, 2012. Available at www.cdc.gov/mmwr/preview/mmwrhtml/mm5932a1.htm?s_cid=mm5932a1_w

Centers for Disease Control and Prevention: Heat-related deaths after an extreme heat event — four states, 2012, and United States, 1999–2009. Morb Mortal Wkly Rep 62:433, June 7, 2013. Accessed July 21, 2013. Available at www.cdc.gov/mmwr/preview/mmwrhtml/mm6222a1.htm?s_cid=mm6222a1_w

Centers for Disease Control and Prevention: Heat stress. Updated May 18, 2012. Accessed October 22, 2012. Available at www.cdc.gov/niosh/topics/heatstress

Centers for Disease Control and Prevention: Nonfatal sports and recreation heat illness treated in hospital emergency departments—United States, 2001–2009. Morb Mortal Wkly Rep 60:977, July 29, 2011. Accessed July 19, 2013. Available at www.cdc.gov/mmwr/preview/mmwrhtml/mm6029a1.htm

Chalupka, S: Tainted water on tap. Am J Nurs 105:40, 2005.

Chepelinsky, AB: Structural function of MIP/aquaporin 0 in the eye lens; genetic defects lead to congenital inherited cataracts. Handb Exp Pharmacol 190:265, 2009.

Consumer Reports. Bottled doesn't mean better. September 2011: 7.

Consumer Reports. Do you know where your bottled water comes from? July 2012: 9. Accessed October 28, 2012. Available at www.consumerreports.org/cro/magazine/2012/07/do-you-know-where-your-bottled-water-comes-from/index.htm

Consumer Reports. Water filters. May, 2010: 33.

Didier, S: Water bottle pollution facts. National Geographic Green Living, undated. Accessed October 18, 2012. Available at greenliving.nationalgeographic.com/water-bottle-pollution-2947.html

Discover Chiropractic: Tap water vs. bottled water. March 4, 2012. Accessed October 20, 2012. Available at dcpdx.com/tap-water-vs-bottled-water

Eckhard, A, Gleiser, C, Arnold, H, et al: Water channel proteins in the inner ear and their link to hearing impairment and deafness. Mol Aspects Med 33:612, 2012.

Esposito, P, Piotti, G, Bianzina, S, et al: The syndrome of inappropriate antidiuresis: Pathophysiology, clinical management and new therapeutic options. Nephron Clin Pract 119:c62, 2011.

Fishman, C: U.S. bottled water sales are booming (again) despite opposition. National Geographic Newswatch, May 17, 2012. Accessed October 18, 2012. Available at http://newswatch.nationalgeographic.com/2012/05/17/u-s-bottled-water-sales-are-booming-again-despite-opposition

Fournier, M: Perfecting your acid-base balancing act. Am Nurse Today 4:17, 2009.

Frouget, T: The syndrome of inappropriate antidiuresis. Rev Med Interne. 33:556, 2012.

Gardner, JW: Death by water intoxication. Mil Med 167:432, 2002.

Giorgianni, A: Bottled water: $346 per year. Tap water: 48 cents. Any questions? Consumer Reports, July 12, 2011. Accessed October 28, 2012. Available at http://news.consumerreports.org/money/2011/07/a-dollar-for-a-bottle-of-water-what-would-martians-think.html

Gorelick, MH, Gould, L, Nimmer, M, et al: Perceptions about water and increased use of bottled water in minority children. Arch Pediatr Adolesc Med 165:928, 2011.

Gropper, SS, and Smith, JL: Advanced Nutrition and Human Metabolism, ed 6. Wadsworth, Belmont, CA, 2013.

Hobson, WL, Knochel, ML, Byington, CL, et al: Bottled, filtered, and tap water use in Latino and non-Latino children. Arch Pediatr Adolesc Med 161:457, 2007.

Holmes, RP: The role of renal water channels in health and disease. Mol Aspects Med 33:547, 2012.

Huang, LH, Anchala, KR, Ellsburg, DL, and George, CS: Dehydration treatment and management. Medscape Reference. Updated March 12, 2012. Accessed December 23, 2012. Available at http://emedicine.medscape.com/article/906999-treatment

Huerta-Saenz, L, Irigoyen, M, Benavides, J, and Mendoza, M: Tap or bottled water: Drinking preferences among urban minority children and adolescents. J Community Health 37:54, 2012.

Institute of Medicine: Dietary Reference Intakes for Water, Potassium, Sodium Chloride, and Sulfate. National Academy Press, Washington, DC, 2004. Accessed October 13, 2012 at www.nap.edu/openbook.php?record_id=10925&page=74

Ishibashi, K, Hara, S, and Kondo, S: Aquaporin water channels in mammals. Clin Exp Nephrol 13:107, 2009.

Ishibashi, K, Kondo, S, Hara, S, and Morishita, Y: The evolutionary aspects of aquaporin family. Am J Physiol Regul Integr Comp Physiol 300:R566, 2011.

Kerr, ZY, Casa, DJ, Marshall, SW, and Comstock, RD: Epidemiology of exertional heat illness among U.S. high school athletes. Am J Prev Med 44:8, 2013.

Knochel, JP: Heatstroke. Merck Manual. February 2010. Accessed October 22, 2012. Available at www.merckmanuals.com/professional/injuries_poisoning/heat_illness/heatstroke.html

Laforenza, U: Water channel proteins in the gastrointestinal tract. Mol Aspects Med 33:642/2012.

Lechtzin, N: Hyperventilation syndrome. Merck Manual. Updated July 2012. Accessed July 25, 2013. Available at www.merckmanuals.com/professional/pulmonary_disorders/symptoms_of_pulmonary_disorders/hyperventilation_syndrome.html?qt=hyperventilation&alt=sh

Leiba, N, Gray, S, and Houlihan, J: EWG bottled water scorecard. 2011. Accessed October 17, 2012. Available at www.ewg.org/bottled-water-2011-summary-findings

Muckelbauer, R, Libuda, L, Clausen, K, et al: Promotion and provision of drinking water in schools for overweight prevention: randomized, controlled cluster trial. Pediatrics 123:e661, 2009. Accessed October 25, 2012. Available at pediatrics.aappublications.org/content/123/4/e661.long

Mueller, FO, and Colgate, B: Annual Survey of Football Injury Research. American Football Coaches Association, Waco, TX, 2010. Accessed October 31, 2012 at www.unc.edu/depts/nccsi/2009AnnualFootball.pdf

Natural Resources Defense Council: Bottled water: Pure drink or pure hype? Executive summary. Revised June 25, 2000. Accessed October 17, 2012 at www.nrdc.org/water/drinking/bw/exesum.asp

Natural Resources Defense Council: Bottled water. Revised April 25, 2008. Accessed October 18, 2012. Available at www.nrdc.org/water/drinking/qbw.asp

O'Brien, KK, Montain, SJ, Corr, WP, et al: Hyponatremia associated with overhydration in U.S. Army trainees. Mil Med 166:405, 2001.

Overgaard-Steensen, C. Initial approach to the hyponatremic patient. Acta Anaesthesiol Scand 55:139, 2011.

Pease, S, Bouadma, L, Kermarrec, N, et al: Early organ dysfunction course, cooling time and outcome in classic heatstroke. Intensive Care Med 35:1454, 2009.

Peate, WF: Hyponatremia in marathon runners [letter]. N Engl J Med 353:427, 2005.

Popkin, BM, D'Anci, KE, and Rosenberg, IH: Water, hydration, and health. Nutr Rev 68:439, 2010.

Scanlon, VC, and Sanders, T: Essentials of anatomy and physiology, ed 6. FA Davis, Philadelphia, 2011.

Sharfstein, JM: Testimony before Committee on Energy and Commerce, U.S. House of Representatives, July 8, 2009. Revised April 19, 2011. Accessed October 18, 2012. Available at www.hhs.gov/asl/testify/2009/07/t20090708a.html

Sterns, RH, Hix, JK, and Silver, S: Treatment of hyponatremia. Curr Opin Nephrol Hypertens 19:493, 2010.

Strauch, KA: Invisible pollution: The impact of pharmaceuticals in the water supply. AAOHN J 59:525, 2011.

U.S. Environmental Protection Agency: Arsenic in drinking water. March 6, 2012. Accessed September 25, 2012. Available at http://water.epa.gov/lawsregs/rulesregs/sdwa/arsenic/index.cfm

U.S. Food and Drug Administration: Disposal of unused medicines: What you should know. Updated July 15, 2013. Accessed July 31, 2013. Available at www.fda.gov/Drugs/ResourcesForYou/Consumers/BuyingUsingMedicineSafely/EnsuringSafeUseofMedicine/SafeDisposalofMedicines/ucm186187.htm

Vaidya, C, Ho, W, and Freda, BJ: Management of hyponatremia: Providing treatment and avoiding harm. Cleve Clin J Med 77:715, 2010.

Vantyghem, MC, Balavoine, AS, Wémeau, JL, and Douillard, C: Hyponatremia and antidiuresis syndrome. Ann Endocrinol (Paris) 72:500, 2011.

Venes, D (ed): Taber's Cyclopedic Medical Dictionary, ed 21. FA Davis, Philadelphia, 2009.

Venes, D (ed): Taber's Cyclopedic Medical Dictionary, ed 22. FA Davis, Philadelphia, 2013.

Verkman, AS: Aquaporins: translating bench research to human disease. J Exp Bio. 212:1701, 2009.

Williams, LS, and Hopper, PD: Understanding Medical Surgical Nursing, ed 4. FA Davis, Philadelphia, 2011.

Xu, M, Su, W, Xu, QP: Aquaporin-4 and traumatic brain edema. Chin J Traumatol 13:103, 2010.

Yool, AJ, Brown, EA, and Flynn, GA: Roles for novel pharmacological blockers of aquaporins in the treatment of brain oedema and cancer. Clin Exp Pharmacol Physiol 37:403, 2010.

Zelenina, M: Regulation of brain aquaporins. Neurochem Int 57:468, 2010.

Chapter 9

Academy of Nutrition and Dietetics: Celiac Disease (CD) Evidence-Based Nutrition Practice Guideline, Accessed April 2013. Available at http:.//andevidencelibrary.com.

Castrogiovanni, A: Communication facts: Special populations: Dysphagia—2008 edition. Accessed April 2013. Available at http://www.asha.org/research/reports/dysphagia/

Colaizzo-Anas, T: Nutrient intake, digestion, absorption, and excretion. In Gottschlich, MM, DeLegge, MH, Mattox, T, et al (eds): The A.S.P.E.N. Nutrition Support Core Curriculum: A Case-Based Approach—The Adult Patient. American Society for Parenteral and Enteral Nutrition, Silver Spring, MD, 2007.

McCallum, SL: The National Dysphagia Diet: Implementation at a regional rehabilitation center and hospital system. J Am Diet Assoc 103:285, 2003.

National Institutes of Health: Celiac Disease Awareness Campaign, December 18, 2012a. Available at www.celiac.nih.gov

National Institutes of Health, National Digestive Diseases Information Clearinghouse: Celiac disease (NIH Pub. No. 08-4269). January 27, 2012b.

National Institutes of Health: Dysphagia (NIH Pub. No. 10-4307). October 2010.

Ojetti, V, Gabrielli, M, Migneco, A, Lauritano, C, et al: Regression of lactose malabsorption in coeliac patients after receiving a gluten-free diet. Scand J Gastroenterol 4:5, 2007.

Scanlon, VC, and Sanders, T: Essentials of Anatomy and Physiology, ed 4. FA Davis, Philadelphia, 2003.

Chapter 10

Adoptive Breastfeeding Resource Website. Accessed December 15, 2012 at www.fourfriends.com/abrw

Agarwal, M, and Phadke, S: Neural tube defects: A need for population-based prevention program. Ind J Hum Genet 18.2:145, 2011.

Allerberger, F, and Wagner, M: Listeriosis: A resurgent foodborne infection. Clin Microbiol Infect 16:16, 2010.

Amar, C., Little, C., Gillespie, L., et al: Keep it cool. Midwives. 13(3):29, 2010.

American Academy of Pediatric Dentistry: Policy on use of fluoride. Revised 2012. Available at www.aapd.org/media/Policies_Guidelines/P_FluorideUse.pdf

American Academy of Pediatrics: AAP reaffirms breastfeeding guidelines. February 27, 2012. Accessed October 23, 2012 at www.aap.org/en-us/about-the-app/aap-press-room/pages/AAPArora, M: Maternal dietary intake of polyunsaturated fatty acids modifies the relationship between lead levels in bone and breast milk. J Nutr 138:73, 2008.

Au, KS, Ashley-Koch, A, and Northrup, H: Epidemiologic and genetic aspects of spina bifida and other neural tube defects. Dev Disabil Res Rev 16:6, 2010.

Bakhireva, LN, and Savage, DD: Focus on: biomarkers of fetal alcohol exposure and fetal alcohol effects. Alcohol Res Health 29, Spring 2011.

Blumenfeld, XJ, Reynolds-May, MF, Altman, RB, and El-Sayed, YY: Maternal-fetal and neonatal pharmacogenomics: a review of current literature. J Perinatol 30:571, 2010.

Bowen, A, and Tumback, L: Alcohol and breastfeeding: Dispelling the myths and promoting the evidence. Nurs Women Health 14:456, 2010–2011.

Casey, G: Breastfeeding and drugs. Kai Taki Nurs N Z 18:20, 2012.

Centers for Disease Control and Prevention: Adolescent and school health. Accessed June 17, 2013. Available at www.cdc.gov/healthyyouth/nutrition/facts.htm

Centers for Disease Control and Prevention: Breastfeeding report card—United States, 2012. Accessed November 1, 2012. Available at www.cdc.gov/breastfeeding/data/reportcard.htm

Centers for Disease Control and Prevention: Alcohol use and binge drinking among women of childbearing age—United States, 2006–2010. Morb Mortal Wkly Rep 61(28), July 20, 2012.

Centers for Disease Control and Prevention: Fetal alcohol spectrum disorders (FASDs). Accessed December 1, 2012. Available at www.cdc.gov/NCBDDD/fasd/alcohol-use.html

Centers for Disease Control and Prevention Grand Rounds: Additional opportunities to prevent neural tube defects with folic acid fortification. Morb Mortal Wkly Rep 59(31), 980, August 13, 2010.

Centers for Disease Control and Prevention: Listeria outbreaks. Accessed November 18, 2012. Available at www.cdc.gov/listeria/outbreaks/index.html

Centers for Disease Control and Prevention: Manifestations of low vitamin B_{12} levels. Accessed October 31, 2012. Available at www.cdc.gov/ncbddd/b12/manifestations.html

Cheung, NW: The management of gestational diabetes. Vasc Health Risk Manage 2009:5: 153, 2009.

Cho, GJ, Shin, J, Yi, KW, et al: Adolescent pregnancy is associated with osteoporosis in postmenopausal women. Menopause 19:456, 2012.

Cooper, MD: Pica. Access. 24(5):39–41, 2010.

Davanzo, R, Copertino, M, De Cunto, A, et al: Antidepressant drugs and breastfeeding: A review of the literature. Breastfeed Med 6:89, 2011.

Dibaba, Y: Child spacing and fertility planning behavior among women in mana district, Jimma Zon, South West Ethiopia. Ethiop J Health Sci 20:83, 2010.

Dror, DK, and Allen, LH: Effects of Vitamin B_{12} deficiency on neurodevelopment in infants: Current knowledge and possible mechanisms. Nutr Rev 66:250, 2008.

Dror, DK, and Allen, LH: Vitamin D inadequacy in pregnancy: Biology, outcomes, and interventions. Nutr Rev 68:465, 2010.

Ettinger, AS, Lamadrid-Figueroa, H, Tellez-Rojo, MM, et al: Effect of calcium supplementation on blood lead levels in pregnancy: A randomized placebo-controlled trial. Environ Health Perspect 117:26, 2009.

Faraz, A. Clinical recommendations for promoting breastfeeding among Hispanics. J Am Acad Nurse Practit 22:292, 2010.

Fehr, KRS, Fehr, KDH, and Penner Protudjer, JL: Knowledge and use of folic acid in women of reproductive age. Can J Dietetic Pract Res 72:197, 2010.

Galloway, R, and McGuire, J: Daily versus weekly: How many iron pills do pregnant women need? Nutr Rev 54:318, 1996.

Garad, R, McNamee, K, Bateson, D, and Harvey, C: Update on contraception. Aust Nurs 20:34, 2012.

Gautam, CS, Saha, L, Kavita, S, and Saha, PK. Iron deficiency in pregnancy and the rationality of iron supplements prescribed during pregnancy. Med J Med 10:283, 2008. Accessed October 31, 2012. Available at www.ncbi.nlm.nih.gov/pmc/articles/PMC2644004/?report=printatble

Giovannini, M, Verduci, E, Salvatici, E, et al: Phenylketonuria: Nutritional advances and challenges. Nutr Metab 9:7, 2012.

Groth, SW, and Kearney, MH: Diverse women's beliefs about weight gain in pregnancy. J Midwifery Women's Health 54:452, 2009.

Guez, S, Chiarelli, G, Menni, F, et al: Severe vitamin B_{12} deficiency in an exclusively breastfed 5-month-old Italian infant born to a mother receiving multivitamin supplementation during pregnancy. BMC Pediatr 12:85, 2012.

Hacker, AN, Fung, EB, and King, JC: Role of calcium during pregnancy: Maternal and fetal needs. Nutr Rev 70:397, 2012.

Institute of Medicine: Weight gain during pregnancy; Reexamining the guidelines. Accessed November 1, 2013. Available at iom.edu/Reports/2009/Weight-Gain-During-Pregnancy-Reexamining-the-Guidelines.aspx

Janevic, T, Stein, CR, Savitz, DA, et al: Neighborhood deprivation and adverse birth outcomes among diverse ethnic groups. Ann Epidemiol 20:445, 2010.

Jordan, SJ, Siskind, V, Green, AC et al: Breastfeeding and risk of epithelial ovarian cancer. Cancer Causes Control 21:109, 2010.

Jones, W, and Breward, S: Drugs and breastfeeding. Commun Pract 83:41, 2010.

Karagus, MR, Choi, AI, Oken, E, et al: Evidence on the human health effects of low-level methylmercury exposure. Environ Health Perspect 120:799, 2012.

Kim, J, Zhao, K, Jiang, P, et al: Transcriptome landscape of the human placent. BMC Genomics 13:115, 2012.

Kotsopoulous, J, Lubinski J, Salmena L, et al: Breastfeeding and the risk of breast cancer in BR,CA1 and BR,CA2 mutation carriers. Breast Cancer Res 14:R42, 2012.

Latva-Pukkila, U, Isolauri, E, and Laitinen, K: Dietary and clinical impacts of nausea and vomiting during pregnancy. J Hum Nutr Diet, 23:69, 2009.

Leung, AM, Pearce, EN, and Braverman, LE: Iodine nutrition in pregnancy and lactation. Endocrinol Metab Clin North Am 40:765, 2011.

Livville, T, Ritchie, S, Novak, D: Vomiting, Failure to thrive in a breastfed infant. Contemp Pediatr 29:32, 2012.

Madadi, P, Moretti, M, Djokanovic, N, et al: Guidelines for maternal codeine use during breastfeeding. Can Fam Physician 55:1077, 2009.

Magee, LA, Abalos, E, von Dadelszen, P, et al: How to manage hypertension in pregnancy effectively. Br J Clin Pharmacol 72:394, 2011.

Mahadevan, S, Kumaravel, V, and Bharath, R: Calcium and bone disorders in pregnancy. Ind J Endocrinol Metab: 16:356, 2012.

Mahffey, DR, Sunderland, EM, Chan, HM, et al: Balancing the benefits of n-3 ployunsaturated fatty acids and the risks of methylmercury exposure from fish consumption. Nutr Rev 69:493, 2011.

Malvasi, A, Tinelli, A, Buia, A, and De Luca, GF: Possible long-term teratogenic effects of isotretinoin in pregnancy. Eur Rev Med Pharmacol Sci 13:393, 2009.

Maslova, E, Bhattacharya, S, Lin, SW, and Michels, KB: Caffeine consumption during pregnancy and risk of preterm birth: A meta-analysis. Am J Clin Nutr 92:1120, 2010.

Mayo Clinic: Pregnancy week by week. 2012. Accessed December 11, 2012. Available at www.mayoclinic.com/health/pregnancy-weight-gain/PR00111/NSECTIONGROUP=2

McArdle, HJ, Lang, C, Hayes, H, and Gambling, L: Role of the placenta in regulation of fetal iron status. Nutr Rev 69(Suppl 1):S17, 2011.

Milman, N: Oral iron prophylaxis in pregnancy: Not too little and not too much. J Pregnancy 2012:514345, 2012.

Mulu, A, Kassu, A, Huruy, K, et al: Vitamin A deficiency during pregnancy of HIV infected and non-infected women in tropical settings of Northwest Ethiopia. BMC Public Health 11:569, 2011.

Mustafa, R, Ahmed, S, Gupta, A, and Venuto, RC: A comprehensive review of hypertension in pregnancy. J Pregnancy 2012:105918, 2012.

National Center on Birth Defects and Developmental Disabilities: Annual report: Folic acid: Reducing folic acid-preventable neural tube defects. Accessed October 12, 2012. Available at http://www.cdc.gov/ncbddd/aboutus/annualreport2012/documents/ncbdddannualrepor2012-full-report.pdf

Nayeri, UA: Hyperemesis in pregnancy: Taking a tiered approach. July 2012. Accessed February 20, 2014. Available at http://digital.healthcaregroup.advanstar.com/nxtbooks/advanstar/obgyn_201207/index.php?startid=22

Pangillnan, F, Molloy, AM, Mills, JL, et al: Evaluation of common genetic variants in 82 candidate genes as risk factors for neural tube defects. BMC Med Genet 13:62, 2012.

Phelan, S, Phipps, MG, Abrams, B, et al: Practitioner advice and gestational weight gain. J Women Health (Larchmt) 20:585, 2011.

Phillips, F: Healthy eating in pregnancy. Pract Nurse 42(1):24–28, 2012.

Picciano, MF, and McGuire, MK: Use of dietary supplements by pregnant and lactating women in North America. Am J Clin Nutr 89(Suppl):663S, 2009.

Pinto, S, and Schub, T: Fetal alcohol syndrome. Cinahl Information Systems, June 2012.

Purnell, LD: Transcultural Health Care: A Culturally Competent Appoach, ed 4. FA Davis, Philadelphia, 2013.

Rahbari, AH, Keshavarz, H, Shojaee, S, et al: IgG avidity EL,ISA test for diagnosis of acute toxoplasmosis in humans. Korean J Parasitol 50:99, 2012.

Ramirez de Arellano, AB: The primacy of prevention: folic acid fortification. P R Health Sci J 29:121, 2012.

Rice, GE, Illanes, SE, and Mitchell, MD: Gestational diabetes mellitus: A positive predictor of type 2 diabetes? Int J Endocrinol 2012;721653, 2012.

Rioux, FM, Belanger-Plourde, J, LeBlanc, CP, and Vigneau, F: Relationship between maternal DH,A and iron status and infants' cognitive performance. Can J Dietetic Pract Res 72, Summer 2011.

Rofail, D, Collins, A, Abetz, L: Factors contributing to the success of folic acid public health campaigns. J. Public Health (Oxf) 34:90, 2012.

Safi, J, Joyeux, L, and Chlauhi, GE: Periconceptional folate deficiency and implications in neural tube defects. J Pregnancy 2012:295083, 2012.

San Joaquin, MA, Molyneux, ME: Malaria and vitamin A deficiency in African children: A vicious circle? Malaria J 8:134, 2009.

Schwartz, J, Drossard, C, Dube, K, et al: Dietary intake and plasma concentrations of PU,FA and LC,-PUFA in breastfed and formula fed infants under real-life conditions. Eur J Nutr 49:189, 2010.

Scholl, TO: Maternal iron status: Relation to fetal growth, length of gestation and the neonate's iron endowment. Nutr Rev 69(Suppl 1):S23, 2011.

Shennan, AH, and Vousden, N: Commentary: nonpharmacological approaches to hypertension in pregnancy need further evaluation. Birth 37: 307, 2010.

Simpson, JL, Shulman, LP, Brown, H, and Holzgreve, W: Closing the folate gap in reproductive aged women. Contemporary OB,/GYN 55:34, 2010.

Smith, MAE, and MacLaurin, TL: Who is telling pregnant women about listeriosis? Can J Public Health 102:441, 2011.

Stillwaggon, E, Carrier, CS, Sautter, M, and McLeod, R: Maternal serologic screening to prevent congenital toxoplasmosis: A decision-analytic economic model. PLoS Negl Trop Dis. 5:e1333, 2011.

Summers, A: Emergency management of hyperemesis gravidarum. Emerg Nurse 20:24, 2012.

The Academy of Breastfeeding Medicine Protocol Committee: ABM Clinical Protocol #21: Guidelines for breastfeeding and the drug-dependent women. Breastfeed Med 4: 225, 2009.

Trottier, M, Erebara, A, and Bozzo, P: Treating constipation during pregnancy. Can Fam Physician 58:836, 2012.

Ural, SH: Prenatal nutrition. 2001. Accessed July 9, 2012. Available at Medscape, http://emedicine.medscape.com/article/259059-overview

U.S. Department of Agriculture: ChooseMyPlate.gov. Accessed November 18, 2012. Available at www.choosemyplate.gov/pregnancy-breastfeeding.html

U.S. Department of Agriculture: The special supplemental nutrition program for women, infants and children, August 2011. Accessed November 18, 2012. Available at www.fns.usda.gov/wic

U.S. Department of Agriculture and U.S. Department of Health and Human Services: Dietary Guidelines for Americans 2010. ed 7. U.S. Government Printing Office, Washington, DC, December 2010.

Uzan, J, Carbonnel, M, Piconne, O, et al: Pre-eclampsia: Pathophysiology, diagnosis, and management. Vasc Health Risk Manage 11:467, 2011.

Wagner, CL, Taylor, SN, Dawodu, A, et al: Vitamin D and its role during pregnancy in attaining optimal health of mother and fetus. Nutrients 4:208, 2012.

Weddig, J, Baker, SS, and Auld, G: Perspectives of hospital-based nurses on breastfeeding initiation best practices. J Obstetr Gynecol Neonatal Nurs 40:166, 2011.

Wegrzyniak, LJ, Repke, JT, and Ural, SH: Treatment of hyperemesis gravidarum. Rev Obstetr Gynecol 5:78, 2012.

World Health Organization: Baby friendly hospital initiative. Accessed November 18, 2012. Available at www.who.int/nutrition/topics/bfhi/en/index.html

Young, G: Leg cramps. Clin Evidence. 3:1113, 2009.

Zera, C, McGirr, S, Oken, E: Screening for obesity in reproductive-aged women. Prev Chronic Sid. 8:A125, 2011. Accessed November 15, 2012. Available at www.cdc.gov/ped/issues/2011/nov/11_0032

Chapter 11

Academy of Nutrition and Dietetics: Feeding vegetarian infants and toddlers (1995–2012). Accessed November 22, 2012. Available at www.eatright.org/Public/content.aspx?id=8060#.UNByM6ytKH8

Afrazi, A, Sodhi, CP, Richardson, W: New insight into the pathogenesis and treatment of necrotizing enterocolitis: toll-like receptors and beyond. Pediatr Res 69:183, 2011.

Alexander, DD, Schmitt, DF, Tran, NL, et al: Partially hydrolyzed 100% whey protein infant formula and atopic dermatitis risk reduction: a systematic review of the literature. Nutr Rev 68:232, 2010.

American Academy of Pediatric Dentistry: Policy on use of fluoride. Reaffirmed 2012. Available at www.aapd.org/media/Policies_Guidelines/P_FluorideUse.pdf

American Academy of Pediatrics. Prevention and treatment of obesity. January, 2011. Accessed November 13, 2012. Available at www2.aap.org/obesity

American Academy of Pediatrics: Vitamin supplements and children. November 5, 2012. Accessed December 18, 2012. Available at www.healthychildren.org/English/ages-stages/gradeschool/nutrition/Pages/Vitamin-Supplements-and-Children.aspx?nfstatus=401&nftoken=00000000-0000-0000-0000-000000000000&nfstatusdescription=ERROR%3a+No+local+token

Anum, EA, Springel, EH, Shriver, MD, and Strauss, JF: Genetic contributions to disparities in preterm birth. Pediatr Res 65:1, 2009.

Aspuru, K, Villa, C, Bermejo, F, et al: Optimal management of iron deficiency anemia due to poor dietary intake. Int J Gen Med 2012:741, 2011.

Ayton, A: Dying to be thin. Your guide to today's mental health issues. Mental Health Today Jan–Feb: 22, 2012.

Bahna, SL: Hypoallergenic formulas: optimal choices for treatment versus prevention. Ann Allergy Asthma Immunol: 101:453, 2008.

Basch, CE: Breakfast and the achievement gap among urban minority youth. J School Health 81:635, 2011.

Bates, B: Failure to thrive symptom demands multifaceted exam. Pediatr News 44:34, 2010.

Beauchamp, GK, and Mennella, JA: Flavor perception in human infants: Development and functional significance. Digestion 83(Suppl 1):1, 2011.

Benjamin-Neelon, SE, and Briley, ME: Position of the American Dietetic Association: Benchmarks for nutrition in child care. J Am Dietetic Assoc 111:607, 2011.

Bhatia, J, and Greer, F: Use of soy protein-based formulas in infant feeding. Pediatrics 121:1062, 2008. Accessed November 14, 2012. Available at pediatrics.aappublications.org/contents/121/5/1062.full.html

Bouchard, C: Childhood obesity: Are genetic differences involved? Am J Clin Nutr 80(Suppl):1494S, 2009.

Bokser, S, Flaherman, VJ, and Newman, TB: First-day newborn weight loss predicts in-hospital weight nadir for breastfeeding infants. Breastfeed Med 5:165, 2010.

Brodribb, WE: Breastfeeding—a framework for educating the primary care medical workforce. Breastfeed Rev 20:25, 2012.

Brook, L: Infant botulism. J Perinatol 27:175, 2007.

Brotanek, JM, Gosz, J, Weitzman, M, and Flores, G: Iron deficiency in early childhood in the United States: Risk factors and racial/ethnic disparities. Pediatrics 120:568, 2007.

Brown, JE (ed): Nutrition Through the Life Cycle, ed 3. Thomson Wadsworth, Belmont, CA, 2008.

Bryant, AS, Worjoloh, A, Caughey, AB, and Washington, AE: Am J Obstetr Gynecol 202:335, 2010.

Burks, AW, Jones, SM, Boyce, JA, et al: NIAID-sponsored 2010 guidelines for managing food allergy: applications in the pediatric population. Pediatrics 128:955, 2011.

Burrows, T, Pursey, K, Neve, M, and Stanwell, P: What are the health implications associated with the consumption of energy drinks? A systematic review. Nutr Rev 70:135, 2013.

Burton-Shepherd, A. Nutritional management of children who follow therapeutic diets for medical reasons. Primary Health Care 22:32, 2012.

Busscher, I, Wapstra, FH, and Veldhuizen, AG: Predicting growth and curve progression in the individual patient with adolescent idiopathic scoliosis; design of a prospective longitudinal cohort study. BMC Musculoskel Disord 11:93, 2010.

Centers for Disease Control and Prevention: Guidelines for evaluation of the nutritional status and growth in refugee children during domestic medical screening examinations. March 28, 2012. Access on December 15, 2012. Available at www.cdc.gov/immigrantrefugeehealth/guidelines/domestic/nutrition-growth.html

Centers for Disease Control and Prevention: Guidelines for the management of acute diarrhea after a disaster. September 14, 2008. Accessed November 12, 2012. Available at http://emergency.cdc.gov/disasters/disease/diarrheaguidelines.asp

Centers for Disease Control and Prevention: Emergency preparedness and response: Botulism. 2011. Accessed October 29, 2012. Available at http://emergency.cdc.gov/disasters/disease/diarrheaguidelines.asp

Centers for Disease Control and Prevention: School health guidelines to promote healthy eating and physical activity: Recommendations and reports. Morb Mortal Wkly Rep 60(RR-5):1, September 15, 2011.

Chandran, A, Fitzwater, S, Zhen, A, and Santosham, M: Prevention of rotavirus gastroenteritis in infants and children: Rotavirus vaccine safety, efficacy, and potential impact of vaccines. Biol Targets Ther 4:213, 2010.

Chaudhry, R: Botulism: A diagnostic challenge. Ind J Med Res 134:10, 2011.

Chauhan, SS, Sarkar, PD, and Bhimte, B: Prematurity and related biochemical outcomes: Study of bone mineralization and renal function parameters in preterm infants. Biochem Res Int. Published online October 18, 2011, doi:10.1155/2011/740370

Chow, CM, Leung, AK, and Hon, KL: Acute gastroenteritis: From guidelines to real life. Clin Exp Gastroenterol 3:97, 2010.

Claud, EC: Neonatal necrotizing enterocolitis-inflammation and immaturity. Antiinflamm Antiallergy Agents Med Chem 8:248, 2009.

Cole, S, and Lanham, JS: Failure to thrive: An update. Am Fam Physician 83:829, 2011.

Corder, K, van Sluijs, MF, Steele, RM, et al: Breakfast consumption and physical activity in British adolescents. Br J Nutr 105:316, 2011.

Critch, JN: Infantile colic: Is there a role for dietary interventions? Paediatr Child Health 16:47, 2011.

Dabas, P, Kumar, A, and Singh, B: Spoon feeding results in early hospital discharge of low birth weight babies. J Perinatology 30:209, 2010.

Da Matta Aprile, M, Feferbaum, R, Andreassa, N, and Leone, C: Growth of very low birth weight infants fed with milk from a human milk bank selected according to the caloric and protein value. Clinics 65:751, 2010.

Deglin, JH, and Vallerand, AH (eds): Davis's Drug Guide for Nurses, ed 11. FA Davis, Philadelphia, 2009.

Dolinsky, DH, Siega-Riz, AM, Perrin, E, and Armstrong, SC: Recognizing and preventing childhood obesity: Challenging pediatricians with averting this epidemic even in their littlest patients. Contemporary Pediatr, January 2011. Accessed March 7, 2014. Available at http://digital.healthcaregroup.advanstar.com/nxtbooks/advanstar/cntped_201101/index.php?startid=32

Droppelmann, K, Navarrete-Dechent, C, Nicklas, C, et al: Comparative study of dietary habits between acne patients and a healthy cohort. Ind J Dermatol Venereol Leprol 78:99, 2012.

Duca, RA: Nutritional considerations in the management of attention deficit hyperactivity disorders. Nutr Perspect 33:5, 2010.

Ducher, G, Turner, AI, Kukuljan, S, et al: Obstacles in the optimization of bone health outcomes in the female athlete triad. Sports Med 41:587, 2011.

Dunbar, H, and Luyt, D: Triggers, clinical features and management of anaphylaxis in children. Nurs Child Young People 23:29, 2011.

Elisia, I, and Kitts, DD: Quantification of hexanal as an index of lipid oxidation in human milk and association with antioxidant components. J Clinical Biochem Nutr 49:147, 2011.

Ferre, C, Handler, A, Hsia, J: Changing trends in low birth weight rates among non-Hispanic infants in the United States, 1991–2004. Matern Child Health J 15:29, 2011.

Food Allergy and Anaphylaxis Network [FANN]: Fomon, SJ: Potential renal solute load: Considerations relating to complementary feedings of breastfed infants. Pediatrics 106(Suppl 4):1284, 2000.

Fomon, SJ: Potential renal solute load: considerations relating to complementary feedings of breastfed infants. Pediatrics 106(Suppl 4):1284, 2000.

Fulkerson, JA, Kubik, MY, Story, M, et al: Are there nutritional and other benefits associated with family meals among at-risk youth? J Adolesc Health 45:389, 2009.

Garver, WS: Gene–diet interactions in childhood obesity. Curr Genomics 12:180, 2011.

Geraghty, SR, Heier, JE, and Rasmussen, KM: Got milk? Sharing human milk via the Internet. Public Health Rep 126:161, 2011.

Gibson-Moore, H: Infant feeding linked to long-term obesity. Nutr Bull 36:95, 2011.

Gopakumar, H, Sivji, R, and Rajiv, PK: Vitamin K deficiency bleeding presenting as impending brain herniation. J Pediatr Neurosci 5:55, 2010.

Gropper, SS, Smith, JL, and Groff, JL: Advanced Nutrition and Human Metabolism, ed 5. Wadsworth, Belmont, CA, 2009.

Haines, J, Gillman, MW, Rifas-Shiman, S, et al: Family dinner and disordered eating behaviors in a large cohort of adolescents. Eating Disord 18:10, 2010.

Hoch, AZ, Pajewski, NM, Moraski, L, et al: Prevalence of the female athlete triad in high school athletes and sedentary students. Clin J Sport Med 19:421, 2009.

Hopkins, KF, DeCristofaro, C, and Elliott, L: How can primary care providers manage pediatric obesity in the real world? J Am Acad Nurse Practit 23:278, 2011.

Hurley, WL, and Theil, PK: Perspectives on immunoglobulins in colostrum and milk. Nutrients 3:442, 2011; doi:10.3390/nu3040442. Printed online at www.mdpi.com/journals/nutrients

Infante, D, Segarra, O, and Le Luyer, B: Dietary treatment of colic caused by excess gas in infants: biochemical evidence. World J Gastroenterol 17:2104, 2011.

Institute of Medicine: Report at a glance: Actions for healthy eating and improved physical activity. June 11, 2010. Accessed December 12, 2002. Availabe at www.iom.edu/Reports/2009/Local-Government-Actions-to-Prevent-Childhood-Obesity/Action-Steps-Local-Government-Actions-to-Prevent-Childhood-Obesity.aspx?page=2

Isaacs, EB, Fischi, BR, Quinn, BT, et al: Impact of breast milk on IQ, brain size and white matter development. Pediatr Res 67:357, 2010.

Ismail, NH, Manaf, ZA, and Azizan, NZ: High glycemic load diet, milk and ice cream consumption are related to acne vulgaris in Malaysian young adults: a case control study. BC Dermatol 12:13, 2012.

Jesitus, J: Food for thought: high glycemic index diet appears to promote acne, physicians says. Dermatol Times 33:S4, 2012.

Johnson, K, and Daitch, L: Peanut allergy awareness. Clin Rev 21:28, 2011.

Katz, DL, Katz, CS, Treu, JA: Teaching healthful food choices to elementary school students and their parents: the nutrition detectives program. J School Health 81:21, 2011.

Kheir, A: Infantile colic, facts and fiction. Ital J Pediatr 38:34, 2012.

Kneepkens, CM. and Meijer, Y: Clinical practice. Diagnosis and treatment of cow's milk allergy. Eur J Pediatr 168:891, 2009.

Labarque, V, Ngo, B, Penders, J, et al: Late vitamin K deficiency bleeding leading to a diagnosis of cystic fibrosis: A case report. Acta Clinica Belgica 66:142, 2011.

Landgren, D, Lundqvist, A, and Hallstrom, I: Remembering the chaos—but life went on and the wound healed. A four year follow up with parents having had a baby with infantile colic. Open Nurs J 6:53, 2012.

Leidy, HJ, and Racki, EM: The additin of a protein-rich breakfast and its effects on acute appetite control and food intake in "breakfast-skipping" adolescents. Int J Obesity 34:1125, 2010.

Long, H, Yi, JM, Li, ZB, et al: Benefits of iron supplementation for low birth weight infants: A systematic review. BMC Pediatr 12:99, 2012.

Martin, JA, Hamilton, BE, Ventura, SJ et al: Births: Final data for 2010. National Vital Statistics Reports 61. National Center for Health Statistics, Hyattsville, MD, 2012.

Mavroudi, A, Xinias, I, Deligiannidis, A, et al: Long term outcome of acquired food allergy in pediatric liver recipients: a single center experience. Pediatr Reports 4:e6, 2012. Published online January 30, 2012. Available at http://www.ncbi.nlm.nih.gov/pmc/articles/PMC3357619

McNeil, ME, Labbok, MH, and Abrahams, SW: What are the risks associated with formula feeding? A re-analysis and review. Birth Issues Perinat Care 37:50, 2010.

Mennella, JA, Forestell, CA, Morgan, LK, and Beauchamp, GK: Early milk feeding influences taste acceptance and liking during infancy. Am J Clin Nutr 90(Ssuppl):780S, 2009.

Minarich, LA, and Silverstein, J: Vitamin D update: Shining light on the debate what the IO,M recommendations really mean for your patients. March 1, 2011. Contemporary Pediatrics. Accessed February 20, 2014. Available at http://contemporarypediatrics.modernmedicine.com/contemporary-pediatrics/news/modernmedicine/modern-medicine-feature-articles/shining-light-vitamin-d

Mitchell, SM, Rogers, SP, Hicks, PD, et al: High frequencies of elevated alkaline phosphatase activity and rickets exist in extremely low birth weight infants despite current nutritional support. BMC Pediatr 9:47, 2009.

Morales, E, Bustamante, M, Gonzalez, JR, et al: Genetic variants of the FA,DS gene cluster and EL,OVL gene family, colostrums LC,-PUFA levels, breastfeeding, and child cognition. PLoS One 6:e17181, 2011.

Moretto, MR, Silva, CC, Kurokawa, CS, et al: Bone mineral density in healthy female adolescents according to age, bone age and pubertal breast staging. Open Orthop J 5:324, 2011.

Murphy, SL, Xu, J, and Kochanek, KD: Deaths: Preliminary data for 2010. National Vital Statistics Reports 60. National Center for Health Statistics, Hyattsville, MD, 2012.

Namiiro, FB, Mugalu, J, McAdams, RM, and Ndeezi, G: Poor birth weight recovery among low birth weight/preterm infants following hospital discharge in Kampalu, Uganda. BMC Pregnancy Childbirth 12:1, 2012.

Noonan, M: Breastfeeding: Is my baby getting enough milk? Br J Midwifery 19:82, 2011.

Nour, NM: Premature delivery and the millennium development goal. Rev Obstetr Gynecol 5:100, 2012.

Oddy, WH: Infant feeding and obesity risk in the child. Breastfeed Rev 20:7, 2012.

Patel, BK, and Shah, JS: Necrotizing enterocolitis in very low birth weight infants: A systemic review. ISRN Gastroenterol 2012; 562594; doi:10.5402/2012/562594.

Picciano, MF, Dwyer, JT, Radimer, KL, et al: Dietary supplement use among infants, children, and adolescents in the United States, 1999–2002. Arch Pediatr Adolesc Med 161:978, 2007.

Porter, RS, and Kaplan, JL (eds): Nutrition in infants. Mereck Manual. 2010–2011. Accessed December 18, 2012. Available at http://www.merckmanuals.com/professional/pediatrics/care_of_newborns_and_infants/nutrition_in_infants.html?qt=nutrition%20in%20infants&alt=sh

Rabbitt, A, and Coyne, I: Childhood obesity: Nurses' role in addressing the epidemic. Br J Nurs 21:731, 2012.

Radauer, C, Adhami, F, Furtler, I, et al: Latex-allergy patients sensitized to the major allergen hevein and hevein-like domains of class 1 chitinases show no increased frequency of latex-associated plant food allergy. Mol Immunol 48:600, 2011.

Rath, M: Energy drinks: What is all the hype? The danger of energy drink consumption. J Am Acad Nurse Practit 24:70, 2012.

Ramirez, DA, and Bahna, SL: Food hypersensitivity by inhalation. Clin Mol Allergy 7:4, 2009.

Rayyan, M, Devlieger, H, Jochum, F, and Allegaert, K: Short-term use of parenteral nutrition with a lipid emulsion containing a mixture of soybean oil, olive oil, medium-chain triglycerides, and fish oil: A randomized double-blind study in preterm infants. J Parenter Enteral Nutr 36(Suppl 1):81S, 2012.

Robinson, J: Assessment and management of atopic eczema in children. Nurs Standard 26:48, 2011.

Rioux, FM, Belanger-Plourde, J, LeBlanc, CP, and Vigneau, F: Relationship between maternal DH,A and iron status and infants' cognitive performance. Can J Diet Pract Res 70:e140, 2011.

Schwartz, J, Drossard, C, Dube, K, et al: Dietary intake and plasma concentrations of PU,FA and LC,-PUFA in breastfed and formula fed infants under real-life conditions. Eur J Nutr 49:189, 2010.

Suh, JS, Hahn, WH, and Cho, BS: Recent advances of oral rehydration therapy. Electrolyte Blood Pres 8:82, 2010.

Smith, HA: Formula supplementation and the risk of cow's milk allergy. Br J Midwifery 20:345, 2012.

Steensma, DP: The kiss of death: A severe allergic reaction to a shellfish induced by a good-night kiss. Mayo Clinic Proc 78:221, 2003.

Stevens, CJ: Obesity prevention interventions for middle school-aged children of ethnic minority: A review of literature. J Spec Pediatr Nurs 15:233, 2010.

Taylor, JA, Geyer, LJ, and Feldman, KW: Use of supplemental vitamin D among infants breastfed for prolonged periods. Pediatrics 125:105, 2010.

Tifanoff, N: Update on early childhood caries since the surgeon general's report. Acad Pediatr 9:396, 2009.

The Food Allergy and Anaphylactic Network: 2012. Accessed March 7, 2014. Available at http://www.foodallergy.org/resources/healthcare-providers

Turocy, P, DePalma, BF, Horswill, CA, et al: National athletic trainers' association position statement: Safe weight loss and maintenance practices in sport and exercise. J Athl Train 46:322, 2011.

U.S. Department of Agriculture: Comparison of previous and current regulatory requirements under final rule "Nutrition Standards in the National School Lunch and School Breakfast Programs" published January 26, 2012. Accessed December 27, 2012. Available at www.usda.gov/healthierschoolday

U.S. Department of Agriculture and U.S. Department of Health and Human Services: Dietary Guidelines for Americans 2010, ed 7. U.S. Government Printing Office, Washington, DC, December 2010.

Valerio, G, Galler, F, Mancusi, C, et al: Pattern of fractures across pediatric age groups: Analysis of individual and lifestyle factors. BMC Public Health 10:656, 2010. Accessed December 16, 2012. Available at www.biomedcentral.com/1471-2458/10/656

Vasquez, Y: Infant botulism: a review of two cases reported in 2008 from El Paso, Texas. J Appl Res 9:52, 2009.

Viehmann, L: Breastfeeding and the use of human milk. Pediatrics 129;e827, February 27, 2012.

Wang, J: Management of the patient with multiple food allergies. Curr Allergy Asthma Rep 10:271, 2010.

Wang, J, and Sampson, HA: Food allergy. J Clin Invest 121:827, 2011.

Warr, BJ, and Woolf, K: The female athlete triad: Patients do best with a team approach to care. J Am Acad Physician Assist 24:50, 2011.

Watkins, AL, and Dodgson, JE: Breastfeeding educational interventions for health professionals: a synthesis of intervention studies. J Spec Pediatr Nurs 15:223, 2010.

Whitney, S: The skinny on breastfeeding. W Virginia Med J 107:39, 2011.

Wittenberg, DF: Management guidelines for acute infective diarrhea/gastroenteritis in infants. S Afr Med J 102:104, 2012.

Xavier, AM, Rai, K, and Hedge, AM: Total antioxidant concentration of breastmilk—an eye-opener to the negligent. J Health Popul Nutr 6:605, 2011.

World Health Organization: Child growth standards. 2012. Accessed December 17, 2012. Available at www.who.int/childgrowth/en

Zanteson, L: Let whole grains, milk and fruit kick start your day. Environ Nutr 35:2, 2012.

Chapter 12

Ahmadieh, H, and Arabi, A: Vitamins and bone health: Beyond calcium and vitamin D. Nutr Rev 69:584, 2011.

Alzheimer's Association: Alzheimer's facts and figures. 2013. Accessed April 4, 2013. Available at www.alz.org/alzheimers_disease_facts_and_figures.asp#quickFacts

American Dietetic Association: Position of the American Dietetic Association: Ethical and legal issues in nutrition, hydration, and feeding. J Am Diet Assoc 108:873, 2008.

Brass, EP, and Sietsema, KE: Considerations in the development of drugs to treat sarcopenia. J Am Geriatr Soc 59:530, 2011.

Callen, BL: Nutritional screening in community dwelling older adults. Int J Older People Nurs 6:272, 2011.

Carlsson, E, Ehnfors, M, and Ehrenberg, A: Multidisciplinary recording and continuity of care for stroke patients with eating difficulties. J Interprof Care 24:298, 2010.

Casey, G: Alzheimer's and other dementias. Kai Taki Nurs N Z 18:20, 2012.

Centers for Disease Control and Prevention: Arthritis. March 26, 2012. Accessed May 2, 2013. Available at www.cdc.gov/arthritis

Centers for Disease Control and Prevention: Hip fractures among older adults. September 20, 2010. Accessed May 2, 2013. Available at www.cdc.gov/HomeandRecreationalSafety/Falls/adulthipfx.html

Centers for Disease Control and Prevention: Leading causes of death. January 13, 2013. Accessed April 17, 2013. Available at www.cdc.gov/nchs/fastats/lcod.htm

Centers for Disease Control and Prevention: Oral health preventing cavities, gum disease, tooth loss, and oral cancers. 2011. Accessed April 18, 2013. Available at www.cdc.gov/chronicdisease/resources/publications/aag/pdf/2011/Oral-Health-AAG-PDF-508.pdf

Centers for Disease Control and Prevention: Oral health. June 29, 2011. Accessed April 18, 2013. Available at www.cdc.gov/chronicdisease/resources/publications/AAG/doh.htm

Centers for Disease Control and Prevention: How much activity do older adults need? December 1, 2011. Accessed May 1, 2013. Available at www.cdc.gov/physicalactivity/everyone/guidelines/olderadults.html

Centers for Disease Control and Prevention. US physical activity statistics. January 14, 2010. Accessed May 6, 2013. Available at apps.nccd.cdc.gov/PASurveillance/DemoCompareResultV.asp?State=0andCat=1andYear=2008andGo=GO#result

Chao, J, Leung, Y, Wang, M, and Chuen-Chung Chang, R: Nutraceuticals and their preventative or potential therapeutic value in Parkinson's disease. Nutr Rev 70(7):373, 2012.

Cole, GM, Ma, QL, and Frautschy, SA: Dietary fatty acids and the aging brain. Nutr Rev 68(Suppl 2):s102, 2010.

Curtis, JR, and Stafford, MM: Management of osteoporosis among the elderly with other chronic medical conditions. Drugs Aging 29:549, 2012.

Dean, WR, Sharkey, JR, and Johnson, CM: Food insecurity is associated with social capital, perceived personal disparity, and partnership status among older and senior adults in a largely rural area of central Texas. J Nutr Gerontol Geriatr 30:169, 2011.

Discovering umami: The fifth taste. Food Insight September 2010(3–4).

Ennis, J: The physiology of ageing. Pract Nurse 43:38, 2013.

Feng, Y, and Wang, X: Antioxidant therapies for Alzheimer's disease. Oxidative Med Cell Longevity 2012(article 472932):1, 2012. Accessed February 20, 2014. Available at http://www.hindawi.com/journals/omcl/2012/472932

Frank, B, Muller, H, Weck, MN, et al: DNA repair gene polymorphisms and risk of chronic atrophic gastritis: A case control study. BMC Cancer 11:440, 2011.

Gaffney-Stomberg, E, Insogna, KL, Rodriguez, NR, and Kerstetter, JE: Increasing dietary protein requirements in elderly people for optimal muscle and bone health. J Am Geriatr Soc 57:1073, 2009.

Gardiner, AB: The effects of ageing on the gastrointestinal system. Nurs Residential Care 15:30, 2013.

Gebhardt, MC, Sims, TT, and Bates, TA: Enhancing geriatric content in baccalaureate nursing programs. Nurs Educ Perspect 30:245, 2009.

Genaro, PS, and Martini, LA: Effect of protein intake on bone and muscle mass in the elderly. Nutr Rev 68:616, 2010.

Green, SM, Martin, HJ, Roberts, HC, and Sayer, AA: A systematic review of the use of volunteers to improve mealtime care of adult patients or residents in institutional settings. J Clin Nurs 20:1810, 2011.

Greenspan, SL, Perera, S, Nace, D, Zukowski, KS, Ferchak, MA, Lee, CL, Nayak, S, and Resnick, NM: FRAX or fiction: Determining optimal screening strategies for treatment of osteoporosis in residents in long-term care facilities. J Am Geriatr Soc 60(4):609, 2012.

Gonoi, W, Abe, O, Yamasue, H, et al: Age-related changes in regional brain volume evaluated by atlas-based method. Neuroradiology 52:865, 2010.

Gowda, C, Hadley, C, and Aiello, AE: The association between food insecurity and inflammation in the US, adult population. Am J Public Health 102:1579, 2012.

Hafsteinsdottir, TB, Mosselman, M, Schoneveld, C, et al: Malnutrition in hospitalized neurological patients approximately doubles in 10 days of hospitalization. J Clin Nurs 19:639, 2012.

Hanson, LC, Carey, TS, Caprio, AJ, et al: Improving decision-making for feeding options in advanced dementia: A randomized, controlled trial. J Am Geriatr Soc 59:2009, 2011.

Hass, R, Maloney, S, Pausenberger, E, et al: Clinical decision making in exercise prescription for fall prevention. Phys Ther 92:666, 2012.

Heisters, D., and Bains, J: Side effects of treatment for Parkinson's disease. Nurs Residential Care 14:230, 2012.

Hines, S, Wilson, J, McCrow, J, Dip, G, Abbey, J, and Sacre, S: Oral liquid nutritional supplements for people with dementia in residential aged care facilities. Int J Evid Based Healthc 8(4):248, 2010.

Jennings, LA, Auerbach, AD, Maselli, J, et al: Missed opportunities for osteoporosis treatment in patients hospitalized for hip fracture. J Am Geriatr Soc 58:650, 2010.

Johnson, R, and Taylor, C: Can playing pre-recorded music at mealtimes reduce the symptoms of agitation for people with dementia? Int J Ther and Rehabil 18(12):700, 2011.

Kaiser, MJ, Bauer, JM, Ramsch, C, et al: Frequency of malnutrition in older adults: A multinational perspective using the mini nutritional assessment. J Am Geriatr Soc 58:1734, 2010.

Kasper, CE: Skeletal muscle and genetics. Ann Rev Nurs Res 29:191, 2011.

Kulminski, AM, Arbeev, KG, Kulminskaya, IV, et al: Body mass index and nine-year mortality in disabled and nondisabled older U.S. individuals. J Am Geriatr Soc 56:105, 2008.

Losing your sense of smell? Harv Health Lett 38:5, 2012.

Li, Z, and Heber, D: Sarcopenic obesity in the elderly and strategies for weight management. Nutr Rev 70:57, 2011.

Nazarko, L: Diabetes, ageing and bladder function. Br J Healthc Assistants 4:352, 2010.

National Institutes of Health and Office of Dietary Supplements: Dietary Fact Sheet: Calcium. March 19, 2013. Assessed May 1, 2013. Available at www.ods.od.nih.gov/factsheets/Calcium-QuickFacts

National Institute on Aging: Exercise & physical activity: Your everyday guide from the National Institute on Aging. Accessed March 7, 2014. Available at www.nia.nih.gov/health/publication/exercise-physical-activity-your-everyday-guide-national-institute-aging-0

Neelemaat, F, Lips, P, Bosmans, JE, Thijs, A, Seidell, JC, and van Bokhorst-de van der Schueren, MAE: Short-term oral nutritional intervention with protein and vitamin D decreases falls in malnourished older adults. J Amer Geriatr Soc 69(4):691, 2012.

New Alzheimer's guidelines define early stages of the disease. Harv Women Health Watch 1991:1, 2011.

Pinheiro C, and Silva, M: Colour, vision and ergonomics. Work 41:5590, 2012.

Posthauer, ME: Nutrition strategies for wound healing. J Legal Nurse Consult 23:15, 2012.

Raghoonandan, P, Cobban, SJ, and Compton, SM: A scoping review of the use of fluoride varnish in elderly people living in long term care facilities. Can J Dent Hygiene 45:217, 2011.

Ross, LJ, Mudge, AM, Yound, AM, and Banks, M: Everyone's problem but nobody's job: Staff perceptions and explanations for poor nutritional intake in older medical patients. Nutr Diet 68:41, 2011.

Shepherd, A: Practical care: Feeding and assisting residents to eat. Nurs Residential Care 13:487, 2011.

Smell: Engaging emotions and memories. Can Nurs Home 19:4, 2008.

Swann, JI: Osteoporosis: The fragile bone disease. Br J Healthc Assist 6:59, 2012.

Tasi, AC, Chou, YT, and Chang, TL: Usefulness of the mini nutritional assessment in predicting the nutrional status of people with mental disorders in Taiwan. J Clin Nurs 20:341, 2011.

Toles, M, Young, HM, and Ouslander, J: Improving care transitions in nursing homes. J Am Soc Aging 36:78, 2012–2013.

Travers, SP, and Geran, LC: Bitter-responsive brainstem neurons: Characteristics and functions. Physiol Behav 97:592, 2009.

Tun, PA, Williams, VA, Small, BJ, and Hafter, ER: The effects of aging on auditory processing and cognition. Am J Audiol 21:344, 2012.

Turner, J. Your brain of food: A nutrient-rich diet can protect cognitive health. J Am Soc Aging 35:99, 2011.

U.S. Department of Health and Human Services, Centers for Disease Control and Prevention, and National Center for Health Statistics: Health, United States, 2011. Accessed March 7, 2014. Available at www.cdc.gov/nchs/data/hus/hus11.pdf#022

U.S. Census Bureau: Current population survey, annual social and economic supplement, 2011. Accessed April 4, 2013. Available at www.census.gov/population/age/data/2011.html

Verdijk, LB, Snijders, T, Beelen, M, et al: Characteristics of muscle fiber type are predictive of skeletal muscle mass and strength in elderly men. J Am Geriatr Soc 58:2069, 2010.

Villarroel, P, Flores, S, Pizarro, F, et al: Effect of dietary protein on heme iron uptake by caco-2 cells. Eur J Nutr 50:637, 2011.

Vitamins unlikely to revitalize the mind. Harv Ment Health Lett, February: 4, 2010.

Ward, J: Sarcopenia and sarcopenic obesity: Is it time the health system accepted fitness of older people as a health responsibility? Australas J Ageing 30:61, 2011.

Walker, R, Davidson, M, and Gray, W: Gender differences in 1-year survival rates after weight loss in people with idiopathic Parkinson's disease. Int J Palliat Nurs 18:35, 2012.

Chapter 13

Academy of Nutrition and Dietetics: Overview of oncology, side effect management, neutropenia. 2012. Accessed March 2013. Available at www.nutritioncaremanual.org

Albrecht, JA, Nagy-Nero, D, and the American Dietetic Association: Position of the American Dietetic Association: Food and water safety. J Am Diet Assoc 109:1449, 2009.

Centers for Disease Control and Prevention: Food safety. September 24, 2012. Accessed March 2013. Available at www.cdc.gov/foodsafety/facts

Centers for Disease Control and Prevention: Estimates of foodborne illness in the United States. February 6, 2013a. Accessed March 2013. Available at www.cdc.gov/foodborneburden/index

Centers for Disease Control and Prevention: Norovirus and working with food. March 21, 2013b. Accessed March 2013. Available at www.cdc.gov/norovirus/food-handlers

Centers for Disease Control and Prevention: BSE (bovine spongiform encephalopathy, or mad cow disease). February 21, 2013c. Accessed March 2013. Available at www.cdc.gov/ncidod/dvrd/bse

Dolan, L, Matulka, RA, and Burdock, GA: Naturally occurring food toxins. Toxins (Basel) 2:2289, 2010.

Environmental Protection Agency: History of food irradiation. June 27, 2012a. Accessed March 2013. Available at www.epa.gov/radiation/sources/food

Environmental Protection Agency: Labeling. June 27, 2012a. Accessed March 2013. Available at www.epa.gov/radiation/sources/food

Food and Drug Administration: Food irradiation: What you need to know. May 9, 2012. Accessed March 2013. Available at www.fda.gov/Food/Resources For You

Foodsafety.gov: Causes of food poisoning. Accessed March 22, 2013. Available at [0]www.foodsafety.gov/poisoning/causes/index.html

Fox, N, and Freifeld, AG: The Neutropenic Diet reviewed: Moving toward a safe food handling approach. Oncology (Williston Park) 26:572, 2012.

Friedman, M, Fleming, LE, Fernandez, M, et al: Ciguatera fish poisoning: Treatment, prevention and management. Mar Drugs 6:456, 2008.

Jubelirer, S: The benefit of the neutropenic diet: fact or fiction? Oncologist April 6, 2011. published online April 2011: 101634/theoncologist.2011.0001

National Institutes of Health: Aflatoxin. January 30, 2013. Accessed March 2013. Available at www.nlm.nih.gov

Scharff, RL: Economic burden from health losses due to foodborne illness in the United States. J Food Prot 75:123, 2012.

Trifilio, S, Helenowski I, Giel M, et al: Questioning the role of a neutropenic diet following hematopoetic stem cell transplantation. Biol Blood Marrow Transplant 18:1385, 2012.

U.S. Department of Health and Human Services: Healthy people 2020. Food safety, 2012. Accessed March 22, 2013. Available at www.healthypeople.gov/2020

U.S. Department of Health and Human Services: Food safety for pregnant women, 2011. Accessed March 2013. Available at www.fda.gov/Food/ResorcesForYou/Consumers/SelectedHealthTopics/ucm312704

World Health Organization: Hepatitis E fact sheet. July 2012. Fact sheet N280. Accessed March 2013. Available at www.who.int/mediacenter/factsheets/fs280/en/

Chapter 14

Academy of Nutrition and Dietetics: Critical Illness Update Evidence-Based Nutrition Practice Guideline, 2012. Accessed August 2012. Available at http://andevidencelibrary.com

American Dietetic Association: International Dietetics and Nutrition Terminology (IDNT) Reference Manual, ed 1. American Dietetic Association, Chicago, 2008.

American Dietetic Association: Manual of Clinical Dietetics, ed 6. American Dietetic Association, Chicago, 2000.

A.S.P.E.N.: Clinical guidelines, nutrition screening, assessment, and intervention in adults. A.S.P.E.N., Silver Spring, MD, 2011.

A.S.P.E.N.: Definition of terms, style, and conventions used in A.S.P.E.N. Board of Directors-approved documents, Silver Spring, MD, May 2012.

A.S.P.E.N.: Position paper: Parenteral nutrition glutamine supplementation, A.S.P.E.N., Silver Spring, MD, 2011.

A.S.P.E.N.: Tube feeding misconnections: Fatal medical mistakes. Press release April 15, 2008. American Society for Parenteral and Enteral Nutrition, Silver Spring, MD, 2008.

Bankhead R, Boullata J, Brantley S, et al: Enteral nutrition practice recommendations. JPEN J Parenter Enteral Nutr 33:122, 2009.

Barker, L, Gout, BS, and Crowe, TC: Hospital malnutrition: Prevalence, identification and impact on patients and the healthcare system. Int J Environ Res Public Health 8:514, 2011.

Blouch, AC, and Mueller, C: Enteral and parenteral nutrition support. In Food, Nutrition and Diet Therapy. Elsevier, Philadelphia, 2004.

Buff, D: Against the flow: Tube feeding and survival in patients with dementia. AAHPM Bull 7:1, Spring 2006.

Butterworth, CE: The skeleton in the hospital closet. Nutr Today 9:8, 1975.

Butterworth, CE, and Blackburn, GL: Hospital malnutrition and how to assess the nutritional status of a patient. Nutr Today 10:8, 1975.

Candy, B, Sampson, EL, and Jones, L: Enteral tube feeding in older people with advanced dementia: Findings from a Cochrane systematic review. Int J Palliat Nurs 15:396, 2009.

Delegge, MH: Tube feeding in patients with dementia: Where are we? Nutr Clin Pract Apr-May;24(2):214-6.: 2009.

Dupertuis, YM: Physical characteristics of total parenteral nutrition bags significantly affect the stability of vitamins C and B_1: A controlled prospective study. J Parenter Enteral Nutr 26:310, 2002.

Falk, A: Evaluating the effectiveness of a micronutrient assessment tool for long-term total parenteral nutrition patients. Nurs Clin Pract 17:240, 2002.

Fessier, T: Malnutrition: A serious concern for hospitalized patients. Today's Dietitian 10:44, 2008.

Gottschlich, MM: The A.S.P.E.N. Nutrition Core Curriculum: A case-based approach—the adult patient. American Society for Parenteral and Enteral Nutrition, Silver Spring, MD, 2007.

McClave, S, Martindale, RG, Vanek, VW, et al: Guidelines for the provision and assessment of nutrition support therapy in the adult critically ill patient: Society of Critical Care Medicine (SCCM) and American Society for Parenteral and Enteral Nutrition (A.S.P.E.N.). JPEN J Parenter Enteral Nutr 33:277, 2009.

Metheny, N, and Titler, MG: Assessing placement of feeding tubes. Am J Nurs 101:36, 2001.

Mirtallo J, Canada T, Johnson D, et al: Safe practices for PN: Administration. JPEN J Parenter Enteral Nutr 28(Suppl):S65, 2004.

Mueller, C, Compher, C, Druyan, ME, et al: A.S.P.E.N. Clinical Guidelines: Nutrition screening, assessment, and intervention in adults. JPEN J Parenter Enteral Nutr 35:16, 2011.

O'Reilly, KB: Feeding tube risks for demential patient often not discussed. American Medical News, May 25, 2011. Accessed March 2013. Available at http://www.amednews.com/article/20110525/profession/305259996/8

Pfau, PR, Rombeau, JL: Nutrition. Med Clin North Am 84:1209, 2000.

Phillips, LD: Manual of Intravenous Therapy, ed 4. FA Davis, Philadelphia, 2006.

Super, J: Tube feedings making you blue? Drug Therapy Topics. University of Washington Medical Center 32:6, 2003.

U.S. Department of Health and Human Services: Healthy people, 2010. U.S. Department of Health and Human Services, Washington, DC, 2000.

U.S. Food and Drug Administration: FDA public health advisory. Reports of blue discoloration and death in patients receiving enteral feedings tinted with the dye, FD and C No. 1. Accessed January 2004. Available at http://www.accessdata.fda.gov/scripts/cdrh/cfdocs/psn/printer.cfm?id=184

Venes, D (ed): Taber's Cyclopedic Medical Dictionary, ed 20. FA Davis, Philadelphia, 2005.

White, J, Guenter, P, Jensen, G, et al: Consensus statement: Academy of Nutrition and Dietetics and American Society for Parenteral and Enteral Nutrition. Characteristics recommended for the identification and documentation of adult malnutrition (undernutrition). JPEN J Parenter Enteral Nutr 36:275, 2012.

Chapter 15

Academy of Nutrition and Dietetics: Vitamin K and prothrombin time. Nutrition Care Manual, Chicago, 2012.

Academy of Nutrition and Dietetics: Supplements and ergogenic aids for athletes. Reviewed January 2013. Accessed March 25, 2013. Available at www.eatright.org/Public/content.aspx?id=7088

Ahn, SC, and Brown, AW: Cobalamin deficiency and subacute combined degeneration after nitrous oxide anesthesia: A case report. Arch Phys Med Rehabil 86:150, 2005.

Aldosary, BM, Sutter, ME, Schwartz, M, and Morgan, BW: Case series of selenium toxicity from a nutritional supplement. Clin Toxicol (Phila) 50:57, 2012.

American College of Preventive Medicine: Over-the-counter medications: use in general and special populations, therapeutic errors, misuse, storage, and disposal, 2011. Accessed March 31, 2013. Available at www.acpm.org/?page=OTCMeds_ClinRefandhhSearchTerms=OTC

American College of Sports Medicine, Sawka, MN, Burke, LM, et al: American College of Sports Medicine position stand. Exercise and fluid replacement. Med Sci Sports Exerc 39:377, 2007.

American Dietetic Association: Position of the American Dietetic Associaton: Integration of medical nutrition therapy and pharmacotherapy. J Am Diet Assoc 110:950, 2010.

American Dietetic Association, Dietitians of Canada, and American College of Sports Medicine, et al: American College of Sports Medicine position stand. Nutrition and athletic performance. Med Sci Sports Exerc 41:709, 2009.

Atwater, J, Montgomery-Salguero, J, and Roll, DB: The USP Dietary Supplement Verification Program: Helping pharmacists and consumers select dietary supplements. US Pharm 6:61, 2005.

American College of Preventive Medicine: Over-the-counter medications: Use in general and special populations, therapeutic errors, misuse, storage and disposal. 2011. Accessed February 27, 2013. Available at www.acpm.org/?OTCMeds_ClinRefv

Ansell, J, McDonough, M, Zhao, Y, et al: The absence of an interaction between warfarin and cranberry juice: A randomized, double-blind trial. J Clin Pharmacol 49:824, 2009.

Arbex, MA, Varella, C, Siqueira, HR, and Mello, FA: Antituberculosis drugs: Drug interactions, adverse effects, and use in special situations. Part 1: First-line drugs. J Bras Pneumol 36:626, 2010. Accessed March 2, 2013. Available at www.ncbi.nlm.nih.gov/pubmed/21085830

Bailey, JL, Sands, JM, and Franch, HA: Water, electrolytes, and acid-base metabolism. In Ross, AC, Caballero, B, Cousins, RJ, et al (eds): Modern Nutrition in Health and Disease, ed 11. Lippincott Williams & Wilkins, Philadelphia, 2014.

Bailey, RL, Gahche, JJ, Miller, PE, et al: Why US adults use dietary supplements. JAMA Intern Med 173:355, 2013.

Bent, S, Goldberg, H, Padula, A, and Avins, AL: Spontaneous bleeding associated with ginkgo biloba: A case report and systematic review of the literature. J Gen Intern Med 20:657, 2005. Accessed March 22, 2013. Available at www.ncbi.nlm.nih.gov/pmc/articles/PMC1490168

Berger, AJ, and Alford, K: Cardiac arrest in a young man following excess consumption of caffeinated "energy drinks." Med J Aust 190:41, 2009.

Bilgi, N, Bell, K, Ananthakrishnan, AN, and Atallah, E: Imatinib and Panax ginseng: A potential interaction resulting in liver toxicity. Ann Pharmacother 44:926, 2010.

Bilgili, SG, Karadag, AS, Calka, O, and Altun, F: Isoniazid-induced pellagra. Cutan Ocul Toxicol 30:317, 2011.

Birks, J, and Grimley Evans, J: Ginkgo biloba for cognitive impairment and dementia. Cochrane Database Syst Rev 21:CD003120, 2009.

Bishop, D: Dietary supplements and team-sport performance. Sports Med 40:995, 2010.

Borrione, P, Spaccamiglio, A, Salvo, RA, et al: Rhabdomyolysis in a young vegetarian athlete. Am J Phys Med Rehabil 88:951, 2009.

Boullata, J: Natural health product interactions with medication. Nutr Clin Pract 20:33, 2005.

Boullata, JI, and Hudson, LM: Drug-nutrient interactions: A broad view with implications for practice. J Acad Nutr Diet 112:506, 2012.

Bradley, JS, Wassel, RT, Lee, L, and Nambiar, S: Intravenous ceftriaxone and calcium in the neonate: Assessing the risk for cardiopulmonary adverse events. Pediatrics 123:e609, 2009. Accessed February 28, 2013. Available at http://pediatrics.aappublications.org/content/123/4/e609.long

Brasseur, A, and Ducobu, J: Severe hypokalemia after holidays return [article in French]. Rev Med Brux 29:490, 2008.

Brown, RO, Minard, G, and Ziegler, TR: Parenteral nutrition. In Ross, AC, Caballero, B, Cousins, RJ, et al (eds): Modern Nutrition in Health and Disease, ed 11. Lippincott Williams & Wilkins, Philadelphia, 2014.

Carlson, J: The role of nutrition in enhancing aerobic training and endurance performance. Presentation at Performance Nutrition for Athletes and Active Individuals. Michigan State University, East Lansing, September 12, 2008.

Carmel, R: Cobalamin (vitamin B_{12}). In Ross, AC, Caballero, B, Cousins, RJ, et al (eds): Modern Nutrition in Health and Disease, ed 11. Lippincott Williams & Wilkins, Philadelphia, 2014.

CBS News: U.S. prescription drug spending drops for first time in 58 years. May 9, 2013. Accessed February 7, 2014. Available at www.cbsnews.com/news/US-prescription-drug-spending-drops-for-first-time-in-58-years/

Centers for Disease Control and Prevention: Lead poisoning associated with Ayurvedic medications—five states, 2000–2003. Morb Mortal Wkly Rep 53:582, July 9, 2004. Accessed March 19, 2013. Available at www.cdc.gov/mmwr/preview/mmwrhtml/mm5326a3.htm

Cereda, E, Barichella, M, and Pezzoli, G: Controlled-protein dietary regimens for Parkinson's disease. Nutr Neurosci 13:29, 2010.

Cermak, NM, and van Loon, LJ: The use of carbohydrates during exercise as an ergogenic aid. Sports Med 43:1139, 2013.

Chan, L-N: Drug-nutrient interactions. In Ross, AC, Caballero, B, Cousins, RJ, et al (eds): Modern Nutrition in Health and Disease, ed 11. Lippincott Williams & Wilkins, Philadelphia, 2014.

Chen, XW, Serag, ES, Sneed, KB, et al: Clinical herbal interactions with conventional drugs: From molecules to maladies. Curr Med Chem 18:4836, 2011.

Cheng, CJ, Chen, YH, Chau, T, and Lin, SH: A hidden cause of hypokalemic paralysis in a patient with prostate cancer. Support Care Cancer 12:810, 2004.

Chicago Academy of Nutrition and Dietetics: Protein supplements for the strength athlete: Weighing the evidence. Undated. Accessed March 26, 2013. Available at http://chicagodieteticassociation.org/protein-supplements-for-the-strength-athlete-weighing-the-evidence

Clauson, KA, Santamarina, ML, and Rutledge, JC: Clinically relevant safety issues associated with St. John's wort product labels. BMC Complement Altern Med 8:42, 2008.

Cluett, J: Muscle of an Olympian. Updated August 17, 2004. Accessed March 28, 2013. Available at orthopedics.about.com/cs/generalinfo6/a/muscle.htm

Cohen, LJ, and Sclar, DA: Issues in adherence to treatment with monoamine oxidase inhibitors and the rate of treatment failure. J Clin Psychiatry 73(Suppl 1):31, 2012.

Consumer Healthcare Products Association: OTC Retail Sales. 2014. Accessed February 7, 2014. Available at www.chpa.org/PR_OTCRetailSales.aspx

Consumer Reports: What's behind our dietary supplements coverage. Updated January 2011. Accessed March 17, 2013. Available at www.consumerreports.org/cro/2012/04/what-s-behind-our-dietary-supplements-coverage/index.htm

Cooper, R, Naclerio, F, Allgrove, J, and Jimenez, A: Creatine supplementation with specific view to exercise/sports performance: An update. J Int Soc Sports Nutr 9:33, 2012. Accessed March 27, 2014. Available at www.ncbi.nlm.nih.gov/pmc/articles/PMC3407788

Custódio das Dôres, SM, Booth, SL, Martini, LA, et al: Relationship between diet and anticoagulant response to warfarin: A factor analysis. Eur J Nutr 46:147, 2007.

Dahmer, S, and Schiller, RM: Glucosamine. Am Fam Physician 78:471, 2008.

Dara, L, Hewett, J, and Lim, JK: Hydroxycut hepatotoxicity: A case series and review of liver toxicity from herbal weight loss supplements. World J Gastroenterol 14:6999, 2008. Accessed March 23, 2013. Available at www.ncbi.nlm.nih.gov/pmc/articles/PMC2773866

Das, R, Parajuli, S, and Gupta, S: A rash imposition from a lifestyle omission: A case report of pellagra [letter]. Ulster Med J 75:92, 2006.

Dhamija, R, Eckert, S, and Wirrell, E: Ketogenic diet. Can J Neurol Sci 40:158, 2013.

Dickerson, RN, Garmon, WM, Kuhl, DA, et al: Vitamin K-independent warfarin resistance after concurrent administration of warfarin and continuous enteral nutrition. Pharmacotherapy 28:308, 2008.

Draves, AH, and Walker, SE: Analysis of the hypericin and pseudohypericin content of commercially available St. John's wort preparations. Can J Clin Pharmacol 10:114, 2003.

Ebrahim, V, Albeldawi, M, and Chiang, DJ: Acute liver injury associated with glucosamine dietary supplement. BMJ Case Rep Dec 13, 2012.

Elinav, E, and Chajek-Shaul, T: Licorice consumption causing severe hypokalemic paralysis. Mayo Clin Proc 78:767, 2003.

Estes, JD, Stolpman, D, Olyaei, A, et al: High prevalence of potentially hepatotoxic herbal supplement use in patients with fulminant hepatic failure. Arch Surg 138:852, 2003.

Fessenden, JM, Wittenborn, W, and Clarke, L: Gingko biloba: A case report of herbal medicine and bleeding postoperatively from a laparoscopic cholecystectomy. Am Surg 67:33, 2001.

Franco, V, Polanczyk, CA, Clausell, N, and Rohde, LE: Role of vitamin K intake in chronic oral anticoagulation: Prospective evidence from observational and randomized protocols. Am J Med 116:651, 2004.

Frost, EA: Herbal medicines and interactions with anesthetic agents. Middle East J Anesthesiol 2006 Jun;18:851–78.

Fugate, SE, and Ramsey, AM: Resistance to oral vitamin K for reversal of overanticoagulation during Crohn's disease relapse. J Thromb Thrombolysis 17:219, 2004.

Gardiner, P, Phillips, R, and Shaughnessy, AF: Herbal and dietary supplement—drug interactions in patients with chronic illnesses. Am Fam Physician 77:73, 2008.

Geyer, H, Parr, MK, Mareck, U, et al: Analysis of non-hormonal nutritional supplements for anabolic-androgenic steroids—results of an international study. Int J Sports Med 25:124, 2004.

Ghobrial, GM, Dalyai, R, Flanders, AE, and Harrop, J: Nitrous oxide myelopathy posing as spinal cord injury. J Neurosurg Spine 16:489, 2012.

Gilmour, J, Harrison, C, and Asadi, L: Natural health product-drug interactions: Evolving responsibilities to take complementary and alternative medicine into account. Pediatrics 128(Suppl 4):S155, 2011. Accessed March 22, 2013. Available at http://pediatrics.aappublications.org/content/128/Supplement_4/S155.long

Gilroy, CM, Steiner, JF, Byers, T, et al: Echinacea and truth in labelling. Arch Intern Med 163:699, 2003.

Goulet, ED: Glycerol-induced hyperhydration: a method for estimating the optimal load of fluid to be ingested before exercise to maximize endurance performance. J Strength Cond Res 24:74, 2010.

Grant, P: Warfarin and cranberry juice: An interaction? J Heart Valve Dis 13:25, 2004.

Grapefruit and drug interactions. Prescrire Int 21:294, 2012.

Griffiths, AP, Beddall, A, and Pegler, S: Fatal hemopericardium and gastrointestinal hemorrhage due to possible interaction of cranberry juice with warfarin. J R Soc Promot Health 128:324, 2008.

Gropper, SS, and Smith, JL: Advanced Nutrition and Human Metabolism, ed 6. Wadsworth, Belmont, CA, 2013.

Gualano, B, Roschel, H, Lancha, AH, Jr, et al: In sickness and in health: The widespread application of creatine supplementation. Amino Acids 43:519, 2012.

Gunturu, KS, Nagarajan, P, McPhedran, P, et al: Ayurvedic herbal medicine and lead poisoning. J Hematol Oncol 4:51, 2011. Accessed March 20, 2013. Available at www.ncbi.nlm.nih.gov/pmc/articles/PMC3259062

Gurley, BJ, Fifer, EK, and Gardner, Z: Pharmacokinetic herb-drug interactions (part 2): Drug interactions involving popular botanical dietary supplements and their clinical relevance. Planta Med 78:1490, 2012. Accessed March 22, 2013. Available at https://www.thieme-connect.com/ejournals/html/10.1055/s-0031-1298331

Haber, SL, Cauthon, KA, and Raney, EC: Cranberry and warfarin interaction: A case report and review of the literature. Consult Pharm 27:58, 2012.

Hafner-Blumenstiel, V: Herbal drug-drug interaction and adverse drug reactions [article in German] Ther Umsch 68:54, 2011.

Hamann, GL, Campbell, JD, and George, CM: Warfarin-cranberry juice interaction. Ann Pharmacother 45:e17, 2011. Accessed March 9, 2013. Available at www.theannals.com/content/45/3/e17.long

Heimbach, JT: Health-benefit claims for probiotic products. Clin Infect Dis 46(Suppl 2):S122, 2008.

Higgins, JP, Tuttle, TD, and Higgins, CL: Energy beverages: Content and safety. Mayo Clin Proc 85:1033, 2010. Accessed March 25, 2013. Available at www.ncbi.nlm.nih.gov/pmc/articles/PMC2966367

Holick, MF, Binkley, NC, Bischoff-Ferrari, HA, et al: Evaluation, treatment and prevention of vitamin D deficiency: An Endocrine Society Clinical Practice Guideline. J Clin Endocrinol Metab 96:1911, 2011.

Huang, S-M, and Cameron, DR: Dietary supplements in adults taking cardiovascular drugs: A comparative effectiveness review. AHRQ CME/CE activity. May 31, 2012.

Hylek, EM: Anticoagulation therapy for atrial fibrillation. Semin Thromb Hemost 39:147, 2013.

Institute of Medicine Committee on the Use of Complementary and Alternative Medicine: Complementary and Alternative Medicine in the United States. National Academy Press, Washington, DC, 2005. Accessed March 18, 2013. Available at www.nap.edu/openbook/0309092701/html

Ize-Ludlow, D, Ragone, S, Bruck, IS, et al: Neurotoxicities in infants seen with the consumption of star anise tea. Pediatrics 114:e653, 2004.

Izzo, AA, and Ernst, E: Interactions between herbal medicines and prescribed drugs: an updated systematic review. Drugs 69:1777, 2009.

Jäger, R, Purpura, M, Shao, A, et al: Analysis of the efficacy, safety, and regulatory status of novel forms of creatine. Amino Acids 40:1369, 2011. Accessed March 25, 2013. Available at www.ncbi.nlm.nih.gov/pmc/articles/PMC3080578

Jeukendrup, AE: Carbohydrate and exercise performance: The role of multiple transportable carbohydrates. Curr Opin Clin Nutr Metab Care 13:452, 2010.

Jeukendrup, A: The new carbohydrate intake recommendations. Nestle Nutr Inst Workshop Ser 75:63, 2013.

Johns, C. Glycyrrhizic acid toxicity caused by consumption of licorice candy cigars. CJEM 11:94, 2009. Accessed March 31, 2013. Available at www.cjem-online.ca/v11/n1/p94

Judkins, C, and Prock, P: Supplements and inadvertent doping—how big is the risk to athletes. Med Sport Sci 59:143, 2012.

Juurlink, DN, Mamdani, MM, Kopp, A, et al: Drug-induced lithium toxicity in the elderly: A population-based study. J Am Geriatr Soc 52:794, 2004.

Karri, SK, Saper, RB, and Kales, SN: Lead encephalopathy due to traditional medicines. Curr Drug Saf 3:54, 2008.

Kaur, S, Goraya, JS, Thami, GP, and Kanwar, AJ: Pellagrous dermatitis induced by phenytoin [letter]. Pediatr Dermatol 19:93, 2002.

Kaye, AD, Kucera, I, and Sabar, R: Perioperative anesthesia clinical considerations of alternative medicines. Anesthesiol Clin N Am 22:125, 2004.

Kennedy, ET, Luo, H, and Houser, RF: Dietary supplement use pattern of U.S. adult population in the 2007–2008 National Health and Nutrition Examination Survey (NHANES). Ecol Food Nutr. 2013;52:76.

Kim, YB, Ko, MJ, Lee, DG, et al: CYP2C9 mutation affecting the individual variability of warfarin dose requirement. Ann Rehabil Med 36:857, 2012. Accessed March 9, 2013. Available at www.ncbi.nlm.nih.gov/pmc/articles/PMC3546190

Kim, Y, and Rho, JM: The ketogenic diet and epilepsy. Curr Opin Clin Nutr Metab Care 11:113, 2008.

Klein, S: POM-boozled: Do health drinks live up to their labels? Health.com. October 27, 2010. Accessed July 27, 2013. Available at www.cnn.com/2010/HEALTH/10/27/health.pom.drink.labels/index.html

Knudsen, JF, and Sokol, GH: Potential glucosamine-warfarin interaction resulting in increased international normalized ratio: Case report and review of the literature and MedWatch database. Pharmacotherapy 28:540, 2008.

Kobayashi, K, Haruta, T, Maeda, H, et al: Cerebral hemorrhage associated with vitamin K deficiency in congenital tuberculosis treated with isoniazid and rifampin. Pediatr Infect Dis J 21:1088, 2002.

Komperda, KE: Potential interaction between pomegranate juice and warfarin. Pharmacotherapy 29:1002, 2009.

Krishna, YR, Mittal, V, Grewal, P, et al: Acute liver failure caused by "fat burners" and dietary supplements: A case report and literature review. Can J Gastroenterol 25:157, 2011. Accessed March 23, 2013. Available at www.ncbi.nlm.nih.gov/pmc/articles/PMC3076034

Lanski, SL, Greenwald, M, Perkins, A, and Simon, HK: Herbal therapy use in a pediatric emergency department population: Expect the unexpected. Pediatrics 111:981, 2003.

Lee, YH, Woo, JH, Choi, SJ, et al: Effect of glucosamine or chondrotin sulfate on the osteoarthritis progression: A meta-analysis. Rheumatol Int 30:357, 2010.

Levy, RG, Cooper, PN, and Giri, P: Ketogenic diet and other dietary treatments for epilepsy. Cochrane Database Syst Rev 3:CD001903, 2012.

Lin, R-J, Chan, H-F, Chang, Y-C, and Su, J-J: Subacute combined degeneration callused by nitrous oxide intoxication: Case reports. Acta Neurol Taiwan 20:129, 2011.

Lin, SH, Yang, SS, Chau, T, and Halperin, ML: An unusual cause of hypokalemic paralysis: Chronic licorice ingestion. Am J Med Sci 325:153, 2003.

Liva, R: Facing the problem of dietary-supplement heavy-metal contamination: How to take responsible action. Int Med 6:36, 2007.

Liwanpo, L, and Hershman, JM: Conditions and drugs interfering with thyroxine absorption. Best Pract Res Clin Endocrinol Metab 23:781, 2009.

Lutas, A, and Yellen, G: The ketogenic diet: Metabolic influences on brain excitability and epilepsy. Trends Neurosci 36:32, 2013.

Lynch, T, and Price, A: The effect of cytochrome P450 metabolism on drug response, interactions, and adverse effects. Am Fam Physician 76:391, 2007.

Lyon, VB, and Fairley, JA: Anticonvulsant-induced pellagra. J Am Acad Dermatol 46:597, 2002.

MacKay, M, Jackson, D, Eggert, L, et al: Practice-based validation of calcium and phosphorus solubility limits for pediatric parenteral nutrition solutions. Nutr Clin Pract 26:708, 2011.

Madden, GR, Schmitz, KH, and Fullerton, K: A case of infantile star anise toxicity. Pediatr Emerg Care 28:284, 2012.

Maughan, RJ, Greenhaff, PL, and Hespel, P: Dietary supplements for athletes: Emerging trends and recurring themes. J Sports Sci 29(Suppl 1):S57, 2011.

Mayo Clinic: Griseofulvin. Health-drug information. Accessed March 1, 2013. Available at www.mayoclinic.com/health/drug-information/DR600735/DSECTION=proper-use

Mazokopakis, EE, and Starakis, IK: Recommendations for diagnosis and management of metformin-induced vitamin B_{12} (Cbl) deficiency. Diabetes Res Clin Pract 97:359, 2012.

McNeely, JK, Buczulinski, B, and Rosner, DR: Severe neurological impairment in an infant after nitrous oxide anesthesia. Anesthesiology 93:1549, 2000.

Meier, C, and Kraenzlin, ME: Antiepileptics and bone health. Ther Adv Musculoskelet Dis 3:235, 2011. Accessed March 12, 2013. Available at www.ncbi.nlm.nih.gov/pmc/articles/PMC3383529

Meisel, C, Johne, A, and Roots, I: Fatal intracerebral mass bleeding associated with Ginkgo biloba and ibuprofen [letter]. Atherosclerosis 167:367, 2003.

Mellen, CK, Ford, M, and Rindone, JP: Effect of high-dose cranberry juice on the pharmacodynamics of warfarin in patients. Br J Clin Pharmacol 70:139, 2010. Accessed March 9, 2013. Available at www.ncbi.nlm.nih.gov/pmc/articles/PMC2909817

Minns, AB, Ghafouri, N, and Clark, RF: Isoniazid-induced status epilepticus in a pediatric patient after inadequate pyridoxine therapy. Pediatr Emerg Care 26:380, 2010.

Mirtallo, JM: Complications associated with drug and nutrient interactions. J Infus Nurs 27:19, 2004.

Morris, CA, and Avorn, J: Internet marketing of herbal products. JAMA 290:1505, 2003.

Morrow, LE, Wear, RE, Schuller, D, and Malesker, M: Acute isoniazid toxicity and the need for adequate pyridoxine supplies. Pharmacotherapy 26:1529, 2006.

Nakasone, Y, Nakamura, Y, Yamamoto, T, and Yamaguchi, H: Effect of a traditional Japanese garlic preparation on blood pressure in prehypertensive and mildly hypertensive adults. Exp Ther Med 5:399, 2013. Accessed March 22, 2013. Available at www.ncbi.nlm.nih.gov/pmc/articles/PMC3570149

National Collegiate Athletic Association: Drug testing. Updated November 29, 2012. Accessed March 25, 2013. Available at www.ncaa.org/wps/wcm/connect/public/NCAA/Health+and+Safety/Drug+Testing

National Collegiate Athletic Association: NCAA banned drug list. Updated January 4, 3013. Accessed March 25, 2013. Available at www.ncaa.org/wps/wcm/connect/public/NCAA/Health+and+Safety/Drug+Testing/Resources/NCAA+banned+drugs+list

National Institutes of Health: Important information to know when you are taking: Coumadin and vitamin K. Warren Grant Magnuson Clinical Center, 2003. Accessed March 31, 2013. Available at http://ods.od.nih.gov/pubs/factsheets/coumadin1.pdf

National Institutes of Health: Using dietary supplements wisely. Updated March 2010. Accessed March 18, 2013. Available at www.nccam.nih.gov/health/supplements/wiseuse.htm#use

Olsen, DP: Ethical issues: Putting the meds in the applesauce. Am J Nurs 112:67, 2012.

Paeng, CH, Sprague, M, and Jackevicius, CA: Interaction between warfarin and cranberry juice. Clin Ther 29:1730, 2007.

Papandreou, D, Pavlou, E, Kalimeri, E, and Mavromichalis, I: The ketogenic diet in children with epilepsy. Br J Nutr 95:5, 2006.

Parr, MK, and Schänzer, W: Detection of the misuse of steroids in doping control. J Steroid Biochem Mol Biol 121:528, 2010.

Peart, DJ, Siegler, JC, and Vince, RV: Practical recommendations for coaches and athletes: a meta-analysis of sodium bicarbonate use for athletic performance. J Strength Cond Res 26:1975, 2012.

Peng, CC, Glassman, PA, Trilli, LE, et al: Incidence and severity of potential drug–dietary supplement interactions in primary care patients: An exploratory study of 2 outpatient practices. Arch Intern Med 164:630, 2004.

Perret, C, Tabin, R, Marcoz, JP, et al: Apparent life-threatening event in infants: Think about star anise intoxication! [article in French]. Arch Pediatr 18:750, 2011.

Petty, HR, Fernando, M, Kindzelskii, AL, et al: Identification of colchicine in placental blood from patients using herbal medicines. Chem Res Toxicol 14:1254, 2001.

Peuscher, R, Dijsselhof, ME, Abeling, NG, et al: The ketogenic diet is well tolerated and can be effective in patients with argininosuccinate lyase deficiency and refractory epilepsy. JIMD Rep 5:127, 2012.

Pierce, SA, Chung, AH, and Black, KK: Evaluation of vitamin B_{12} monitoring in a veteran population on long-term, high-dose metformin therapy. Ann Pharmacother 46:1470, 2012.

Pritchett, K, and Pritchett, R: Chocolate milk: A post-exercise recovery beverage for endurance sports. Med Sport Sci 59:127, 2013.

Pronsky, ZM, and Crowe, JP: Food Medication Interactions, ed 17. Food-Medication Interactions, Birchrunville, PA, 2012.

Qato, DM, Alexander, GC, Conti, RM, et al: Use of prescription and over-the-counter medications and dietary supplements among older adults in the United States. JAMA 300:2867, 2008. Accessed February 27, 2013. Available at www.ncbi.nlm.nih.gov/pmc/articles/PMC2702513

Quinn, E: Fast and slow twitch muscle fibers. About.com Guide. Updated October 1, 2012. Accessed March 27, 2013. Available at http://sportsmedicine.about.com/od/anatomyandphysiology/a/MuscleFiberType.htm

Rahimi, R, and Abdollahi, M: An update on the ability of St. John's wort to affect the metabolism of other drugs. Expert Opin Drug Metab Toxicol 8:691, 2012.

Ray, KK, Dorman, S, and Watson, RDS: Severe hyper-kalemia due to the concomitant use of salt substitutes and ACE inhibitors in hypertension: A potentially life threatening interaction. J Hum Hypertens 13:717, 1999.

Reinstatler, L, Qi, YP, Williamson, RS, et al: Association of biochemical B_{12} deficiency with metformin therapy and vitamin B_{12} supplements: the National Health and Nutrition Examination Survey, 1999–2006. Diabetes Care 35:327, 2012.

Richmond, J, Hunter, D, Irrgang, J, et al: Treatment of osteoarthritis of the knee (nonarthroplasty). J Am Acad Orthop Surg 17:591, 2009. Accessed March 23, 2013. Available at www.ncbi.nlm.nih.gov/pmc/articles/PMC3170838

Rindone, JP, and Murphy, TW: Warfarin-cranberry juice interaction resulting in profound hypoprothrombinemia and bleeding. Am J Ther 13:283, 2006.

Ringdahl, E, and Pandit, S: Treatment of knee osteoarthritis. Am Fam Physician 83:1287, 2011. Accessed March 23, 2013. Available at www.aafp.org/afp/2011/0601/p1287.html

Roberge, RJ, Rao, P, Miske, GR, and Riley, TJ: Diarrhea-associated over-anticoagulation in a patient taking warfarin: Therapeutic role of cholestyramine. Vet Hum Toxicol 42:351, 2000.

Rohde, LE, de Assis, MC, and Rabelo, ER: Dietary vitamin K intake and anticoagulation in elderly patients. Curr Opin Clin Nutr Metab Care 10:1, 2007.

Rodriguez, NR, DiMarco, NM, Langley, S, et al: Position of the American Dietetic Association, Dietitians of Canada, and the American College of Sports Medicine: Nutrition and athletic performance. J Am Diet Assoc 109:509, 2009.

Roland, PD, and Nergård, CS: Ginkgo biloba—effect, adverse events and drug interaction [article in Norwegian]. Tidsskr Nor Laegeforen 132:956, 2012.

Roman, GC: Nutritional disorders of the nervous system. In Ross, AC, Caballero, B, Cousins, RJ, et al (eds): Modern Nutrition in Health and Disease, ed 11. Lippincott Williams & Wilkins, Philadelphia, 2014.

Rosenbloom, C: Food and fluid guidelines before, during, and after exercise. Nutr Today 47:63, 2012.

Rosener, M, and Dichgans, J: Severe combined degeneration of the spinal cord after nitrous oxide anesthesia in a vegetarian [letter]. J Neurol Neurosurg Psychiatry 60:354, 1996.

Sandon, L: Sports nutrition for an adult female endurance athlete. Cyberounds CME, January 10, 2011.

Saper, RB, Phillips, RS, Sehgal, A, et al: Lead, mercury, and arsenic in US- and Indian-manufactured ayurvedic medicines sold via the Internet. JAMA 300:915, 2008. Accessed March 19, 2013. Available at www.ncbi.nlm.nih.gov/pmc/articles/PMC2755247

Sarino, LV, Dang, KH, Dianat, N, et al: Drug interaction between oral contraceptives and St. John's Wort: appropriateness of advice received from community pharmacists and health food store clerks. J Am Pharm Assoc 47:42, 2007.

Schmidt, LE, and Dalhoff, K: Food–drug interactions. Drugs 62:1481, 2002.

Schultz, H: Supplement sales hit $11.5 billion in U.S. report says. William Reed Business Media, 2013. Accessed February 27, 2013. Available at www.nutraingredients-usa.com/Industry/Supplement-sales-hit-11.5-billion-in-U.S.-report-says?utm_source=copyright&utm_medium=OnSite&utm_campaign=copyright

Schwarz, UI, Ritchie, MD, Bradford, Y, et al: Genetic determinants of response to warfarin during initial anticoagulation. N Engl J Med 358:999, 2008.

Schwellnus, MP: Cause of exercise associated muscle cramps (EAMC)—altered neuromuscular control, dehydration or electrolyte depletion? Br J Sports Med 43:401, 2009.

Schwellnus, MP, Drew, N, and Collins, M. Increased running speed and previous cramps rather than dehydration or serum sodium changes predict exercise-associated muscle cramping: A prospective cohort study in 210 Ironman triathletes. Br J Sports Med 45:650, 2011.

Sehnert, S: Fueling the strength and power athlete. Presentation at Performance Nutrition for Athletes and Active Individuals. Michigan State University, East Lansing, September 12, 2008.

Selzer, RR, Rosenblatt, DS, Laxova, R, and Hogan, K: Adverse effect of nitrous oxide in a child with 5,10-methyletetrahydofolate reductase deficiency. N Eng J Med 349:45, 2003.

Shi, S, and Klotz, U: Drug interactions with herbal medicines. Clin Pharmacokinet 51:77, 2012.

Silverberg, NB: Whey protein precipitating moderate to severe acne flares in 5 teenaged athletes. Cutis 90:70, 2012.

Simonart, T: Acne and whey protein supplementation among bodybuilders. Dermatology 225:256, 2012.

Spaccarotella, KJ, and Andzel, WD: Building a beverage for recovery from endurance activity: A review. J Strength Cond Res 25:3198, 2011.

Srinivasan, VS: Challenges and scientific issues in the standardization of botanicals and their preparations. United States Pharmacopeia's dietary supplement verification program—a public health program. Life Sciences 78:2039, 2006.

Stack, G, for the Education Committee of the Academy of Clinical Laboratory Physicians and Scientists: Pathology consultation on warfarin pharmacogenetic testing. Am J Clin Pathol 135:13, 2011. Accessed March 9, 2013. Available at ajcp.ascpjournals.org/content/135/1/13.long

Stickel, F, Kessebohm, K, Weimann, R, and Seitz, HK: Review of liver injury associated with dietary supplements. Liver Int 31:595, 2011.

Suvarna, R, Pirmohamed, M, and Henderson, L: Possible interaction between warfarin and cranberry juice. BMJ 327:1454, 2003. Accessed March 9, 2013. Available at www.ncbi.nlm.nih.gov/pmc/articles/PMC300803

Swanson, CA, Thomas, PR, and Coates, PM: The evolving science of dietary supplements. In Ross, AC, Caballero, B, Cousins, RJ, et al (eds): Modern Nutrition in Health and Disease, ed 11. Lippincott Williams & Wilkins, Philadelphia, 2014.

Taylor, JR, and Wilt, VM: Probable antagonism of warfarin by green tea. Ann Pharmacother 33:426, 1999.

Thorsteinsdottir, B, Grande, JP, and Garovic, VD: Acute renal failure in a young weight lifter taking multiple food supplements, including creatine monohydrate. J Ren Nutr 16:341, 2006.

Tipton, KD: Protein nutrition and exercise: What's the latest? Scan's Pulse, Spring 2011.

Tsai, HH, Lin, HW, Simon Pickard, A: Evaluation of documented drug interactions and contraindications associated with herbs and dietary supplements: A systematic literature review. Int J Clin Pract 66:1056, 2012.

U.S. Food and Drug Administration: Ceftriaxone (marketed as Rocephin and generics). Safety alerts. Updated: June 11, 2009. Accessed February 28, 2013. Available at www.fda.gov/Safety/MedWatch/Safety Information/SafetyAlertsforHumanMedicalProducts/ucm136533.htm

U.S. Food and Drug Administration: Dietary Supplement Health and Education Act of 1994. Updated May 20, 2009. Accessed March 18, 2013. Available at www.fda.gov/RegulatoryInformation/Legislation/Federal FoodDrugandCosmeticActFDCAct/Significant AmendmentstotheFDCAct/ucm148003.htm

U.S. Food and Drug Administration: Dietary supplements—Q&A. Updated March 14, 2013. Accessed March 18, 2013. Available at www.fda.gov/Food/DietarySupplements/QADietarySupplements/ucm191930.htm#FDA_role

U.S. Food and Drug Administration: FDA issues advisory on "teas." September 10, 2003. Accessed March 18, 2013. Available at www.fda.gov/ICECI/Enforcement Actions/EnforcementStory/EnforcementStoryArchive/ucm095929.htm

U.S. Food and Drug Administration: FDA warns consumers about "total body formula" and "total body mega formula." May 1, 2008. Accessed March 18, 2013. Available at www.fda.gov/NewsEvents/Newsroom/PressAnnouncements/2008/ucm116892.htm

U.S. Food and Drug Administration: Guidance for Industry: Current Good Manufacturing Practice in Manufacturing, Packaging, Labeling, or Holding Operations for Dietary Supplements; Small Entity Compliance Guide, December 2010. Accessed March 18, 2013. Available at www.fda.gov/Food/GuidanceRegulation/Guidance DocumentsRegulatoryInformation/DietarySupplements/ucm238182.htm#III

U.S. Food and Drug Administration: KG Enterprises LLC, Inc. issues a voluntary nationwide recall of all Maxidus pills, a product marketed as a dietary supplement. Updated December 14, 2010. Accessed March 20, 2013. Available at www.fda.gov/Safety/Recalls/ArchiveRecalls/2008/ucm112415.htm

U.S. Food and Drug Administration: TWC Global LLC, Inc. issues a voluntary nationwide recall of Axcil and Desirin products marketed as dietary supplements. Updated June 18, 2009. Accessed March 20, 2013 at www.fda.gov/Safety/Recalls/ArchiveRecalls/2007/ucm112274.htm

U.S. National Library of Medicine: MTHFR. Genetics Home Reference. Updated July 11, 2011. Accessed March 16, 2013. Available at ghr.nlm.nih.gov/gene/MTHFR

U.S. Pharmacopeial Convention: USP verification services for dietary supplements, 2013. Accessed March 19, 2013. Available at www.usp.org/dietary-supplements/verification-services

Vallerand, AH, Sanoski, CA, and Deglin, JH: Davis's Drug Guide for Nurses, ed 13. FA Davis, Philadelphia, 2013.

van der Watt, JJ, Harrison, TB, Benatar, M, and Heckmann, JM: Polyneuropathy, anti-tuberculosis treatment and the role of pyridoxine in the HIV/AIDS era: A systematic review. Int J Tuberc Lung Dis 15:722, 2011.

van Rosendal, SP, Osborne, MA, Fassett, RG, and Coombes, JS: Guidelines for glycerol use in hyperhydration and rehydration associated with exercise. Sports Med 40:113, 2010.

Van Strater, AC, and Bogers, JP: Interaction of St. John's wort (Hypericum perforatum) with clozapine. Int Clin Psychopharmacol 27:121, 2012.

Vaysse, J, Balayssac, S, Gilard, V: Analysis of adulterated herbal medicines and dietary supplements marketed for weight loss by DOSY 1H-NMR. Food Addit Contam Part A Chem Anal Control Expo Risk Assess 27:903, 2010.

Vermaak, I, Viljoen, A, and Lindström, SW: Hyperspectral imaging in the quality control of herbal medicines—the case of neurotoxic Japanese star anise. J Pharm Biomed Anal 75:207, 2013.

Williams, MH: Sports nutrition. In Ross, AC, Caballero, B, Cousins, RJ, et al (eds): Modern Nutrition in Health and Disease, ed 11. Lippincott Williams & Wilkins, Philadelphia, 2014.

Woolf, AD, Hussain, J, McCullough, L, et al: Infantile lead poisoning from an Asian tongue powder: a case report and subsequent public health inquiry. Clin Toxicol (Phila) 46:841, 2008.

World Anti-Doping Agency: Prohibited list. 2013. Accessed March 25, 2013. Available at www.wada-ama.org/en/World-Anti-Doping-Program/Sports-and-Anti-Doping-Organizations/International-Standards/Prohibited-List

Yasue, H, Itoh, T, Mizuno, Y, and Harada, E: Severe hypokalemia, rhabdomyolysis, muscle paralysis, and respiratory impairment in a hypertensive patient taking herbal medicines containing licorice. Intern Med 46:575, 2007.

Zhou, SF, Liu, JP, and Chowbay, B: Polymorphism of human cytochrome P450 enzymes and its clinical impact. Drug Metab Rev 41:89, 2009.

Chapter 16

Adams, TD, Davidson, LE, Litwin, SE, et al: Health benefits of gastric bypass surgery after 6 years. JAMA 308:1122, 2012.

Annesi, JJ, and Marti, CN: Path analysis of exercise treatment-induced changes in psychological factors leading to weight loss. Psychol Health 26:1081, 2011.

Baugh, E, Mullis, Ron, Mullis, A, et al: Ethnic identity and body image among black and white college females. J Am College Health 59:105, 2010.

Bezerra, IN, Curioni, C, and Sichieri, R: Association between eating out of home and body weight. Nutr Rev 70:65, 2012.

Brown, J, and Wimpenny, P: Developing a holistic approach to obesity management. Int J Nurs Pract 17:9, 2011.

Burke, LE, and Wang, J: Treatment strategies for overweight and obesity. J Nurs Scholar 43:368, 2011.

Campbell, H: Managing emotional eating. Ment Health Pract 15:84, 2012.

Centers for Disease Control and Prevention: Overweight and obesity. 2012. Accessed January 4, 2013. Available at www.cdc.gov/obesity/data/adult.html

Centers for Disease Control and Prevention: Overweight and obesity: Causes and consequences. 2012. Accessed February 25, 2013. Available at www.cdc.gov/obesity/adult/causes/index.html

Clifton, PM: Low-carbohydrate diets for weight loss: The pros and cons. J Hum Nutr Diet 24:523, 2011.

Disordered eating in midlife and beyond. Harv Women Health Watch 19:1, 2012.

Furtado, LC: Nutritional management after roux-en-y gastric bypass. Br J Nurs 19:428, 2010.

Furtado, LC: Procedure and outcomes of roux-en-y gastric bypass. Br J Nurs 19:307, 2010.

Grossniklaus, DA, Gary, RA, Higgins, MK, and Dunbar, SB: Biobehavioral and psychological differences between overweight adults with and without waist circumference risk. Res Nurs Health 33:539, 2010.

Holtcamp, W: Obesogens: An environmental link to obesity. Environ Health Perspect 120:A23, 2012.

Keyes, A, Brozek, J, and Henschel, A: The Biology of Human Starvation, 2 vols. University of Minnesota Press, Minneapolis, 1950.

Klempel, MC, and Varady, KA: Reliability of leptin, but not adiponectin, as a biomarker for diet-induced weight loss in humans. Nutr Rev 26:145, 2011.

Moss, C, Dhillo, WS, Frost, G, and Hickson, M: Gastrointestinal hormones: the regulation of appetite and the anorexia of ageing. J Hum Nutr Diet 25:3, 2012.

National Institutes of Health: Weight control information network: Understanding obesity. Accessed February 17, 2013. Available at win.niddk.nih.gov/publications/understanding.htm#measured

National Institute of Health: Assessing your weight and health risks. Accessed February 9, 2014. Available at www.nhlbi.nih.gov/health/public/heart/obesity/lose_wt/risk.htm

National Institutes of Health and National Heart, Lung, and Blood Institute: Calculating your body mass index. Accessed February 9, 2013. Available at www.nhlbisupport.com/bmi

National Institutes of Health and National Heart, Lung, and Blood Institute: Clinical guidelines on the identification, evaluation, and treatment of overweight and obesity in adults. NIH, Bethesda, MD, June 1998.

National Weight Control Registry: Research findings. Accessed March 5, 2013. Available at www.nwcr.ws/Research/default.htm

Ohsiek, S, and Williams, M: Psychological factors influencing weight loss maintenance: An integrative literature review. J Am Acad Nurse Practit 23:592, 2011.

Polivy, J (1996). Psychological consequences of food restriction. J Amer Diet Assoc 96:589.

Rooney, BL, Mathiason, MA, and Schauberger, CW: Predictors of obesity in childhood, adolescence, and adulthood in a birth cohort. Matern Child Health J 15:1166, 2011.

Shay, LE, Shobert, JL, Seibert, D, and Thomas, LE: Adult weight management: Translating research and guidelines into practice. J Am Acad Nurse Practit 21:197, 2009.

Shikany, JM, Desmond, R, McCubrey, R, and Allison, DB: Meta-analysis of studies of a specific delivery mode for a modified-carbohydrate diet. J Hum Nutr Diet 24:525, 2011.

Stubbs, J, Whybrown, S, and Lavin, J: Dietary and lifestyle measures to enhance satiety and weight control. Nutr Bull 35:113, 2010.

Swann, J: Understanding bariatrics. Br J Healthc Assist 4:338, 2010.

Taber, DR, Stevens, J, Evenson, KR, Ward, DS, Poole, C, Maciejewski, ML, Murray, DM, and Brownson, RC: State policies targeting junk food in schools: Racial/ethnic differences in the effect of policy change on soda consumption. Amer J Pub Health 101(9):1769, 2011.

Wolf, C: Physician assistant students' attitudes about obesity and obese individuals. J Physician Assist Educ 21:37, 2010.

Wozniak, G, Rekleiti, M, and Roupa, Z: (April–June, 2012). Contribution of social and family factors in anorexia nervosa. Health Sci J 6(2): 257, 2012.

Chapter 17

American Diabetes Association: Nutrition recommendations and interventions for diabetes: A position statement of the American Diabetes Association. Diabetes Care 31:S61, 2008.

American Diabetes Association and American Dietetic Association: Choose your foods: Exchange lists for diabetes. 2009.

American Diabetes Association: Diagnosis and classification of diabetes mellitus. Care.diabetesjournals.org. 35, January 2012a.

American Diabetes Association: Standards of medical care in diabetes—2012. Care.diabetesjournals.org 35, January 2012b.

American Diabetes Association: Standards of medical care in diabetes—2013. Diabetes Care 36 2013a.

American Diabetes Association: Create your plate. 2013b. Accessed February 18, 2013. Available at www.diabetes.org/food-and-fitness/food/planning-meals

American Diabetes Association: Economic costs of diabetes in the US in 2012. 2013c. Care.diabetesjournals.org, March 6, 2013.

Basu, S, Yoffe, P, Hills, N, and Lustig, RH: The relationship of sugar to population-level diabetes prevalence: an econometric analysis of repeated cross-sectional data. PloS ONE 2, E57873. Dol:10.1371 February 2013.

Centers for Disease Control and Prevention: National diabetes fact sheet, 2011. Accessed February 2013. Available at http://www.cdc.gov/diabetes/pubs/pdf/ndfs_2011.pdf

Chen, SM, Creedy, D, Lin, HS, and Willin, J: Effects of motivational interviewing intervention on self-management, psychological and glycemic outcomes in type 2 diabetics: A randomized controlled trial. Int J Nurs Stud, 49:637, 2012.

Diabetes Control and Complication Trial Research Group: Influence of intensive treatment on quality-of-life outcomes in the diabetes control and complications trial. Diabetes Care 19:195, 1993.

Diabetes Control and Complication Trial Research Group: The effect of intensive treatment of diabetes on the development and progression of long-term complications in insulin-dependent diabetes mellitus. N Engl J Med 329:977, 1998.

Dugdale, D, and Zieve, D: Mediterranean Diet. National Institutes of Health, Bethesda, MD, 2012. Accessed June 2013. Available at www.nim.nih.gov/medlineplus/ency/patientinstructions/000110.htm

Fagherazzi, G, Vilier, A, Saes Sartorelli, D, et al: Consumption of artificially and sugar-sweetened beverages and incident type 2 diabetes in the Etude Epidémiologique auprès des femmes de la Mutuelle Générale de l'Education Nationale—European Prospective Investigation into Cancer and Nutrition cohort. Am J Clin Nutr 97:517, 2013.

Goran, M, Ulijaszek, SJ, and Ventura, EE: High fructose corn syrup and diabetes prevalence: A global perspective. Global Public Health, 2012. doi:10.1080

Kirpitch, A, and Maryniuk, MD: The 3 R's of glycemic index: Recommendations, research, and the real world. Clin Diabetes 29:155, 2011.

Magaji, V, and Johnston, J: Inpatient management of hyperglycemia and diabetes. Clin Diabetes 3:29 2011.

Natural Medicines Comprehensive Database: Natural product effectiveness checker, diabetes. Accessed through the Academy of Nutrition and Dietetics Practice Group. Dietitians in Integrative and Functional Medicine (DIFM), January 23, 2013. Available at http://naturaldatabase.therapeuticresearch.com/

National Diabetes Information Clearinghouse: Hypoglycemia (NIH Pub. No. 09-3926), October 2008, updated November 6, 2012. Accessed February 2013. Available at http://diabetes.niddk.niu.gov/dm/pubs/hypoglycemia

Shane-McWhorter, L: Dietary supplements and probiotics for diabetes. Am J Nurs 112(7):47,2012.

U.S. National Library of Medicine, National Institutes of Health: First-Ever Guidelines Issued for Treating Type 2 Diabetes in Kids. January 28, 2013. Accessed January 2013. Available at www.nlm.nih.gov/medlineplus/news/fullstory_133483.html

UKPDS Group. Intensive blood-glucose control with sulphonylureas or insulin compared with conventional treatment and risk of complications in patients with type 2 diabetes (PKPDS 33). Lancet 352:837, 1998.

University of Sydney. The glycemic index. Accessed February 18, 2013. Available at www.glycemicindex.com.

Visalli, M: Mediterranean Diet bests Low-Fat Diet for CVD Prevention in PREDIMED. Clin Insights Diabetes 14(1), 2013.

Wirström, T, Hilding, A, Gu, HF, et al: Consumption of whole grain reduces risk of deteriorating glucose tolerance, including progression to prediabetes. Am J Clin Nutr 97:179, 2013.

Zimmerman, G, Olsen, CG, and Boswoth, MF: A "stages of change" approach to helping patients change behavior. Am Fam Physician Mar 1;61(5):1409, 2000.

Chapter 18

Aglony, M, Acevedo, M, and Ambrosio, G: Hypertension in adolescents. Expert Rev Cardiovasc Ther 7:1595, 2009.

Ambrose, JA, and Barua, RS: The pathophysiology of cigarette smoking and cardiovascular disease: An update. J Am Coll Cardiol 43:1731, 2004.

American Dietetic Association: Disorders of lipid metabolism evidence-based nutrition practice guideline. 2008a. Accessed March 2013. Available at http://andevidencelibrary.com

American Dietetic Association: Heart failure evidence-based nutrition practice guideline. 2008b. Accessed March 2013. Available at http://andevidencelibrary.com

American Dietetic Association: Hypertension evidence-based nutrition practice guideline. 2008c. Accessed March 2013. Available at http://andevidencelibrary.com

American Dietetic Association: Position of the American Dietetic Association: Vegetarian diets. J Am Diet Assoc, 109:1266, 2009.

American Heart Association: Iron and heart disease. 2000. Accessed June 5, 2000. Available at http://www.americanheart.org/Heart_and_Stroke_Z_ZGuideline.iron.html

American Heart Association: Fish and omega-3 fatty acids. 2008. Accessed October 13, 2008. Available at http://www.heart.org/HEARTORG/GettingHealthy/NutritionCenter/HealthyDietGoals/Fish-and-Omega-3-Fatty-Acids_UCM_303248_Article.jsp

American Heart Association: Homocysteine, folic acid and cardiovascular disease. Updated January 2012. Accessed January 2013. Available at http://www.heart.org/HEARTORG/GettingHealthy/NutritionCenter/Homocysteine-Folic-Acid-and-Cardiovascular-Disease_UCM_305997_Article.jsp

American Heart Association: 2020 goal, 2013 statistical fact sheet. Accessed January 2013. Available at www.heart.org/idc/groups/heart-public/@wcm/@sop/@smd/documents/downloadable/ucm_319831.pdf.

American Heart Association: Lifestyle changes and cholesterol. Updated May 1, 2013a. Accessed June 2013. Available at www.heart.org/HEARTORG/Conditions/Cholesterol/PreventionTreatmentofHighCholesterol/Prevention-and-Treatment-of-High-Cholesterol_UCM_001215_Article.jsp.

American Heart Association: Vitamin supplements, healthy or hoax? Updated February 26, 2014, 2013b. Accessed March 9, 2014. Available at www.heart.org/HEARTORG/GettingHealthy/NutritionCenter/HealthyEating/Vitamin-Supplements-Healthy-or-Hoax_UCM_432104_Article.jsp.

American Heart Association and American Stroke Association: Heart disease and stroke statistics. 2008. Updated 2009. Available at http://circ.ahajournals.org/content/119/3/e21.full.pdf

American Heart Association and American Stroke Association: Heart disease and stroke statistics—2012 update. Circulation, 125:2, 2012.

American Stroke Association: Impact of stroke (stroke statistics). Updated May 1, 2012. Accessed January 2013. Available at www.strokeassociation.org/STROKEORG/

AboutStroke/Impact-of-Stroke_UCM_310728_Article.jsp.

Appel, LJ, and Anderson, CAM: Compelling evidence for public health action to reduce salt intake. N Engl J Med 362:650, 2010.

Appel, LJ, Frohlich, ED, Hall, JE, et al: The importance of population-wide sodium reduction as a means to prevent cardiovascular disease and stroke: A call to action from the American Heart Association. Circulation, 123:1138, 2011.

Arnett, DK, Baird, AE, Barkley, RA, et al: Relevance of genetics and genomics for prevention and treatment of cardiovascular disease: A scientific statement from the American Heart Association Council on Epidemiology and Prevention, the Stroke Council, and the Functional Genomics and Translational Biology Interdisciplinary Working Group. Circulation 115:2878, 2007.

Barker, DJP: Fetal origins of cardiovascular disease. Ann Med 31(Suppl 1):3, 1999.

Bonita, JS, Mandarano, M, Shuta, D, Vinson, J, et al: Coffee and cardiovascular disease: In vitro, cellular, animal, and human studies. Pharmacol Res 55:187, 2007.

Bonomini, F, Tengattini, S, Fabiano, A, et al: Atherosclerosis and oxidative stress. Histol Histopathol 23:381, 2008.

Brannon, C: Is wine a functional food? Diet Integ Functional Med 13:1, 2011.

Brown, JE: Nutrition Through the Life Cycle, ed 3. Thomson Wadsworth, Belmont, CA, 2008.

Brunzell, JD: Hypertriglyceridemia. N Engl J Med 357:1009, 2007.

Catalgol, B, Batirel, S, Taga, Y, and Ozer, NK: Resveratrol: French paradox revisited. Front Pharmacol 3:141, 2012.

Centers for Disease Control and Prevention: Disparities in screening for and awareness of high blood cholesterol—United States, 1999–2002. Morb Mortal Wkly Rep 54:117, 2005. Accessed October 10, 2008. Available at www.cdc.gov/mmwr/preview/mmwrhtml/mm5405a2.htm

Centers for Disease Control and Prevention: Stroke fact sheet. June 25, 2008a. Accessed October 2008. Available at www.cdc.gov/DHDSP/library/fs

Centers for Disease Control and Prevention: Heart disease fact sheet. July 1, 2008b. Accessed October 2008. Available at www.cdc.gov/DHDSP/library/fs

Centers for Disease Control and Prevention: Heart failure fact sheet. January 25, 2010. Accessed October 2008. Available at www.cdc.gov/DHDSP/library/fs

Centers for Disease Control and Prevention: Screening for lipid disorders among adults—National Health And Nutrition Examination Survey, United States 2005–2008. Morb Mortal Wkly Rep 62(02):26, 2012.

Centers for Disease Control and Prevention: High Blood Pressure Facts, March 20, 2013, Accessed August 27, 2013. Available at www.cdc.gov/bloodpressure/facts.htm

Consumer Lab: Vegetarian sources of omega-3 fatty acids. Accessed August 17, 2012 at www.consumerlab.com/reviews/Omega-3fattyacids_Review/

Consumer Lab: Resveratrol supplements. Accessed August 17, 2012 at www.consumerlab.com/reviews/Resveratrol_Review/Resveratrol_Red_Wine/

Consumer Lab: Omega-3 fatty acids. Accessed August 1, 2013. Available at www.consumerlab.com

Cornelis, MC, El-Sohemy, A, Kabagambe, EK, and Campos, H: Coffee, CYP1A2 genotype, and risk of myocardial infarction. JAMA 295:1135, 2006.

Daniels, SR, and Greer, FR: Lipid screening and cardiovascular health in childhood. Pediatrics 122:198, 2008.

de Ferranti, S, and Washington, RL: NHLBI guidelines on cholesterol in kids: What's new and how does this change practice? AAP News, 33:1, 2012.

Delanghe, JR, Langlois, MR, De Buyzere, ML, and Torck, MA: Vitamin C deficiency and scurvy are not only a dietary problem but are codetermined by the haptoglobin polymorphism. Clin Chem 53:1397, 2007.

Dietary Management of Hyperlipoproteinemias: A Handbook for Physicians and Dietitians. U.S. Department of Health, Education, and Welfare, Bethesda, MD, 1980.

Din, JN, Newby, DE, and Flapan, AD: Omega 3 fatty acids and cardiovascular disease—fishing for a natural treatment. BMJ 328:30, 2004.

Ding, EL, and Mozaffarian, D: Optimal dietary habits for the prevention of stroke. Semin Neurol 26:11, 2006.

Epstein, D, Sherwood, A, Smith, PJ, et al: Determinants and consequences of adherence to the dietary approaches to stop hypertension diet in African-American and White adults with high blood pressure: Results from the ENCORE trial. J Acad Nutr Diet 112:1763, 2012.

Eriksson, JG: The role of genes in growth and later health. Nestle Nutr Workshop Ser Pediatr Program 61:69, 2008.

Expert Panel on Detection, Evaluation, and Treatment of High Blood Cholesterol in Adults: Executive summary of the third report of the Expert Panel on Detection, Evaluation, and Treatment of High Blood Cholesterol in Adults (Adult Treatment Panel III). JAMA 285:2486, 2001.

Fang, J, Yang, Q, Hong, Y, and Loustalot, F: Status of cardiovascular health among adult Americans in the 50 states and the District of Columbia, 2009. J Am Heart Assoc, 112.005371, 2012.

Fauci, AS, Braunwald, E, Isselbacher, KJ, et al (eds): Harrison's Principles of Internal Medicine Companion Handbook. McGraw-Hill, New York, 1998.

Ferrieres, J: The French paradox: Lessons for other countries. Heart 90:107, 2004.

George, MG, Tong, X, McGruder, H, et al: Paul Coverdell National Acute Stroke Registry surveillance—four states, 2005–2007. Morb Mortal Wkly Rep 58:SS-7, 2009. Accessed March 3, 2010. Available at www.merck.com/mmpe/sec12/ch159b.

Godfrey, KM, and Barker, DJ: Fetal programming and adult health. Public Health Nutr 4:611, 2001.

Goldberg, AC: Dyslipidemias. Merck Manual, September 2008. Accessed March 2010 at: www.merk.com/mmpe/se12/ch159b.htm

Greenberg, JA, Dunbar, CC, Schnoll, R, et al: Caffeinated beverage intake and the risk of heart disease mortality in the elderly: A prospective analysis. Am J Clin Nutr 85:392, 2007.

Gropper, SS, Smith, JL, and Groff, JL: Advanced Nutrition and Human Metabolism, ed 5. Wadsworth, Belmont, CA, 2009.

Grundy, SM: Nutrition in the management of disorders of serum lipids and lipoproteins. In Shils, ME, Shike, M, Ross, AC, and Caballero, MD (eds): Modern Nutrition in Health and Disease, ed 10. Lippincott Williams & Wilkins, Philadelphia, 2006.

Grundy, SM, Cleeman, JI, Merz, CN, et al: Implications of recent clinical trials for the National Cholesterol Education Program Adult Treatment Panel III guidelines. Circulation 110:227, 2004.

Hausenloy, DJ, and Yellon, DM: Targeting residual cardio-vascular risk: Raising high-density lipoprotein cholesterol levels. Heart 94:706, 2008.

He, FJ, Nowson, CA, and MacGregor, GA: Fruit and vegetable consumption and stroke: Meta-analysis of cohort studies. Lancet 367:320, 2006.

Hofman, PL, Jackson, WE, and Knight, DB: Premature birth and later insulin resistance. N Engl J Med 351:2179, 2004.

Horowitz, CR, Rein, SB, and Leventhal, H: A story of maladies, misconceptions and mishaps: Effective management of heart failure. Soc Sci Med 58:631, 2004.

Holvoet, P: Relations between metabolic syndrome, oxidative stress and inflammation and cardiovascular disease. Verh K Acad Geneeskd Belg 70:193, 2008.

Hoyert, DL, and Xu, J: Deaths: Preliminary data for 2011. Natl Vital Stat Rep 61(6), October 10, 2012. Accessed January 2013. Available at www.cdc.gov/nchs/data/nvsr/nvsr61/nvsr61_06.pdf

Jawalekar, S: The hyperlipoproteinemia—an approach to diagnosis and classification. Biochem Physiol 1(1), 2012. Available at http://dx.doi.org/10.4172/2168-9652.1000e105

Keenan, N, and Rosendorf, K: Prevalence of hypertension and controlled hypertension—United States, 2005–2008. Centers for Disease Control and Prevention. Morb Mortal Wkly Rep 60(1):94, 2011.

Klipstein-Grosbusch, K, Grobbee, DE, den Breeijen, JH, et al: Dietary iron and risk of myocardial infarction in the Rotterdam Study. Am J Epidemiol 149:421, 1999.

Kotchen, TA, and Kotchen, JM: Nutrition, diet, and hypertension. In Shils, ME, Shike, M, Ross, AC, and Caballero, MD (eds): Modern Nutrition in Health and Disease, ed 10. Lippincott Williams & Wilkins, Philadelphia, 2006.

Lichtenstein, AH, Appel, LJ, Brands, M, et al: Diet and lifestyle recommendations revision 2006: A scientific statement from the American Heart Association Nutrition Committee. Circulation 114:82, 2006.

Lopez-Garcia, E, van Dam, RM, Willett, WC, et al: Coffee consumption and coronary heart disease in men and women: A prospective cohort study. Circulation 113:2045, 2006.

Love, JA, and Prusa, KJ: Nutrient composition and sensory attributes of cooked ground beef: Effects of fat content, cooking method, and water rinsing. J Am Diet Assoc 92:1367, 1992.

Matsuura, E, Hughes, GR, and Khamashta, MA: Oxidation of LDL and its clinical implication. Autoimmun Rev 7:558, 2008.

Michaelsson, K, Melhus, H, Warensjö Lemming, E, et al: Long term calcium intake and rates of all cause and cardiovascular mortality: Community based prospective longitudinal cohort study. BMJ 346:f228, 2013.

Miller, M, Stone, NJ, Ballantyne, C, et al: Triglycerides and cardiovascular disease: A scientific statement from the American Heart Association. Circulation 123:2291, 2011.

Natural Medicines Comprehensive Database: Resveratrol. Accessed December 2012. Available at http://natural-database.therapeuticresearch.com

Mostofsky, E, Rice, MS, Levitan, EB, and Mittleman, MA: Habitual coffee consumption and risk of heart failure: A dose-response meta-analysis. Circ Heart Failure 112, 2012. doi: 10.1161/CIRCHEARTFAILURE.112967299

Mukamal, K: Alcohol intake and noncoronary cardiovascular diseases. Ann Epidemiol 17:S8, 2007.

National Heart Lung and Blood Institute, National Institute of Health: Integrated guidelines for cardiovascular health and risk reduction in children and adolescents. Accessed August 2013a. Available at www.nhlbi.nih.gov/guidelines/cvd_ped/

National Heart Lung and Blood Institute, National Institute of Health: How to prevent and control coronary heart disease risk factors. Accessed August 2013b. Available at www.nhlbi.nih.gov/health/health-topics/topics/hd/prevent.html

National Heart Lung and Blood Institute, National Institute of Health: What is the DASH eating plan? Accessed December 2012. Available at www.nhlbi.nih.gov/health/health-topics/topics/dash/

National Institutes of Health: The DASH diet. Press Release, April 3, 1997.

National Institutes of Health: A Pocket Guide to Blood Pressure Measurement in Children (NIH Publication 07-5268). May 2007.

Nygård, O, Nordrehaug, JE, Refsum, H, et al: Plasma homocysteine levels and mortality in patients with coronary artery disease. N Engl J Med 337:230, 1997.

O'Callaghan, P: Homocysteine—is it the end of the line? Br J Cardiol 14:69, 2007.

Parikh, A, Lipsitz, SR, and Natarajan, S: Association between a DASH-like diet and mortality in adults with hypertension: Findings from a population-based follow-up study. Am J Hypertens 22:409, 2009.

Patel, MD, and Thompson, PD: Phytosterols and vascular disease. Atherosclerosis 186:12, 2006.

Petrone, A, Weir, N, Hanson, NQ, et al: Omega-6 fatty acids and risk of heart failure in the Physicians' Healthy Study. Am J Clin Nutr 97:66, 2012.

Qureshi, AI, Suri, MF, Kirmani, JF, and Divani, AA: Prevalence and trends of prehypertension and hypertension in United States: National Health and Nutrition Examination Surveys 1976 to 2000. Med Sci Monit 11:CR403-9.

Rader, DJ: Illuminating HDL—is it still a viable therapeutic target? N Engl J Med 357:2180, 2007.

Refsum, H, Smith, AD, Ueland, PM, et al: Facts and recommendations about total homocysteine determinations: An expert opinion. Clin Chem 50:3, 2004.

Salonen, JT, Nyyssönen, K, Korpela, H, et al: High stored iron levels are associated with excess risk of myocardial infarction in Eastern Finnish men. Circulation 86:803, 1992.

Scanlon, VC, and Sanders, T: Essentials of Anatomy and Physiology, ed 5. FA Davis, Philadelphia, 2007.

Serra-Majem, L, Ribbas, L, Tsesserras, R, et al: How could changes in diet explain changes in coronary heart disease mortality in Spain? The Spanish paradox. Am J Clin Nutr 61(Suppl):1351S, 1995.

Sofi, F, Conti, AA, Gori, AM, et al: Coffee consumption and risk of coronary heart disease: A meta-analysis. Nutr Metab Cardiovasc Dis 17:209, 2007.

Sperling, MA: Prematurity—a window of opportunity? N Engl J Med 351:2229, 2004.

Sports, Cardiovascular, and Wellness Nutrition: Functional Foods and Dietary Management of LDL Cholesterol. 2 2009.

Sports, Cardiovascular, and Wellness Nutrition: The Role of Soy in the Performance of Active and Athletic Americans. 4 2012.

Tanne, D, Haim, M, Goldbourt, U, et al: Elevated homocysteine in heart patients linked with higher stroke risk. Stroke 34 (Rapid Access Issue), February 21, 2003.

The Academy of Nutrition and Dietetics: Disorders of lipid metabolism. Academy Evidence-Based Practice Guidelines, Washington, DC, 2011.

Theuwissen, E, and Mensink, RP: Water-soluble dietary fibers and cardiovascular disease. Physiol Behav 94:285, 2008.

Thies, F, Garry, JM, Yaqoob, P, et al: Association of n-3 polyunsaturated fatty acids with stability of atherosclerotic plaques: A randomized controlled trial. Lancet 361:477, 2003.

Tomkins, CC: Does fetal under-nutrition predispose disease in adult offspring? Alberta Health Sci J 4:16, 2007. Accessed February 8, 2014. Available at www.uahsj.ualberta.ca/files/Issues/4-1/pdf/16.pdf

Tuomainen, TP, Punnonen, K, Nyyssönen, K, and Salonen, JT: Association between body iron stores and the risk of acute myocardial infarction in men. Circulation 97:1461, 1998.

Tzonou, A, Lagiou, P, Trichopoulou, A, et al: Dietary iron and coronary heart disease risk: A study from Greece. Am J Epidemiol 147:161, 1998.

U.S. Department of Agriculture: Dietary Guidelines for Americans, 2010. Accessed October 2012. Available at www.usda.gov/dietaryguidelines/dga

U.S. Department of Health and Human Services: The seventh report of the Joint National Committee on Prevention, Detection, Evaluation, and Treatment of High Blood Pressure. National Institutes of Health, Washington, DC, 2003.

U.S. Department of Health and Human Services: Healthy people 2020. Accessed March 2013. Available at www.healthypeople.gov/2020

U.S. Food and Drug Administration: FDA allows foods containing psyllium to make health claim on reducing risk of heart disease. U.S. Department of Health and Human Services, Rockville, MD, February 17, 1998.

U.S. Food and Drug Administration: FDA approves new health claim for soy protein and coronary heart disease. U.S. Department of Health and Human Services, Rockville, MD, October 20, 1999.

Vasan, RS, Beiser, A, D'Agostino, RB, et al: Plasma homocysteine and risk for congestive heart failure in adults without prior myocardial infarction. JAMA 289:1251, 2003.

Vollset, SE, Refsum, H, Tverdal, A, et al: Plasma total homocysteine and cardiovascular and noncardiovascular mortality: The Hordaland Homocysteine Study. Am J Clin Nutr 74:130, 2001.

Wierzbicki, AS: Homocysteine and cardiovascular disease: A review of the evidence. Diab Vasc Dis Res 4:143, 2007.

Yancy, CW, Jessup, M, Bozkurt, B, et al: 2013 ACCF/AHA Guidelines for the management of heart failure: A report of the American College of Cardiology Foundation/American Heart Association Task Force on practice guidelines. Circulation 128:1810, 2013.

Yoon, SS, Burt, V, Louis, T, and Carroll, MD: Hypertension among adults in the United States, 2009–2010 (NCHS Data Brief 107). Centers for Disease Control and Prevention, Atlanta, GA, October 2012. Accessed February 7, 2013. Available at www.cdc.gov/nchs/data/databriefs/db107.htm

Chapter 19

Academy of Nutrition and Dietetics Practice Guidelines: CKD evidence-based nutrition practice guidelines. 2010. Accessed April 10, 2013. Available at www.eatright.org

Beto, JA, and Bansal, VK: Medical nutrition therapy in chronic kidney failure: Integrating clinical practice guidelines. J Am Diet Assoc 104:404, 2004.

Moore, MC: Mosby's Pocket Guide to Nutrition and Care, ed 6. Mosby Year Book, St. Louis, 2009.

National Institutes of Health: Nutrition for Advanced Chronic Kidney Disease in Adults (NIH Publication No. 11-5572). Accessed April 2011a. Available at http://kidney.niddk.nih.gov/kudiseases/pubs/NutritionAdvancedCKD/Nutrition_Advanced_CKD_Adult_508.pdf

National Institutes of Health, and National Kidney Disease Education Program: Chronic kidney disease (CKD) and diet: Assessment, management, and treatment. Treating CKD patients who are not on dialysis. September 2011b.

National Institutes of Health: Diet for Kidney Stone Prevention. National Institute of Diabetes and Digestive and Kidney Diseases (NIH Publication No. 13-6425). Accessed February 2013. http://kidney.niddk.nih.gov/kudiseases/pubs/NutritionAdvancedCKD/Nutrition_Advanced_CKD_Adult_508.pdf

National Kidney Foundation: K/DOQI clinical practice guidelines for chronic kidney disease: Evaluation, classification and stratification. Am J Kidney Dis 39(Suppl 1):S1, 2002.

National Kidney Foundation: Kidney Disease Outcomes Quality Initiative (KDOQI) clinical practice guidelines for diabetes and CKD. Am J Kidney Dis 49, 2007.

National Kidney Foundation: Kidney Disease Outcomes Quality Initiative clinical practice guidelines for diabetes and CKD: 2012 update. Am J Kidney Dis 60:850, 2012.

National Kidney Foundation: About chronic kidney disease. Accessed April 5, 2013a. Available at www.kidney.org/kidneydisease/aboutckd.cfm

National Kidney Foundation: Phosphorus and your CKD diet. Accessed April 21, 2013b. Available at www. kidney.org/atoz/content/phosphorus.cfm

Pennington, JA, and Souglass, JA: Bowers and Churches Food Values of Portions Commonly Used, ed 18. Lippincott Williams & Wilkins, Baltimore, 2004.

Scanlon, VD, and Sanders, T: Essentials of Anatomy and Physiology, ed 5. FA Davis, Philadelphia, 2007.

Venes, D (ed): Taber's Cyclopedic Medical Dictionary, ed 21. FA Davis, Philadelphia, 2010.

U.S. Department of Agriculture: Dietary guidelines for Americans, 2010. Accessed March 2013. Available at www.usda.gov/dietaryguidelines/dga

Chapter 20

Academy of Nutrition and Dietetics: Fiber-restricted nutrition therapy. Nutrition Care Manual, Academy of Nutrition and Dietetics, Chicago, 2012a.

Academy of Nutrition and Dietetics: Gastroesophageal re-flux disease (GERD) nutrition therapy. Nutrition Care Manual, Academy of Nutrition and Dietetics, Chicago, 2012b.

Academy of Nutrition and Dietetics: Nutrition therapy for inflammatory bowel disease. Nutrition Care Manual, Chicago, 2012c.

Alame, AM, and Bahna, H: Evaluation of constipation. Clin Colon Rectal Surg 25:5, 2012. Accessed May 11, 2013. Available at www.ncbi.nlm.nih.gov/pmc/articles/ PMC3348731

Alastair, F, Emma, G, and Emma, P: Nutrition in inflamma-tory bowel disease. JPEN J Parenter Enteral Nutr 35:571, 2011.

Ambühl, PM: Protein intake in renal and hepatic disease. Int J Vitam Nutr Res 81:162, 2011.

American Society of Anesthesiologists Committee on Standards and Practice Parameters: Practice guidelines for preoperative fasting and the use of pharmacologic agents to reduce the risk of pulmonary aspiration: Application to healthy patients undergoing elective procedures. Anesthesiology 114:495, 2011. Accessed April 20, 2013. Available at http://journals.lww.com/ anesthesiology/Citation/2011/03000/Practice_ Guidelines_for_Preoperative_Fasting_and.13.aspx

Anderson, M, and Comrie, R: Adopting preoperative fasting guidelines. AORN J 90:73, 2009.

Au, DH, Kivlahan, DR, Bryson, CL, et al: Alcohol screening scores and risk of hospitalizations for GI conditions in men. Alcohol Clin Exp Res 31:443, 2007.

Bakris, GL: Postprandial hypotension. Merck Manual, May 2007. Accessed August 8, 2013. Available at www.merckmanuals.com/home/heart_and_blood_ vessel_disorders/low_blood_pressure/postprandial_ hypotension.html

Barrett, JS: Extending our knowledge of fermentable, short-chain carbohydrates for managing gastrointestinal symptoms. Nutr Clin Pract 28:300, 2013.

Barrett, JS, and Gibson, PR: Fermentable oligosaccharides, disaccharides, monosaccharides and polyols (FODMAPs) and nonallergic food intolerance: FODMAPs or food chemicals? Therap Adv Gastroenterol 5:261, 2012.

Accessed May 5, 2013. Available at www.ncbi. nlm.nih.gov/pmc/articles/PMC3388522

Bastida, G, and Beltrán, B: Ulcerative colitis in smokers, non-smokers and ex-smokers. World J Gastroenterol 17: 2740, 2011. Accessed April 23, 2013. Available at www.ncbi.nlm.nih.gov/pmc/articles/PMC3122262

Behari, A, and Kapoor, VK: Asymptomatic gallstones (AsGS)—to treat or not to? Ind J Surg 74:4, 2012. Accessed April 30, 2013. Available at www.ncbi. nlm.nih.gov/pmc/articles/PMC3259178

Beier, JI, Landes, S, Mohammad, M, and McClain, CJ: Nutrition in liver disorders and the role of alcohol. In Ross, AC, Caballero, B, Cousins, RJ, et al (eds): Modern Nutrition in Health and Disease, ed 11. Lippincott Williams & Wilkins, Philadelphia, 2014.

Bell, RC, Mavrelis, PG, Barnes, WE, et al: A prospective multicenter registry of patients with chronic gastro-esophageal reflux disease receiving transoral incisionless fundoplication. J Am Coll Surg 215:794, 2012.

Bémeur, C, Desjardins, P, and Butterworth, RF: Role of nu-trition in the management of hepatic encephalopathy in end-stage liver failure. J Nutr Metab, published online December 22, 2010. 2010:489823. Accessed May 12, 2013. Available at www.ncbi.nlm.nih.gov/pmc/articles/ PMC3017957

Bernstein, CN: New insights into IBD epidemiology: Are there any lessons for treatment? Dig Dis 28:406, 2010.

Blachier, F, Davila, AM, Mimoun, S, et al: Luminal sulfide and large intestine mucosa: Friend or foe? Amino Acids 39:335, 2010.

Boyle, MP, and Elborn, S: Modulating CFTR: Can it be clinically efficacious in cystic fibrosis? Medscape CME. November 11, 2011. Accessed April 25, 2012. Available at www.medscape.org/viewprogram/32332

Boyle, MP, and McColley, SA: Where do we go after newborn screening for cystic fibrosis? Medscape CME. November 11, 2011. Accessed April 25, 2012. Available at www.medscape.org/viewprogram/32332

Boyle, MP, and McKone, EF: Ivacaftor in CF: What do we know in 2012? Medscape CME. June 15, 2012. Ac-cessed May 11, 2013. Available at www.medscape. org/viewarticle/765699_transcript

Boyle, MP, and Singh, CM: Vitamin D and pulmonary exacerbations: A multipronged approach to CF care. Medscape CME. November 11, 2011. Accessed April 9, 2012. Available at www.medscape.org/viewprogram/ 32332

Brady, M, Kinn, S, Ness, V, et al: Preoperative fasting for preventing perioperative complications in children. Cochrane Database Syst Rev 4:CD005285, 2009.

Brady, M, Kinn, S, and Stuart, P: Preoperative fasting for adults to prevent perioperative complications. Cochrane Database Syst Rev 4:CD005285, 2003.

Braga, M: Perioperative immunonutrition and gut function. Curr Opin Clin Nutr Metab Care 15:485, 2012.

Brown, AC, Rampertab, SD, and Mullin, GE: Existing dietary guidelines for Crohn's disease and ulcerative colitis. Expert Rev Gastroenterol Hepatol 5:411, 2011.

Brown, AC, and Roy, M: Does evidence exist to include diet therapy in the treatment of Crohn's disease? Expert Rev Gastroenterol Hepatol 4:191, 2010.

Burden, S, Todd, C, Hill, J, and Lal, S: Pre-operative nutrition support in patients undergoing gastrointestinal surgery. Cochrane Database Syst Rev Nov 14;11: CD008879, 2012.

Cabada, MM, and White, AC, Jr: Travelers' diarrhea: An update on susceptibility, prevention, and treatment. Curr Gastroenterol Rep 10:473, 2008.

Cabré, E, and Domènech, E: Impact of environmental and dietary factors on the course of inflammatory bowel disease. World J Gastroenterol 18:3814, 2012. Accessed April 23, 2013. Available at www.ncbi.nlm.nih.gov/pmc/articles/PMC3413052

Calabrese, E, Yanai, H, Shuster, D, et al: Low-dose smoking resumption in ex-smokers with refractory ulcerative colitis. J Crohns Colitis 6:756, 2012.

Cameron, C, Lodes, MW, and Gershan, WM: Facial nerve palsy associated with a low serum vitamin A level in an infant with cystic fibrosis. J Cyst Fibros 6:241, 2007.

Camilleri, M, Bharucha, AE, and Farrugia, G: Epidemiology, mechanisms and management of diabetic gastroparesis. Clin Gastroenterol Hepatol 9: 5, 2011. Accessed April 14, 2013. Available at www.ncbi.nlm.nih.gov/pmc/articles/PMC3035159

Camilleri, M, Parkman, HP, Shafi, MA, et al: Clinical guideline: Management of gastroparesis. Am J Gastroenterol 108:18, 2013. Accessed August 7, 2013. Available at www.ncbi.nlm.nih.gov/pmc/articles/PMC3722580

Carbonero, F, Benefiel, AC, Alizadeh-Ghamsari, AH, and Gaskins, HR: Microbial pathways in colonic sulfur metabolism and links with health and disease. Front Physiol 3:448, 2012.

Centers for Disease Control and Prevention: Notes from the field: Deaths from acute hepatitis B virus infection associated with assisted blood glucose monitoring in an assisted-living facility—North Carolina, August–October 2010. Morb Mortal Wkly Rep 60:182, February 18, 2011. Accessed May 11, 2013. Available at www.cdc.gov/mmwr/preview/mmwrhtml/mm6006a5.htm

Centers for Disease Control and Prevention: Inflammatory Bowel Disease (IBD). Updated July 15, 2011. Accessed April 24, 2013. Available at www.cdc.gov/ibd

Centers for Disease Control and Prevention: Sexual transmission of hepatitis C virus among HIV-infected men who have sex with men—New York City, 2005–2010. Morb Mortal Wkly Rep 60:945, July 22, 2011. Accessed May 11, 2013. Available at http://www.cdc.gov/mmwr/preview/mmwrhtml/mm6028a2.htm?s_cid=mm6028a2_e&source=govdelivery

Centers for Disease Control and Prevention: Notes from the field: Transplant-transmitted hepatitis B virus—United States, 2010. Morb Mortal Wkly Rep 60:1087 August 19, 2011. Accessed March 11, 2014. Available at http://www.cdc.gov/mmwr/preview/mmwrhtml/mm6032a4.htm?s_cid=mm6032a4_e&source=govdelivery

Centers for Disease Control and Prevention: Transmission of Hepatitis C Virus Through Transplanted Organs and Tissue—Kentucky and Massachusetts, 2011. Morb Mortal Wkly Rep 60:1697, December 23, 2011. Accessed May 11, 2013. Available at www.cdc.gov/mmwr/preview/mmwrhtml/mm6050a1.htm?s_cid=mm6050a1_w

Centers for Disease Control and Prevention: Multiple outbreaks of hepatitis B virus infection related to assisted monitoring of blood glucose among residents of assisted living facilities—Virginia, 2009–2011. Morb Mortal Wkly Rep 61:339, May 18, 2012. Accessed May 11, 2013. Available at www.cdc.gov/mmwr/preview/mmwrhtml/mm6119a3.htm?s_cid=mm6119a3_e

Centers for Disease Control and Prevention: Viral hepatitis surveillance—United States, 2010. Updated June 5, 2012. Accessed April 26, 2013. Available at www.cdc.gov/hepatitis/Statistics/2010Surveillance/Commentary.htm

Cersosimo, MG, and Benarroch, EE: Pathological correlates of gastrointestinal dysfunction in Parkinson's disease. Neurobiol Dis 46:559, 2012.

Charoenkwan, K, Phillipson, G, and Vutyavanich, T: Early versus delayed (traditional) oral fluids and food for reducing complications after major abdominal gynaecologic surgery. Cochrane Database Syst Rev 4:CD004508, 2007.

Chiba, M, Abe, T, Tsuda, H, et al: Lifestyle-related disease in Crohn's disease: Relapse prevention by a semi-vegetarian diet. World J Gastroenterol 16:2484, 2010. Accessed April 24, 2013. Available at www.ncbi.nlm.nih.gov/pmc/articles/PMC2877178

Chiossi, G, Neri, I, Cavazzuti, M, et al: Hyperemesis gravidarum complicated by Wernicke encephalopathy: Background, case report, and review of the literature. Obstet Gynecol Surv 61:255, 2006.

Cho, JH, and Brant, SR: Recent insights into the genetics of inflammatory bowel disease. Gastroenterology 140:1704, 2011.

Choung, RS, Locke, GR, III, Schleck, CD, et al: Risk of gastroparesis in subjects with type 1 and 2 diabetes in the general population. Am J Gastroenterol 107:82, 2012. Accessed April 15, 2013. Available at www.ncbi.nlm.nih.gov/pmc/articles/PMC3280088

Cohen, S: Peptic ulcer disease. Merck Manual, 2007, Modified 2012. Accessed April 15, 2013. Available at www.merckmanuals.com/professional/gastrointestinal_disorders/gastritis_and_peptic_ulcer_disease/peptic_ulcer_disease.html?qt=peptic ulcer disease&alt=sh

Connor, BA: Chronic diarrhea in travelers. Curr Infect Dis Rep 15:203, 2013.

ConsumerLab: Probiotics for adults, children, and pets. Accessed March 19, 2014. Available at www.consumerlab.com/reviews/Probiotic_Supplements_Lactobacillus_acidophilus_Bifidobacterium/probiotics/

Cooper, A, Mones, RL, and Heird, WC: Nutritional management of infants and children with specific diseases and other conditions. In Ross, AC, Caballero, B, Cousins, RJ, et al (eds): Modern Nutrition in Health and Disease, ed 11. Lippincott Williams & Wilkins, Philadelphia, 2014.

Craft, L, and Prahlow, JA: From fecal impaction to colon perforation. Am J Nurs 111:38, 2011.

Crenshaw, JT: Preoperative fasting: Will the evidence ever be put into practice? Am J Nurs 111:10, 38, 2011.

Cunningham, E: Are low-residue diets still applicable? J Acad Nutr Diet 112:960, 2012.

Cystic Fibrosis Foundation: About cystic fibrosis. Undated. Accessed May 2, 2013. Available at www.cff.org/AboutCF

Czinn, SJ, and Blanchard, S: Gastroesophageal reflux disease in neonates and infants: When and how to treat. Paediatr Drugs 15:19, 2013.

Dasenbrook, EC, Checkley, W, Merlo, CA, et al: Association between respiratory tract methicillin-resistant Staphylococcus aureus and survival in cystic fibrosis. JAMA 303:2386, 2010.

de Aguilar-Nascimento, JE, and Dock-Nascimento, DB: Reducing preoperative fasting time: A trend based on evidence. World J Gastrointest Surg 2: 57, 2010. Accessed April 22, 2013. Available at www.ncbi.nlm.nih.gov/pmc/articles/PMC2999216

de la Cabada Bauche, J, and DuPont, HL: New developments in traveler's diarrhea. Gastroenterol Hepatol (NY) 7:88, 2011. Accessed April 19, 2013. Available at www.ncbi.nlm.nih.gov/pmc/articles/PMC3061023

Delegge, MH: Esophagus and stomach. In Ross, AC, Caballero, B, Cousins, RJ, et al (eds): Modern Nutrition in Health and Disease, ed 11. Lippincott Williams & Wilkins, Philadelphia, 2014.

Douglas, LC, and Sanders, ME: Probiotics and prebiotics in dietetics practice. J Am Diet Assoc 108:510, 2008.

Drago, L, Rodighiero, V, and Celeste, T, et al: Microbiological evaluation of commercial probiotic products available in the USA in 2009. J Chemother 22:373, 2010.

Dryden, GW, and Seidner, DL: Nutrition in inflammatory bowel disease: Implications for its role in the management of Crohn disease and ulcerative colitis. In Ross, AC, Caballero, B, Cousins, RJ, et al (eds): Modern Nutrition in Health and Disease, ed 11. Lippincott Williams & Wilkins, Philadelphia, 2014.

Dugdale, DC, III: Low-residue fiber diet. Updated November 12, 2011. Accessed April 11, 2013. Available at www.nlm.nih.gov/medlineplus/ency/patientinstructions/000200.htm

Engfer, EM, Green, CJ, and Silk, DB: Systematic review and meta-analysis: The clinical and physiological effects of fibre-containing enteral formulae. Aliment Pharmacol Ther 27:120, 2008. Accessed April 20, 2013. Available at onlinelibrary.wiley.com/doi/10.1111/j.1365-2036.2007.03544.x/full

Etzioni, DA, Mack, TM, Beart, RW Jr, and Kaiser, AM: Diverticulitis in the United States: 1998–2005: Changing patterns of disease and treatment. Ann Surg 249:210, 2009.

Ezri, J, Marques-Vidal, P, and Nydegger, A: Impact of disease and treatments on growth and puberty of pediatric patients with inflammatory bowel disease. Digestion 85:308, 2012. Accessed April 24, 2013. Available at www.karger.com/Article/FullText/336766#SC8

Fujiwara, Y, Arakawa, T, and Fass, R: Gastroesophageal reflux disease and sleep disturbances. J Gastroenterol 47:760, 2012.

Feinstein, LB, Holman, RC, Yorita Christensen, KL, et al: Trends in hospitalizations for peptic ulcer disease, United States, 1998–2005. Emerg Infect Dis 16: 1410, 2010. Accessed April 15, 2013. Available at www.ncbi.nlm.nih.gov/pmc/articles/PMC3294961

Festi, D, Scaioli, E, Baldi, F, et al: Body weight, lifestyle, dietary habits and gastroesophageal reflux disease. World J Gastroenterol 15:1690, 2009. Accessed May 8, 2013.

Available at www.ncbi.nlm.nih.gov/pmc/articles/PMC2668774/#B142

Ford, AC, Chey, WD, Talley, NJ, et al: Yield of diagnostic tests for celiac disease in individuals with symptoms suggestive of irritable bowel syndrome: Systematic review and meta-analysis. Arch Intern Med 169:651, 2009.

Freedman, SD: Chronic pancreatitis. Merck Manual. November 2012. Accessed May 1, 2013. Available at www.merckmanuals.com/professional/gastrointestinal_disorders/pancreatitis/chronic_pancreatitis.html?qt=chronic pancreatitis&alt=sh

Friedman, G: The role of probiotics in the prevention and treatment of antibiotic-associated diarrhea and Clostridium difficile colitis. Gastroenterol Clin North Am 41:763, 2012.

Ghoshal, UC, Daschakraborty, SB, and Singh, R: Pathogenesis of achalasia cardia. World J Gastroenterol 18: 3050, 2012. Accessed April 12, 2013. Available at www.ncbi.nlm.nih.gov/pmc/articles/PMC3386318

Gibson, PR, and Shepherd, SJ: Evidence-based dietary management of functional gastrointestinal symptoms: The FODMAP approach. J Gastroenterol Hepatol 25:252, 2010.

Green, PH, and Jabri, B: Celiac disease. Annu Rev Med 57:207, 2006.

Griffiths, AM: Growth retardation in early-onset inflammatory bowel disease: should we monitor and treat these patients differently? Dig Dis 27:404, 2009.

Guimarães, EV, Schettino, GC, Camargos, PA, and Penna, FJ: Prevalence of hyponatremia at diagnosis and factors associated with the longitudinal variation in serum sodium levels in infants with cystic fibrosis. J Pediatr 161:285, 2012.

Hajar, N, Castell, DO, Ghomrawi, H, et al: Impedance pH confirms the relationship between GERD and BMI. Dig Dis Sci 57:1875, 2012.

Halme, L, Paavola-Sakki, P, Turunen, U, et al: Family and twin studies in inflammatory bowel disease. World J Gastroenterol 12:3668, 2006. Accessed April 23, 2013. Available at www.wjgnet.com/1007-9327/full/v12/i23/3668.htm

Hamid, B, and Khan, A: Cerebral hemorrhage as the initial manifestation of cystic fibrosis. J Child Neurol 22:114, 2007.

Harris, LA: Diagnosing irritable bowel syndrome: challenges in primary care. Medscape CME. March 30, 2012. Accessed April 6, 2012. Available at www.medscape.org/viewarticle/760639

Eating can cause low blood pressure. Harvard Health Letter, July 2010. Accessed April 18, 2013. Available at www.health.harvard.edu/newsletters/Harvard_Heart_Letter/2010/July/eating-can-cause-low-blood-pressure

Hempel, S, Newberry, S, Ruelaz, A, et al: Safety of Probiotics to Reduce Risk and Prevent or Treat Disease, Evidence Report/Technology Assessment Number 200 (Pub. No. 11-E007). Agency for Healthcare Research and Quality, Rockville, MD, April 2011.

Heuschkel, R, Salvestrini, C, Beattie, RM, et al: Guidelines for the management of growth failure in childhood inflammatory bowel disease. Inflamm Bowel Dis 14:839, 2008.

Heymann, DL (ed): Control of Communicable Diseases Manual, ed 19. American Public Health Association, Washington, DC, 2008.

Hill, DR, and Beeching, NJ: Travelers' diarrhea. Curr Opin Infect Dis 23:481, 2010.

Hinson, JA, Roberts, DW, and James, LP: Mechanisms of acetaminophen-induced liver necrosis. Handb Exp Pharmacol 196:369, 2010. Accessed April 26, 2013. Available at www.ncbi.nlm.nih.gov/pmc/articles/PMC2836803

Jantchou, P, Morois, S, Clavel-Chapelon, F, et al: Animal protein intake and risk of inflammatory bowel disease: The E3N prospective study. Am J Gastroenterol 105:2195, 2010.

Jeejeebhoy, KN: Short bowel syndrome. In Ross, AC, Caballero, B, Cousins, RJ, et al (eds): Modern Nutrition in Health and Disease, ed 11. Lippincott Williams & Wilkins, Philadelphia, 2014.

Johnston, BC, Goldenberg, JZ, Vandvik, PO, et al: Probiotics for the prevention of pediatric antibiotic-associated diarrhea. Cochrane Database Syst Rev 2011 Nov 9(11): CD004827.

Johnston, BC, Ma, SS, Goldenberg, JZ, et al: Probiotics for the prevention of Clostridium difficile–associated diarrhea: A systematic review and meta-analysis. Ann Intern Med 157:878, 2012.

Jones, C, Badger, SA, and Hannon, R: The role of carbohydrate drinks in preoperative nutrition for elective colorectal surgery. Ann R Coll Surg Engl 93:504, 2011. Accessed April 22, 2013. Available at www.ncbi.nlm.nih.gov/pmc/articles/PMC3604918

Jones, DT, Osterman, MT, Bewtra, M, and Lewis, JD: Passive smoking and inflammatory bowel disease: A meta-analysis. Am J Gastroenterol 103:2382, 2008. Accessed April 24, 2013. Available at www.ncbi.nlm.nih.gov/pmc/articles/PMC2714986

Jowett, SL, Seal, CJ, Pearce, MS, et al: Influence of dietary factors on the clinical course of ulcerative colitis: A prospective cohort study. Gut 53:1479, 2004. Accessed April 24, 2013. Available at www.ncbi.nlm.nih.gov/pmc/articles/PMC1774231

Jussila, A, Virta, LJ, Salomaa, V, et al: High and increasing prevalence of inflammatory bowel disease in Finland with a clear North–South difference. J Crohns Colitis 7:e256, 2013

Kale-Pradhan, PB, Jassal, HK, and Wilhelm, SM: Role of Lactobacillus in the prevention of antibiotic-associated diarrhea: A meta-analysis. Pharmacotherapy 30:119, 2010.

Kalnins, D, and Wilschanski, M: Maintenance of nutritional status in patients with cystic fibrosis: new and emerging therapies. Drug Des Devel Ther 6:151, 2012. Accessed May 2, 2013. Available at www.ncbi.nlm.nih.gov/pmc/articles/PMC3392141/#b75-dddt-6-151

Keld, R, Kinsey, L, Athwal, V, and Lal, S: Pathogenesis, investigation and dietary and medical management of gastroparesis. J Hum Nutr Diet 24:421, 2011.

Khalili, H, Huang, ES, Ananthakrishnan, AN, et al: Geographical variation and incidence of inflammatory bowel disease among US women. Gut 61:1686, 2012.

Khor, B, Gardet, A, and Xavier, RJ: Genetics and pathogenesis of inflammatory bowel disease. Nature 474:307, 2011. Accessed April 22, 2013. Available at www.ncbi.nlm.nih.gov/pmc/articles/PMC3204665

Kim, KE: Strategies for identifying and screening patients at risk for HBV infection. Medscape Continuing Education. October 13, 2011. Accessed April 27, 2012. Available at www.medscape.org/viewprogram/32175

Kollaritsch, H, Paulke-Korinek, M, and Wiedermann, U: Traveler's diarrhea. Infect Dis Clin North Am 26:691, 2012.

Krawczyk, M, Wang, DQ, Portincasa, P, and Lammert, F: Dissecting the genetic heterogeneity of gallbladder stone formation. Semin Liver Dis 31:157, 2011.

Kudsk, KA: Nutrition support for the patient with surgery, trauma, or sepsis. In Ross, AC, Caballero, B, Cousins, RJ, et al (eds): Modern Nutrition in Health and Disease, ed 11. Lippincott Williams & Wilkins, Philadelphia, 2014.

Latella, G, Fiocchi, C, and Caprili, R: News from the 5th International Meeting on Inflammatory Bowel Diseases, CAPRI 2010. J Crohns Colitis 4:690, 2010.

Lawrence, R: How to treat dehydration caused by vomiting or diarrhea. Alaska Family Doctor, January 24, 2011. Accessed October 21, 2013. Available at http://alaskafamilydoctor.tumblr.com/post/2921401281/how-to-treat-dehydration-caused-by-vomiting-or-diarrhea

Lembke, A, Bradley, KA, Henderson, P, et al: Alcohol screening scores and the risk of new-onset gastrointestinal illness or related hospitalization. J Gen Intern Med 26: 777, 2011. Accessed April 28, 2013. Available at www.ncbi.nlm.nih.gov/pmc/articles/PMC3138581

Leung, AA, McAlister, FA, Rogers, SO Jr, et al: Preoperative hyponatremia and perioperative complications. Arch Intern Med 172:1474, 2012.

Levison, ME: Aminoglycosides. Merck Manual. February 2012. Accessed April 23, 2013. Available at www.merckmanuals.com/professional/infectious_diseases/bacteria_and_antibacterial_drugs/aminoglycosides.html?qt=aminoglycosides&alt=sh#Indications

Lionetti, E, Francavilla, R, Castellazzi, AM, et al: Probiotics and Helicobacter pylori infection in children. J Biol Regul Homeost Agents 26(Suppl 1):S69, 2012.

Liu, Ye, Gong, YH, Sun, LP, et al: The relationship between H. pylori virulence genotypes and gastric diseases. Pol J Microbiol 61:147, 2012. Accessed April 15, 2013. Available at www.ncbi.nlm.nih.gov/pubmed/23163215

London, WT: Increasing awareness and decreasing the burden of HBV-related disease. Medscape Continuing Education. October 13, 2011. Accessed April 9, 2012. Available at www.medscape.org/viewprogram/32175

Luciano, GL, Brennan, MJ, and Rothberg, MB: Postprandial hypotension. Am J Med 123:281.e1, 2010.

Magee, EA, Edmond, LM, Tasker, SM, et al: Associations between diet and disease activity in ulcerative colitis patients using a novel method of data analysis. Nutr J 4:7, 2005. Accessed April 24, 2013. Available at www.ncbi.nlm.nih.gov/pmc/articles/PMC549081/#S5

Manolakis, AC, Kapsoritakis, AN, Kapsoritaki, A, et al: Readressing the role of Toll-like receptor-4 alleles in inflammatory bowel disease: Colitis, smoking, and seroreactivity. Dig Dis Sci 58:371, 2013.

Marcason, W: What is the FODMAP diet? J Acad Nutr Diet 112:1696, 2012.

Markland, AD, Palsson, O, Goode, PS, et al: Association of low dietary intake of fiber and liquids with constipation: Evidence from the National Health and Nutrition Examination Survey. Am J Gastroenterol 108:796, 2013.

Mayo Foundation for Medical Education and Research: Low-fiber (low-residue) diet. August 13, 2011. Accessed April 11, 2013. Available at www.mayoclinic.com/health/low-fiber-diet/my00744

McCabe, H: Riboflavin deficiency in cystic fibrosis: Three case reports. J Hum Nutr Diet 14:365, 2001.

McCabe, MA, Toughill, EH, Parkhill, AM, et al: Celiac disease: A medical puzzle. Am J Nurs 112:34, 2012.

McGowan, KE, Castiglione, DA, and Butzner, JD: The changing face of childhood celiac disease in North America: Impact of serological testing. Pediatrics 124:1572, 2009. Accessed April 20, 2013. Available at http://pediatrics.aappublications.org/content/124/6/1572.long

Medani, M, Collins, D, Docherty, NG, et al: Emerging role of hydrogen sulfide in colonic physiology and pathophysiology. Inflamm Bowel Dis 17:1620, 2011.

Muls, V, Eckardt, AJ, Marchese, M, et al: Three-year results of a multicenter prospective study of transoral incisionless fundoplication. Surg Innov 20:321, 2013.

National Digestive Diseases Information Clearinghouse: Celiac disease. National Institute of Diabetes and Digestive and Kidney Diseases, January 27, 2012. Accessed April 20, 2013. Available at http://digestive.niddk.nih.gov/ddiseases/pubs/celiac/index.aspx

National Digestive Diseases Information Clearinghouse: Crohn's disease. National Institute of Diabetes and Digestive and Kidney Diseases. Updated January 18, 2013. Accessed November 6, 2008. Available at http://digestive.niddk.nih.gov/ddiseases/pubs/crohns

National Digestive Diseases Information Clearinghouse: Heartburn, gastroesophageal reflux (GER), and gastroesophageal reflux disease (GERD). National Institute of Diabetes and Digestive and Kidney Diseases. Updated April 30, 2012. Accessed May 8, 2013. Available at http://digestive.niddk.nih.gov/ddiseases/pubs/gerd/#3

National Digestive Diseases Information Clearinghouse: Irritable bowel syndrome. National Institute of Diabetes and Digestive and Kidney Diseases, July 2, 2012. Accessed April 19, 2013. Available at http://digestive.niddk.nih.gov/ddiseases/pubs/ibs

National Digestive Diseases Information Clearinghouse: Ulcerative colitis. National Institute of Diabetes and Digestive and Kidney Diseases. Updated November 15, 2011. Accessed May 4, 2013. Available at http://digestive.niddk.nih.gov/ddiseases/pubs/colitis/#cancer

Nespoli, L, Coppola, S, and Gianotti, L: The role of the enteral route and the composition of feeds in the nutritional support of malnourished surgical patients. Nutrients 4:1230, 2012. Accessed April 4, 2013. Available at www.ncbi.nlm.nih.gov/pmc/articles/PMC3475233

Ness-Jensen, E, Lindam, A, Lagergren, J, and Hveem, K: Weight loss and reduction in gastroesophageal reflux. A prospective population-based cohort study: The HUNT study. Am J Gastroenterol 108:376, 2013.

Ngo, B, Van Pelt, K, Labarque, V, et al: Late vitamin K deficiency bleeding leading to a diagnosis of cystic fibrosis: A case report. Acta Clinica Belgica 66:142, 2011.

NIDDK Gastroparesis Clinical Research Consortium: Dietary intake and nutritional deficiencies in patients with diabetic or idiopathic gastroparesis. Gastroenterology 141:486, 2011. Accessed April 15, 2013. Available at www.ncbi.nlm.nih.gov/pmc/articles/PMC3499101

Nitsche, C, Simon, P, Weiss, FU, et al: Environmental risk factors for chronic pancreatitis and pancreatic cancer. Dig Dis 29:235, 2011.

Nurse Courtney: Oral rehydration solution recipe. March 12, 2012. Accessed October 20, 2013. Available at www.nursecourtney.com/2012/03/12/homemade-pedialyte

O'Brien, CP: The CAGE questionnaire for detection of alcoholism. JAMA 300:2054, 2008.

Ogershok, PR, Rahman, A, Nestor, S, and Brick, J: Wernicke encephalopathy in nonalcoholic patients. Am J Med Sci 323:107, 2002.

Ohge, H, Furne, JK, Springfield, J, et al: Association between fecal hydrogen sulfide production and pouchitis. Dis Colon Rectum 48:469, 2005.

Ong, DK, Mitchell, SB, Barrett, JS, et al: Manipulation of dietary short chain carbohydrates alters the pattern of gas production and genesis of symptoms in irritable bowel syndrome. J Gastroenterol Hepatol 25:1366, 2010.

Overmier, JB, and Murison, B: Restoring Psychology's Role in Peptic Ulcer. Appl Psychol Health Well Being 5:5, 2013. Accessed April 15, 2013. Available at www.ncbi.nlm.nih.gov/pmc/articles/PMC3613748

Paredes-Paredes, M, Flores-Figueroa, J, and Dupont, HL: Advances in the treatment of travelers' diarrhea. Curr Gastroenterol Rep 13:402, 2011.

Parkman, HP, Yates, KP, and Hasler, WL: Dietary intake and nutritional deficiencies in patients with diabetic or idiopathic gastroparesis. Gastroenterology 141:486, 2011.

Patel, MR, Eppolito, AL, and Willingham, FF: Hereditary pancreatitis for the endoscopist. Therap Adv Gastroenterol 6: 169, 2013. Accessed May 1, 2013. Available at www.ncbi.nlm.nih.gov/pmc/articles/PMC3589131

Patel, NM, and Johnson, MM: Nutrition in respiratory diseases. In Ross, AC, Caballero, B, Cousins, RJ, et al (eds): Modern Nutrition in Health and Disease, ed 11. Lippincott Williams & Wilkins, Philadelphia, 2014.

Popkin, BM, D'Anci, KE, and Rosenberg, IH: Water, hydration, and health. Nutr Rev 68:439, 2010.

Raina, A, and O'Keefe, JD: Nutrition in pancreatic diseases. In Ross, AC, Caballero, B, Cousins, RJ, et al (eds): Modern Nutrition in Health and Disease, ed 11. Lippincott Williams & Wilkins, Philadelphia, 2014.

Ramsey, BW, Davies, J, McElvaney, G, et al: A CFTR potentiator in patients with cystic fibrosis and the G551D mutation. N Engl J Med 365:1163, 2011.

Rayner, CK, and Horowitz, M: Physiology of the ageing gut. Curr Opin Clin Nutr Metab Care 16:33, 2013.

Richter, J, Balfe, LM, and Greene, L: Updates on the comparative effectiveness of management strategies for adults with gastroesophageal reflux disease. Agency for Healthcare Research and Quality: Prime Education CME/CE, October 31, 2011.

Ritchie, ML, and Romanuk, TN: A meta-analysis of probiotic efficacy for gastrointestinal diseases. PLoS One 7:e34938, 2012. Accessed April 16, 2013. Available at www.ncbi.nlm.nih.gov/pmc/articles/PMC3329544

Roncone, DP: Xerophthalmia secondary to alcohol-induced malnutrition. Optometry 77:124, 2006.

Ros, E: Health benefits of nut consumption. Nutrients 2:652, 2010. Accessed April 30, 2013. Available at www.ncbi.nlm.nih.gov/pmc/articles/PMC3257681

Rosenstein, BJ: Cystic fibrosis. Merck Manual. 2012. Accessed May 4, 2013. Available at www.merckmanuals.com/professional/pediatrics/cystic_fibrosis_cf/cystic_fibrosis.html?qt=cystic fibrosis&alt=sh#Diagnosis

Rowan, FE, Docherty, NG, Coffey, JC, and O'Connell, PR: Sulphate-reducing bacteria and hydrogen sulphide in the aetiology of ulcerative colitis. Br J Surg 96:151, 2009.

Rubio-Tapia, A, Ludvigsson, JF, Brantner, TL et al: The prevalence of celiac disease in the United States. Am J Gastroenterol 107:1538, 2012.

Ruiz, AT: Short bowel syndrome. Merck Manual. August 2012. Accessed April 25, 2013. Available at www.merckmanuals.com/professional/gastrointestinal_disorders/malabsorption_syndromes/short_bowel_syndrome.html?qt=short bowel syndrome&alt=sh

RxList: Gallstones, 2013. Accessed May 1, 2013. Available at www.rxlist.com/gallstones/page9.htm

Sanyal, AJ, Mullen, KD, and Bass, NM: The treatment of hepatic encephalopathy in the cirrhotic patient. Gastroenterol Hepatol (NY) 6(4 Suppl 8): 1, 2010. Accessed April 29, 2013. Available at www.ncbi.nlm.nih.gov/pmc/articles/PMC2886485

Schwartz, L, and Semrad, CE: Irritable bowel syndrome and diverticular disease. In Ross, AC, Caballero, B, Cousins, RJ, et al (eds): Modern Nutrition in Health and Disease, ed 11. Lippincott Williams & Wilkins, Philadelphia, 2014.

Schwartz, SM: Pediatric gastroesophageal reflux. Medscape Essential Updates in Gastroenterology, May 8. 2013. Accessed May 8, 2013. Available at http://emedicine.medscape.com/article/930029-overview?src=wnl_ref_prac_gast&uac=30801BJ

Semrad, CE: Celiac disease. In Ross, AC, Caballero, B, Cousins, RJ, et al (eds): Modern Nutrition in Health and Disease, ed 11. Lippincott Williams & Wilkins, Philadelphia, 2014.

Setty, M, Hormaza, L, and Guandalini, S: Celiac disease: Risk assessment, diagnosis, and monitoring. Mol Diagn Ther 12:289, 2008.

Shield, KD, Gmel, G, Kehoe-Chan, T, et al: Mortality and potential years of life lost attributable to alcohol consumption by race and sex in the United States in 2005. PLoS One. 2013; 8: e51923. Accessed April 27, 2013. Available at www.ncbi.nlm.nih.gov/pmc/articles/PMC3534703

Smith, MM: Emergency: Variceal hemorrhage from esophageal varices associated with alcoholic liver disease. Am J Nurs 110:32, 2010.

Snydman, DR: The safety of probiotics. Clin Infect Dis 46(Suppl 2): S104, 2008. Accessed April 15, 2013.

Available at http://cid.oxfordjournals.org/content/46/Supplement_2/S104.long

Stickel, F, Buch, S, Lau, K, et al: Genetic variation in the PNPLA3 gene is associated with alcoholic liver injury in Caucasians. Hepatology 53:86, 2011.

Stickel, F, and Hampe, J: Genetic determinants of alcoholic liver disease. Gut 61:150, 2012.

Stinton, LM, and Shaffer, EA: Epidemiology of gallbladder disease: Cholelithiasis and cancer. Gut Liver 6: 172, 2012. Accessed April 30, 2013. Available at www.ncbi.nlm.nih.gov/pmc/articles/PMC3343155

Stokes, CS, Krawczyk, M, and Lammert, F: Gallstones: Environment, lifestyle and genes. Dig Dis 29:191, 2011.

Stover, PJ, and Gu, Z: Genetic variation: Effect on nutrient utilization and metabolism. In Ross, AC, Caballero, B, Cousins, RJ, et al (eds): Modern Nutrition in Health and Disease, ed 11. Lippincott Williams & Wilkins, Philadelphia, 2014.

Strate, LL: Lifestyle factors and the course of diverticular disease. Dig Dis 30:35, 2012.

Strate, LL, Erichsen, R, Baron, JA, et al: Heritability and familial aggregation of diverticular disease: A population-based study of twins and siblings. Gastroenterology 144:736, 2013.

Subrahmanyam, M, and Venugopal, M: Perioperative fasting: A time to relook. Indian J Anaesth. 2010 Sep–Oct; 54: 374, 2010. Accessed April 5, 2013. Available at www.ncbi.nlm.nih.gov/pmc/articles/PMC2991644

Sultan, M, Werlin, S, and Venkatasubramani, N: Genetic prevalence and characteristics in children with recurrent pancreatitis. J Pediatr Gastroenterol Nutr 54:645, 2012.

Tejero, S, Rowland, IR, Rastal, R, and Gibson, GR: Probiotics and prebiotics as modulators of the gut microbiota. In Ross, AC, Caballero, B, Cousins, RJ, et al (eds): Modern Nutrition in Health and Disease, ed 11. Lippincott Williams & Wilkins, Philadelphia, 2014.

Tekeuchi, Y, Kobayashi, G, Matui, Y, et al: Outbreak of food–borne infection with hepatitis A virus. Jpn J Infect Dis 59:346, 2006.

Thomas, DW, Greer, FR, American Academy of Pediatrics Committee on Nutrition, and American Academy of Pediatrics Section on Gastroenterology, Hepatology, and Nutrition: Probiotics and prebiotics in pediatrics. Pediatrics 126:1217, 2010. Accessed April 16, 2013. Available at pediatrics.aappublications.org/content/126/6/1217.long

Thomas, JR, Nanda, R, and Shu, LH: A FODMAP diet update: Craze or credible? Prac Gastroenterol December: 37, 2012.

Thomson, AD, Guerrini, I, and Marshall, EJ: The evolution and treatment of Korsakoff's syndrome: Out of sight, out of mind? Neuropsychol Rev 22:81, 2012. Accessed April 27, 2013. Available at www.ncbi.nlm.nih.gov/pmc/articles/PMC3545191

Tilg, H, and Kaser, A: Diet and relapsing ulcerative colitis: Take off the meat? Gut 53:1399, 2004. Accessed April 24, 2013. Available at www.ncbi.nlm.nih.gov/pmc/articles/PMC1774255

Toneva, GD, Dierhoi, RJ, Morris, M, et al: Oral antibiotic bowel preparation reduces length of stay and readmissions after colorectal surgery. J Am Coll Surg 216:756, 2013.

Trad, KS, Turgeon, DG, and Deljkich, E: Long-term outcomes after transoral incisionless fundoplication in patients with GERD and LPR symptoms. Surg Endosc 26:650, 2012. Accessed May 10, 2013. Available at www.ncbi.nlm.nih.gov/pmc/articles/PMC3271216

Triggs, CM, Munday, K, Hu, R, et al: Dietary factors in chronic inflammation: Food tolerances and intolerances of a New Zealand Caucasian Crohn's disease population. Mutat Res 690:123, 2010.

U.S. Food and Drug Administration: FDA defines "gluten-free" for food labeling. August 2, 2013. Accessed August 6, 2013. Available at www.fda.gov/NewsEvents/Newsroom/PressAnnouncements/ucm363474.htm

Vallerand, AH, Sanoski, CA and Deslin, JH: Davis's Drug Guide for Nurses, ed 13. FA Davis, Philadelphia, 2013.

VandenBranden, S: A nurse's perspective on advances in care for cystic fibrosis. Medscape Continuing Education. July 15, 2011. Accessed April 8, 2012. Available at www.medscape.org/viewprogram/32086

Vandenplas, Y, Salvatore, S, Vieira, M, et al: Probiotics in infectious diarrhoea in children: Are they indicated? Eur J Pediatr 166:1211, 2007.

Vandenplas, Y, Veereman-Wauters, G, De Greef, E, et al: Probiotics and prebiotics in prevention and treatment of diseases in infants and children. J Pediatr (Rio J) 87:292, 2011.

Videlock, EJ, and Cremonini, F: Meta-analysis: Probiotics in antibiotic-associated diarrhoea. Aliment Pharmacol Ther. 2012 Jun;35(12):1355, 2012.

Weizman, AV, and Nguyen, G: Diverticular disease: Epidemiology and management. Can J Gastroenterol 25:385, 2011. Accessed April 26, 2013. Available at www.ncbi.nlm.nih.gov/pmc/articles/PMC3174080

Wheble, GA, Knight, WR, and Khan, OA: Enteral vs total parenteral nutrition following major upper gastrointestinal surgery. Int J Surg 10:194, 2012.

Wheeler, C, Vogt, TM, Armstrong, GL, et al: An outbreak of hepatitis A associated with green onions. N Engl J Med 353:890, 2005.

Wilkins, T, Khan, N, Nabh, A, and Schade, RR: Diagnosis and management of upper gastrointestinal bleeding. Am Fam Physician 85:469, 2012. Accessed April 15, 2013. Available at www.aafp.org/afp/2012/0301/p469.html#afp20120301p469-b7

Williams, LS, and Hopper, PD: Understanding Medical Surgical Nursing, ed 4. FA Davis, Philadelphia, 2011.

Williams, NT: Probiotics. Am J Health Syst Pharm 67:449, 2010.

Wilson, K, Mudra, M, Furne, J, and Levitt, M: Differentiation of the roles of sulfide oxidase and rhodanese in the detoxification of sulfide by the colonic mucosa. Dig Dis Sci 53:277, 2008.

Witteman, BPL, Strijkers, R, de Vries, E, et al: Transoral incisionless fundoplication for treatment of gastroesophageal reflux disease in clinical practice. Surg Endosc 26:3307, 2012. Accessed May 10, 2013. Available at www.ncbi.nlm.nih.gov/pmc/articles/PMC3472060

Wolvers, D, Antoine, JM, Myllyluoma, E, et al: Guidance for substantiating the evidence for beneficial effects of probiotics: Prevention and management of infections by probiotics. J Nutr 140:698S, 2010. Accessed May 12, 2013. Available at http://jn.nutrition.org/content/140/3/698S.long

World Gastroenterology Organization: Acute diarrhea in adults and children: A global perspective, February 2012. Accessed April 19, 2013. Available at www.worldgastroenterology.org/acute-diarrhea-in-adults.html

Yan, F, and Polk, DB: Probiotics: Progress toward novel therapies for intestinal diseases. Curr Opin Gastroenterol 26:95, 2010. Accessed April 16, 2013. Available at www.ncbi.nlm.nih.gov/pmc/articles/PMC3036989/#R53

Yang, YJ, and Sheu, BS: Probiotics-containing yogurts suppress Helicobacter pylori load and modify immune response and intestinal microbiota in the Helicobacter pylori-infected children. Helicobacter 17:297, 2012.

Yi, F, Ge, L, Zhao, J, et al: Meta-analysis: Total parenteral nutrition versus total enteral nutrition in predicted severe acute pancreatitis. Intern Med 51:523, 2012. Accessed May 1, 2013. Available at www.jstage.jst.go.jp/article/internalmedicine/51/6/51_6_523/_article

Chapter 21

Albert-Puleo, M: Physiological effects of cabbage with reference to its potential as a dietary cancer-inhibitor and its use in ancient medicine. J Ethnopharmacol 9:261, 1983.

Alpha-tocopherol, Beta-carotene Cancer Prevention Study Group: Effect of vitamin E and beta-carotene on the incidence of lung cancer and other cancers in male smokers. N Engl J Med 330:1029, 1994.

American Cancer Society: Cancer facts and figures, 2013. Accessed May 20, 2013. Available at www.cancer.org/research/cancerfactsstatistics/cancerfactsfigures2013/index

American Cancer Society: Guidelines on nutrition and physical activity for cancer prevention. Revised August 20, 2012. Accessed March 2, 2014. Available at www.cancer.org/acs/groups/cid/documents/webcontent/002577-pdf.pdf

American Institute for Cancer Research: Cancer experts issue "5-steps" warning on grill safety. May 6, 2013. Accessed May 22, 2013. Available at www.aicr.org/press/press-releases/5-steps-warning-grilling-safety.html

American Institute for Cancer Research: Soy is safe for breast cancer survivors. Cancer Research Update, November 21, 2012. Accessed June 2, 2013. Available at www.aicr.org/cancer-research-update/2012/november_21_2012/cru-soy-safe.html

August, DA, and Huhmann, M: Nutritional support of the patient with cancer. In Ross, AC, Caballero, B, Cousins, RJ, et al (eds): Modern Nutrition in Health and Disease, ed 11. Lippincott Williams & Wilkins, Philadelphia, 2014.

Barbir, A, Linseisen, J, Hermann, S, et al: Effects of phenotypes in heterocyclic aromatic amine (HCA) metabolism-related genes on the association of HCA intake with the risk of colorectal adenomas. Cancer Causes Control 23:1429, 2012.

Bian, Q, Gao, S, Zhou, J, et al: Lutein and zeaxanthin supplementation reduces photooxidative damage and modulates the expression of inflammation-related genes in retinal pigment epithelial cells. Free Radic Biol Med 53:1298, 2012.

Burstein, HJ, and Schwartz, RS: Molecular origins of cancer. N Engl J Med 358:527, 2008. Accessed June 1, 2013. Available at www.nejm.org/doi/full/10.1056/NEJMe0800065

Campbell, PT, Patel, AV, Newton, CC, et al: Associations of recreational physical activity and leisure time spent sitting with colorectal cancer survival. J Clin Oncol 31:876, 2013.

Chang, ET, and Adami, HO: The enigmatic epidemiology of nasopharyngeal carcinoma. Cancer Epidemiol Biomarkers Prev 15:1765, 2006.

Chiou, HL, Wu, MF, Chien, WP, et al: NAT2 fast acetylator genotype is associated with an increased risk of lung cancer among never-smoking women in Taiwan. Cancer Lett 223:93, 2005.

Cramp, F, and Byron-Daniel, J: Exercise for the management of cancer-related fatigue in adults. Cochrane Database Syst Rev 11:CD006145, November 14, 2012.

Cuyun Carter, GB, Katz, ML, Ferketich, AK, et al: Dietary intake, food processing, and cooking methods among Amish and non-Amish adults living in Ohio Appalachia: Relevance to nutritional risk factors for cancer. Nutr Cancer 63:1208, 2011. Accessed March 2, 2014. Available at www.ncbi.nlm.nih.gov/pmc/articles/PMC3800012/

Da Costa, LA, Badawi, A, and El-Sohemy, A: Nutrigenetics and modulation of oxidative stress. Ann Nutr Metab 60 Suppl 3:27, 2012.

Da Silva, TD, Felipe, AV, de Lima, JM, et al: N-Acetyltransferase 2 genetic polymorphisms and risk of colorectal cancer. World J Gastroenterol 17:760, 2011. Accessed May 21, 2013. Available at www.ncbi.nlm.nih.gov/pmc/articles/PMC3042654

D'Elia, L, Rossi, G, Ippolito, R, et al: Habitual salt intake and risk of gastric cancer: A meta-analysis of prospective studies. Clin Nutr 31:489, 2012.

De Stefani, E, Boffetta, P, Ronco, AL, et al: Processed meat consumption and risk of cancer: A multisite case–control study in Uruguay. Br J Cancer 107:1584, 2012. Accessed March 2, 2014. Available at www.nature.com/bjc/journal/v107/n9/full/bjc2012433a.html

Eggert, J: The biology of cancer: What do oncology nurses really need to know. Semin Oncol Nurs 27:3, 2011.

Erinosho, TO, Moser, RP, Oh, AY, et al: Awareness of the fruits and veggies—more matters campaign, knowledge of the fruit and vegetable recommendation, and fruit and vegetable intake of adults in the 2007 Food Attitudes and Behaviors (FAB) Survey. Appetite 59:155, 2012.

Evans, WJ: Skeletal muscle loss: Cachexia, sarcopenia, and inactivity. Am J Clin Nutr 91:1123S, 2010. Accessed June 2, 2013. Available at http://ajcn.nutrition.org/content/91/4/1123S.long

Fox, N, and Freifeld, AG: The neutropenic diet reviewed: Moving toward a safe food handling approach. Oncology (Williston Park) 26:572, 2012.

Fulop, T, Larbi, A, Kotb, R, et al: Aging, immunity, and cancer. Discov Med 11:537, 2011. Accessed June 1, 2013. Available at www.discoverymedicine.com/Tamas-Fulop/2011/06/24/aging-immunity-and-cancer

Ge, S, Feng, X, Shen, L, et al: Association between habitual dietary salt intake and risk of gastric cancer: A systematic review of observational studies. Gastroenterol Res Pract 2012;2012:808120. Accessed May 14, 2013. Available at www.ncbi.nlm.nih.gov/pmc/articles/PMC3485508

Gullett, NP, Mazurak, V, Hebbar, G, and Ziegler, TR: Nutritional interventions for cancer-induced cachexia. Curr Probl Cancer 35:58, 2011. Accessed June 1, 2013. Available at www.ncbi.nlm.nih.gov/pmc/articles/PMC3106221

Hesketh, J: Personalized nutrition: How far has nutrigenomics progressed? Eur J Clin Nutr 67:430, 2013.

Ibrahim, EM, and Al-Homaidh, A: Physical activity and survival after breast cancer diagnosis: Meta-analysis of published studies. Med Oncol 28:753, 2011.

Isaacson, C: The change of the staple diet of black South Africans from sorghum to maize (corn) is the cause of the epidemic of squamous carcinoma of the oesophagus. Med Hypotheses 64:658, 2005.

Isaak, CK, and Siow, YL: The evolution of nutrition research. Can J Physiol Pharmacol 91:257, 2013.

Jackson, CL, Szklo, M, Yeh, HC, et al: Black–White disparities in overweight and obesity trends by educational attainment in the United States, 1997–2008. J Obes 2013:140743, 2013.

Kamat, AM, and Lamm, DL: Chemoprevention of bladder cancer. Urol Clin North Am 29:157, 2002.

Kandala, V, and Playfor, S: Massive tongue swelling following the use of synthetic saliva. Paediatr Anaesth 13:827, 2003.

Kenfield, SA, Stampfer, MJ, Giovannucci, E, and Chan, JM: Physical activity and survival after prostate cancer diagnosis in the health professionals follow-up study. J Clin Oncol 29:726, 2011. Accessed May 30, 2013. Available at www.ncbi.nlm.nih.gov/pmc/articles/PMC3056656

Kushi, LH, Doyle, C, McCullough, M, et al: American Cancer Society Guidelines on nutrition and physical activity for cancer prevention: Reducing the risk of cancer with healthy food choices and physical activity. CA Cancer J Clin 62:30, 2012. Accessed May 23, 2013. Available at onlinelibrary.wiley.com/doi/10.3322/caac.20140/full#sec1-6

Larsson, SC, Bergkvist, L, and Wolk, A: Processed meat consumption, dietary nitrosamines and stomach cancer risk in a cohort of Swedish women. Int J Cancer 119:915, 2006.

Levine, M, and Padayatty, SJ: Vitamin C. In Ross, AC, Caballero, B, Cousins, RJ, et al (eds): Modern Nutrition in Health and Disease, ed 11. Lippincott Williams & Wilkins, Philadelphia, 2014.

Lin, J, Kamat, A, Gu, J, et al: Dietary intake of vegetables and fruits and the modification effects of GSTM1 and NAT2 genotypes on bladder cancer risk. Cancer Epidemiol Biomarkers Prev 18:2090, 2009. Accessed May 21, 2013. Available at http://cebp.aacrjournals.org/content/18/7/2090.long

Magee, PJ, and Rowland, I: Soy products in the management of breast cancer. Curr Opin Clin Nutr Metab Care 15:586, 2012.

Meyerhardt, JA: Beyond standard adjuvant therapy for colon cancer: Role of nonstandard interventions. Semin Oncol 38:533, 2011. Accessed June 1, 2013. Available at www.ncbi.nlm.nih.gov/pmc/articles/PMC3150459

Milner, J, Toner, C, and Davis, CD: Functional foods and nutraceuticals in health promotion. In Ross, AC, Caballero, B, Cousins, RJ, et al (eds): Modern Nutrition in Health and Disease, ed 11. Lippincott Williams & Wilkins, Philadelphia, 2014.

MRC Vitamin Study Research Group: Prevention of neural tube defects: Results of the Medical Research Council Vitamin Study. Lancet 338:131, 1991.

National Institutes of Health: Cancer. Updated March 29, 2013. Accessed May 31, 2013. Available at http://report.nih.gov/NIHfactsheets/ViewFactSheet.aspx?csid=75

Nechuta, S, Shu, X-O, Li, H-L, et al: Prospective cohort study of tea consumption and risk of digestive system cancers: Results from the Shanghai Women's Health Study. Am J Clin Nutr 96:1056, 2012.

Omenn, GS, Goodman G, Thornquist M, et al: The Beta-Carotene and Retinol Efficacy Trial (CARET) for chemoprevention of lung cancer in high risk populations: Smokers and asbestos-exposed workers. Cancer Res 54:2038S, 1994. Accessed May 23, 2013. Available at http://cancerres.aacrjournals.org/content/54/7_Supplement/2038s.long

Omenn, GS, Goodman, GE, Thornquist, MD, et al: Risk factors for lung cancer and for intervention effects in CARET, the Beta-Carotene and Retinol Efficacy Trial. J Natl Cancer Inst 98:1550, 1996. Accessed May 23, 2013. Available at http://jnci.oxfordjournals.org/content/88/21/1550.long

Ong, DK, Mitchell, SB, Barrett, JS, et al: Manipulation of dietary short chain carbohydrates alters the pattern of gas production and genesis of symptoms in irritable bowel syndrome. J Gastroenterol Hepatol 25:1366, 2010.

Ong, TP, Moreno, FS, and Ross, SA: Targeting the epigenome with bioactive food components for cancer prevention. J Nutrigenet Nutrigenomics 4:275, 2012. Accessed May 21, 2013. Available at www.ncbi.nlm.nih.gov/pmc/articles/PMC3388269

Pawelec, G, Derhovanessian, E, and Larbi, A: Immunosenescence and cancer. Crit Rev Oncol Hematol 75:165, 2010.

Patterson, RE, Cadmus, LA, Emond, JA, and Pierce, JP: Physical activity, diet, adiposity and female breast cancer prognosis: a review of the epidemiologic literature. Maturitas 66:5, 2010.

Pelletier, JE, Laska, MN, Neumark-Sztainer, D, and Story, M: Positive attitudes toward organic, local, and sustainable foods are associated with higher dietary quality among young adults. J Acad Nutr Diet 113:127, 2013.

Pierce, JD, McCabe, S, White, N, and Clancy, RL: Biomarkers: An important clinical assessment tool. Am J Nurs 112:52, 2012.

Pisanò, M, Mezzolla, V, Galante, MM, et al: A new mutation of BRCA2 gene in an Italian healthy woman with familial breast cancer history. Fam Cancer 10:65, 2011.

Pronsky, ZM, and Crowe, JP: Food Medication Interactions, ed 17. Food-Medication Interactions, Birchrunville, PA, 2012.

Protani, M, Coory, M, and Martin, JH: Effect of obesity on survival of women with breast cancer: Systematic review and meta-analysis. Breast Cancer Res Treat 123:627, 2010.

Purnell, LD: Transcultural Health Care: A Culturally Competent Appoach, ed 4. FA Davis, Philadelphia, 2013.

Raina, A, and O'Keefe, SJD: Nutrition in pancreatic diseases. In Ross, AC, Caballero, B, Cousins, RJ, et al (eds): Modern Nutrition in Health and Disease, ed 11. Lippincott Williams & Wilkins, Philadelphia, 2014.

Redlich, CA, Blaner, WS, Van Bennekum, AM, et al: Effect of supplementation with beta-carotene and vitamin A on lung nutrient levels. Cancer Epidemiol Biomarkers Prev 7:211, 1998. Accessed May 28, 2013. Available at http://cebp.aacrjournals.org/content/7/3/211.long

Rock, CL, Doyle, C, Demark-Wahnefried, W, et al: Nutrition and physical activity guidelines for cancer survivors. CA Cancer J Clin 62:242, 2012. Accessed May 23, 2013. Available at http://onlinelibrary.wiley.com/doi/10.3322/caac.21142/full

Tan, HL, Thomas-Ahner, JM, Grainger, EM, et al: Tomato-based food products for prostate cancer prevention: what have we learned? Cancer Metastasis Rev 29:553, 2010.

Tantamango-Bartley, Y, Jaceldo-Siegl, K, Fan, J, and Fraser, G: Vegetarian diets and the incidence of cancer in a low-risk population. Cancer Epidemiol Biomarkers Prev 22:286, 2013.

van Dalen, EC, Mank, A, Leclercq, E, et al: Low bacterial diet versus control diet to prevent infection in cancer patients treated with chemotherapy causing episodes of neutropenia. Cochrane Database Syst Rev. 2012 Sep 12;9:CD006247

Visich, KL, and Yeo, TP: The prophylactic use of probiotics in the prevention of radiation therapy-induced diarrhea. Clin J Oncol Nurs 14:467, 2010.

Wallace, TA, Martin, DN, and Ambs, S: Interactions among genes, tumor biology and the environment in cancer health disparities: Examining the evidence on a national and global scale. Carcinogenesis 32:1107, 2011. Accessed May 20, 2013. Available at www.ncbi.nlm.nih.gov/pmc/articles/PMC3149201

Ward, KK, Shah, NR, Saenz, CC, et al: Cardiovascular disease is the leading cause of death among endometrial cancer patients. Gynecol Oncol 126:176, 2012.

Wheatley, KE, Nogueira, LM, Perkins, SN, and Hursting, SD: Differential effects of calorie restriction and exercise on the adipose transcriptome in diet-induced obese mice. J Obes 2011:265417, 2011. Accessed May 27, 2013. Available at www.ncbi.nlm.nih.gov/pmc/articles/PMC3092555

Willett, WC, and Giovannucci, E: Epidemiology of diet and cancer risk. In Ross, AC, Caballero, B, Cousins, RJ, et al (eds): Modern Nutrition in Health and Disease, ed 11. Lippincott Williams & Wilkins, Philadelphia, 2014.

Wolin, KY, Schwartz, AL, Matthews, CE, et al: Implementing the Exercise Guidelines for Cancer Survivors. J Support Oncol 10: 171, 2012. Accessed May 30, 2013.

Available at www.ncbi.nlm.nih.gov/pmc/articles/
PMC3543866

Wu, P, Zhao, XH, Ai, ZS, et al: Dietary intake and risk for
reflux esophagitis: A case-control study. Gastroenterol
Res Pract 2013:691026, 2013. Accessed May 27, 2013.
Available at www.ncbi.nlm.nih.gov/pmc/articles/
PMC3652144

Chapter 22

Academy of Nutrition and Dietetics: What is the effect of
enteral nutrition versus parenteral nutrition on the cost
medical care in critically ill patients? February 15,
2011. Accessed May 26, 2013. Available at http://
andevidencelibrary.com/evidence.cfm?evidence_
summary_id=16&auth=1ns.

Aversa, Z, Alamdari, N, and Hasselgren, P: Molecules
modulating gene transcription during muscle wasting in
cancer, sepsid, and other critical illness. Crit Rev Clin
Lab Sci 48:71, 2011.

Barnett, M: Providing nutritional support for patients with
COPD. J Commun Nurs 25:4, 6, 8, 2011.

Dahl, D, Wajtal, GG, Breslow, MJ, et al: The high cost of
low-acuity ICU outliers. J Healthc Manage 57: 421,
2012.

McClave, SA, Martindale, RG, Vanek, VW, et al: Guidelines
for the provision and assessment of nutrition support
therapy in the adult critically ill patient. J Parenter
Enteral Nutr 33:290, 2009.

Makic, MB, VonRueden, KT, Rauen, CA, and Chadwick, J:
Evidence-based practice habits: Putting more sacred
cows out to pasture. Crit Care Nurse 31:38, 2011.

Qaseem, A, Humphrey, LL, Chou, R, et al: Use of intensive
insulin therapy for the management of glycemic control
in hospitalized patients: A clinical practice guideline
from the American College of Physicians. Ann Int Med
154:260, 2011.

Robson, W, and Daniels, R: Diagnosis and management of
sepsis in adults. Nurs Prescrib 11:76, 2013.

Rojas, Y, Finnerty, CC, Radhakrishnan, RS, and Herndon,
DN: Burns: An update on current pharmacotherapy.
Exp Opin Phamacother 13:2485, 2012.

Rowley-Conway, G: Management of major burns in the
emergency department. Nurs Standard 27:62, 2013.

Shepherd, A: The nutritional management of COPD: An
overview. Br J Nurs 19:559, 2010.

Sinno, S, Lee, DS, and Khachemoune, A: Vitamins and
cutaneous wound healing. J Wound Care 20:287,
2011.

Ziegler, TR: Parenteral nutrition in the critically ill patient.
N Engl J Med 361:1088, 2009.

Chapter 23

American Dietetic Association: Position of the American
Dietetic Association: Nutrition intervention and human
immunodeficiency virus infection. J Am Diet Assoc
110:1105, 2010.

Cahill, S, and Valadez, R: Growing older with HIV/AIDS:
New public health challenges. Am J Pub Health 103:e7,
2013.

Centers for Disease Control: Basic information on HIV/
AIDS. April 11, 2012. Accessed March 14, 2013.
Available at www.cdc.gov/hiv/topics/basic/#origin

Centers for Disease Control and Prevention. HIV
Surveillance Report 23, 2011. Published February 2013.
Accessed March 10, 2013. Available at www.cdc.gov/
hiv/topics/surveillance/resources/reports

Eyawo, O, Fernandes, KA, Brandson, EK, et al: Suboptimal
use of HIV drugs resistance testing in a universal
health-care setting. AIDS Care 23:42, 2011.

Gagnon, M, and Holmes, D: Bodies in mutation: Understanding liposystrophy among women living with
HIV/AIDS. Res Theory Nurs Pract 25:23, 2011.

Kondro, W: Tuberculosis infection rate declining. Can Med
Assoc J 184(17): E898, 2012.

Kirk, JB, and Bidwell-Goetz, M: Human immunodeficiency
virus in an aging population, a complication of success.
J Am Geriatr Soc 57: 2129, 2009.

Mehta, S, Mugusi, FM, Spiegelman, D, et al: Vitamin D
status and its association with morbidity including
wasting and opportunistic illness in HIV-infected
women in Tanzania. AIDS Patient Care STDs 25: 579,
2011.

Mohandas, A, Reifsnyder, J, Jacobs, M, and Fox, T: Current
and future directions in frailty research. Popul Health
Manag 14:277, 2011.

Moss, JA: HIV/AIDS review. Radiol Technol 84:247, 2012.

Neurological disorders strikingly high among HIV/AIDS
patients. AIDS Alert 26:121, 2011.

Ramsuran, V, Kulkarni, H, He, W, et al: Duffy-null-associated
low neutrophil counts influence HIV-1 susceptibility in
high-risk South African Black women. Clin Infect Dis
52:1248, 2011.

Shah, K, Hilton, TN, Myers, L, et al: A new frailty syndrome: Central obesity and frailty in older adults with
the human immunodeficiency virus. Am Geriatr Soc
60:545, 2012.

U.S. Department of Health and Human Services, AIDS.gov:
Signs and symptoms. June 6, 2012. Accessed February
27, 2013. Available at www.aids.gov/hiv-aids-basics/
hiv-aids-101/signs-and-symptoms

U.S. Department of Health and Human Services, AIDS.gov:
Panel on Antiretroviral Guidelines for Adults and Ado-
lescents. Guidelines for the use of antiretroviral agents in
HIV-1-infected adults and adolescents. Department of
Health and Human Services. Accessed March 20, 2013.
Available at aidsinfo.nih.gov/contentfiles/lvguidelines/
AdultandAdolescentGL.pdf

U.S. National Library of Medicine and National Institute of
Health: AIDS. April 30, 2012. Accessed March 14, 2013.
Available at www.nlm.nih.gov/medlineplus/ency/article/
000594.htm

U.S. Preventative Service Task Force: Screening for HIV.
April 2013. Accessed July 23, 2013. Available at www.
uspreventiveservicestaskforce.org/uspstf13/hiv/
hivfinalrs.htm

World Health Organization: Global summary of the AIDS
epidemic. 2011. Accessed March 7, 2013. Available at
www.who.int/hiv/data/2012_epi_core_en.png

Wyndham, H: Fungal infections. Pract Nurse 42:24,
2012.

World Health Organization: WHO welcomes news that a child born with HIV now appears "functionally cured" through early antiretroviral treatment. Accessed March 17, 2013. Available at www.who.int/hiv/mediacentre/hiv_child_20130305/en/index.html

Chapter 24

American Dietetic Association: Position of the American Dietetic Association: Ethical and legal issues in nutrition, hydration, and feeding. J Am Diet Assoc 108:873, 2008.

Barrocas, A, Geppert, C, Durfee, SM, et al: A.S.P.E.N. ethics position paper. Nutr Clin Pract 25:672, 2010.

Couch, E, Mead, JM, and Walsh, MM: Oral health perceptions of paediatric palliative care nursing staff. Int J Palliat Nurs 19:9, 2013.

Cowdell, F: Care and management of patients with pruritus. Nurs Older People 21:35, 2009.

Davies, A, and Hall, S: Salivary gland dysfunction (dry mouth) in patients with advanced cancer. Int J Palliat Nurs 17:477, 2011.

Fuhrman, MP: Nutrition at the end of life: A critical decision. Today's Dietitian 10:68, 2008.

Hipp, B, and Letizia, MJ: Understanding and responding to the death rattle in dying patients. Medsurg Nurs 18:17, 2009.

Kompanje, EJ, van der Hoven, B, and Bakker, J: Anticipation of distress after discontinuation of mechanical ventilation in the ICU at the end of life. Intensive Care Med 34:1593, 2008.

National Hospice and Palliative Care Organization: NHPCA facts and figures. 2012 edition. Accessed March 23, 2013. Available at www.nhpco.org/sites/default/files/public/Statistics_Research/2012_Facts_Figures.pdf

Parker, M, and Power, D: Management of swallowing difficulties in people with an advanced dementia. Nurs Older People 25:26, 2013.

Ruxton, C: Promoting and maintaining healthy hydration in patients. Nurs Standard 26:50, 2012.

U.S. Department of Health and Human Services: Medicare hospice benefits. January, 2013. Accessed March 21, 2013. Available at www.medicare.gov/publications/Pubs/pdf/02154.pdf

World Health Organization: Essential medicines in palliative care (2013, January). Accessed March 21, 2013. Available at www.who.int/selection_medicines/committees/expert/19/applications/PalliativeCare_8_A_R.pdf

Index

Note: Page numbers followed by *b* refer to boxes; *f*, figures; *t*, tables.

Respiratory function, impaired nutritional status and, 525
Respiratory system, acid-base balance and, 183
Resting energy expenditure, 87–88
Retina, 100
Retinoic acid syndrome, 221
Retinol, 98
Retinol activity equivalents, 98
Retinopathy, diabetes and, 394
Rhabdomyolysis, 354
Rheumatoid arthritis, older adults and, 279
Rhodopsin, 100
Riboflavin, 118–119
Ribonucleic acid (RNA), 74
Rickets, vitamin D and, 105–106
Rickets, Vitamin D resistant, 145
Rifampin, 334
Rotavirus, 252
Roux-en-Y, 376–377
Rugae, 201

S

Saccharin, 37
Salivary glands, 199
Salmonella infection, 290, 291t
Salmonellosis, 290
Salt intake, hypertension and, 418
Salt substitutes, 344–345
Sapropterin dihydrochloride, 70
Saquinavir, 350
Sarcomas, 496
Sarcopenia, 273b
Satiety, cancer patients and, 509
Satiety value, fats and, 52
Saturated fats, 51, 425, 447
Saturated fatty acids, 49–50
Scar tissue, 66b
Schizophrenia, 119
School-age child (ages 6 to 12 years)
    good nutrition indications and, 259t
    meal patterns and behaviors, 259
    MyPlate serving guidelines and, 259t
    nutritional needs and concerns, 259
    physical growth and development and, 258
    psychosocial development and, 258
    school nutrition and, 259–260, 260b
School foods, 260b
Scombroid fish poisoning, 295
Screening. *see* Nutrition screening
Scurvy, 114–115
Seafood, toxic, 295
Secondary diabetes, 390
Secondary hypertension, 413
Secretion, tubular, 437, 438f
Secretions, digestion and, 198–199
Seizure control, ketogenic diet for, 336
Selegiline, 336t, 342
Selenium
    deficiency and toxicity, 163
    intakes and sources, 163
    toxicity and, 143t
Self-care, diabetes and, 406–407
Self-feeding, 315
Self-monitoring
    blood glucose and, 395–396
    weight management and, 376b

Semisolid food introduction, infants and, 246–248
Senior Farmer's Market Nutrition Program, 280
Sensible water losses, 185–186
Sensory system, older adults and, 271–272
Sepsis, burn patients and, 520–521
Set point theory, obesity and, 373
Sex hormones, 262
Shellfish, 226
Shortness of breath, 122
Sibutramine, 377t
Sickle cell disease, 67
Sildenafil, 348
Silicon, 166
Simple carbohydrates, 34–35
Simvastatin, 336t, 337
Sitosterolemia, 425
Skin
    nutritional status and, 16
    synthesis of, 106–107
    Vitamin D, as source of, 106–107
Slower eating, weight management and, 376b
Small intestine
    absorption and, 204–206
    carbohydrate digestion and, 202
    cross-section of, 206f
    fat digestion and, 202–204
    protein digestion and, 204
Smell, older adults and, 272
Social consequences, obesity and, 369
Sodium
    calcium balance and, 138
    deficiency and, 146
    dietary reference intakes, 145–146
    fluids and lithium and, 344
    fresh and processed foods and, 147t
    hyponatremia and, 146
    kidney disease and, 444
    kidney failure and, 440
    mean intake of, 146f
    older adults and, 278t
    sodium pumps, 179
    table salt, 145
    toxicity and, 142t, 146
Sodium-controlled diets, 427–429, 430t–431t
    labeling requirements and, 429t
    sample menus for, 430t–431t
    sodium content in beverages, 430t
Soft cheeses, 225
Solubility, 38
Soluble fiber, 39
Solutes, 175
Somatostatin, 391
South Beach diet, 379t
Soy protein, 245, 427
Spare body protein, 39
Special diets, 310
Special formulas, 245
Specific dynamic action, 88
Specific gravity, 190, 344
Sphincters, 197
Spina bifida, 220
Spores, 241
St. John's wort, 347, 349–350, 349t
Standard feedings, 317

Standard formulas, 316
Staph infection, 292
Staphylococcus aureus, 292
Starch/bread exchange list, 42, 563
Starches, 21–22, 34, 37–38, 41–42
Starvation
    critical care and, 516–518
    fuel consumption during, 517f
    gluconeogenesis and, 516–517
    glycogenolysis and, 516
    ketosis and, 517
    lipolysis and, 517
    prolonged, 517–518
    refeeding syndrome and, 527
    uncomplicated, 516
Steatorrhea, 139, 209
Sterols, 48
Stevia, 37
Stimulus control, weight management and, 376b
Stoma, 478
Stomach
    food pathway and, 201
    full stomach and breathing, 274
Stomach disorders
    delayed gastric emptying, 464–465
    dumping syndrome, 467, 469t
    gastritis, 464, 464f
    peptic ulcers, 465–467
    postprandial hypotension, 467–468
    vitamin B$_{12}$ deficiency and, 124
Stomatitis, 440, 509, 550b
Strokes, 415, 432
Subjective data, nutritional assessment and, 14
Sucralose, 37
Sucrase, 202
Sucrose, 36
Sugars
    added sugar in U.S. diet, 36, 36b
    carbohydrates and, 41
    converting grams into teaspoons of, 36
    in foods, 36
    sugar alcohols, 36–37
    sugar-free beverages, 36
Sulfonylureas, 398t
Sulfur, 142t, 150
Supplemental feedings, 315–316
Supplemental food assistance, 224
Surgery
    dietary considerations, 455
    postoperative nutrition, 459–460
    preoperative nutrition, 456–459
    weight management and, 376–378
Survival skills, diabetes and, 399
Swallowing difficulty, cancer patients and, 510
Sweat, 185–186
Symptom control, dietary management for, 548
Syndrome of inappropriate antidivresis (SIAD), 181
Systolic pressure, 180, 413

T

T-lymphocytes, 511
Table salt, 145